Handbook of
Neuropsychology and Aging

CRITICAL ISSUES IN NEUROPSYCHOLOGY

Series Editors

Antonio E. Puente
University of North Carolina, Wilmington

Cecil R. Reynolds
Texas A&M University

Current Volumes in this Series

BEHAVIORAL INTERVENTIONS WITH BRAIN-INJURED CHILDREN
A. MacNeill Horton, Jr.

CLINICAL NEUROPSYCHOLOGICAL ASSESSMENT:
A Cognitive Approach
Edited by Robert L. Mapou and Jack Spector

CONTEMPORARY APPROACHES TO NEUROPSYCHOLOGICAL
ASSESSMENT
Edited by Gerald Goldstein and Theresa M. Incagnoli

FAMILY SUPPORT PROGRAMS AND REHABILITATION:
A Cognitive–Behavioral Approach to Traumatic Brain Injury
Louise Margaret Smith and Hamish P. D. Godfrey

HANDBOOK OF CLINICAL CHILD NEUROPSYCHOLOGY, Second Edition
Edited by Cecil R. Reynolds and Elaine Fletcher-Janzen

HANDBOOK OF NEUROPSYCHOLOGY AND AGING
Edited by Paul David Nussbaum

NEUROPSYCHOLOGICAL EXPLORATIONS OF
MEMORY AND COGNITION:
Essays in Honor of Nelson Butters
Edited by Laird S. Cermak

NEUROPSYCHOLOGICAL TOXICOLOGY:
Identification and Assessment of Human Neurotoxic Syndromes, Second Edition
David E. Hartman

THE PRACTICE OF FORENSIC NEUROPSYCHOLOGY:
Meeting Challenges in the Courtroom
Edited by Robert J. McCaffrey, Arthur D. Williams, Jerid M. Fisher,
and Linda C. Laing

PRACTITIONER'S GUIDE TO CLINICAL NEUROPSYCHOLOGY
Robert M. Anderson, Jr.

A Continuation Order Plan is available for this series. A continuation order will bring delivery
of each new volume immediately upon publication. Volumes are billed only upon actual
shipment. For further information please contact the publisher.

Handbook of
Neuropsychology and Aging

Edited by

Paul David Nussbaum

Lutheran Affiliated Services
Aging Research and Education Center
Mars, Pennsylvania

Plenum Press • New York and London

Library of Congress Cataloging-in-Publication Data

Handbook of neuropsychology and aging / edited by Paul David Nussbaum.
      p.   cm. -- (Critical issues in neuropsychology)
   Includes bibliographical references and index.
   ISBN 0-306-45460-2
   1. Geriatric neuropsychiatry. 2. Geriatric neurology.
3. Clinical neuropsychology.   I. Nussbaum, Paul David. II. Series.
RC451.4.A5H39   1997
   618.97'68--dc21   97-12001
                                                         CIP

ISBN 0-306-45460-2

© 1997 Plenum Press, New York
A Division of Plenum Publishing Corporation
233 Spring Street, New York, N. Y. 10013

http://www.plenum.com

10 9 8 7 6 5 4 3 2 1

Printed in the United States of America

To Ryan Paul

Contributors

Daniel N. Allen • Psychology Service, Highland Drive Veterans Affairs Medical Center, Pittsburgh, Pennsylvania 15206

Kathryn A. Bayles • National Center for Neurogenic Communication Disorders, University of Arizona, Tucson, Arizona 85721

James T. Becker • Department of Psychiatry, University of Pittsburgh School of Medicine, Pittsburgh, Pennsylvania 15213

Pelagie M. Beeson • National Center for Neurogenic Communication Disorders, University of Arizona, Tucson, Arizona 85721

David A. Bennett • Rush Institute on Aging, Rush Alzheimer's Disease Center, and Rush Presbyterian-St. Luke's Medical Center, Chicago, Illinois 60612

Julie Berkey • Allegheny General Hospital/Allegheny Neuropsychiatric Institute, Pittsburgh, Pennsylvania 15212

Erin D. Bigler • Department of Psychology, Brigham Young University, Provo, Utah 84602; and LDS Hospital, Salt Lake City, Utah 84103

Mark W. Bondi • Department of Psychiatry, School of Medicine, University of California, San Diego, La Jolla, California 92093-0948; and San Diego Department of Veterans Affairs Medical Center, San Diego, California 92161

Jennifer J. Bortz • Barrow Neurological Institute, St. Joseph's Hospital and Medical Center, Phoenix, Arizona 85013-4496

Jon Brillman • Allegheny General Hospital, Pittsburgh, Pennsylvania 15212

Meryl A. Butters • Department of Psychiatry, University of Pittsburgh School of Medicine, Pittsburgh, Pennsylvania 15213

Frederick W. Bylsma • Department of Psychiatry and Behavioral Sciences, Division of Medical Psychology, The Johns Hopkins University School of Medicine, Baltimore, Maryland 21287

Jeffrey L. Cummings • Department of Neurology, University of California, Los Angeles, School of Medicine, Los Angeles, California 90024; and West Los Angeles Veterans Affairs Medical Center, Los Angeles, California 90095-1769

Louis F. Damis • Private Practice, Clinical and Health Psychology, Orlando, Florida 32803

Richard C. Delaney • Neuropsychology Section, Psychology Service, Veterans Affairs Medical Center, West Haven, Connecticut 06516

Denise L. Evert • Laboratory of Neuropsychology, Division of Psychiatry, and Department of Neurology, Boston University School of Medicine, Boston, Massachusetts 02118; and Psychology Research Service, Department of Veterans Affairs Medical Center, Boston, Massachusetts 02130

Robert B. Fields • Department of Psychiatry, Allegheny General Hospital, and Allegheny University of the Health Sciences, Pittsburgh, Pennsylvania 15212

Gerald Goldstein • Highland Drive Veterans Affairs Medical Center, Pittsburgh, Pennsylvania 15206; and Departments of Psychiatry and Psychology, University of Pittsburgh, Pittsburgh, Pennsylvania 15213

Anthony J. Goreczny • Department of Behavioral Sciences, University of Indianapolis, Indianapolis, Indiana 46227

George Grossberg • Division of Geriatric Psychiatry, Department of Psychiatry and Human Behavior, St. Louis University, St. Louis, Missouri 63104

Alfred W. Kaszniak • Department of Psychology, University of Arizona, Tucson, Arizona

Harold G. Koenig • Duke University Medical Center, Durham, North Carolina 27710

Daniel A. Krauss • Department of Psychology, University of Arizona, Tucson, Arizona 85721

Rhonda K. B. Landis • Behavioral Health Services, DuBois Regional Medical Center, DuBois, Pennsylvania 15801

Asenath La Rue • Department of Psychiatry, University of New Mexico, Albuquerque, New Mexico 87131; and Department of Psychiatry and Biobehavioral Sciences, University of California, Los Angeles, Los Angeles, California 90024-1759

Mark R. Lovell • Division of Neuropsychology, Henry Ford Hospital, Detroit, Michigan 48202

David C. Martin • Division of Geriatric Medicine, Shadyside Hospital, Pittsburgh, Pennsylvania 15232; and Departments of Medicine, Psychiatry, and Health Services Administration, University of Pittsburgh, Pittsburgh, Pennsylvania 15260

Harry W. McConnell • Institute of Epileptology, Maudsley Hospital, London SE5 8AZ, England

Michael McCue • Center for Applied Neuropsychology, Pittsburgh, Pennsylvania 15222

Susan E. McPherson • Department of Psychiatry and Biobehavioral Sciences, University of California, Los Angeles, School of Medicine, Los Angeles, California 90024; and Cedars Sinai Alzheimer's Disease Research and Treatment Center, Los Angeles, California 90024

Benoit H. Mulsant • Western Psychiatric Institute and Clinic and Department of Psychiatry, University of Pittsburgh School of Medicine, Pittsburgh, Pennsylvania 15213

Jodi D. Nadler • Medical Psychology Section, Florida Hospital Health Center, Orlando, Florida 32803

Paul David Nussbaum • Aging Research and Education Center, Lutheran Affiliated Services, Mars, Pennsylvania 16046; and Department of Neurology, University of Pittsburgh School of Medicine, Pittsburgh, Pennsylvania 15261

Kevin P. O'Brien • Barrow Neurological Institute, St. Joseph's Hospital and Medical Center, Phoenix, Arizona 85013-4496

Marlene Oscar-Berman • Laboratory of Neuropsychology, Division of Psychiatry, and Department of Neurology, Boston University School of Medicine, Boston, Massachusetts 02118; and Psychology Research Service, Department of Veterans Affairs Medical Center, Boston, Massachusetts 02130

Linda Peterson • Department of Psychology, Barry University, Miami Shores, Florida 33161

Lisa D. Ravdin • Department of Neurology and Neuroscience, The New York Hospital-Cornell Medical Center, New York, New York 10021

Emily D. Richardson • Yale University School of Medicine, Adler Geriatric Center, Yale-New Haven Hospital, New Haven, Connecticut 06504

Linda S. Rockey • Geriatric Care Services, Lutheran Affiliated Services, Mars, Pennsylvania 16046-0928

Fred H. Rubin • Department of Medicine, Shadyside Hospital, Pittsburgh, Pennsylvania 15232; and Department of Medicine, University of Pittsburgh, Pittsburgh, Pennsylvania 15260

Bruce D. Sales • Department of Psychology, University of Arizona, Tucson, Arizona 85721

David P. Salmon • Department of Neurosciences, School of Medicine, University of California, San Diego, La Jolla, California 92093-0948

Carol J. Schramke • Psychology Service, Highland Drive Veterans Affairs Medical Center, Pittsburgh, Pennsylvania 15206; and Departments of Neurology and Psychiatry, University of Pittsburgh, Pittsburgh, Pennsylvania 15213

Gregory T. Slomka • Western Psychiatric Institute and Clinic, Pittsburgh, Pennsylvania 15213

Stanley S. Smith • Department of Psychiatry, Medical College of Pennsylvania and Hahnemann University–Allegheny Campus, Pittsburgh, Pennsylvania 15212

Bonnie Lynn Snyder • School of Social Work Graduate Program, University of Pittsburgh, Pittsburgh, Pennsylvania

Peter J. Snyder • Department of Neurology, Medical College of Pennsylvania and Hahnemann University–Allegheny Campus, Pittsburgh, Pennsylvania 15212

Elizabeth Soety • Department of Psychiatry, University of Pittsburgh School of Medicine, Pittsburgh, Pennsylvania 15213

Christopher Starratt • Department of Psychology, Barry University, Miami Shores, Florida 33161

Rex Swanda • Veterans Affairs Medical Center, Albuquerque, New Mexico 87108

Andrea Swartzendruber • Rush Institute on Aging, Rush Alzheimer's Disease Center, and Rush Presbyterian-St. Luke's Medical Center, Chicago, Illinois 60612

John A. Sweeney • Western Psychiatric Institute and Clinic and Department of Psychiatry, University of Pittsburgh School of Medicine, Pittsburgh, Pennsylvania 15213

Alexander I. Tröster • Department of Neurology, University of Kansas Medical Center, Kansas City, Missouri 66160-7314

Mahmood A. Usman • The Alzheimer Center of Pittsburgh, Pittsburgh, Pennsylvania 15205

James Valeriano • Department of Neurology, Medical College of Pennsylvania and Hahnemann University–Allegheny Campus, Pittsburgh, Pennsylvania 15212

Sharon M. Wallsten • Duke University School of Nursing, Duke University Medical Center, Durham, North Carolina 27710

Robert S. Wilson • Rush Institute on Aging, Rush Alzheimer's Disease Center, and Rush Presbyterian-St. Luke's Medical Center, Chicago, Illinois 60612

Ben Zimmer • Geriatric Psychiatry Program, Department of Psychiatry, and Allegheny Neuropsychiatric Institute, Medical College of Pennsylvania and Hahnemann University–Allegheny Campus, Pittsburgh, Pennsylvania 15212

Foreword

As larger numbers of persons survive into older age, biobehavioral scientists and health care professionals have become more aware of the unique needs of older adults. This awareness is reflected in a dramatic increase in the publication of both basic and applied research concerned with aging and age-related disorders. Nowhere has this been more true than within those various disciplines that contribute to our understanding of the neuropsychology of aging. Disorders of the central nervous system in older age are a cause of considerable disability and suffering, and there is widespread recognition of the need to better understand the psychological consequences of these disorders. Similarly, there is increasing recognition of the contributions to both diagnosis and intervention being made by clinical neuropsychologists with expertise in aging. For example, neuropsychological consultation now plays a critical role in the early identification of progressive dementia, contributes to differential neurologic and neuropsychiatric diagnosis of the many possible causes of dementia, and aids in the treatment and clinical management of dementing illness. Similar contributions are being made in regard to a variety of other (e.g., focal cerebrovascular) neurobehavioral syndromes that are prevalent among older adults.

Particular challenges face the clinician or investigator who wishes to become better informed about research and clinical application in this area. The neuropsychology of aging is a fundamentally interdisciplinary field of study, with neuropsychology, behavioral neurology, neuropsychiatry, speech and language science, and various other neurobehavioral and neurobiological disciplines playing necessary roles. Complex interactions exist between fundamental changes in the aging brain, neurological and systemic illnesses, age-related changes in pharmacokinetics and pharmacodynamics, and a variety of psychological and social factors that influence the occurrence and nature of both cognitive and affective symptoms in older adults. It is not surprising therefore to find that relevant research and clinical scholarship are published across a wide range of journals and books. For both neophyte and seasoned clinician or investigator, there is a need for authoritative reference sources that critically review, summarize, integrate, and abstract the most important clinical applications of this increasingly large body of work.

Over the past decade, a small number of excellent books have been published that partially fill this need by providing integrative overviews of the clinical neuropsychology of aging (e.g., Albert & Moss, 1988; La Rue, 1992) or by focusing on particular problems in the neuropsychological assessment of older adults (e.g., Poon, 1986; Storandt & VandenBos, 1994). However, none of these previous volumes has provided the scope or depth of this handbook. Dr. Nussbaum has brought together an outstanding multidisciplinary group of authors, many of whom are recognized as the nation's leading researchers and clinicians in neuropsychological aspects of aging. The topics covered by these authorities represent the scope of knowledge that is critical to fully understanding this field. The range of neuropsychological and psychiatric disorders most frequently seen among elderly persons is given comprehensive review. It is noteworthy that chapters are included that review areas of newly emerging research (e.g., frontal lobe dementias, neuropsychological aspects of late-life depression), as well as those clinical problems that typically are given insufficient consideration (e.g., seizure disorders, head injury, mental retardation) in other sources. An adequate understanding of the psychological consequences of these disorders is, of course, not possible without an appreciation of the neuro-anatomical, neurophysiological, cognitive, personality, and psychosocial aspects of normal aging, and this volume covers these areas in good detail. In reviewing assessment procedures that contribute to the clinical evaluation of older persons with known or suspected neuropsychological disorder, the volume makes a significant contribution by bringing together in one place discussions of neurological, brain imaging, electrophysiological, neuropsychological, and functional approaches. The breadth of approaches described again underscores the inherently multidisciplinary nature of clinical assessment in this area.

A quite unique aspect of this handbook, among other volumes concerned with neuropsychological aspects of aging, is its comprehensive review of clinical intervention. The neuropsychology of aging has recently moved beyond an exclusive focus on descriptive and diagnostic efforts in its clinical application, and the handbook reflects this current status. Developments in psychotherapeutic, behavioral, psychopharmacologic, and electroconvulsive interventions are described and critically evaluated, as are those in the new and growing area of cognitive rehabilitation. In addition, consideration is given to clinically critical issues concerning both guardianship and caregiving.

Dr. Nussbaum and the authors he has gathered together have made a major contribution to this area of growing clinical and research importance. This *Handbook of Neuropsychology and Aging* will serve as an indispensable resource as new clinicians and investigators from various disciplines become attracted to the neuropsychology of aging and as experienced professionals look to expand and update their expertise.

Alfred W. Kaszniak
University of Arizona

References

Albert, M. S., & Moss, M. B. (Eds.). (1988). *Geriatric neuropsychology*. New York: Guilford Press.

La Rue, A. (1992). *Aging and neuropsychological assessment*. New York: Plenum Press.

Poon, L. W. (Ed.). (1986). *Handbook for the clinical memory assessment of older adults*. Washington, DC: American Psychological Association.

Storandt, M., & VandenBos, G. R. (Eds.). (1994). *Neuropsychological assessment of dementia and depression in older adults: A clinician's guide*. Washington, DC: American Psychological Association.

Preface

The ongoing demographic revolution in the United States represents a tremendous opportunity and responsibility for the health care system. Indeed, by the year 2010, the baby boom generation, estimated to number 75 million, will begin to turn 65 years of age. Clinicians and researchers interested in the field of aging need to prepare for this growth. Specific agendas might include development of a vision of health care and research in aging, education of society about the facts of aging, and creation of new models of training and clinical philosophy. Indeed, a progressive model of health care, based on wellness and prevention rather than the current disease-based approach, might be a starting point worthy of critical analysis. There is clear need to highlight the many positive attributes of aging, emphasizing the later years of life to be a productive and natural part of the life span. Finally, there is a tremendous need for well-trained geriatricians and allied health professionals to meet the growing medical, psychological, and social needs of the older adult population.

Within this context, clinical neuropsychology can contribute significantly, both from a clinical and scientific perspective. There is a need to establish specialized training in geriatric neuropsychology with consideration for board certification status. Continued illumination of brain–behavior relations with advancing age remains a high priority of research, particularly with models of normal aging. Clinical neuropsychology can advance the study of preclinical markers for progressive dementias such as Alzheimer's disease. The clinical neuropsychologist can also contribute significantly to our understanding of why some older adults thrive while others isolate. These and many other areas of study in aging require continued investigation and development. Clinical neuropsychology can be a leader in this regard, helping to map the frontiers of clinical care and research of aging into the 21st century.

This volume does not provide answers to all of the critical issues raised here. However, it attempts to provide a comprehensive text on aging that can be used by both the clinician and scientist. The handbook is meant to build upon the excellent works of La Rue (1992) and Albert and Moss (1988), who initiated the discussion on integrating neuropsychology and gerontology. A main purpose of the handbook is to provide an overview of neuropsychology and aging that will accentuate the importance of geriatric neuropsychology and serve as a comprehensive reference.

The volume follows a scientist-practitioner model and is divided into five broad parts: Normal Aging, Psychiatric Disorders of Late Life, Neuropsychological Disorders of Late Life, Assessment Procedures and the Older Patient, and Treatment Interventions and the Older Patient. Normal aging is the first part because, in the opinion of the editor, it is the most important area of study for neuropsychology and gerontology and deserves increased attention. The other parts are significant in that they are meant to provide a review of current knowledge as well as direction for future clinical investigation. Some of the chapters, such as those covering epilepsy, head injury, legal issues, and personality, highlight areas that have not received much attention in the literature and, as such, may not be readily familiar to clinicians who examine and treat older adults.

This handbook is written for all students and professionals interested in the aging process. It is meant to serve as a useful reference source and teaching guide that promotes progressive ideas regarding the attitudes and care of aging individuals in our society. The knowledge presented in each chapter is not meant to be conclusive, but a catalyst for continued investigation and question.

Paul David Nussbaum

ACKNOWLEDGMENTS

This volume reflects the hard work of many individuals, including Melinda Gatesman, Connie Peterson, and Tammy Sherrick. Mary Butler, in particular, proved herself invaluable with many hours of excellent proofreading. Thanks also go to Eliot Werner and Mariclaire Cloutier, Senior Editors; their professionalism and advice made my work much easier. As with any of my small professional successes, none is achieved without the guidance of my primary mentor Alfred W. Kaszniak and secondary mentor Gerald Goldstein. Much appreciation and gratitude is also directed to Michael Hendrickson and Grady Hunter for their vision and leadership and for giving me the opportunity to succeed. I wish to thank the many students whom I have had the pleasure of teaching; their enthusiasm and critical questions have provided fuel for my own investigative efforts. Finally, special thanks to Kim.

Contents

IV. Assessment Procedures and the Older Patient

V. Treatment Interventions and the Older Patient

Handbook of
Neuropsychology and Aging

1

Introduction

PAUL DAVID NUSSBAUM

Clinical neuropsychology involves the study of brain–behavior relations and has emerged as an important discipline within health care. There are several subspecializations within neuropsychology, including pediatrics, head injury, and behavioral epilepsy. The study of aging also represents a subspecialization and is the topic of this handbook. Indeed, integration of neuropsychology and gerontology represents a relatively new area of study that is critical given the ongoing demographic revolution in the United States. The *Handbook of Neuropsychology and Aging* is meant to inspire a critical review of the aging process in the United States. While the focus of this text is clinical in nature, it is clear that the expanding older adult population will influence not only health care, but also political, social, and economic issues.

Demographics

It is clear that a demographic revolution has begun in the United States, yielding a significant increase in the number of older adults, defined as those 65 years of age and older. At present, approximately 12% (34 million) of the United States population is "older." This percentage will increase to 17% by the turn of the century and to 20% by the middle of the 21st century (La Rue, 1992). Perhaps more striking is the fact that those 85 years of age and older comprise the fastest growing segment of the population. At present, approximately 2.5 million individuals are 85 years of age or older, and this

PAUL DAVID NUSSBAUM • Aging Research and Education Center, Lutheran Affiliated Services, Mars, Pennsylvania 16046; and Department of Neurology, University of Pittsburgh School of Medicine, Pittsburgh, Pennsylvania 15261.

number will increase to 16 million (5% of the total population) by the year 2050 (La Rue, 1992). In the year 2010, the baby boom generation, comprising 76 million individuals born between 1945 and 1964, will begin to turn 65, yielding an unprecedented aging of America (Baltes & Baltes, 1993).

The demographic revolution has already begun to affect society. Health care expenditures for older adults continue to grow, representing at least one third of the personal expenditures in the United States (La Rue, 1992). Medicare and Medicaid, two government-sponsored programs that affect the elderly, are presently under scrutiny by politicians. There is a growing belief that these programs will be reengineered, perhaps terminated, for more cost-effective health care programs within a capitated managed care system. Social Security, another government-sponsored program, is perhaps the most controversial issue affecting the older adult population. Otto Von Bismarck of Germany (19th century) is typically given credit for the idea of granting social benefits to those over the age of 64. Incredibly, although the idea originated over a century ago, age 65 remains the standard threshold for granting specific social benefits in the United States. The appropriateness of age 65 as a cutoff for Social Security is challenged on two points: First, individuals are living longer and can remain productive in the work force until later in life, an issue that has direct psychosocial and perhaps physiological consequence; second, the economic costs of Social Security demand that the age threshold for receipt of benefits be increased.

These social and political issues have implications for all Americans and will force the country to address the issue of aging in a new and perhaps more comprehensive manner. This includes a redefinition of what it means to be "old" with perhaps less focus on chronological age and more on functional capacity. A serious overview of retirement needs to be made in the context of the import of occupation to identity, sense of role, and self-esteem for Americans. Removal of occupation potentially exacerbates the inability to thrive for individuals who derive their general well-being from work. Individuals who fail to thrive will create an increased economic hardship for themselves and the health care system. Finally, social policy with regard to education of our youth on aspects of aging might be considered as one method to confront and defeat ageism.

Challenges for Neuropsychology and the Health Care System

For clinical neuropsychology, the demographic revolution raises several challenges. First, there are not enough neuropsychologists with expertise in aging to handle the burgeoning health care demands of older adults. This is equally true for all medical disciplines. Indeed, according to the American Geriatrics Society, there are approximately 6,800 board-certified geriatricians in the United States, certainly not enough to meet the overwhelming health care needs of the aging population. The fact that older adults suffer from Alzheimer's disease (see Salmon and Bondi, Chapter 10 of this volume), stroke (see Delaney, Chapter 21), cardiac illness, and cancer, all of which have or can have devastating effects on the central nervous system, underscores the need for neuropsychological expertise at an unprecedented rate. Other disorders, considered somewhat nontraditional for clinicians who treat older adults, are no less devastating nor less demanding of neuropsychology. These include head injury (see Fields, Chapter 19), epilepsy (see Snyder, Chapter 18), and substance abuse (see Allen, Chapter 9). In order to meet the increased demand for neuropsychological services, consideration must be given to development of specialized training and board certification in geriatric neuropsychology. Undergraduate and graduate programs should begin to provide curricula focusing on the multiple aspects of aging. Internships and fellow-

ships might provide formalized tracks in geriatrics and gerontology, and a curriculum that integrates the clinical aspects of geriatrics with managed care is vital.

Innovative clinical research represents a second major challenge for neuropsychology and the health care system. The need to bridge laboratory-based research findings to clinical practice is a high priority. Pure experimental neuropsychology remains important to the development of our understanding of aging, but clinical research that can be applied will likely become increasingly important and necessary. Research domains important for neuropsychology will likely include development of new models of health care, preventative care, identification of clinical correlates of functional capacity, identification of preclinical markers of disease, and use of advanced technology with cognitive rehabilitation and design of community-based residential settings. Neuropsychologists have the opportunity to play important roles in defining health care models for the older adult. This will include establishing integrated continuum-of-care models as an alternative to acute care settings. Indeed, neuropsychology will need to position itself as a leader in community-based health care delivery to survive the decreased utility of traditional hospital-based models of care. Within this context, the understanding and articulation of managed care as the primary system for care for the older adult is both needed and ripe for neuropsychologists. Managed care involves concepts of standardization, protocol development, managing the care, not the payment, of the older adult, comprehensive assessment, measurement of outcome, and team approaches that are integrated and focused on patient care. These are domains of expertise that should be familiar to neuropsychologists given the nature of their training. Overall, neuropsychology can assist in the creation of innovative health care delivery systems that will serve as alternatives to the current fragmented hospital-based/disease-based model.

Education in the area of aging is a third challenge that confronts the health care system. Clinical neuropsychology can contribute to many areas of education, including presenting current research, training clinicians, disputing myths of aging, and pioneering a new paradigm of aging, one that is based on wellness and not on disease. Neuropsychology has the opportunity to promote the study and understanding of normal aging, create systems of preventative care, and develop new settings for care of the elderly that are community-based and not confined to hospitals. This type of educational input represents a paradigm shift that is necessary given the trends in health care and the demographic revolution. Certainly, society must not only provide education and training to clinicians, but also begin to create innovative models of care and progressive methods of thinking about the older adult. Curriculums on aging might begin in elementary schools with emphasis on normal aging, methods of enhancing wellness across the life span, caregiving, and financial planning. Education of youth on the social and health issues of aging is a proactive method of enhancing factual knowledge and dispelling myths.

This handbook, therefore, represents an attempt to promote the specialization of aging as a high priority for the field of neuropsychology and health care in general. Continued publication of material specific to aging is necessary to maintain a critical assessment of the care of elderly in the United States. The current position of health care, both in terms of paradigm status and human resources, is not adequate to meet the demands posed by the aging population. A new vision of health care for the older adult is certainly needed, one that deviates from the pure "medical model" of the past and instead approaches the older adult from a more comprehensive perspective. Attitudes on aging must be challenged and systems of care developed that are based on sound empirical research, not on speculation. Neuropsychologists have been trained as scientist practitioners who can educate, train, and create. As such, the field of neuropsychology is well positioned to be a leader in the development of a vision of care for the aging population. This challenge, however, is not unique to neuropsychology. Indeed, all health care providers are confronted with the need to adopt new ways of thinking, something that is not only difficult, but likely to meet much resistance. This handbook underscores the importance of the demographic revolution and the need to change archaic, highly routinized clinical approaches; adopt new innovative methods of care;

and create a new paradigm for aging in the Untied States.

Aging in the 21st Century

An argument can be made that the current fragmented, negative and dependency-driven model of health care for the older adult needs to be critically challenged, particularly as we enter the 21st century with more older individuals living than at any time in our history. As an attempt to discuss the need for change, several ideas are proposed for consideration.

1. Convert the current disease-based approach of care for the older individual to a wellness-based perspective, focusing on preserved capacity, not limitations. This will enhance independence, not dependence. Much can be learned from those who have aged successfully.

2. Create integrated continuum-of-care delivery systems that are community-based, and employ acute care hospitals as one point on the continuum rather than as the only setting for older adult care. Indeed, a primary goal of any health care team should be to keep individuals out of the hospital.

3. Realign the focus of care away from the physician/clinician and toward the patient or resident. Further, operationalize clinical teams as medical directors who appreciate the complexities of aging from a physiological, functional, psychosocial, and family perspective.

4. Integrate the new vision of care into higher education in order to train the next generation of health care providers. This includes managed care curriculum and interdisciplinary clinical experience in community-based settings.

5. Attempt to link health care systems with advanced technologies to create viable community-based alternatives to nursing homes. This author supports the viewpoint that hospitals and nursing homes are the "dinosaurs" of health care.

6. Educate the media and youth on the facts of aging. This alone will assist in breaking down the unnecessary fear of aging that exists in our country. Lobby for standardization of grade school curriculum on the facts of aging and financial planning as a practical means of accomplishing the same. Where nursing homes exist, placement of familiar corporations such as McDonald's will also help to provide a symbol of safety for young children and grandchildren who visit relatives. Other such innovative intergenerational programs are needed.

7. Create social vehicles for the older individual to remain integrated in society. If occupations are to be removed because of age, we are obligated to provide options for individuals to maintain a sense of role and import. Further, older adults can benefit all of society with their wisdom, experience, and knowledge.

8. Remove the authority of social policy-based legislation from politicians who generally are not expert in the complexities of aging. At a minimum, legislatures need to be more informed about the challenges that Americans will confront with regard to the expanding older population.

References

Baltes, P. B., & Baltes, M. M. (1993). *Successful aging*. New York: Cambridge University Press.

La Rue, A. (1992). *Aging and neuropsychological assessment*. New York: Plenum.

I

Normal Aging

2

Age-Related Change in Cognitive Function

ROBERT S. WILSON, DAVID A. BENNETT,
AND ANDREA SWARTZENDRUBER

Introduction

This chapter considers cognitive functioning in persons age 65 or older. Persons within this age group commonly report difficulty with memory and other cognitive abilities compared to an earlier period. These perceptions may contribute to concern about Alzheimer's disease (AD) and other dementing illnesses. In view of the prevalence of AD and other conditions that affect cognition in this age group (e.g., Parkinson's disease, stroke), such concern is understandable. Indeed, impaired cognitive function in older persons is associated with loss of independence, increased morbidity and mortality, and reduced quality of life. Not surprisingly, therefore, considerable scientific effort has been expended in attempts to understand age-related cognitive decline, its neural bases, and factors which may modify or delay it.

At present, there is no general agreement about which aspects of decline in cognitive abilities are due to "normal" aging and which are due to an early dementing illness such as AD. We have chosen to focus, therefore, on the difficult issue of identification of impaired cognition in elderly persons. First, we outline current evidence regarding loss of cognitive abilities among older persons. Next, we consider neuropsychological approaches to determining cognitive impairment in elderly per-

sons in light of cognitive aging research. In the final section, we discuss directions for future research and clinical practice.

Age-Related Cognitive Impairment

Methodological issues loom large in the study of age-related cognitive impairment. Many of these issues are not peculiar to cognition, but are critical for studies of many conditions related to aging. One especially important issue, in our view, is the use of longitudinal studies. Because cognitive abilities are related to many factors, in addition to age, inferences about cognitive impairment from cross-sectional data are often based on uncertain assumptions and involve substantial risk of bias. For example, although the average score on many neuropsychological tests is lower in older than in younger people, there is typically more variability in the older age group, with some persons performing better than persons in the younger age group, and a subset performing relatively poorly. Studies that attempt to understand interindividual variability in cognitive abilities are of major importance. Direct measurement of change in cognitive function is the best way to understand person-specific patterns of cognitive decline. Although cross-sectional studies can show differential associations of specific cognitive functions with age and possible neural bases of such impairment, longitudinal studies are required to gain a fuller understanding of individual patterns of change in specific cognitive functions, as well as

ROBERT S. WILSON, DAVID A. BENNETT, AND ANDREA SWARTZENDRUBER • Rush Institute on Aging, Rush Alzheimer's Disease Center, and Rush Presbyterian-St. Luke's Medical Center, Chicago, Illinois 60612.

antecedents, consequences, and neural bases of such change.

Longitudinal cognitive research is complex, time-consuming, and costly. In addition, it poses a number of difficult operational, psychometric, and analytic challenges. Perhaps not surprisingly, therefore, relatively little longitudinal cognitive research has been published. Further, findings of many published studies are hard to interpret due to attrition, floor or ceiling effects on cognitive measures, and questionable analytic strategies. Fortunately, recent analytic advances and their successful application to longitudinal studies of other age-related conditions have made this approach to the study of cognitive aging more feasible (Evans, 1991; Rogosa, 1988).

Another methodological concern is the need to investigate at least some issues in cognitive aging among people drawn from defined populations. Use of population-based samples permits the study of the full spectrum of cognitive abilities exhibited by older persons. Findings from studies of volunteers may be difficult to interpret when older age groups are selected to be equivalent to younger age groups on variables which are known to be related to age on a population basis (e.g., education, health, medication use).

Perhaps the most basic question is whether cognitive decline occurs regularly among persons age 65 or older. Cross-sectional studies consistently report an inverse correlation between age and performance on most cognitive tasks (Lindenberger, Mayr, & Kliegl, 1993; Scherr et al., 1988; Wechsler, 1987). These studies also stress substantial individual differences in cognitive function exhibited by older persons, ranging from levels equivalent or superior to those seen in younger persons to clinically manifest dementia. Longitudinal studies suggest similar conclusions. Two recent longitudinal studies are notable for (a) use of population-based samples and (b) high rates of initial and follow-up participation (Colsher & Wallace, 1991; Evans et al., 1993). Decline on a 10-item mental status test (Pfeiffer, 1975) was observed over an interval of approximately 3 years in one study (Evans et al., 1993) and 6 years in the other (Colsher & Wallace, 1991), and age was associated with degree of decline in each study.

Although there is consensus that cognitive decline occurs in many older persons, there is limited knowledge of the factors that contribute to individual differences in decline. A number of potential risk factors are currently under investigation, including education and other markers of socioeconomic status, gender, race, smoking, parkinsonism, volume of the hippocampus on magnetic resonance imaging (MRI), and presence of one or two apolipoprotein E ϵ4 alleles. Of these factors, only education has been shown to predict rate of cognitive decline in population studies (Colsher & Wallace, 1991; Evans et al., 1993). That is, persons with few years of formal education show a relatively greater rate of cognitive decline than do more educated persons. Although level of education has long been recognized as a factor affecting cognitive and neuropsychological performance tests, the association of education with change in cognitive function is not likely to be artifactual since any biases associated with education would presumably be equivalent at each measurement point. The meaning of the association between education and cognitive decline is uncertain. Education might directly affect cognition, or the correlation might reflect some other variable(s) related to both education and cognitive decline. Of course, it is reasonable to assume that a substantial amount of decline observed in population-based samples may be due to common clinical conditions (e.g., AD) known to cause cognitive impairment in this age range. However, even when persons with such conditions are excluded, substantial age-related differences in cognitive functioning remain.

Much scientific effort has been devoted to the study of differential association of age with specific forms of cognition. Although age-related differences are clearly more pronounced on some tests than on others, virtually all cognitive performance measures show such differences. Indeed, even abilities considered relatively impervious to age-related decline like reading, word knowledge, and implicit memory have been shown to be correlated with age in prior research (Chiarello & Hoyer, 1988; Fromm, Holland, Nebes, & Oakley, 1991; Salthouse, 1993). Below we briefly discuss declarative memory, working memory, and perceptual speed, functions which show pronounced age-related differences and are critical to any neuropsychological understanding of aging.

Perhaps the most widely recognized cognitive

consequence of aging is decline in ability to explicitly learn and retain new information. This impairment, in what may be termed *declarative* (or episodic) *memory*, is evident on explicit tests of recall or recognition of previously presented information. Pronounced age group differences are usually observed on such declarative memory tasks (Craik, Byrd, & Swanson, 1987; Scherr et al., 1988; Verhaeghen & Marcoen, 1993). Two relevant population-based longitudinal studies have also been published. In one study (Colsher & Wallace, 1991), decline in free recall of word lists was observed over a 6-year interval; in the other study (Evans et al., 1993) decline in recall of narrative material was observed over a 3-year interval. In both studies, advancing age and limited education were associated with more pronounced decline.

Cross-sectional studies suggest that impairment is most pronounced on declarative tasks that mainly involve internally generated strategies (Craik, 1986). Thus, age-related differences are typically more pronounced when retention is assessed with free recall rather than cued recall or recognition, which are thought to be less demanding of limited processing resources. The neural bases of age-related changes in declarative memory are incompletely understood, but degenerative changes involving hippocampal-diencephalic networks seem likely to be involved (Squire & Zola-Morgan, 1991) and have been implicated in imaging studies (Golomb et al., 1993, 1994).

Pronounced age-related differences are also seen in what may be termed strategic or working memory (Baddeley & Hitch, 1974). Working memory has been defined and operationally decomposed in several ways (Baddeley & Hitch, 1994; Gathercole, 1994; Moscovitch, 1994). Most approaches require participants to simultaneously retain and process information. Dual-task procedures have been used with some success but are unwieldy for clinical use. Fortunately, a variety of span techniques have been developed and used successfully in this age group (Cooper & Sagar, 1993; Craik, 1986; Salthouse & Babcock, 1991). Substantial age-related differences are seen on such measures (Foos, 1989; Light & Anderson, 1985; Salthouse, Babcock, & Shaw, 1991). The limited available longitudinal evidence also supports the view that working memory declines with age (Hultsch, Hertzog, Small, McDonald-Miszczak, & Dixon, 1992). Further, working memory impairment is believed to contribute to performance on most declarative memory tasks, especially those with high processing demands on which age-related differences are most pronounced (Salthouse, 1991). The neural bases of working memory are uncertain, though neural networks within the striatum and prefrontal cortex have been implicated (Gabrieli, 1994; Moscovitch, 1994).

In cross-sectional studies, the largest age group differences are usually seen on measures of perceptual speed. Perceptual speed refers to the speed with which simple perceptual comparisons can be performed. It is typically measured with timed tasks requiring symbol substitution or same/different judgments about pairs of visually presented stimuli. Digit Symbol from the Wechsler Adult Intelligence Scale-Revised (Wechsler, 1981) and the Symbol Digit Modalities Test (Smith, 1982) are two widely used neuropsychological measures of perceptual speed. Although these tasks also make motoric and mnemonic demands, age-related differences have been shown to persist when these demands are substantially reduced (Salthouse, 1992).

In cross-sectional studies, age group differences in perceptual speed emerge early and seem to reflect a broad segment of those who are studied rather than a subset of poor performers (Salthouse, 1991, 1992). Decline in perceptual speed is also observed in longitudinal studies of volunteer cohorts (Schaie, 1989). When age-related differences in perceptual speed are controlled analytically, age group differences on some explicit memory and higher order cognitive tasks, including many standard neuropsychological tests, are reduced or eliminated (Salthouse, 1991, 1993). Although such correlational evidence does not mean that reduced perceptual speed explains other cognitive impairments, it does underscore the importance of perceptual speed for any understanding of cognitive aging. The neural bases of perceptual speed are uncertain.

In summary, there is firm agreement about several important issues in cognitive aging: (a) Many older persons experience decline in cognitive function; (b) diseases which impair cognitive function account for some portion of this decline; (c) level of formal education is also related to cognitive decline; and (d) cognitive decline is especially evident in declarative memory and in processing abilities, like perceptual speed and working memory. Much remains to be learned, however, about person-specific patterns of change in specific forms of cognition, the neural bases of such changes, or factors which may mediate or modify such cognitive changes.

Neuropsychological Determination of Cognitive Impairment among Older Persons

The central aim of most neuropsychological assessments of older persons is determining the presence or absence of cognitive impairment. Cognitive impairment refers to substantial decline from a previously higher level of function. In the absence of longitudinal data, prior functional level is unknown and must be estimated, implicitly or explicitly. Further, as reviewed in the preceding section, some cognitive decline will frequently occur prior to the onset of clinically manifest dementia. Thus, identification of cognitive impairment due to AD or another medical condition is challenging. Clinical determination of cognitive impairment is typically based on the following categories of evidence: (a) change in cognitively mediated social or occupational functioning, (b) discrepancy between current test performance and demographically based estimates of past performance, and (c) discrepancy between current performance on "age-sensitive" and "age-insensitive" tests. In the remainder of this section, we consider each of these sources of information regarding cognitive impairment.

A careful history of cognitively mediated aspects of social and occupational functioning is an essential component of any evaluation of cognitive impairment. A variety of structured interview procedures and questionnaires are available for measuring current competence in selected daily living activities and subtle changes in level of competence (Bennett & Knopman, 1994; Sano et al., 1995). In evaluating persons with known or suspected cognitive impairment, a knowledgeable informant, typically a spouse or child, should be the primary source of these historical data. Informants are often reluctant to lodge complaints about the patient and may need to be interviewed separately. In persons

with cognitive impairment, self-report about current and past behavior is of limited value for purposes of clinical classification. Even in the absence of cognitive impairment, self-appraisal of cognitive functioning is at best weakly related to current performance (Zelinski & Gilewski, 1988) and has not been shown to predict cognitive decline (Flicker, Ferris, & Reisberg, 1993; Taylor, Miller, & Tinklenberg, 1992; Youngjohn & Crook, 1993). Report from a knowledgeable informant of decline in cognitively mediated aspects of social/occupational function should be considered strong evidence in favor of cognitive impairment. Indeed, some diagnostic systems (e.g., *Diagnostic and Statistical Manual of Mental Disorders*, fourth edition) require evidence of such impact on real-world functioning for the diagnosis of dementia. Assessment of functional competence is no panacea, however, since decline still must be inferred from one data collection point, and functional impairment may result from a wide variety of other age-related neurologic and non-neurologic conditions. Further, in comparison to observer ratings, performance-based tests are widely believed to provide psychometrically superior measures of cognitive functioning. Absence of informant report of decline, therefore, does not prove that decline has not occurred.

The cornerstone of any neuropsychological conception of cognitive impairment is a comparison between an observed test score and an estimate of past performance on that test. Past performance is usually inferred from the distribution of scores within some normative reference group. A subset of the reference group, specified by one or more demographic variables (e.g., age, gender, education), is used, with the aid of normative tables or regression equations, to specify confidence intervals within which the observed score should fall. If the observed score falls below that range, impairment is inferred.

The adequacy of these estimates of impairment rests heavily on the adequacy of the normative group. Yet, few cognitive tests have norms which extend beyond age 75, though normative studies of this age range have recently begun to emerge (Ivnik et al., 1990, 1992a, 1992b; Ryan, Paolo, & Brungardt, 1990). There are two particularly difficult issues for normative studies within this age range. The first is defining *eligibility*. Implicitly or explicitly, most normative studies exclude persons whose cognitive function is not normal. Yet, there is limited consensus on how this should be done. The decision takes on special importance because of the striking increase in cognitive impairment among the oldest old, with estimates of dementia increasing from about 3% of persons ages 65–74 to nearly 50% of persons ages 85 and older in one population-based study (Evans et al., 1989). Depending on how eligibility is defined, level of cognitive function within an 85 and older group is likely to vary considerably, as will demographically based estimates of cognitive impairment. Second, since cross-sectional studies consistently show that older persons do not perform as well as younger persons on cognitive tests, age-adjusted norms implicitly assume that an average amount of impairment is "normal," and "impairment" is reserved for only those people who are more impaired than the average. However, impaired cognition is likely to be equally problematic for all persons within this age range, and it is not altogether certain that definitions of cognitive impairment should depend on age.

Prediction of performance within the reference group is usually maximized by inclusion of multiple demographic variables, which in turn should enhance detection of cognitive impairment by improving the estimate of past performance level. In practice, however, incorporation of demographically based estimates of past performance to guide interpretation of current performance does not appear to alter determinations of cognitive impairment as much as might be expected (e.g., Stern et al., 1992). One factor may be that demographic prediction errors are most apt to occur in persons with extreme levels of premorbid ability, the persons who are most difficult to classify in the first place.

Another means of estimating cognitive impairment involves contrasting performance on cognitive measures thought to be especially vulnerable to age-related decline with performance on less sensitive measures. This ipsative approach is based on the widespread observation that some forms of cognitive functioning are especially affected by age and age-related diseases whereas other cognitive functions are relatively less sensitive to these factors. In the absence of cognitive impairment, it is presumed that performance on sensitive and insensitive measures will be equivalent; if performance on the sensitive measure is substantially below that on the insensitive measure, cognitive impairment is inferred.

There are numerous examples of the ipsative approach to identifying cognitive impairment in older persons, some of which date back several decades (Babcock, 1930; Nelson, 1982; Wechsler, 1939). The principal difficulty with the approach (see Yates, 1956, for review) is that decline with advancing age is seen on virtually all cognitive performance measures, including very brief mental status tests (Colsher & Wallace, 1991; Evans et al., 1993), measures of practiced verbal skills (Fromm et al., 1991), and measures of relatively automatic cognitive processes (Chiarello & Hoyer, 1988). Pre-existing or disease-induced differences in the configuration of cognitive abilities may contribute further error. Perhaps not surprisingly, there is limited empirical support for this ipsative approach (Fromm et al., 1991; Patterson, Graham, & Hodges, 1994; Wilson, Rosenbaum, & Brown, 1979; Yates, 1956). Nonetheless, most neuropsychological test interpretation takes into consideration the differential impact of age and specific neurologic disorders on cognitive function and attempts to use this information clinically to differentiate spared and impaired cognition.

In summary, it is clear that clinical differentiation of normal and impaired cognition in elderly persons is complex and difficult. Substantial progress will require longitudinal studies of samples from defined populations. Such research can provide a more detailed picture of age-related change in cognition, antecedents and consequences of such change, and factors which may identify persons who have experienced, or are at risk to experience, substantial cognitive decline.

In the uncertain interval before such studies are accomplished, what can be done to improve clinical decision-making about cognitive impairment in elderly persons? In our view, it is important to structure those aspects of the evaluation that are amenable to control. Thus, reliance on a routine set of tests and structured interview procedures is recommended. A core set of tests should be selected to measure the cognitive domains of interest. In addition to the usual psychometric and neuropsychological factors used to guide test selection, prior use in clinical gerontological research and practice should be considered. The Mini-Mental State Examination (Tombaugh & McIntyre, 1992), for example, is not especially sensitive to cognitive impairment and provides minimal localizing information. On the other hand, because it has been widely used in population-based and longitudinal studies, it can provide useful descriptive information about the global level of cognitive functioning, and, in the event of follow-up evaluation, change in cognitive function. A range of cognitive measures specifically designed for use with older persons is available (Albert et al., 1991; Mattis, 1988; Morris et al., 1989; Rosen, Mohs, & Davis, 1984) and should be carefully considered for inclusion in a core set of tests or as supplements to more traditional neuropsychological tests.

Substantial and potentially controllable sources of variance in judgment about cognitive impairment include the number of tests used to measure a given ability, the level of performance chosen to separate normal from impaired scores, and the method of resolving discrepant test results. That is, determinations about memory impairment, for example, depend, inter alia, on how many memory tests are given, where cutoff scores are placed (e.g., 10th vs. 20th percentile), and specification of the proportion of impaired tests needed to conclude that memory is impaired. In the absence of absolute answers to these issues, it is important to adopt a structured, consistent approach which can be amended as new information becomes available.

In view of the difficulty in determining presence or absence of cognitive impairment, we recommend that the judgment always be considered a probabilistic one. Importantly, we advocate that a category of "possibly impaired" be included between "not impaired" and "probably impaired." Inclusion of an uncertain category reflects clinical reality and provides an impetus to the clinician and the participant to repeat testing at some future date(s) in order to gather more definitive evidence. The most secure approach in doubtful cases is to repeat testing, usually at annual intervals, until a clearer answer emerges. At intervals less than 1 year, level of change expected rarely exceeds the test's standard error of measurement. Although alternative forms are available for some tests, repeated administration of the same form is the most reliable approach to measuring change in cognitive function.

Summary

In summary, declining cognitive function threatens the well-being, independence, and longevity of elderly persons. The problem is likely to increase in the next century with the projected aging of the population in the United States and many other industrialized societies. Advances in our understanding of cognitive decline will require substantial scientific effort. Longitudinal studies of samples from defined populations are especially needed in order to characterize the full spectrum of cognitive change, describe its neural bases, and identify factors that may mediate change, especially factors that are potentially modifiable. Several such studies are currently in progress and should contribute substantially to our knowledge of person-specific patterns of cognitive change within this age group.

Differentiation of "normal" and "pathological" cognitive functioning in elderly persons is a complex and imperfect process, and currently there is no firm agreement about the optimal approach. In making this determination, the neuropsychologist typically relies heavily on normative data to make inferences about cognitive impairment. Fortunately, normative data for this age group are increasingly becoming available for many traditional neuropsychological tests. Further, a number of cognitive measures designed specifically for use in this age range have extensive normative information available.

Normative information, whatever its strengths and limitations may be, is only a part, albeit a visible part, of the clinical determination of cognitive impairment. Normative information provides a means of quantifying the likelihood that a given test performance is impaired. It is still uncertain, however, how much deviation in test performance constitutes impairment, how multiple indicators of impairment should best be used to make inferences about an ability, which and how many abilities should be assessed, and how comparisons between tests or domains can be used to support clinical decisions. Research on these difficult issues is needed. In the meantime, we advocate development of highly structured approaches to data collection and interpretation. In some circumstances, it may be feasible to formalize interpretation of neuropsychological tests by constructing algorithms which convert individual test performances into decisions about presence/absence of impairment in a given ability (Stern et al., 1992). Given limitations in current knowledge and the complexity of decisions, such algorithms are unlikely to substitute for clinical decision-making. Rather, they can provide a framework that provides rigor and consistency to these difficult determinations, reserving for the clinician the final decision, which may incorporate more qualitative historical information, other test findings not included in the algorithm, observations about level of cooperation with test procedures, information about sensory or motor impairment, current medications, and other medical conditions.

Acknowledgments

This work was supported in part by National Institute on Aging grants P30 AG10161 and P01 AG09466.

References

Albert, M. S., Smith, L. A., Scherr, P. A., Funkenstein, H. H., Taylor, J. O., & Evans, D. A. (1991). Use of brief cognitive tests to identify individuals in the community with clinically diagnosed Alzheimer's disease. *International Journal of Neuroscience, 57,* 167–178.

Babcock, H. (1930). An experiment in the measurement of mental deterioration. *Archives of Psychology, 117,* 1–105.

Baddeley, A. D., & Hitch, G. J. (1974). Working memory. In G. Bower (Ed.), *The psychology of learning and motivation* (Vol. 8, pp. 47–90). San Diego, CA: Academic Press.

Baddeley, A. D., & Hitch, G. J. (1994). Developments in the concept of working memory. *Neuropsychology, 8,* 485–493.

Bennett, D. A., & Knopman, D. S. (1994). Alzheimer's disease: A comprehensive approach to patient management. *Geriatrics, 49,* 20–26.

Chiarello, C., & Hoyer, W. J. (1988). Adult age differences in implicit and explicit memory: Time course and encoding effects. *Psychology and Aging, 3,* 358–366.

Colsher, P. L., & Wallace, R. B. (1991). Longitudinal application of cognitive function measures in a defined population of community-dwelling elders. *Annals of Epidemiology, 1,* 215–230.

Cooper, J. A., & Sagar, H. J. (1993). Incidental and intentional recall in Parkinson's disease: An account based on diminished attentional resources. *Journal of Clinical and Experimental Neuropsychology, 15,* 713–731.

Craik, F. I. M. (1986). A functional account of age differences in memory. In F. Klix & H. Hagendorf (Eds.), *Human memory and cognitive capabilities—Mechanisms and performance*

(pp. 409–422). North-Holland: Elsevier Science Publishers B.V.

Craik, F. I. M., Byrd, M., & Swanson, J. M. (1987). Patterns of memory loss in three elderly samples. *Psychology and Aging, 2,* 79–86.

Evans, D. A. (1991). Why should we study change in cognitive function? *Annals of Epidemiology, 1,* 283–284.

Evans, D. A., Funkenstein, H. H., Albert, M. S., Scherr, P. A., Cook, N. R., Chown, M. J., Hebert, L. E., Hennekens, C. H., & Taylor, J. O. (1989). Prevalence of Alzheimer's disease in a community population of older persons—higher than previously reported. *Journal of the American Medical Association, 262,* 2551–2556.

Evans, D. A., Beckett, L. A., Albert, M. S., Hebert, L. E., Scherr, P. A., Funkenstein, H. H., & Taylor, J. O. (1993). Level of education and change in cognitive function in a community population of older persons. *Annals of Epidemiology, 3,* 71–77.

Flicker, C., Ferris, S. H., & Reisberg, B. (1993). A longitudinal study of cognitive function in elderly persons with subjective memory complaints. *Journal of the American Geriatrics Society, 41,* 1029–1032.

Foos, P. W. (1989). Adult age differences in working memory. *Psychology and Aging, 4,* 269–275.

Fromm, D., Holland, A. L., Nebes, R. D., & Oakley, M. A. (1991). A longitudinal study of word-reading ability in Alzheimer's disease: Evidence from the National Adult Reading Test. *Cortex, 17,* 367–376.

Gabrieli, J. D. E. (1994). Contributions of the basal ganglia to skill learning and working memory in humans. In J. C. Houk, J. L. Davis, & D. G. Beiser (Eds.), *Models of information processing in the basal ganglia* (pp. 277–294). Cambridge, MA: MIT Press.

Gathercole, S. E. (1994). Neuropsychology and working memory: A review. *Neuropsychology, 8,* 494–505.

Golomb, J., de Leon, M. J., Kluger, A., George, A. E., Tarshish, C., & Ferris, S. H. (1993). Hippocampal atrophy in normal aging: An association with recent memory impairment. *Archives of Neurology, 50,* 967–976.

Golomb, J., Kluger, A., de Leon, M. J., Ferris, S. H., Convit, A., Mittelman, M. S., Cohen, J., Rusinek, H., De Santi, S., & George, A. E. (1994). Hippocampal formation size in normal human aging: A correlate of delayed secondary memory performance. *Learning & Memory, 1,* 45–54.

Hultsch, D. F., Hertzog, C., Small, B. J., McDonald-Miszczak, L., & Dixon, R. A. (1992). Short-term longitudinal change in cognitive performance in later life. *Psychology and Aging, 7,* 571–584.

Ivnik, R. J., Malec, J. F., Tangalos, E. G., Petersen, R. C., Kokmen, E., & Kurland, L. T. (1990). The Auditory-Verbal Learning Test (AVLT): Norms for ages 55 years and older. *Psychological Assessment: A Journal of Consulting and Clinical Psychology, 2,* 304–312.

Ivnik, R. J., Malec, J. F., Smith, G. E., Tangalos, E. G., Petersen, R. C., Kokmen, E., & Kurland, L. T. (1992a). Mayo's Older Americans Normative Studies: WAIS-R norms for ages 56 to 97. *The Clinical Neuropsychologist, 6,* 1–30.

Ivnik, R. J., Malec, J. F., Smith, G. E., Tangalos, E. G., Petersen, R. C., Kokmen, E., & Kurland, L. T. (1992b). Mayo's Older

Americans Normative Studies: WMS-R norms for ages 56 to 94. *The Clinical Neuropsychologist, 6*, 49–82.

Light, L. L., & Anderson, P. A. (1985). Working memory capacity, age, and memory for discourse. *Journal of Gerontology, 40*, 737–747.

Lindenberger, U., Mayr, U., & Kliegl, R. (1993). Speed and intelligence in old age. *Psychology and Aging, 8*, 207–220.

Mattis, S. (1988). *Dementia Rating Scale (DRS)*. Odessa, FL: Psychological Assessment Resources.

Morris, J. C., Heyman, A., Mohs, R. C., Hughes, J. P., van Belle, G., Fillenbaum, G., Mellits, E. D., Clark, C., & the CERAD Investigators. (1989). The Consortium to Establish a Registry for Alzheimer's Disease (CERAD). Part I. Clinical and neuropsychological assessment of Alzheimer's disease. *Neurology, 39*, 1159–1165.

Moscovitch, M. (1994). Cognitive resources and dual-task interference effects at retrieval in normal people: The role of the frontal lobes and medial temporal cortex. *Neuropsychology, 8*, 524–534.

Nelson, H. E. (1982). *Nelson Adult Reading Test manual*. London: the National Hospital for Nervous Diseases.

Patterson, K., Graham, N., & Hodges, J. R. (1994). Reading in dementia of the Alzheimer type: A preserved ability? *Neuropsychology, 8*, 395–407.

Pfeiffer, E. (1975). A short portable mental status questionnaire for the assessment of organic brain deficit in elderly patients. *Journal of the American Geriatrics Society, 23*, 433–439.

Rogosa, D. (1988). Myths about longitudinal research. In K. W. Schaie, R. T. Campbell, W. Meredith, & S. C. Rawlings (Eds.), *Methodological issues in aging research* (pp. 171–209). New York: Springer.

Rosen, W. G., Mohs, R. C., & Davis, K. L. (1984). A new rating scale for Alzheimer's disease. *American Journal of Psychiatry, 141*, 1356–1364.

Ryan, J. J., Paolo, A. M., & Brungardt, T. M. (1990). Standardization of the Wechsler Adult Intelligence Scale-Revised for persons 75 years and older. *Psychological Assessment: A Journal of Consulting and Clinical Psychology, 2*, 404–411.

Salthouse, T. A. (1991). Mediation of adult age differences in cognition by reductions in working memory and speed of processing. *Psychological Science, 2*, 179–183.

Salthouse, T. A. (1992). What do adult age differences in the Digit Symbol Substitution Test reflect? *Journal of Gerontology: Psychological Sciences, 47*, P121–P128.

Salthouse, T. A. (1993). Speed and knowledge as determinants of adult age differences in verbal tasks. *Journal of Gerontology, 48*, 29–36.

Salthouse, T. A., & Babcock, R. L. (1991). Decomposing adult age differences in working memory. *Developmental Psychology, 27*, 763–776.

Salthouse, T. A., Babcock, R. L., & Shaw, R. J. (1991). Effects of adult age on structural and operational capacities in working memory. *Psychology and Aging, 1*, 118–127.

Sano, M., Devanand, D. P., Richards, M., Miller, L. W., Marder, K., Bell, K., Dooneief, G., Bylsma, F. W., Lafleche, G., Albert, M., Folstein, M., & Stern, Y. (1995). A standardized technique for establishing onset and duration of symptoms of Alzheimer's disease. *Archives of Neurology, 52*, 961–966.

Schaie, K. W. (1989). Perceptual speed in adulthood: Cross-sectional and longitudinal studies. *Psychology and Aging, 4*, 443–453.

Scherr, P. A., Albert, M. S., Funkenstein, H. H., Cook, N. R., Hennekens, C. H., Branch, L. G., White, L. R., Taylor, J. O., & Evans, D. A. (1988). Correlates of cognitive function in an elderly community population. *American Journal of Epidemiology, 128*, 1084–1101.

Smith, A. (1982). *Symbol Digit Modalities Test (SDMT) Manual* (Rev.). Los Angeles: Western Psychological Services.

Squire, L. R., & Zola-Morgan, S. (1991). The medial temporal lobe memory system. *Science, 20*, 1380–1386.

Stern, Y., Andrews, H., Pittman, J., Sano, M., Tatemichi, T., Lantigua, R., & Mayeux, R. (1992). Diagnosis of dementia in a heterogeneous population—Development of a neuropsychological paradigm-based diagnosis of dementia and quantified correction for the effects of education. *Archives of Neurology, 49*, 453–460.

Taylor, J. L., Miller, T. P., & Tinklenberg, J. R. (1992). Correlates of memory decline: A 4-year longitudinal study of older adults with memory complaints. *Psychology and Aging, 7*, 184–193.

Tombaugh, T. N., & McIntyre, N. J. (1992). The Mini-Mental State Examination: A comprehensive review. *Journal of the American Geriatrics Society, 40*, 922–935.

Verhaeghen, P., & Marcoen, A. (1993). More or less the same? A memorability analysis on episodic memory tasks in young and older adults. *Journal of Gerontology: Psychological Sciences, 48*, P172–P178.

Wechsler, D. (1939). *The measurement of adult intelligence*. Baltimore: Williams & Wilkins.

Wechsler, D. (1981). *Wechsler Adult Intelligence Scale-Revised Manual*. New York: Psychological Corporation.

Wechsler, D. (1987). *Wechsler Memory Scale-Revised Manual*. New York: Psychological Corporation.

Wilson, R. S., Rosenbaum, G., & Brown, G. (1979). The problem of premorbid intelligence in neuropsychological assessment. *Journal of Clinical Neuropsychology, 1*, 49–53.

Yates, A. (1956). The use of vocabulary in the measurement of intellectual deterioration—A review. *Journal of Mental Science, 102*, 409–440.

Youngjohn, J. R., & Crook, T. H., III. (1993). Stability of everyday memory in age-associated memory impairment: A longitudinal study. *Neuropsychology, 7*, 406–416.

Zelinski, E. M., & Gilewski, M. J. (1988). Assessment of memory complaints by rating scales and questionnaires. *Psychopharmacology Bulletin, 24*, 523–529.

3

Personality and Normal Aging

CHRISTOPHER STARRATT AND LINDA PETERSON

Introduction

At first glance, a chapter on theories of personality and aging may seem misplaced in a text on geriatric neuropsychology. Cognition, after all, represents the construct of particular interest for clinical and experimental investigation within neuropsychology. We are developing an ever growing understanding of the age-related effects on various cognitive processes such as attention and concentration, sensorimotor integration, visual perception and construction, new learning and memory, language, novel problem-solving, and cognitive flexibility. We are attuned to the potential age-related effects associated with the psychometric evaluation of cognitive processes. Although extensive age-related norms for many of our clinical measures of cognitive functioning are still lacking, it is an issue that is well recognized and directly addressed in the literature. There are ongoing efforts to provide age-appropriate norms or other correction procedures that can be applied to our cognitive data. We are also in an exciting era where neuroanatomical and neuropsychological correlates are more readily available, even to the day-to-day clinician. Procedures such as computed tomography (CT), magnetic resonance imaging (MRI), positron emission tomography (PET), single photon emission computed tomography (SPECT), and electroencephalogram (EEG)/event–related potentials (ERP) have not only given us the opportunity to understand the structural and functional processes of neuropathological conditions, but have also allowed us to investigate the relationship between brain structure,

CHRISTOPHER STARRATT AND LINDA PETERSON • Department of Psychology, Barry University, Miami Shores, Florida 33161.

brain function, and cognition among normal, non-brain-injured individuals.

Although not universally accepted, neuropsychological evaluation typically includes the discrete measurement of specific cognitive components or combinations of such components. This is generally followed by an evaluation of the absolute and relative level of performance within and across functional domains in order to discern a pattern that is more or less typical of a neurological disorder. Within such a context, the relatively global, "soft" construct of personality indeed does seem out of place. This is not to imply that there is no interest in "noncognitive" behaviors. In fact, dimensions that traditionally would be thought of as related to personality figure prominently in the evaluation and diagnosis of numerous neurological disorders. There have been efforts to describe personality changes as an important feature of conditions such as frontal lobe dysfunction (e.g., Miller, Cummings, Villanueva-Mayer, & Boone, 1991), temporal lobe dysfunction (Neppe & Tucker, 1992), and traumatic brain injury (Silver, Hales, & Yudofsky, 1992), as well as Pick's disease (Whitehouse, Friedland, & Strauss, 1992), Huntington's disease (Whitehouse et al., 1992), and Alzheimer's disease (Cummings, 1992). These efforts, however, rarely are embedded within the context of more general theories of personality. We will take the position in this chapter that the neuropsychological evaluation of older individuals can be enhanced by considering both cognitive and noncognitive factors that might be affected by neurological impairment. While there are a number of conceptual schemes that can be used to organize these noncognitive domains, we will focus on theories of normal personality. Our basic premise is that in order to make sense of observed or described personality changes in older individuals who present for neuropsychological evaluation, we need to know something about the construct of personality itself, how it can be measured, and how it is related to the aging process. Specifically, we will review the major current models of personality, with a focus on trait theories and biological theories, and review the literature on personality and aging with a focus on issues of stability and change in personality among normal elders across the life span. Much of what we know about normal aging, in general, has been gathered through several well-known longitudinal studies such as the Duke project (Palmore, Busse, Maddox, Nowlin, & Siegler, 1985), the Baltimore project (Shock et al., 1984), the Institute of Human Development project (Eichorn, Clausen, Haan, Honzig, & Mussen, 1981), and the Kelly Longitudinal project (Conley, 1985). While many of the ideas presented in this chapter have their origin in the work of investigators involved in these projects, they will not be reviewed in detail, but rather integrated into a broader overview of personality and life span development.

Trait Theories of Personality

The study of personality has taken many forms over the years. Scholars have tried to explain the structure, dynamics, development, and deviances of the relatively enduring, characteristic ways in which we relate to our interpersonal world. Much of the current literature in personality research has focused on a specific aspect of personality, that is, those behavioral tendencies that we call traits. Life span studies of normal personality, in particular, have relied heavily on the assessment of traits. Due to their current status within the personality literature and, as we shall see later, because of the relationship to biological models of personality, personality traits as they relate to the process of normal aging will be the emphasis of this chapter.

Allport defined personality as "the dynamic organization within the individual of those psychophysical systems that determine his unique adjustments to his environment" (Allport, 1937, p. 48). In the same vein, Pervin (1970) said that "personality represents those structural and dynamic properties of an individual or individuals as they reflect themselves in characteristic responses to situations" (p. 2). Personality theorists have constructed a large number of theories describing what the structural components of personality are and how these structures relate to each other. Traits figure prominently among the proposed structures. Virtually all trait theorists agree that individuals possess traits to varying degrees, that these traits are related somehow to behavior, and that traits can be measured.

Until recently, however, there has been little agreement on which traits are central to the structure of personality. There has been some consensus that traits do not include talents and abilities, but do include the inclination to engage in skill-related behaviors (Watson, Clark, & Harkness, 1994). Intelligence, while arguably a major component of personality, has generally been left out of trait measures and placed under the heading of "cognition."

Overview of Trait Theories

The use of traits to describe behavior is an approach familiar to most people. The notion that language embodies important aspects of personality led to an interest in a lexical approach for the evaluation of fundamental aspects or dimensions of personality. The first major endeavor in this area was conducted by Allport and Odbert (1936) who reviewed a standard edition of the dictionary and extracted 18,000 terms, 4,500 of which were classified as trait words, descriptive of personality. Subsequently, Cattell reduced the list to 35 representative terms. Factor analysis yielded 12 clusters which Cattell identified as 12 personality factors (Cattell, 1943, 1945a, 1945b). At about the same time, Eysenck identified three enduring factors of personality: neuroticism, extraversion, and psychoticism as central or core factors in personality (Eysenck & Eysenck, 1964, 1975). Guilford (1959) and Guilford and Zimmerman (1956) proposed yet another factor analytic model, this one with 14 factors. Despite the variety in number and content of the proposed personality factors, some consistent results were beginning to be found even at this early date. Fiske (1949) obtained a five-factor solution using a subset of the Cattell data. Furthermore, the solution was replicable. In an analysis of Air Force personnel data, Tupes and Christal (1961) also obtained five replicable and meaningful factors. In 1963, Norman published his replication of the five-factor structure as well. The convergence of these studies was largely ignored until Goldberg (1981) labeled them the "Big Five." (See McCrae & John, 1992, for a more detailed historical review.) Since that time, the five-factor model of personality has received considerable attention among personality theorists.

During the 1980s, numerous studies were published demonstrating that the five-factor structure could be obtained from a variety of data, both old and new. For example, Digman and Takemoto-Chock (1981) reanalyzed the data from six major studies and obtained the five-factor structure, while Goldberg (1990) found a similar structure using a subset of Norman's adjectives and a sample of 187 college students. Similar factor structures have been replicated in a German sample (Ostendorf, 1990) and at least partially replicated in a Chinese sample (Yang & Bond, 1990) suggesting the cross-cultural relevance of the Big Five.

The five factors that have emerged from these studies have been defined by Costa and McCrae (1987) who developed the NEO Personality Inventory to measure them. They label the five factors as neuroticism (as opposed to emotional stability), extraversion or surgency, openness to experience, agreeableness (as opposed to antagonism), and conscientiousness (as opposed to undirectedness). The traits which compose the five factors are sometimes surprising such as the finding that dominance, energy, and sociability all tend to covary across individuals and load on the extraversion (surgency) factor. The five factors thus represent a higher level of abstraction than traits (John & Robins, 1993).

Costa and McCrae are of the opinion that consensus in the field of personality has been reached with regard to the five factors (McCrae & Costa, 1986), which, in their view, "offer a universal and comprehensive framework for the description of individual personality differences" (p. 1001). Certainly there are many adherents to and defenders of the five-factor model (see Goldberg & Saucier, 1995, or Costa & McCrae, 1995, for a defense of the model), but there is disagreement as to whether a consensus has been reached (Block, 1995; Pervin, 1994; Waller & Ben-Porath, 1987). Both Block (1995) and Pervin (1994) raise concerns regarding theoretical assumptions, or the lack thereof, underlying the five-factor model, the use of factor analysis, and the selection of adjectives used by many of the studies. Other researchers have made attempts to integrate the five-factor model with other approaches (Benjamin, 1994; Johnson & Ostendorf, 1993).

Despite the ongoing controversy regarding the status of the five-factor model as delineating the most important features of personality, this model may be useful for clinicians who wish to add an evaluation of normal personality to their armament of usual cognitive measures.

Stability of Personality Traits among Adults

Personality change is an issue about which there is little agreement (Heatherton & Weinberger, 1994). Personality theorists have postulated various theories about the stability of personality once it is formed. Freud believed that personality formation was complete during early childhood, usually by the end of the phallic stage (3–5 years), and that one's personality would not undergo radical change unless there were extraordinary circumstances, one of which was psychoanalysis (Freud, 1933). James (1950), more expansive in his time limits, set the age for the solidification of personality at about age 30, but concurred that there was little or no change to be expected after that. On the other hand, Erikson's stage theory of personality delineated developmental tasks that occur throughout the life span (Erikson, 1950). Despite Erikson's view, the general opinion that permeated the field of personality was that one's personality underwent little change beyond ordinary maturation. This assumption of stability, indeed, inability to change, was made in spite of the fact that there was little or no empirical evidence. In fact, Kelly (1955) had to argue, presumably as clinical psychology was coming into its own as a field, that personality change was even possible. The assumption that personality was stable, even unchanging, remained unchallenged and largely untested until the 1960s.

In 1968, Mischel suggested that personality stability is illusory and that behavior is far less stable than we believe. Consistencies in personality ratings, such as peer ratings, arise from either rater-constructed views of the person being observed or from regularities in the individual's social roles, environmental contexts, and stable routines (p. 70). Mischel seemed to suggest that personality, per se, does not exist and, at best, descriptions like " hostile" and "aggressive" are useful only for screening purposes. According to Mischel it is far better to focus on specific contingencies and discriminative conditions than on trait or disposition words.

Mischel (1968) helped to ignite the person/ situation argument which formed the research in personality for the next 15 years. While this controversy stimulated much research, the end result appears to have been to reinforce the idea for researchers that the context in which behavior occurs is important when trying to predict individual behavior. In their discussion of what is to be learned from the person/situation controversy, Kendrick and Funder (1988) list five ways in which persons and situations interact. Included in the list are the ideas that traits can influence behavior only when the situation is relevant and that traits are more easily expressed in some situations than others.

The relevance of both traits and situations has important ramifications for evaluation. Some of the reported failure to demonstrate consistency in personality may have come from the fact that either the situations were not relevant to the individual or that the personality constructs (traits) had differential relevance to individuals (Britt, 1993). Although psychologists have assumed that people can define themselves on all the theoretical constructs presented to them, Baumeister (as cited in Britt, 1993) has noted that some individuals may not even possess a particular trait.

One of the strengths of the five-factor approach to personality is the number of characteristics associated with each of the five factors. Assessment based on this approach should be broad enough to capture traits that people possess. Rather than expecting that someone will be extraverted in the same way all one's life, we can expect that there will be some change in the way extraversion is expressed, depending on life circumstances, with perhaps less change in the overall measure of extraversion. The model, therefore, allows for growth and change within the context of a stable personality structure. The extravert may always be extraverted but may express it differently over time. Kroessler (1990) notes that the same thing may occur with regard to pathological traits, noting that the elderly are rarely

diagnosed with personality disorders. He suggests that this is because the diagnostic criteria are not adjusted to reflect changes that occur with age. Rosowsky and Gurian (1992) concur that the underlying pathology does not change but that the expression of it may, as when an individual engages in self-injurious behavior as a young adult and anorexic behavior during old age.

Clinicians working with older individuals obviously must address the issue of whether observed behavior reflects a lifelong pattern, normal aging, or a possible pathologic condition. The experimental personality research may be of assistance to us as we try to distinguish between these alternatives. Studies that have looked at the longitudinal stability of personality characteristics have generally found a fairly high level of stability. Costa, McCrae, and Arenberg (1980) found high correlations (in the 0.7 to 0.8 range) for 10 characteristics over 6- and 12-year intervals. They concluded that the stability of these traits was high by young adulthood. Interestingly, they found lower psychometric stability for the trait of emotionality. Costa et al. (1980) suggest that either affective traits are harder to measure or that persons who score higher on neurotic traits are more likely to change. There is also evidence of a common core of traits in measures of morale, well-being, and personal adjustment to aging. Costa, McCrae, and Norris (1981) used measures of neuroticism and extraversion to predict adjustment in the elderly over periods ranging from 2 to 10 years. Results support the notion of stability in both extraversion and neuroticism scores although the latter were again less stable. In contrast to the Costa et al. (1980, 1981) studies, Levenson, Aldwin, Bosse, and Spiro (1988) found evidence for stability of negative affect. Emotionality and extraversion predicted 25% of the variance in mental health in men 10 years later.

An important issue in the stability of personality research has been the effect of self-report (Mischel, 1968). Do self-report measures reflect consistency because that is how the person wishes to present himself or herself or is there actually some consistency? Studies using both self-reports and reports by knowledgeable others have found substantial convergent and divergent validity. Conley (1985) demonstrated consistency in personality over five decades using a combination of self-reports and ratings by acquaintances and marriage partners. He found consistency for neuroticism, social extraversion, and impulse control for both men and women. Agreeableness had more mixed results. Costa and McCrae (1988) demonstrated consistency in neuroticism, extraversion, and openness to experience over a 5-year period based on spouse and self-ratings. Agreeableness and conscientiousness proved stable over a 3-year period.

Even those studies which posit change have found only a small degree of fluctuation. Specifically, change in the expression of traits has been posited as a negatively accelerating slope with a positive gradient for most traits (Bloom, 1964). This model has been supported for a number of traits (e.g., Finn, 1986). Exceptions to this pattern of change were demonstrated in depression and neurasthenic somatization which may be regarded more as affective states than personality traits in the usual sense. In another cross-sectional sample, Eysenck (1987) noted changes in neuroticism, psychoticism, and extraversion in adult samples ranging in age from 16–19 to 60–69, although the magnitude of change was generally quite small.

Summary

The conclusion that can be drawn from these studies, and the most important one from our perspective, is that personality, while sometimes indicating change, is relatively consistent across the life span. We can, however, expect some change to occur in situations where there is a traumatic or major precipitating event. Otherwise, changes are likely to be quite small and to occur over a long period of time, best measured in years. Pervin (1993) rightly notes that how much change or stability a particular researcher finds depends largely on definitions of change, the time period over which the data are gathered, and the method of measurement. Stability can mean that over time one maintains one's relative position in the group. The most extraverted stays the most extraverted within the group, regardless of whether the group as a whole has changed. Alternatively, stability can mean that the score obtained on some measure has stayed the same from one testing to the next. For our purposes, it is sufficient to recognize that measurable changes over shorter periods of time are unlikely and that

changes in scores on personality characteristics will remain at consistent levels. When changes in personality ratings do occur, it is appropriate to seek sources of these changes in processes other than those that occur in the normal course of aging.

The general stability of personality has important ramifications for the measurement of personality. Specifically, personality changes that are noticeable clearly have meaning and signal an event which is potentially of clinical relevance. Indeed, in the diagnosis of clinical disorders, personality changes are often the first markers that are noticed by either the patient or significant others. In the evaluation of the effects of neurological conditions, however, neuropsychology has focused on cognitive factors and how they have changed. In terms of diagnosis and treatment, personality changes may be as important, if not more important, than cognitive changes.

Biological Theories of Personality

Efforts to explain the biological underpinnings of personality are not new. Most scholars and students of personality trace these efforts back to Hippocrates and Galen. In fact, the most prominent current theorist on the biological basis of personality, Hans J. Eysenck (1967), traces his own theory of personality back to the concepts of these early thinkers. Most basic personality texts remind us that Galen inferred from his observations of everyday behavior that there were four basic types of individuals and that these types were based on individual differences in bodily fluids. While modern theorists have discarded its biological underpinnings, the concept of a finite number of fundamental personality characteristics, or traits, remains popular. In fact, trait theories are enjoying a resurgence of interest, though not uncontested, among personality scholars.

Currently, biologically based explanations of personality are best represented by the works of Eysenck (1967) and Gray (1970). More recently, Damasio, Tranel, and Damasio (1991) have proposed a neuroanatomical model of behavior that is relevant to the study of personality. None of these authors has written extensively about the applications of their theories to the life span. In fact, only recently has Eysenck directly addressed this issue

(Eysenck, 1987). Despite the dearth of literature on the longitudinal aspects of the biological bases of personality, a brief review of these theories seems warranted given the interest in neuropsychology in basic brain–behavior relationships.

Eysenck's Theory of Personality: Extraversion and Neuroticism

The most comprehensive biologically based theory of personality is that of Eysenck (1967). It has been refined and extended over more than 40 years of conceptual and empirical work. The interested reader is referred to several of Eysenck's writings for a complete presentation of his theory (Eysenck, 1967, 1981; Eysenck & Eysenck, 1985). The development of this theory of personality has been described as progressing through a series of stages over the past 40 years (Brocke & Battmann, 1992; Monte, 1995). Briefly, Eysenck began with a descriptive theory of personality based on two orthogonal personality dimensions: introversion versus extraversion and neuroticism versus stability. The quadrants formed by these dimensions yield four basic personality types: neurotic introvert, neurotic extravert, stable introvert, and stable extravert. Each of these types has associated descriptors. Neurotic introverts are described as anxious, serious, worried, suspicious, and thoughtful. Neurotic extraverts are considered quickly aroused, egocentric, hot-headed, and histrionic. Stable introverts are calm, reasonable, controlled, and persistent. Finally, stable extraverts are regarded as playful, easygoing, carefree, sociable, and contented (Eysenck, 1967). His more recent work has described other personality dimensions including one termed "psychoticism." All of these dimensions can be measured using the Eysenck Personality Questionnaire (EPQ; Eysenck & Eysenck, 1976), a self-report instrument.

Since these early descriptive efforts, Eysenck has worked toward describing, and empirically demonstrating, the putative biological (i.e., neurological) underpinnings of these two dimensions of personality. He proposes two distinct, but interacting, neurological systems associated with the expression of the personality dimensions of introversion–extraversion and neuroticism–stability.

Further, interindividual variation in these neural systems largely accounts for individual differences in the associated personality dimensions. Detailed descriptions of this aspect of Eysenck's theory can be found elsewhere (Brocke & Battmann, 1992; Eysenck, 1967). Briefly, an individual's position on the introversion–extraversion dimension is related to the amount of endogenous cortical activation associated with the functioning of the ascending reticular formation or, more commonly, the ascending reticular activating system (ARAS). Individuals with greater resting-state ARAS levels are more cortically aroused and can process external stimuli of minimal intensity with considerable efficiency. Extraverts, on the other hand, because of lower levels of endogenous cortical tone, require more intense external stimuli in order to engage in maximally efficient processing.

Neuroticism is proposed to be associated with the functioning of the "visceral brain system" or limbic system (Eysenck, 1967, p. 230). This system is proposed to be specific to emotionally relevant stimuli. Neurotic or emotionally unstable individuals have lower thresholds for emotional stimuli than emotionally stable individuals and will, therefore, be more reactive to emotionally laden events. Additionally, since there are afferent pathways between the limbic system and the ARAS, limbic activation due to exposure to emotional stimuli can produce increased ARAS arousal.

Further, a curvilinear relationship between arousal and behavioral performance is proposed. Commonly described as the "inverted U," level of performance increases as level of arousal increases to an optimal point. However, as arousal levels increase beyond this point, performance begins to show steady decline (Hebb, 1955).

In simplified form, these postulates lead to specific predictions about the type of behavior to expect from the four fundamental personality types (neurotic introvert, neurotic extravert, stable introvert, stable extravert). In the extreme, neurotic introverts would be expected to be the most avoidant of excessive external stimulation, while stable introverts would be expected to be most active in pursuit of external stimulation.

Considerable research has been conducted to evaluate the theoretical relationship between Eysenck's descriptive personality dimensions and the proposed underlying neural substrate. As Brocke and Battmann (1992) have noted, much of this work relied upon indirect measures of neural functioning such as conditionability (Eysenck & Eysenck, 1985; O'Gorman, 1977), vigilance (Eysenck, 1982), and drug use (Eysenck, 1983). However, there have been studies that have used more direct measures of conceptual nervous system (CNS) functioning such as EEG indices (see Gale, 1981, for a review). More recent work in this area has focused on the relationship between event-related potentials (ERP) and introversion–extraversion. In general, a number of studies have found characteristic ERP wave form differences between introverts and extraverts (Stelmack, 1990). Specifically, introverts have been noted to show larger N1-P2 amplitudes (e.g., De-Pascalis & Montirosso, 1988) as well as larger P3 amplitudes (Daruna, Karrer, & Rosen, 1985), although these differences are not uniformly found (e.g., Polich & Martin, 1992; Rust, 1975).

A fewer number of studies have investigated the relationship between Eysenck's personality dimensions and functional brain measures such as regional cerebral brain flow (rCBF; e.g., Stenberg, Risberg, Warkentin, & Rosen, 1990), positron emission tomography (PET; e.g., Haier, Sokolski, Katz, & Buchsbaum, 1987), and single photon emission computed tomography (SPECT; e.g., Ebmeier et al., 1994). Again, the general finding is of one of systematic differences in brain function between groups of introverts and extraverts. Differences have been observed in brain regions such as the temporal lobes (Stenberg et al., 1990), hippocampus, cingulate, putamen, and caudate (Haier et al., 1987). The study by Ebmeier et al. (1994) is of particular interest because the subjects were normal, healthy, elderly volunteers. The principal finding from this study was a positive relationship between the personality dimension of extraversion and brain activity in the cingulate region. Additionally, a negative relationship was reported between age and both extraversion and cingulate activity, although the relationship between extraversion and cingulate activity remained significant even after statistically controlling for age.

As mentioned previously, Eysenck (1987) presented a brief paper that reviews the cross-sectional normative data from the EPQ manual and proposes some interesting implications for personality and aging. In general, he notes that absolute scores on the EPQ steadily decline for all three of his personality dimensions (extraversion, neuroticism, and psychoticism) for every age decade between 16 years of age (16–19 years) and 69 years of age (60–69 years). The rate of change varies by personality dimension and gender. For example, males show the most dramatic age-related decline on the dimension of extraversion while females demonstrate a more gradual decline. The net result is a pattern where males are higher than females in extraversion during the early adult years, approximately equivalent during the middle age years, and lower than females in extraversion during the early-old years. The pattern for neuroticism, on the other hand, is marked by a parallel decline among males and females across the decades, with females demonstrating consistently higher neuroticism scores. Eysenck suggests that these findings are consistent with a pattern of lessened emotional variability among older individuals. That is to say, as individuals age they are likely to experience less intensity and variability in emotion and behavior. Specifically, he states that "older people are less variable in their conduct and their moods" (Eysenck, 1987, p. 19). We will present additional perspectives regarding the impact of aging on emotions in the next section.

In summary, Eysenck has proposed one of the few biologically based theories of personality and one that has been the basis for an extensive number of empirical investigations. Despite the description of fundamental postulates of his theory that implicate specific regions of the CNS (i.e., ARAS and limbic system), there have been only a relatively limited number of direct studies of the relationship between these, or any other neural systems, and the overt behavioral manifestations that are theoretically related to these neural systems. The results from these studies are generally, but not uniformly, consistent with Eysenck's biological theory of personality. More to the point for present purposes, we have not found any reported studies, neither cross-sectional nor longitudinal, that have sought to determine the stability or change associated with these neurobehavioral relationships across the life span.

Gray's Theory of Personality: Anxiety and Impulsivity

Gray offers a somewhat more delimited model of personality with roots in the neuroanatomical and neurophysiological underpinnings of anxiety (Gray, 1982). Much of the empirical work upon which his theory is based is derived from both animal and human studies of the effects of anxiolytics on learning. A number of Gray's writings provide a full explanation of his theoretical position along with detailed descriptions of proposed neural mechanisms as well as supportive empirical evidence (Gray, 1970, 1976, 1982, 1991).

Basically, Gray proposes two orthogonal dimensions to personality: anxiety and impulsivity. These two dimensions are subserved by different neural systems. The most extensively investigated and clearly articulated of these systems, the behavioral inhibition system or BIS, is proposed as being responsible for the subjective experience of anxiety. This system is activated by four types of external stimuli: impending punishment, frustrative nonreward, novelty, and innate fear. An individual who has an extremely sensitive BIS, therefore, will respond with anxiety when exposed to any of the aforementioned stimuli. Anxiolytics serve to block or attenuate the intensity of BIS activation thereby allowing the sufferer to deal with ongoing daily events with less distress.

Although initially developed to address conditions associated with clinical anxiety, Gray has extended his theory to address normal personality. He proposes that there are individual differences in the strength of response of the BIS leading to the personality dimension of trait anxiety (Diaz & Pickering, 1993; Gray, 1982). The neural structures associated with the BIS are clearly articulated by Gray (1982) and include:

> ... the septal area, the hippocampal formation, and their interconnections (i.e. the septo-hippocampal system); the 'Papez circuit', running from the subicular area in the hippocampal formation to the mammillary bodies, anterior thalamus, cingulate cortex, and back to the subicular area; the neocortical inputs to the septo-hippocampal system from the entorhinal area and prefrontal cortex; the ascending noradrenergic and serotonergic inputs to the septo-hippocampal system; the dopaminergic ascending input to the prefrontal cortex; an ascending cholinergic input to the septo-hippocampal system; the noradrenergic innervation of the hypothalamus; and perhaps (underlying the autonomic outflow of the behavioral inhibition system) the descending noradrenergic fibres of the locus coeruleus ... (p. 459)

The behavioral approach system (BAS), also referred to as the behavioral activation system, is Gray's second dimension of personality. This is a relatively newer construct with less description in the literature. In contrast to the BIS, the behavioral activation system is associated with learned conditions of reward. Revelle (1995) described this system as the "engine of behavior" (and the BIS as the "braking system") (p. 312). In the extreme, impulsive behavior is associated with activation of this system (Gray, 1994; Zinberg & Revelle, 1989). It is a dimension that has also been associated with the experience of positive affect (Watson, Clark, & Harkness, 1994) and novelty seeking (Cloninger, 1987). As with the BIS, Gray (1994) is specific about the neural substrate of the behavioral approach system which includes:

> ... the basal ganglia (the dorsal and ventral striatum, and dorsal and ventral pallidum); the dopaminergic fibers that ascend from the mesencephalon (substantia nigra and nucleus A 10 in the ventral tegmental area) to innervate the basal ganglia; thalamic nuclei closely linked to the basal ganglia; and similarly, neocortical areas (motor, sensorimotor, and prefrontal cortex) closely linked to the basal ganglia. (p. 41)

Compared to Eysenck's, Gray's model provides much more specific neuroanatomical detail, but the psychometric evaluation of the dimensions is less well established. Diaz and Pickering (1993) note fairly recent efforts to develop self-report measures of Gray's dimensions (e.g., MacAndrew & Steele, 1991; Wilson, Gray, & Barrett, 1990). Other investigators of this model have opted to use Eysenck's measures (e.g., Wallace & Newman, 1990). They are able to use this method because Gray (1982) has specified the theoretical relationship between his two dimensions of personality (anxiety and impulsivity) and Eysenck's (introversion and neuroticism). Psychometrically, Gray's dimensions diagonally bisect Eysenck's dimensions (e.g., Eysenck & Eysenck, 1985, pp. 209–212). Essentially, Gray proposes that Eysenck's neurotic introvert is an individual who is high on his dimension of anxiety. A stable extravert, on the other hand, would be low on the dimension of anxiety. The relationship between the personality dimensions associated with these theories remains far from clear and continues to be an issue of active debate (e.g., Diaz & Pickering, 1993; Eysenck & Eysenck, 1985).

We have been unable to find any published reports of the direct application of Gray's model to the issues of personality and normal aging. This is unfortunate because his theory provides a well-articulated, empirically testable formulation of the neural substrates of normal personality as well as specific pathological conditions such as anxiety, phobias, and obsessive-compulsive disorders. His emphasis on the septo-hippocampal and basal ganglia systems are of particular interest within the context of the neuropsychology of aging especially given the association of these regions with age-related disorders such as Alzheimer's disease and Parkinson's disease. For this reason, we look forward to life span studies of Gray's model of personality.

Damasios' Somatic Theory

Within the past few years, the Damasios have formulated an interesting theory in an attempt to explain the disruptions in socially skilled behavior that they have observed among their patients with frontal lobe impairment (Damasio et al., 1991). While this theory is not necessarily presented by the authors as a model for understanding normal personality, it does offer an intriguing neurologically based explanation for the mechanisms associated with our ability to relate to our social world in an effective manner. As opposed to Eysenck or Gray, who use a trait model of personality, the Damasios present a more cognitively based model of personality. That is, they follow the more recent trend among both personality theorists and cognitive psychologists in attempting to explain the underlying cognitive operations that cause an individual to interact effectively (or ineffectively) with his or her social environment. The Damasios, however, have taken these efforts one step further and have suggested an underlying neural mechanism which can account for the dysfunctional social interactions often encountered among individuals with frontal lobe abnormalities.

According to their view, the minimal requirements for social behavior include the ability to (1) accurately evaluate a social situation, (2) select from one's past experiences an array of potential response alternatives, (3) assess the value or valence (positive or negative) associated with each alternative (based on prior experience), and finally, (4) select the single alternative that is most likely to lead to the desired outcome. It is assumed that some form of parallel distributed neural process is required to elicit and sustain all of the cognitive operations required to accomplish such a task. Within this framework, it is suggested that frontal lobe patients have specific difficulty with the selection of the most adaptive response alternative. The reason for this problem in response selection is due to a "defect in the activation of somatic markers that must accompany the internal and automatic processing of possible response options" (p. 220).

The authors propose a neural system that includes the bilateral ventromedial frontal cortex, the amygdala and related structures, and the cortical and projection areas responsible for the processing of somatosensory information. In brief, the ventromedial frontal regions receive and consolidate input from all sensory systems as well as the somatic states that have been previously associated with that particular pattern of sensory input. This input generates an output from the ventromedial frontal region to the amygdala. Activation of the amygdala, consequently, produces the experience of the somatic marker associated with that set of sensory events. Hence, a certain social situation can evoke a "feeling" about which several possible response alternatives represent the best course of action. For frontal lobe patients, it is this inability to "automatically" choose the correct course of action in a real-life social situation that creates the most difficulty. They are "disconnected" from the subcortical inputs that provide valence information from prior experience which could be useful in a new situation.

Damasios' theory is clearly of relevance to those age-related disorders that include frontal lobe involvement. However, as with Gray's theory, we have been unable to find any direct reference regarding the application of this model to normal personality among the elderly. In addition, while the Damasios have focused on the role of the frontal lobes, it would be of interest to determine the effect of disruption in other components of the "somatic marker" system on social behavior or personality.

Summary

While we must remain cautious in our expectations of finding easily discernible relationships between the construct of personality and putative underlying neurological mechanisms (e.g., Amelang & Ullwer, 1991), the work reviewed here should give cause for encouragement. Each of these investigators has provided us with a distinct model of the relationship between those aspects of behavior that we generally construe as related to personality and an associated neural system. At the very least, these models permit us to move beyond the realm of traditional neurophysiological evaluation in that they offer a conceptual framework for considering the role of various neural systems in the production of complex interpersonal behaviors.

The role of aging in the relationship between personality and neural systems, however, remains sparsely investigated. Katzman and Terry (1992) note that there are virtually no longitudinal studies, and only a few cross-sectional studies which focus on the neurology of normal aging. However, as we use procedures such as CT, MRI, PET, and SPECT to gather more information about the neuroanatomy and neurophysiology of normal aging, we will be in a better position to evaluate more directly the existing biological models of personality and develop life span models as well.

Evaluation of Personality

The assessment of personality following a neurological insult poses several unique problems. First, depending on the site of lesion, the cognitive deficits associated with an injury may render an individual unable to answer a self-report instrument. For those who are able to answer for themselves, a difficulty in interpretation arises. Specifically, premorbid personality status is difficult to ascertain. For most, there is no baseline against which to compare their results beyond reports of spouses, children, or significant others. Since our emphasis is on normal personality, we will briefly

review the primary assessment instrument for the five-factor trait theory, that is, the NEO Personality Inventory (Costa & McCrae, 1985). We will also present a brief review of a newer personality instrument that has its roots in geriatric neurophysiology, the Neuropsychological Behavior and Affect Profile (Nelson et al., 1989). Finally, since the Minnesota Multiphasic Personality Inventory (MMPI) still represents probably the most widely used personality instrument in the market, we will summarize the evidence related to the use of the MMPI and MMPI-2 across the life span.

The NEO Personality Inventory

The NEO-PI, which was developed by Costa and McCrae (1985) specifically to measure the five-factor model of personality, is an evaluation instrument that may have some utility with a neurologically compromised sample. The test comprises a self-report version as well as one to be completed by a person who knows the target individual well. Comparisons of observer and self-ratings have been demonstrated to show substantial agreement on all five factors (McCrae & Costa, 1987). This level of agreement lends support to the use of third party informants to gain information regarding personality change. It also may be of benefit to use both the self-report and observer report versions to look for discrepancies in current behavior. Further, the authors suggest that the use of a measure of normal personality, in conjunction with clinical assessment, can provide clinicians with a richer, more complete understanding of the individual (Costa and McCrae, 1992). However, the NEO-PI still provides no direct measure of premorbid functioning, and personality change must be inferred.

The Neuropsychology Behavior and Affect Profile

Nelson et al. (1989) have developed the Neuropsychological Behavior and Affect Profile (NBAP) as a proposed solution to some of the problems associated with personality assessment among the neurologically impaired. This instrument was designed based on existing research and clinical observation of specific neurological groups and provides a way to assess psychological changes in personality, affect, and behavior among the neuro-logically impaired. In addition to the more tradi-tional assessment of cognitive changes, it allows the clinician to obtain a more complete picture of the individual's behavioral functioning and the changes therein. The NBAP is completed twice by an indi-vidual who knows the patient well. In the first as-sessment, the respondent answers questions from the perspective of premorbid functioning. The sec-ond assessment concerns the current functioning of the patient. The profile yields five scales: (a) indif-ference, described as a tendency to minimize the disability; (b) inappropriateness, described as ex-hibiting behavior that is inappropriate to the con-text; (c) depression; (d) mania consisting of ele-vated or expansive mood and sustained high energy; and (e) pragnosia, described as a defect in commu-nicative style.

The NBAP has been validated with several patient groups. In a comparison of normal elders and dementing elders, Nelson et al. (1989) found significant discriminative validity on all scales ex-cept mania. In a comparison of premorbid scores between the two groups they found no differences in scale scores, although the dementing group tended to have higher scores in general. These researchers speculated that perhaps subtle behavioral signs of dementia occur before cognitive symptoms are ob-served. In contrast, Nelson, Cicchetti, Satz, Sowa, and Mitrushina (1994) noted elevations in the pre-morbid scale scores of stroke patients as compared to normal elders. These results, while requiring fur-ther confirmation, are intriguing because they sug-gest the potential differential utility of premorbid personality factors in predicting the vulnerability of an individual to various neurological conditions.

Nelson and colleagues (Nelson, Mitrushina, Satz, Sowa, & Cohen, 1993) have also demonstrated postmorbid discriminative validity between stroke patients and normal elders using the NBAP. The factors of indifference, depression, and pragnosia all distinguished between stroke patients and nor-mal elders on postmorbid ratings. In contrast, inap-propriateness and mania did not distinguish be-tween these two samples, suggesting that the NBAP may be able to distinguish between clinical syn-dromes as well as pre- to postmorbid states.

The NBAP has also been shown to be useful in monitoring emotional changes in stroke patients.

Nelson, Cicchetti, et al. (1993) were able to empiri-cally measure changes in depression from the pre-morbid to poststroke period. In addition, they were able to demonstrate differences in the level of both depression and indifference depending on the hemi-sphere in which the lesion occurred. Specifically, depression was noted with strokes to either hemi-sphere whereas increased indifference was noted among left hemisphere stroke patients. It is of inter-est to note that aphasics could be included in this study since the NBAP is completed by significant others.

Longitudinal follow-up of this same sample (Nelson et al., 1994) enabled these researchers to chart changes in depression over time, which re-sulted in the identification of a differential pattern of recovery depending on the hemisphere in which the lesion occurred.

The MMPI and MMPI-2

The use of the MMPI and MMPI-2 with older populations has been extensively investigated and is presented elsewhere (see Taylor, Strassberg, & Turner, 1989, for a thorough review). Briefly, there is considerable evidence (e.g., Colligan & Offord, 1992; Schenkenberg, Gottfredson, & Christensen, 1984) that specific MMPI clinical scales tend to be more elevated in normal elderly samples as com-pared to normal younger adult groups. Scale eleva-tions are reported for the following: 1 (hypo-chondriasis), 2 (depression), 3 (hysteria), and 0 (social introversion). Other scales tend to be lower in older groups, such as scales 4 (psychopathic deviate), and 9 (hypomania). Butcher et al. (1991), however, suggest that these differences are typically small and probably not of clinical relevance, are reflected on scales that contain a number of physical health items, and may be the result of cohort, and not generational, differences. Butcher et al. (1991) also report similar findings with the MMPI-2. Sig-nificant age-related differences were obtained for depression, hypomania, psychopathic deviate, and social introversion. Again, these were relatively small, approximately 5 points, and were not consid-ered clinically significant by the authors. They did not recommend the need for MMPI-2 geriatric norms.

Another approach using the MMPI with neurological groups has been to establish scoring correction methods to account for the physical symptom items in order to facilitate the interpretation of psychopathology when clinically relevant scale elevations are present. Gass and Lawhorn (1991) explored the effect of the endorsement of neurological items on the MMPI profiles of stroke patients with no premorbid history of psychopathology and found that correction for the items identified as having neurological content resulted in 38% fewer subjects with high scores on the neurotic triad. To adequately assess patients with neurological compromise, these authors recommend that scores be corrected. As with the NEO-PI, there remains the question of premorbid functioning, although we are more used to using other clinical information to ascertain level of psychopathology prior to neurological insult. In addition, as with all self-report instruments, the patient must be able to understand and respond to questionnaire items.

In general, the MMPI continues to be one of the most extensively used self-report instruments of personality. Age-related changes on both the MMPI and MMPI-2 are consistently reported on specific clinical subscales. However the magnitude of the age-related effects tends to be fairly small, usually on the order of 5 to 6 points. In addition, the meaning of these elevations, in terms of reflecting actual changes in psychopathology versus generational differences in response to health-related items, continues to be debated. Finally, since the MMPI is primarily intended as a measure of psychopathology, it may not be as sensitive to some of the more subtle changes in characteristic patterns of behavior as measures intended to evaluate normal personality structure.

Emotion and Aging

We spend much of our life engaging in the process of experiencing and expressing our own emotions in addition to trying to understand the emotional expressions of others. Within a clinical context, alterations in emotional experience or expression can represent either primary or secondary features of a neuropsychiatric disorder. When working with older individuals, the same question we

asked of personality can be asked of emotion: What is "normal"? Are there age-related changes in the structure, experience, or expression of emotion? Without this knowledge, interpretation of clinical observations or family reports of change in the emotional life of an elderly patient may be misleading.

We offer this brief section on emotion and aging in a chapter on personality largely because of the ubiquitous nature of the emotional alterations seen in neuropsychiatric conditions. Since the traditional literature on personality rarely addresses directly the issue of emotion (Izard, 1991), we will highlight the research on emotion and normal aging as presented in the recent gerontological literature.

Lawton, Kleban, Rajagopal, and Dean (1992) recently conducted a cross-sectional study of the modes of experiencing emotion using a 71-item, self-report instrument. They distinguish between actually experiencing an emotion and the self-monitoring of the emotional experience. That is, this self-monitoring can occur along a number of dimensions, and it is these dimensions that are the focus of study. Eleven dimensions are evaluated, including affect intensity; leveling of positive affect (adaptation to the environment with minimal emotional arousal to novelty and concomitant boredom); psychophysiological responsiveness; emotional maturity through moderation (based on life experiences, we learn not to respond to events in an emotionally extreme manner); and affective variability.

Responses of young, middle-aged, and older adults were compared. Age-related differences were obtained both in the interrelationship among dimensions as well as on the mean level of the dimensional scores. Specifically, when cross-sectionally compared to younger groups, older individuals appear to become more moderate and self-regulated in their emotional experiences, at least upon self-appraisal.

In a follow-up study, Lawton, Kleban, and Dean (1993) investigated the actual factoral structure of affect among different age groups using a 46-item list of affective terms representing a multidimensional model of affect. The current factor analytic literature of emotion suggests that two emotion factors can be consistently replicated: a pleasantness factor, which is bipolar (pleasantness–

unpleasantness), and a level of activation factor, which is unipolar (e.g., Russell, 1980). Others suggest that a more refined description of the dimensions of emotion are required (e.g., Izard, 1991). Whether 2 or 10 emotions best capture the range of emotional experience, the issue of interest to Lawton et al. (1993) was whether the structure of emotion and the frequency of various emotions vary across age groups. Respondents indicated how frequently they had experienced each of the 46 emotions over the past year. Exploratory factor analysis yielded a six-factor solution for all age groups and a seventh factor that emerged for the young and old age groups. The six factors common to all groups included positive affect, anxiety-guilt, contentment, depression, hostility, and shyness. The seventh factor was labeled interpersonal warmth. Despite the similarities in the derived factors for each group, there were age-related differences within factors. In general, the size of the factor loadings were most different between the younger and older group. For example, younger subjects had stronger loadings on items reflecting intensity of arousal on the positive affect dimension. As the authors note, it appears that emotional arousal is more salient and more positively interpreted by younger than older individuals. In contrast, older individuals seemed to experience stronger direct feelings of anxiety (fearful, scared) on the anxiety-guilt factor, while younger adults focus more on the cognitive mediators of guilt.

Interestingly, evaluation of the level of emotion across groups (i.e., the frequency with which the emotion was experienced over the past year) indicated that there is no difference in the frequency of the experience of positive emotions across the age groups, but that the frequency of experiencing negative emotions decreased as a function of age. The older group reported fewer experiences of depression, anxiety-guilt, hostility, and shyness. It does not appear, therefore, that these are the types of emotional complaints that we should expect to hear from normal, well-functioning older adults.

The overall structure of emotion remains fairly stable across the life span, although the strength of the relationship among emotions and the frequency of emotional experience may vary, at least based on cross-sectional investigation. Is there any evidence that the physiological correlates of emotional experience vary with age? A recent study by Levenson, Carstensen, Friesen, and Ekman (1991) has addressed this issue. These authors extend their earlier work that demonstrates specific autonomic nervous system patterns of response to different basic emotions. Young and old subjects engaged in a directed facial expression task and a relived emotional experience task while heart rate, skin conductance, finger temperature, and general somatic activity were recorded. Both young and old subjects demonstrated similar emotion-specific patterns of physiological activity, although the magnitude of the physiological changes were considerably smaller. For example, both groups showed an increase in heart rate when experiencing anger, fear, and sadness, but not disgust. The younger subjects, however, experienced an average of between four and nine beats per minute, whereas the significant changes among the elderly were under two beats per minute.

In summary, it appears that there is a fair amount of stability in the structure of emotions across the life span, both at the level of self-report and physiologically. If anything, older adults have a tendency to experience less intensity in their emotional life. This may help to explain why many older individuals find the affective dysregulation associated with some neurological disorders so troubling.

Summary

We began this chapter with the goal of presenting a brief excursion into the world of normal personality as it relates to aging. With several goals in mind, we were fairly selective in the theories of personality that we surveyed. First, we wanted to include current empirically based personality research with potential relevance to life span development. Second, we attempted to restrict our review to approaches that might pique the interest of clinicians and researchers in the neurosciences. As a result, there are a number of models of personality as well as numerous empirical investigations that are not covered here. Within these limits, we hope to have encouraged consideration of the role of normal personality theory and assessment when confronting the changes in behavior that often accompany age-related neurological conditions.

If nothing else, we hope the reader has gained a greater appreciation of the impressive stability in fundamental behavioral tendencies across the adult life span. Whereas specific expressions of these tendencies, that is traits, may vary according to environmental influences, radical change in fundamental characteristics of an individual should be regarded as atypical. Beyond anecdotal family reports of personality change, we are also able to assess these characteristics with the same level of sophistication that we use to evaluate the cognitive dimensions of the older individual who presents with possible neurological dysfunction. Additionally, links between normal personality and underlying neural systems have also been proposed. Elaboration of these models and extension of them across the life span are formidable challenges but ones that are increasingly attainable as we become more involved in interdisciplinary investigations of human behavior.

References

Allport, G. (1937). *Personality: A psychological interpretation.* New York: Holt.

Allport, G., & Odbert, H. (1936). Trait names: A psycho-lexical study. *Psychological Monographs, 47,* (1, Whole No. 211).

Amelang, M., & Ullwer, U. (1991). Correlations between psychometric measures and psychophysiological as well as experimental variables in studies of extraversion and neuroticism. In J. Strelau & A. Angleitner (Eds.), *Explorations in temperament: International perspectives on theory and measurement* (pp. 297–315). London: Plenum.

Benjamin, L. S. (1994). SASB: A bridge between personality theory and clinical psychology. *Psychological Inquiry, 5,* 273–316.

Block, J. (1995). A contrarian view of the five-factor approach to personality description. *Psychological Bulletin, 117,* 187–215.

Bloom, B. S. (1964). *Stability and change in human characteristics.* New York: Wiley.

Britt, T. W. (1993). Metatraits: Evidence relevant to the validity of the construct and its implications. *Journal of Personality and Social Psychology, 65,* 554–562.

Brocke, B., & Battmann, W. (1992). The arousal-activation theory of extraversion and neuroticism: A systematic analysis and principal conclusions. *Advances in Behaviour Research and Therapy, 14,* 211–246.

Butcher, J. N., Aldwin, C. M., Levenson, M. R., Ben-Porath, Y. S., Spiro, A., III, & Boss, R. (1991). Personality and aging: A study of the MMPI-2 among older men. *Psychology and Aging, 6,* 361–370.

Cattell, R. B. (1943). The description of personality: Basic traits resolved into clusters. *Journal of Abnormal and Social Psychology, 38,* 476–506.

Cattell, R. B. (1945a). The description of personality: Principles and findings in a factor analysis. *American Journal of Psychology, 58,* 69–90.

Cattell, R. B. (1945b). The principal trait clusters for describing personality. *Psychological Bulletin, 42,* 129–161.

Cloninger, C. R. (1987). A systematic method for clinical description and classification of personality variants. *Archives of General Psychiatry, 44,* 573–588.

Colligan, R. C., & Offord, K. P. (1992). Age, stage, and the MMPI: Changes in response patterns over an 85-year age span. *Journal of Clinical Psychology, 48,* 476–493.

Conley, J. J. (1985). Longitudinal stability of personality traits: A multitrait-multimethod-multioccasion analysis. *Journal of Personality and Social Psychology, 49,* 1266–1282.

Costa, P. T., Jr., & McCrae, R. R. (1985). *The NEO Personality Inventory manual.* Odessa, FL: Psychological Assessment Resources.

Costa, P. T., Jr., & McCrae, R. R. (1987). Validation of the five-factor model of personality across instruments and observers. *Journal of Personality and Social Psychology, 52,* 81–90.

Costa, P. T., Jr., & McCrae, R. R. (1988). Personality in adulthood: A six year longitudinal study of self-reports and spouse ratings on the NEO Personality Inventory. *Journal of Personality and Social Psychology, 54,* 853–863.

Costa, P. T., Jr., & McCrae, R. R. (1992). Normal personality assessment in clinical practice: The NEO Personality Inventory. *Psychological Assessment, 4,* 5–13.

Costa, P. T., Jr., & McCrae, R. R. (1995). Solid ground in the wetlands of personality: A reply to Block. *Psychological Bulletin, 117,* 216–220.

Costa, P. T., Jr., McCrae, R. R., & Arenberg, D. (1980). Enduring dispositions in adult males. *Journal of Personality and Social Psychology, 38,* 793–800.

Costa, P. T., Jr., McCrae, R. R., & Norris, A. H. (1981). Personal adjustment to aging: Longitudinal prediction from neuroticism and extraversion. *Journal of Gerontology, 36,* 78–85.

Cummings, J. L. (1992). Neuropsychiatric aspects of Alzheimer's disease and other dementing disorders. In S. C. Yudofsky & R. E. Hales (Eds.), *Textbook of neuropsychiatry* (2nd ed., pp. 605–620). Washington, DC: American Psychiatric Press.

Damasio, A. R., Tranel, D., & Damasio, H. C. (1991). Somatic markers and the guidance of behavior: Theory and preliminary testing. In H. S. Levin, H. M. Eisenberg, & A. L. Benton (Eds.), *Frontal lobe function and dysfunction* (pp. 217–229). New York: Oxford University Press.

Daruna, J. H., Karrer, R., & Rosen, A. J. (1985). Introversion, attention, and the late positive component of event related potentials. *Biological Psychology, 20,* 249–259.

DePascalis, V., & Montirosso, R. (1988). Extroversion, neuroticism and individual differences in event-related potentials. *Personality and Individual Differences, 9,* 353–360.

Diaz, A., & Pickering, A. D. (1993). The relationship between Gray's and Eysenck's personality spaces. *Personality and Individual Differences, 15,* 297–305.

Digman, J. M., & Takemoto-Chock, N. K. (1981). Factors in the natural language of personality: Re-analysis, comparison, and interpretation of six major studies. *Multivariate Behavioral Research, 16,* 149–170.

Ebmeier, K. P., Deary, I. J., O'Carroll, R. E., Prentice, N., Moffoot, A. P. R., & Goodwin, G. M. (1994). *Personality and Individual Differences, 17,* 587–595.

Eichorn, D. H., Clausen, J. A., Haan, N., Honzig, M. P., & Mussen, P. H. (Eds.). (1981). *Present and past middle life.* San Diego, CA: Academic Press.

Erikson, E. H. (1950). *Childhood and society.* New York: Norton.

Eysenck, H. J. (1967). *The biological basis of personality.* Springfield, IL: Charles C. Thomas.

Eysenck, H. J. (1981). *A model for personality.* New York: Springer.

Eysenck, H. J. (1983). Psychopharmacology and personality. In W. Janke (Ed.), *Response variability to psychotropic drugs.* London: Pergamon.

Eysenck, H. J. (1987). Personality and ageing: An exploratory analysis. *Journal of Social Behavior and Personality, 3,* 11–21.

Eysenck, H. J., & Eysenck, M. W. (1985). *Personality and individual differences: A natural science approach.* New York: Plenum.

Eysenck, H. J., & Eysenck, S. B. G. (1964). *Manual of the Eysenck Personality Inventory.* London: University Press.

Eysenck, H. J., & Eysenck, S. B. G. (1975). *Manual of the Eysenck Personality Inventory.* San Diego, CA: EDITS.

Eysenck, M. W. (1982). *Attention and arousal.* New York: Springer.

Finn, S. (1986). Stability of personality self-ratings over thirty years: Evidence for age/cohort interaction. *Journal of Personality and Social Psychology, 50,* 813–818.

Fiske, D. W. (1949). Consistency of the factorial structures of personality ratings from different sources. *Journal of Abnormal and Social Psychology, 44,* 329–344.

Freud, S. (1964). New introductory lectures on psychoanalysis. In J. Strachey (Ed. and Trans.), *The standard edition of the complete psychological works of Sigmund Freud* (Vol. 22). London: Hogarth. (Original work published 1933)

Gale, A. (1981). EEG studies of extraversion-introversion: What's the next step? In R. Lynn (Ed.), *Dimensions of personality: Papers in honour of H. J. Eysenck* (pp. 181–207). Oxford: Pergamon.

Gass, C., & Lawhorn, L. (1991). Psychological adjustment following stroke: An MMPI study. *Psychological Assessment, 3,* 628–633.

Goldberg, L. R. (1981). Language and individual differences: The search for universals in personality lexicons. In L. Wheeler (Ed.), *Review of personality and social psychology* (Vol. 2, pp. 131–165). Beverly Hills, CA: Sage.

Goldberg, L. R. (1990). An alternative "description of personality": The big five factor structure. *Journal of Personality and Social Psychology, 59,* 1216–1229.

Goldberg, L. R., & Saucier, G. (1995). So what do you propose we use instead? A reply to Block. *Psychological Bulletin, 117,* 221–225.

Gray, J. A. (1970). The psychophysiological basis of introver-sion-extraversion. *Behaviour Research and Therapy, 8,* 249–266.

Gray, J. A. (1976). The behavioural inhibition system: A possible substrate for anxiety. In M. P. Feldman & A. M. Broadhurst (Eds.), *Theoretical and experimental bases of behaviour modification* (pp. 3–41). Chichester, United Kingdom: Wiley.

Gray, J. A. (1982). *The neuropsychology of anxiety: An enquiry into the functions of the septo-hippocampal system.* New York: Oxford University Press.

Gray, J. A. (1991). Neural systems, emotion and personality. In J. Madden (Ed.), *Neurobiology of learning, emotion, and affect.* New York: Raven.

Gray, J. A. (1994). Framework for a taxonomy of psychiatric disorder. In S. H. M. van Goozen, N. E. van de Poll, & J. Sergeant (Eds.), *Emotions: Essays on emotion theory* (pp. 29–59). Hillsdale, NJ: Erlbaum.

Guilford, J. P. (1959). *Personality.* New York: McGraw-Hill.

Guilford, J. P., & Zimmerman, W. S. (1956). Fourteen dimensions of temperament. *Psychological Monographs, 70,* (10, Whole No. 417).

Haier, R. J., Sokolski, K., Katz, M., & Buchsbaum, M. S. (1987). The study of personality with positron emission tomography. In J. Strelau & H. J. Eysenck (Eds.), *Personality dimensions and arousal* (pp. 267–351). New York: Plenum.

Heatherton, T. F., & Weinberger, J. L. (1994). *Can personality change?* Washington, DC: American Psychological Association.

Hebb, D. O. (1955). Drives and the C.N.S. (conceptual nervous system). *Psychological Review, 62,* 243–254.

Izard, C. E. (1991). *The psychology of emotions.* New York: Plenum.

James, W. (1950). *The principles of psychology.* New York: Dover Press.

John, O. P., & Robins, R. W. (1993). Gordon Allport: Father and critic of the five-factor model. In K. Craik, R. Hogan, & R. Wolfe (Eds.), *Fifty years of personality psychology.* New York: Plenum.

Johnson, J. A., & Ostendorf, F. (1993). Clarification of the five-factor model with the abridged big five dimensional circumplex. *Journal of Personality and Social Psychology, 65,* 563–576.

Katzman, R., & Terry, R. (1992). Normal aging of the nervous system. In R. Katzman & J. W. Rowe (Eds.), *Principles of geriatric neurology* (pp. 18–46). Philadelphia: F. A. Davis.

Kelly, E. L. (1955). Consistency of the adult personality. *American Psychologist, 10,* 659–681.

Kendrick, D., & Funder, D. (1988). Profiting from controversy: Lessons from the person-situation debate. *American Psychologist, 43,* 23–34.

Kroessler, D. (1990). Personality disorder in the elderly. *Hospital and Community Psychiatry, 41,* 1325–1329.

Lawton, M. P., Kleban, M. H., Rajagopal, D., & Dean, J. (1992). Dimensions of affective experience in three age groups. *Psychology and Aging, 7,* 171–184.

Lawton, M. P., Kleban, M. H., & Dean, J. (1993). Affect and age: Cross-sectional comparisons of structure and prevalence. *Psychology and Aging, 8,* 165–175.

Levenson, M. R., Aldwin, C. M., Bosse, R., & Spiro, A., III.

(1988). Emotionality and mental health: Longitudinal findings from the normative aging study. *Journal of Abnormal Psychology, 97,* 94–96.

Levenson, R. W., Carstensen, L. L., Friesen, W. V., & Ekman, P. (1991). Emotion, physiology, and expression in old age. *Psychology and Aging, 6,* 28–35.

MacAndrew, C., & Steele, T. (1991). Gray's behavioral inhibition system: A psychometric examination. *Personality and Individual Differences, 12,* 157–171.

McCrae, R. R., & Costa, P. T., Jr. (1986). Clinical assessment can benefit from recent advances in personality psychology. *American Psychologist, 41,* 1001–1003.

McCrae, R. R., & Costa, P. T., Jr. (1987). Validation of the five-factor model of personality across instruments and observers. *Journal of Personality and Social Psychology, 52,* 81–90.

McCrae, R., & John, O. (1992). An introduction to the five-factor model and its applications. *Journal of Personality, 60,* 175–215.

Miller, B. L., Cummings, J. L., Villanueva-Mayer, J., & Boone, K. (1991). Frontal lobe degenerations: Clinical, neuropsychological and SPECT characteristics. *Neurology, 41,* 1374–1382.

Mischel, W. (1968). *Personality and assessment.* New York: Wiley.

Monte, C. F. (1995). *Beneath the mask: An introduction to theories of personality* (5th ed.). Fort Worth, TX: Harcourt Brace College Publishers.

Nelson, L. D., Cicchetti, D., Satz, P., Sowa, M., & Mitrushina, M. (1994). Emotional sequelae of stroke: A longitudinal perspective. *Journal of Clinical and Experimental Neuropsychology, 16,* 796–806.

Nelson, L. D., Cicchetti, D., Satz, P., Stern, S., Sowa, M., Cohen, S., Mitrushina, M., & Van Gorp, W. (1993). Emotional sequelae of stroke. *Neuropsychology, 7,* 553–560.

Nelson, L. D., Mitrushina, M., Satz, P., Sowa, M., & Cohen, S. (1993). Cross-validation of the Neuropsychology Behavior and Affect Profile in stroke patients. *Psychological Assessment, 5,* 374–376.

Nelson, L. D., Satz, P., Mitrushina, M., Van Gorp, W., Cicchetti D., Lewis, R., & Van Lancker, D. (1989). Development and validation of the neuropsychology behavior and affect profile. *Journal of Consulting and Clinical Psychology, 1,* 266–272.

Neppe, V. M., & Tucker, G. J. (1992). Neuropsychiatric aspects of seizure disorders. In S. C. Yudofsky & R. E. Hales (Eds.), *Textbook of neuropsychiatry* (2nd ed., pp. 397–426). Washington, DC: American Psychiatric Press.

Norman, W. T. (1963). Toward an adequate taxonomy of personality attributes: Replicated factor structure in peer nomination personality ratings. *Journal of Abnormal and Social Psychology, 66,* 574–583.

O'Gorman, J. G. (1977). Individual differences in habituation of human physiological responses: A review of theory, method, and findings in the study of personality correlates in nonclinical population. *Biological Psychology, 5,* 257–318.

Ostendorf, F. (1990). *Sprache und Persoenlichkeitsstruktur: zur Validitaet des funf-faktoren-Modells der Persoenlichkeit* [Language and personality structure: On the validity of the five-factor model of personality]. Regensburg, Germany: S. Roderer Verlag.

Palmore, E., Busse, W. W., Maddox, G. L., Nowlin, J. B., & Siegler, I. C. (Eds.). (1985). *Normal Aging III.* Durham, NC: Duke University Press.

Pervin, L. (1970). *Personality: Theory, assessment and research.* New York: John Wiley & Sons.

Pervin, L. (1993). Personality stability, personality change, and the question of process. In T. F. Heatherton & J. L. Weinberger (Eds.), *Can personality change?* Washington, DC: American Psychological Association.

Pervin, L. (1994). A critical analysis of current trait theory. *Psychological Inquiry, 5,* 103–113.

Polich, J., & Martin, S. (1992). P300, cognitive capability, and personality: A correlational study of university undergraduates. *Personality and Individual Differences, 13,* 533–543.

Revelle, W. (1995). Personality processes. *Annual Review of Psychology, 46,* 295–328.

Rosowsky, E., & Gurian, B. (1992). Impact of borderline personality disorder in late life on systems of care. *Hospital and Community Psychiatry, 43,* 386–389.

Russell, J. A. (1980). A circumplex model of affect. *Journal of Personality and Social Psychology, 39,* 1161–1178.

Rust, J. (1975). Cortical evoked potentials, personality and intelligence. *Journal of Comparative and Physiological Psychology, 89,* 1220–1226.

Schenkenberg, T., Gottfredson, D. K., & Christensen, P. (1984). Age differences in MMPI scale scores from 1,189 psychiatric patients. *Journal of Clinical Psychology, 40,* 1420–1426.

Shock, N. W., Gruelich, R. C., Andres, R., Arenberg, D., Costa, P. T., Lakkata, E. G., & Tobin, J. D. (Eds.). (1984). *Normal human aging: The Baltimore longitudinal study of aging* (NIH Publication No. 84-2450). Washington, DC: U.S. Government Printing Office.

Silver, J. M., Hales, R. E., & Yudofsky, S. C. (1992). Neuropsychiatric aspects of traumatic brain injury. In S. C. Yudofsky & R. E. Hales (Eds.), *Textbook of neuropsychiatry* (2nd ed., pp. 363–396). Washington, DC: American Psychiatric Press.

Stelmack, R. M. (1990). Biological basis of extraversion: Psychophysiological evidence. *Journal of Personality, 58,* 293–311.

Stenberg, G., Risberg, J., Warkentin, S., & Rosen, I. (1990),. Regional patterns of cortical blood flow distinguish extraverts from introverts. *Personality and Individual Differences, 11,* 663–673.

Taylor, J. R., Strassberg, D. S., & Turner, C. W. (1989). Utility of the MMPI in a geriatric population. *Journal of Personality Assessment, 53,* 665–676.

Tupes, E. C., & Christal, R. E. (1961). Recurrent personality factors based on trait ratings (USAF ASD Technical Report No. 61-97). Lackland Air Force Base, TX: U.S. Air Force, reprinted in *Journal of Personality, 1992, 60,* 225–251.

Wallace, J. F., & Newman, J. P. (1990). Differential effects of reward and punishment cues on response speed in anxious and impulsive individuals. *Personality and Individual Differences, 11,* 999–1009.

Waller, N. G., & Ben-Porath, Y. S. (1987). Is it time for clinical psychology to embrace the five-factor model of personality? *American Psychologist, 42,* 887–889.

Watson, D., Clark, L. A., & Harkness, A. R. (1994). Structures of personality and their relevance to psychopathology. *Journal of Abnormal Psychology, 103,* 1–14.

Whitehouse, P. J., Friedland, R. P., & Strauss, M. E. (1992). Neuropsychiatric aspects of degenerative dementias associated with motor dysfunction. In S. C. Yudofsky & R. E. Hales (Eds.), *Textbook of neuropsychiatry* (2nd ed., pp. 585–604). Washington, DC: American Psychiatric Press.

Wilson, G. D., Gray, J. A., & Barrett, P. T. (1990). A factor analysis of the Gray-Wilson Personality Questionnaire. *Personality and Individual Differences, 11,* 1037–1045.

Yang, K., & Bond, M. H. (1990). Exploring implicit personality theories with indigenous or imported constructs: The Chinese case. *Journal of Personality and Social Psychology, 58,* 1087–1095.

Zinberg, R., & Revelle, W. (1989). Personality and conditioning—a test of 4 models. *Journal of Personality and Social Psychology, 57,* 301–314.

4

Anatomy and Physiology of the Aging Human Brain

DAVID C. MARTIN AND FRED H. RUBIN

Introduction

Acceptance of cultural myth, whether it involves sexism, racism, or ageism has a stifling effect on human potential. Almost no aspect of ageism is as pernicious as thinking of the old as intellectually dulled or equating the senium with senility. Consider the experience of one of the great theoretical physicists of the 20th century.

> When I was a young fellow in the 1940's and 50's there was a myth around that theoretical physics can only be done by young people. The reason was historical—that relativity and quantum mechanics had recently been developed by young men. If you look at the history of older discoveries, you find it isn't really true, and if you look at mathematics in particular, you would find that there were many mathematicians who were quite old and still doing fine, original work. I hadn't read the history then, and I sort of believed the myth. But I kept going. (Feynman, 1994, p. 120)

It was fortunate indeed for us all that Richard Feynman did keep going—going on to exploit the path-integral method of calculation, to invent the famous diagrams which bear his name, and to build a theory of quantum electrodynamics for which he

DAVID C. MARTIN • Division of Geriatric Medicine, Shadyside Hospital, Pittsburgh, Pennsylvania 15232; and Departments of Medicine, Psychiatry, and Health Services Administration, University of Pittsburgh, Pittsburgh, Pennsylvania 15260. **FRED H. RUBIN** • Department of Medicine, Shadyside Hospital, Pittsburgh, Pennsylvania 15232; and Department of Medicine, University of Pittsburgh, Pittsburgh, Pennsylvania 15260.

was ultimately awarded the Nobel Prize for physics in 1962.

A difficulty in dealing with a topic such as the physiology of the aging brain is the very complexity of the organ itself. There is simply no arguing from a set of first principles. Most reviews of this topic often leave the reader unsatisfied in that the review can almost always be characterized as idiosyncratic and less than exhaustive. With due apologies to the reader, this review is no exception. We only hope that our own idiosyncratic view helps to set a useful frame for the subsequent chapters in this book. If we spark someone's interest to pursue one of the many underdeveloped areas in the knowledge base of this topic, then that would be an unexpected reward.

Compared to the knowledge of physiology in disease states, knowledge of the aging normal brain is sparse. Indeed research related to aging is ironically one of the younger areas of inquiry. Research into aging received a tremendous boost in the mid-1970s with the creation of the National Institutes on Aging, the Center on Aging of the National Institute of Mental Health, and the Geriatric Research and clinical Centers of the Veterans Administration. Indeed, much of what follows has been garnered by research initiatives sponsored by these centers.

Brain changes occur on a continuum of young to old. It might be best to think of age-related changes as progressively later stages of development rather than a comparison of "young" versus "old" physiology. One should also keep in mind the inability of medical science to completely filter out changes which may be due to pathological states (especially in preclinical phases). Few studies are technically able to restrict investigation to just primary aging. Thus we are often able to approach the "truth" as to what constitutes primary aging only as an approximation.

Anatomical Changes of Aging

Measurements of the gross weights and volumes of the human brain were among some of the earliest anatomical measurements performed. Modern work on this topic dates back some 150 years to the measurements of Esquirol in *Des Maladies Mentalis*, published in 1838 (as cited in Scheibel & Scheibel, 1975). Since those early measurements of Esquirol, in numerous studies involving thousands of subjects one of the most consistent findings has been an almost linear decrease in brain weight occurring with increasing age beyond the age of 20.

At birth, the brain weighs approximately 350 g and increases to a mean of 1,375 g at around age 20. One of the larger series surveyed 20,000 autopsy reports and selected for study nearly 5,000 cases which were free of pathological lesions. This study found that the largest increases in brain weight occurred in the first 3 years of life, during which there was a quadrupling in size. Brain weight decline began at about 45 to 50 years of age and decreased by 11% from its maximal weight in young adulthood (Dekaban & Sadowsky, 1978).

Katzman and Terry (1992) have correctly pointed out that there have been large variations in attempts to measure brain weight, and many studies are flawed in that there is often no record of psychological testing before death to ascertain that the individual did not have a late-life brain disease. Corsellis (1978) and others (Coleman & Flood, 1987) have additionally pointed out the importance of a cohort effect, in that persons born in the early part of the century tend to have brain weights which are significantly lower than persons born later in the century. To avoid the problem of the variability of brain weight, two investigators compared the ratio of the brain volume to the volume of the cranium. They found that ratio to be stable at 0.92 until age 55 and then to decline to a ratio of 0.83 by age 90 (Davis & Wright, 1977). This provided quite sound evidence for brain atrophy. Still, this technique does not take into consideration increasing ventricular size and may therefore underestimate the degree of volume loss.

Tissue loss is manifest on the surface of the brain by shrinkage of the convolutions or gyri and widening of the grooves, or sulci, between the gyri. These changes are more prominent in the forebrain and less so in the cerebellum and are observable on computed tomography (CT) or magnetic resonance imaging (MRI) scanning. The third and lateral ventricles undergo modest dilation with less notable change in the aqueduct and fourth ventricle. Corsellis (1978) and colleagues compared the ratio of total cortex to white matter as a function of age and found that not only was this nonlinear but it also formed a J-shaped curve. In the young brain, the ratio of gray matter to white matter was 1:28 and this declined to 1:13 in brains of subjects in their sixties and then increased back to 1:55 by age 90. Thus they concluded that there was an initial loss of gray matter over white matter followed by a complete reversal of this trend.

Neuronal Changes

The brain is composed of literally billions of cells and billions more of glial cells which nourish and support the neural structure. These glial cells are also involved in reaction to injury and disease and are responsible for the production and maintenance of myelin.

The body of the cell is where most of the metabolic reactions occur. Branching out from the cell body are numerous processes which form the interconnections with other neurons. Numerous dendrites form the processes carrying incoming signals from other neurons while the axon directs outgoing information either to other cells in the network or out of the brain and spinal column entirely to connect with distant muscle cells.

Each cell receives an enormous amount of input from thousands of interconnections with other cells. These contacts are being made, not only upon each dendrite, but also at its secondary and tertiary branches. Thus, the input is more complex than it first appears, once these second- and third-order connections are considered.

The makeup of the human nervous system has often invited comparisons to modern computers.

Such metaphors should not be surprising since von Neumann and other pioneers of modern computing patterned the handling of working memory after their conception of the human nervous system. With neurons being modulated by input from thousands of dendritic connections, the signal processing is massively parallel and has an analog quality about it. The distinction between analog and digital is somewhat artificial in that at some fundamental level all information is received as a singular packet, whether that may be the release of a neuro-transmitter packet or the alteration of a single ion channel.

Contacts between neurons are separated by a cleft of 10 to 20 nm width. Stimulation of one neuron by another is accomplished by the release of packets of neurotransmitter enveloped in membrane into the synaptic cleft. These packets diffuse across the gap to bind to postsynaptic receptors. There they alter the permeability of ion channels to affect the electrical transmissibility of the neuron. The trans-mitters may be excitatory, inhibitory, or modulating in their effects.

Actual quantification of changes in numbers of specific types of neurons has been hampered by the technical difficulty of performing the measures and the application of disparate and perhaps not compa-rable techniques. There is currently evidence to suggest that neurons are either lost through cell death, or that great numbers of the larger (> 90 μm^2) neurons shrink in size, and that synaptic con-tacts are lost, gained, or altered with aging. There are also concomitant increases, decreases, or alter-ations in neurotransmitters. These important issues will each be treated in turn.

Brain Stem

Most regions in the brain stem that have been investigated do not demonstrate a decrease in cell number with increasing age. This includes a number of the cranial nerve nuclei and the inferior olivary nucleus. Brain stem structures are more easily quan-tified than cortical structures because they are tech-nically much easier to examine. Often it is possible to visualize the entire structure and do a complete cell count (Poirier & Finch, 1994). In general, youn-ger brains show shorter cranial nerve nuclei with stable populations of cells. In more aged brains, the nuclei tend to be longer but the cell numbers remain

the same. This has been observed in the facial nerve nucleus (Van Buskirk, 1945), the ventral cochlear nucleus (Konigsmark & Murphy, 1970), and the trochlear and abducens nuclei (Vijayashankar & Brody, 1977).

Not all deep structures are resistant to cell loss, however. Structures which consistently do show cell loss include the locus ceruleus (Vijayashankar & Brody, 1979), the substantia nigra (Mann, Yates, & Marcyniuk, 1984; McGeer, McGeer, & Suzuki, 1977), and the hippocampus. The hippocampus has been studied more than any other subcortical struc-ture, and age-related neuronal cell losses are on the order of 3% to 9% per decade (Coleman & Flood, 1987).

Cerebral Cortex

Knowledge of neuronal cell loss of the cere-brum in the human dates back to the mid-1950s when Brody (1955) performed painstaking manual cell counts on multiple regions of the cerebral cor-tex in human subjects ranging in age from 0 months to 95 years. Cell loss was a consistent phenomenon in all cortical areas. The greatest decrease in cell numbers occurred in the superior temporal gyrus followed by the precentral gyrus and then the area striata. Brody also noted that granular layers were particularly affected, and that in older age groups there was a shift from granular to pyramidal cells. He also observed something which was to presage later findings: Between certain ages, the cell loss was apparent rather than real.

Some 25 years later, this study was repeated using more modern techniques of computer image analysis, and the results were similar, with the addi-tional finding that cell loss seemed to be greater (up to 60%) among the larger neurons (Henderson, Tomlinson, & Gibson, 1980). Little change was noted in the glia.

Devaney and Johnson (1980) approached this question by using cell suspensions and counting cells by a hemacytometer. They reported results quite similar to the hand counting techniques which had been employed earlier, that is, a nearly 50% decline of neurons per gram of tissue from age 20 to age 80. Although this study was restricted to the visual cortex, it confirmed earlier findings through a totally separate technique.

Terry, DeTeresa, and Hansen (1987) examined

51 brains from clinically normal individuals ranging in age from 24 to 100 years. They used an image-analysis technique and found that the aging effects were most prominent in the frontal and parietal lobes. Most importantly they also noted that neuronal loss was much less than previous estimates, and that the main cause of diminished cortical weight and volume might be due to a shrinkage in the size of the larger (those greater than 90 μm^2) neurons. They noted an increase in the number of glial cells. Katzman (1995) has pointed to the paucity of findings for neuronal cell death in that there seems to be no evidence in the aging brain of cellular inflammation or karyorrhexis, and the neurons "seem to disappear without a trace." Shrinkage rather than cell death would fit these observations.

In spite of these intriguing findings, however, a thorough review of the data concluded that the bulk of evidence indicates an age-related decrease in density of neurons at the same time that cortical volume is decreasing. This suggests neuronal loss in excess of that predicted by density measures alone (Coleman & Flood, 1987).

Along with changes in cell size and possibly cell number due to aging effects, there are also changes in the dendritic arborization. The Scheibels (1975) carefully evaluated dendritic changes using the Golgi method and identified a sequence of changes that consisted of swelling and lumpiness in the outline of the neurons' soma and proximal dendrites. This was followed by progressive loss of horizontally oriented dendrites, especially the basilar shafts, and eventual loss of apical shafts just preceding cell death. They attached special significance to the loss of horizontal dendrites as these receive synaptic terminals from intracortical loops, and their loss would have an especially negative effect on the modulatory aspects of cortical activity and a deterioration of psychomotor performance.

The issue of synaptic density raised by the Scheibels is a crucial one. Synaptic density in the diseased brain was found to correlate most strongly of all physiologic parameters with the degree of dementia (Dekosky & Scheff, 1990; Terry et al., 1991). Using immunolabeling for synaptophysin to quantify synaptic density, Masliah, Mallory, Hensen, DeTeresa, and Terry (1993) found that individuals without dementia who were over 60 years of age had an average of 20% less presynaptic terminal density than individuals younger than 60 years.

Conversely, using a phosphotungstic acid method, other researchers found little change in synaptic density from age 16 to 72 and only a slight decrease from age 74 to 90 (Huttenlocher, 1979).

Data gathered with a computer-microscope system actually showed that normal elderly individuals had longer and more branched dendrites than either young adults or individuals with Alzheimer's disease (AD). This study was performed on the parahippocampal gyrus, and the investigators interpreted these intriguing results as an example of plasticity in the human brain (Buell & Coleman, 1981).

The hippocampus shows age-related reductions in synaptic density (Haug & Eggers, 1991) and is a structure that is particularly affected in Alzheimer's disease. Cell loss in the hippocampus with normal aging appears to be region-specific and distinct from AD. In particular the CA1 region shows no loss of nerve cells (West, Coleman, Flood, & Troncosos, 1994) with normal aging nor a reduction in dendritic length. This is not true, however, in AD, where there does seem to be selective loss in this region.

Cytostructural and Extracellular Changes

Lipofuchsin has been dubbed the "aging pigment" or the "wear and tear pigment" because of its frequent association with aging. Lipochromes (which are yellow, green, or brown fluorescing pigments) consist of coarse, insoluble, granular material composed of complex oxidized lipids. They are highly cross-linked and are polymerized with proteins. Lipochromes are bounded by membrane and also contain iron, zinc, and hydrolytic enzymes.

Evidence suggests that this pigment may begin to accumulate at an early age and fill a large percentage of cells. It was once felt that the accumulation of this pigment might impair the metabolic functioning of a cell and lead to cell senescence. It is now felt that this is not so (Katzman & Terry, 1992). In fact, speculation has it that precursors of lipofuchsin may be toxic, and creation of pigment is the cells' way of rendering it nontoxic. Thus pigment may identify cells with an intact protective mechanism which would confer a survival advantage to those cells (Brody, 1992).

Other cytoskeletal changes which are commonly seen in aging are the granulovacuolar changes of Simchowitz, composed of tubulin and seen more prominently in the hippocampus and Hirano bodies which are made up of products of actin (Katzman & Terry, 1992; Scheibel & Scheibel, 1975). In addition to these inclusions are others which are spherical and composed mainly of polysaccharides with small amounts of protein. These are found mainly in astrocytes in subependymal regions of the brain (Katzman & Terry, 1992). The precise functional significance of these inclusions remains unelucidated. Cytoplasm can fill with bundles of helically wound protein filaments called neurofibrillary tangles. Although large numbers of these are associated with AD, their presence in smaller numbers in the brains of individuals who seem clinically free of disease remains unexplained.

Areas between neurons also undergo changes with aging. Spherical deposits which Simchowitz named the *senile plaque* accumulate in the extracellular spaces of the hippocampus, cerebral cortex, and other brain regions. These are composed primarily of aggregates of a small molecule, the beta-amyloid protein, whose role in normal physiology is unknown (Selkoe, 1992).

Again there is overlap between what appears to be successful aging and late-life brain disease where senile plaques may be present in smaller numbers in individuals with normal mentation. Some have suggested that AD, just like many other illnesses, represents a threshold phenomenon, wherein the disease is not made manifest clinically until a critical threshold has been crossed. If some individuals have a richer neural network, either through inheritance, or through anatomic changes caused by learning, then this might "raise the bar" on the threshold effect. On the other hand, Mackenzie (1994) recently noted that although the prevalence of senile plaques in the neocortex correlated with age, the mean number or density did not increase with advancing age. This suggests that senile plaques may develop over a limited period of time after which their number stabilizes. Alzheimer's disease may be a qualitatively different process altogether.

Radiographic Changes

Rapid progress in neuroimaging technologies has created an entirely new way to investigate aging changes and confirm previous anatomic studies of changes in brain morphology. Techniques of MRI or CT can be used to eliminate such variables as postmortem changes, changes due to illness, and selection bias which have plagued previous morphologic studies. Brain imaging has in fact confirmed the previous morphologic studies which showed dilation of cortical sulci and enlargement of ventricles with advancing age (DeCarli, Kaye, Horwitz, & Rapoport, 1990).

Neuroimaging, however, also has the added potential to examine changes serially over time within individual subjects and to examine such previously unmeasurable parameters as tissue density changes, cerebral blood flow and metabolism, and cerebrospinal fluid (CSF) dynamics. Through nuclear magnetic resonance (NMR) analysis of protons and high-energy phosphate bonding, it has even become possible to take snapshots of what is occurring at a chemical level in neural tissue with aging.

Coffey and colleagues (1992) performed MRI scanning on 76 volunteers ranging in age from 30 to 91. They presented their data as a logarithmic transform which showed a volume loss of 0.55% per year in the frontal lobes, 0.28% per year in the temporal lobes, and 0.30% per year in the amygdala–hippocampal complex. The odds that the patient would show cortical atrophy rose by 8.9% per year, and the odds that a subject would show subcortical hyperintensity in deep white matter rose by 6.3% per year.

Cortical gray matter tissue density declines after age 60 as measured by CT, and there is speculation that this finding parallels a decline in cortical synaptic density (Meyer et al., 1994). Complementing this result is the finding that MRI-derived proton T1 values decrease in the cortical gray matter with increasing age (Steen, Gronemeyer, & Taylor, 1995).

There is a strong correlation between increased CSF volume and increasing age (Malko, Hoffman, & Green, 1991), and patients with AD show greater annual increases in CSF than controls (Shear et al., 1995). On the other hand, the rate of cerebrospinal fluid production does not seem to be influenced by age (Gideon, Thomsen, Stahlberg, & Hendriksen, 1994), nor do flow rates in the aqueduct (Barkhof et al., 1994).

The prevalence of white matter lucencies and

patchy white-matter lucencies, which Hachinski, Potter, and Mersky (1987) have termed "leuko-araiosis," increases with advancing age and correlates with mean arterial blood pressure (Yamashita, Kobayashi, Fukada, Yamaguchi, & Hiromi, 1992). The finding of frontal leukoaraiosis correlates strongly with cortical atrophy and reduction in cerebral perfusion (Kawamura et al., 1993) and may manifest clinically as slowing of motor performance and diminished attentiveness (Ylikoski et al., 1993).

Using ^{31}P NMR spectroscopy, Pettegrew, Withers, and Panchalingam (1990) found that phosphomonoesters were elevated in immature, developing brains of animals during periods of elaboration of dendritic processes. Similar elevations were later found in subjects with Alzheimer's disease. This might be taken as evidence of neural plasticity and attempts at repair in the diseased brain. Similar technology using proton spectra showed that there are lower levels of choline and creatine in cortical and subcortical gray matter with aging (Charles et al., 1994).

Neurochemical Changes

Changes in neurotransmitters with aging is a crucial area of research. The cholinergic hypothesis of memory and the identification of the central role of the nucleus basalis in the etiology of memory disorders make this research a high priority. Progress has been hampered, however, by technical difficulties, especially those surrounding the rapid postmortem changes in many neurochemicals. Results have often been conflicting, and little can be stated with certainty at this point.

Neuropeptides, in particular, undergo rapid autolysis, and little may be stated with confidence about changes in their concentrations with aging. Short peptides such as carnosine and glutathione are made enzymatically with synthetases while larger peptides such as nerve growth factor (NGF) are made by way of a prohormone through the usual translation of messenger ribonucleic acid (RNA) (Poirier & Finch, 1994). Neuropeptides seem to play a particularly important role in the control of sympathetic output, and there are several modulating pathways arising in the hypothalamus and the medulla (Benarroch, 1994).

A great deal of interest has recently surrounded nerve growth factor, in particular, because of its effect on the cholinergic system. High-affinity receptors for this compound exist on the basal forebrain cholinergic neurons, and these undergo increasing axonal arborization in response to NGF. Intracerebral NGF has recently been shown to enhance both synthesis and release of acetylcholine (although aged animals responded less predictably than young animals) (Rylett, Goddard, Schmidt, & Williams, 1993). This leads to the possibility of treatment of memory disorders which may be caused by a state of cholinergic deficit.

Cholinergic System

Forebrain cholinergic and glutaminergic neurons are believed to play a central role in memory and cognition. The seminal work of Drachman and Leavitt (1974), which showed that the administration of scopolamine induced memory deficits which were similar to those seen with aging, drew attention to the role of the cholinergic system in disease states. This was coupled with findings of marked reductions of choline acetyltransferase (CAT) in victims of Alzheimer's disease, along with a reduction of cells in the nucleus basalis which provides much of the cholinergic input to the cortical mantle.

Although profound changes in the cholinergic system have been found in disease states, the effects of aging seem to be much less. This is true both of the integrity of the nucleus basalis itself (Whitehouse et al., 1983) and loss of cholinergic function in general (Decker, 1987; Poirier & Finch, 1994). McGeer and colleagues (1977) found noticeable declines in (CAT), particularly in the cortex but less so in extrapyramidal and rhinencephalic structures. On the other hand, Court and colleagues (1993) found just the opposite. Hippocampal levels of CAT declined after age 40 to 50 whereas frontal cortical levels remained constant.

Glutamate is the neurotransmitter of numerous clinically important pathways including corticocortical association pathways, and both afferent and efferent hippocampal pathways. Recent work has focused on the possibility that glutamate may act as an excitotoxin and lead to cell injury and death (Greenamyre & Porter, 1994). Unfortunately there is no chemical marker (such as CAT in cholinergic neurons) for glutaminergic neurons. However, when ligands binding to glutamate receptors were used as an assay for activity in this system, there was little loss in hippocampal regions until after the seventh decade. Conversely, in the frontal cortex, there was a 50% loss from age 40 to age 100 (Court et al., 1993).

There may be a significant reduction of central muscarinic cholinergic receptors with aging (Decker, 1987) and a reduction in nicotinic receptors in the cortex (Poirier & Finch, 1994). Recent animal data suggest an age-related decline in cholinergic synaptic transmission in the hippocampus (Taylor & Griffith, 1993).

Catecholamines, Serotonin, Monoamine Oxidase Inhibitor, and γ-Aminobutyric Acid

The family of catecholamines in the central nervous system (CNS) consists of three distinct neurotransmitters: dopamine, norepinephrine, and serotonin. Dopamine is a precursor of norepinephrine, and norepinephrine is a precursor of epinephrine, yet each has distinct anatomic localization and receptor effects. The ascending biogenic amine pathways seem to affect attentiveness, modulate affect, and control visceral functions. Serotonin is involved in central regulatory processes such as temperature, sleep, and heart rate.

The noradrenergic system arises from a pigmented nucleus, the locus ceruleus, and projects diffusely throughout the cortex. A variety of both alpha- and beta-adrenergic receptors are present throughout the cortex, and these show regional declines with aging. There appears to be a linear loss of noradrenergic neurons after the age of 40 with losses sustained in the locus ceruleus of greater than 30% (Mann et al., 1984). A relationship has been established between the noradrenergic system and affective disorders such as depression. Depression which commonly coexists with dementia may be related to loss of neurons in the locus ceruleus (Zubenko, Moosy, & Kopp, 1990).

There is a progressive loss of neurons in the substantia nigra with aging (McGeer et al., 1977), and levels of tyrosine hydroxylase, dopa decarboxylase, and dopamine show regional decline with aging. The decline in tyrosine hyroxylase in the caudate, putamen, and nucleus accumbens was es-

pecially striking in one study (McGeer, 1978). At least two types of dopamine receptors have been studied in the aging striatum. The D1 receptor is positively linked to adenylate cyclase activity while the D2 receptor is negatively coupled (Poirier & Finch, 1994). Dopamine receptor density (D1 receptors) increased with aging in one study and correlated inversely with dopamine content in the putamen (Morgan et al., 1987). This has led to speculation that D1 receptors are upregulated in response to declines in brain dopamine. The age-related changes in the dopaminergic system are of particular interest in neurology, because of the overlap between Parkinson's disease and motor changes which are commonly witnessed in advanced age (i.e., increased muscle tonus and stooped posture) (Katzman, 1995). Development of idiopathic Parkinson's disease might again represent a threshold effect in similar fashion to the development of dementia. Subjects who live to a very advanced age, or undergo an earlier insult which accelerates loss of neurons in the region of the substantia nigra, would be more likely to cross this threshold and develop symptomatic Parkinson's disease.

Serotonin production is centered in the dorsal raphe nucleus in the midline of the midbrain and pons. Tryptophan hydroxylase, the key enzyme in the production of serotonin, is unstable in tissue preparations, and successful assays are lacking (McGeer, 1978). Limited data do suggest a gradual loss of serotonin production and serotonin receptor density with aging (Powers, 1994).

Catecholamines are metabolized by catechol-O-methyltransferase (COMT) and monoamine oxidase (MAO). The data on COMT are mixed, whereas there is good convergence of opinion from many investigators that levels of MAO rise with increasing age (McGeer, 1978).

Glutamic acid decarboxylase (GAD), which synthesizes γ-aminobutyric acid (GABA), is a widely dispersed enzyme that has been studied much less than others. One study which sampled 56 brain areas found a curvilinear correlation between age and GAD activity such that the loss was most significant in younger age groups (McGeer & McGeer, 1976).

The neuroanatomical and neurochemical changes which have been discussed thus far form the physiologic substrate for the cognitive and behavioral manifestations which will be discussed in subsequent chapters. One final important question, however, remains for consideration: What are the causes of the changes which occur with aging? This of course takes us to the heart of the causation of aging and aging theories in general.

Genetics and Aging

Many theories have been put forth to explain the decline in function in organ systems, which has come to be referred to as primary aging. With these decrements in function come decreased ability to maintain homeostasis and an increased susceptibility to the forces of mortality. This may be taken as the very definition of aging. As scientists become clever enough to experimentally peel away the layers of organ system changes which are due to disease (secondary aging), that which is left and which may be attributed to primary aging becomes smaller and smaller.

Some theories have postulated that the aging nervous system is actually the pacemaker of aging in general. These theories speculate that neurally mediated alterations of neuroendocrine function lead to incremental loss of organ function (Finch, 1987). Other theories postulate that cellular damage occurring over time (i.e., accumulations of toxic waste products, damage to deoxyribonucleic acid [DNA] cross-links by background radiation, or the chemical damage wrought by free radicals) account for aging changes. Yet, at the heart of all this, there seems to be a more fundamental pacemaker for aging which resides in the genome itself. Hayflick and Moorhead (1961) first showed a finite and fixed number of cell doublings in human fibroblasts. Later, this work was extended to show an almost predetermined numerical cellular doubling potential which seemed to be species-specific. These findings became an early foundation for the genetic theories of aging. More recently the actual "biological clock" residing in the genome that is the basis of this observation may have been located. This biologic clock involves a progressive shortening of specific sequences of DNA at the ends of DNA strands (known as telomeres) which may serve to protect or "harden" the ends of the DNA strands (Haber, 1995).

Perhaps the most encompassing of the theories of aging then is that which postulates that cells senesce because of deficits which slowly accrue in their DNA. This lowers the quantity and quality of critical molecules such as proteins and leads eventually to malfunction and death. Initial focus of these genetic theories has been on the chromosomal DNA. It has been found by some that the enzymatic machinery necessary to excise and repair faulty DNA becomes less efficient in late life, and the cellular controls governing genetic activity become more relaxed. Methylation of DNA through attachment of residues such as 5-methylcytosine also leads to subtle inactivation of genes (Farrer, 1994). Subba Rao and Loeb (1992) collected data from numerous studies and concluded that a preponderance of evidence suggested increasing levels of DNA damage with increasing age, but that there was no clear direction on whether or not there was decline in DNA repair capacity with aging. In a later work Subba Rao (1993) speculated that DNA repair in the brain must be a "highly discrete process" that is barely detectable.

A very exciting line of work, alluded to earlier, is investigation of the role of telomeres in senescence and cancer. Telomeres were originally suspected to exist functionally when it was found that the broken ends of DNA strands are normally quite unstable. These DNA strands tend to fuse end to end or form ring structures leading to unstable chromosome formations. Chemical analyses revealed guanine-rich repeating structures at the ends of chromosomes which were highly conserved and helped to lend stability to the ends of the chromosomes. These structures permitted the chromosome to be replicated without the loss of 5′ terminal bases at the end of the DNA strands. (Some writers have likened telomeres to the plastic ends of shoelaces which prevent the laces from unravelling).

Telomeres are highly conserved sequences of nucleotides (AGGGTT in the human) which are repeated from a few hundred to a few thousand times at the ends of DNA strands. These seem to be critical in maintaining chromosomal integrity. Some 50 to 200 base pairs are lost from the end of the DNA molecule with each cell division, and some 4,000 are lost by the time of cellular senescence (Harley, Futcher, & Greider, 1990). Indeed, victims of progeria have been found to have shortening of telomeres (Harley et al., 1990). An enzyme, telomerase (whose gene has not yet been isolated in humans), serves to preserve the telomere by rebuilding it. The balance between telomere shortening through cell division and the rebuilding by the telomerase may actually be what determines senescence. Expression of telomerase has recently been found to be a feature of cancer cells and may account for the "escape" from the normal biological clock which propels these cells into immortality (Counter, Hirte, Bacchetti, & Harley, 1994).

Evidence that telomeres might be related to senescence also comes from the study of the ciliated protozoan *Tetrahymena*. Overexpression of a mutant telomerase gene in this organism was found to lead to telomere shortening and senescence (Blackburn, 1991). Telomeres have also been found to shorten with the aging of human fibroblasts, and the total quantity of telomeric DNA likewise decreases (Harley et al., 1990). In fact, telomere length correlates better with replicative capacity of human fibroblasts than the chronological age of the donor (Allsopp et al., 1992). The presence of telomerase may confer immortality upon cell lines. The enzyme has been detected in HeLa cells and, in another study, was found in 98 of 100 immortal cell lines and in none of 22 mortal cell lines (Kim, Piatyszck, & Prowse, 1994). Other have found that progression of tumors may be dependent on telomerase, and telomerase inhibition could have an antitumor effect (Counter et al., 1994).

If neurons are postmitotic, then how could a mechanism such as telomere shortening play a role in neuronal senescence? Selkoe (1992) has emphasized the potential role of mitochondrial DNA and its contribution to cellular senescence. Mitochondrial DNA codes for 13 proteins needed for energy production by the cell (Anderson et al., 1981). Because mitochondrial DNA does remain genetically active, then one might postulate that neuronal senescence is mediated through such a mechanism as telomere degradation of mitochondrial DNA. In fact, there are recent reports of late-onset mitochondrial encephalomyopathies which have been related to clonal expansions of muscle fibrils containing mitochondrial DNA deletions (Johnston, Karpati, Carpenter, Arnold, & Shoubridge, 1995). Ragged red fibers, which are a marker for mitochondrial disease, have also been found to

be higher in aging, possibly reflecting age-related decline in muscle oxidative metabolism (Rifai, Welle, Kamp, & Thornton, 1995).

Mitochondrial DNA seems even more vulnerable to degradation than chromosomal DNA. This may be due in part to less efficient maintenance of integrity by organelles, or due to the fact that free radicals are present in greater concentration around the mitochondria, as these free radicals are a by-product of the reactions involved in energy production.

Posttranslational modifications of proteins may also occur and lead to abnormal structure and metabolism. Oxidation, glycosylation, and cross-linking have all been shown to occur over time and to corrupt protein structure. Antioxidants such as vitamin E and vitamin C may aid in protecting the brain from oxidants. An important and recently discovered new line of defense is the antioxidant capacity of indole melatonin, which is produced in the pineal gland (Pierpaoli, 1994; Reiter, 1995). This chemical has been found to decline markedly with age (Reiter, 1994, 1995).

Chemical destruction of enzymes, neurotransmitters, and receptors has received scrutiny because of the central role of these entities in neural function. Proteases (which are an important line of defense against this corruption of proteins) themselves undergo oxidation leading to diminished activity. This effect is exaggerated by parallel declines of catalase and superoxide dismutase and less efficient clearing of free radicals.

What is the link then between all of these anatomic and chemical effects seen with aging and function of the nervous system? Systematic assessment of global neurologic examinations of the very old (Nichols et al., 1993) has demonstrated diminished attentiveness among sexagenarians and octagenarians and a decline in free recall beginning after the sixth decade. Only centenarians demonstrated significant decline in language function and visuospatial deterioration beginning after the seventh decade. In addition to cognitive changes, decrease in visual acuity, upward eye gaze, auditory acuity, movement speed and accuracy, and gait stability were noted. Other investigators (Kaye et al., 1994) have found that deficits in olfaction, balance, and visual pursuit discriminate best between the healthy young and old. Some have found that primitive reflexes increase with age (Odenheimer et al., 1994) whereas others have not (Nichols et al., 1993). Still others have pointed to the extrapyramidal quality of gait and postural changes which occur with aging and have speculated as to whether this represents primary or secondary aging (Katzman, 1995) or whether idiopathic Parkinson's disease results from discrete events or a more long-term process (Calne, 1994).

Another defensible answer to the question posed above may be that there is very little clinically relevant effect of aging at all. It will be seen in subsequent chapters that, although there is fairly universal slowing of processing speed, in the absence of disease, human intellect remains largely intact across the life span. As Selkoe (1992) has correctly pointed out, losses of the magnitude of 20% to 30% in cell numbers, protein levels, and enzyme activity seem to have few effects on functional significance. This is very likely due to the fact that the brain, like most other organ/systems, has substantial built-in physiologic reserve.

Future Directions

It seems likely that the study of the brain will be subjected to the same paradigm shifts that are being wrought upon all of the other life sciences by the spectacular advances in molecular genetics. Work will proceed on identifying what is primary aging and what is secondary aging, and inroads may be made on ways to modify both. One often thinks of medical science as addressing only the latter, however recent advances may hold clues to ways to actually alter primary aging. For example, it is now known that the G-rich strand of the telomere is synthesized in a unique way by the copying of a separate RNA sequence (Blackburn, 1991). If indeed programmed senescence is mediated by telomere length and this is under control of a unique process, then it is not a great leap of imagination to foresee a possible alteration in this process. "Usual aging" may be thought of as distinct from "successful aging," and the goal of medical science might be to confer the same preservation of function and compression of morbidity which is currently only enjoyed by a few.

Another approach of medical science might be to use the physiologic reserve discussed above to better advantage. Even if it should prove impossible to definitively "cure" late-life brain disease, one could hope to retard its progression, raise the threshold of symptoms, or shift the dynamic plasticity in the direction of repair to delay the onset of functional decline. As has been noted by others, if the onset of Alzheimer's disease could be delayed in the population at risk by 5 years, the prevalence of the disorder would be halved (Katzman, 1993). If such a goal could be achieved, think not of just the reduction of individual misery and tragedy, think also of the societal resources reclaimed.

> Intelligence and reflection and judgement reside in old men, and if there had been none of them, no states could exist at all.
>
> —*Cicero*

References

Allsopp, R., Vaziri, H., Patterson, C., Goldstein, S., Younglai, E., Futcher, A., Greider, C., & Harley, C. (1992). Telomere length predicts replicative capacity of human fibroblasts. *Proceedings of the National Academy of Sciences, USA, 89*, 10114–10118.

Anderson, S., Bankier, A., Barrel, B., de Bruijn, M., Coulson, A., Drouin, J., Eperon, I., Nierlich, D., Roe, B., Sanger, F., Shreier, P., Smith, A., Staden, R., & Young, I. (1981). Sequence and organization of the human mitochondrial genome. *Nature, 290*, 457–465.

Barkhof, F., Kouwenhoven, M., Scheltens, P., Sprenger, P., Algra, P., & Valk, J. (1994). Phase-contrast cine MR imaging of normal CSF aqueductal CSF flow. *Acta Radiologica, 35*, 123–130.

Benarroch, E. (1994). Neuropeptides in the sympathetic system: Presence, plasticity, modulation, and implications. *Annals of Neurology, 36*, 6–13.

Blackburn, E. (1991). Structure and function of telomeres. *Nature, 350*, 569–573.

Brody, H. (1955). Organization of the cerebral cortex. III. A study of aging in the human cerebral cortex. *Journal of Comparative Neurology, 102*, 511–556.

Brody, H. (1992). The aging brain. *Acta Neurologica Scandanavia Suppl. 137*, 40–44.

Buell, S., & Coleman, P. (1981). Quantitative evidence for selective dendritic growth in normal human aging but not in senile dementia. *Brain Research, 214*, 23–41.

Calne, D. (1994). Is idiopathic parkinsonism the consequence of an event or a process? *Neurology, 44*, 5–10.

Charles, H., Lazeyras, F., Rama Krishnan, K., Boyko, O., Patterson, L., Doraiswamy, P., & McDonald, W. (1994). Proton spectroscopy of human brain: Effects of age and sex. *Progress in Neuro-Psychopharmacology and Biological Psychiatry, 18*, 995–1004.

Coffey, C., Wilkinson, W., Parashos, I., Soady, S., Sullivan, R., Patterson, L., Figiel, G., Webb, M., Spritzer, C., & Djang, W. (1992). Quantitative cerebral anatomy of the aging human brain. *Neurology, 42*, 527–536.

Coleman, P., & Flood, D. (1987). Neuron numbers and dendritic extent in normal aging and Alzheimer's disease. *Neurobiology of Aging, 8*, 521–545.

Corsellis, J. (1978). Discussion. In R. Katzman, R. Terry, & K. Bick (Eds.), *Alzheimer's disease: Senile dementia and related disorders* (p. 397). New York: Raven Press.

Counter, C., Hirte, H., Bacchetti, S., & Harley, C. (1994). Telomerase activity in human ovarian carcinoma. *Proceedings of the National Academy of Sciences, 91*, 2900–2904.

Court, J., Perry, E., Johnson, M., Piggot, M., Kerwin, J., Perry, R., & Ince, P. (1993). Regional patterns of cholinergic and glutamate activity in the developing and aging human brain. *Developmental Brain Research, 74*, 73–82.

Davis, P., & Wright, E. (1977). A new method for measuring cranial cavity volume and its application to the assessment of cerebral atrophy at autopsy. *Neuropathology and Applied Neurobiology, 3*, 341–358.

DeCarli, C., Kaye, J., Horwitz, B., & Rapoport, S. (1990). Critical analysis of the use of computer-assisted transverse axial tomography to study human brain in aging and dementia of the Alzheimer type. *Neurology, 40*, 872–883.

Decker, M. (1987). The effects of aging on hippocampal and cortical projections of the forebrain cholinergic system. *Brain Research Reviews, 12*, 423–438.

Dekaban, A., & Sadowsky, D. (1978). Changes in brain weights during the span of human life: Relation of brain weights to body heights and body weights. *Annals of Neurology, 4*, 345–356.

Dekosky, S., & Scheff, S. (1990). Synapse loss in frontal cortexbiopsies in Alzheimer's disease: Correlation with cognitive severity. *Annals of Neurology, 27*, 457–464.

Devaney, K., & Johnson, H. (1980). Neuron loss in the aging visual cortex of man. *Journal of Gerontology, 35*, 836–841.

Drachman, D., & Leavitt, J. (1974). Human memory and the cholinergic system. *Archives of Neurology, 30*, 113–131.

Farrer, L. (1994). Neurogenetics of aging. In M. Albert & J. Knoefel (Eds.), *Clinical neurology of aging* (pp. 136–155). New York: Oxford University Press.

Feynman, R. (1994). Feynman. In C. Sykes (Eds.), *No ordinary genius* (p. 120). New York: W. W. Norton & Co.

Finch, C. (1987). Neural and endocrine determinants of senescence: Investigation of causality and reversibility by laboratory and clinical interventions. In H. Warner, R. Butler, R. Sprott, & E. Schneider (Eds.), *Modern biological theories of aging* (pp. 261–308). New York: Raven Press.

Gideon, P., Thomsen, C., Stahlberg, F., & Hendriksen, O. (1994). Cerebrospinal fluid production and dynamics in normal aging: A MRI phase-mapping study. *Acta Neurologica Scandinavica, 89*, 362–366.

Greenamyre, J., & Porter, R. (1994). Anatomy and physiology of glutamate in the CNS. *Neurology, 44 (Suppl. 8)*, S7–S13.

Haber, D. (1995). Telomeres, cancer, and immortality. *New England Journal of Medicine, 332*(14), 955–956.

Hachinski, V., Potter, P., & Mersky, H. (1987). Leuko-araiosis. *Archives of Neurology, 44*, 21–23.

Harley, C., Futcher, A., & Greider, C. (1990). Telomeres shorten during aging of human fibroblasts. *Nature, 345*, 458–460.

Haug, H., & Eggers, R. (1991). Morphometry of the human cortex cerebri and corpus striatum during aging. *Neurobiology of Aging, 12*, 336–338.

Hayflick, L., & Moorhead, P. (1961). The serial cultivation of human diploid cell strains. *Experimental Cell Research, 25*, 585.

Henderson, G., Tomlinson, B., & Gibson, P. (1980). Cell counts in human cerebral cortex in normal adults throughout life using an image analysis computer. *Journal of Neuroscience, 46*, 113–136.

Huttenlocher, P. (1979). Synaptic density in human frontal cortex—Developmental changes and effects of aging. *Brain Research, 163*, 195–205.

Johnston, W., Karpati, G., Carpenter, S., Arnold, D., & Shoubridge, E. (1995). Late-onset mitochondrial myopathy. *Annals of Neurology, 37*, 16–23.

Katzman, R. (1993). Education and the prevalence of dementia and Alzheimer's disease. *Neurology, 43*, 13–20.

Katzman, R. (1995). Human nervous system. In E. Masoro (Ed.), *Aging* (pp. 325–344). New York: Oxford University Press.

Katzman, R., & Terry, R. (1992). Normal aging of the nervous system. In R. Katzman & J. Rowe (Eds.), *Principles of geriatric neurology* (pp. 18–46). Philadelphia: F. A. Davis.

Kawamura, J., Terayama, Y., Takashima, S., Obara, K., Pavol, M., Meyer, J., Mortel, K., & Weathers, S. (1993). Leukoaraiosis and cerebral perfusion in normal aging. *Experimental Aging Research, 19*, 225–240.

Kaye, J., Oken, B., Howieson, D., Howieson, J., Holm, L., & Dennison, K. (1994). Neurological evaluation of the optimally healthy oldest old. *Archives of Neurology, 51*, 1205–1211.

Kim, N., Piatyszck, M., & Prowse, K. (1994). Specific association of human telomerase activity with immortal cells and cancer. *Science, 266*, 2011–2015.

Konigsmark, B., & Murphy, E. (1970). Neuronal populations in the human brain. *Nature, 228*, 1335–1336.

Mackenzie, I. (1994). Senile plaques do not progressively accumulate with normal aging. *Acta Neuropathologica, 87*, 520–525.

Malko, J., Hoffman, J., Jr., & Green, R. (1991). MR measurement of intracranial CSF volume in 41 elderly normal volunteers. *American Journal of Neuroradiology, 12*, 371–374.

Mann, D., Yates, P., & Marcyniuk, B. (1984). Monoaminergic neurotransmitter systems in presenile Alzheimer's disease and senile dementia of the Alzheimer type. *Clinical Neruopathology, 3*, 199–205.

Masliah, E., Mallory, M., Hansen, L., DeTeresa, R., & Terry, R. (1993). Quantitative synaptic alterations in the human neocortex during normal aging. *Neurology, 43*, 192–197.

McGeer, E. (1978). Aging and neurotransmitter metabolism in the human brain. In R. Katzman, R. Terry, & K. Bick (Eds.), *Alzheimer's disease, senile dementia and related disorders* (pp. 427–440). New York: Raven Press.

McGeer, E., & McGeer, P. (1976). Neurotransmitter metabolism in the aging brain. In R. Terry & S. Gershon (Eds.), *Aging* (pp. 389–403). New York: Raven Press.

McGeer, P., McGeer, E., & Suzuki, J. (1977). Aging and extrapyramidal function. *Archives of Neurology, 34*, 33–35.

Meyer, J., Takashima, S., Terayama, Y., Obara, K., Muramatsu, K., & Weathers, S. (1994). CT changes associated with normal aging of the human brain. *Journal of Neuroscience, 123,* 200–208.

Morgan, D., Marcusson, J., Nyberg, P., Wester, P., Winblad, B., Gordon, M., & Finch, C. (1987). Divergent changes in D-1 and D-2 dopamine binding sites in human brain during aging. *Neurobiology of Aging, 8,* 195–201.

Nichols, M., Meador, K., Loring, D., Poon, L., Clayton, G., & Martin, P. (1993). Age-related changes in the neurologic examination of healthy sexagenarians, octogenarians, and centenarians. *Journal of Geriatric Psychiatry and Neurology, 6,* 1–7.

Odenheimer, G., Funkenstein, H., Beckett, L., Chown, M., Pilgrim, D., Evans, D., & Albert, M. (1994). Comparison of neurologic changes in "successfully aging" persons vs. the total aging population. *Archives of Neurology, 51,* 573–580.

Pettegrew, J., Withers, G., & Panchalingam, K. (1990). ³¹P NMR of brain aging and Alzheimer's disease. In J. Pettegrew (Ed.), *NMR: Principles and applications to biomedical research* (pp. 204–254). New York: Springer-Verlag.

Pierpaoli, W. (1994). The pineal gland as ontogenic scanner of reproduction, immunity, and aging. *Annals of the New York Academy of Sciences, 741,* 46–49.

Poirier, J., & Finch, C. (1994). Neurochemistry of the aging human brain. In W. Hazzard, E. Bierman, J. Blass, W. Ettinger, & J. Halter (Eds.), *Principles of geriatric medicine and gerontology* (pp. 1005–1012). New York: McGraw-Hill.

Powers, R. (1994). Neurobiology of aging. In C. Coffey, J. Cummings, M. Lovell, & G. Pearlson (Eds.), *Textbook of geriatric neuropsychiatry.* Washington, DC: American Psychiatric Press, Inc.

Reiter, R. (1994). Pineal function during aging: Attenuation of the melatonin rhythm and its neurobiological consequences. *Acta Neurobiologiae Experimentalis, 54 (Suppl.),* 31–39.

Reiter, R. (1995). Oxidative processes and antioxidative defense mechanisms in the aging brain. *FASEB Journal, 9,* 526–533.

Rifai, Z., Welle, S., Kamp, C., & Thornton, C. (1995). Ragged red fibers in normal aging and inflammatory myopathy. *Annals of Neurology, 37,* 24–29.

Rylett, R., Goddard, S., Schmidt, B., & Williams, L. (1993). Acetylcholine synthesis and release following continuous intracerebral administration of NGF in adult and aged Fischer-344 rats. *Journal of Neuroscience, 13*(9), 3956–3965.

Scheibel, M., & Scheibel, A. (1975). Structural changes in the aging brain. In H. Brody, D. Harman, & J. Ordy (Eds.), *Clinical morphologic, and neurochemical aspects in the aging central nervous system. Aging series* (pp. 11–37). New York: Raven Press.

Selkoe, D. (1992). Aging brain, aging mind. *Scientific American, 267*(3), 134–142.

Shear, P., Sullivan, E., Mathalon, D., Lim, K., Avis, L., Yesavage, J., Tinklenberg, J., & Pfefferbaum, A. (1995). Longitudinal volumetric computed tomographic analysis of regional brain changes in normal aging and Alzheimer's disease. *Archives of Neurology, 52,* 392–402.

Steen, R., Gronemeyer, S., & Taylor, J. (1995). Age-related changes in proton T1 values of normal human brain. *Journal of Magnetic Resonance Imaging, 5,* 43–48.

Subba Rao, K. (1993). Genomic damage and its repair in young and aging brain *Molecular Neurobiology, 7*(1), 23–48.

Subba Rao, K., & Loeb, L. (1992). DNA damage and repair in brain: Relationship to aging. *Mutation Research, 275,* 317–329.

Taylor, L., & Griffith, W. (1993). Age-related decline in cholinergic synaptic transmission in hippocampus. *Neurobiology of Aging, 14,* 509–515.

Terry, R., DeTeresa, R., & Hansen, L. (1987). Neocortical cell counts in normal human adult aging. *Annals of Neurology, 10,* 184–192.

Terry, R., Masliah, E., Salmon, D., Butters, N., DeTeresa, R., Hill, R., Hansen, L., & Katzman, R. (1991). Physical basis of cognitive alterations in Alzheimer's disease: Synapse loss is the major correlate of cognitive impairment. *Annals of Neurology, 30,* 572–580.

Van Buskirk, C. (1945). The seventh nerve complex. *Journal of Comparative Neurology, 82,* 303–333.

Vijayashankar, N., & Brody, H. (1977). A study of aging in the human abducens nucleus. *Journal of Comparative Neurology, 173,* 433–438.

Vijayashankar, N., & Brody, H. (1979). A quantitative study of the pigmented neurons in the nuclei locus coeruleus and sub coeruleus in man as related to aging. *Journal of Neuropathology and Experimental Neurology, 38,* 490–497.

West, M., Coleman, P., Flood, D., & Troncosos, J. (1994). Differences in the pattern of hippocampal neuronal loss in normal ageing and Alzheimer's disease. *Lancet, 344,* 769–772.

Whitehouse, P., Parhad, I., Hedreen, J., Clark, A., White, C., III, Struble, R., & Price, D. (1983). Integrity of the nucleus basalis of Meynert in normal aging. *Neurology, 33 (Suppl. 2),* 159.

Yamashita, K., Kobayashi, S., Fukada, H., Yamaguchi, S., & Hiromi, K. (1992). Leuko-araiosis and event-related potentials (P300) in normal aged subjects. *Gerontology, 38,* 233–240.

Ylikoski, R., Ylikoski, A., Erkinjuntti, T., Sulkava, R., Raininko, R., & Tilvis, R. (1993). White matter changes in healthy elderly persons correlate with attention and speed of mental processing. *Archives of Neurology, 50,* 818–824.

Zubenko, G., Moosy, J., & Kopp, U. (1990). Neurochemical correlates of major depression in primary dementia. *Archives of Neurology, 47,* 209–215.

5

Psychosocial Aspects of Aging

JODI D. NADLER, LOUIS F. DAMIS, AND EMILY D. RICHARDSON

Introduction

The process of aging into the elderly years (i.e., 65 years and older) often involves a number of progressive physiological changes. Within the context of these changes, and often related to them, prominent issues of psychological and social adjustment emerge. Such issues include coping with declines in physical and functional abilities, changing social relationships and roles, and dealing with multiple losses. Throughout this period of life, which presents individuals with an increasing number of life stressors and adjustments, elderly people strive to maintain a sense of purpose and well-being. This chapter will familiarize the reader with major psychosocial changes and adjustments that occur with aging. Areas of discussion include life satisfaction, retirement, marriage, sexuality, and bereavement. The chapter concludes with a discussion of successful aging.

Life Satisfaction

Life satisfaction is an area of research that has been studied extensively in elderly populations. It is often used as an index of successful aging and sometimes considered synonymous with mental health. However, life satisfaction is more accurately

JODI D. NADLER • Medical Psychology Section, Florida Hospital Health Center, Orlando, Florida 32803. LOUIS F. DAMIS • Private Practice, Clinical and Health Psychology, Orlando, Florida 32803. EMILY D. RICHARDSON • Yale University School of Medicine, Adler Geriatric Center, Yale-New Haven Hospital, New Haven, Connecticut 06504.

conceptualized as a component of the larger construct of *subjective well-being*. This broader construct also includes measures of morale and mood. George (1981, 1986) defines life satisfaction as a global assessment of life quality, derived from comparison of one's aspirations to his or her actual conditions of life. Moreover, she emphasizes that life satisfaction is a cognitive evaluation of the discrepancy between one's life achievements and aspirations. In contrast to measures of mood, an emotional judgment of current state, life satisfaction is a more stable judgment of one's overall status in life. Consequently, measures of life satisfaction tend to be less affected by short-term or contemporaneous psychosocial events that readily alter indices of mood.

Examinations of levels of life satisfaction in elderly populations reveal that most individuals, 85% or more, describe themselves as satisfied or very satisfied with their lives (George, 1981; Larson, 1978; Sauer & Warland, 1982). Moreover, comparisons of levels of life satisfaction across age groups typically reveal that older adults are at least as satisfied with their lives as their middle-aged and younger counterparts (Campbell, Converse, & Rodgers, 1976; Herzog & Rodgers, 1981). The work of Campbell et al. (1976) also revealed that whereas levels of happiness were higher in young adults in comparison to elderly individuals, the reverse was true for life satisfaction. George (1986) interpreted these findings to suggest that "euphoria is the prerogative of youth, whereas contentment is the reward of old age" (p. 6).

Gender differences in the determinants of life satisfaction have been observed by several researchers. Lubben (1989) found that for men, family relationships were more strongly related to well-being than peer relationships and that the opposite was true for women. Moreover, the results of his study revealed that the psychological and physical well-being of married women were negatively affected by the burden of caring for physically ill, dependent husbands. Furthermore, Quirouette and Pushkar-Gold (1992) found that spousal variables of husbands' health, positive well-being, and perception of marriage predicted significantly wives' well-being but that these spousal variables did not predict husbands' well-being.

Life satisfaction has been examined extensively in reference to its potential objective determinants. Health status has been found to be one of the strongest predictors of life satisfaction relative to other psychosocial variables (Bowling & Brown, 1991; Bowling, Farquhar, & Brown, 1991; Gupta & Korte, 1994; Lubben, 1989). This is not surprising in that physical problems and associated functional disability interfere with participation in daily activities and social interactions, two variables also predictive of life satisfaction (Bowling, Farquhar, Grundy, & Formby, 1993). Along with better health, higher levels of social support/integration, activity, and socioeconomic status are associated with greater levels of life satisfaction (Collette, 1984; Markides & Martin, 1979).

Social isolation has been assumed to be related to decreased life satisfaction, loneliness, and poor health in elderly individuals. In this respect, Gupta and Korte (1994) found that both confidant and peer group variables contributed equally to well-being and health in their study of elderly people. However, Chappell and Badger (1989) cite evidence for the differential impact of subjective versus objective aspects of isolation, noting that emotional isolation (absence of a confidant) is more detrimental than social isolation (limited social network contacts). Moreover, in a study of community dwelling Canadians ages 60 years and older, Chappell and Badger (1989) found that the number of contacts participants had with other people was unrelated to several measures of well-being. In contrast, they found that not having a confidant was related to ratings of less happiness and lower life satisfaction scores. Consequently, Chappell and Badger caution that quantitative measures of social contact as indices of social isolation may not be related to well-being and that qualitative measures are needed to

adequately assess social isolation as a risk factor in elderly adults.

Life satisfaction has also been examined in relation to loss and transitioning of social roles in later life. Adelmann (1994), in her review of this literature, noted that well-being is higher for adults participating in multiple social roles. However, little research has specifically examined the effects of multiple roles in elderly individuals. One such study found that increasing participation in up to eight different social roles was associated with higher levels of present life satisfaction and self-efficacy along with lower levels of depression in a sample of adults ages 60 years and older (Adelmann, 1994). In addition, Krause (1994) found, in a sample of individuals ages 65 years and older, that stressors occurring in salient roles detracted more from feelings of life satisfaction than stressors occurring in less valued roles. Moreover, Adelmann (1994) noted that results of her study along with other accumulating evidence provide support for the importance of enhancing role participation and maintaining activity levels as a means of promoting well-being in later life.

In their review of the relationships among religiosity, aging, and life satisfaction, Markides, Levin, and Ray (1987) and Levin (1989) noted that participation in organized religious activities has shown repeated associations with better health and well-being. Moreover, results of the Markides et al. (1987) longitudinal study of religious activity in elderly individuals revealed that religiosity remains fairly stable over time, that there is a decrease in religious attendance due to declining health, and that the association between religious attendance and well-being is at least partly related to the tendency of both of these variables to be influenced by functional health. In contrast, they noted that higher levels of nonorganizational religious involvement (e.g., private prayer) were inversely related to well-being in older adults. However, this contradiction is explained by the tendency of elderly people with failing health to compensate for decreased church attendance by increasing nonorganizational religious involvement.

When controlling for functional health and other demographic variables, Markides et al. (1987) found a modest association between religious attendance and life satisfaction. Similarly, Levin, Chatters, and Taylor (1995) reported on the positive relationship between both organizational (e.g., church attendance) and subjective (e.g., self-report of religious conviction) religiosity and life satisfaction after controlling for health status. In addition, Levin and Markides (1986) found that religious attendance was associated with improved health even after controlling for social support. Consequently, religious attendance is not considered a proxy for either functional health or social support, and it is likely that various forms of religious involvement offer some degree of protection from the stressors of aging in terms of life satisfaction and health.

In summary, measures of life satisfaction are commonly used indicators of well-being in elderly populations. These measures have been explored relative to many objective determinants and have been found to be positively associated with measures of health, income, activity levels, social support, marital satisfaction, and religious involvement. Research in this area has benefited from the use of multivariate designs controlling for indirect effects of health, functional status, and gender as well as other confounding variables. With respect to assessment of elderly individuals and related policy decisions, it should be noted that life satisfaction is only one dimension of well-being that can be quite insensitive to other important dimensions of mental health, well-being, and successful aging (Euler, 1992; George, 1986).

Retirement

Retirement has been viewed in the aging literature as an event, a status, and a process. Retirement is an event that occurs when a person definitively stops working and withdraws from the formal labor market (Atchley, 1976). It most commonly occurs during the seventh decade of life. With regard to status, retirement represents an achievement and completion of one's role as a productive laborer. It is seen as a legitimate nonworking status that is entered voluntarily and represents a time of entitlement for rest after a life of work. The process of retirement involves a transition from employment to nonemployment and from adulthood to old age.

Henry (1971) suggested that work provides the most central social and psychological framework during adulthood. As retirement represents the point of termination of one's role as a productive worker, it can involve multiple and significant losses. Such losses include important social relationships, productive activity, a consistent structure or routine, responsibility, professional identity, and income. Because of the substantial number of losses associated with retirement, it has been suggested that retirement leads to an increase in psychosocial distress. Moreover, the degree of satisfaction with retirement depends to a large extent on how the process is experienced. Theories examining concepts of retirement, aging, and productive activity have described the experience in different ways.

Disengagement theory (Cummings & Henry, 1961) views retirement as the first step in a progressive decrease in interaction between an aging individual and society. An individual's withdrawal from participation in societal functions is seen as a natural part of her or his aging process. Moreover, it is viewed as something beneficial to the individual and the social structure of society. Disengagement theory has provided support for policies promoting early and mandatory retirement at specified ages. However, little empirical support for this theory as an optimal model of adjustment exists (Adelmann, 1995; Hochschild, 1975). For example, Pohjolainen (1991) found declines in social participation with increasing age, but these declines were likely related to poor physical health.

In contrast to disengagement theory, activity theory (Havighurst & Albrecht, 1953) views retirement as a crisis wherein loss of work must be replaced by other productive activity. The theory postulates that productive activity is central to one's sense of self-worth and is necessary for life satisfaction. A related theory, the continuity theory (Atchley, 1976, 1989), proposes that attitudes and activities undergo a minimal amount of change after retirement. The theory holds that rather than developing new roles, retired individuals seek to increase time in their remaining roles to make their time before and after retirement as similar as possible. Long (1987) suggested that those who adjust most successfully to retirement have made the least changes in their lives. Studies documenting the continuation of work and/or productive activity in older adults provide support for both the activity and continuity theories (Glass, Seeman, Herzog, Kahn, & Berkman, 1995; Parnes & Sommers, 1994). Glass et al. (1995), for example, reported that 12.7% of their MacArthur Successful Aging cohort (ages 70 to 79 years) increased their level of productive activity over a 3-year period. In addition, Parnes and Sommers (1994) found that 16.6% of their sample of elderly males ages 69 to 84 years maintained employment, with a 20% employment rate for men ages 69 to 74 years.

Retirement has been viewed as a stressful life change that has the potential to adversely affect life satisfaction, physical health, psychological status, and social adjustment. However, many individuals make the transition constructively and adjust well to retirement. For example, Bosse, Aldwin, Levenson, and Workman-Daniels (1991) found that among individuals participating in their Normative Aging Study, only 30% rated retirement as stressful. Moreover, when recent retirees were asked to rate the degree of stress associated with 31 different life events, they rated their own and their spouse's retirement as the two least stressful events. Retirement-related hassles also were less frequently reported and were rated less stressful than the work-related hassles of men still employed. Matthews, Brown, Davis, and Denton (1982) also reported that retirement was ranked among the least stressful of 34 events rated by their subjects.

Consistent with the finding that retirement is not universally a stressful experience, one longitudinal study found stability in morale from pre- to postretirement (George & Maddox, 1977). Furthermore, Palmore, Fillenbaum, and George (1984) found no relationship between retirement and feelings of usefulness, morale, or life satisfaction. Palmore, Burchett, Fillenbaum, George, and Wallman (1985) similarly found no significant differences in well-being between retired and nonretired subjects in longitudinal comparisons. Along these same lines, George, Fillenbaum, and Palmore (1984) found no evidence that a retiree's subjective well-being was influenced by his or her retirement. In the same study these authors found that life satisfaction increased significantly after retirement in one sample of married men.

In contrast, studies examining relations between retirement and physical health have consistently shown significant associations between retirement and health problems (Bosse, Aldwin, Levenson, & Ekerdt, 1987; Tuomi, Jarvinen, Eskelinen, Llmarinen, & Klockars, 1991). Moreover,

Bosse et al. (1987) reported more severe physical illness in retirees than in workers, even when controlling for age. Retirees also were found to make greater use of medical services (Boaz & Muller, 1989). However, health status has not been found to be significantly different between retirees and workers when preretirement health status has been controlled (Crowley, 1985; Ekerdt, Baden, Bosse, & Dibbs, 1983; Palmore et al., 1984). Furthermore, a longitudinal study by Mattila, Joukamaa, and Salokangas (1989) found no significant changes in number or degree of physical diseases over a 4-year period in retirees. These latter observations suggest that retirement does not function as a causal factor in poor health, but may more likely serve as a variable contributing to the decision to retire.

Activity levels in elderly individuals also have been examined in relation to retirement and health status. Rogers, Meyer, and Mortel (1990) demonstrated that retirees who maintained an active lifestyle were similar on cerebral blood flow studies across a 4-year period to those elderly individuals who continued to work. In contrast, inactive retirees showed declines in cerebral blood flow. Active retirees also outperformed inactive retirees on cognitive testing after the 4th year of follow-up. These findings suggest that although inactivity in retirement may be associated with health declines, retirement per se, does not contribute to poor health.

Early studies examining the effects of retirement on psychological status showed decreased levels of functioning. It was estimated that up to a third of retirees had difficulty adjusting to retirement (Atchley, 1976; Elwell & Maltbie-Crannell, 1981; Kimmel, Price, & Walker, 1978). Bosse et al. (1987) examined psychological symptoms in older male participants in the Normative Aging Study. These results revealed that retirees reported more psychological distress than did workers, even after controlling for physical health status. Retirement also has been seen as an important factor leading to depression (Portnoi, 1983; Stenback, 1980) and suicide (Kirsling, 1986; Minkler, 1981; Rothberg, Ursano, & Holloway, 1987; Seiden, 1981) in elderly individuals. Atchley (1976) proposed that a period of disenchantment after retirement could account, at least in part, for these psychological declines as individuals adjust to changing social roles.

In contrast to findings noted above, more recent research by Tuomi et al. (1991) found very few changes in the prevalence of mental disorders after retirement regardless of previous work category or type of retirement. Moreover, in the group of individuals who did report mental disorders, increased prevalence of similar problems was seen in the preretirement period. Similar to the relationship between health and retirement, it appears that greater degrees of mental illness in retirees may be related to the presence of such disorders prior to and unrelated to retirement.

Further support for this contention is provided by Midanik, Soghikian, Ransom, and Tekawa (1995). They assessed the short-term effects of retirement on health behaviors and mental health in members (ages 60–66 years) of a health maintenance organization. Controlling for age, gender, marital status, and education, these researchers demonstrated that retired members, in comparison to nonretired members, were more likely to have lower stress levels and to engage in regular exercise. Retired women also were less likely to report problems with alcohol. Furthermore, there were no differences between the groups on self-reported mental health status, coping, depression, smoking, or alcohol use.

With regard to social losses, Wan and Odell (1983) found that retirement was associated with decreased formal and informal social interactions. Palmore et al. (1984) examined the consequences of retirement on social interaction in six longitudinal studies. Across studies, these researchers found conflicting evidence for increases, decreases, and stability in social interactions following retirement. In the context of the Normative Aging Study, Bosse, Aldwin, Levenson, Workman-Daniels, and Ekerdt (1990) found that long-term retirees reported less quantitative social support from previous coworkers than workers or recent retirees. However, retirees did not evidence a decrease in overall qualitative support. Similarly, Bosse, Aldwin, Levenson, Spiro, and Mroczek (1993) found that retirees reported less quantitative social support but evidenced no differences in qualitative support. Both workers and retirees looked to family and friends in times of need, suggesting that the quality of support is maintained in retirement.

Studies examining predictors of good adaptation to retirement have identified health, educational attainment, income, and social support as important factors. For example, Szinovacz and Washo (1992) found that individuals with higher levels of educational attainment and those without health problems adapted better to retirement than did persons with lower levels of educational attainment and those with health problems. For longer-term retirees, significant predictors of retirement adaptation were income, health, visiting friends, and residence in an extended-family household. Again, individuals with higher incomes and better health showed better retirement adaptation. Frequent visits with friends also contributed to positive retirement adaptation. Bosse et al. (1991) examined stress related to the retirement transition and found that the only consistent predictors of retirement-related stress in retirees were poor health and family finances. Furthermore, Riddick (1985) found that subjective health and financial indicators were significant predictors of retirement satisfaction.

In summary, it appears that retirement is a multidimensional process that cannot be accounted for by any single, unidimensional theory. Good health remains a major factor in determining adaptation to retirement and life satisfaction in elderly individuals. Once health status is controlled, it can be seen that psychosocial variables such as income, level of educational attainment, ability to participate in multiple social roles, social support, and maintenance of activity levels during retirement make meaningful contributions to constructive adjustment to retirement. Further study of the factors involved in successful adjustment to retirement, as well as the relationships among these factors, is needed.

Marriage

The quality of the marital relationship is a crucial component of personal well-being (Depner & Ingersoll-Dayton, 1985). Married persons tend to be happier and healthier and live longer than widowed or divorced persons (Gove, Hughes, & Style, 1983). Although adult children and friends also can be important sources of emotional, financial, and instrumental support for older adults, the marital relationship is generally believed to contribute the most to well-being (Alwin, Converse, & Martin, 1985; Gove, Style, & Hughes, 1990; Mancini &

Blieszner, 1989). Moreover, marriage tends to constitute a primary source of social and emotional support.

Marital satisfaction has been studied extensively in younger populations, but less often in elderly individuals. The limited representation of older adult marriages in the literature may be due, in part, to fewer marriages surviving to old age given the shorter life spans of elderly individuals. However, increased life span statistics and recent projections estimate that one of every five marriages will survive to the 50th wedding anniversary (Gilford, 1986). Moreover, Gilford noted that although aging married cohorts become depleted over the years due to death and divorce, more than half of Americans over the age of 65 are married and living with a spouse in an independent household. As such, it is essential to study the quality and psychosocial impact of these important relationships.

Studies that have examined the status of elderly marriages generally reflect a positive interaction between aging and the marital relationship. Older adults report higher levels of marital satisfaction than do middle-aged adults, although not as high as newly married younger adults (Anderson, Russell, & Schumm, 1983; Gilford & Bengtson, 1979; Rollins & Feldman, 1970; Troll, Atchley, & Miller, 1979). Moreover, elderly married individuals report high levels of happiness (Glenn, 1975) and greater satisfaction with family and friends (Uhlenberg & Myers, 1981) than unmarried persons. Another indirect indicator of the quality of marriages among the elderly is the low rate of divorce in this population. Only 1.3% of 2.4 million people receiving a divorce in 1985 were above age 65 (Uhlenberg, Cooney, & Boyd, 1990). Thus, available data generally support a positive association between marriage and emotional well-being in elderly individuals. However, the high level of marital satisfaction in later life can also be attributed to lessened demands placed on older couples due to reduced social roles, such as parenthood and employment (Lee, 1988). It should also be noted that the high prevalence of satisfactory marriages in later life may be due, in part, to a survivor effect of better functioning relationships. That is, ineffective or dissatisfying relationships are more likely to terminate prior to old age leaving only the better functioning marriages for study.

Atchley (1985) described three major functions of marriages that may account for the positive effects of the marital relationship on older couples. These functions include intimacy, defined as the mutual affection, regard, trust, and love within the relationship; interdependence, which involves sharing of housework, income, and other resources; and a sense of belonging, which involves identification with couplehood, sharing of values and perspectives, and a routine source of comfortable interaction and socialization. These functions may serve to increase feelings of emotional support within a marriage and may account for higher levels of reported well-being for married versus unmarried individuals (Gove et al., 1983). Therefore, it is not surprising that marriage for older adults has been reported to minimize the negative impact of significant life events, such as retirement, reduced income, and declining functional capacity that can occur with advancing age (Gilford, 1986).

Some investigators have questioned the stability of marital satisfaction across the elderly life course (e.g., Gilford, 1986; Herman, 1994). Gilford (1986) suggested, for example, that levels of reported marital satisfaction in older couples do not necessarily persist throughout the marital career. On the contrary, she reported that spouses at younger and older extremes of old age report considerably lower marital satisfaction than do spouses at the middle stage of old age (Gilford, 1984). Given the increased life span and longer duration of later-life marriage, the elderly marital relationship and marital satisfaction continues to be examined across substages of later life.

One such study conducted by Herman (1994) surveyed older married adults ages 55 to 88 to examine their marital relationships, degree of marital satisfaction, and sources of marital dissatisfaction across age-defined substages of later life. Subjects were categorized into four age groups: 55–62 years, 63–69 years, 70–77 years, and 78 years or older. His results demonstrated no significant changes in marital satisfaction from adulthood to old age or across later-life substages. Moreover, levels of reported marital satisfaction were not indicative of significant disturbance in marital satisfaction in later years. Furthermore, marital dissatisfaction was found to be associated with lower levels of satisfaction with sexual relations and communication. Unlike Gilford's (1986) study, these findings suggest relative stability across substages of later-life marriage. A possible reason for the differential findings between Gilford (1986) and Herman (1994) is the lack of correspondence between the substage age classifications across studies.

There are multiple factors that affect marital satisfaction in elderly individuals. Physical health and gender are most frequently reported. In general, marital status appears to have a positive effect on physical health, especially in elderly individuals (Verbrugge, 1979). Although spousal illness has been reported to have a detrimental effect on both wives' and husbands' psychological well-being, Johnson (1985) found that elderly couples showed adequate adaptation to changes imposed by physical impairments, thereby limiting potential negative effects on marital satisfaction. Studies examining gender differences in marital satisfaction in later life indicate that elderly men are more satisfied with their marriages than elderly women (Antonucci & Akiyama, 1987; Bernard, 1973; Gilford, 1984; Lurie, 1974). Possible reasons posited for these gender differences have included additional demands placed on women due to traditional female roles (Quirouette & Pushkar-Gold, 1992) and lower levels of perceived social support by wives from their husbands (Depner & Ingersoll-Dayton, 1985). However, at least one study found that observed gender differences in marital satisfaction in elderly individuals were accounted for by differences in self-esteem rather than marriage, per se (Herman, 1994).

In summary, marital relationships in older adults are generally rated as satisfactory, often constitute the primary social relationship and source of support in the elderly person's life, and provide notable benefit in terms of health and well-being. Although these results reflect a positive interplay between aging and marital relations, they may actually reflect, to some degree, a survivor effect. Future research in this area is needed to analyze marital functioning through later ages. In addition, because of the apparently positive effects of marriage in later life, continued study of predictive factors of successful and lasting marriages, as well as methods for ameliorating specific marital problems encountered by older couples, is needed.

Sexuality

Sexual functioning in elderly individuals is usually described with reference to disease and dysfunction. Physiological changes, ill health, and medication use have been documented to adversely affect sexual functioning in older adults. There also are well-documented psychological and social issues that affect sexual functioning in elderly individuals. Loss of one's primary sexual partner, feelings of decreased attractiveness, and incorporation of negative societal attitudes toward sexuality in older adults can all contribute to reduced sexual interest and activity.

Over the past few decades, studies have documented changes in sexual behavior in aging individuals. Kinsey, Pomeroy, and Martin (1948) found a steady decline in sexual activity and capability from adolescence to old age and attributed these results to diminished physical functioning as well as emotional issues, such as boredom. Pfeiffer, Verwoerdt, and Wang (1968) similarly found that levels of sexual activity and interest decreased with advancing age in many, but not all, older subjects. In addition, they noted that levels of sexual activity and interest were essentially the same for both married and unmarried men. Martin (1981) also observed an age-related decrease in sexual activity and noted that physiological variables, such as metabolic rate and serum cholesterol, were significantly related to amount of sexual activity reported. Marsiglio and Donnelly (1991) likewise reported age-related decreases in sexual activity, although approximately 53% of their elderly sample reported having had sexual relations at least one time within the past month.

In contrast, a few studies have reported no substantial changes in sexual behavior with age (George & Weiler, 1981; Mulligan & Palguta, 1991; Pfeiffer, Verwoerdt, & Davis, 1974). For example, in the Duke Longitudinal Study, patterns of sexual interest and activity in married couples remained fairly stable over time, with males reporting higher levels of sexual interest and activity than females (George & Weiler, 1981). Younger cohorts of respondents also reported higher rates of sexual activity than older cohorts. Whereas the relatively lower rate of decline in sexual interest and activity seen in this study may be related to the presence of a regular partner, age-related declines have been reported in the context of stable relationships (Schiavi, 1992). Mulligan and Palguta (1991) studied residents in a nursing home and reported that sexual intercourse occurred at least monthly among 17%, while other forms of sexual contact, such as hugging and kissing, occurred at least monthly among 73% of the sample.

Steinke (1994) conducted studies to explore differences between elderly males and females on their sexual knowledge, attitudes, and behavior. These results revealed comparable levels of sexual knowledge and attitudes for women and men. Sexual activity occurred an average of 4 times per month and ranged from 0 to 30 times per month. Bretschneider and McCoy (1988) examined sexual interest and behavior in males and females ages 80 to 102 years living in residential retirement facilities. For both males and females, the most common activity reported was touching and caressing without sexual intercourse, followed by sexual intercourse. Furthermore, touching and caressing showed a significant decline with age.

With regard to physiology, a number of regular age-related changes occur in sexual response systems of men and women. In men, a prolonged excitement phase creates a longer period before full erection is obtained and greater physical stimulation is required to produce erections. Orgasms tend to become less frequent and the refractory phase is greatly prolonged so that once an erection is terminated, the erectile capacity may be inhibited for hours. Similarly, women experience prolonged excitement and refractory phases. In addition, women have reduced orgasmic vigor along with decreased vulvovaginal sensitivity and sexual lubrication. On the other hand, sexuality can be enhanced by reduced fear of pregnancy and prolonged excitement phase.

In addition to normal age-related changes, medical problems that commonly occur with aging can contribute to alterations in sexual patterns. Renal disease, for example, may result in reduced sexual potency (Wise, Epstein, & Ross, 1992). Studies of patients after myocardial infarction have revealed sexual problems including orgasmic difficulties in women and erectile dysfunction and premature ejaculation in men (Wise et al., 1992). Moreover, the anxiety and depression often associated with cardiac episodes also can inhibit sexual desire and functioning (Wise et al., 1992). Insulin-dependent diabetes mellitus can diminish sexual functioning in women and men (Felstein, 1983; Wise et al., 1992). Renshaw (1981) suggested that damage to the autonomic nervous system in male stroke patients can lead to erectile difficulties, impaired ejaculation, or total impotency, and in female patients, to decreased lubrication. Strokes also can interfere with sensory appreciation, motor activity, and verbalization, making sexual activity difficult and less rewarding (Felstein, 1983). In patients with pulmonary disease, loss of sexual desire can occur from low levels of testosterone related to chronic arterial hypoxia (Wise et al., 1992). In addition, respiratory difficulties may limit one's physical ability to engage in sexual activity (Wise et al., 1992). In cancer patients, sexual functioning may be affected by physical aspects of neoplasms, side effects of treatment, and psychological factors.

Related to the higher incidence of medical illnesses in elderly individuals compared to younger adults is an increase in the use of medications. Given their aging sexual physiology, elderly individuals become particularly vulnerable to adverse effects of medications on sexual functioning. Deamer and Thompson (1991) reported that psychotropic (i.e., antipsychotic and antidepressant medications) and antihypertensive drugs are often associated with such detrimental effects. In this regard, antihypertensive drugs are a major contributor to impotency and may adversely affect the female libido. In addition, diuretics can also inhibit sexual desire.

Psychological and social issues relating to sexuality in elderly individuals also contribute to changes in sexual patterns that occur with aging. It has been suggested that cohort effects may be responsible for the more conservative sexual behavior and attitudes in the present generation of older adults (O'Donohue, 1987). In addition, the socially defined role of older people as not sexual may affect sexual feelings and activity levels (O'Donohue, 1987). Feelings of decreased sexual attractiveness (Cameron, 1970; Kaas, 1978; Ludeman, 1981) as well as negative attitudes toward sexuality in older adults (Cameron, 1970; LaTorre & Kear, 1977) also may contribute to lessened sexual interest and activity among elderly individuals. In addition, Pfeiffer et al. (1968) reported that past sexual experiences, subjective and objective health factors, and social class were significant predictors of sexual behavior in elderly individuals. Moreover, an individual's prior attitude toward sexuality is an important determinant of subsequent functioning (Wise et al., 1992).

To summarize, despite a number of changes in sexual behavior associated with physiology, physical illness, medication use, and psychosocial influences in older adults, a sizeable proportion of the elderly population continues to enjoy and actively participate in sexual activities. More research is needed to identify the components of optimal sexual functioning and advance treatment of sexual dysfunction in older adults.

Grief and Loss

Old age is a time of multiple and continued losses that may include the death of one's spouse, siblings, peers, and with increased life expectancy, possibly one's children. The process of aging is also imbued with a much wider and often unappreciated range of losses including retirement and associated loss of occupational status, reduced income, decrements in sensory and physical functioning, loss of home and neighborhood, loss of possessions, and loss of one's pet through death or the individual's inability to care for the pet (Smyth, 1994). Death of one's spouse is often a very difficult loss because it involves the loss of one's confidant, sexual partner, and companion.

Although considerable research has been conducted on the course of bereavement and grief in young adult populations, relatively little work has addressed grief in old age (Fasey, 1990; Sable, 1991). In his review of the literature, Fasey (1990) concludes that elderly individuals experience phases of grief similar to those described in the literature on younger adults: numbness, depression, and resolution. The phase of numbness is characterized by shock, an unwillingness to accept the loss, emotional dullness, and episodes of distress and autonomic arousal. The phase of depression follows the initial stage of shock and is associated with full emotional expression of loss that may include crying, low mood, sleep disturbance, an-

orexia, resentment, anger, and guilt. In this phase it also is common for individuals to be preoccupied with understanding or contemplating the reason or meaning of the loss. The final phase of resolution brings about an acceptance of the death or loss along with a return to normal levels of function and affect. Although description of the phases of the grieving process can facilitate an understanding of the grief-stricken individual's symptoms and may enhance her or his experience of control by being able to predict shifts in symptoms, it should be noted that such "stages" are not as apparent in the elderly bereaved as in younger adults (Brink, 1985; Parkes, 1972). Moreover, an empirical repeated measures examination of five clusters of different grief-related symptoms revealed that changes in symptoms were continuous and gradual (Lund, Caserta, & Dimond, 1986). In addition, these authors noted that bereavement in both men and women is characterized by a complex and often competing array of symptoms.

The time course of grief resolution is quite variable. As such, it is common for individuals to experience recurrences of sadness, distressing recollections, and episodic yearning for the deceased for several years after the loss. Assessment of depressive symptomatology associated with widowhood revealed that widows returned to prebereavement levels within 12 months of the death of their spouse (Harlow, Goldberg, & Comstock, 1991). Moreover, the notion of any type of absolute resolution of a loss is unlikely and acceptance is more a reintegration into a new life without the deceased (Garrett, 1987; Sable, 1991). Although the duration of the grieving process is uncertain, Garrett (1987) delineated common signs of resolution: the ability to recall both positive and negative aspects of the deceased as opposed to idealized recollections characteristic of earlier phases; the ability to console others experiencing grief in contrast to prior preoccupation with personal loss; and reinvestment in new relationships, revival of old friendships, and development of new interests.

Whereas Fasey (1990) reported that grief is a serious problem with a definite associated psychiatric morbidity and mortality, he noted that the process may be less severe for individuals over 65 years of age. Similarly, Brink (1985) agreed with this contention and cited Ball (1976), indicating that age predicted early, successful resolution of widows' grief. However, Sable (1991) found that elderly widows do not tolerate or adapt to bereavement more successfully than younger women. Moreover, Lund et al. (1986) found in their 2-year longitudinal study of the bereavement process in men and women that bereavement is a long-term process that does not end at 2 years. This is consistent with Carey's (1979) report that bereavement extends well beyond the first year. Furthermore, due to the complication of multiple losses in old age, elderly individuals may develop chronic grief (Garrett, 1987; Parkes, 1992).

Normal bereavement reactions have much in common with depressive disorders. Anorexia, insomnia, difficulty with concentration, and dysphoria are frequently occurring symptoms. As noted in the *Diagnostic and Statistical Manual of Mental Disorders (DSM-III-R)* of the American Psychiatric Association (1987), the identification of abnormal grieving processes is often difficult due to substantial individual and cultural variations in adjustment to bereavement. However, the authors of *DSM-III-R* noted that bereavement can be complicated by depression and with the recent revision of the manual (*DSM-IV*, American Psychiatric Association, 1994), the diagnosis of major depression can now be made as early as 2 months following the onset of bereavement. Furthermore, Breckenridge, Gallagher, Thompson, and Peterson (1986) confirmed earlier findings that normal bereavement is not associated with the presence of notable self-deprecatory cognitions. A recent study by Prigerson et al. (1995) empirically distinguished complicated grief from bereavement-related depression. These researchers found that a set of symptoms indicative of complicated bereavement (that is, searching for the deceased, yearning for the deceased, preoccupation with thoughts of the deceased, crying, disbelief regarding the death, feeling stunned by the death, and lack of acceptance of the death) at 3 to 6 months after the deaths of their subjects' spouses was distinct from bereavement-related depressive symptoms in a principal components analysis. Furthermore, they found that scores on this set of complicated grief symptoms predicted global functioning, depressed mood, self-reported sleep quality, and self-esteem at the 18-month follow-up whereas scores on the depression-related bereavement set of symptoms only predicted degree of medical illness burden at follow-up.

As noted by Fasey (1990), grief in elderly individuals has been associated with mortality and psychiatric morbidity. In this respect, a study by Young, Benjamin, and Wallis (1963) found a significant increase in mortality in the first 6 months of widowhood, accounted for by males dying from vascular disease, along with a return to normal rates of mortality within 2 years of bereavement. Moreover, in an epidemiological study of married and widowed individuals ages 60 years or older, Li (1995) found that risk of suicide for widowed men was 3.3 times as high as that for married men. In addition, he noted that risk for suicide in widowed women was no greater than that for married women. Furthermore, he recommends that elderly widowed men should be considered prime targets for suicide prevention.

With respect to psychiatric morbidity related to bereavement, Parkes (1992), in his review of the literature, noted that there is a substantial minority of bereaved individuals who develop depressive disorders or experience exacerbations of premorbid conditions including substance abuse and anxiety disorders. Hays, Kasl, and Jacobs (1994) found that a past personal history of dysphoric mood was associated with elevated levels of depressive symptoms, general anxiety, and hopelessness/helplessness through 25 months postbereavement. In contrast to the increased mortality in men, Lund et al. (1986) did not find gender differences in depression, life satisfaction, or grief-related symptom profiles in their 2-year longitudinal study of bereavement in the individuals.

Optimal adjustment to widowhood has been associated with presence of perceived social support (Dimond, Lund, & Caserta, 1987; Prigerson, Frank, Reynolds, George, & Kupfer, 1993), good physical health, and adequate mental health (Brink, 1985). In contrast, factors associated with poorer bereavement outcomes include greater caregiver strain prior to the death of a loved one (Bass & Bowman, 1990), bereavement support from family members who inappropriately give advice and encourage recovery (Lehman, Ellard, & Wortman, 1986), perceived non-supportiveness of others (Maddison & Walker, 1967), loss of the deceased through suicide (Farberow, Gallagher-Thompson,

Gilewski, & Thompson, 1992), and additional concurrent losses (Herth, 1990).

Fasey (1990) notes that "most bereaved individuals neither want nor require professional help, and through individual coping mechanisms and social networks, deal with the loss and may even be strengthened by it" (p. 72). He goes on to describe the goal of grief work as "accepting the loss and adapting to it such that life can be reestablished, albeit, perhaps, different from that before the loss" (p. 72). He also indicates that many forms of treatment have been found beneficial including individual and group formats. Moreover, the common ingredient to successful interventions is positive encouragement to discuss the deceased rather than avoidance of the loss. In their study of what bereaved individuals found to be helpful, Lehman et al. (1986) reported that contacts with similar others and the opportunity to express feelings were most frequently mentioned. In addition, Caserta and Lund (1993) found that bereaved older adults who rated themselves low on personal competencies (related to adaptation and resiliency) benefited most from group participation.

It should also be noted that the bereaved elderly may demonstrate atypical reactions such as inhibited grief or delayed grief patterns (Fasey, 1990). This minority of individuals may not evince symptoms of grief or emotional distress and may not receive needed attention from caregivers. The status of these individuals should be monitored, and emergence of delayed depressive symptomatology should be interpreted in the context of a grieving process to promote optimal outcomes.

To summarize, the elderly years are associated with multiple losses ranging from death of close family members and peers to loss of health, functional ability, and personal property. Although much remains to be learned about grief processes among elderly individuals, recent findings indicate that adjustment to significant losses in this population is associated with distress equal to or greater than that for younger individuals, lengthy adjustment periods that are often complicated by other concurrent losses, and a notable increase in risk for suicide and mortality from other causes, particularly for men. Moreover, the decreasing range of intra- and interpersonal resources available to older adults places them at risk for developing chronic grief reactions or other atypical grief syndromes that warrant special attention. In contrast, optimal adjustment appears to be associated with the presence of adequate social support, the opportunity to express feelings, contact with others dealing with similar losses, and the avoidance of inappropriate advice-giving or pressure to recover too quickly. Although many older adults seem to adjust to the losses associated with aging in a veiled manner, dealing with grief is a significant emotional burden of aging that warrants further attention.

Successful Aging

Successful aging is a rapidly growing area of gerontological research (Birren & Schaie, 1985; Butt & Beiser, 1987; Eisdorfer, 1983; Rowe & Kahn, 1987). It has been defined as a relatively high level of physical health, psychological well-being, and competence in adaptation (Wong, 1989). The notion of successful aging is based on the recognition of heterogeneity among older adults (Rowe & Kahn, 1987). The concept of successful aging has allowed aging research to extend beyond the often inadequate impaired/nonimpaired dichotomy to include identification of individuals who have aged particularly well (Rowe & Kahn, 1987). It also expands the concept of aging beyond the simplistic view of declining health and limited resources (Garfein & Herzog, 1995). Garfein and Herzog (1995) note that the emphasis on aging well is consistent with the World Health Organization's definition of health as a state of complete physical, mental, and social well-being, rather than merely the absence of disease.

Wont (1989) reviewed the importance of personal meaning in promotion of health and successful aging. He defined personal meaning as an individually constructed cognitive system grounded in subjective values and capable of endowing life with personal significance and satisfaction. Studies examining the relationship of personal meaning to successful aging reveal that successful agers are more likely to show existential acceptance of things that cannot be changed, are more inclined to attach meaning and purpose to undesirable life events, and are more likely to report personal meaning as a source of happiness (Wong, 1989). Likewise, Reker,

Peacock, and Wong (1987) found positive associations between indices of personal meaning and perceived well-being.

Berkman, Seeman, and Albert (1993) identified correlates of successful aging in the MacArthur Successful Aging Study sample. Factors related to successful aging included health status, level of attained educational achievement, income, volunteer activities, lack of psychiatric symptoms, and personality characteristics of self-efficacy and mastery. However, their epidemiological study employed a cross-sectional methodology. Supporting possible causal relationships among similar variables, a longitudinal study of successful aging (Roos & Havens, 1991) found that self-reported health, absence of certain chronic conditions, and not losing a spouse to death or institutionalization were significant predictors of maintained functional independence.

Garfein and Herzog (1995) examined the interrelationships among four multicategory definitions of robust (successful) aging: productive involvement, affective status, functional status, and cognitive status. Using a sample of older adults, ages 60 years and older, they found several personal characteristics that distinguished robustly aging individuals from less well-functioning age-matched peers. The most robustly aging individuals reported greater social contact, better health and vision, and fewer significant life events in the past 3 years than their age counterparts. Whereas these data did reveal a linear age-related decrease in the proportion of respondents found in the most robust aging categories, membership in the oldest-old cohort did not preclude the presence of robust aging. Overall, these findings support the notion that presumed losses and ill effects of aging are not universal occurrences.

Baltes and Baltes (1990) described the model of *selective optimization with compensation* as a strategy of successful aging. Selection refers to the adaptive task of the person and society to concentrate on those domains that are of high priority and that suit their skills and situations. Optimization reflects the view that people will have become skilled at maximizing their chosen life courses with regard to quantity and quality. Compensation, like selection, results from restrictions in the range of adaptive potentials, and it involves aspects of both

mind and technology. As a combined strategy, selective optimization with compensation allows elderly people to engage in life tasks that are important to them despite reductions in physiological, cognitive, and social resources. A recent study investigating this approach with aging individuals in the workplace demonstrated its usefulness as a strategy for older workers (Abraham & Hansson, 1995).

Future research will need to further define and study the determinants of successful aging. As in other aging areas, much of the information available to date has been obtained with cross-sectional methodologies, thereby limiting the potential for causal inferences and increasing the likelihood of confounding cohort effects. A number of longitudinal studies (e.g., the MacArthur Successful Aging Study) are currently under way to investigate factors that facilitate successful aging. In addition to psychosocial variables, these studies are investigating the impact of such factors as mobility, exercise, physical health, and educational attainment on maintenance of functional and cognitive independence in later life. These investigations will provide useful information on possible protective mechanisms as well as potential intervention strategies that may enhance the process of aging.

References

Abraham, J. D., & Hansson, R. O. (1995). Successful aging at work: An applied study of selection, optimization, and compensation through impression management. *Journal of Gerontology: Psychological Sciences, 50,* 2, P94–P103.

Adelmann, P. K. (1994). Multiple roles and psychological well-being in a national sample of older adults. *Journal of Gerontology: Social Sciences, 49,* S277–S285.

Alwin, D. F., Converse, P. E., & Martin, S. S. (1985). Living arrangements and social integration. *Journal of Marriage and the Family, 47,* 319–334.

American Psychiatric Association. (1994). *Diagnostic and statistical manual of mental disorders* (3rd ed.). Washington, DC: Author.

American Psychiatric Association. (1987). *Diagnostic and statistical manual of mental disorders* (4th ed., revised). Washington, DC: Author.

Anderson, S. A., Russell, C. S., & Schumm, W. A. (1983). Perceived marital quality and the family life cycle categories: A further analysis. *Journal of Marriage and the Family, 95,* 127–139.

Antonucci, T. C., & Akiyama, H. (1987). An examination of sex differences in social support among older men and women. *Sex Roles, 17,* 737–749.

Atchley, R. C. (1976). *The sociology of retirement.* Cambridge, MA: Schenkman.

Atchley, R. C. (1985). *Social forces in aging* (4th ed.). Belmont, CA: Wadsworth.

Atchley, R. C. (1989). A continuity theory of normal aging. *The Gerontologist, 29,* 183–190.

Ball, J. F. (1976). Widow's grief: The impact of age and mode of death. *Omega, 7,* 307–333.

Baltes, P. B., & Baltes, M. M. (1990). Psychological perspectives on successful aging: The model of selective optimization with compensation. In P. B. Baltes & M. M. Baltes (Eds.), *Successful aging: Perspectives from the behavioral sciences* (pp. 1–34). Cambridge, United Kingdom: Cambridge University Press.

Bass, D. M., & Bowman, K. (1990). The transition from caregiving to bereavement: The relationship of care-related strain and adjustment to death. *The Gerontologist, 30,* 35–42.

Berkman, L. F., Seeman, T. E., & Albert, M. (1993). High, usual, and impaired functioning in community-dwelling older men and women: Findings from the MacArthur Foundation Research Network on Successful Aging. *Journal of Clinical Epidemiology, 46,* 1129–1140.

Bernard, J. (1973). *The future of marriage.* New York: Bantam Books.

Birren, J. E., & Schaie, K. W. (1985). *Handbook of the psychology of aging* (2nd ed.). New York: Van Nostrand Reinhold.

Boaz, R. F., & Muller, C. F. (1989). Does having more time after retirement change the demand for physician services? *Medical Care, 27,* 1–15.

Bosse, R., Aldwin, C. M., Levenson, M. R., & Ekerdt, D. J. (1987). Mental health differences among retirees and workers: Findings from the normative aging study. *Psychology and Aging, 2,* 383–389.

Bosse, R., Aldwin, C. M., Levenson, M. R., Workman-Daniels, K., & Ekerdt, D. J. (1990). Differences in social support among retirees and workers: Findings from the normative aging study. *Psychology and Aging, 5,* 41–47.

Bosse, R., Aldwin, C. M., Levenson, M. R., & Workman-Daniels, K. (1991). How stressful is retirement? Findings from the Normative Aging study. *Journal of Gerontology: Psychological Sciences, 46,* P9–P14.

Bosse, R., Aldwin, C. M., Levenson, M. R., & Spiro, A., III, & Mroczek, D. K. (1993). Change in social support after retirement: Longitudinal findings from the normative aging study. *Journal of Gerontology: Psychological Sciences, 48,* P210–P217.

Bowling, A., & Brown, P. (1991). Social networks, health, and emotional well-being among the oldest old in London. *Journal of Gerontology: Social Sciences, 46,* S20–S32.

Bowling, A., Farquhar, M., & Brown, P. (1991). Life satisfaction and associations with social network and support variables in three samples of elderly people. *International Journal of Geriatric Psychiatry, 6,* 549–566.

Bowling, A., Farquhar, M., Grundy, E., & Formby, J. (1993). Changes in life satisfaction over a two and a half year period among very elderly people living in London. *Social Science Medicine, 36,* 641–655.

Breckenridge, J. N., Gallagher, D., Thompson, L. W., & Peterson, J. (1986). Characteristic depressive symptoms of bereaved elders. *Journal of Gerontology, 41,* 163–168.

Bretschneider, J. G., & McCoy, N. L. (1988). Sexual interest and behavior in healthy 80- to 102-year-olds. *Archives of Sexual Behavior, 17,* 109–129.

Brink, T. L. (1985). The grieving patient in later life. *Psychotherapy-Patient, 2,* 117–127.

Butt, D. S., & Beiser, M. (1987). Successful aging: A theme for international psychology. *Psychology and Aging, 2,* 87–94.

Cameron, P. (1970). The generation gap: Beliefs about sexuality and reported and self-reported sexuality. *Developmental Psychology, 3,* 272.

Campbell, A., Converse, P. E., & Rodgers, W. (1976). *The quality of American life.* New York: Russell Sage Foundation.

Carey, R. G. (1979). Weathering widowhood: Problems and adjustments of the widowed during the first year. *Omega, 10,* 163–174.

Caserta, M., & Lund, D. (1993). Intrapersonal resources and the effectiveness of self-help groups for bereaved older adults. *The Gerontologist, 33,* 619–629.

Chappell, N. L., & Badger, M. (1989). Social isolation and well-being. *Journal of Gerontology, 44,* S169–S176.

Collette, J. (1984). Sex differences in life satisfaction: Australian data. *Journal of Gerontology, 39,* 243–245.

Crowley, J. E. (1985). Longitudinal effects of retirement on men's psychological and physical well-being. In H. S. Parnes, J. E. Crowley, R. J. Haurin, L. J. Less, W. R. Morgan, F. L. Mott, & G. Nestel (Eds.), *Retirement among American men* (pp. 147–173). Lexington, MA: Lexington Books.

Cummings, E., & Henry, W. H. (1961). *Growing old: The process of disengagement.* New York: Basic Books.

Deamer, R. L., & Thompson, J. F. (1991). The role of medications in geriatric sexual functioning. *Geriatric Sexuality, Clinics in Geriatric Medicine, 7,* 95–111.

Depner, C. E., & Ingersoll-Dayton, B. (1985). Conjugal social support: Patterns in later life. *Journal of Gerontology, 40,* 761–766.

Dimond, M., Lund, D., & Caserta, M. (1987). The role of social support in the first two years of bereavement in an elderly sample. *The Gerontologist, 27,* 599–604.

Eisdorfer, C. (1983). Conceptual models of aging. *American Psychologist, 38,* 197–202.

Ekerdt, D. J., Baden, L., Bosse, R., & Dibbs, E. (1983). The effect of retirement on physical health. *American Journal of Public Health, 73,* 779–783.

Elwell, F., & Maltbie-Crannell, A. D. (1981). The impact of role loss upon coping resources and life satisfaction of the elderly. *Journal of Gerontology, 36,* 223–232.

Euler, B. (1992). A flaw in gerontological assessment: The weak relationship of elderly superficial life satisfaction to deep psychological well-being. *International Journal of Aging and Human Development, 34,* 299–310.

Farberow, N., Gallagher-Thompson, D., Gilewski, M., & Thompson, L. (1992). Changes in grief and mental health of bereaved spouses of older suicides. *Journal of Gerontology, 47,* P357–P366.

Fasey, C. N. (1990). Grief in old age: A review of the literature. *International Journal of Geriatric Psychiatry, 5,* 67–75.

Felstein, I. (1983). Dysfunction: Origins and therapeutic approaches. In R. Weg (Ed.), *Sexuality in the later years*. New York: Academic Press.

Garfein, A. J., & Herzog, A. R. (1995). Robust aging among the young-old, old-old, and oldest-old. *Journal of Gerontology: Social Sciences, 50*, S77–S87.

Garrett, J. E. (1987). Multiple losses in older adults. *Journal of Gerontological Nursing, 13*, 8–12.

George, L. K. (1981). Subjective well-being: Conceptual and methodological issues. In C. Eisdorfer, (Ed.), *Annual review of gerontology and geriatrics* (Vol. 2). New York: Springer.

George, L. K. (1986). Life satisfaction in later life. *Generations, Spring*, 5–8.

George, L. K., & Maddox, G. L. (1977). Subjective adaptation to loss of the work role: A longitudinal study. *Journal of Gerontology, 32*, 456–462.

George, L. K., & Weiler, S. J. (1981). Sexuality in middle and late life. *Archives of General Psychiatry, 38*, 919–923.

George, L. K., Fillenbaum, G. G., & Palmore, E. (1984). Sex differences in the antecedents and consequences of retirement. *Journal of Gerontology, 39*, 364–371.

Gilford, R. (1984). Contrasts in marital satisfaction throughout old age: An exchange theory analysis. *Journal of Gerontology, 39*, 325–333.

Gilford, R. (1986). Marriages in later life. *Generations, Summer*, 16–20.

Gilford, R., & Bengtson, V. (1979). Measuring marital satisfaction in three generations: Positive and negative dimensions. *Journal of Marriage and the Family, 41*, 387–398.

Glass, T. A., Seeman, T. E., Herzog, A. R., Kahn, R., & Berkman, L. F. (1995). Change in productive activity in late adulthood: MacArthur studies of successful aging. *Journal of Gerontology: Social Sciences, 50*, S65–S76.

Glenn, N. (1975). The contribution of marriage to the psychological well-being of males and females. *Journal of Marriage and the Family, 37*, 594–601.

Gove, W., Hughes, M., & Style, C. (1983). Does marriage have positive effects on the psychological well-being of the individual? *Journal of Health and Social Behavior, 24* (June), 122–131.

Gove, W., Style, C., & Hughes, M. (1990). Effects of marriage on the well-being of adults. *Journal of Family Issues, 11*, 4–35.

Gupta, V., & Korte, C. (1994). The effects of a confidant and a peer group on the well-being of single elders. *International Journal of Aging and Human Development, 39*, 293–302.

Harlow, S. D., Goldberg, E. L., & Comstock, G. W. (1991). A longitudinal study of the prevalence of depressive symptomatology in widowed and married women. *Archives of General Psychiatry, 48*, 1065–1068.

Havighurst, R. J., & Albrecht, R. (1953). *Older people*. New York: Longmans, Green.

Hays, J. C., Kasl, S., & Jacobs, S. (1994). Past personal history of dysphoria, social support, and psychological distress following conjugal bereavement. *Journal of the American Geriatric Society, 42*, 712–718.

Henry, W. E. (1971). The role of work in structuring the life cycle. *Human Development, 14*, 125–131.

Herman, S. M. (1994). Marital satisfaction in the elderly. *Gerontology and Geriatrics Education, 14*, 69–79.

Herth, K. (1990). Relationship of hope, coping styles, concurrent losses, and setting to grief resolution in the elderly widow(er). *Research in Nursing and Health, 13*, 109–117.

Herzog, A. R., & Rodgers, W. L. (1981). Age and satisfaction: Data from several large surveys. *Research on Aging, 7*, 209–233.

Hochschild, A. R. (1975). Disengagement theory: A critique and proposal. *American Sociological Review, 40*, 553–569.

Johnson, C. (1985). The impact of illness on late-life marriages. *Journal of Marriage and the Family, 47*, 165–172.

Kaas, M. J. (1978). Sexual expression of the elderly in nursing homes. *The Gerontologist, 18*, 372–378.

Kimmel, D. C., Price, K. F., & Walker, J. W. (1978). Retirement choice and retirement satisfaction. *Journal of Gerontology, 33*, 575–585.

Kinsey, A. C., Pomeroy, W. B., & Martin, C. E. (1948). *Sexual behavior in the human male*. Philadelphia: Saunders.

Kirsling, R. A. (1986). Review of suicide among elderly persons. *Psychological Reports, 59*, 359–366.

Krause, N. (1994). Stressors in salient social roles and well-being in later life. *Journal of Gerontology, 49*, S137–S148.

Larson, R. (1978). Thirty years of research on the subjective well-being of older Americans. *Journal of Gerontology, 33*, 109–125.

LaTorre, R. A., & Kear, K. (1977). Attitudes toward sex in the aged. *Archives of Sexual Behavior, 6*, 203–213.

Lee, G. R. (1988). Marital satisfaction in later life: The effects of nonmarital roles. *Journal of Marriage and the Family, 50*, 775–783.

Lehman, D. R., Ellard, J. H., & Wortman, C. B. (1986). Social support for the bereaved: Recipients' and providers' perspectives on what is helpful. *Journal of Consulting and Clinical Psychology, 54*, 438–446.

Levin, J. S. (1989). Religious factors in aging, adjustment, and health: A theoretical overview. In W. M. Clements (Ed.), *Religion, aging, and health: A global perspective*. New York: The Hawthorne Press.

Levin, J. S., & Markides, K. S. (1986). Religious attendance and subjective health. *Journal of the Scientific Study of Religion, 25*, 31–40.

Levin, J. S., Chatters, L. M., & Taylor, R. J. (1995). Religious effects on health status and life satisfaction among black Americans. *Journal of Gerontology: Social Sciences, 50B*, S154–S163.

Li, G. (1995). The interaction effect of bereavement and sex on the risk of suicide in the elderly: An historical cohort study. *Social Science Medicine, 40*, 825–828.

Long, J. (1987). Continuity as a basis for change: Leisure and male retirement. *Leisure Studies, 6*, 55–70.

Lubben, J. E. (1989). Gender differences in the relationship of widowhood and psychological well-being among low income elderly. *Women and Health, 14*, 161–189.

Ludeman, K. (1981). The sexuality of the older person: Review of the literature. *The Gerontologist, 21*, 203–208.

Lund, D. A., Caserta, M. S., & Dimond, M. F. (1986). Gender differences through two years of bereavement among the elderly. *The Gerontologist, 26*, 314–320.

Lurie, E. E. (1974). Sex and stage differences in perceptions of marital and family relationships. *Journal of Marriage and the Family, 36*, 260–269.

Maddison, D., & Walker, W. (1967). Factors affecting the outcome of conjugal bereavement. *The British Journal of Psychiatry, 113*, 1057–1067.

Mancini, J. A., & Blieszner, R. (1989). Aging parents and adult children: Research themes in intergenerational relations. *Journal of Marriage and the Family, 51*, 275–290.

Markides, K. S., & Martin, H. W. (1979). A causal model of life satisfaction among the elderly. *Journal of Gerontology, 34*, 86–93.

Markides, K. S., Levin, J. S., & Ray, L. A. (1987). Religion, aging, and life satisfaction: An eight-year, three-wave longitudinal study. *The Gerontologist, 27*, 660–665.

Marsiglio, W., & Donnelly, D. (1991). Sexual relations in later life: A national study of married persons. *Journal of Gerontology: Social Sciences, 46*, S338–S344.

Martin, C. E. (1981). Factors affecting sexual functioning in 60–79 year old married males. *Archives of Sexual Behavior, 10*, 399–420.

Matthews, A. M., Brown, K. H., Davis, C. K., & Denton, M. A. (1982). A crisis assessment technique for the evaluation of life events: Transition to retirement as an example. *Canadian Journal on Aging, 1*, 28–39.

Mattila, V. J., Joukamaa, M. I., & Salokangas, R. K. R. (1989). Retirement, aging, psychosocial adaptation, and mental health. Findings of the TURVA project. *Acta Psychiatrica Scandinavica, 80*, 356–367.

Midanik, L. T., Soghikian, K., Ransom, L. J., & Tekawa, I. S. (1995). The effect of retirement on mental health and health behaviors: The Kaiser Permanente retirement study. *Journal of Gerontology: Social Sciences, 50*, S59–S61.

Minkler, M. (1981). Research on the health effects of retirement: An uncertain legacy. *Journal of Health and Social Behavior, 22*, 117–130.

Mulligan, T., & Palguta, R. F. (1991). Sexual interest, activity, and satisfaction among male nursing home residents. *Archives of Sexual Behavior, 20*, 199–204.

O'Donohue, W. T. (1987). The sexual behavior and problems of the elderly. In L. L. Carstenson, & B. A. Edelstein (Eds.), *Handbook of clinical gerontology*, New York: Pergamon Books, Inc.

Palmore, E. B., Fillenbaum, G. G., & George, L. K. (1984). Consequences of retirement. *Journal of Gerontology, 39*, 109–116.

Palmore, E. B., Burchett, B. M., Fillenbaum, G. G., George, L. K., & Wallman, L. M. (1985). *Retirement: Causes and consequences*. New York: Springer.

Parkes, C. M. (1972). *Bereavement: Studies of adult grief*. New York: International Universities Press.

Parkes, C. M. (1992). Bereavement and mental health in the elderly. *Reviews in Clinical Gerontology, 2*, 45–51.

Parnes, H. S., & Sommers, D. G. (1994). Shunning retirement: Work experience of men in their seventies and early eighties. *Journal of Gerontology: Social Sciences, 49*, S117–S124.

Pfeiffer, E., Verwoerdt, A., & Davis, G. C. (1974). Sexual behavior in middle-life. In E. Palmore (Ed.), *Normal aging II*. Durham, NC: Duke University Press.

Pfeiffer, E., Verwoerdt, A., & Wang, H. S. (1968). Sexual behavior in aged men and women. *Archives of General Psychiatry, 19*, 753–758.

Pohjolainen, P. (1991). Social participation and life-style: A longitudinal and cohort study. *Journal of Cross-Cultural Gerontology, 6*, 109–117.

Portnoi, V. A. (1983). Postretirement depression: Myth or reality. *Comprehensive Therapy, 9*, 31–37.

Prigerson, H. G., Frank, E., Reynolds, C. F., III, George, B. S., & Kupfer, D. J. (1993). Protective psychosocial factors in depression among spousally bereaved elders. *The American Journal of Geriatric Psychiatry, 1*, 296–309.

Prigerson, H. G., Frank, E., Kasl, S. V., Reynolds, C. F., III, Anderson, M. S., Zubenko, G. S., Houck, P. R., George, C. J., & Kupfer, D. J. (1995). Complicated grief and bereavement-related depression as distinct disorders: Preliminary empirical validation in elderly bereaved spouses. *American Journal of Psychiatry, 152*, 22–30.

Quirouette, C., & Pushkar-Gold, D. (1992) Spousal characteristics as predictors of well-being in older couples. *International Journal of Aging and Human Development, 34*, 257–269.

Reker, G. T., Peacock, E. J., & Wong, P. T. P. (1987). Meaning and purpose in life and well-being: A life-span perspective. *Journal of Gerontology, 42*, 44–49.

Renshaw, D. (1981). Pharmacotherapy and female sexuality. *British Journal of Sexual Medicine, 71*, 34–37.

Riddick, C. C. (1985). Life satisfaction for older female homemakers, retirees, and workers. *Research on Aging, 7*, 383–393.

Rogers, R. L., Meyer, J. S., & Mortel, K. F. (1990). After reaching retirement age physical activity sustains cerebral perfusion and cognition. *Journal of the American Geriatrics Society, 38*, 123–128.

Rollins, B., & Feldman, H. (1970). Marital satisfaction over the family life cycle. *Journal of Marriage and the Elderly, 32*, 20–28.

Roos, N. P., & Havens, B. H. (1991). Predictors of successful aging: A twelve-year study of Manitoba elderly. *American Journal of Public Health, 81*, 63–68.

Rothberg, J. M., Ursano, R. J., & Holloway, H. C. (1987). Suicide in the United States military. *Psychiatric Annals, 17*, 545–548.

Rowe, J. W., & Kahn, R. L. (1987). Human aging: Usual and successful. *Science, 237*, 143–149.

Sable, P. (1991). Attachment, loss of spouse, and grief in elderly adults. *Omega, 23*, 129–142.

Sauer, W. J., & Warland, R. (1982). Morale and life satisfaction. In D. J. Mangen, & W. A. Peterson, (Eds.), *Research instruments in social gerontology: Clinical and social psychology*. Minneapolis, MN: University of Minnesota Press.

Schiavi, R. C. (1992). Normal aging and the evaluation of sexual dysfunction. *Psychiatric Medicine, 10*, 217–225.

Seiden, R. H. (1981). Mellowing with age: Factors influencing the nonwhite suicide rate. *International Journal of Aging and Human Development, 13*, 265–284.

Smyth, K. (1994). Activity and loss. In B. R. Bonder & M. B.

Wagner (Eds.), *Functional performance in older adults*. Philadelphia: F. A. Davis Company.

Steinke, E. E. (1994). Knowledge and attitudes of older adults about sexuality in ageing: A comparison of two studies. *Journal of Advanced Nursing, 19*, 477–485.

Stenback, A. (1980). Depression and suicide behavior in old age. In J. E. Birren & R. B. Sloane (Eds.), *Handbook of mental health and aging* (pp. 616–652). Englewood Cliffs, NJ: Prentice Hall.

Szinovacz, M., & Washo, C. (1992). Gender differences in exposure to life events and adaptation to retirement. *Journal of Gerontology: Social Sciences, 47*, S191–S196.

Troll, L., Atchley, R., & Miller, S. (1979). *Families in later life*. Belmont, CA: Wadsworth.

Tuomi, K., Jarvinen, E., Eskelinen, L., Llmarinen, J., & Klockars, M. (1991). Effect of retirement on health and work ability among municipal employees. *Scandinavian Journal of Work and Environmental Health, 17* (Suppl. 1), 75–81.

Uhlenberg, P., & Myers, M. (1981). Divorce and the elderly. *The Gerontologist, 21*, 276–282.

Uhlenberg, P., Cooney, T., & Boyd, R. (1990). Divorce for women after midlife. *Journal of Gerontology: Social Sciences, 45*, S3–S11.

Verbrugge, L. (1979). Marital status and health. *Journal of Marriage and the Family, 41*, 267–285.

Walls, N., & Meyers, A. (1985). Outcome in group treatments for bereavement: Experimental results and recommendations for clinical practice. *International Journal of Mental Health, 13*, 126–147.

Wan, T. T. H., & Odell, B. G. (1983). Major role losses and social participation of older males. *Research on Aging, 50*, 173–196.

Weishaus, S., & Field, D. (1988). A half century of marriage: Continuity or change? *Journal of Marriage and the Family, 50*, 763–774.

Wise, T. N., Epstein, S., & Ross, R. (1992). Sexual issues in the medically ill and aging. *Psychiatric Medicine, 10*, 169–180.

Wong, P. T. P. (1989). Personal meaning and successful aging. *Canadian Psychology, 30*, 516–525.

Young, M., Benjamin, B., & Wallis, C. (1963). The mortality of widowers. *The Lancet, 2*, 454–456.

II

Psychiatric Disorders of Late Life

6

Mood Disorders

HAROLD G. KOENIG

This chapter examines the epidemiology of mood disorders, the effects of mood disorders on cognitive function, the factors affecting vulnerability to late-life depression, and psychopharmacological interventions for these disorders. The importance of this topic is underscored by the fact that depression and mania are among the most treatable psychopathological conditions in late life. They are also a major cause for cognitive impairment, which may improve with treatment of the underlying mood disorder. Thus, recognition and differentiation of depression and mania from other late-life psychiatric disorders is of the utmost importance.

Epidemiology

Aging is frequently accompanied by loss and unwanted change in health, functional independence, social relationships, and economic circumstances. These psychosocial changes, along with brain changes from cerebrovascular and other age-related diseases, increase an older person's vulnerability to depression. Nevertheless, recent epidemiological surveys report that most older adults (at least in this cohort) have low rates of diagnosable major depression and bipolar disorder. The National Institute of Mental Health (NIMH) Epidemiologic Catchment Area (ECA) studies and other national surveys have documented a progressive decrease in the prevalence of major depression with age (Kessler et al., 1994; Weissman et al., 1988). The ECA studies found the lowest rates (0.4–1.4%) of major depression with the oldest cohorts and the highest

rates (1.6–4.8%) among young adults (Weissman et al., 1988). The same trend was found for bipolar disorder. Only 0.1% of 5,507 persons over age 65 met criteria for bipolar disorder within the past year, compared to 0.4% of persons age 45 to 64 years, and 1.4% of those ages 18 to 44 years (Weissman et al., 1988). The high rates of mood disorders, alcoholism, and drug abuse in younger adults have been at least partly attributed to changes in social and family values, which played an important role in stabilizing emotional development among members of the present cohort of older adults (Klerman & Weissman, 1989; Koenig, 1994).

Low rates of diagnosable major depression in the elderly, however, may also be attributed to higher rates of subsyndromal depressions. Older patients frequently complain to their physicians about symptoms like insomnia, anergia, impaired concentration, anxiety, somatization, and a whole host of other physical and emotional discomforts. While these symptoms may not meet the threshold for a formal psychiatric disorder, they cause substantial disability and morbidity (Broadhead, Blazer, George, & Tse, 1990). Blazer, Hughes, and George (1987) found that while less than 1% of 1,300 older adults fulfilled criteria for a major depression, 27% had depressive symptoms that caused social or occupational impairment.

There are certain subpopulations of older adults that have higher rates of depression than others. While only 1% of community dwelling adults have a major depressive disorder, 10–13% or more of acutely hospitalized elders do so and an additional 30% may have subsyndromal or minor depressive disorders (Koenig, Meador, Cohen, & Blazer, 1988a; Koenig et al., 1991; Koenig, O'Connor, Guarisco, Zabel, & Ford, 1993). Likewise, high

HAROLD G. KOENIG • Duke University Medical Center, Durham, North Carolina 27710.

rates of major depression have been documented in medical outpatients (7–15%) (Borson et al., 1986; Coulehan, Schulberg, Block, Janosky, & Arena, 1990; Perez-Stable, Miranda, Munos, & Ying, 1990) and nursing home patients (10–16%) (Parmelee, Katz, & Lawton, 1989; Rovner et al., 1991; Weissman, Bruce, Leaf, Florio, & Holzer, 1991). It is unfortunate that the vast majority of depressed older patients in medical settings are neither diagnosed nor treated, despite the ready availability of instruments to screen for these disorders (Koenig, Cohen, Blazer, Meador, & Westlund, 1992; Koenig, Meador, Cohen, & Blazer, 1988b; Rapp, Walsh, Parisi, & Wallace, 1988).

As noted earlier, bipolar disorder is less common in persons over age 65 than in younger age groups; this may result partly from a failure to diagnose the disorder because of unusual presentation. When bipolar disorder occurs in later life, the presentation is frequently atypical, with a mixture of manic, cognitive, and dysphoric symptoms (Post, 1978; Spar, Ford, & Liston, 1979). Euphoria is less common in older adults than in younger persons. An episode of mania in older adults is often associated with changes in cognitive function. "Manic delirium" is a term sometimes used to describe the altered state of consciousness experienced by such patients. The condition is difficult to distinguish from the agitation associated with dementia or schizophrenia (Shulman, 1986). When younger patients with bipolar disorders are followed over time (retrospectively), they show a pattern of increasing episodes in mid-life followed by decreasing manic episodes thereafter (Winokur, 1975). One study of elderly bipolars found that only 8% experienced their first manic episode before the age of 40 (Shulman & Post, 1980). The association between life events and the onset of a first manic episode is not as strong in late-onset cases where organic factors (cerebrovascular events, head trauma, other neurological disorders) play a more important role (Shulman, 1989).

Cognitive Effects of Major Depression

Major depression has long been known to have adverse effects on cognition, called the "dementia syndrome of depression" (Folstein & McHugh,

1978). In fact, it may be difficult to distinguish a primary depressive disorder from dementia in older adults (Post, 1951; Roth & Morrissey, 1952; Wells, 1979). Between 5% and 8% of elderly patients originally diagnosed with dementia have a reversible depressive disorder (Kendell, 1974; Nott & Fleminger, 1975; Smith & Kiloh, 1981). On the other hand, older persons in the early stages of a dementing illness frequently experience depression when they become aware of memory deficits and lose their ability to function; nearly one quarter of patients with dementia have clinically significant depressive disorder (Reifler, Larson, & Henley, 1982).

Cognitive deficits in depression frequently are related to attention and memory functions, as well as to information processing speed (Miller, 1975). Some studies of neuropsychological function have found right-hemispheric deficits in patients with depression (Kronfol, Hansher, Digre, & Waziri, 1978). Finally, studies have reported both verbal and nonverbal memory deficits in depressed patients, although these results may be partly attributed to reduced motivation, poor ability to sustain attention, or other memory-related functions (Roy-Byrne, Weingartner, Bierer, Thompson, & Post, 1986).

Factors Affecting Vulnerability to Late-Life Depression

Geriatric depression is a multifactorial disorder. It represents a common end point for a number of physical and psychosocial disorders. A wide range of genetic, demographic, psychological, social, and biological factors contribute to the onset of depression in later life. It is difficult to determine whether psychosocial, genetic, or acquired biological changes play a stronger role. We do know that biological changes in the brain influence emotions, just as psychological experiences cause changes in brain chemistry (see below) (Post, 1992).

Theoretical Model

Figure 1 displays the multiple causal pathways that may be involved in the genesis of late-life depressive disorders (Koenig, Blazer, & Hocking, 1995). Genetic factors are largely responsible for a person's basic temperament. The emotional stabil-

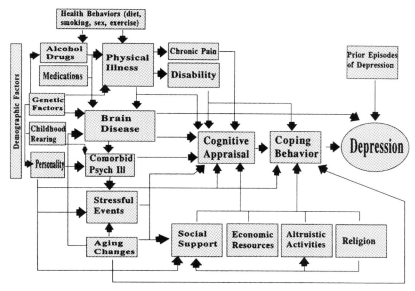

FIGURE 1. Causal model of late-life depression. Reproduced with permission from Koenig, Blazer, & Hocking (1995).

ity of primary caregivers (also partly genetically determined) affects the quality of childhood experiences. The fit of the child's temperament with his or her interpersonal environment helps to form personality which will define habitual ways of adapting to both internal and external stressors. Personality is further formed by life events and the successes or failures of coping responses. Coping responses receive their greatest test in later life when issues of control and dependency left unresolved since childhood may flare up. Genetic factors and/or childhood experiences affect vulnerability to comorbid psychiatric illness (schizophrenia, anxiety disorder, organic mental disorder, etc.) which acts as another stressor that must be adapted to and may further complicate adjustments to aging.

Physical health plays a central role in this model and is largely determined by current and past habits, health behaviors, accidents, and genetically determined susceptibilities. Exercise and healthy dietary habits influence physical health in a positive way, whereas alcohol or drug abuse can either directly result in adverse health outcomes or complicate the management of comorbid medical conditions. Physical illness further contributes to mood disorder by inducing brain changes that increase vulnerability to depression or mania: by causing disability,

forced dependency, and disturbing physical symptoms; by impairing cognitive flexibility necessary for effective adaptation; and by restricting the range of coping options. Disability often evokes humiliation and shame, which then compound the psychological distress of physical symptoms and induce feelings of helplessness and loss of control.

In this model, cognitive appraisal and coping responses are key intervening variables that largely determine the effects which disability, physical symptoms, and other concurrent life stressors have on mood. If psychological, social, and economic resources are inadequate to counteract hopelessness, particularly in the presence of predisposing brain changes, then the susceptibility to depression or other mood disorders will be high.

Genetic Factors

Both twin and family studies indicate that genetic factors play a role in mood disorders (Egeland et al., 1987; Slater & Cowie, 1971). That contribution, however, appears to be less for late-life depression than for mood disorders presenting earlier in life (Hopkinson, 1964; Maier et al., 1991; Mendlewicz, 1976). Studies indicate a history of depression in only 5–8% of relatives of patients with late-onset depression, compared with 20% of relatives of younger depressed patients (Hopkinson, 1964; Stenstedt, 1969). Some studies have found decreased levels of serotonin and norepinephrine and increased monoamine oxidase in brains of older persons, biological changes that would seem to increase the likelihood of emotional disorders in late life (Robinson, Davies, Nies, Rqavaris, & Sylwester, 1971).

Depressed patients have been found to have increased cortisol excretion throughout the day and night (Sachar, 1975). Rosenbaum and colleagues (1984), in a study of normal persons ages 20 to 78, found that 18% of those over age 65 were nonsuppressors of cortisol after a dexamethasone suppression test; younger subjects were only half (9%) as likely to demonstrate nonsuppression. This represents either a general dysregulation of the hypothalamic-pituitary axis in later life or an age-related effect on how the body handles dexamethasone. Changes in thyroid function with aging have also been reported and may contribute to the development of depression in later life. There is a blunting in response to the administration of thyrotropin-releasing hormone (TRH) both in normal elderly and in depressed patients (Snyder & Utiger, 1972; Targum, Sullivan, & Byrnes, 1982). Elderly patients with depressed mood and thyroid-stimulating hormone levels above 3 or 4 should probably have thyroid supplementation with thyroxin to treat subclinical hypothyroidism.

Demographic Factors

There is at least a 2:1 female–male ratio in geriatric depression (Weissman et al., 1988). This sex difference persists even after other psychosocial variables are controlled. Whether or not women are truly more likely than men to become depressed or whether they are simply more likely to complain about dysphoria is unclear. Given the high rate of alcoholism and suicide in elderly men, it may be that men deal with feelings differently (and perhaps less effectively) than do women.

Personality

Personality disorder increases the risk of late-life depression. In one of the few studies on this topic, Schneider, Zemansky, Bender, and Sloane (1992) studied personality traits of depressed and nondepressed elderly patients. Antisocial, borderline, histrionic, narcissistic, avoidant, dependent, obsessive–compulsive, and passive–aggressive traits were significantly more common among recovered depressed elders than nondepressed controls. In general, however, late-onset depression is not as likely to be associated with personality abnormalities as are early-onset disorders (Brodaty et al., 1991; Fogel & Westlake, 1990). Almost 50% of older adults with both depression and axis II disorders have compulsive personality disorder, and compulsive traits are thought to increase with age (Fogel & Westlake, 1990).

Health Behaviors

Diet, exercise, smoking habits, and sexual practices throughout the adult years may affect vulnerability to geriatric depression by a cumulative impact on physical health. Malnutrition, deconditioning, chronic lung diseases, and sexually transmitted diseases (AIDS, syphilis, genital herpes) can all affect mood. Vitamin B deficiencies (thiamine, riboflavin, pyridoxine, cobalamin) can impair cognitive status and induce depression (Bell et al., 1991; Lindenbaum et al., 1988; Smidt, Cremin, Grivetti, & Clifford, 1991). A number of studies have now shown that aerobic exercise enhances life satisfaction and reduces depression in elderly persons (McMurdo & Burnett, 1992; McMurdo & Rennie, 1993). Smoking may increase the risk of depression either directly or as a consequence of adverse effects on health (Green et al., 1992).

Specific Medical Illnesses

Hyperthyroidism and hypothyroidism are commonly associated with depression. Hypothyroidism produces a syndrome associated with dysphoric affect, psychomotor retardation, and cognitive changes that treatment with T4 (thyroxin) often reverses. Likewise, hyperparathyroidism associated with hypercalcemia can cause both cognitive changes and poor motivation or loss of interest. Patients with pancreatic or lung cancer have reported depressive symptoms even before the cancer was diagnosed; this effect may be mediated by neuroendocrine substances released from tumors. In any case, nearly 25% of all cancer patients experience depression (Massie & Holland, 1990). The mood disturbance, however, does not always reflect a direct physiological effect of tumor-related neuroendocrine substances on the brain. More often, mood changes result from difficulties coping with the psychological effects of cancer, of going through rigorous treatment regimens, and of experiencing progressive disability and worsening physical symptoms.

Cerebrovascular disease induces brain changes that are likely to increase susceptibility to depression. During the first year after a hemispheric stroke, depression is a common diagnosis (up to 50% of cases). According to Robinson, Morris, and Fedoroff (1990), the likelihood of depression is increased if the stroke is in the left frontal cortex. Other investigators disagree, arguing that it is not the site of the lesion that determines vulnerability to depression, but rather, the extent of disability induced by the stroke. For example, Sharpe and coworkers (1990) did not find an association between lesion location and depression in 60 elderly stroke patients; they did, however, find higher depression rates in patients with larger strokes and greater associated disability.

Parkinson's disease is also associated with high rates of depression. The symptoms of this disease frequently mimic depression (flat affect, psychomotor retardation, social withdrawal). Levodopa, the main treatment for Parkinson's disease, is likewise associated with a wide range of cognitive and depressive side effects (Guze & Barrio, 1991; Mayeux, 1990).

As noted above, dementing disorders like Alzheimer's disease are often accompanied by depression, just as depression is frequently associated with cognitive impairment. Elderly persons who present with a combination of cognitive and depressive symptoms often have an underlying dementing disorder that the depression has unmasked. Alexopoulos, Meyers, and Young (1993) followed 23 elderly depressed patients who were diagnosed with "reversible dementia" and 34 depressed elders without cognitive impairment; irreversible dementia developed in 43% of the depressed group with reversible dementia, but it developed in only 12% of those with depression alone. It is of note that as cognitive impairment progresses, patients lose insight into their illness, and depressive symptoms may improve (Reifler et al., 1982).

Myocardial infarction is frequently followed by anxiety and depressive symptoms. Dovenmuehle and Verwoerdt (1962) found that 64% of cardiac patients experienced symptoms of dysphoria and lowered self-esteem and anxiety, although biological symptoms of depression (weight loss, insomnia, psychomotor retardation) were frequently not present. In a follow-up study of 283 patients who had suffered myocardial infarction, Schleifer and colleagues (1989) found that 45% of patients were depressed 8 to 10 days following the event; furthermore, 3 to 4 months after discharge, 33% were depressed, including over three quarters of those initially diagnosed with major depression.

Chronic obstructive pulmonary disease (COPD) is likewise associated with high rates of depression and anxiety disorders. The prevalence of COPD-associated major depression may be as high as 20% (Light, Merrill, Despairs, Gordon, & Mutalipassi, 1985). In a study of hospitalized elderly veterans, we found that patients with pulmonary disorders were more likely than any other medical group to experience depression (Koenig, Goli, et al., 1992). Treatment of mood disorder in these patients leads to improvement in both psychological and physiological parameters (Borson et al., 1992).

Drugs

Medications play an important role in treating physical illnesses that predispose patients to depression. The number of medications taken, however, has been associated with depression and cognitive disturbances in older persons (Chrischilles et al., 1992). Cardiovascular drugs may interfere with neurotransmitter availability or receptor sensitivity in the brain. Especially culpable in this regard are antihypertensives such as reserpine, beta-blockers, clonidine, methyldopa, prazosin, and guanethidine. Central nervous system drugs may also affect mood state, including antiparkinsonian drugs, benzodiazepines, neuroleptics, alcohol, and stimulants (rebound effects). Cancer drugs like tamoxifen, vincristine, L-asparaginase, and interferon have all been associated with depression. Likewise, dexamethasone, prednisone, estrogen, and progesterone preparations are known to affect mood, inducing depressive as well as manic states.

Brain Diseases

Tumors, cysts, infections, or other central nervous system lesions can increase intracranial pressure and/or interfere with frontal lobe functioning, resulting in disinterest, reduced drive, and loss of pleasure (Barclay, Blass, & Lee, 1984; Meyers, 1984). As noted earlier, dementing illnesses often mimic depression (Alexopoulos, Young, & Shindledecker, 1992). Cerebrovascular disorders produce changes in brain structure not only in the frontal lobes but also in subcortical periventricular, hippocampal, and basal ganglia areas that may predispose patients to depression (Alexopoulos et al., 1992; Coffey et al., 1993; Krishnan, 1993; Krishnan et al., 1991; Lesser, Hill-Gutierrez, Miller, & Boone, 1993).

Physical Impairment and Illness Severity

A number of studies have examined correlates of depression in elderly patients with physical illnesses severe enough to require hospitalization (Kitchell, Barnes, Veith, Okimoto, & Raskind, 1982; Koenig et al., 1988a; Koenig et al., 1991; Koenig, O'Connor, et al., 1993; Rapp, Parisi, & Walsh, 1988). In almost every one of these studies, severity of illness or functional disability was strongly related to depressive disorder. When followed over time, depressive symptoms track closely with functional impairment, improving when impairment improves and worsening as physical function declines. Depression that occurs in this setting and that is closely linked with physical illness severity is difficult to treat with conventional therapies (Cole, 1985; Koenig, Cohen, Blazer, Pieper, et al., 1992).

Sensory Loss

Visual and hearing impairment commonly cause impaired functioning and mood changes in older persons. Treatment of sensory loss has been associated with improved mood and life satisfaction. For example, Mulrow and colleagues (1990), and Mulrow, Tuley, and Aguilar (1992) examined 192 hearing-impaired elders at 4-month intervals

after they had received a hearing aid. They found that depressive symptoms, social withdrawal, and communication difficulties all improved significantly during the 1-year follow-up.

Pain

The physical symptom of pain, particularly when it is chronic and difficult to control, is invariably accompanied by anxiety and depression (Magni, Schifano, & de Leo, 1985; Moss, Lawton, & Glicksman, 1991; Romano & Turner, 1985). Furthermore, patients with depression frequently complain of pain. For example, Magni and colleagues examined the prevalence of pain in 51 depressed elders and 71 age-matched nondepressed controls, finding moderate to severe pain in 72% of depressed patients compared to 34% of controls. Likewise, Williamson and Schulz (1992) found a strong correlation between physical illness, functional disability, pain, and depressive symptoms in 288 community dwelling older outpatients. They found that functional disability, rather than the specific physical illness, mediated the relationship between pain and mood state. These investigators concluded that the extent to which pain or physical illness causes functional disability is the primary factor leading to depression.

Chronic pain plays a central role in our theoretical formulation of how depression develops in later life. Physical illnesses that cause chronic pain (or breathlessness) are also those frequently associated with depression (arthritis, cancer, diabetic neuropathy, multiple sclerosis, spinal stenosis, chronic lung disease). These illnesses often manifest themselves through symptoms that mimic those of primary depression; if depression does occur, it can magnify the experience of pain or other physical symptoms. Pain, in turn, can disrupt sleep, enhance irritability, exaggerate fatigue, and impair concentration. These symptoms, then, may interfere with interpersonal relationships and disrupt social networks. Thus, a vicious cycle can be created that leads to increasing depression, suffering, and social isolation.

Prior Depressive Episodes

Studies show that the majority of mood disorders in older persons begin after the age of 60 (late-onset depression) (Meyers, Kalayam, & Mei-Tal, 1984); a significant minority of elderly persons, however, do have a history of recurrent mood disorders dating back to young adulthood or middle age. Older persons with a history of depression, anxiety, bipolar disorder, or other psychiatric disorder are particularly vulnerable to depression in late life as they encounter role changes, loss of loved ones, and changes in health (Koenig et al., 1991). Once an episode of depression or mania occurs, whether it is the first episode or an exacerbation of a disorder beginning earlier in life, the risk of having another episode is increased. According to Post, prior episodes of depression and mania increase the risk of future episodes (Post, 1993; Post, Rubinow, & Ballenger, 1986), underscoring the need for monitoring and treatment.

Nonaffective Psychiatric Illness

Late-life psychoses (schizophrenia, delusional disorders, organic mental disorders), anxiety disorders, and other psychiatric conditions frequently increase the older person's susceptibility to depression. Because of their impact on social roles and interpersonal relationships, nonaffective psychiatric disorders can act as psychosocial stressors in the same way that bereavement or health problems do.

Alcoholism and Drug Abuse

Alcoholism and prescription drug abuse are frequently associated with late-life depression; substance abuse may be an attempt to treat an underlying mood disorder or may itself induce depression by its physiological effects on the brain. When uncontrolled drinking begins for the first time after the age of 60 (late-onset alcoholism), the likelihood of an associated mood disorder is high, since the changing pattern of alcohol consumption is often a response to problems with family, job, or health (Finlayson, Hurt, Davis, & Morse, 1988). According to Jinks and Raschko (1990), one third or more of elderly alcoholics have a primary depression or mood disorder that underlies and precedes their alcohol abuse. Alcoholism as a primary disorder frequently leads to emotional disturbance because of its destructive effects on occupational, family, and physical functioning. Among elderly chronic alcoholics admitted to the hospital, fully one half have evidence of organic brain syndrome (Finlayson et al., 1988).

Stressful Life Experiences

Negative life events frequently precede the development of depression in the elderly (Blazer et al., 1987). Examples of negative events include bereavement, death of friends, sickness of a close family member, divorce or separation, relocation, retirement, and worsening financial situation. Nearly 15% of bereaved adults experience a depressive disorder that requires some type of treatment (Clayton, 1990). Brink (1985) reviews the stages of grief involved in the experience of negative life events and discusses the grieving process as it relates to losses in late life. As noted earlier, work by Robert Post (1992) suggests a link between stressful life events and biological changes in the brain that increase the risk of depression. According to this hypothesis, negative life events cause chemical changes in the brain by inducing the protooncogene c-fos and related transcription factors which then interfere with the expression of neurotransmitters, receptors, and neuropeptides that regulate mood.

Cognitive Appraisal of Events

In order for stressful life events, changes in health, disability, pain, or other experiences to induce depression, they must be understood and defined by the person as negative, threatening, or having a particular onerous implication. Richard Lazarus (1974) notes that it is not the particular stress itself that determines the degree to which it will be experienced as threatening; instead, it is the person's cognitive appraisal of the event. Bereavement for an older person who interprets the event as disastrous and intolerable will be more stressful than for the person who sees it as unfortunate, but not an end to joy and pleasure in life. One's life history and world view create a pattern of underlying assumptions and thoughts that determine how events are interpreted. Personal resources like health and socioeconomic reserves affect both the way events are appraised and the choice of strategies to cope with them. Attitudes toward self and personal goals also influence appraisal. The older person who sees his or her value in terms of the ability to remain active and productive will experience a disabling physical illness as much more stressful than the person whose self-esteem is based on factors unrelated to physical functioning. A number of studies have shown that physical illness can give rise to dysfunctional attitudes and negative interpretations that both precipitate and maintain mood disorder (Bombardier, D'Amico, & Jordan, 1990; Holroyd & Lazarus, 1982; Olinger, Kuiper, & Shaw, 1987). This is particularly true for persons with chronic pain, where catastrophizing and overgeneralization can quickly lead to helplessness and more disability than would be predicted by the severity of pain alone (Holroyd & Andrasik, 1982; Smith, Follick, Ahern, & Adams, 1986).

Choice of Coping Strategy

Coping involves all "cognitive and motor activities which a sick person employs to preserve his bodily and psychic integrity, to recover reversibly impaired function and compensate to the limit for any irreversible impairment" (Lipowski, 1970). Healthy coping involves the appropriate match of a behavior to a situation. For instance, active problem-solving behaviors are healthy and appropriate in situations where a particular action can help solve the problem or favorably change the circumstance. On the other hand, in situations that are completely out of the person's control and about which nothing can be done, the healthiest coping behavior might be distraction or denial. For instance, a person whose spouse just died may distract himself or herself by staying busy in volunteer work, personal hobbies, or social relationships. Religious beliefs or behaviors may be used quite effectively in coping with chronic medical conditions and disability, particularly those that are out of the individual's control (see below). Unhealthy coping behaviors in most circumstances include total denial of the situation, projection of feelings onto others, exhausting physical activity, alcohol abuse, or abuse of prescription medications.

Social Support

Until now, the discussion has focused on factors that increase the older person's vulnerability to depression. I will now examine factors that either help prevent the development of mood disorder or facilitate its resolution. Psychiatrist Elaine Murphy (1982) has emphasized that depression in later life often has social origins. As a person grows older and experiences fewer contacts with friends and family because of death, relocation, disability, or lack of transportation, his or her social network may begin to shrink. This can result in intense feelings of loneliness, isolation, worthlessness, and uselessness. If a mood disorder develops, it can cause the older person to further withdraw and even shun contact with others. This tendency toward isolation may be counteracted by support from family, friends, or even health professionals.

A number of studies have now shown that strong social support may help protect older adults from experiencing depressive illness (Blazer, 1983; Blazer et al., 1987; George, Blazer, Hughes, & Fowler, 1989; Goldberg, Van Natta, & Comstock, 1985; Koenig et al., 1991; Murphy, 1982; Murrell, Himmelfarb, & Wright, 1983; Stallones, Marx, & Garrity, 1990; Surtees, 1980; Winefield, 1979). This is particularly true when stressful life events threaten emotional stability. Pfifer and Murrell (1986) examined the relationship between stressful life events and social resources in a sample of 1,200 community dwelling older adults. They found that health and social support played both an additive and an interactive role in the onset of depressive symptoms, while other life events had only weak effects. In other words, older persons with physical health problems and poor social support were much more likely to be depressed. Several studies have now demonstrated that only certain types of social support are effective in buffering against depression. Homogeneity of the support network, number of confidants, level of intimacy in social relationships, and subjective perception of the adequacy of support are more likely to be related to life satisfaction and well-being than the size of the support network or even marital status (George et al., 1989; Goldberg et al., 1985).

In one of the few interventional studies that have tested the hypothesized effects of social support on mood, Ong, Maritean, Lloyd, and Robbins (1987) randomly assigned 20 hospitalized depressed elders to either a support group or no support group after hospital discharge. They discovered that not one of the 10 patients in the support group had to be readmitted to the hospital in the following 9 months, compared with six of the control group ($p < .01$). Social support, then, may affect both the development and resolution of mood disorders in late life. A brief- 11-item social support scale has now been developed specifically for use in physically ill older adults that may facilitate future research in this area (Koenig, Westlund, George, Hughes, & Hybels, 1993).

Religious Beliefs and Activities

Cultural factors have long been known to affect health practices and use of health services. Judeo-Christian religious beliefs and behaviors are prevalent among the current cohort of older adults in the United States. Studies have shown that older adults use religion to help them understand, cope with, and adapt to a wide range of interpersonal and health problems. Between one quarter and one third of unselected older adults will spontaneously give religious answers to open-ended questions about how they cope with stress (Koenig, Meador, Goli, et al., 1992; Koenig, George, & Siegler, 1988; Rosen, 1982). There have been recent reports that church attendance, scripture reading, personal prayer, and intrinsic religious attitudes among older adults are associated with higher life satisfaction, well-being, and less frequent depression (Idler, 1987; Koenig, Kvale, & Ferrel, 1988; Pressman, Lyons, Larson, & Strain, 1990).

This relationship may be particularly strong in older persons with chronic or acute health problems. One study found that use of religion as a coping behavior was associated with fewer depressive symptoms and lower rates of major depressive disorder in a sample of 850 hospitalized elderly veterans (Koenig, 1994; Koenig, Meador, Goli, et al., 1992). Likewise, Idler (1987), reporting from the Yale Health and Aging project, found that at any given level of chronic medical illness, older men who were religious were less likely than their nonreligious peers to view themselves as disabled. If disabled, religious elders were also less likely to be depressed. These data indicate that Judeo-Christian religious beliefs and practices may affect the way older persons view physical illness and the level of both physical and psychological disability related to specific disease states. The cognitive aspects of religious belief appear to be especially important in conveying these effects (Koenig, George, & Siegler, 1988; Koenig, Cohen, Blazer, Kudler, et al., 1995).

Besides enabling older adults to cognitively reframe and appraise their circumstances in a more positive light, religion may also affect mental health in a positive way through its social aspects. Studies indicate that one of the most common sources of social support for older persons outside of their immediate family is the church (Tobin, Ellor, & Anderson-Ray, 1986). The elderly are more often involved in church groups than in all other voluntary forms of social activity combined (Cutler, 1976; Mayo, 1951). One study found that over half of all older patients attending a geriatric medicine clinic indicated that 80% to 100% of their closest friends came from their local church (Koenig, Moberg, & Kvale, 1988). Churches and synagogues, then, provide a readily available, acceptable, and inexpensive source of support for many older persons.

Economic Resources

Most studies report that mood disorders are more common among older adults with lower incomes (Blazer et al., 1987; Blazer, Burchett, Service, & George, 1991; Goldberg et al., 1985; Murrell et al., 1983; Stallones et al., 1990). The availability of financial resources affects the range of coping options available to the older adult when stressful life circumstances call for adaptation. The financially secure elder who is suddenly disabled by a stroke can decide to hire a nurse to care for him or her at home rather than be forced to move to a nursing home. Furthermore, economic resources will allow the purchase of adaptive devices (e.g., motorized wheelchair, specially designed automobile, etc.) that will enable the disabled elder to maintain his or her independence. Finally, older persons with financial resources will have a wider choice of recreational activities with which to occupy themselves and enhance their life satisfaction.

Diagnostic Evaluation

Differential Diagnosis

Depression subtypes and other psychiatric disorders that mimic depression must be distinguished.

The Diagnostic and Statistical Manual of Mental Disorders, fourth edition (*DSM-IV*) describes a number of depressive subtypes ranging from severe major depression with psychosis that requires emergent treatment to normal bereavement or simple grief (Lindemann, 1944) that requires no intervention other than the passage of time. Other subtypes of depression include organic mood syndrome (when depression or mania results from the direct physiological effects of medical illness or drugs), seasonal affective disorder (Jacobsen, Wehr, Sack, James, & Rosenthal, 1987), dysthymia (sometimes called chronic, neurotic, or characterological depression) (Verwoerdt, 1976), adjustment disorder with depressed mood (minor depression occurring within 6 months of a psychosocial stressor), and depression not otherwise specified (catch-all category of minor depression).

Besides dementia, a number of other psychiatric disorders in late life can mimic mood disorders. Because treatment of these conditions differs from that of depression or bipolar disorder, their identification is of the utmost importance. Older adults may exhibit psychotic features during an episode of major depression (Meyers et al., 1984). This condition may be difficult to distinguish from late-onset schizophrenia or delusional disorder. However, older adults with late-life schizophrenia are not usually profoundly depressed. Instead, they are *distressed* by an imagined hostile external environment. These patients usually exhibit bizarre delusions of influence and report elaborate preparations to ensure their safety. Late-life delusional disorder usually presents with paranoid symptoms and delusions that are more plausible than those reported by schizophrenics.

Hypochondriasis frequently confounds depression in older adults. While a depressed mood can be experienced by the hypochondriacal elder, the main feature of the disorder that distinguishes it from primary depression is an unrealistic interpretation of physical sensations as abnormal, which in turn leads to a preoccupation with the fear or belief that one is suffering from a serious illness (De Alarcon, 1964). The differentiation of depression from primary anxiety states (as with generalized anxiety disorder and adjustment disorder with anxious mood) is difficult because of the frequent coexistence of anxiety (including panic disorder) in late-life depression (Blazer, Hughes, & Fowler, 1989). Symptoms of alcoholism often mimic depression and include cognitive changes, disturbed sleep, chronic fatigue, weight loss, and even suicidal thoughts. Alcohol abuse or other substance abuse may coexist with depression, and as noted earlier, many late-onset alcoholics use alcohol as a form of self-medication for their depressive symptoms. A diagnosis of depression in an alcoholic patient, however, should not be made until the patient has been sober for 2 weeks or longer and withdrawal symptoms have passed.

Laboratory Evaluation

Lab tests necessary to rule out organic causes for mood disorders in older adults include thyroid function studies (T4, TSH), complete blood count (CBC), serum electrolytes, Vitamin B_{12} level, and prescription drug levels. Vitamin B_{12} deficiency may present with cognitive impairment, depressive symptoms, or both in a patient with a normal serum B_{12} level or CBC (Lindenbaum et al., 1988). While a computed tomography (CT) or magnetic resonance imaging (MRI) scan can rule out brain tumors, the yield from these tests is low unless the history is suggestive or the neurological exam is abnormal. If antidepressants or electroconvulsive therapy (ECT) are possible treatment options, an electrocardiogram, as well as renal and liver function tests, should be obtained.

Psychopharmacological Interventions

Once a correct diagnosis is made, medical illnesses are ruled out or stabilized, and the patient's safety is ensured, management should include psychological support, psychotherapy, pharmacotherapy, and/or ECT. All depressed elders require psychological support. This involves attentive listening, demonstration of empathy, and expression of sincere concern, which are the hallmarks of good clinical care. Patients with less severe forms of depression frequently improve with this intervention alone.

Psychotherapy avoids the side effects frequently seen with antidepressants (Koenig & Breitner, 1990; Koenig, Goli, Shelp, Kudler, Cohen,

Meador, & Blazer, 1989). Cognitive behavioral therapy (CBT), administered individually or in a group setting, will train elders to identify and correct negative thinking and dysfunctional behaviors which either cause or perpetuate the depressive state (Beck, Rush, & Shaw, 1979). Cognitive appraisal plays a central role in the causal path that leads to depression (see Figure 1). The effectiveness of short-term CBT in the treatment of late-life depression has been demonstrated, with response rates comparable to those achieved with biological interventions (Arean et al., 1993; Marmar, Horowitz, Weiss, Wilner, & Kaltreider, 1988; Thompson, Gallagher, & Breckenridge, 1987).

Even when psychotherapy is the primary mode of therapy, drug treatment should always be considered as well. The three classes of psychopharmacologic drugs used to treat mood disorders are (1) tricyclic and newer antidepressants, (2) monoamine oxidase (MAO) inhibitors, and (3) mood stabilizers such as lithium and the anticonvulsants. While second generation tricyclic antidepressants (nortriptyline or desipramine) remain the drugs of choice for severe late-life depressions (Salzman, 1992), the selective serotonin reuptake inhibitors (SSRIs) and bupropion may soon take their place in this regard. Nortriptyline, desipramine, and doxepin are effective and relatively safe when used with caution in older adults with endogenous-type depressions. The doses of these compounds must be substantially lower than those used in younger adults. Doses of 10 to 30 mg of nortriptyline or 25 to 75 mg of desipramine are frequently adequate to treat depression in frail, elderly patients with concurrent medical problems.

If there is a lack of response after 4 to 6 weeks of treatment at therapeutic blood levels, then a number of strategies may be tried, including (1) augmenting with low doses of lithium (300 to 600 mg/day) or cytomel (T3); (2) adding an SSRI (5–10 mg of paroxetine or 25–50 mg of sertraline); or (3) switching to a different drug class (SSRI or bupropion). When initiating treatment with an SSRI, doses should be small (10 mg/day or 10 mg every other day for fluoxetine, 25–50 mg/day for sertraline, and 5–10 mg/day for paroxetine) to prevent excessive agitation or gastrointestinal effects that limit compliance. Bupropion is another alternative, particularly if orthostasis and cardiovascular

side effects need to be avoided or loss of sexual interest is a problem; doses are usually initiated at 75 mg/day and increased up to a maximum of 300–375 mg/day in divided doses. Toxicity is indicated by tremor, unpleasant gastrointestinal side effects, or visual hallucinations.

While the newer antidepressants are generally void of the orthostatic, anticholinergic, and cardiac side effects associated with tricyclics, they have their own set of adverse effects that frequently limit their use in older patients: excessive stimulation and agitation, tremor and dysequilibrium, akathesia (for SSRIs), insomnia, gastrointestinal side effects, and weight loss. Paroxetine is a safer drug than fluoxetine to use in older adults because of the half-life of these drugs (1 day for paroxetine vs. 10 to 14 days for fluoxetine). Furthermore, fluoxetine has been associated with serious weight loss (Brymer & Winograd, 1992) and fatal cardiac arrhythmias (Spier & Frontera, 1991) when used in older patients with multiple medical problems. Paroxetine, however, must be discontinued slowly because of its short half-life and propensity to cause withdrawal reactions. Patients with agitated depressions or those with significant sleep disturbances will often benefit from trazodone alone or in combination with other antidepressants (Gerner, Estabrook, Steuer, & Jarvik, 1980). At doses between 50 and 300 mg/day, trazodone has virtually no anticholinergic side effects. When used alone, however, its antidepressant potency at tolerable doses is questionable, and side effects such as excessive drowsiness, orthostasis, and priapism can be prohibitive.

Frequently effective in older adults with resistant depression is the combination of an SSRI and a tricyclic or trazodone. All SSRIs may interfere with the hepatic metabolism of tricyclics and will increase blood levels up to three times in some cases (sertraline may be an exception in this regard). Therefore, when an SSRI is added to nortriptyline or desipramine, the dose of the latter should be reduced by at least 50% and blood levels carefully monitored. Another favorite combination is trazodone and an SSRI, since each tends to counteract the negative effects of the other. Monoamine oxidase inhibitors are as effective as tricyclic antidepressants for treating geriatric depression (Georgotas, McCue, Friedman, & Cooper, 1989), although they are difficult to use in older adults who often have comorbid medical conditions and are taking medications that might interact with this drug class. Given the high rate of relapse after treatment of geriatric patients with depression, some experts now recommend that after one or more episodes of major depression, older adults should continue on lifelong maintenance therapy at therapeutic doses (Greden, 1993).

Lithium carbonate remains the drug of choice for older patients with bipolar disorder and may be useful in preventing the recurrence of unipolar depression. Lithium itself is a poor antidepressant, but as noted earlier, it may be used to augment the effects of other antidepressants (Finch & Katona, 1989). Lithium must be used cautiously in older patients with medical illness (Morton, Sonne, & Lydiard, 1993). Some elders tolerate doses of only 300 to 600 mg/day before experiencing tremor and other neurotoxic side effects; lithium levels of 0.4 to 0.8 meg/L are often sufficient to prevent recurrence of mania. The anticonvulsants carbamazepine and valproic acid are especially useful in patients with rapidly cycling or dysphoric mania; valproic acid may be particularly safe when used in older adults, although drug levels require careful monitoring (McFarland, Miller, & Straumfjord, 1990).

Benzodiazepines are useful in treating manic patients because they facilitate sleep and allow for lower doses of neuroleptics. Except in certain circumstances, this is not true for depressed patients. While the benzodiazepine alprazolam is reported to have antidepressant properties at doses of 2 to 4 mg/day, it can easily cause dependence in older adults if the drug is used regularly for several weeks or longer; tapering such patients off alprazolam can be difficult and take months. Benzodiazepines should not be used as a primary treatment for depression in older adults since they can cause excess sedation, worsen confusion, precipitate falls, and worsen the depressive state (Greenblatt, Shader, & Abernathy, 1983; Tyrer & Murphy, 1987).

Stimulants like methylphenidate may be used effectively in older patients with multiple concurrent health problems to enhance appetite and reduce apathy (Katon & Raskin, 1980). At doses of 5 to 15 mg three times per day, side effects are rare and abuse is uncommon. Dependence may occur with the use of stimulants, requiring doses to be increased to maintain the desired effect. Patients with unstable angina or labile blood pressure should probably avoid these drugs.

For severe, delusional, or refractory depressions, ECT is often the most effective form of treatment (Benbow, 1989). Despite remarkable effectiveness and safety in older adults, ECT is typically performed only after other methods have failed. Electroconvulsive therapy is a first-line treatment for depressions that are life-threatening, for older patients who have responded well to this treatment previously, and for those who prefer ECT to drugs or psychotherapy. In older drug-nonresponders, ECT is effective 60% to 80% of the time. However, if patients do not receive maintenance ECT or prophylactic treatment with antidepressants, over 50% will relapse within one year.

Summary and Conclusions

Depressive disorders are among the most treatable of all psychiatric conditions in late life. Many older adults, particularly those with comorbid medical illness, experience depressive symptoms that impair quality of life, decrease compliance, and increase both health service use and mortality (Koenig, Shelp, Goli, Cohen, & Blazer, 1989). The clinical presentation of depression overlaps heavily with dementia as well as other medical and psychiatric conditions. The onset and maintenance of depression in later life is influenced by a wide range of biological, psychological, and social factors that have cumulative effects over a lifetime. These factors have been described and modeled, and the research linking them with depression reviewed. Knowledge about risk factors is necessary to identify individuals who are particularly vulnerable. By reducing risk factors, along with early recognition and treatment, we hope to either help prevent or stall the progression of these disorders. Combinations of psychosocial and biological treatments now exist that can reverse geriatric depression in at least 80% of cases (Reynolds et al., 1992; Scogin & McElreath, 1994). Thus, diagnostic and therapeutic nihilism is no longer tenable.

Directions for Research

According to the National Institutes of Health Consensus Development Panel (1992) there are several questions that need to be answered with regard to late-life depression: (1) How does depression in late life differ from depressions that occur at earlier ages, and what are the sources of heterogeneity? (2) How prevalent is depression in older persons and what are its risk factors? (3) What are safe and efficacious treatments for late-life depression, and what are indications and contraindications for specific treatments? (4) What are the patterns of health service use and obstacles to provision of appropriate services? (5) What are the benefits of (and consequences of not) recognizing and treating late-life depressions?

The sixth question deals with avenues for future research: improving diagnosis and identification of elders likely to benefit from specific treatments; clarifying the relationships between subcortical brain changes, cognitive and depressive symptoms, and early versus late-onset depression; exploring pharmacokinetic changes in the very old; metabolic subtyping; conducting prospective cross-sequential studies to identify general risk factors of depression onset and course; assessing risk factors for suicide in late life; examining ECT as continuation and maintenance treatment; exploring psychotherapeutic and psychopharmacologic treatments for grief; conducting clinical trials and observational studies in elderly subgroups (very old, minorities, underserved communities, nursing homes, elders with medical illness); developing and evaluating psychosocial treatments and relating them to biological treatments; initiating demonstration projects to enhance service delivery (effectiveness research); and conducting long-term clinical trials to assess outcomes to determine benefits to society of effective recognition and treatment of late-life depression. While much has been accomplished, a great deal remains to be done to push forward the frontiers of knowledge in the area of geriatric mood disorders.

ACKNOWLEDGMENTS

This work was supported by a NIMH Clinical Mental Health Academic Award (MH01138).

References

Alexopoulos, G. S, Young, R. C., & Shindledecker, R. D. (1992). Brain computed tomography findings in geriatric depression and primary degenerative dementia. *Biological Psychiatry, 31,* 591–599.

Alexopoulos, G. S., Meyers, B. S., & Young, R. C. (1993). The course of geriatric depression with "reversible dementia": A controlled study. *American Journal of Psychiatry, 150,* 1693–1699.

Arean, P. A., Perri, M. G., Nezu, A. M., Schein, R. L., Christopher, F., & Joseph, T. X. (1993). Comparative effectiveness of social problem-solving therapy and reminiscence therapy as treatments for depression in older adults. *Journal of Consulting and Clinical Psychology, 61,* 1003–1010.

Barclay, L. L., Blass, J. P., & Lee, R. E. (1984). Cerebral metastases mimicking depression in a "forgetful" attorney. *Journal of the American Geriatrics Society, 32,* 866–867.

Beck, A. T., Rush, J., & Shaw, B. (1979). *Cognitive therapy of depression.* New York: Guilford.

Bell, I. R., Edman, J. S., Marrow, F. D., Marby, D. W., Marages, S., Perrone, G., Kayne, H. L., & Cole, J. O. (1991). B complex vitamin patterns in geriatric and young adult inpatients with major depression. *Journal of the American Geriatrics Society, 39,* 252–257.

Benbow, S. M. (1989). The role of electroconvulsive therapy in the treatment of depressive illness in old age. *British Journal of Psychiatry, 155,* 147–152.

Blazer, D. G. (1983). Impact of late-life depression on the social network. *American Journal of Psychiatry, 140,* 162–166.

Blazer, D. G., Hughes, D. C., & George, L. K. (1987). The epidemiology of depression in an elderly community population. *The Gerontologist, 27,* 281–287.

Blazer, D. G., Hughes, D. C., & Fowler, N. (1989). Anxiety as an outcome symptom of depression in elderly and middle-aged adults. *International Journal of Geriatric Psychiatry, 4,* 273–278.

Blazer, D., Burchett, B., Service, C., & George, L. K. (1991). The association of age and depression among the elderly: An epidemiologic exploration. *Journal of Gerontology, 46,* M210–M215.

Bombardier, C., D'Amico, C., & Jordan, J. (1990). The relationship of appraisal and coping to illness adjustment. *Behavioral Research and Therapy, 28,* 297–304.

Borson, S., Barnes, R. A., Kukul, W. A., Okimoto, J. T., Veith, R. C., Inui, T. S., Carter, W., & Raskind, M. A. (1986). Symptomatic depression in elderly medical outpatients. *Journal of the American Geriatrics Society, 34,* 341–347.

Borson, S., McDonald, G. J., Gayle, T., Deffebach, M., Lakshminarayan, S., & Van Tuinen, C. (1992). Improvement in mood, physical symptoms, and function with nortriptyline for depression in patients with chronic obstructive pulmonary disease. *Psychosomatics, 33,* 190–201.

Brink, T. L. (1985). The grieving patient in later life. *Psychotherapy Patient, 2,* 117–127.

Broadhead, W., Blazer, D., George, L., & Tse, C. (1990). Depression, disability days, and days lost from work in a prospective epidemiological survey. *Journal of the American Medical Association, 264,* 2524–2528.

Brodaty, H., Peters, K., Boyce, P., Hickie, I., Parker, G., Mitchell, P., & Wilhelm, K. (1991). Age and depression. *Journal of Affective Disorders, 23,* 137–149.

Brymer, C., & Winograd, C. H. (1992). Fluoxetin in elderly patients. Is there cause for concern? *Journal of the American Geriatrics Society, 40,* 902–905.

Chrischilles, E. A., Foley, D. J., Wallace, R. B., Lemke, J. H.,

Semla, T. P., Hanlon, J. T., Glynn, R. J., Ostfeld, A. M., & Guralnik, J. M. (1992). Use of medications by persons 65 and over. Data from the established populations for epidemiologic studies of the elderly. *Journal of Gerontology, 47,* M137–M144.

Clayton, P. (1990). Bereavement and depression. *Journal of Clinical Psychiatry, 51*(Suppl. 7), 34–38.

Coffey, C. E., Wilkinson, W. E., Weiner, R. D., Parashos, I. A., Djang, W. T., Webb, M. C., Figiel, G. S., & Spritzer, C. E. (1993). Quantitative cerebral anatomy in depression: A controlled resonance imaging study. *Archives of General Psychiatry, 50,* 7–16.

Cole, M. G. (1985). The course of elderly depressed outpatients. *Canadian Journal of Psychiatry, 30,* 217–220.

Coulehan, J. L,. Schulberg, H. C., Block, M. R., Janosky, J. E., & Arena, V. C. (1990). Medical comorbidity of major depressive disorder in a primary medical practice. *Archives of Internal Medicine, 150,* 2363–2367.

Cutler, S. (1976). Membership in different types of voluntary associations and psychological well being. *The Gerontologist, 16,* 335–339.

De Alarcon, R. (1964). Hypochondriasis and depression in the aged. *Gerontologia Clinica, 6,* 266–277.

Dovenmuehle, R. H., & Verwoerdt, A. (1962), Physical illness and depressive symptomatology. *Journal of the American Geriatrics Society, 10,* 932–947.

Egeland, J. A., Gerhard, D. S., Pauls, D. L., Sussex, J. N., Kidd, K. K., Allen, C. R., Hostetter, A. M., & Housman, D. E. (1987). Bipolar affective disorders linked to DNA markers on chromosome 11. *Nature, 325,* 783–787.

Finch, E. J. L., & Katona, C. L. E. (1989). Lithium augmentation in the treatment of refractory depression in old age. *International Journal of Geriatric Psychiatry, 4,* 41–46.

Finlayson, R. E., Hurt, R. D., Davis, L. J., & Morse, R. M. (1988). Alcoholism in elderly persons. *Mayo Clinic Proceedings, 63,* 761–768.

Fogel, B. S., & Westlake, R. (1990). Personality disorder diagnoses and age in patients with major depression. *Journal of Clinical Psychiatry, 51,* 232–235.

Folstein, M. F., & McHugh, P. R. (1978). Dementia syndrome of depression. In R. Katzman, R. D. Terry, & K. L. Bick (Eds.), *Alzheimer's disease: Senile dementia and related disorders* (pp. 87–93). New York: Raven Press.

George, L. K., Blazer, D. G., Hughes, D. C., & Fowler, N. (1989). Social support and the outcome of major depression. *British Journal of Psychiatry, 154,* 478–485.

Georgotas, A., McCue, R. E., Friedman, E., & Cooper, T. B. (1989). A placebo-controlled comparison of nortriptyline and phenelzine in maintenance therapy of elderly depressed patients. *Archives of General Psychiatry, 46,* 783–786.

Gerner, R., Estabrook, W., Steuer, J., & Jarvik, L. (1980). Treatment of geriatric depression with trazodone, imipramine, and placebo: A double-blind study. *Journal of Clinical Psychiatry, 41,* 216–220.

Goldberg, E. L., Van Natta, P., & Comstock, G. W. (1985). Depressive symptoms, social networks, and social support of elderly women. *American Journal of Epidemiology, 121,* 448–456.

Greden, J. F. (1993). Antidepressant maintenance medications: When to discontinue and how to stop. *Journal of Clinical Psychiatry, 54*(Suppl. 8), 39–45.

Green, B. H., Copeland, J. R., Dewey, M. E., Sharma, V., Sunders, P. A., Davidson, I. A., Sullivan, C., & McWilliam, C. (1992). Risk factors for depression in elderly people: A prospective study. *Acta Psychiatrica Scandinavica, 86,* 213–217.

Greenblatt, D. J., Shader, R. I., & Abernathy, D. R. (1983). Current status of benzodiazepines: Clinical use of benzodiazepines. *New England Journal of Medicine, 309,* 410–415.

Guze, B. H., & Barrio, J. C. (1991). The etiology of depression in Parkinson's disease patients. *Psychosomatics, 32,* 390–395.

Holroyd, K., & Andrasik, F. (1982). Do the effects of cognitive therapy endure? A two-year follow-up of tension headache sufferers treated with cognitive therapy or biofeedback. *Cognitive Therapy and Research, 6,* 325–334.

Holroyd, K., & Lazarus, R. (1982). Stress, coping and somatic adaptation. In L. Goldberger & S. Breznitz (Eds.), *Handbook of stress.* New York: Freepress.

Hopkinson, G. (1964). A genetic study of affective illness in inpatients over 50. *British Journal of Psychiatry, 110,* 244–254.

Idler, E. (1987). Religious involvement and health of the elderly: Some hypotheses and an initial test. *Social Forces, 66,* 226–238.

Jacobsen, F. M. ,Wehr, T. A., Sack, D. A., James, S. P., & Rosenthal, N. E. (1987). Seasonal affective disorder: A review of the syndrome and its public health implications. *American Journal of Public Health, 77,* 57–60.

Jinks, M. J., & Raschko, R. R. (1990). A profile of alcohol and prescription drug abuse in a high-risk community-based elderly population. *Geriatrics and Gerontology, 24,* 971–975.

Katon, W., & Raskin, M. (1980). Treatment of depression in the medically ill elderly with methylphenidate. *American Journal of Psychiatry, 137,* 963–965.

Kendell, R. E. (1974). The stability of psychiatric diagnoses. *British Journal of Psychiatry, 124,* 352–356.

Kessler, R. C., McGonagle, K. A., Zhao, S., Nelson, C. B., Hughes, M., Eschleman, S., Wittchen, H. U., & Kendler, K. S. (1994). Lifetime and 12-month prevalence of DSM-III-R psychiatric disorders in the United States. *Archives of General Psychiatry, 51,* 8–19.

Kitchell, M., Barnes, R., Veith, R. ,Okimoto, J., & Raskind, M. (1982). Screening for depression in hospitalized geriatric patients. *Journal of the American Geriatrics Society, 30,* 174–177.

Klerman, G. L., & Weissman, M. M. (1989). Increasing rates of depression. *Journal of the American Medical Association, 261,* 2229–2235.

Koenig, H. G. (1994). *Aging and God.* New York: Haworth Press.

Koenig, H. G., Blazer, D. G., & Hocking, L. B. (1995). Depression, anxiety and other affective disorders. In C. K. Cassell et al. (Eds.), *Geriatric medicine* (3rd ed.). New York: Springer-Verlag.

Koenig, H. G., & Breitner, J. C. S. (1990). Antidepressant use in the medically ill older person. *Psychosomatics, 31,* 22–32.

Koenig, H. G., Cohen, H. J., Blazer, D. G., Kudler, H. S., Krishnan, K. R. R., & Sibert, T. E. (1995). Cognitive symptoms of depression and religious coping in elderly medical patients. *Psychosomatics, 36,* 369–375.

Koenig, H. G., Cohen, H. J., Blazer, D. G., Meador, K. G., & Westlund, R. (1992). A brief depression scale for detecting major depression in the medically ill hospitalized patient. *International Journal of Psychiatry in Medicine, 22*, 183–195.

Koenig, H. G., Cohen, H. J., Blazer, D. G., Pieper, C., Meador, K. G., Shelp, F., Goli, V., & DiPasquale, R. (1992). Religious coping and depression in elderly hospitalized medically ill men. *American Journal of Psychiatry, 149*, 1693–1700.

Koenig, H. G., Ford, S. M., & Blazer, D. G. (1993). Should physicians screen for depression in elderly medical inpatients?: Results of a decision analysis. *International Journal of Psychiatry in Medicine, 23*, 239–263.

Koenig, H. G., George, L. K., & Siegler, I. (1988). The use of religion and other emotion-regulating coping strategies among older adults. *The Gerontologist, 28*, 303–310.

Koenig, H. G., Goli, V., Shelp, F., Kudler, H. S., Cohen, H. J., & Blazer, D. G. (1992). Major depression in hospitalized medically ill men: Documentation, treatment, and prognosis. *International Journal of Geriatric Psychiatry, 7*, 25–34.

Koenig, H. G., Goli, V., Shelp, F., Meador, K. G., & Blazer, D. G. (1989). Antidepressant use in older medically ill inpatients: Lessons from an attempted clinical trial. *Journal of General Internal Medicine, 4*, 498–505.

Koenig, H. G., Kvale, J. N., & Ferrel, C. (1988). Religion and well-being in later life. *The Gerontologist, 28*, 18–28.

Koenig, H. G., Meador, K., Cohen, H. J., & Blazer, D. (1988a). Depression in elderly men hospitalized with medical illness. *Archives of Internal Medicine, 148*, 1929–1936.

Koenig, H. G., Meador, K. G., Goli, V., Shelp, F., Cohen, H. J., & Blazer, D. G. (1992). Self-rated depressive symptoms in medical inpatients. Age and racial differences. *International Journal of Psychiatry in Medicine, 22*, 11–31.

Koenig, H. G., Meador, K. G., Shelp, F., Goli, V., Cohen, H. J., & Blazer, D. G. (1991). Depressive disorders in hospitalized medically ill patients: A comparison of young and elderly men. *Journal of the American Geriatrics Society, 39*, 881–890.

Koenig, H. G., Meador, K. G., Cohen, H. J., & Blazer, D. G. (1988b). Detection and treatment of major depression in older hospitalized patients with medical illness. *International Journal of Psychiatry in Medicine, 18*, 17–31.

Koenig, H. G., Moberg, D. O., & Kvale, J. N. (1988). Religious activities and attitudes of older adults in a geriatric assessment clinic. *Journal of the American Geriatrics Society, 35*, 362–374.

Koenig, H. G., O'Connor, C., Guarisco, S., Zabel, M., & Ford, S. (1993). Depressive disorder in elderly inpatients admitted to general medicine and cardiology services at a private hospital. *American Journal of Geriatric Psychiatry, 1*, 197–210.

Koenig, H. G., Shelp, F., Goli, V., Cohen, H. J., & Blazer, D. G. (1989). Survival and healthcare utilization in elderly medical inpatients with major depression. *Journal of the American Geriatrics Society, 37*, 599–606.

Koenig, H. G., Westlund, R. E., George, L. K., Hughes, D. C., & Hybels, C. (1993). Abbreviating the Duke Social Support Index for use in chronically ill older adults. *Psychosomatics, 34*, 61–69.

Krishnan, K. R. (1993). Neuroanatomic substrates of depression in the elderly. *Journal of Geriatric Psychiatry and Neurology, 6*, 39–58.

Krishnan, K. R., Doraiswamy, M. P., Figiel, G. S., Hussain, M. M., Shah, S. A., Na, C., Boyko, O. B., McDonald, W. M., Nemeroff, C. B., & Ellinwood, E. H. (1991). Hippocampal abnormalities in depression. *Journal of Neuropsychiatry and Clinical Neurosciences, 3*, 387–391.

Kronfol, Z., Hansher, K., Digre, K., & Waziri, R. (1978). Depression and hemispheric functions: Changes associated with unilateral ECT. *British Journal of Psychiatry, 132*, 560–567.

Lazarus, R. (1974). Psychological stress and coping in adaptation and illness. *International Journal of Psychiatry in Medicine, 5*, 321–333.

Lesser, I. M., Hill-Gutierrez, E., Miller, B. L., & Boone, K. B. (1993). Late-onset depression with white matter lesions. *Psychosomatics, 34*, 364–367.

Light, R. W., Merrill, E. J., Despairs, J. A., Gordon, G. H., & Mutalipassi, L. R. (1985). Prevalence of depression and anxiety in patients with COPD. *Chest, 87*, 35–38.

Lindemann, E. (1944). Symptomatology and management of acute grief. *American Journal of Psychiatry, 101*, 141–148.

Lindenbaum, J., Healton, E. B., Savage, D. G., Brust, J. C. M., Garrett, T. J., Podell, E. R., Marcell, P. D., Stabler, S. P., & Allen, R. H. (1988). Neuropsychiatric disorders caused by cobalamin deficiency in the absence of anemia or microcytosis. *New England Journal of Medicine, 318*, 1720–1728.

Lipowski, Z. (1970). Physical illness, the individual and the coping processes. *International Journal of Psychiatry in Medicine, 1*, 91–102.

Magni, G., Schifano, F., & de Leo, D. (1985). Pain as a symptom in elderly depressed patients: Relationship to diagnostic subgroups. *European Archives of Psychiatry and the Neurological Sciences, 235*, 143–145.

Maier, W., Lichtermann, D., Minges, J., Heun, R., Hallmayer, J., & Klingler, T. (1991). Unipolar depression in the aged: Determinants of familial aggregation. *Journal of Affective Disorder, 23*, 53–61.

Marmar, C. R., Horowitz, M. J., Weiss, D. S., Wilner, N. R., & Kaltreider, N. B. (1988). A controlled trial of brief psychotherapy and mutual-help group treatment of conjugal bereavement. *American Journal of Psychiatry, 145*, 203–209.

Massie, M. J., & Holland, J. C. (1990). Depression and the cancer patient. *Journal of Clinical Psychiatry, 51*, (Suppl. 7), 12–17.

Mayeux, R. (1990). Depression in the patient with Parkinson's disease. *Journal of Clinical Psychiatry, 51*,(Suppl. 7), 20–23.

Mayo, S. C. (1951). Social participation among the older population in rural areas of Wake County, NC. *Social Forces, 30*, 53–59.

McFarland, B. H., Miller, M. R., & Straumfjord, A. A. (1990). Valproate use in the older manic patient. *Journal of Clinical Psychiatry, 51*, 479–481.

McMurdo, M. E., & Burnett, L. (1992). Randomised controlled trial of exercise in the elderly. *Gerontology, 38*, 292–298.

McMurdo, M. E., & Rennie, L. (1993). A controlled trial of exercise by residents of old people's homes. *Age and Aging, 22*, 11–15.

Mendlewicz, J. (1976). The age factor in depressive illness: Some genetic considerations. *Journal of Gerontology, 31*, 300–303.

Meyers, B. S. (1984). Increased intracranial pressure and depression in the elderly. *Journal of the American Geriatrics Society, 32*, 936–938.

Meyers, B. S., Kalayam, B., & Mei-Tal, V. (1984). Late-onset delusional depression: A distinct clinical entity? *Journal of Clinical Psychiatry, 45*, 347–349.

Miller, W. R. (1975). Psychological deficit in depression. *Psychological Bulletin, 82*, 238–260.

Morton, W. A., Sonne, S. C., & Lydiard, R. B. (1993). Lithium side effects in the medically ill. *International Journal of Psychiatry in Medicine, 23*, 357–382.

Moss, M. S., Lawton, M. P., & Glicksman, A. (1991). The role of pain in the last year of life of older persons. *Journal of Gerontology, 46*, P51–P57.

Mulrow, C. D., Aguilar, C., Endicott, J. E., Tuley, M. R., Velex, R., Charlip, W. S., Rhodes, M. C., Hill, J. A., & DeNino, L. A. (1990). Quality of life changes and hearing impairment: A randomized trial. *Annals of Internal Medicine, 113*, 188–194.

Mulrow, C. D., Tuley, M. R., & Aguilar, C. (1992). Sustained benefits of hearing aids. *Journal of Speech and Hearing Research, 35*, 1402–1405.

Murphy, E. (1982). Social origins of depression in old age. *British Journal of Psychiatry, 141*, 135–142.

Murrell, S. A., Himmelfarb, S., & Wright, K. (1983). Prevalence of depression and its correlates in older adults. *American Journal of Epidemiology, 117*, 173–185.

National Institutes of Health Consensus Development Panel (1992). Diagnosis and treatment of depression in late life. *Journal of the American Medical Association, 268*, 1018–1024.

Nott, P. N., & Flemminger, J. J. (1975). Presenile dementia: The difficulties of early diagnosis. *Acta Psychiatrica Scandinavica, 51*, 210–217.

Olinger, L., Kuiper, N., & Shaw, B. (1987). Dysfunctional attitudes and stressful life events: An interactive model of depression. *Cognitive Therapy and Research, 11*, 25–40.

Ong, Y. K., Maritean, F., Lloyd, C., & Robbins, I. (1987). A support group for the depressed elderly. *International Journal of Geriatric Psychiatry, 2*, 119–123.

Parmelee, P. A., Katz, I. R., & Lawton, M. P. (1989). Depression among institutionalized aged: Assessment and prevalence estimation. *Journal of Gerontology, 44*, M22–M29.

Perez-Stable, E. J., Miranda, J., Munos, R. F., & Ying, Y. (1990). Depression in medical outpatients. *Archives of Internal Medicine, 150*, 1083–1088.

Pfifer, J. F., & Murrell, S. A. (1986). Etiologic factors in the onset of depressive symptoms in older adults. *Journal of Abnormal Psychology, 95*, 282–291.

Post, F. (1951). The outcome of mental breakdown in old age. *British Medical Journal, 1*, 436–448.

Post, F. (1978). The functional psychoses. In A. D. Isaacs & F. Post (Eds.), *Studies in geriatric psychiatry*. New York: Wiley.

Post, R. M. (1992). Transduction of psychosocial stress into the neurobiology of recurrent affective disorder. *American Journal of Psychiatry, 149*, 999–1010.

Post, R. M. (1993). Mechanisms underlying the evolution of affective disorders: Implications for long-term treatment. In L. Grunhaus & J. F. Greden (Eds.), *Progress in psychiatry: Severe depressive disorders*. Washington, DC: American Psychiatric Press.

Post, R. M., Rubinow, D. R., & Ballenger, J. C. (1986). Conditioning and sensitisation in the longitudinal course of affective illness. *British Journal of Psychiatry, 149*, 191–201.

Pressman, P., Lyons, J., Larson, D., & Strain, J. (1990). Religious belief, depression, and ambulation status in elderly women with broken hips. *American Journal of Psychiatry, 147*, 758–760.

Rapp, S., Parisi, S., & Walsh, D. (1988). Psychological dysfunction and physical health among elderly medical inpatients. *Journal of Consulting and Clinical Psychology, 56*, 851–855.

Rapp, S. R., Walsh, D. A., Parisi, S. A., & Wallace, C. E. (1988). Detecting depression in elderly medical inpatients. *Journal of Consulting and Clinical Psychology, 56*, 509–513.

Reifler, B. V., Larson, E., & Henley, R. (1982). Coexistence of cognitive impairment and depression in geriatric outpatients. *American Journal of Psychiatry, 39*, 623–626.

Reynolds, C. F., Fran, E., Perel, J. M., Imber, S. D., Cornes, C., Morycz, R. K., Mazumdar, S., Miller, M. D., Pollock, B. G., Rifai, A. H., Stack, J. A., George, C. J., Houck, P. R., & Kupfer, D. J. (1992). Combined pharmacotherapy and psychotherapy in the acute and continuation treatment of elderly patients with recurrent major depression: A preliminary report. *American Journal of Psychiatry, 149*, 1687–1692.

Robinson, D. S., Davies, J. M., Nies, A., Rqavaris, C. L., & Sylwester, D. (1971). Relation of sex and aging to monoamine oxidase activity of human plasma and platelets. *Archives of General Psychiatry, 24*, 536–541.

Robinson, R. G., Morris, P. L. P., & Fedoroff, J. P. (1990). Depression and cerebrovascular disease. *Journal of Clinical Psychiatry, 51*(Suppl. 7), 26–31.

Romano, J. M., & Turner, J. A. (1985). Chronic pain in depression: Does the evidence support a relationship? *Psychological Bulletin, 97*, 18–34.

Rosen, C. C. (1982). Ethnic differences among impoverished rural elderly in use of religion as a coping mechanism. *Journal of Rural and Community Psychology, 3*, 27–34.

Rosenbaum, A. H., Schatzberg, A. F., MacLaughlin, M. S., Snyder, K., Jian, N. S., Ilstrup, D., Rothschild, A. J., & Kliman, B. K. (1984). The DST in normal control subjects: A comparison of two assays and the effects of age. *American Journal of Psychiatry, 141*, 1550–1555.

Roth, M., & Morrissey, J. D. (1952). Problems in the diagnosis and classification of mental disorders in old age. *Journal of Mental Science, 98*, 66–80.

Rovner, B. W., German, P., Brant, L. J., Clark, R., Burton, L., & Folstein, M. F. (1991). Depression and mortality in nursing homes. *Journal of the American Medical Association, 265*, 993–996.

Roy-Byrne, P. P., Weingartner, H., Bierer, L. M., Thompson, K., & Post, R. M. (1986). Effortful and automatic cognitive process in depression. *Archives of General Psychiatry, 43*, 265–267.

Sachar, E. J. (1975). Neuroendocrine abnormalities in depressive illness. *Topics in psychoendocrinology*. New York: Grune & Stratton.

Salzman, C. (1992). *Clinical geriatric psychopharmacology* (2nd ed., p. 145). Baltimore: Williams & Wilkins.

Schleifer, S., Macari-Hinson, M., Coyle, D., Salter, W. R., Kahn, M., Gorlin, R., & Zucker, H. (1989). The nature and course of depression following myocardial infarction. *Archives of Internal Medicine, 149*, 1785–1789.

Schneider, L. S., Zemansky, M. F., Bender, M., & Sloane, R. B. (1992). Personality in recovered depressed elderly. *International Psychogeriatrics*, *4*, 177–185.

Scogin, F., & McElreath, L. (1994). Efficacy of psychosocial treatments for geriatric depression: A quantitative review. *Journal of Consulting and Clinical Psychology*, *62*, 69–74.

Sharpe, M., Hawton, K., House, A., Molyneux, A., Sandercock, P., Bamford, J., & Warlow, C. (1990). Mood disorder in long-term survivors of stroke. Associations with brain lesion location and volume. *Psychological Medicine*, *20*, 815–828.

Shulman, K. I. (1986). Mania in old age. In E. Murphy (Ed.). *Affective disorders in the elderly*. Edinburgh, Scotland: Churchill Livingstone.

Shulman, K. I. (1989). The influence of age and ageing on manic disorder. *International Journal of Geriatric Psychiatry*, *4*, 63–65.

Shulman, K., I., & Post, F. (1980). Bipolar affective disorder in old age. *British Journal of Psychiatry*, *136*, 26–32.

Slater, E., & Cowie, V. (1971). *The genetics of mental disorder*. London: Oxford University Press.

Smidt, L. J., Cremin, F. M., Grivetti, L. E., & Clifford, A. J. (1991). Influence of thiamine supplementation on the health and general well-being of an elderly Irish population with marginal thiamin deficiency. *Journal of Gerontology*, *46*, M16–M22.

Smith, J. S., & Kiloh, L. G. (1981). The investigation of dementia: Results in 200 consecutive admissions. *Lancet*, *1*, 824–827.

Smith, T., Follick, M., Ahern, D., & Adams, A. (1986). Cognitive distortion and disability in chronic low back pain. *Cognitive Therapy and Research*, *10*, 201–210.

Snyder, P. J., & Utiger, R. D. (1972). Response to thyrotropin releasing hormone (TRH) in normal man. *Journal of Clinical Endocrinology and Metabolism*, *34*, 380–385.

Spar, J. E., Ford, C. V., & Liston, E. H. (1979). Bipolar affective disorder in aged patients. *Journal of Clinical Psychiatry 1979*, *40*, 504–507.

Spier, S. A., & Frontera, M. A. (1991). Unexpected deaths in depressed medical inpatients treated with fluoxetine. *Journal of Clinical Psychiatry*, *52*, 377–382.

Stallones, L., Marx, M. B., & Garrity, T. F. (1990). Prevalence and correlates of depressive symptoms among older U.S. adults. *American Journal of Preventive Medicine*, *6*, 295–303.

Stenstedt, A. (1959). Involutional melancholia: An etiologic, clinical and social study of endogenous depression in later life, with special reference to genetic factors. *Acta Psychiatrica Neurologica Scandinavica*, *127*(Suppl.), 5–71.

Surtees, P. G. (1980). Social support, residual adversity and depressive outcome. *Social Psychiatry*, *15*, 71–80.

Targum, S. D., Sullivan, A. C., & Byrnes, S. M. (1982). Neuroendocrine relationships in major depressive disorder. *American Journal of Psychiatry*, *139*, 282–286.

Thompson, L. W., Gallagher, D., & Breckenridge, J. S. (1987). Comparative effectiveness of psychotherapies for depressed elders. *Journal of Consulting and Clinical Psychology*, *55*, 385–390.

Tobin, S. S., Ellor, J., & Anderson-Ray, S. M. (1986). *Enabling the elderly: Religious institutions within the community service system*. Albany, NY: State University of New York Press.

Tyrer, P., & Murphy, S. (1987). The place of benzodiazepines in psychiatric practice. *British Journal of Psychiatry*, *151*, 719–723.

Verwoerdt, A. (1976). *Geropsychiatry*. Baltimore: Williams & Wilkins.

Weissman, M., Leaf, P., Tischler, G., Blazer, D., Karno, M., Bruce, M., & Lorio, L. (1988). Affective disorders in five United States communities. *Psychological Medicine*, *18*, 141–153.

Weissman, M. M., Bruce, M. L., Leaf, P. J., Florio, L. P., & Holzer, C. (1991). Affective disorders. In L. N. Robins & D. A. Regier (Eds.), *Psychiatric disorders in America: The Epidemiologic Catchment Area study* (p. 53). New York: Free Press.

Wells, C. E. (1979). Pseudodementia. *American Journal of Psychiatry*, *136*, 896–900.

Williamson, G. M., & Schulz, R. (1992). Pain, activity restriction, and symptoms of depression among community-residing elderly adults. *Journal of Gerontology*, *47*, P367–P372.

Winefield, H. R. (1979). Social support and social environment of depressed and normal women. *Australian and New Zealand Journal of Psychiatry*, *13*, 35–39.

Winokur, G. (1975). The Iowa 500: Heterogeneity and course in manic-depressive illness (bipolar). *Comprehensive Psychiatry*, *16*, 125–131.

7

Anxiety Disorders

CAROL J. SCHRAMKE

Introduction

Although symptoms of anxiety are more prevalent than affective symptoms in later life (Matt, Dean, Wang, & Wood, 1992), a review of the anxiety and aging literature as well as the anxiety and cognitive dysfunction literature reveals that much less attention has been focused on anxiety than on depression. It is estimated that 20% of elderly adults have "pathologic levels of anxiety" with even higher rates among the "old old" (Raj, Corvea, & Dagon, 1993), suggesting the need for health care providers of older adults to address anxiety. Neuropsychologists are asked to evaluate a variety of patients, some of whom, in the course of the evaluation, may reveal symptoms suggestive of an anxiety disorder. Although complaints of anxiety in older adults are not uncommon, appropriate treatment of these complaints seems to be rare, as suggested by studies examining prevalence and treatment rates in older community dwelling samples (Flint, 1994; Lindesay, 1991). Given the responsiveness of anxiety and depressive disorders to treatment, unlike many of the other disorders neuropsychologists are likely to diagnose, accurate identification of these disorders offers a unique opportunity for intervention which may greatly enhance the patient's quality of life.

Numerous studies suggest that although many elderly with psychiatric complaints are treated regularly by physicians, both anxiety and depressive disorders may be missed or misdiagnosed by primary care providers. While Barbee and McLaulin (1990) report that the highest prescription rate of benzodiazepines in a Danish study of general practitioners was for patients in the 60- to 69-year-old group, only a quarter of those had a psychiatric diagnosis. Lindesay (1991) found that of those elderly phobic patients who were provided with treatment for an anxiety disorder, few were likely to be provided with the most efficacious medication or psychotherapy for this disorder. These two studies support the need for intervention, both to ensure appropriate treatment and to prevent inappropriate treatment. The neuropsychologist, who may be the first or only mental health professional an older client encounters, may be the older adult's best hope for accurate diagnosis. In addition, while identification of previously unidentified psychiatric difficulties can be important no matter what the age of the patient, development of specific anxiety disorders after early or middle adulthood is uncommon and may be a sign of a neurologic or medical disorder.

Assessment of anxiety symptoms is crucial for an accurate diagnosis of these disorders. Unfortunately, accurate diagnoses may not be easy to establish. Ouslander (1984) observes that psychiatric symptoms may be manifestations of physical illness, physical symptoms can be manifestations of psychiatric illness, and physical illness can cause stress which can cause psychiatric decompensation. In addition, physical conditions as well as psychiatric conditions can present atypically in the elderly (e.g., pneumonia can occur without fever or cough, and myocardial infarction can occur without pain). Recognizing atypical presentations of psychiatric and neurologic disorders, as well as understanding the many factors which can contribute to the devel-

CAROL J. SCHRAMKE • Psychology Service, Highland Drive Veterans Affairs Medical Center, Pittsburgh, Pennsylvania 15206; and Departments of Neurology and Psychiatry, University of Pittsburgh, Pittsburgh, Pennsylvania 15213.

opment and expression of these disorders, is essential for the accurate identification and treatment of these illnesses.

This chapter reviews the difficulties associated with defining and conceptualizing anxiety, as well as the concepts of state and trait anxiety and adaptive versus pathological anxiety in older adulthood. The definitions of the *Diagnostic and Statistical Manual of Mental Disorders*, fourth edition (*DSM-IV*) anxiety disorders and their relationship to aging, medical and neurologic conditions associated with increased anxiety and the role of the brain and brain disorders in anxiety symptoms are discussed. Relevant research investigating the influence of anxiety and anxiety disorders on cognition and neuropsychological test performance are also examined, followed by a brief review of the literature investigating treatment of anxiety disorders in the elderly. Finally, implications of this information for neuropsychologists and additional areas of research through which neuropsychologists can contribute to our understanding of anxiety will be outlined.

What Is Anxiety?

Anxiety is a concept not easily defined, which in turn complicates attempts to determine whether an individual is anxious and attempts to measure the intensity of an individual's anxiety. Separating anxiety into how anxious one feels at the moment (state anxiety) versus how one normally or usually feels (trait anxiety) may be most frequently assessed, in psychological research, with the Spielberger State-Trait Anxiety Inventory (Spielberger, 1982). Fairly compelling evidence exists that individuals differ with regard to how sensitive they are to anxiety-arousing situations. Whether this is due primarily to physiologic differences or differences in coping and cognition remains to be determined. Clinically, a number of popular measures of depression are available, while fewer anxiety measures exist, and there is less consensus regarding their utility. A number of studies have suggested that there is a great deal of overlap between scales designed to measure depression and anxiety. This has resulted in some researchers arguing that self-report scales are measuring a more general level of distress which may reflect anxiety, depression, and/or situational

stress (e.g., Fechner-Bates, Coyne, & Schwenk, 1994); others argue that this only highlights the need for developing better measures of these two constructs (e.g., Endler, Cox, Parker, & Bagby, 1992).

Sheikh (1991) notes most anxiety scales are designed and normed initially for use with younger adults. Additional research needs to be completed to determine whether these measures are appropriate for use with the elderly. Some of these scales (e.g., the Beck Anxiety Inventory and Self Rating Anxiety Scales) have normative data available for older adults, but research with these instruments in older populations is limited. When evaluating this literature and its implications for the elderly, a number of concerns become apparent. Most surveys of psychopathology exclude institutionalized elderly, which may not be a problem when accurately representing the "young" old, since they are infrequently institutionalized. This may be more important in understanding the "old" old, or individuals over 75, who are more likely to be residing in an institution (Flint, 1994). It has also been suggested that symptoms endorsed in interviews or on questionnaires, which are indicative of anxiety in younger adults, may only reflect normal aging in an elderly sample. This argues for norming measures on the elderly and additional examination of how we define pathology in older adults (Matt et al., 1992).

While overattending to normal age-related somatic changes (e.g., alterations in sleep patterns and lower levels of energy) may lead to pathologizing normal aging, ignoring or failing to ask about somatic symptoms, particularly in an elderly patient who may feel more comfortable admitting to physical rather than psychological distress (Flint, 1994), can result in clinicians failing to identify anxiety and depressive disorders. It also has been suggested that older adults, because of memory difficulties, may be less reliable in their report of symptoms (Flint, 1994), which could influence both reliability and validity of measures of distress. Additional studies establishing reliability and validity of these measures, with specific subgroups of older adults, need to be accomplished before clinicians can use them with confidence.

A review of the literature on prevalence of anxiety disorders in the general population reveals significant variability between studies. Closer inspection of this literature reveals that this is due, at least in part, to differences in how patients are evaluated for anxiety symptoms. Matt et al. (1992) note that although self-report questionnaires such as the Symptoms Checklist-42 (SCL-42) may identify most subjects who meet criteria for psychiatric diagnoses, they also note limitations of these measures. For example, subjects may vary with regard to their comfort level in admitting symptoms and may answer questions differently due to subtle changes in phrasing, and older adults may interpret questions differently than younger adults. A number of older adults in our clinic initially reported nervousness or anxiety in themselves or their spouse, but with additional questioning it became apparent this was due to "shakiness" or a tremor, rather than an internal feeling of anxiety. More simply, variability in defining cut off scores for severity and variations in survey instruments used, even with similar methodologies, can result in pronounced differences in incidence figures. This has led some researchers to suggest that separating "cases" of anxiety from "noncases" may be less helpful than looking at anxiety on a continuum (Flint, 1994).

Focusing on anxiety or depressive disorders alone, or on a specific anxiety or depressive disorder, may also be difficult and misleading. Studies suggest significant comorbidity between anxiety and depression; that anxiety and depressive disorders may respond to the same medications, have overlapping symptoms, and share common etiologic (i.e., biologic) factors; and that prominence of different symptoms may change over time (Alexopoulos, 1991). Matt et al. (1992) found in a community-based sample that more than half the subjects who reported depressive symptoms also reported significant anxiety, and the majority of subjects who endorsed symptoms of anxiety reported symptoms of more than one anxiety disorder. Gurian and Miner (1991) argue that the concept of anxiety in the elderly may be less helpful than such terms as "dysphoria" or "subjective distress" and a focus on the specific and particular symptoms of the individual patient. Flint (1994) notes, while significant comorbidity of anxiety and depressive disorders has been demonstrated in younger adults with prevalence figures ranging from 20% to 30%, much less research has looked at comorbidity of these disorders in the elderly. He concludes that rates appear to be similar in younger and older adults, but in most cases anxiety appears to be secondary to depression rather than vice versa.

With older adults in particular, determining whether certain psychological responses to stress are normal, or possibly even adaptive, can be complicated. Older adults may have more reasons to feel anxious given their increased social isolation, need for reliance on others, financial difficulties, health problems, and proximity to death (Flint, 1994). Verwoerdt (1980) argues that anxiety is the expected response to stress, and in old age, depletion anxiety, which refers to anxiety resulting from expected loss, is the most common. He argues that how one copes with stress changes as one ages, and he points to research which suggests that older adults may show smaller but longer lasting physiologic responses to stress for support of this contention. He contends that increased anxiety is related to the fear of being a burden to others, fear of abandonment, and loneliness.

Health professionals also may see adaptive or normal responses to aging as "pathological." Shamoian (1991) notes that an older adult who is constantly worried about falling and being mugged and who lives in a high-rise in an area with a high crime rate could meet criteria for generalized anxiety disorder, but treating this anxiety pharmacologically may not be efficacious. Similarly, the older adult who is losing peers to death and who acknowledges that his or her own death is more likely may talk more about death. Practitioners who are inexperienced with this population may misinterpret this as death anxiety or depression (Shamoian, 1991). While noting that anxiety and fearfulness may be a normal reaction to stress, Verwoerdt (1980) also notes that anxiety can be a first symptom of dementia, with patients presenting with "delusional fears, persecutory anxieties and paranoid fears" (p. 371).

Neuropsychologists may be better diagnosticians if they are aware of factors associated with an increased risk for development of anxiety disorders. For example, women consistently report more anxiety than men, physical illness is associated with an increased incidence of anxiety, and early parental loss is associated with development of phobic disorders, as well as depression (Flint, 1994). Hearing loss, visual impairment, and dementia also appear to be associated with a greater incidence of anxiety (Cohen, 1991; Gurian & Miner, 1991). At least one study found lower levels of anxiety among men who were institutionalized compared to those who resided in the community, but the opposite pattern was found in institutionalized women who reported higher levels of anxiety compared to the household sample (Flint, 1994). Gurian and Miner (1991) suggest that anxiety is common in personality disorders, particularly narcissistic, paranoid, and obsessive–compulsive personality disorders, and older adults who may initially present with anxiety symptoms may fail to respond to treatment due to these underlying traits. Awareness of these risk factors, as well as factors predictive of poor response to some forms of treatment, can help the interviewer in obtaining clinical information necessary for relevant and appropriate treatment recommendations.

Diagnostic and Statistical Manual of Mental Disorders Fourth Edition (DSM-IV) Anxiety Disorders

An exhaustive and detailed description of anxiety disorders is outside the realm of this chapter, and interested readers would be better served by referring to the most recent edition of the *DSM* or *DSM-IV* (American Psychiatric Association, 1994) for a review of anxiety disorders and their diagnostic criteria. In this section, each of the anxiety disorders are reviewed briefly, focusing specifically on information relevant to diagnosing these disorders in the elderly and prevalence rates of these disorders throughout the life span.

Obsessive–Compulsive Disorder

According to the *DSM-IV*, obsessive–compulsive disorder (OCD) is characterized by recurrent obsessions or compulsions that are ego-dystonic and time-consuming and that interfere with normal functioning. Obsessions refer to thoughts, ideas, or images which reoccur and are distressing or unwanted. Compulsions or compulsive behavior may result when patients engage in repetitive behavior in an attempt to reduce anxiety or cope with these obsessive thoughts.

The prevalence rate of OCD is not known exactly since patients with this disorder may be secretive about their symptoms and avoid seeking help (Rasmussen & Tsuang, 1984). Studies suggest that OCD typically begins in childhood, adolescence, or early adulthood (Jenike, 1983; Rasmussen & Tsuang, 1984). Epidemiologic studies examining the incidence of OCD have found that older adults are less likely, relative to younger adults, to meet diagnostic criteria for OCD. Prevalence rates for individuals over the age of 65 are estimated to be just under 1%, compared to just over 2% for 18- to 44-year-olds and just over 1% for 44- to 65-year-olds, with the data in general suggesting that the risk of developing OCD declines as one ages (Anthony & Aboraya, 1992). However, there is some suggestion that a closer examination of these rates may lead to different conclusions, with women showing a somewhat greater risk of developing OCD in later life (Anthony & Aboraya, 1992). Some studies suggest that OCD is associated with higher IQ, but much of this is based on clinical impression rather than systematic measurement (Rasmussen & Tsuang, 1984). Most studies have found that the severity of OCD lessens across the life span (Jenike, 1983; Rasmussen & Tsuang, 1984). Given the low incidence of onset after age 35 and reports of OCD being associated with neurologic illness, Jenike (1983) argues for full neurologic work-up of late-onset OCD patients. Data are conflicting on how depression and OCD symptoms interact, with some studies finding worsening depression associated with exacerbation of symptoms and others suggesting a decline in obsessions with worsening mood. (Jenike, 1983).

Anthony and Aboraya (1992) suggest that some checking behavior may be a way to cope with declining cognitive abilities in the cognitively impaired and in the elderly. They contend that this may, in part, explain the greater incidence in women, who are more likely to be engaging in behaviors that, if left unchecked or forgotten, could have more serious consequences (e.g., stoves left unattended or turned on).

Posttraumatic Stress Disorder and Acute Stress Disorder

According to the *DSM-IV* posttraumatic stress disorder (PTSD) and acute stress disorder (ASD) differ from other anxiety disorders in that they can be diagnosed only in individuals who have experienced an identifiable and severe stressor before the development of the characteristic symptoms of these disorders. Typically PTSD involves fear, helplessness, or horror in response to the trauma, followed by recurring memories of the event, attempts to avoid anything which reminds one of the event, and persistent increased arousal. Patients typically report feeling numb or removed and having difficulties feeling emotionally close to others or interested in previously pleasurable activities. Patients may complain of difficulty concentrating and may report amnesia or difficulty recalling details about the traumatic event.

Acute stress disorder was first introduced as a diagnosable anxiety disorder in the *DSM-IV*. It differs from PTSD primarily with regard to onset and duration of symptoms. Patients are given the diagnoses of ASD if distress occurs within 1 month of the stressor and lasts for a minimum of 2 days and if symptoms resolve within 4 weeks of the trauma. In addition, dissociation, derealization, and depersonalization seem to be more common as an acute reaction to an extreme stressor. When symptoms persist more than 1 month PTSD is diagnosed. Given the recency of the ASD diagnosis, very little research has been conducted involving patients identified with this disorder, and no data are available about how it varies across the life span.

Although it is the Vietnam Era veteran who has received the most attention with regard to PTSD, more recently, older adults, many of whom were exposed to combat during World War II or the Korean War, have been scrutinized for the presence of this disorder. It was estimated that up to 25% of all males who were over the age of 65 in 1994 were exposed to combat, which is clearly associated with an increased incidence of PTSD (Spiro, Schnurr, & Aldwin, 1994). The incidence of PTSD may vary with degree of combat exposure; veterans who saw heavy to moderate combat were 13 times more likely to endorse PTSD symptoms, even when measured 45 years following exposure (Spiro et al., 1994). This underscores the need for assessment of past traumatic experiences as well as recent life stressors in patients with anxiety symptoms.

Hermann and Eryavec (1994) found, in an institutionalized setting for veterans, that only 10% were on disability pensions due to wartime injuries, yet there was a 23% lifetime prevalence of PTSD, with 57% of those reporting chronic symptoms. Kaup, Ruskin, and Nyman (1994) found these symptoms were likely to be exacerbated by the common life stressors faced by the elderly such as retirement, loss of loved ones, and deteriorating health. Although an assessment of military experience may be fairly common in a Department of Veterans Affairs medical facility, it is less likely in other settings and may be less common, in both settings, during a neuropsychological as opposed to a psychiatric evaluation. Previously cited studies suggest that combat exposure or a history of other trauma may be widespread in other settings that treat older adults, particularly among World War II veterans who frequently receive health care outside the Department of Veterans Affairs medical system.

Clinicians also need to be aware that patients with a history of other significant trauma, such as being a prisoner of war (POW), are at extremely high risk for PTSD as well as other psychiatric disorders, with PTSD prevalence rates varying from 46% to 90% (Hermann & Eryavec, 1994). Physical trauma, including malnutrition and head injuries, as a result of these experiences also may need to be assessed. One recent study focusing on memory, attention, and executive deficits substantiated previous research and found that POWs showed compromised performance on neuropsychological test measures. These investigators then specifically examined whether starvation and psychological trauma contributed separately to this impairment (Sutker, Vasterling, Brailey, & Allain, 1995). They concluded that severe weight loss during captivity is associated with mild learning and memory deficits that resemble the pattern seen in Korsakoff's syndrome, with relative sparing of executive functions. Stress-related psychopathology or anxiety disorders appeared to be associated with deficits in attention and mental tracking, which they conclude is likely due to disruption in the arousal system and changes in the neurochemical systems resulting from prolonged exposure to stress.

While POW experiences may be relatively rare, other serious traumas during childhood or early adulthood should not be overlooked, given the significant impact these events can have on both psychological and neurological functioning later in life.

Phobias

Agoraphobia, specific (formerly called simple) phobias, and social phobia all involve intense fear and anxiety and result in avoidance of fear-provoking situations or stimuli. Agoraphobia, or anxiety in situations in which escape might be difficult or embarrassing or in which help may not be available, is typically manifested in avoidance of open spaces, being alone, crowds, and traveling. It may occur with or without panic attacks and differs from social phobia, where avoidance is limited to social situations and is related to fears of embarrassment. Specific phobia is much more circumscribed—fear is generated in response to a specific and identifiable stimulus (e.g., an object or a situation). Patients generally recognize these fears as unreasonable, and these fears only warrant a diagnosis when they cause significant impairment in functioning.

Although prevalence estimates of phobic disorders in older adults are slightly lower than those for the population in general (i.e., 5% vs. 6%), these disorders are not uncommon in the elderly (Anthony & Aboraya, 1992). However, older adults may neglect to talk about these embarrassing symptoms, or at least may not volunteer symptoms unless specifically asked (Lindesay, 1991). Lindesay and Banerjee (1993) noted that prevalence rates can vary between 4% and 26% within the same sample depending on the diagnostic system used. They also suggest that phobic symptoms, if not sufficient for a convincing diagnosis of a formal phobic disorder, are relatively common. Of all types of phobias surveyed, after the age of 65, simple or specific phobias are most common followed by agoraphobia and social phobias. Phobias also are unique in that, compared to many other psychiatric disorders in which incidence of onset varies across the life span, risk of developing a phobia seems to be as great late in life as during younger adulthood (Anthony & Aboraya, 1992). However, at least one study suggests that the type of phobia one develops may vary depending on age, with older adults more likely to develop situational agoraphobia and less likely to develop classic agoraphobia (Eaton & Keyl, 1990). The most common fears reported by older adults (i.e., animals, heights, and enclosed spaces) are likely to be lifelong fears, rather than phobias that necessarily have a late-life onset (Lindesay, 1991).

Many subjects link development of their phobias, particularly agoraphobia, to specific and traumatic life events such as episodes of physical illness, falls, or muggings (Flint, 1994). Agoraphobia, unlike simple phobias, seems more likely to have a late-life onset (Lindesay, 1991). Illnesses commonly reported as precursors to development of phobias include myocardial infarctions, respiratory symptoms, fractures, stroke, sudden onset of visual difficulties, and elective surgical procedures (Lindesay, 1991). Concomitant panic disorder, which is common in younger adults, is apparently rare in older adults (Flint, 1994). In contrast, a prior history of psychiatric disorder and concomitant depression is common in late-life onset of phobia (Lindesay, 1991). Subjects with phobias also report more physical symptoms such as palpitations, dyspnea, giddiness, and tinnitus (Lindesay, 1991).

Panic Disorder

Panic disorder is diagnosed when a patient suffers a panic attack and as a result develops significant anxiety about these attacks or significantly alters his or her behavior. The *DSM-IV* identifies 13 possible symptoms of a panic attack, the majority of which are somatic and include traditional anxiety symptoms such as fear and trembling as well as chest pain, nausea, and chills or hot flashes. Panic disorder may or may not be associated with agoraphobia.

The overall prevalence rate of panic disorder for adults older than 65 seems to be extremely small (i.e., 0.1%), and panic disorder is most likely to develop before the age of 65; however, certain medical disorders, particularly cardiovascular disorders, may predispose an older adult to the development of this symptom cluster later in life (Anthony & Aboraya, 1992). In a number of epidemiological studies, all cases identified as developing in late life were in females (Flint, 1994). Raj et al. (1993) argue that these prevalence studies seriously underestimate the incidence and importance of panic disorder in the elderly, since elderly subjects with panic disorder symptoms are not included in these statistics if an identifiable physical cause can contribute to the disorder. They retrospectively examined records of patients over 60 years of age who were referred to a university psychiatric geriatric service and found that approximately 6% were discharged with this diagnosis. They further conclude that stress, cardiac disease, Parkinson's disease, chronic obstructive pulmonary disease, and other stressful life events play a role in the development of this disorder in late life. While *DSM-IV* criteria would argue against diagnosing panic disorder in individuals who develop panic symptoms as a result of a medical condition, this does not mean the symptoms are not disruptive to the patient's functioning or amenable to treatment.

Generalized Anxiety Disorder

Generalized anxiety disorder (GAD) is a chronic condition in which patients report significant anxiety, the majority of the time for a period of at least 6 months. In addition, in order to meet *DSM-IV* criteria for this disorder, patients must endorse symptoms such as restlessness, fatigue, sleep disturbance, irritability, and muscle tension. This anxiety disorder differs from other anxiety disorders in that the anxiety is free-floating and not limited to a specific situation or condition. Although *DSM-IV* indicates that patients do not have to experience this anxiety as "excessive," the anxiety about specific situations, upcoming events, or the likelihood of a negative outcome must be grossly out of proportion to the actual likelihood of a negative event. Physical conditions which are caused or worsened by stress, such as headaches and irritable bowel syndrome, are common in patients diagnosed with GAD. In addition, Barbee and McLaulin (1990) cite studies suggesting that the most frequent finding in anxious older adults may be an abnormal liver function test related to these patients "secretly drink(ing) too much," in attempt to self-medicate their anxiety.

Epidemiological data on incidence of GAD suggest a prevalence rate between 1% and 7% for the elderly, a rate not substantially different for ranges reported for all adults over the age of 18 (Flint, 1994). There is some suggestion that GAD is not likely to develop after the age of 65. Blazer, George, & Hughes (1991) report that only 3% of elderly patients with GAD develop this disorder after the age of 65. Patients frequently describe suffering from this disorder most of their lives, but this disorder is apparently exacerbated by stress (American Psychiatric Association, 1994). Patients

who previously coped with anxiety through high levels of activity or other outlets when they were young may have more difficulty when age or disability prevents or interferes with these coping strategies.

Anxiety Disorder Due to General Medical Conditions and Adjustment Disorder with Anxiety

The *DSM-IV* indicates that anxiety disorder due to a general medical condition is the appropriate diagnosis when anxiety symptoms are the direct result of a medical condition which can be verified by physical exam, history, or laboratory findings. If anxiety results from the stress of being ill rather than the physical illness per se, then the correct diagnosis would be adjustment disorder. Although medical illness is common in older adults, there has been remarkably little research on anxiety in older, physically ill subjects (Flint, 1994).

Medical illness and concomitant disability may increase vulnerability to anxiety disorders (Lindesay, 1993). On the other hand, anxiety may be the first symptom of a medical illness. Sklar (1978) followed 300 patients over the age of 65 who were diagnosed with psychogenic gastric complaints for at least a year and found that 44% eventually were given diagnoses indicating that physical factors were playing a role in their complaints. "Dread, bewilderment, weakness, dizziness, respiratory distress, and/or sweating" are common as initial signs of myocardial infarction and following myocardial infarction (Cohen, 1991). Anxiety also is common with thyroid and endocrine problems, vitamin deficiencies, hypoglycemia, and pancreatic carcinoma (Cohen, 1991). Up to 75% of patients with pancreatic cancer exhibit both anxiety and depression as well as anorexia, back pain, and weight loss (Ouslander, 1984). Barbee and McLaulin (1990) list a number of cardiovascular disorders, respiratory disorders, endocrine disorders, and neurologic disorders that are known to cause anxiety symptoms. Specific anxiety disorders seem to be particularly problematic with certain medical conditions. Probable or definite panic disorder is described in as many as 83% of patients with cardiomyopathy, 16% of patients waiting for a new heart, 21% of patients with Parkinson's disease, and 16% of hospitalized chronic pain patients; it has also been described in epilepsy patients (Cassem, 1990).

In addition, because of the increased incidence of physical illness among the elderly, older adults are more likely to be taking prescription medications. The 1988 *Physicians' Desk Reference* (*PDR*) lists 150 medications that could cause anxiety as a side effect and 90 medications with a potential side effect of agitation (Cohen, 1991). Withdrawal from sedative-hypnotics, caffeine, and nicotine, as well as ingestion of stimulants, anorectics, analgesics, anticholinergics, sympathomimetics, neuroleptics, and diuretics, can all cause anxiety symptoms (Barbee and McLaulin, 1990). Screening for these causes of anxiety is necessary before diagnosing an anxiety disorder in any patient, but given the increased risk of side effects from medication in the elderly, concerns about iatrogenic causes of anxiety are particularly relevant.

Neurologic Disorders, Specific Brain Areas, and Anxiety Symptoms

Medical disorders in general increase risk of anxiety disorders and anxiety symptoms. Conditions affecting the central nervous system may have the greatest probability of causing psychological and behavioral changes, with specific conditions and specific brain areas being associated with predictable changes indicative of anxiety or "anxiety-like" symptoms. Following frontal lobe damage, repetitive behavior, even to the point of apparent obsessive-compulsive disorder, is not uncommon. Ames, Cummings, Wirshing, Quinn, and Mahler (1994) found that 78% of a sample of 46 "proven pathologic cases" of frontal lobe degeneration exhibited repetitive and compulsive behaviors. Typically these behaviors were not the presenting behavioral symptoms of this disorder and, on average, began approximately 3 years after other behavioral symptoms. However, in one case the compulsive behaviors were the first indication of a problem, preceding other behavioral changes by 2 years. They suggest, based on their review of the literature on frontal lobe degeneration, that these symptoms may be underassessed in this population. Further, they conclude that these behaviors are most likely to occur in cases of combined damage to the frontal

lobe, caudate nucleus, and globus pallidus. Specific disorders noted to be associated with obsessive–compulsive symptomatology include Huntington's disease, Parkinson's disease, neurocanthocytosis, hypoxic-ischemic caudate necrosis, Sydenham's chorea, progressive supranuclear palsy, carbon monoxide poisoning, anoxic-ischemic pallidal injury, manganese intoxication, encephalitis, diabetes insipidus, and head injury (Ames et al., 1994; Hollander, DeCaria, & Liebowitz, 1989; Jenike, 1983).

Orsillo and McCaffrey (1992) describe two patients who presented with anxiety symptoms that were later discovered to be the result of a right temporal lobe meningioma in one case and a left frontoparietal lobe glioblastoma in another. They also note the similarity in fear symptoms associated with some seizure activity and panic attacks. This may be indicative of a common neurologic mechanism underlying this type of anxiety reaction, but clinicians who treat these populations should be aware of the distinguishing factors in these two conditions (Orsillo & McCaffrey, 1992). A specific physical cause for panic attack or severe anxiety reaction is more likely to be found in patients with no personal or family history of psychiatric disorder, onset of symptoms after age 35, atypical and variable symptoms, an abnormal electroencephalogram (EEG), poor response to anxiolytics, and a positive response to anticonvulsants (Orsillo & McCaffrey, 1992).

Traumatic brain injury (TBI), in addition to causing OCD symptoms as noted above, can cause a variety of psychiatric symptoms. Both increased and decreased anxiety have been described following TBI, with both types of changes likely to result in poorer functioning for the patient. The patient may be easier to get along with and emotionally more stable. However, as Lezak (1995) notes, most patients who report better functioning due to decreased anxiety have family members or coworkers who are alarmed by the patient's lack of concern and or anxiety about things which normally provoke anxiety. In patients with increased anxiety it can be difficult to determine whether this is biologically based or the result of the stress associated with acquired disability, and research to date suggests that both factors may be important (Lezak, 1995).

Much less research has focused on the recovery curve or time course for psychological changes other than cognitive changes. At least one study suggests that anxiety and depression may actually become more prominent over time. For example, Fordyce, Roueche, and Prigatano (1983) found that patients who had sustained head injuries more than 6 months before the assessment reported greater distress than patients who were tested acutely (i.e., less than 6 months) after head injury.

The psychiatric manifestations of some specific neurologic conditions are well known. Psychiatric symptoms associated with Parkinson's disease are frequently described in the literature, and while a few authors review cases of obsessive-compulsive or anxiety symptoms, most have focused on depression and affective symptoms. While some studies have suggested prevalence rates of depression as high as 70%, others have found rates as low as 4% with a mean prevalence rate of 43%. Hantz, Caradoc-Davies, Caradoc-Davies, Weatherall, and Dixon (1994) contend that these rates are no greater than appropriately age- and sex-matched physically disabled controls. Additional research is needed to accurately characterize the frequency and nature of anxiety and depressive symptoms in this population.

The dementias and psychiatric and behavioral disturbances that can develop are familiar to most neuropsychologists who have had any exposure to these patients. Systematic study of affective and anxiety symptoms is difficult in this population due to communication and memory problems. It is not uncommon, in our clinic, to see a demented patient who the family describes as anxious or even frankly paranoid at home. During a clinical interview this same patient may appear calm and deny all distress. Likewise, increased agitation and anxiety in the clinical setting, as a reaction to this unfamiliar and threatening environment, is not surprising and should not be overinterpreted. One study examining premorbid anxiety and anxiety following development of senile dementia of the Alzheimer's type (SDAT) found no clear pattern or predictive factors to determine which patients would become more anxious (Yesavage & Taylor, 1991). In addition, these researchers found that a significant proportion of patients became less anxious than they were premorbidly after developing SDAT. Experience in our clinic suggests that this may be true in other types of dementia as well. One patient, an ex-POW

treated for many years for severe PTSD, became noticeably less anxious and stopped having nightmares as he became progressively more cognitively impaired due to a vascular dementia.

Although the majority of research on psychological difficulties following stroke has focused on depression, a study by Federoff et al. (1991) indicates that both depression and anxiety disorders are more common following stroke than in other serious and disabling medical conditions. Subsequent research, in which over 300 inpatients who were admitted with a diagnosis of stroke were administered a semi-structured clinical interview, revealed that approximately one quarter met criteria for GAD, and an additional 14% were classified as "worried," although they did not meet full criteria for GAD (Castillo, Starkstein, Federoff, Price, & Robinson, 1993). Similar to the findings in the stroke and depression literature, this study found that development of anxiety was related to specific brain areas affected by stroke, with specific symptom clusters more likely to be found with certain lesions. Castillo et al. (1993) concluded that anxiety without depression was more likely with right hemisphere lesions, while anxiety with concomitant depression was more commonly associated with left hemisphere lesions. Within the right hemisphere group, GAD was associated with posterior lesions while "worry" was associated with anterior lesions. In contrast to the findings in the depression and stroke literature, larger lesions did not appear to increase the likelihood of anxiety symptoms.

While psychiatric symptoms may be the direct result of changes in the central nervous system, life changes associated with these diseases also may contribute to the development of these disorders. Psychological reactions to neuropsychological deficits or to the injury that caused the deficits are prevalent. McCaffrey, Rapee, Gansler, and Barlow (1990) describe two cases of "space phobia" in which patients had an exaggerated fear of falling without support or in open spaces. They conclude that subtle disturbances in visuospatial functioning contributed to the development of this disorder. In our clinic, we have seen numerous anxiety reactions including panic attacks when falling asleep in a young adult patient who had an aneurysm rupture while sleeping; an avoidance of cars or extreme anxiety in cars following motor vehicle accidents;

and both PTSD and agoraphobia in a patient who sustained a closed head injury while in a large bunker during a SCUD missile attack.

Blanchard, Hickling, Taylor, Loos, and Gerardi (1994) found that nearly half of 50 patients who sought medical treatment following a motor vehicle accident met criteria for PTSD, and half of those met criteria for major depression as well. Another 20% had PTSD symptoms, without meeting criteria for this diagnosis. In our clinic, we treated an elderly patient who had suffered a mild closed head injury in a plane crash during World War II. Although he apparently had mild PTSD symptoms throughout his adult life, the PTSD symptoms worsened and he developed OCD after age 60. A computerized tomography (CT) scan and neuropsychological testing were suggestive of early vascular dementia. Similarly, Cassidy and Lyons (1992) present a case study of a World War II combat veteran who developed PTSD symptoms, including dissociative episodes and intrusive thoughts following a stroke. These cases suggest that acquired neuropsychological deficits in combination with premorbid characteristics and life experiences can contribute to development of psychiatric symptoms.

The role of brain abnormalities in the etiology of specific anxiety disorders has been suggested for many years. The many case reports of OCD following recovery from encephalitis described in the early part of this century led to the hypothesis that all cases of OCD are neurologic, rather than psychodynamic in origin. In addition, patients diagnosed with OCD have been found to be more likely to show soft signs of neurologic abnormalities, including abnormalities in fine motor coordination and visuospatial functioning and involuntary motor movements (Aronowitz et al., 1994; Hollander et al., 1989; Jenike, 1983). Cingular lesions have been found to be associated with an improvement in OCD symptoms, leading to suggestions that an overactive cingulum is responsible for this disorder (Jenike, 1983). For the most part nonpsychotic patients with OCD have normal EEGs, and no differences have been consistently demonstrated in MRIs (Kellner et al., 1991). Most reviews of this literature suggest that abnormalities in the frontal, cingulate, limbic, and basal ganglia areas are implicated in OCD (Aronowitz et al., 1994).

While older adults may be at an increased risk of developing OCD symptoms, given their increased risk of the many neurologic disorders noted to cause these symptoms, age-associated brain changes may result in a lower risk for development of other anxiety symptoms. Flint (1994) cites studies implicating the limbic system and brain stem in anxiety disorders. Other studies suggest that there is a significant loss of cells in the locus ceruleus and decreased noradrenaline and increased monoamine oxidase in normal aging. In addition, panic attacks, thought to be related to levels of monoamine neurotransmitters, may be less common in later adulthood due to age-associated declines in these neurotransmitters (Anthony & Aboraya, 1992).

Sunderland, Lawlor, Martinez, and Molchan (1991) conclude after reviewing the literature on the neurobiology of anxiety and aging that it is inappropriate to assume that neurobiological factors influence anxiety in the same manner across the life span. They note that neurotransmitters are important in both anxiety and in changes seen in normal aging. However, they also recognize that there is no single neurotransmitter system and that it is not simply the level of neurotransmitters that accounts for symptoms of anxiety and changes linked to normal aging, but the balance between these systems.

The Influence of Anxiety on Neuropsychological Test Performance

There exists a fairly convincing body of evidence that anxiety influences cognition, but controversy remains regarding how and to what extent it influences cognition. Anxiety often causes subjects to perform most tasks more slowly and less accurately. However, in some situations, for example when a narrow focus and ignoring irrelevant information are beneficial, anxious subjects may do better than control subjects (Leon, 1989). Leon's (1989) study, as well as other studies she cites, suggests that anxious subjects may generate internal task-irrelevant information which may strain memory capacity, or for some other reason, they may not allocate all their attentional resources to the task at hand. Overall the literature suggests that working memory and initial encoding of information are most affected by anxiety, while more automatic tasks are not affected (e.g., Bradley, Mogg, & Williams, 1994; Darke, 1988; Hill & Vandervoort, 1992; MacLeon & Donnellan, 1993).

A number of studies suggest that increased anxiety results in a decline in performance, while others find that anxiety is most strongly associated with self-reported deficits rather than documented impairment. West, Boatwright, and Schlesler (1984) had elderly subjects rate anxiety, depression, and memory abilities and administered tests of memory to them. While both anxiety and depression rating scales were strongly associated with ratings of memory performance, they were not correlated with actual memory performance. In another study with cardiac patients, anxiety was associated with an increase in reports of cognitive dysfunction, while neuropsychological test performance was not significantly related to increased anxiety or depression (Newman et al., 1989).

King, Hannay, Masek, and Burns (1978) found a significant correlation between self-reported anxiety and performance on two timed tasks, the finger tapping and form board tests, but only for female college students. Although this result may be related to actual gender differences in the way anxiety influences performance, they note that only the female subjects in their study endorsed significant anxiety symptoms. Although many studies have found a relationship between distress ratings and performance, there may be an equal number of studies that fail to find a relationship. At a minimum, we must conclude that anxiety does not negatively influence all cognitive tasks in all individuals, and complaints of cognitive dysfunction may be a symptom of psychological distress rather than a sign of compromised functioning in at least some patients who complain of anxiety and depressive symptoms.

While there may be some similarities in how depression and anxiety influence cognitive performance, there also are significant differences. While the Yerkes Dodsen Law and its prediction that there is a curvilinear relationship between anxiety and performance is well known, there are no suggestions that there is a curvilinear relationship between depression and cognitive function. In addition, unlike depressed patients who are more likely to recall negative or depressing information, patients with anxiety are not more likely to recall anxiety-provoking information (Bradley et al., 1994; Foa, McNally, & Murdock, 1989; Mogg, Mathews, & Weinman, 1987).

After reviewing the arousal literature, Talland (1968) suggested that the elderly were more susceptible to interfering effects of anxiety on cognition and more likely to benefit from attempts to reduce anxiety associated with testing situations. However, the degree to which differences in anxiety explain age differences remains controversial. Although they failed to find that older adults are more susceptible to deleterious effects of anxiety on reasoning and problem-solving, La Rue and D'Elia (1985) found that both middle-aged and older adults showed an inverse relationship between performance and reports of anxiety. Research has shown that depressive and anxiety symptoms frequently occur together, but virtually no research has examined whether anxiety symptoms, depressive symptoms, or a combined index of distress is the best predictor of how an individual will perform on cognitive tests.

Specific anxiety disorders have been hypothesized to be associated with specific deficits on neuropsychological tests. Various studies examining neuropsychological functioning in patients with OCD have found impairment in set shifting, set maintenance, establishing set, visuospatial and visuoconstructional abilities, attention, speeded tasks, and memory (Aronowitz et al., 1994; Zielinski, Taylor, & Juzwin, 1991). Gordon (1985) notes that patients with OCD tend to make decisions much more slowly, and in contrast to patients with phobia and a normal control group, they tended to make decisions even more slowly in reaction to stress. This research is not without controversy. Zielinski et al. (1991) found patients with OCD to show greater deficits on nonverbal tasks and to score equal to or better than controls on language tasks and "measures of frontal lobe functioning," whereas other studies suggest impairment on frontal/executive tasks and verbal memory tasks.

Aronowitz et al. (1994) note inconsistent findings among studies examining the influence of OCD on neuropsychological test performance. They criticize this research for methodological problems, including small sample sizes, heterogeneity within the sample, and a lack of comprehensiveness within the evaluations. Their study, with a larger sample and well-matched controls, supported previously noted deficits in set shifting, set maintenance, establishing set, visuospatial and visuoconstructional abilities, attention, and memory. They also found that these deficits were more prominent in males.

The variability within these patients and the notion that there may be subgroups within this diagnosis is supported by studies in which OCD patients were divided into groups depending on whether they had a history of impulsiveness (Hoehn-Saric & Barksdale, 1983). They found impulsiveness and acting out (i.e., behavior described as potentially harmful to the patient and/or society, such as sexual excesses, spending sprees, and excessive drinking) typically predated the onset of OCD symptoms. They suggest that, for this impulsive subgroup, OCD symptoms may have developed as an attempt by patients to cope with fears of losing control of their behavior. Rasmussen (1994) also argues for existence of different subgroups of patients with OCD. He describes one subgroup as having co-morbid tics, low anxiety, and more compulsive personality traits and suffering from "incompleteness" or a need to have things "perfect or just so." Another subgroup has high anxiety, developmental history of behavioral inhibition, and comorbidity of other anxiety disorders. His experience leads him to suggest that these two groups also differ in their response to serotonin reuptake inhibitors and therefore may differ at the neurotransmitter level.

Patients with diagnosis of PTSD often complain of memory and concentration difficulties. Most studies examining neuropsychological test performance in patients with PTSD have focused on memory and attention tasks, and some of these have found abnormalities in patients with PTSD compared to controls; no significant differences were found on tests of general intellectual abilities (e.g., Bremner et al., 1993; Uddo, Vasterling, Brailey, & Sutker, 1993). However, other studies have found either no or only small differences between patients with this diagnosis and a control group (e.g., Dalton, Pederson, & Ryan, 1989; Zalewski, Thompson, & Gottesman, 1994). These inconsistencies seem to be related to both sampling differences and the cognitive tests chosen to evaluate for deficits.

One study comparing combat veterans with and without PTSD for neurologic soft signs and neuropsychological test performance is particularly thought-provoking (Gurvitz et al., 1993). They found that Vietnam Era veterans with PTSD had significantly more neurologic soft signs than similar veterans without PTSD, and that these soft signs correlated significantly with neuropsychological test performance (Gurvitz et al., 1993). While they argue that these signs represent acquired neurologic impairment, they acknowledge that it is equally plausible that these neurologic abnormalities increase risk of development of PTSD. It may be that these preexisting factors or interaction between these preexisting factors and this psychiatric disorder result in memory and attention deficits.

Age-Related Cognitive Differences and Anxiety

One proposed explanation for age-related cognitive differences is that older adults are more anxious in a psychological testing situation than their younger counterparts, and this anxiety interferes with both attention and memory (e.g., Craik, 1980; Eysenck, 1979; Smith, 1980). Differences between anxiety levels have not been substantiated as a sufficient explanation for age-related memory differences. Consistent between-group differences have been found even when younger and older adults are matched for anxiety and when younger adults are more anxious than the older adult sample (Poon, 1985).

This is not to say anxiety plays no role in cognition or performance on cognitive tasks in the elderly adult. Yesavage and Jacob's (1984) study with older adults suggested that neither training in mnemonic techniques nor relaxation training alone had positive effects on their memory and attention task, but a positive effect was demonstrated when these two forms of training were combined. Their study, as well as others they cite, demonstrated that relaxation training and concomitant anxiety reduction can have a positive influence on some cognitive tasks in both younger and older adults. In an earlier study relaxation alone resulted in improvement in memory performance in older adults with higher levels of anxiety, while the performance on memory tasks declined among subjects with lower levels of anxiety following relaxation training (Yesavage, 1984). They also maintain that learning complicated mnemonics can provoke anxiety in older adults, which is why older adults benefited from relaxation training prior to teaching the mnemonic.

Treatment of Anxiety in the Elderly

A brief review of the treatment literature seems relevant since the neuropsychologist who identifies an older adult with an anxiety disorder may have more training in psychiatric diagnosis and treatment than other health professionals who will see this patient. Therapists and other clinicians who are treating the patient also may turn to the neuropsychologist with questions about the client's ability to understand concepts and instructions that are an integral part of the therapeutic process. Increased awareness about possible interventions, (e.g., simple environmental alterations, pharmacological treatment, and behavioral interventions) can greatly enhance the neuropsychologist's ability to assist the patient, other health care providers, and the patient's family in locating and providing the best possible care for the patient.

Unfortunately, this literature is somewhat limited. In general, older adults, like younger adults, should benefit from both pharmacotherapy and psychotherapy (Verwoerdt, 1976). Although appropriate cautions are given regarding use of these powerful medications and the greater risk of side effects in older adults, there has been little research focusing on the efficacy of treatment of the elderly or neurologically compromised patients using either medication or psychotherapy. For neuropsychologists who are asked to provide treatment recommendations for patients with both anxiety symptoms and compromised cognitive abilities, there are few studies examining the degree to which cognitive impairment interferes with efficacy of psychotherapy; the literature on how this might be done or might be different from working with younger and neurologically normal clients is limited. Treatment approaches clearly will vary depending on the types of problems present in the patient. Patients who feel comfortable with an examiner after a lengthy neuropsychological evaluation may confide details about life situations that may be remedied or altered to

decrease anxiety. Verwoerdt (1980) notes that treatment may begin with identifying ways to provide support or assistance in such basic areas as finances, housekeeping, legal aid, or social contacts. He also suggests the need to balance this assistance such that sufficient support is provided to minimize realistic anxiety, but not so much support that regression would be encouraged. Neuropsychologists, given their knowledge of the patient's strengths and limitations, and by using information gained through reassessments to document changes in cognitive functioning, can provide useful information regarding what is enough support and may be able to alert care providers when additional support is needed.

There are few studies specifically examining the efficacy of either behavioral or psychodynamic treatment for anxiety in the elderly, but there is a convincing body of evidence that behavioral techniques can significantly decrease anxiety. Kooken and Hayslip (1984) found that elderly students benefited from both stress inoculation and an attention placebo, compared to a wait list control group, and showed the greatest reduction in anxiety with the stress inoculation treatment. Johnson (1991) provides case studies suggesting that psychotherapy can be used effectively with both neurologically normal and mildly demented elderly to reduce anxiety.

Specific anxiety disorders and treatment in the elderly have been examined. For example, older adults tend to have a poorer outcome when diagnosed with GAD, but this may be related to the elderly receiving worse care rather than a relative ineffectiveness of treatment in this population (Lindesay, 1993). Not surprisingly, given the relative rarity of OCD, few controlled studies have been conducted specifically examining treatment efficacy in the elderly. Calamari, Faber, Hitsman, and Poppe (1994) review case studies published on elderly subjects with OCD and conclude that older adults respond similarly to pharmacotherapy, with the caution that older adults may be at greater risk for side effects. They note that there exists almost no literature on the efficacy of psychotherapy alone, but they do cite a few case studies describing successful outcomes with elderly patients with OCD treated with both medication and behavioral therapy. Reviews of the literature on behavioral and pharmacologic treatment of OCD and agoraphobia consistently indicate that medications are easy to prescribe, use, and monitor but they also have side effects, and patients tend to relapse when medication is discontinued; behavioral treatments are described as taking more time for the professional, causing greater discomfort for the patient, more difficult to monitor, but more likely to produce lasting change (Cottraux, 1989; Marks, 1986; Marks & O'Sullivan, 1988). Marks and O'Sullivan (1988) argue for the use of medication only as a last resort, when patients fail or refuse behavioral approaches.

The tendency of physicians to quickly prescribe pharmacologic treatment rather than psychotherapy (Lindesay, 1993) may be related in part to beliefs that memory impairment or other cognitive difficulties prevent effective psychotherapy in older adults and particularly in cognitively impaired older adults. The well-known increased susceptibility of older adults to medication side effects provides a compelling argument, at a minimum, for a trial of nonpharmacologic treatment since behavioral treatments are unlikely to result in physical dependence, increased cognitive impairment, drowsiness, and incontinence, which have all been reported with benzodiazepine use in the elderly (Lindesay, 1993). However, Gurian and Miner (1991) suggest that patients may respond best to the treatment approach that they have the most confidence in, and older adults, like younger adults, should be informed of treatment options and be allowed to choose for themselves. In addition, Barbee and McLaulin (1990), in their review of the literature on safety of pharmacotherapy with the elderly, contend that there is no evidence of increased susceptibility to dependence or greater risk of complications following cessation of benzodiazepines.

Salzman (1991) has reviewed the literature examining efficacy of pharmacologic treatment of anxiety with the elderly and identified 19 studies on benzodiazepines. However, he notes that it is difficult to conclude much from these studies given the vague use of the term anxiety and the difficulty in diagnosing an anxiety disorder. In addition, almost all studies included hospitalized or nursing home patients, most subjects were not asked or were unable to describe subjective changes, and there was no distinction between primary anxiety and anxiety as part of another medical or psychiatric condition. Given the lack of controlled studies, it is difficult to make recommendations regarding medication of the older adult patient for anxiety symptoms. Pomara, Deputla, Singh, and Monroy (1991), in a review of the literature on the cognitive effects of benzodiazepines, conclude that the elderly are not necessarily more susceptible to cognitive side effects, but partial tolerance seems to develop. However, as in younger adults, memory, attention, and motor skills are affected by these drugs, and these difficulties persist even after several weeks and are measurable in the morning, even among patients taking these medications only in the evening.

Given concerns about side effects of medications and skepticism about the feasibility of behavioral techniques with cognitively impaired clients, there may be a temptation to forego attempts at treating an anxiety disorder. Although most of us do not think of anxiety as lethal, Cohen (1991) and Shamoian (1991) cite studies that suggest that increased anxiety is associated with higher mortality, although underlying factors for this association remain unclear. Cohen (1991) concludes that the cases in which psychological intervention following heart attacks and surgery results in better outcomes and shorter hospital stays indicate that anxiety may be an "aggravating factor" in these physical illnesses. These studies suggest that appropriate treatment of anxiety may not only enhance a patient's quality of life but also maximize the use of increasingly limited health care dollars.

Summary and Implications for Clinicians and Researchers

A better understanding of the nature of anxiety and anxiety disorders in older adults offers opportunities for neuropsychologists to improve diagnostic accuracy, enhance clinical care, and conduct additional research.

The clinician attempting to identify cognitive dysfunction and establish the etiology of the identified deficits needs to consider the role of anxiety in this dysfunction. Talland (1968) suggests that older adults are likely to benefit from efforts to reduce anxiety and arousal in the test-taking situation. Some of Bolton's (1978) suggestions for enhancing the elderly student's performance in the classroom are relevant for the testing laboratory as well. Such things as allowing sufficient time to master new test procedures and instructions, minimizing negative feedback, and praising effort should have a beneficial effect on all examinees, but may be particularly helpful with older adults. Kooken and Hayslip (1984) cite studies that suggest that older adults react more strongly (i.e., show greater performance decrements) and react more negatively to failure, which they contend results in greater anxiety. Recognizing the older adult's greater susceptibility to the interfering effects of anxiety and minimizing this anxiety should provide assessments that are a better reflection of the older adult's optimal level of functioning.

Recognizing anxiety and the possibility of an anxiety disorder is a necessary first step in making an accurate diagnosis. Gathering sufficient information, or even recommending additional tests before diagnosing or dismissing symptoms, could be crucial in assuring appropriate intervention and preventing inappropriate and possibly harmful treatment. Neuropsychologists need to ensure that an assessment of anxiety symptoms is a standard part of any neuropsychological evaluation.

Clinical neuropsychologists asked to make treatment recommendations have the opportunity to address both cognitive and noncognitive factors that can influence the client's ability to benefit from and participate in treatment. Reducing anxiety in the elderly can result in older adults learning mnemonic techniques, and this notion is relevant for clinicians attempting to teach older adults other information that may enhance their physical or psychological health. While some neuropsychologists evaluate and treat patients, most will refer some, if not all, clients to other clinicians for treatment of psychological disorders. These clinicians need to be educated about the influence of anxiety on cognition before attempting interventions that require elderly patients to learn how to use memory aids, alter cognitions to reduce anxiety or depression, or use medical equipment. Noncompliance in patients is frustrating to all health care professionals and is likely to result in less than optimal treatment outcome.

Neuropsychologists may assist patients by informing other health care providers about a patient's cognitive and psychiatric difficulties which may limit or interfere with the patient's ability to comprehend and follow treatment recommendations.

Particularly with elderly patients who appear anxious, clinicians may want to ensure that anxiety is minimized before initiating training or giving instructions. In addition, they may want to provide instructions in writing or give them to a family member in order to enhance the likelihood of compliance. Ley (1979) examined the influence of many factors, including age and anxiety, on recall of medical information. He concludes that age is not consistently related to rate of recall, while anxiety appears to have a curvilinear relationship. Even when working with normal elderly, an awareness of how anxiety can affect compliance is important.

Neuropsychologists involved in research also benefit from a broader knowledge base and understanding of anxiety disorders. Most studies of anxiety disorders in the elderly begin by excluding those who are cognitively impaired (e.g., Lindesay, 1991), both when focusing on the description of anxiety in the elderly and when examining the efficacy of treatment. Neuropsychologists, with their access to neurologically impaired and anxious patients, can contribute in a variety of ways. Basic research is needed to better determine how anxiety presents in neurologically impaired patients and to evaluate whether current measures of anxiety reliably and validly assess anxiety in this population. Neuropsychologists can suggest treatment approaches, assist with research to determine whether these therapies can be modified to treat patients who are both anxious and brain impaired, and document the effectiveness of these interventions. In addition, measures of anxiety need to be routinely included in drug studies with which neuropsychologists are likely to be involved. Research investigating influence of pharmacological interventions with demented patients, even when targeting cognitive abilities, have found that these treatments may influence anxiety without affecting cognitive abilities (Ferris, Sathananthan, Gershon, & Clark, 1977). Future medication studies, designed to measure changes in cognition or affect, may be improved by the inclusion of measures of anxiety.

Anxiety is clearly a significant problem throughout the life span and provides both challenges and opportunities for clinicians and researchers. By taking advantage of opportunities for intervention and research, neuropsychologists can significantly improve patient care and contribute to our knowledge of the causes and remedies for anxiety in the older adult.

References

Alexopoulos, G. S. (1991). Anxiety and depression in the elderly. In C. Salzman & B. Lebowitz (Eds.), *Anxiety in the elderly: Treatment and research* (pp. 63–77). New York: Springer.

American Psychiatric Association. (1994). *Diagnostic and statistical manual of mental disorders* (4th ed.). Washington, DC: Author.

Ames, D., Cummings, J. L., Wirshing, W. C., Quinn, B., & Mahler, M. (1994). Repetitive and compulsive behaviors in frontal lobe degeneration. *Journal of Neuropsychiatry, 6,* 100–113.

Anthony, J. C., & Aboraya, A. (1992). The epidemiology of selected mental disorders in later life. In J. E. Birren, R. B. Sloane, G. D. Cohen, N. R. Hooyman, B. D. Lebowirtz, M. H. Wyle, & D. E. Deutschman (Eds.), *Handbook of mental health and aging* (2nd ed.). San Diego: Academic Press.

Aronowitz, B. R., Hollander, E., DeCaria, C., Cohen, L., Saoud, J. B., Stein, D., Liebowitz, M. R., & Rosen, W. G. (1994). Neuropsychology of obsessive compulsive disorder. *Neuropsychiatry, Neuropsychology, and Behavioral Neurology, 7,* 81–86.

Barbee, J. G., & McLaulin, J. B. (1990). Anxiety disorders: Diagnosis and pharmacotherapy in the elderly. *Psychiatric Annals, 20,* 439–445.

Blanchard, E. B., Hickling, E. J., Taylor,, A. E., Loos, W. R., & Gerardi, R. J. (1994). Psychological morbidity associated with motor vehicle accidents. *Behavior Research and Therapy, 32,* 283–290.

Blazer, D., George, L. K., & Hughes, D. (1991). The epidemiology of anxiety disorders: An age comparison. In C. Salzman & B. Lebowitz (Eds.), *Anxiety in the elderly: Treatment and research* (pp. 17–30). New York: Springer.

Bolton, E. B. (1978). Cognitive and noncognitive factors that affect learning in older adults and their implications for instruction. *Educational Gerontology, 3,* 331–344.

Bradley, B. P., Mogg, K., & Williams, R. (1994). Implicit and explicit memory for emotional information in non-clinical subjects. *Behavior Research and Therapy, 32,* 65–78.

Bremner, J. D., Scott, T. M., Delaney, R. C., Southwick, S. M., Mason, J. W., Johnson, D. R., Innis, R. B., McCarthy, G., & Charney, D. S. (1993). Deficits in short term memory in posttraumatic stress disorder. *American Journal of Psychiatry, 150,* 1015–1019.

Calamari, J. E., Faber, S. D., Hitsman, B. L., & Poppe, C. J. (1994). Treatment of obsessive compulsive disorder in the elderly: A review and case example. *Journal of Behavior Therapy and Experimental Psychiatry, 25,* 95–104.

Cassem, E. H. (1990). Depression and anxiety secondary to medical illness. *Psychiatric Clinics of North America, 13,* 597–612.

Cassidy, K. L., & Lyons, J. A. (1992). Recall of traumatic memories following cerebral vascular accident. *Journal of Traumatic Stress, 5,* 627–631.

Castillo, C. S., Starkstein, S. E., Federoff, J. P., Price, T. R. & Robinson, R. G. (1993). Generalized anxiety disorder after stroke. *Journal of Nervous and Mental Disease, 181,* 100–106.

Cohen, G. D. (1991). Anxiety and general medical disorders. In C. Salzman, & B. Lebowitz (Eds.), *Anxiety in the elderly: Treatment and research* (pp. 47–62). New York: Springer.

Cottraux, J. (1989). Behavioral psychotherapy for obsessive-compulsive disorder. *International Review of Psychiatry, 1,* 227–234.

Craik, F. I. M. (1980). Age differences in memory: The role of attention and depth of processing. In L. W. Poon, J. L. Fozard, L. S. Cermack, D. Arenberg, & L. W. Thompson (Eds.), *New directions in memory and aging: Proceedings of the George A. Talland Memorial Conference.* Hillsdale, NJ: Lawrence Erlbaum Associates.

Dalton, J. E., Pederson, S. L., & Ryan, J. L. (1989). Effects of posttraumatic stress disorder on neuropsychological test performance. *International Journal of Clinical Neuropsychology, 11,* 121–124.

Darke, S. (1988). Effects of anxiety on inferential reasoning task performance. *Journal of Personality and Social Psychology, 55,* 499–505.

Davidson, H. A., Dixon, R. A., & Hultsch, D. F. (1991). Memory anxiety and memory performance in adulthood. *Applied Cognitive Psychology, 5,* 423–433.

Eaton, W. W. & Keyl, P. M. (1990). Risk factors for the onset of DIS/DSM-III agoraphobia in a prospective population based study. *Archives of General Psychiatry, 47,* 819–824.

Endler, N. S., Cox, B. J., Parker, J. D., & Bagby, R. M. (1992). Self reports of depression and state-trait anxiety: Evidence for differential assessment. *Journal of Personality and Social Psychology, 63,* 832–838.

Eysenck, M. W. (1979). Anxiety, learning, and memory: A reconceptualization. *Journal of Research in Personality, 13,* 363–385.

Fechner-Bates, S., Coyne, J. C., & Schwenk, T. L. (1994). The relationship of self-reported distress to depressive disorders and other psychopathology. *Journal of Consulting and Clinical Psychology, 62,* 550–559.

Federoff, J. P., Lipsey, J. R., Starkstein, S. E., Forrester, A., Price, T. R., & Robinson, R. G. (1991). Phenomenological comparisons of major depression following stroke, myocardial infarction, and spinal cord lesions. *Journal of Affective Disorders, 22,* 83–89.

Ferris, S. H., Sathananthan, G., Gershon, S., & Clark, S. (1977). Senile dementia: Treatment with deanol. *Journal of the American Geriatrics Society, 25,* 241–244.

Flint, A. J. (1994). Epidemiology and comorbidity of anxiety disorders in the elderly. *American Journal of Psychiatry, 151,* 640–649.

Foa, E. B., McNally, R., & Murdock, T. B. (1989). Anxious mood and memory. *Behavior Research and Therapy, 27,* 141–147.

Fordyce, D. J., Roueche, J. R., & Prigatano, G. P. (1983). Enhanced emotional reactions in chronic head trauma patients. *Journal of Neurology, Neurosurgery, and Psychiatry, 46,* 620–624.

Gordon, P. K. (1985). Allocation of attention in obsessional disorder. *British Journal of Clinical Psychology, 24,* 101–107.

Gurian, B. S., & Miner, J. H. (1991). Clinical presentation of anxiety in the elderly. In C. Salzman & B. Lebowitz (Eds.), *Anxiety in the elderly: Treatment and research* (pp. 31–44). New York: Springer.

Gurvitz, T. V., Lasko, N., Schacter, S. C., & Kuhne, A. A., Orr, S. P., & Pittman, R. K. (1993). Neurological status of Vietnam veterans with chronic posttraumatic stress disorder. *Journal of Neuropsychiatry and Clinical Neurosciences, 5,* 183–188.

Hantz, P., Caradoc-Davies, G., Carodoc-Davies, T., Weatherall, M., & Dixon, G. (1994). *American Journal of Psychiatry, 151,* 1010–1014.

Hermann, N., & Eryavec, G. (1994). Posttraumatic stress disorder in institutionalized World War II veterans. *American Journal of Geriatric Psychiatry, 2,* 324–331.

Hill, R. D., & Vandervoort, D. (1992). The effects of state anxiety on recall performance in older learners. *Educational Gerontology, 18,* 597–605.

Hoehn-Saric, R., & Barksdale, V. C. (1983). Impulsiveness in obsessive-compulsive patients. *British Journal of Psychiatry, 143,* 177–182.

Hollander, E., DeCaria, C., & Liebowitz, M. R. (1989). Biologic aspects of obsessive compulsive disorder. *Psychiatric Annals, 19,* 80–87.

Jenike, M. A. (1983). Obsessive compulsive disorder. *Comprehensive Psychiatry, 24,* 99–115.

Johnson, F. A. (1991). Psychotherapy of the elderly anxious patient. In C. Salzman & B. Lebowitz (Eds.), *Anxiety in the elderly: Treatment and research* (pp. 215–248). New York: Springer.

Kaup, B. A., Ruskin, P. E., & Nyman, G. (1994). Significant life events and PTSD in elderly World War II veterans. *American Journal of Geriatric Psychiatry, 2,* 239–243.

Kellner, C. H., Jolley, R. R., Holgate, R. C., Austin, L., Lydiard, R. B., Laraia, M., & Ballenger, J. C. (1991). Brain MRI in obsessive-compulsive disorder. *Psychiatry Research, 36,* 45–49.

King, G. D., Hannay, H. J., Masek, B. J., & Burns, J. W. (1978). Effects of anxiety and sex on neuropsychological tests. *Journal of Consulting and Clinical Psychology, 46,* 375–376.

Kooken, R. A., & Hayslip, B., Jr. (1984). The use of stress inoculation in the treatment of test anxiety in older students. *Educational Gerontology, 10,* 39–58.

La Rue, A., & D'Elia, L. F. (1985). Anxiety and problem solving in middle-aged and elderly adults. *Experimental Aging Research, 11,* 215–220.

Leon, M. R. (1989). Anxiety and inclusiveness of information processing. *Journal of Research in Personality, 23,* 85–98.

Ley, P. (1979). Memory for medical information. *British Journal of Clinical Psychology, 18,* 245–255.

Lezak, M. D. (1995). *Neuropsychological assessment.* New York: Oxford University Press.

Lindesay, J. (1991). Phobic disorders in the elderly. *British Journal of Psychiatry, 159,* 531–541.

Lindesay, J. (1993). Neurotic disorders in the elderly. *International Review of Psychiatry, 5,* 461–467.

Lindesay, J., & Banerjee, S. (1993). Phobic disorders in the elderly: A comparison of three diagnostic systems. *International Journal of Geriatric Psychiatry, 8,* 387–393.

MacLeod, C., & Donnellan, A. M. (1993). Individual differences in anxiety and the restriction of working memory capacity. *Personality and Individual Differences, 15,* 163–173.

Marks, I. (1986). Behavioral and drug treatment of phobic and obsessive-compulsive disorders. *Psychotherapy and Psychosomatics, 46,* 35–44.

Marks, I., & O'Sullivan, G. (1988). Drugs and psychological treatment for agoraphobia/panic and obsessive–compulsive disorders: A review. *British Journal of Psychiatry, 153,* 650–658.

Matt, G. E., Dean, A., Wang, B., & Wood, P. (1992). Identifying clinical syndromes in a community sample of elderly persons. *Psychological Assessment, 4,* 174–184.

McCaffrey, R. J., Rapee, R. M., Gansler, D. A., & Barlow, D. H. (1990). Interaction of neuropsychological and psychological factors in "space phobia." *Journal of Behavioral Therapy and Experimental Psychiatry, 2,* 113–120.

Mogg, K., Mathews, A., & Weinman, J. (1987). Memory bias in clinical anxiety. *Journal of Abnormal Psychology, 96,* 94–98.

Newman, S., Klinger, L., Venn, G., & Smith, P., Harrison, M., & Treasure, T. (1989). Subjective reports of cognition in relation to assessed performance following coronary artery bypass surgery. *Journal of Psychosomatic Research, 33,* 227–233.

Orsillo, S. M., & McCaffrey, R. J. (1992). Anxiety disorders. In A. E. Puente & R. J. McCaffrey (Eds.), *Handbook of neuropsychological assessment.* New York: Plenum.

Ouslander, J. G. (1984). Psychiatric manifestations of physical illness in the elderly. *Psychiatric Medicine, 1,* 363–387.

Pomara, N., Deputla, D., Singh, R., & Monroy, C. A. (1991). Cognitive toxicity of benzodiazepines in the elderly. In C. Salzman & B. D. Lebowitz (Eds.), *Anxiety in the elderly: Treatment and research* (pp. 175–196). New York: Springer.

Poon, L. W. (1985). Differences in human memory with aging: Nature, causes, and clinical implication. In J. E. Birren & K. W. Schaie (Eds.), *Handbook of the psychology of aging* (2nd ed., pp. 427–462). New York: Van Nostrand Reinhold Company.

Raj, B. A., Corvea, M. H., & Dagon, E. M. (1993). The clinical characteristics of panic disorder in the elderly: A retrospective study. *Journal of Clinical Psychiatry, 54,* 150–155.

Rasmussen, S. A. (1994). Obsessive compulsive spectrum disorders. *Journal of Clinical Psychiatry, 55,* 89–91.

Rasmussen, S. A., & Tsuang, M. T. (1984). The epidemiology of obsessive compulsive disorder. *Journal of Clinical Psychiatry, 45,* 450–457.

Salzman, C. (1991). Pharmacologic treatment of the anxious elderly patient. In C. Salzman & B. Lebowitz (Eds.), *Anxiety in the elderly: Treatment and research* (pp. 17–30). New York: Springer.

Shamoian, C. A. (1991). What is anxiety in the elderly? In C. Salzman & B. Lebowitz (Eds.), *Anxiety in the elderly: Treatment and research* (pp. 3–15). New York: Springer.

Sheikh, J. I. (1991). Anxiety rating scales for the elderly. In C. Salzman & B. Lebowitz (Eds.), *Anxiety in the elderly: Treatment and research* (pp. 251–265). New York: Springer.

Sklar, M. (1978). Gastrointestinal diseases in the aged. In W. Reichel (Ed.), *Clinical aspects of aging.* Baltimore: Williams & Wilkins.

Smith, A. D. (1980). Age differences in encoding, storage, and retrieval. In L. W. Poon, J. L. Fozard, L. S. Cermack, D. Arenberg, & L. W. Thompson (Eds.), *New directions in memory and aging: Proceedings of the George A. Talland Memorial Conference*. Hillsdale, NJ: Lawrence Erlbaum Associates.

Spielberger, V. D. (1983). *Manual for the State-Trait Anxiety Inventory STAI* (Form Y). Palo Alto, CA: Consulting Psychologists Press.

Spiro, A., Schnurr, P. P., & Aldwin, C. M. (1994). Combat-related post traumatic stress disorder symptoms in older men. *Psychology and Aging, 9*, 17–26.

Sunderland, T., Lawlor, B. A., Martinez, R. A., & Molchan, S. E. (1991). Anxiety in the elderly: Neurobiological and clinical interface. In C. Salzman & B. Lebowitz (Eds.), *Anxiety in the elderly: Treatment and research* (pp. 17–30). New York: Springer.

Sutker, P. B., Vasterling, J. J., Brailey, K., & Allain, A. N. (1995). Memory, attention, and executive deficits in POW survivors: Contributing biological and psychological factors. *Neuropsychology, 9*, 118–125.

Talland, G. A. (1968). *Human aging and behavior: Recent advances in research and theory*. New York: Academic Press.

Uddo, M., Vasterling, J. J., Brailey, K., & Sutker, P. (1993). Memory and attention in combat related PTSD. *Journal of Psychopathology and Behavioral Assessment, 15*, 43–52.

Verwoerdt, A. (1976). *Clinical geropsychiatry*. Baltimore: Waverly Press.

Verwoerdt, A. (1980). Anxiety, dissociative and personality disorders in the elderly. In E. W. Busse & D. G. Blazer (Eds.), *Handbook of geriatric psychiatry* (pp. 368–380). New York: Van Nostrand Reinhold Company.

West, R. L., Boatwright, L. K., & Schlesler, R. (1984). The link between memory performance, self-assessment, and affective status. *Experimental Aging Research, 10*, 197–200.

Yesavage, J. A. (1984). Relaxation and memory training in 39 elderly patients. *American Journal of Psychiatry, 141*, 778–781.

Yesavage, J. A., & Jacob, R. (1984). Effects on relaxation and mnemonics on memory, attention, and anxiety in the elderly. *Experimental Aging Research, 10*, 211–214.

Yesavage, J. A., & Taylor, B. (1991). Anxiety and dementia. In C. Salzman & B. Lebowitz (Eds.), *Anxiety in the elderly: Treatment and research* (pp. 79–85). New York: Springer.

Zalewski, C., Thompson, C., & Gottesman, W. (1994). Comparison of neuropsychological test performance in PTSD, generalized anxiety disorder, and control Vietnam veterans. *Assessment, 1*, 133–142.

Zielinski, C. M., Taylor, M. A., & Juzwin, K. R. (1991). Neuropsychological deficits in obsessive-compulsive disorder. *Neuropsychiatry, Neuropsychology, and Behavioral Neurology, 4*, 110–126.

8

Psychotic Disorders in Late Life

GERALD GOLDSTEIN

Definitions

The term "psychosis" has changed over time and become more specific. The earlier *Diagnostic and Statistical Manuals of Mental Disorders (DSM-I and DSM-II)* (American Psychiatric Association, 1952, 1968) made a distinction between "psychotic" and "nonpsychotic" organic brain syndromes based mainly upon severity. That terminology was abandoned in the initial version of *DSM-III* (American Psychiatric Association, 1980) and has not been restored. Thus, some patients we would now diagnose as having dementia would have been diagnosed as having a "psychotic" condition if the dementia was severe. It is interesting to note the further progression of this redescriptive process in *DSM-IV* (American Psychiatric Association, 1994). Here, the term dementia is not abandoned, but is characterized as a cognitive disorder. This definition takes us even further from the concept of psychosis as it is generally understood, implying severe disorganization of the personality. The term psychosis in current usage is now mainly restricted to schizophrenia and bipolar disorder. The *DSM-IV* does not specifically characterize bipolar disorder as psychotic and limits that term to schizophrenic, schizoaffective, and delusional disorders. This chapter adopts that convention, but we will briefly consider psychotic features, notably delusions and hallucinations, that are frequently associated with some forms of dementia. We will deal largely with schizophrenia. A detailed presentation of late-onset psychotic conditions and schizophrenia in old age is contained in a volume by Miller and Cohen (1987) to which the reader is referred for more detailed information than can be presented here. It is noted that while schizophrenia may be a life-shortening disease, many schizophrenic patients live relatively long lives and may continue to suffer from symptoms of the disorder throughout those lives.

The Course of Schizophrenia

It is particularly interesting to observe that just as severe dementia was characterized as psychosis, schizophrenia was once called dementia. Its original name, coined by Morel (1860), was *dementia-praecox*, and the condition was later divided into dementia-praecox and manic–depressive psychosis by Kraepelin. Eugen Bleuler (1952) first introduced the term "schizophrenia." The term dementia-praecox was devised because of the commonly observed poor outcome of the disorder. It was therefore initially considered to be a progressive, degenerative dementia, with the term praecox added because of its early onset relative to the presenile and senile dementias. The issue that concerns us is just that matter. Is schizophrenia a form of abnormal or premature aging?

Research addressing this matter has involved clinical, epidemiological, and neuropsychological approaches. The epidemiological and clinical studies appear to have reached the consensus that schizophrenia is not, for the most part, a degenerative progressive disorder. The impression that it was may have been created by an observer artifact since clinicians located in institutional settings only saw patients who relapsed and required further inpatient

GERALD GOLDSTEIN • Highland Drive Veterans Affairs Medical Center, Pittsburgh, Pennsylvania 15206; and Departments of Psychiatry and Psychology, University of Pittsburgh, Pittsburgh, Pennsylvania 15213.

care, but they did not see other patients initially treated for schizophrenia who remained clinically stable in the community for many years, if not indefinitely (Bleuler, 1978). Thus, the patients who were seen constituted a biased sample, and one can see how the impression of deterioration may have been created.

A number of extensive epidemiological studies have indicated that the outcome of schizophrenia is better than initially thought, and that while patients do not become "cured" of the disorder, they may maintain life in the community over long time periods, particularly if they comply with medication schedules and other treatments, as indicated. Current concepts of the course of schizophrenia largely involve matters of episodes and relapse. Many, if not most, schizophrenic patients have an initial episode of psychosis manifested largely by the positive symptoms of the disorder (e.g., hallucinations, delusions), recover from that episode, and are then described as stabilized. Stabilization usually implies absence of frank psychotic symptoms and capability of leaving an institutional setting and returning to reasonably independent living in the community. At some later time symptoms may reappear and the individual is said to have relapsed. A major cause of relapse is thought to be noncompliance with medication, but it is apparently not the only cause (Hogarty, Goldberg, Schooler, & Ulrich, 1974). Much research effort has been spent on attempting to predict when an individual may relapse, so that preventive measures can be taken (van Kammen et al., 1995).

Thus, it is currently reasonably well accepted that schizophrenia is not a degenerative dementia, but rather an episodic disorder marked by intermittent appearance of symptoms, sometimes requiring rehospitalization, separated by sometimes lengthy periods of stability marked by the absence of prominent symptoms. It is assumed that the schizophrenia is still there during the periods of stability, but is not active. This point is unfortunately often illustrated when individuals fail to comply with medication schedules and relapse. There is a point of view that individuals with schizophrenia are particularly sensitive to stress, and that medication may serve to relieve that sensitivity (van Kammen et al., 1995). A more general theory of schizophrenia, "vulnerability theory," maintains that schizophrenia is a condi-

tion of increased vulnerability to stress (Zubin & Spring, 1977). Some of that vulnerability may be inherited, while some of it may be acquired. The proposed neurobiology of the course of schizophrenia suggests that it is produced by an event that occurs relatively early in life that generates dysfunction in some crucial area of the brain, perhaps the prefrontal region (Goldberg & Weinberger, 1988; Goldberg, Weinberger, Berman, Pliskin, & Podd, 1987; Weinberger, Berman, & Zec, 1986) or the left temporal-limbic system (Gruzelier, 1991). The event is time-limited and is not progressive. Individuals with schizophrenia are therefore thought to have a static encephalopathy that is nonprogressive yet permanent. The details of this process is a mystery since we don't know what produces it or what constitutes its specific nature. Nevertheless, these considerations help to explain why middle-aged and elderly individuals with schizophrenia often do not show the memory failure and other cognitive losses of individuals with Alzheimer's disease. Obviously, a major exception is those individuals with schizophrenia who also have Alzheimer's disease or organic dementias associated with other causes. Comorbidity with substance abuse, notably alcoholism, is not infrequent among schizophrenic patients (Alterman, 1985).

Some Exceptions

While schizophrenia is usually described as nondegenerative, episodic, and beginning during young adulthood, there are several important exceptions. Jeste (1993) has recently suggested that schizophrenia that begins during the second half of life may be more common than was once believed. With regard to age of onset, the disorder known as *paraphrenia* has to be considered. This disorder has been thoroughly reviewed by Roth (1987), but briefly, paraphrenia is a disorder with onset past age 55 and is primarily manifested by paranoid symptoms. Historically, it has been characterized as "presenile delusional insanity," and its relationship with schizophrenia has been debated over the years. Apparently, there are some resemblances and some differences. Roth has made the following distinctions within paraphrenia, as follows: (1) late paranoia, characterized by growing suspiciousness and persecutory delusions; (2) late paraphrenia with "reactive" features in which there are bizarre delusions and hallucinations; and (3) "endogenous" late paraphrenia which is marked by symptoms that resemble paranoid schizophrenia in early life, such as persecutory and erotic delusions, auditory hallucinations, and passivity feelings. Interestingly, individuals with these disorders frequently have sensory loss, mainly deafness. An exemplary case of paraphrenia was observed by Goldstein (unpublished observations). The patient was an elderly man, who after retirement from a long, successful career developed the belief that he was being pursued by invisible men who were harassing him and stealing his property. During conversations with him on topics other than this belief, he was entirely normal. However, the belief was unshakable, and he was entirely unresponsive to pharmacological treatment with regard to abandoning the belief.

The other major exception is a subgroup of schizophrenic individuals who have been described as having Kraepelinian or poor-outcome schizophrenia (Keefe et al., 1987). The group is a small one, representing no more than 15% of the schizophrenic population. These patients are described as "Kraepelinian" because they apparently have a course consistent with Kraepelin's views concerning the outcome of dementia-praecox. More specifically, they have a 5-year history of continuous hospitalization or an inability to provide themselves with the basic necessities of living. These patients do not demonstrate the more typical course of partial or total remission intermixed with relapse. It is thought that their course is, in fact, a deteriorating one.

A third possible exception to the rule concerning a stable course is the late-life improvement seen in some schizophrenic patients. This area has been reviewed by McGlashan (1987) who quotes M. Bleuler's remark: "In old age, schizophrenics may not only become less excited, less aggressive, and less active regarding their delusions, but many of them start to develop an active inner life, true interests, and a sounder activity than before." McGlashan, using data from the Chestnut Lodge follow-up study, concluded that a small group of patients with chronic schizophrenia do improve, the extent of improvement ranging from amelioration of disruptive behaviors to significant, but not total, return of normal function.

Psychotic Behaviors in Nonschizophrenic Elderly Individuals

The *DSM-IV* indicates that delusions are common in dementia and that hallucinations may occur in any sensory modality, however, they are mainly visual. The delusions are generally persecutory (things stolen, relatives after money) and typically do not have a bizarre quality. The hallucinations are not well understood and may sometimes be a function of neurological visual gnostic disturbances producing distorted or incomplete recognition of objects. Hallucinations have also been described as a form of "sensory tic" or recurrent somatic sensation (Koziol & Stout, 1994). Such tics in the visual or auditory system may be experienced as hallucinations, but they can be understood within the framework of the neuropathology of dementia. Delusions are far more common than hallucinations in dementia. Cummings (1985) identified delusions in half of a sample of patients with Alzheimer's disease or multi-infarct dementia. Consistent with the *DSM-IV* he indicates that most of the delusions found in patients with cortical dementias are of the simple paranoid type (theft or infidelity), but patients with subcortical dementias (e.g., Huntington's disease) are more likely to have complicated delusions. In most cases, these phenomena are not of sufficient magnitude to call for the diagnosis of psychotic disorder.

In the *DSM-IV*, it is possible to make the diagnosis of dementia of the Alzheimer's type with delusions (290.20), vascular dementia with delusions (290.42), or psychotic disorder due to a general medical condition (293.81 or 293.82). In this last condition, there must be prominent delusions (293.81) or hallucinations (293.82) produced by a general medical condition. Psychotic behavior can also be seen during the course of delirium, which may be superimposed on a preexisting dementia, but these symptoms should disappear when the delirium is resolved.

Schizophrenia and Aging: Neuropsychological Investigations

While schizophrenia may be a life-shortening disease (Allebeck, 1989), with improved health care and advances in medical research, it is likely that increasing numbers of individuals with schizophrenia will live a full life span. It therefore becomes important to know what the schizophrenic faces in old age and what health care resources may be required. One crucial issue is the matter raised above concerning cognitive deterioration in schizophrenia. While the clinical evidence suggests that schizophrenia is, for the most part, not a progressive dementia, the point can be better documented through established aging or age-difference research methods, using objective tests of cognitive function. These studies may be longitudinal or cross-sectional in design, but since each method has its own deficiencies, it would probably be best to draw conclusions based on a combination of longitudinal and cross-sectional studies.

It is well established that most schizophrenic individuals perform more poorly than normal controls on most cognitive tests. This phenomenon, commonly characterized as the "general deficit syndrome" (Chapman & Chapman, 1973), apparently occurs in schizophrenia across ages and from the time of onset of the illness. Apparently, the neurobiological changes that produce these deficits have done their work prior to appearance of the clinical phenomenology of the illness, and indeed, preliminary suggestions of cognitive inefficiencies may be observed retrospectively from early in life, or they may be seen in a reduced form in relatives of schizophrenic patients (Condray, Steinhauer, & Goldstein, 1992). From the standpoint of aging research, the schizophrenic, at some beginning marker age, starts from a different baseline than the normal individual. Thus, an assessment of the elderly schizophrenic that produces abnormal findings may be mistaken as evidence of deterioration when, in fact, the patient's performance reflects the patient's baseline combined with whatever changes may be anticipated on the basis of normal aging. Some years ago, a major distinction was proposed between good and poor premorbid schizophrenia or process and reactive schizophrenia (Garmezy, 1970), and even earlier, E. Bleuler coined the term *propfschizophrenie* to describe a group of patients in whom the schizophrenia appeared to be "grafted" onto mental retardation. These developmental considerations would appear to have clear implications for outcome. Furthermore, Waddington (1993) has

indicated that the subtle effects of normal aging may interact in schizophrenia with an already developmentally compromised brain giving the appearance of deterioration when, in fact, there is no evidence of an active progressive disease associated with the original event that produced the schizophrenia.

The matter of whether aging in schizophrenia is normal can be investigated with longitudinal or cross-sectional research in which the interaction between age and group membership (schizophrenic or appropriate control in this case) can be examined. In an extensive literature review, Heaton and Drexler (1987) inferred that "cognitive functioning in schizophrenia is not abnormally or dramatically affected by age" (p. 161). However, that conclusion was not based entirely on studies using this design. Heaton and collaborators (1994) confirmed that view in a study that compared patients with schizophrenia and patients with Alzheimer's disease using an expanded Halstead-Reitan neuropsychological test battery (HRB) (Reitan & Wolfson, 1993).

Differences between Young and Old Schizophrenic Patients: The Goldstein and Zubin Study

The premature aging or interaction design was directly implemented in a large-sample cross-sectional study by Goldstein and Zubin (1990). The investigation used data from the Halstead-Reitan neuropsychological test battery (HRB) (Reitan & Wolfson, 1993) and the Wechsler Adult Intelligence Scale (WAIS) (Wechsler, 1955). Subjects were divided into relatively young and old groups based upon a median split, and schizophrenic subjects were compared with a sample of patient controls. The younger subjects averaged about 30 years of age while the older subjects averaged about 52 years of age. The schizophrenic patients were subdivided into a group with neurological comorbidity and a group without neurological comorbidity. Neurological comorbidity was defined as the presence of a neurological disorder other than schizophrenia or neurological dysfunction as manifested by some diagnostic procedure (e.g., abnormal electroencephalogram [EEG] or positive findings on the neurological examination). The controls consisted of patients with a variety of medical and psychiatric disorders and were also divided into subgroups consisting of patients with and without neurological disorders. While numerous significant differences were found between young and old subjects, and between schizophrenic and nonschizophrenic subjects regardless of age, the findings of greatest interest are in the interactions. In the case of the schizophrenics without neurological comorbidity, of the 23 HRB and WAIS variables considered, there were only two significant interactions. Among the schizophrenic subjects with neurological comorbidity, there were 10 significant interactions. The characteristic pattern obtained is illustrated in Figure 1, using Halstead Category Test data. The Category Test has been reported to be highly correlated with age in non-brain damaged samples, and that seems to be the case here. The old controls made many more errors than the young controls. It has also been reported that individuals with schizophrenia do more poorly on this test than do normals (Braff et al., 1991), a finding that also exists here. However, the curves are almost exactly parallel, with no indication of an interaction. Thus, there is no evidence of a disproportionate age difference in schizo-

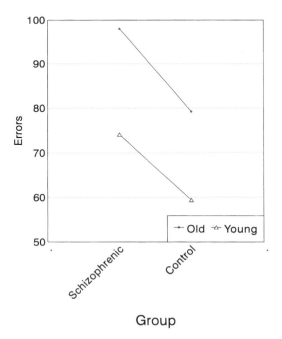

FIGURE 1. Halstead Category Test results for old and young schizophrenic subjects.

phrenic patients, but only the anticipated difference in level of performance across ages. As indicated, this pattern emerged in all but two of the tests.

The findings for the schizophrenic patients with neurological comorbidity had a different pattern. There were many significant interactions, but they existed almost exclusively on tests involving language specifically or those with an important linguistic component. These significant interactions were found for all of the WAIS verbal subtests except for Digit Span, for the Picture Completion and Block Design subtests, and for the Speech Perception, Trail Making B, and Aphasia Screening tests from the HRB. With the exception of Block Design, there were no significant interactions for complex, nonverbal problem-solving tests from the WAIS or the HRB.

It was concluded from this study that there does not appear to be an abnormal deterioration of cognitive abilities in neurologically intact schizophrenic patients. This conclusion was based on the relatively consistent absence of a significant interaction between age and diagnostic group across numerous tests of cognitive function. The second major conclusion was that certain cognitive tests produced an interaction between group and age in the schizophrenic patients with neurological comorbidity. The nature of these relationships is illustrated in Figure 2. The WAIS Arithmetic subtest was used as an example because it produced a significant interaction in the comorbid but not in the neurologically intact schizophrenic group. The figure shows that there is no age-related effect on this test in the neurologically intact control group. There are moderate effects in the neurologically impaired control group and the intact schizophrenic group, as well as a large effect, reaching statistical significance, in the schizophrenic group with neurological comorbidity.

While the study involved a cross-sectional design, it was felt that a cohort effect was not a major influence for several reasons. First, the samples were drawn from a very homogeneous population of male veterans hospitalized at Department of Veterans Affairs medical facilities. Second, a cohort phenomenon would not be consistent with the differences found between neurologically impaired and intact schizophrenic patients. Third, Heaton and Drexler (1987) indicated that their final conclusion

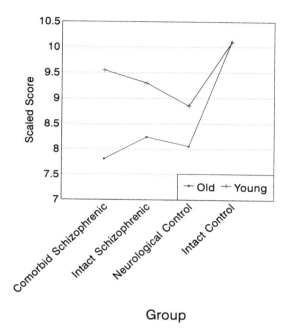

FIGURE 2. Wechsler Adult Intelligence Scale (WAIS; Wechsler, 1955) Arithmetic subtest results for old and young schizophrenic subjects with and without comorbidity, and for controls with and without neurological dysfunction.

A Possible Cohort Effect: The WAIS Comprehension Subtest

The two significant interactions between age and group for the neurologically intact schizophrenic group were for Part B of the Trail Making test and the WAIS Comprehension subtest. The latter finding, illustrated in Figure 3, was of particular interest for two reasons. First, performance on Comprehension has not been found to be age-related, but is more associated with education. Educational differences were not found in the Goldstein and Zubin study. Second, in the neurologically intact control group, the old group obtained a slightly higher mean score than the young group (10.80 vs. 10.56). These considerations would suggest that the obtained interaction may not be a true age-related effect, but may be a cohort effect. That is, the level of social cognition or judgment that this test is thought to assess may vary among schizophrenic veterans across generations.

The large majority of the patients in the Goldstein and Zubin study were assessed between 1965

about the absence of remarkable age-related deterioration in schizophrenic individuals was based upon both cross-sectional and longitudinal studies.

It would seem that there is good agreement among clinical, longitudinal, and neuropsychological studies regarding the absence of abnormal deterioration across a large part of the schizophrenia spectrum. The main proviso we would add is that maintenance of neurological health is an important consideration. When neurological dysfunction is present, there may be significant deterioration, perhaps more related to the neurological disorder itself than the schizophrenia. This relationship between schizophrenia and health, however, is not completely straightforward because schizophrenia may be a risk factor for a variety of medical disorders. We will not document the relevant epidemiology here, but only take note of the commonly observed co-occurrence of schizophrenia with a substance use disorder and the propensity of schizophrenic individuals, particularly in noninstitutional settings, to acquire infectious and diet-related disorders.

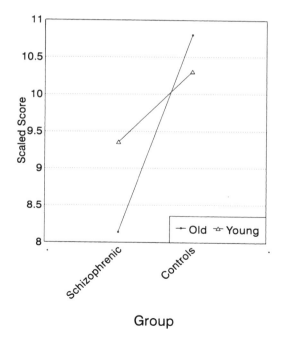

FIGURE 3. WAIS Comprehension subtest results for old and young schizophrenic subjects.

and 1975. Thus, the old group (mean age = 52) would have been born between the world wars. They would be mainly World War II veterans. The members of the younger group (mean age = 30) were born mainly during or after World War II, and many of them were therefore Vietnam Era veterans. Many of them would be classified as baby boomers for whatever cultural significance that might have.

Since the publication of the Goldstein and Zubin study, we have had the opportunity to assess a new cohort of schizophrenic patients tested during the 1990 to 1994 period. A median split of these 86 patients did not produce the same wide age disparity as in the original study, but the findings were nevertheless of interest. The old group had a mean age of 49 while the young group had a mean age of 36. The relatively old group then consisted largely of Vietnam Era veterans, while the relatively young group would typically have been too young to serve in Vietnam and were mainly peacetime veterans. The results comparing this new cohort with various subgroups in the Goldstein and Zubin study are presented in Figure 4. The most remarkable finding is that the young group in the new cohort performed

significantly less well on WAIS Comprehension than did the old group. The difference was statistically significant [$t(80) = 2.24$, $p = .03$], and it was the only significant difference among all of the WAIS Verbal subtests. Looking at level of performance, the old group had about the same mean score as the old schizophrenics in the Goldstein and Zubin study, but there was a dramatic difference between the young cohorts (9.33 vs. 6.76). It therefore seems clear that the results for the Comprehension subtest cannot be viewed as age-related with respect to cognitive decline, but appear to reflect the performance of varying cohorts of veterans on this measure of social cognition and judgment. Whether or not this phenomenon is specific to schizophrenia, or even more specific to schizophrenic veterans, can only be obtained following collection of appropriate control data.

In the Goldstein and Zubin paper, we suggested that whatever abnormal cognitive deterioration occurs in schizophrenic individuals seems to mainly affect semantic knowledge abilities that are influenced by sociocultural stimulation. These abilities tend to remain stable across age in normal individuals, and, in fact, diminished only slightly in the neurologically intact schizophrenics. The new data suggest that group differences on tests of these abilities may not be specifically age-associated, but may reflect levels of sociocultural stimulation in different cohorts. However, taking all of the data together, it seems necessary to postulate a complex model involving an interaction among neuropsychology-related considerations, age, history of environmental stimulation, and neurological comorbidity. One possible explanation is that schizophrenic individuals brought up during a generation characterized by strong environmental stimulation and support will not show age-associated deterioration of semantic knowledge unless they acquire neurological comorbidity. However, schizophrenic individuals may demonstrate poor semantic knowledge abilities regardless of age or presence of comorbidity, if they were brought up in an unsupportive atmosphere. Thus, the mean WAIS Comprehension score of our young subjects in the 1990 cohort (6.76) was lower than the comparable mean score (8.03) for the subjects with comorbidity in the 1965–1975 cohort. An alternative view that the 1990 cohort simply consisted of more impaired patients was not

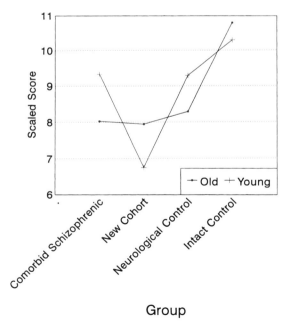

FIGURE 4. WAIS Comprehension subtest results for old and new cohorts of schizophrenic subjects and controls.

supported by examination of data from some of the complex problem-solving tests contained in the HRB. The mean scores in the younger and older groups for the Category and Tactual Performance tests, for example, were almost identical to those obtained in the original study. Thus, differences in generalized cognitive deficit do not appear to explain these findings.

Age, Schizophrenia, and Institutionalization

Another form of cohort effect may be iatrogenic in nature. For many centuries, individuals with the disorder now known as schizophrenia were frequently restricted to institutions following onset of the illness, often until death. Even in the most benign and sophisticated of these institutional settings, it was proposed by a number of clinicians and social scientists that institutionalization, particularly long stays in what were described as total institutions, was in and of itself detrimental to outcome. A forceful and effective program of advocacy, probably culminating in the publication of Goffman's book *Asylums: Essay on the social situation of mental patients and other inmates* (1961), led to the deinstitutionalization movement marked by large-scale discharge of schizophrenic patients from mental hospitals and development of the community mental health center as a more ideal treatment modality. Currently, many of the older large mental hospitals have closed or are only minimally used, and the length of hospitalization for schizophrenia is quite brief, rarely lasting beyond the reduction of acute symptoms and stabilization on medication.

While this program went forward, dramatically altering the face of treatment of schizophrenia, the underlying assumption regarding the detrimental effects of prolonged institutionalization was never carefully, scientifically evaluated. The common wisdom was that the effect was pervasive, involving morale, motivation, self-esteem, development of inordinate dependency, and possibly, cognitive ability. Thus, the possibility was raised that the cognitive deterioration originally attributed to the schizophrenia was, in fact, largely a product of living for many years in a total institution, a term

suggesting provision by the institution of all one's needs, with very little time spent outside of its walls. We therefore have a possible cohort effect in which only schizophrenics institutionalized over a long time period will show a pattern of cognitive deterioration previously thought be to produced by the schizophrenia itself. Individuals not part of a cohort institutionalized for many years, although schizophrenic, may not show such deterioration. Furthermore, nonschizophrenic individuals incarcerated for long time periods may develop some of the symptoms typically associated with schizophrenia. Indeed, the question has been asked whether prisoners develop behaviors that look like the so-called negative symptoms generally associated with schizophrenia (Zubin, 1985).

Unfortunately for advocates of these views, the small amount of data available are not particularly confirmatory. Johnstone, Owens, Gold, Crow, and Macmillan (1981) compared changes in cognitive test scores in groups of schizophrenic individuals who were in or out of hospitals over the same time period between assessments. Cognitive deficits were found in both groups, but no more so in one group than in the other. Similarly, Harrow, Marengo, Pogue-Geile, and Pawelski (1987) found no cognitive differences between continuously hospitalized and intermittently hospitalized schizophrenic patients. Goldstein and Halperin (1977) found that schizophrenic patients with more than 1 year of hospitalization performed more poorly on the HRB than a group hospitalized less than 1 year, but that finding was not confirmed by Goldstein, Zubin, and Pogue-Geile (1991). These investigators, also using measures from the HRB, found that apparently detrimental effects associated with length of hospitalization disappeared when chronological age was taken into consideration. That is, the cognitive deterioration found in long-term hospitalized schizophrenic patients appeared to be no greater than what could be anticipated on the basis of chronological age.

With regard to the negative or deficit symptoms of schizophrenia, Zubin (1985) has suggested that these symptoms are not intrinsic to schizophrenia, but rather are "secondary disabilities" associated with premorbid personality or result from the social and medical consequences of being ill. He suggests that they are not indigenous to schizophrenia but may be found in association with depression or in non-patients who are isolated or incarcerated for long periods of time. The basic issue is the modifiability of the symptoms with treatment or environmental change. For example, these kinds of symptoms may disappear in prisoners shortly after they are released, but may not disappear in schizophrenic patients following completion of an episode and discharge from a hospital.

It seems that long-term institutionalization does not make an independent contribution to cognitive deterioration. That is not to say that it may not have other detrimental consequences, perhaps in interaction with premorbid personality characteristics. However, in contemporary treatment, it is often necessary to weigh these possible negative consequences against what may occur in a sometimes unsupportive community environment. Various solutions have been offered to this dilemma, including sheltered living arrangements, such as halfway houses or community nursing homes, respite programs, and perhaps the least desirable alternative, continued hospitalization in a long-term care facility. The respite programs are of particular interest. These programs were initiated originally to help relieve the family burden for individuals with dementia. The relative with dementia would be housed in a sheltered setting while the family took its vacation or conducted business necessitating leaving home. It has recently been applied to schizophrenic individuals and is used in part for family respite, but also for patients who appear to be approaching relapse or who have had a relapse not requiring acute care. These patients are briefly hospitalized and may receive supportive treatment or adjustment of their medication. They typically return to community living following discharge.

Despite these progressive efforts, there remains a residual population of primarily elderly schizophrenic patients who remain in long-term care psychiatric facilities. These are the patients who do not do well in sheltered living or nursing home facilities largely because of behavioral problems associated with their psychoses. Informal observation of these patients and some formal testing suggest that these patients have a number of common characteristics. Many of them would meet diagnostic criteria for the residual subtype of schizophrenia, with some exceptions. They have predominantly negative symptoms, but may maintain their odd beliefs and some degree of bizarre language. However, they appear to require continued psychiatric hospitalization because of potentially disruptive behaviors, notably unprovoked shouting, or poor self-care activities of daily living. They are rarely aggressive, but tend to have poor social skills, and they may not have the preserved social amenities often seen in even very deteriorated patients with Alzheimer's disease. It is suspected that many of them have significant neurological comorbidity, often as a result of substance abuse, progressive dementia, or other medical conditions. The proportion of these patients who have the biological basis for Kraepelinian or poor-outcome schizophrenia is an interesting but unanswered question.

Heterogeneity of Outcome

It is apparent from all of these considerations that schizophrenia in old age may show many faces, from the individual with late-life remission who functions effectively and independently in the community to the severely disabled individual who cannot survive outside of a psychiatric care facility. Reasons for optimism about the course of schizophrenia have been based upon observation of individuals of the first type, and treatment and management efforts may be effectively directed toward achieving that kind of possible outcome. Important considerations include a supportive environment, maintenance of medication schedules and other treatments, maintenance of neurological good health, the availability of respite care, and a treatment philosophy based on the view that relapses are likely to occur, but that they have a beginning and end and do not necessitate prolonged hospitalization. Prevention of relapse through appropriate intervention has become a major treatment issue. The investigation of the conditions that precipitate or at least precede relapses with the aim of forestalling them has become a major research effort.

If the individual is endowed with a high premorbid level of functioning and does not sustain severe neurological damage in association with the etiological event for schizophrenia, those considerations also help. Concepts such as "brain reserve" and threshold theory (Satz, 1993) may ultimately be useful in reaching a further understanding of schizophrenia in individual cases. It now seems well established with advanced magnetic resonance imaging technologies that there are substantial correlations between quantitative measures of brain volume and cognitive function in schizophrenia (Kareken et al., 1995). Several investigators have proposed that there are subtypes of schizophrenia based upon severity of cognitive dysfunction (Goldstein, 1994). In our own work, we have tried to show that schizophrenia is a cognitively heterogeneous disorder, with varying levels and patterns of cognitive function (Goldstein, 1990). It would therefore appear that the varied outcome in schizophrenia may be determined in part by neurobiological events that are as yet poorly understood, but may also be influenced by appropriate treatment and management.

Schizophrenia or psychosis in general in the elderly is best understood as a life span phenomenon. In that way, these disorders are quite different from Alzheimer's disease in which there may be a perfectly normal life until symptoms begin to appear in late-middle or old age. The shock of seeing an intact, productive individual rather abruptly losing the ability to communicate or remember often experienced with the onset of Alzheimer's disease may not occur, or at least not as dramatically, with schizophrenic individuals. Perhaps that is the reason why little attention has been paid to the problem of schizophrenia in the elderly. The individual with schizophrenia typically has it for most of her or his adult life and does not become suddenly ill toward the end of the life span. At the other extreme, schizophrenia is different from the pervasive developmental disorders, consisting mainly of mental retardation and autism, in which the disorder is generally disabling from early childhood on (Minshew, Goldstein, Muenz, & Payton, 1992). Many schizophrenic patients have a relatively normal childhood and may not become ill until they are over 30 years of age. Their developmental course is therefore more like that of the individual with multiple sclerosis or Huntington's disease, with the major exception that these are inexorably progressive disorders, while schizophrenia is not, at least in most cases.

The paraphrenias appear to represent an exception to these developmental considerations, since they appear to occur in the elderly without warning. In his review, however, Roth (1987) points out that premorbid personality traits, including hostile, suspicious, and unsympathetic characteristics, are common in this disorder. There is also a potential hereditary component, since in about one fifth of patients with the disorder, there is a first-degree relative with a frank schizophrenic illness. Roth favors the view that paraphrenia is a form of schizophrenia, based on numerous considerations of phenomenology, treatment response, and course, and therefore it may also be viewed as a life span disorder. He tentatively suggests that the late manifestation of the disorder may relate to personality features that allow for avoidance of exposure to emotionally stressful interpersonal situations. Social isolation is a major factor.

Summary and Conclusions

We would suggest that there is nothing particularly unique or specific about psychosis in the elderly. Furthermore, the research literature strongly suggests that there is nothing substantially abnormal about the aging process in schizophrenia. Most psychoses are developmental episodic or chronic disorders that typically persist into old age and may remain at a stable level of severity or get better or worse. Winokur, Behar, and Schlesser (1980) expressed the belief that depression in the elderly is not strikingly different from depression in the younger adult. We would suggest that the same is true for schizophrenia. The elderly schizophrenic is apparently not a separate species. If Roth is correct, even paraphrenia is really late-onset schizophrenia that occurs in individuals uniquely suited to avoid a psychotic breakdown during the earlier years of adulthood. As we have tried to show, outcome of schizophrenia in old age is extremely heterogeneous. We seem to have some degree of understanding of several of the factors that may contribute to this heterogeneity, at least at a descriptive level, but many other influences are far from being understood.

A topic worthy of extensive consideration, but not touched upon here, is how individuals with schizophrenia perceive their own aging. Perhaps one of the most profound treatments of this topic is to be found in an unpublished manuscript by Joseph Lyons called "The Psychology of Angels." Lyons takes the view that schizophrenics experience themselves and behave as though they were immortal. They therefore do not have the conventional view of death and dying and do not behave in a manner that bespeaks any degree of urgency. Thus, the perception of old age as a time for confronting one's mortality and "winding things up" may not be shared by the schizophrenic individual. The patient with dementia may have lost the conceptual ability to understand impending death, but mortality and its consequences may never have been part of the schizophrenic individual's experience or consciousness. Clinically, it may therefore be important to understand that the elderly schizophrenic's experience of impending death may be different from our own.

In numerous places, we have contrasted outcome in schizophrenia with outcome in dementia. Nevertheless, schizophrenia is not known to be protective against senile dementia, and it is likely that the proportion of individuals with schizophrenia who develop senile dementia or Alzheimer's disease is not substantially different from what occurs in the general population. However, there may be major differential diagnostic problems as evidenced by the effort in past years to find tests or test profiles that differentiate between "organics" and "schizophrenics" (Goldstein, 1978, 1986). Thus, in the absence of biological markers for Alzheimer's disease and schizophrenia in living individuals, differential diagnosis becomes difficult if only clinical phenomenology is available. Current neuroimaging procedures may also be insufficient for differential diagnostic purposes. The problem may not be clinically relevant for most treatment and management purposes but would be important for long-term planning, and if there is further development of cognition-enhancing medication. In that case, there would have to be some evaluation of the efficacy of these drugs in patients with dual diagnoses and of possible interactions between them and antipsychotic agents. Thus, further research in this difficult area would be desirable.

In conclusion, we would reemphasize the point that, unlike in many other neurobehavioral disorders, outcome of schizophrenia in the elderly is highly variable. Like normal individuals, people with schizophrenia may live through their later years in a highly satisfactory manner, while others experience a devastating, unhappy old age. The difference appears to relate to a number of influences including personality and constitutional factors, maintenance of health and treatment regimes, degree of support in the environment, and severity of the schizophrenia and associated cognitive dysfunction. We would emphasize that this variability in outcome is substantial, ranging the full gamut from independent life in the community to total institutionalization. Thus, the dismal outcome previously forecast for all of schizophrenia does not appear to occur in many cases. This contemporary view of schizophrenia may aid in improving outcome since it does not assume progressive deterioration, understands relapses as recoverable episodes rather than evidence of progression of the disorder, and therefore encourages maintenance of aggressive treatment over the typically lengthy course of the illness.

ACKNOWLEDGMENTS

Indebtedness is expressed to the Department of Veterans Affairs for support of this work.

References

Allebeck, P. (1989). Schizophrenia: A life shortening disease. *Schizophrenia Bulletin, 15,* 81–89.

Alterman, A. I. (1985). Substance abuse in psychiatric patients: Etiological, developmental, and treatment considerations. In A. I. Alterman (Ed.), *Substance abuse and psychopathology* (pp. 121–136). New York: Plenum.

American Psychiatric Association. (1952). *Diagnostic and statistical manual of mental disorders.* Washington, DC: Author.

American Psychiatric Association. (1968). *Diagnostic and statistical manual of mental disorders* (2nd ed.). Washington, DC: Author.

American Psychiatric Association. (1980). *Diagnostic and statistical manual of mental disorders* (3rd ed.). Washington, DC: Author.

American Psychiatric Association. (1994). *Diagnostic and statistical manual of mental disorders* (4th ed.). Washington, DC: Author.

Bleuler, E. (1952). *Dementia praecox or the group of schizophrenias.* New York: International Universities Press.

Bleuler, M. (1978). *The schizophrenic disorders: Long term patient and family studies.* New Haven, CT: Yale University Press.

Braff, D., Heaton, R., Kuck, J., Cullum, M., Moranville, J., Grant, I., & Zisook, S. (1991). The generalized pattern of neuropsychological deficits in outpatients with chronic schizophrenia with heterogeneous Wisconsin card sorting test results. *Archives of General Psychiatry, 48*, 891–898.

Chapman, L. J., & Chapman, J. P. (1973). *Disordered thought in schizophrenia.* Englewood Cliffs, NJ: Prentice-Hall.

Condray, R., Steinhauer, S., & Goldstein, G. (1992). Language comprehension in schizophrenics and their brothers. *Biological Psychiatry, 32*, 790–802.

Cummings, J. L. (1985). Organic delusions: Phenomenology, anatomical correlation, and review. *British Journal of Psychiatry, 146*, 184–197.

Garmezy, N. (1970, Fall). Process and reactive schizophrenia: Some conceptions and issues. *Schizophrenia Bulletin*, 30–74.

Goffman, E. (1961). *Asylums: Essay on the social situation of mental patients and other inmates.* New York: Aldine.

Goldberg, T. E., & Weinberger, D. R. (1988). Probing prefrontal function in schizophrenia with neuropsychological paradigms. *Schizophrenia Bulletin, 14*, 179–183.

Goldberg, T. E., Weinberger, D. R., Berman, K. F., Pliskin, N. H., & Podd, M. H. (1987). Further evidence for dementia of the prefrontal type in schizophrenia? *Archives of General Psychiatry, 44*, 1008–1014.

Goldstein, G. (1978). Cognitive and perceptual differences between schizophrenics and organics. *Schizophrenia Bulletin, 4*, 160–185.

Goldstein, G. (1986). The neuropsychology of schizophrenia. In I. Grant & K. Adams (Eds.), *Neuropsychological assessment of neuropsychiatric disorders* (pp. 147–171). New York: Plenum.

Goldstein, G. (1990). Neuropsychological heterogeneity in schizophrenia: A consideration of abstraction and problem solving abilities. *Archives of Clinical Neuropsychology 5*, 251–264.

Goldstein, G. (1994). Cognitive heterogeneity in psychopathology: The case of schizophrenia. In P. Vernon (Ed.), *The neuropsychology of individual differences* (pp. 209–233). New York: Academic Press.

Goldstein, G., & Halperin, K. M. (1977). Neuropsychological differences among subtypes of schizophrenia. *Journal of Abnormal Psychology, 86*, 34–40.

Goldstein, G., & Zubin, J. (1990). Neuropsychological differences between young and old schizophrenics with and without associated neurological dysfunction. *Schizophrenia Research, 3*, 117–126.

Goldstein, G., Zubin, J., & Pogue-Geile, M. F. (1991). Hospitalization and the cognitive deficits of schizophrenia: The influences of age and education. *Journal of Nervous and Mental Disease, 179*, 202–206.

Gruzelier, J. H. (1991). Hemispheric imbalance syndromes of schizophrenia, premorbid personality, and neurodevelopmental influences. In S. R. Steinhauer, J. Gruzelier, & J. Zubin (Eds.), *Handbook of schizophrenia* (pp. 599–650). London: Elsevier.

Harrow, M., Marengo, J., Pogue-Geile, M. F., & Pawelski, T. J. (1987). Schizophrenic deficits in intelligence and abstract thinking: Influence of aging and long-term institutionalization. In N. E. Miller & G. D. Cohen (Eds.), *Schizophrenia and aging* (pp. 133–144). New York: Guilford.

Heaton, R. K., & Drexler, M. (1987). Clinical neuropsychological findings in schizophrenia and aging. In N. E. Miller & G. D. Cohen (Eds.), *Schizophrenia and aging* (pp. 145–161). New York: Guilford.

Heaton, R. K., Paulsen, J. S., McAdams, L. A., Kuck, J., Zisook, S., Braff, D., Harris, J., & Jeste, D. V. (1994). Neuropsychological deficits in schizophrenia. Relationship to age, chronicity, and dementia. *Archives of General Psychiatry, 51*, 469–476.

Hogarty, G. E., Goldberg, S. C., Schooler, N. R., & Ulrich, R. F. (1974). Drug and sociotherapy in the aftercare of schizophrenic patients. II. Two year relapse rates. *Archives of General Psychiatry, 31*, 603–608.

Jeste, D. V. (1993). Late-life schizophrenia: Editor's introduction. *Schizophrenia Bulletin, 19*, 687–689.

Johnstone, E. C., Owens, D. G. C., Gold, A., Crow, T. J., & Macmillan, J. F. (1981). Institutionalization and the defects of schizophrenia. *British Journal of Psychiatry, 139*, 195–203.

Kareken, D. A., Gur, R. C., Mozley, P. D., Mozley, L. H., Saykin, A. J., Shtasel, D. L., & Gur, R. E. (1995). Cognitive functioning and neuroanatomic volume measures in schizophrenia. *Neuropsychology, 9*, 211–219.

Keefe, R. S. E., Mohs, R. C., Losonczy, M. F., Davidson, M., Silverman, J. M., Kendler, K. S., Horvath, T. B., Nora, N., & Davis, K. L. (1987). Characteristics of very poor outcome schizophrenia. *American Journal of Psychiatry, 144*, 889–895.

Koziol, L. F., & Stout, C. E. (1994). *The neuropsychology of mental disorders.* Springfield, IL: C. C. Thomas.

Kraepelin, E. (1913). *Dementia praecox and paraphrenia* (R. M. Barclay, trans.). Edinburgh: Livingstone.

McGlashan, T. H. (1987). Late onset improvement in chronic schizophrenia: Characteristics and prediction. In N. E. Miller & G. D. Cohen (Eds.), *Schizophrenia and aging* (pp. 61–73). New York: Guilford.

Miller, N. E., & Cohen, G. D. (1987). *Schizophrenia and aging.* New York: Guilford.

Minshew, N. J., Goldstein, G., Muenz, L. R., & Payton, J. B. (1992). Neuropsychological functioning in non-mentally retarded autistic individuals. *Journal of Clinical and Experimental Neuropsychology, 14*, 749–761.

Morel, B. (1860). *Traités des maladies mentales.* Paris: Masson.

Reitan, R. M., & Wolfson, D. W. (1993). *The Halstead Reitan Neuropsychological Battery* (2nd ed.). Tucson, AZ: Neuropsychology Press.

Roth, M. (1987). Late paraphrenia: Phenomenology and etiological factors and their bearing upon problems of the schizophrenic family of disorders. In N. E. Miller & G. D. Cohen (Eds.), *Schizophrenia and aging* (pp. 217–234). New York: Guilford.

Satz, P. (1993). Brain reserve capacity on symptom onset after brain injury: A formulation and review of evidence for threshold theory. *Neuropsychology, 7*, 273–295.

van Kammen, D. P., Kelley, M. E., Gurklis, J. A., Gilbertson, M. W., Yao, J. K., & Peters, J. L. (1995). Behavioral vs. biochemical prediction of clinical stability following haloperidol withdrawal in schizophrenia. *Archives of General Psychiatry, 52*, 673–678.

Waddington, J. L. (1993). Neurodynamics of abnormalities in cerebral metabolism and structure in schizophrenia. *Schizophrenia Bulletin, 19*, 55–69.

Wechsler, D. (1955). *Wechsler Adult Intelligence Scale manual.* New York: Psychological Corporation.

Weinberger, D., Berman, K., & Zec, R. (1986). Physiological dysfunction of dorsolateral prefrontal cortex in schizophrenia: I. Regional cerebral blood flow evidence. *Archives of General Psychiatry, 43*, 114–125.

Winokur, G., Behar, D., & Schlesser, M. (1980). Clinical and biological aspects of depression in the elderly. In J. O. Cole & J. E. Barrett (Eds.), *Psychopathology in the aged* (pp. 145–153). New York: Raven Press.

Zubin, J. (1985). Negative symptoms: Are they indigenous to schizophrenia? *Schizophrenia Bulletin, 11*, 461–469.

Zubin, J., & Spring, B. (1977). Vulnerability: A new view of schizophrenia. *Journal of Abnormal Psychology, 86*, 103–126.

9

Substance Abuse in Elderly Individuals

DANIEL N. ALLEN AND RHONDA K. B. LANDIS

Introduction

Individuals over the age of 65 currently comprise 12% of the U.S. population, and this figure is projected to reach 18% by the year 2020 and 20% by the year 2030 (La Rue, 1992; Spencer, 1989). This marked change in demographics reflects the aging of the baby boom generation. In the year 2010, the eldest of the 76 million baby boomers will start to turn 65. So, while the current number of individuals over the age of 65 is 30 million, by the year 2020, this number will increase to 52 million. This general aging trend within our society, combined with the fact that substance abuse and, more specifically, alcohol abuse is the single most prevalent psychiatric disorder among males suggests that management of substance use disorders in elderly individuals will emerge as a critical area of health care delivery.

However, within the more general substance use disorder literature, studies examining substance use among elderly individuals are limited. There is only limited information regarding prevalence of substance abuse and dependence in individuals over the age of 65. Some of the existing information probably significantly underestimates prevalence of drug abuse and dependence among the elderly because of methodological limitations. These methodological limitations account, at least in part, for the significant differences between studies examining rates of substance abuse among the elderly. Within the more general geriatric substance abuse literature, information on neuropsychological profiles of long-term substance abusers is even more limited. One exception to this general paucity of information is within the area of alcohol abuse and dependence and, to a lesser extent, benzodiazepine abuse and dependence. Of the existing literature, relatively more studies provide prevalence estimates of elderly alcoholism, investigate neuropsychological sequelae of chronic alcoholism, and provide recommendations for treatment of elderly alcoholics. However, even in the cases of alcohol and benzodiazepines, existing information is quite limited.

In this chapter, we will summarize the available information on geriatric substance use disorders, with particular emphasis on the neuropsychological concomitants of these disorders. The majority of the discussion will focus on alcohol and benzodiazepines, as these have been the most extensively studied and most frequently used. However, we will also discuss some of the methodological limitations of existing studies, including limitations of current diagnostic criteria. In addition, we will discuss prevalence rates of alcohol and drug use disorders and several factors that increase elderly individuals' risk or potential for developing these disorders. Finally, we will make recommendations for assessment and treatment of elderly individuals with substance abuse disorder and dependence.

DANIEL N. ALLEN • Psychology Service, Highland Drive Veterans Affairs Medical Center, Pittsburgh, Pennsylvania 15206. RHONDA K. B. LANDIS • Behavioral Health Services, DuBois Regional Medical Center, DuBois, Pennsylvania 15801.

Definitions

There is currently no universally accepted definition of substance use disorders. Because of this, clinicians and researchers define these disorders using a number of methods and criteria. The two most popular systems that provide specific diagnostic criteria are those promulgated by the *Diagnostic and Statistical Manual of Mental Disorders*, fourth edition (*DSM-IV*; American Psychiatric Association [APA], 1994) and the Research Diagnostic Criteria (RDC; Spitzer, Endicott, & Robins, 1978). The *DSM-IV* category of substance-related disorders is broadly defined to include abuse of specific substances (e.g., alcohol, cannabis, opiates, etc.), medication side effects, and exposure to toxins. In the *DSM-IV* nomenclature, substance-related disorders are further broken down into two categories: (a) substance use disorders, including substance abuse and substance dependence; and (b) substance-induced disorders. The latter category includes disorders resulting from misuse of medications.

In contrast to diagnostic systems such as the *DSM-IV* and *RDC*, there are also numerous self-report measures used to diagnose alcohol use disorders such as the CAGE questionnaire (Ewing, 1984; Mayfield, McLeod, & Hall, 1974) and the Michigan Alcohol Screening Test (MAST; Selzer, 1971). These self-report questionnaires are brief and assess a range of alcohol symptomatology. They have defined cutoff scores demonstrated to accurately classify a significant proportion of alcoholics. Of the two instruments, we recommend use of the MAST for screening elderly individuals because it detects more individuals who actually have diagnoses of alcohol use disorders than does the CAGE (Fulop et al., 1993). In many instances, these measures are used as screening devices to identify individuals who are at high risk for alcohol or drug abuse. After identification is made, further evaluation of symptomatology is conducted through clinical or standardized interviews before a final diagnosis is made.

In this chapter, we will discuss substance abuse and dependence with the *DSM-IV* definition in mind. However, we recognize that many definitions have been developed to diagnose substance abuse and dependence. We also recognize the limitations of any specific definition of substance abuse and dependence, particularly as these definitions apply to elderly individuals. We will discuss these limitations later in the chapter. Our discussion will focus primarily on substance abuse and dependence, with less emphasis on substance-related disorders resulting from substance misuse and adverse side effects.

Potential for Abuse and Dependence among Elderly Individuals

Although individuals over the age of 65 make up only 12% of the U.S. population, estimates suggest that the elderly consume approximately 30% of all prescribed drugs taken each year, making them the largest consumers of legal drugs in this country (Baum, Kennedy, & Forbes, 1984). Elders are also the largest consumers of nonprescribed over-the-counter (OTC) medications (Kofoed, 1984). When considering all types of OTC medication, estimates suggest that two thirds of all individuals over the age of 60 take at least one medication daily for treatment of arthritis, constipation, or insomnia (Abrams & Alexopoulos, 1988). Several studies have further investigated the drug use characteristics of hospitalized and community dwelling elderly. Ellor and Kurz (1982) conducted a drug survey of 41 patients (75% female) in a general and rehabilitation hospital who were between 62 and 83 years of age. Overall, 134 drugs were prescribed with an average of 3.1 drugs per person (range = 0–8 drugs/person). For community dwelling elderly individuals, prevalence rates of prescribed drug use ranged between 2.1 and 4.5 medications per person, while use of OTC medication ranged between 2.3 and 3.4 drugs per person (Darnell, Murray, Martz, & Weinberger, 1986; Pollow, Stoller, Forster, & Duniho, 1994). In these studies, the combined average number of prescribed and OTC medications ranged between 4.4 and 7.9 per person (Darnell et al., 1986; Pollow et al., 1994). Outside of any other considerations, the large number of medications taken by elderly individuals increases the potential for drug misuse, abuse, and dependence.

Research also suggests that many elderly individuals do not take their medications as directed (Darnell et al., 1986; Ellor & Kurz, 1982). Ellor and Kurz (1982) reported that individuals in their study missed doses of medications and none remembered receiving instructions from health care professionals about the appropriate action to take if they missed doses. Twenty-two (53.6%) admitted that they would skip doses. Six individuals (14.6%) who missed doses took double the amount the next time. Darnell et al. (1986) found that only 49.3% of the individuals in their study reported taking all their prescribed drugs correctly. Most instances of noncompliance were due to omitted doses, but 7.5% admitted to adding doses. Men were more compliant than women, but they were also taking less medication. Overall, they found that compliance was inversely related to the number of drugs prescribed. Another finding from these studies was the underreporting of nonprescription drugs taken by these individuals.

In addition to increased risk resulting from increased use of and access to prescription medications, elderly individuals may also be at higher risk because of age-related changes in physiology that cause drugs to be more potent or less predictable. Pollow et al. (1994) point out that the physiological effects of aging, including changes in body composition and vital organ function, cause changes in "the distribution, metabolism and excretion of drugs" (p. 44). These factors account for the observation that, after consuming similar amounts of alcohol, blood alcohol levels are lower in younger individuals compared to older individuals (Vestal et al., 1977).

When considered in light of the number of medications that elderly individuals take, age-related changes in physiology and pharmacokinetics, and the potential for abuse in this age group, it is clear that elderly individuals are also at a higher risk for adverse drug reactions. Pollow and colleagues (1994) reported that out of 667 community dwelling individuals 65 years of age or older, 65.8% were taking at least one medication combination that put them at risk for experiencing an adverse drug reaction over the preceding month. Of these 667 individuals, 10.6% (n = 71) had taken psychoactive medications over the past month. Individuals who had taken psychoactive medications were at highest risk for possible adverse drug reactions, with 98.6% identified as taking at least one drug combination that had the potential to produce an adverse reaction. This last point is particularly salient, as prescription drugs with the highest potential for abuse and dependence are classified as psychoactive.

In summary then, the potential for abuse of prescription and nonprescription medications is higher for elderly individuals because of the increased prescription of medications that are potentially addictive (e.g., benzodiazepines), poor understanding of medication effects and interactions, inadequate education and/or misconceptions regarding proper use of medications, decreased cognitive abilities, increased physical symptoms, and age-related changes in physiology.

Prevalence of Alcohol and Drug Abuse among the Elderly

Despite increased potential for abuse, current estimates of drug and alcohol use disorders in elderly individuals suggest that these conditions are less prevalent than in younger individuals. However, there is some reason to believe that current information may significantly underestimate the prevalence of drug and alcohol use disorders in the elderly. In the following sections, we will discuss prevalence rates of drug and alcohol use disorders, as well as some of the methodological limitations of current studies.

Current Estimates

There is some disagreement regarding incidence of alcohol abuse and dependence in individuals over age 65. After a thorough review of the literature, Liberto, Oslin, and Ruskin (1992) report that incidence of heavy drinking (12–21 drinks per week) in elderly individuals ranges between 3% and 9%. However, incidence of alcohol abuse and dependence is much lower than incidence of heavy consumption, with 1-month prevalence rates of alcohol abuse and dependence for elderly individuals ranging from 0.9% (Regier et al., 1988) to 1.4% (Helzer, Burnam, & McEvoy, 1991) to 2.2% (Baily, Haberman, & Alksne, 1964). Men have higher 1-year prevalence rates of alcohol abuse and dependence than women (3.1% vs. 0.46%, respectively; Helzer et al., 1991) and higher lifetime prevalence rates (14.0% vs. 1.5%, respectively; Helzer & Burnam, 1991).

The rates for individuals over age 65 are in contrast to the rates for younger individuals. Using the *DSM-III* (APA, 1980) criteria, Regier and colleagues (1988) reported that 1-month prevalence rates of alcohol abuse and dependence for individuals 18–24 years of age was 4.1%. It is also apparent from Regier's data that males at all ages exhibit higher rates of alcohol abuse and dependence than do females. For males 18–24 years old, the 1-month prevalence rate of alcohol abuse and dependence was 6.0%, compared to 1.8% for males 65 years of age and older. The comparable rates for females were 2.3% and 0.3%, respectively.

Although incidence is low in community dwelling elderly, hospitalized patients show a marked increase in the incidence of alcohol abuse. Incidence of alcohol abuse in elderly patients admitted to hospitals ranges widely, from 5% to 50% (see Liberto et al., 1992, for review). These differences are undoubtedly accounted for by differences in types of hospital admission (e.g., psychiatric vs. surgical) and by criteria used to define alcohol abuse. However, it does appear that incidence of alcohol abuse is significantly higher for elderly patients admitted to hospitals than for the population at large.

It also appears that drug abuse and dependence are less prevalent in the elderly than in younger individuals. In the Epidemiology Catchment Area study, Regier and colleagues (1988) reported a 1-month drug abuse/dependence (*DSM-III* criteria) prevalence rate of 3.5% for individuals 18–24 years old, but less than one tenth of 1.0% (reported percentage $< 0.0\%$) for individuals older than 65. A study by Solomon and Stark (1993) found that only 2 of 26 elderly men in a substance abuse program had ever used illicit drugs. In comparison to younger men in the study, older addicts were more likely to abuse prescription drugs by taking more than the prescribed dose. As with alcohol use disorders, some groups of elderly individuals exhibit higher rates of drug abuse and dependence. A study of high-risk community dwelling elderly evaluated at a mental health clinic found that prescription drug abuse constituted approximately 5% of the average caseload (Jinks & Raschko, 1990). The most commonly misused prescription drugs were sedative-hypnotics, antianxiety agents, and analgesics.

Benzodiazepines are one of the most widely prescribed medications in the world (APA, 1990), and the elderly receive almost 40% of these prescriptions (Thompson, Moran, & Neis, 1983). Because these drugs can lead to psychological and physical dependence, there is great potential for abuse and addiction (Juergens, 1993). Prevalence rates of benzodiazepine abuse among elderly individuals are not clear at this time, although some studies indicate the rate of abuse may be quite high. For example, in a randomly selected group of over 1,000 community dwelling elderly individuals, Morgan, Dallosso, Ebrahim, Arie, and Fentem (1988) found approximately 16% used hypnotics for sleep the night prior to the interview. Of these individuals, 19% reported using hypnotics for 5 to 10 years, and 25% reported using hypnotics for more than 10 years.

Available studies do suggest the following: (a) Substance use disorders decrease with increasing age; (b) prevalence of substance use disorders is higher among men than women; and (c) certain groups of elderly individuals have higher rates of substance use disorders.

Factors Contributing to Decreased Prevalence

"Maturing Out" Theory

One of the most popular theories to explain the apparent decrease in substance use disorders among the elderly was proposed by Winick (1962) and is referred to as the "maturing out" theory. To summarize, Winick proposed that the number of narcotic addicts decreased with age because of factors associated with the aging process and length of abuse. These factors include passing from one developmental stage to the next and succumbing to adverse consequences of substance use disorders.

Although this explanation remains controversial (see Petersen, 1988), it does have support. Studies examining mortality rates among alcohol abusers have generally found an increased risk of mortality that is anywhere from two to five times higher when compared to age- and sex-matched peers (for reviews see Finney & Moos, 1991; Moos, Brennan, & Mertens, 1994). Additionally, individuals who abuse drugs have a higher risk of mortality than individuals who abuse alcohol (Engstrom, Adamsson, Allebeck, & Rydberg, 1991). In one of the few studies examining mortality rates in elderly substance abusers, Moos and colleagues (1994) found that out of approximately 98,000 inpatients with diagnoses of substance abuse treated at Department of Veterans Affairs medical centers in fiscal year 1987, 21,139 were 55 years of age or older. Over the next 4 years, mortality rates of these patients were, on the average, 2.64 times higher than expected when compared to the general population (matched for age, sex, and race). Increased mortality rates declined from 3.02 to 2.25 to 1.66 in the 55–64, 65–74, and 75+ age groups, respectively. Also, mortality rates were somewhat higher among those patients diagnosed with drug dependence or psychosis compared to patients with alcohol dependence diagnoses (2.93 vs. 2.42, respectively). Although the increased mortality rates associated with substance abuse decrease with age, it is worth noting that mortality rates remain significantly higher than the general population even in the oldest group of individuals with substance use disorders (Moos et al., 1994).

Underdetection of Elderly Substance Abusers

In addition to decreased prevalence rates that may result from "maturing out," at least three other factors may play a role in underdetection of substance abuse in elderly patients. These factors include inadequate or inappropriate definitions of substance abuse for elderly individuals, abuse of prescription medications, and late-life onset of substance abuse in elderly individuals.

Inadequate Definitions of Substance Use Disorders. Several authors suggest that studies examining prevalence rates of substance use disorders among the elderly significantly underestimate the widespread nature of the problem because of inadequacies in currently existing psychiatric definitions of substance use disorders, including *DSM-III-R* (APA, 1987) criteria (Ellor & Kurz, 1982; King, VanHasselt, Segal, & Hersen, 1994; Miller, Belkin, & Gold, 1991). These authors have criticized current diagnostic strategies because they

were not developed with the elderly in mind, and they are not adequately validated with elderly individuals.

Development and validation of standard substance abuse criteria specifically for elderly individuals with substance use disorders is necessary because of obvious age-related differences between individuals across the life span. Factors such as physical health, age-appropriate life tasks, and socioeconomic resources vary with age. These and other factors contribute to diagnosis of abuse and dependence, but are typically based on young and/or middle-aged individuals. As a result, current diagnostic criteria have limited utility when applied to elders. In order to understand the way in which age influences current diagnostic criteria for substance abuse, one need only consider definitions of substance abuse and dependence contained in the *DSM-IV* (APA, 1994). The first *DSM-IV* criterion for substance dependence is *increased tolerance* to effects of the substance, so that increased consumption is necessary. In elderly individuals, tolerance for substances (including alcohol) is often decreased due to changes in physiology and altered pharmacokinetics. As a result, an older individual dependent on alcohol may consume less alcohol over time but continue to become intoxicated. Similarly, examples of adverse consequences listed as possible indicators of substance abuse include repeated absences or poor work performance; substance-related absences, suspensions, or expulsions from school; and neglect of children or household (APA, 1994, p. 182).

On brief reflection, it is clear that these consequences pertain to young and middle-aged individuals with substance use disorders, more so than elders. As Miller and colleagues (1991) point out, elderly individuals often do not have the same vulnerability to social consequences as do their younger counterparts, since older adults are often unemployed and live alone. As a result, one would expect to observe fewer instances of adverse consequences on occupational performance and family functioning in the elderly. Rather, substance use disorders in the elderly will more often present as medical or psychiatric conditions (Miller et al., 1991). Because current diagnostic criteria do not adequately characterize substance abuse and dependence in the elderly, it is likely that substance use disorders are underidentified.

Misuse versus Abuse. The issue of "misuse" versus "abuse" is also sometimes obfuscated by current definitions of substance abuse. Ellor and Kurz (1982) define drug abuse as use of a drug for other than the intended purpose. In contrast, drug misuse refers to underuse, overuse, or erratic use of a drug. Ellor and Kurz (1982) correctly point out that, within the elderly population, drug abuse may constitute extreme cases of drug misuse. The *DSM-IV* has included criteria for substance misuse as part of its diagnostic nomenclature. Several studies suggest that substance abuse problems in the elderly result from misuse and abuse of prescription or OTC medications. This fact distinguishes them from younger substance abusers, who most often abuse illicit drugs. By drawing a distinction between misuse and abuse, it becomes clear that elders may use substances in a maladaptive manner not because of positive psychogenic side effects typically associated with drug abuse and dependence or because of physiological and psychological dependence associated with some substances, but, rather, because they cannot remember proper dosages, they have misconceptions about the need to continue to take medications after initial symptoms have resolved, they do not understand the ways in which medications work (e.g., if one dose is good, two doses must be better), and/or they are unable to read medication labels.

To illustrate, we consider the way in which labeling deficiencies affect compliance among elderly individuals with decreased visual acuity. Often, labels on prescriptions are crowded with information unrelated to proper use of the medication. Script is sometimes light and typeface is often exceedingly small and condensed (this is particularly true for OTC medications). It is unlikely that an elderly individual with decreased visual acuity will take medications as prescribed, based solely on this information. When this situation is multiplied by the number of prescription and OTC medications taken by elderly individuals (4.4–7.9; Darnell et al., 1986; Pollow et al., 1994), the potential for misuse leading to abuse is high.

Prescription Substance Use Disorders. With regard to prescription drug abuse, there is often substantial underdetection of elderly prescription substance abuse (Buchsbaum, Boling, & Groh, 1987; Finlayson, Hurt, Davis, & Morse, 1988; Whitcup & Miller, 1987). Dependence on medications often goes unrecognized by health care providers, including physicians (McInnes & Powell, 1994). In fact, dependence on prescription medications, such as benzodiazepines, is sometimes not detected until withdrawal from medication is precipitated by hospitalization for another medical condition. At that time, symptoms of withdrawal become apparent and often cause significant complications in the treatment process. At least one factor contributing to this underdetection is the masking of symptoms associated with dependence by coexisting psychiatric disorders. Finlayson and colleagues (1988) found that approximately 14% of 216 patients being treated for alcohol abuse or dependence had coexisting diagnoses of drug dependence. Whitcup and Miller (1987) report a similar finding after reviewing cases of 90 patients treated for psychiatric disorders. Approximately 21% of their patients had coexisting drug dependence diagnoses. Whitcup and Miller (1987) go on to point out that over 50% of individuals with drug dependence were not identified as being dependent on a prescribed medication.

Development of Substance Use Disorders in Late Life. Because of late-life onset of substance abuse, health care providers may not be as likely to detect substance abuse in elderly individuals simply because these elders have no prior history of substance abuse. While it appears that elderly individuals use alcohol less frequently than younger individuals and that heavy alcohol use decreases with age (Liberto et al., 1992; Regier et al., 1988), a significant number of elderly individuals begin to abuse alcohol or experience deleterious effects of alcohol use after age 65. A number of studies have examined incidence of late-life onset problem drinking in individuals reporting for treatment of alcohol use disorders. These studies have found that between 15% and 68% of elderly individuals treated for alcohol problems were late-onset drinkers (Atkinson, Tolson, & Turner, 1990; Finlayson et al., 1988; Schonfeld & Dupree, 1991; Wiens, Menustik, Miller, & Schmitz, 1982–1983; Zimberg, 1979). Without intervention, incidence of late-life onset alcohol abuse and dependence will increase as the population ages and as advancing medical technology prolongs the average life span. In this sense, the decrease in older substance abusers caused by "maturing out" (Winick, 1962) could be countered by a "maturing in" process, whereby the unique and novel challenges of late life combined with increased access to prescription psychogenic agents and increased potency secondary to physiological changes that accompany the aging process lead to an increased incidence of substance use disorders among the elderly.

Reasons for onset of substance use disorders in late life have not been systematically investigated. Jinks and Raschko (1990) reported that drug abuse was more common among women, those who lived alone, those who had a greater number of physical illnesses, and those who took multiple prescription drugs simultaneously. Jinks and Raschko's (1990) report was partially supported by a recent review which suggests that predictors of late-life substance abuse vary based on gender (Gomberg, 1995). In contrast to men, older women who abuse alcohol are more often widowed. Also, older women appear to abuse prescribed psychoactive agents more often than men. In addition to factors that contribute to late-onset alcohol abuse and dependence, Atkinson et al. (1990) suggest factors that are not likely to be responsible for development of substance use disorders in the elderly. These include severe and persistent psychiatric illness and genetic influences. In our clinical experience, we have found that loss of loved ones, loss of social status, decreased activity level due to retirement, stress caused by decreased financial resources, and increased use of prescription medications for medical conditions are all contributing factors to the onset of or increase in substance abuse.

Assessment of Substance-Induced Cognitive Deficits

Although the elderly take multiple medications that have potential for misuse, abuse, and dependence, there are relatively few studies examining drug effects on cognitive abilities in the elderly. Research conducted to date has focused almost exclusively on alcohol and benzodiazepine use in older adults. This research has typically examined cognitive functioning of groups of individuals with substance use disorders. The following sections provide descriptions of neuropsychological functioning in *groups* of geriatric substance abusers. Considerable variation in cognitive functioning exists from one individual to the next as a result of the interaction of multiple factors that produce cognitive deficits. Prior to discussing specific substance-induced cognitive deficits, we discuss a number of factors that influence neuropsychological test performance in the elderly.

General Considerations

Clinicians and researchers need to consider a number of factors that distinguish elderly individuals with substance use disorders from their younger counterparts when conducting neuropsychological assessment. These factors arise from two general sources: (a) *client* characteristics and (b) instrument and test *environment* characteristics. Others have provided excellent discussions of factors that arise from these two sources as they pertain to the general elderly population (Crook, 1979; Storandt, 1994; Zarit, Eiler, & Hassinger, 1985) and to elderly individuals with severe cognitive impairment (Nussbaum & Allen, in press). We encourage readers interested in further review of general issues in geriatric assessment to consult these reviews. However, we will mention a few factors that we feel are of particular relevance when assessing cognition in elderly individuals with substance use disorders, including chronic medical conditions, prescription and nonprescription drug effects, and comorbid psychiatric disorders.

First, it is important to consider the impact that chronic physical illnesses have on test performance. For individuals older than 65, there is ample evidence indicating that 80% have at least one chronic medical condition, and that by age 85, 29% have severe disabilities (Kunkel & Applebaum, 1992). Arthritis, hearing impairment, orthopedic impairment, and tinnitus are among the 10 most common health problems for individuals 65 years of age and older (Adams & Benson, 1992). It is necessary to evaluate these conditions when assessing elderly individuals because these chronic medical conditions can cause impairment of sensory and motor functions, which, in turn, can adversely affect performance on tests designed to assess cognitive functioning. Impairment of sensory and motor functions secondary to chronic medical conditions are not always apparent during neuropsychological evaluation, and one cannot expect patients to spontaneously report these conditions. As a result, a thorough medical history is imperative in an evaluation of elderly substance abusers.

Second, because of the high rate of medication use among elderly, it is also important to evaluate medication profiles in addition to evaluating characteristic patterns of substance use. This evaluation should include both prescription and OTC medications. It is important to consider not only possible negative effects of single medications, but also synergistic effects of multiple medications on cognitive processes.

Third, some psychiatric disorders that are accompanied by cognitive deficits have a high rate of comorbidity with alcoholism. These conditions include depression, anxiety, and antisocial personality disorder (Hesselbrock, Meyer, & Keener, 1985; Ross, Glaser, & Germanson, 1988). If clinicians do not adequately assess these variables when evaluating cognitive functioning in elderly substance abusers, these variables may significantly influence results of testing.

Two other points relating to neuropsychological assessment and cognitive impairment are worth mentioning. First, there are vagaries inherent in evaluating cognitive dysfunction in elderly individuals with substance abuse disorders. A specific cognitive profile produced by any neuropsychological assessment procedure is the result of multiple factors. For elderly individuals with substance abuse disorders, some of these factors include short-versus long-term consequences of substance abuse, physiological states that occur at each stage of the substance use process, cognitive deficits induced by comorbid or preexisting psychiatric disorders, medical conditions caused by substance use disorders (e.g., cirrhosis of the liver) and their resulting cognitive deficits, variability in response to medications resulting from altered pharmacokinetics, and effects of substance use on cognition versus declines in cognitive functioning due to aging. Because of the multiple factors that influence cognitive functioning, trying to determine the etiology of cognitive

deficits in this group is a complex and sometimes daunting process.

The second point is that even when etiology, type, and severity of cognitive deficits are quantified by administration of neuropsychological and other laboratory tests, determining the impact of the identified cognitive deficits on daily functioning can be problematic. If one has a memory deficit on neuropsychological testing but is able to meet day-to-day life challenges, the question "What is the significance of these quantified memory deficits?" comes to the fore. From this discussion, we hope that the readers have gained a basic understanding of the many issues involved in cognitive functioning in elderly individuals as well as the complexity of interactions between these factors that, in the end, produce neuropsychological profiles and behavioral repertoires of elderly substance abusers.

Alcohol Abuse and Dependence

Characteristics and Side Effects

Alcohol is the most often used depressant in the United States. Acute alcohol intoxication affects neurological, behavioral, and psychological functioning. The most common neurological symptoms of alcohol intoxication include ataxia, slurred speech, incoordination, and nystagmus. Behavioral symptoms include increased aggression. Psychological symptoms include mood fluctuations and impairment across several cognitive domains such as memory, attention, and judgment. Physiological dependence on alcohol develops only after prolonged heavy consumption. Withdrawal effects usually occur soon after drinking cessation (4–12 hours) and almost always occur within 48 hours. The majority of withdrawal symptoms typically resolve within the first week after drinking cessation. Symptoms indicative of withdrawal are quite varied in severity. Mild symptoms, such as anxiety, restlessness, irritability, perspiration, increased heart rate, and insomnia are by far the most common withdrawal symptoms. However, in a small minority of cases, more severe symptoms, such as grand mal seizures, hallucinations, and delirium can develop. Also, Brower, Mudd, Blow, Young, and Hill (1994) recently reported that when compared to younger individuals with similar recent drinking histories, elderly individuals experience significantly more symptoms of withdrawal, and these symptoms last for significantly longer time periods. Additionally, elderly individuals appear more susceptible to impairment in cognitive functioning than younger alcoholics during withdrawal (Brower et al., 1994). As a result, it is necessary to closely monitor symptoms of alcohol withdrawal when a history of alcohol dependence is expected.

Cognitive Deficits in Alcoholics

Neuropsychological deficits among alcoholics is by far the most extensive body of literature investigating neuropsychological sequelae of substance use disorders. As such, neuropsychological profiles of geriatric alcoholics are the most clearly defined. Despite this fact, there is some disagreement among investigators regarding the exact profile of cognitive deficits.

Methodological Limitations

Factors endemic to individuals who abuse alcohol as well as methodological limitations inherent in conducting research with this group account for the majority of inconsistencies between studies. With regard to *endemic* factors, it is often impossible to adequately control for neurological risk factors that could adversely influence cognitive functioning in alcoholics. For example, it is often not possible to accurately measure the number of mild-moderate head injuries sustained by chronic alcoholics, as these individuals may well have no memory of the incident due to intoxication and/or unconsciousness and they may not receive medical intervention for these injuries. A second endemic factor is that cognitive deficits arising from other chronic medical conditions (e.g., cirrhosis of the liver) often go undetected, even though these conditions may significantly influence cognitive functioning. We discuss hepatic encephalopathy more fully later in this chapter because of its prevalence in alcoholics and the significant impact it can have on cognitive functioning. Third, transient biochemical disturbances (such as vitamin deficiencies) can have long-lasting effects on cognitive functioning but may have little relation to drinking history. Fourth,

decreased cognitive functioning may result from some predispositional factors that contribute to development of alcoholism, so that cognitive deficits are present before onset of alcohol abuse and dependence. Studies have implicated such childhood factors as poor educational achievement, childhood minimal brain dysfunction, and attention deficit hyperactivity disorder as contributing to cognitive deficits typically observed in alcoholics, although contribution of some of these factors has not been consistently demonstrated (Eckardt, Stapleton, Rawlings, Davis, & Grodin, 1995). Finally, as previously mentioned, research indicates that psychiatric disorders that have concomitant cognitive deficits (depression, anxiety, and antisocial personality disorder) also have a high rate of comorbidity with alcohol use disorders (Eckardt et al., 1995; Hesselbrock, Weidenman, & Reed, 1985; Ross et al., 1988).

From a *methodological* standpoint, factors that influence the results of studies examining neuropsychological functioning in alcoholics include sampling bias, drinking history, and time since drinking cessation. First, although it is obvious that sampling from an older, more chronic population would produce biased results that could not be generalized to the more general population of individuals with alcohol use disorders, more subtle and as yet not fully understood biases also exist. A dramatic example of this was recently reported by Tivis, Parsons, Glenn, and Nixon (1993), who found that even after other significant factors were controlled (e.g., depression, anxiety, race, socioeconomic status, alcohol use history, medical conditions, motivation, family history of alcoholism, etc.), significant differences in neuropsychological test performance remained between patients in a Department of Veterans Affairs medical center treatment program and patients in community-based treatment programs. Veterans exhibited more severe cognitive deficits.

A second methodological factor is varying levels of chronicity between alcoholic populations participating in research. In one way or another, all studies rely on alcoholics' self-reports about their drinking to establish drinking history. While some may find it easy to report drinking history for 1 month or possibly 1 year, one must wonder about the validity of estimated alcohol intake over the course of 10 to 40 years. Similarly, denial or minimization of severity of problems associated with alcoholism may also influence reporting of long-term alcohol use. As a result, chronicity is often difficult to assess. Third, it is clear that, in the case of alcohol, time since abstinence is a significant predictor of cognitive impairment as assessed by neuropsychological tests. The longer the period of abstinence, the greater the improvement in some cognitive abilities (Goldman, 1986). However, in longitudinal studies (6–12 months), this variable is also typically determined by self-report and, as such, is subject to factors like denial, underreporting, and outright deception.

Despite these methodological problems, the literature is unequivocal in reporting that patients do exhibit neuropsychological correlates of cerebral dysfunction in a variety of ability areas. This literature has portrayed a fairly consistent pattern of neuropsychological deficits. It is also apparent that while some deficits recover as a function of time, others do not.

Etiology of Cognitive Deficits in Alcoholics

Investigators have gained some insight into expected types of cognitive deficits accompanying alcohol use disorders by examining etiologies of cognitive deficits common to this group. At least six types of etiologic factors contribute to varying profiles of cognitive impairment that occur in chronic alcohol abusers. Reitan and Wolfson (1985) categorize etiologic factors that cause cognitive deficits as follows: (1) acute alcohol intoxication, (2) withdrawal effects resulting from abstinence, (3) diseases of the nervous system due to malnutrition, (4) conditions associated with alcoholism in which the etiology is uncertain, (5) neurological disorders secondary to alcohol-induced cirrhosis of the liver, and (6) teratogenic abnormalities such as fetal alcohol syndrome (Reitan & Wolfson, 1985, p. 269; cf. Tarter & Ryan, 1986, and Goldstein, 1987b). The lifetime pattern of alcohol consumption often dictates incidence and severity of cognitive disorders because the aforementioned etiologic factors result either directly or indirectly from amount of alcohol ingested over time. However, as surmised from Reitan and Wolfson's categorization of etiologic factors, this is not always the case. Teratogenic abnormalities (such as fetal alcohol syndrome) are the most obvious category in which cognitive deficits are not related to lifetime pattern of alcohol consumption. In this case, the lifetime pattern of consumption has little relevance as the cognitive deficits are not in the chronic alcohol abuser but the child.

There is also disagreement as to whether alcohol has neurotoxic effects. This is because it appears that white matter losses often reported in recently detoxified alcoholics resolve over time. One recent serial magnetic resonance imaging (MRI) study reported that after approximately 105 days of abstinence, patients exhibited white matter volume increases and cerebral spinal fluid volume reductions (Shear, Jernigan, & Butters, 1994). These changes were not present in individuals who resumed drinking between MRI scans (Shear et al., 1994). One of the strongest opponents of neurotoxicity of alcohol has been Victor (1994), who contends that the large majority of suspected cases of alcohol-induced cognitive deficits resolve over time. Those that are more severe and that are typically described as alcohol dementia can be explained more adequately by other disorders (most notably Korsakoff's disorder) rather than as a result of neurotoxic effects of alcohol. Victor's (1994) review does provide a concise and insightful discussion of this issue and does summarize the literature supporting the view that alcohol has no neurotoxic effects.

However, it appears that neurotoxic effects of alcohol that are not apparent at a structural level may become more obvious when techniques are used that assess brain metabolic functions, (e.g., positron emission tomography [PET]), electrophysiological functioning, and density of synaptic receptors. At least one group of investigators has found that neuropsychological impairment is associated with hypometabolism (as measured by PET) in the medial frontal cortex and that this hypometabolism is not solely the result of tissue loss (Adams et al., 1993). Similarly, Parsons and colleagues (Glenn, Parsons, & Sinha, 1994; Parsons, 1994) reported that electrophysiological evaluations of abstinent alcoholics revealed deficits in evoked related potentials that did not improve over time. Finally, brain autopsy studies have found that alcoholics have significant (40%) decreases in muscarinic cholinergic receptors in frontal and temporal cortex and putamen, as well as decreased benzodiazepine receptors in the frontal cortex (30%) and hippocampus (25%) (Freund & Ballinger, 1991). These decreases were found in the absence of Wernicke's encephalopathy. These studies suggest that, while improved volumetric changes in white matter may occur as a result of abstinence, impairment in brain metabolism and electrophysiological functioning persists and there are significant decreases in synaptic receptors.

Of the etiologic factors suggested by Reitan and Wolfson (1985), cognitive deficits most often observed in geriatric substance abusers result from diseases of the nervous system due to malnutrition, neurological disorders secondary to alcohol-induced cirrhosis of the liver, and disorders whose etiology is unclear. Specific disorders resulting from malnutrition and cirrhosis of the liver include Wernicke-Korsakoff syndrome, Marchiafava-Bignami disease, hepatic encephalopathy, and pellagrous encephalopathy. Researchers have identified other disorders but we will limit our discussion to Wernicke-Korsakoff syndrome and hepatic encephalopathy because these are most common. More research has focused on determining type and prevalence of specific cognitive deficits in individuals who chronically abuse alcohol. Many of these more general studies have not attempted to identify a specific etiology for observed cognitive deficits. However, they provide valuable information regarding types and severity of cognitive deficits in the more general alcoholic population. In the following sections, we discuss the general pattern of cognitive deficits among alcoholics, differential improvement in cognitive function resulting from abstinence, as well as typical cognitive deficits in individuals with specific disorders and syndromes.

General Cognitive Deficits

Types of Deficits. As the specific nature of neuropsychological deficits resulting from chronic alcohol abuse has been reviewed extensively elsewhere (Ellis & Oscar-Berman, 1989; Parsons & Nixon, 1993; Salmon, Butters, & Heindel, 1993; Tarter & Ryan, 1986), only a summary of this research is provided. Studies conducted over the past 30 years are generally consistent in reporting that individuals who chronically abuse alcohol retain general cognitive functioning as assessed by standardized intelligence tests. However, on more sensitive tests of specific ability areas, they exhibit deficits in areas of verbal and nonverbal memory (O'Mahony & Doherty, 1993; Ryan & Butters, 1986; Tarter, 1980; Wilson, Kolb, Odland, & Wishaw, 1987), visuospatial abilities (O'Mahony & Doherty, 1993; Ryan & Butters, 1986; Wilson et al., 1987), visuoperceptual abstraction (Donovan, Queisser, & O'Leary, 1976), conceptual learning (Adams et al., 1993; Fitzhugh, Fitzhugh, & Reitan, 1965; Tarter & Parsons, 1971), problem-solving abilities (Braun & Richer, 1993; Grant, Adams, & Reed, 1984), and perceptual-motor skills (Fabian & Parsons, 1983). Impairment of these abilities appears to be most prominent directly following detoxification, and, while resolution of some of the aforementioned deficits occurs as a function of length of abstinence, recovery of function may not occur in all cases without some type of rehabilitative intervention. Abstraction and visuospatial abilities are reported as most consistently impaired. Goldman (1990) has suggested that the cognitive deficits noted in alcoholics may be caused by a single factor (such as impaired attention) although other factors, such as impaired sensory processing, may also play a role.

Resolution of Deficits. A number of studies have suggested tentative time periods in which resolution of cognitive deficits occurs after detoxification. During the first 2 weeks following drinking cessation, performance improves on tasks assessing overall intellectual functioning, short-term memory, and visual motor skills (Goldman, 1986). Other deficient cognitive abilities, including abstract problem-solving, perceptual motor abilities, learning, memory, and attention, improve more slowly, if at all. Yohman, Parsons, and Leber (1985) reported that even after 13 months of abstinence, chronic alcoholics' performance differed significantly from age- and education-matched controls on tests requiring abstract problem-solving and perceptual-motor abilities. Additionally, nonsignificant but consistent differences were evident between controls and alcoholics on learning and memory tests. Verbal comprehension was the only ability in which alcoholics' performance was similar to that of controls at 13 months. Brandt, Butters, Ryan, and Bayog (1983) reported that even after 5 years of abstinence, alcoholics may continue to experience decreased performance on tasks requiring short-term memory, attention, and visuospatial abilities. One study of younger alcoholics (ages 18–35) with shorter drinking histories (average of 6 years) who were abstinent an average of 39 days was unable to find significant cognitive impairment in areas of language, intelligence, motor abilities, memory, or problem-solving abilities (Eckardt et al., 1995). This is consistent with the observation that many cognitive deficits exhibited by alcoholics do improve with abstinence, and that cognitive deficits that do not resolve in chronic alcohol abusers result from cumulative effects of a lifetime pattern of alcohol abuse. Eckardt and colleagues (1995) found that, even in their younger group, individuals who consumed more alcohol over the course of their lives performed more poorly on neuropsychological measures and that individuals who were abstinent for longer periods of time performed better on neuropsychological tests. Improvement in cognitive abilities following cessation of alcohol consumption may result from a number of factors, including abstinence and improved nutrition (Goldstein, 1987a).

Goldman (1990) has further addressed the process of cognitive recovery in alcoholics by distinguishing between *experience-dependent recovery*, that is, recovery of cognitive abilities directly resulting from external intervention, and *time-dependent recovery*, that is, recovery of cognitive functions that occurs spontaneously or as a function of length of abstinence. This categorization of recovery is suggestive of at least two types of cognitive deficits: those that improve of their own accord and those that require specific intervention in order to improve. It should be noted that a third category of deficits may also exist, namely, abilities that are permanently impaired or irremediable. Inability to learn new information, which is observed in individuals suffering from Korsakoff's syndrome, is one example of such irremediable deficits.

Inconsistencies in studies examining recovery of specific cognitive abilities over time probably result from the methodological limitations and factors endemic to alcoholic populations that we discussed earlier. However, of particular relevance to studies examining improvement in cognitive function over time are methodological issues related to

longitudinal research. As with all research that spans extended time periods, factors such as subject maturation and subject attrition almost certainly affect results but are difficult to control experimentally.

Specific Disorders and Syndromes Associated with Alcohol Use Disorders

Hepatic Encephalopathy. As many as 30% of individuals who abuse alcohol go on to develop cirrhosis of the liver. A growing body of research implicates cirrhosis of the liver in producing cognitive deficits among alcoholics. In fact, some authors suggest that cirrhosis of the liver and other medical conditions, if not controlled, may cause the weak correlations between cognitive impairment and chronicity of consumption (Arria, Tarter, Starzl, & VanThiel, 1991). The exact mechanisms underlying cognitive deficits observed in individuals with cirrhosis of the liver are not thoroughly understood. However, it does appear that increases in nitrogenous compounds (e.g., gamma-aminobutyric acid) and decreases in protein synthesis, which are indicators of different aspects of liver dysfunction, are significantly correlated with different types of cognitive impairment (Moss, Tarter, Yao, & VanThiel, 1992). These results suggest that cognitive impairment produced by hepatic dysfunction is a multiply determined and complex phenomenon.

Early studies in this area indicated that alcoholics with cirrhosis performed worse on some tests of cognitive functioning than did alcoholics without cirrhosis, even though the two groups had similar histories of alcohol consumption (Gilberstadt et al., 1980; Smith & Smith, 1977). However, Tarter and colleagues have provided convincing evidence to date of the negative impact of cirrhosis on cognitive functions (Arria et al., 1991; Moss et al., 1992; Tarter, Moss, Arria, & VanThiel, 1990; Tarter, Switala, Lu, & VanThiel, 1995; Trzepacz et al., 1994). In their series of investigations, Tarter and coworkers (Tarter et al., 1990) noted that neuropsychological performance of individuals with cirrhosis due to alcohol abuse was remarkably similar to that of individuals with cirrhosis due to other factors, although individuals with alcohol-induced cirrhosis also performed worse on tests of short-term memory, eye tracking, and hand-eye coordination. This suggests that hepatic encephalopathy significantly contributes to level of neuropsychological impairment experienced by cirrhotic alcoholics. While many of these deficits appear to resolve following liver transplantation, memory capacity does not appear to improve (Arria et al., 1991).

Tarter and coworkers have also reported that liver dysfunction that does not present with typical alterations in mood, cognition, and consciousness associated with hepatic encephalopathy can still produce significant neuropsychological impairment (Moss et al., 1992). Furthermore, they report that different biochemical indices of liver dysfunction are associated with specific types of cognitive dysfunction. Elevations in nitrogenous compounds (in serum) were associated with impairment of visuospatial abilities, while impaired protein synthesis was associated with impaired psychomotor ability, language efficiency, and perceptual abilities. Also, decreased hepatic blood flow was related to decreases in language efficiency. Although these correlations were significant, various measures of liver functioning accounted for a relatively small proportion of overall variance in neuropsychological test scores, suggesting that other, as yet undetermined factors significantly contribute to cognitive functioning in patients with subclinical hepatic encephalopathy. Despite apparent deficits caused by cirrhosis of the liver, other abilities, such as abstraction abilities, do not appear to be adversely affected in these subclinical patients (Tarter et al., 1995).

Finally, there is some evidence that has localized the areas of the cerebrum that are most susceptible to effects of hepatic dysfunction. Trzepacz et al. (1994) utilized single photon emission computed tomography (SPECT) scanning to examine regional cerebral blood flow (rCBF) in six subjects who exhibited subclinical hepatic encephalopathy and were in the end stage of cirrhosis. When compared to six control subjects, cirrhotic subjects had decreased rCBF in the right basal ganglia and decreased rCBF bilaterally in the frontotemporal regions. These decreases in rCBF were consistent with the cirrhotic subjects' neuropsychological test performance as they also exhibited deficits on tasks requiring visuopractic abilities.

These studies suggest that liver function is an important factor to consider when attempting to determine etiology of cognitive deficits in alcoholic patients. This is particularly true for elderly alcoholics who have prolonged histories of alcohol consumption and an increased risk of hepatic dysfunction. Also, these studies make it clear that cognitive impairment due to liver dysfunction may occur even though the typical pattern of symptomatology associated with hepatic encephalopathy is absent.

Wernicke-Korsakoff Syndrome.   Oscar-Berman and colleagues have discussed Wernicke-Korsakoff syndrome elsewhere in this volume (see Chapter 14). Wernicke-Korsakoff syndrome is caused by a deficiency in thiamine (vitamin B; Victor, Adams, & Collins, 1989). Compared to other populations, alcoholics are particularly susceptible to Wernicke-Korsakoff syndrome because of poor dietary practices. In most cases, Wernicke-Korsakoff syndrome occurs following prolonged periods of drinking during which the alcoholic becomes malnourished. Thiamine deficiency resulting from poor nutrition causes hemorrhages in white matter structures (specifically, the third and fourth ventricles and the aqueduct of Sylvius). Lesions produced by this hemorrhaging result in impairment of motor and cognitive functioning. Typically, ataxic gait, nystagmus, and opthalmoplegia are noted along with a confused state during the acute phase of the disorder. This encephalopathy improves within 4 weeks if patients are administered large doses of thiamine. Most patients who survive Wernicke's encephalopathy go on to develop Korsakoff's syndrome. Korsakoff's syndrome is characterized by impairment in several areas of cognitive functioning, including executive functions (Pollux, Wester, & De Haan, 1995). Prominent deficits are in memory functioning. Memory deficits produce severe retrograde and anterograde amnesias (see Salmon et al., 1993, for review). While some studies suggest that medications (e.g., fluvoxamine) can cause some improvement in amnesia (Martin et al., 1995), these findings remain controversial, and amnesia is typically considered irreversible. Retrograde amnesia can affect recall of information as much as 20 years prior to onset of the encephalopathy, while anterograde amnesia significantly impairs ability to acquire new information. In contrast, general intellectual functioning and semantic memory are typically preserved. While related to length of drinking history, this disorder is not confined to older alcoholics. In our work with patients who are dependent on alcohol, we have treated individuals in their early forties with Wernicke-Korsakoff syndrome. Because of the severe and debilitating cognitive deficits characteristic of Wernicke-Korsakoff syndrome, clinicians treating elderly alcoholics need to be acutely aware of the nutritional status of their patients and may consider giving thiamine prophylactically to all patients who are being treated for alcohol dependence or abuse.

Alcoholic Dementia.   There is controversy regarding the etiology of alcoholic dementia. However, one report indicates that alcohol-related dementias account for 1.0% of cases of dementia in community dwelling elderly over 65 years of age (N = 1,070) followed over 6 years (Copeland et al., 1992). Other reports indicate that as many as 25% of elderly alcoholic patients have alcohol dementia (Finlayson et al., 1988) and that 24% of institutionalized elderly have alcohol-related dementia (Carlen et al., 1994). Because many individuals with histories of chronic alcohol consumption do go on to develop a dementia syndrome, we discuss it here. The *DSM-IV* has included diagnosis of alcohol-induced persisting dementia in recognition of this syndrome. While this diagnosis does acknowledge presence of a dementia syndrome in individuals who have chronically abused alcohol, it does not specify whether the dementia is induced specifically by neurotoxic effects of alcohol or if it results from other problems associated with alcohol abuse, such as hemorrhaging with Wernicke-Korsakoff syndrome. As with other forms of dementia, cognitive impairment in alcohol dementia is severe enough to significantly interfere with occupational and social functioning.

Similar to Wernicke-Korsakoff syndrome, cognitive impairment noted in alcohol dementia is a permanent condition that persists long after consumption of alcohol has ceased and after spontaneous recovery of cognitive functioning noted in less severely cognitively impaired alcoholics has occurred. In contrast to Wernicke-Korsakoff syndrome, onset of alcohol dementia is slow and progressive (Goldstein, 1985). Patients with alcohol-induced dementia exhibit a broad range of cognitive dysfunction that affects general intellectual abilities

as well as memory. Memory deficits noted in patients with alcohol dementia are not more severe than other cognitive deficits that accompany this type of dementia. Studies that examined severity of memory impairment in patients with alcohol dementia suggest that these memory deficits can be just as severe as those noted in Wernicke-Korsakoff syndrome (Lishman, 1990). In addition to memory deficits, patients with alcohol dementia also exhibit impairment of other abilities including visuospatial abilities (Goldstein, 1985; Seltzer & Sherwin, 1978) and abstraction and problem-solving abilities (Jones & Parsons, 1972; Martin, Adinoff, Weingartner, Mukherjee, & Eckardt, 1986; Shelly & Goldstein, 1976).

Because of the prevalence of alcohol dementia, it is important to distinguish it from other forms of dementia, particularly dementia of the Alzheimer's type. One area that remains relatively well preserved in patients with alcohol dementia is language abilities (Goldstein, 1985). In fact, because they do not exhibit the typical aphasic language disturbances which are cardinal features of Alzheimer's dementia (Cummings & Benson, 1992), this may help distinguish between patients with alcohol-related dementia and Alzheimer's dementia.

Benzodiazepine Abuse and Dependence

Although the elderly take multiple medications that have the potential for abuse and misuse, relatively few studies have examined drug effects on neuropsychological performance in the elderly. Research has focused almost exclusively on benzodiazepine use in older adults. As such, this discussion is focused on benzodiazepines.

Drug Characteristics and Side Effects

Benzodiazepines are classified as sedative-hypnotics and are used frequently to treat anxiety, insomnia, and agitation in the elderly. Because of their calming and sometimes euphoric effects, particularly when used in combination with alcohol (Juergens, 1993), use of benzodiazepines can lead to psychological dependence. Long-term use of benzodiazepines can lead to development of tolerance to their therapeutic effects, and physiological dependence can appear after only a few days or weeks of daily administration (APA, 1990).

Normal side effects of benzodiazepine use include sedation, ataxia, dysarthria, incoordination, diplopia, vertigo, dizziness, and less frequently, hostility and depression (APA, 1990). The elderly have been shown to have greater incidence of side effects because of increased sensitivity to these drugs (Higgit, 1992). Even small single doses in elderly hospitalized patients can cause a distinct syndrome characterized by reversible delirium, anterograde amnesia, and automatic movements (Patterson, 1987). Closser (1991) describes several pharmacokinetic changes due to normal aging that may explain this increased sensitivity. Factors that may account for an enhanced response include (a) decreased plasma clearance of benzodiazepines, (b) increased drug volume of distribution, and (c) greater increases in gamma-aminobutyric acid (GABA) binding and neuronal inhibition.

Elderly individuals also appear to experience greater withdrawal effects. Sudden discontinuance from benzodiazepines often causes confusion in older adults (Closser, 1991). Juergens (1993) describes common symptoms of withdrawal which include anxiety, irritability, insomnia, fatigue, headache, muscle twitching or aching, tremor, shakiness, sweating, dizziness, concentration difficulties, nausea, loss of appetite, depression, derealization, increased sensory perception, seizures, tinnitus, delirium, and confusion. These withdrawal effects are often increased and more intense when shorter-acting benzodiazepines are discontinued abruptly (Woods & Winger, 1995). Abrupt discontinuance has been shown to cause seizures within the first 1 to 3 days of stopping the drug (APA, 1990). This most often occurs with long half-life benzodiazepines such as diazepam. Gradual tapering is the preferred treatment for benzodiazepine dependence, and the standard regimen is to reduce the dose by one fourth each week over 4 to 6 weeks (Hommer, 1991).

Because the elderly are more sensitive to daytime sedation and are at increased risk for falls from benzodiazepine use, a task force recommended that three long-acting benzodiazepines, chlordiazepoxide, diazepam, and flurazepam, be entirely avoided in patients who are 65 years or older (Beers et al.,

1991). The APA (1990) also notes that they are especially hazardous for elderly and goes on to recommend that these drugs not be used for long-term treatment of insomnia.

Cognitive Deficits

A number of investigators have examined cognitive changes due to benzodiazepine use in adult samples, and several of these studies have compared elderly individuals to younger individuals. Pomara et al. (Pomara, Deptula, Medel, Block, & Greenblatt, 1989; Pomara, Deptula, Rubinstein, Stanley, & Stanley, 1988; Pomara et al., 1985) have conducted several controlled studies on the effects of diazepam on neuropsychological test performance in the elderly. The first of these studies (Pomara et al., 1985) examined the effect of a 2.5 mg dose of diazepam on test performance in 12 young (ages 20–36) and 12 older adults (ages 60–77). Subjects were administered diazepam or placebo orally under double-blind conditions. Blood plasma concentrations and neuropsychological testing were completed at baseline, at 1 hour, and at 3 hours following drug administration. Results showed that in comparison to placebo, the 2.5 mg of diazepam significantly affected performance in the elderly group but not in the younger group. Diazepam impaired both immediate and delayed recall on the Buschke Selective Reminding Task, delayed recall on a visual memory task, and reaction time. Immediate visual memory recall, digit span, and critical flicker fusion showed no significant effects of the acute dose of diazepam in the elderly. These authors concluded that in the elderly (a) long-term memory and psychomotor speed are most susceptible to the effects of diazepam; (b) even a low dose of diazepam causes cognitive impairment; and (c) there may be an age-related increase in sensitivity to diazepam's effects on learning and retention of new information.

In another study on these same 24 subjects, Pomara and colleagues (1988) assessed the effects of diazepam on intrusion errors using the Buschke Selective Reminding Task. Three dose levels (2.5 mg, 5.0 mg, and 10 mg) were compared to placebo within the elderly group. Young subjects were only given 2.5 mg or placebo. For the elderly, a 5 mg dose produced a significant increase in intrusion errors at 1 hour after drug administration and a significant increase with 10 mg at both 1 and 3 hours. This increase was found to be positively correlated with drug plasma concentrations. Neither group had a significant increase in intrusions with the 2.5 mg dose on the immediate recall task, but 2.5 mg produced significant increases on the delayed recall task for the elderly. One curious result was that 5 mg and 10 mg doses in the elderly did not significantly increase intrusion errors on delayed recall.

A third study conducted by Pomara et al. (1989) examined the effects of chronic administration of diazepam in the elderly. Using a double-blind counterbalanced design, these authors compared the effect of placebo, 2.5 mg and 10 mg doses, and chronic administration on recall and intrusions in 45 elderly and 44 young volunteers. They also examined whether acute effects of a dose of diazepam would change following 3 weeks of chronic administration and whether tolerance develops to the acute side effects of diazepam on memory. Subjects were screened for any significant cognitive or memory impairment prior to inclusion in the study. Acute effects of diazepam were assessed by a neuropsychological test battery which was administered immediately before the dose and 1.5 and 3 hours following ingestion. After the acute drug sessions, subjects were given a supply of diazepam (2.5 or 10 mg) or placebo for chronic administration.

Results of acute drug trials showed that a 10 mg dose of diazepam impaired recall performance significantly more than placebo or 2.5 mg at both 1.5 and 3 hours following drug administration, and that young and elderly were not differentially affected by the drug. After a 2.5 mg dose, no impairment in recall performance was found as in the 1985 study, but this may have been caused by several methodological differences. In addition, the elderly produced more intrusion errors at baseline than the young and made more intrusions in response to diazepam. After chronic administration, 10 mg of diazepam were found to produce significantly greater impairment in recall than placebo for both groups, but the magnitude of impairment was smaller than in the acute phase. In addition, when given an acute rechallenge after 3 weeks of use, total recall was significantly decreased with 10 mg as compared to placebo, but again, the decrement was smaller than observed with just acute adminis-

tration. After chronic administration, both the young and older groups showed a significant increase in number of intrusion errors in comparison to placebo. These results suggest that after chronic administration of diazepam for 3 weeks, some tolerance to its effects may occur. Also it appears that the elderly demonstrate higher sensitivity to some of diazepam's acute deleterious cognitive effects (intrusion errors) but not to others (recall). Partial tolerance appears to develop to the drug's adverse effects on memory with chronic administration. Results of this study (Pomara et al., 1989) also showed that the pattern of response on recall of verbal material to diazepam was similar for the young and elderly with 10 mg of diazepam, but baseline performance was substantially lower for the elderly. This suggests that drug-induced impairment may be more noticeable and of greater clinical significance for older adults.

The results of Pomara and coworkers have been replicated by others. Hinrichs and Ghoneim (1987) used a double-blind controlled group design to compare 36 subjects comprising three age groups: young (ages 19–28), middle-aged (ages 40–45) and elderly (ages 61–73). Subjects were given placebo or a dose of diazepam dependent upon body weight (10, 5, 4, or 2 mg). They were tested on six different tasks at baseline and at 65 and 155 minutes after drug administration. Overall, they found that diazepam produced significant impairment over all groups on measures of memory and psychomotor performance, and the pattern of response and impairment produced by diazepam was similar for all age groups. From this they concluded that differences in "baseline performance may make equal decrements more noticeable and more serious in older individuals. A modest decline in cognitive or psychomotor abilities of a younger person may have little or no effect on that person's activities. The same loss of ability in an older individual who is already performing at a low level or exerting more effort to maintain comparable behavior may have serious subjective and clinical consequences" (p. 105).

Other investigators have extended the results to shorter-acting benzodiazepines. Lawlor and coworkers (1992) examined effects of lorazepam on attention and recent memory in elderly adults. These investigators employed a within-subject double-blind placebo controlled research design to investigate effects of lorazepam and buspirone on attention and verbal memory. Ten adults (mean age = 62.5 ± 2.6) were randomly administered lorazepam or buspirone or placebo on three separate occasions. Tests of attention and memory were given approximately 90 minutes following drug administration. Results indicated that relative to placebo, subjects performed significantly worse on tests requiring attention and exhibited a trend toward poorer performance on tasks requiring recent memory after they were administered lorazepam. As expected, these results extend those of previous studies of the cognitive effects of lorazepam in younger individuals.

Two studies were found that examined the effect of benzodiazepine discontinuance on cognition. In a study of adverse drug reactions in outpatients being evaluated for dementia, Larson, Kukull, Buchner, and Reifler (1987) found that sedative-hypnotics, especially benzodiazepines, were the most common drugs associated with cognitive impairment. After discontinuing these drugs, even individuals with diagnosed dementia showed some improvement in cognitive functioning. Interestingly, the authors note that many patients in this study had been using benzodiazepines for years and developed cognitive impairment insidiously as a late complication of their use. This may lend support to Hinrichs and Ghoneim's statement (1987) that cognitive deficits from prolonged benzodiazepine use do not become apparent until combined with the effects of aging. However, there is also initial evidence suggesting that cognitive deficits produced by long-term benzodiazepine use may not improve even after a substantial time period has elapsed. Recently, Tata, Rollings, Collins, Pickering, and Jacobson (1994) reported that, relative to controls (age- and IQ-matched), patients withdrawn from diazepam exhibited deficits in verbal memory, visuospatial abilities, and psychomotor abilities when tested prewithdrawal, postwithdrawal, and at 6-months follow-up. Because the average age of patients was 44.4 (±9.4), they cannot be considered geriatric patients. However, it is reasonable to expect that a similar course in the resolution of deficits would be present in elderly individuals because existing literature suggests that the elderly are more sensitive to acute and chronic effects of benzodiazepine use on cognition.

From the results of these studies, it is apparent that benzodiazepines (including diazepam and lorazepam) produce significant changes in cognitive functioning in the elderly. Studies investigating the acute and chronic effects of benzodiazepine use have found that even a small single dose of diazepam can cause some impairment in memory and psychomotor performance although tolerance to some of these effects may develop with chronic use. Differing methodologies make the results of existing studies difficult to compare. In addition, since many elderly patients are placed on diazepam for long-term treatment of sleep and anxiety disorders, longitudinal research that follows patients over longer time periods is required. One study examining the effects of discontinuance on cognitive functioning suggested that cognitive functioning improved in the elderly after discontinuation of benzodiazepines, while a second study suggested that cognitive impairment persisted following benzodiazepine withdrawal in younger individuals. Further investigation is required to identify factors that cause persisting cognitive deficits and improvement in cognitive functioning following discontinuation of long-term benzodiazepine use. It may be that individuals who are already demonstrating some cognitive impairment (elderly individuals with mild dementia) exhibit improvement following benzodiazepine withdrawal, even though they do not ever regain previous levels of functioning, that is, continue to exhibit benzodiazepine-induced cognitive deficits. This effect would be more clearly demonstrated in patients without cognitive impairment (see Tata et al., 1994) and is consistent with results of two studies on the effects of benzodiazepine withdrawal (Hinrichs & Ghoneim, 1987; Tata et al., 1994).

Treatment of Substance Use Disorders

Although information on prevalence of substance use disorders among elderly individuals is limited, sufficient information exists to dispel the myth that these disorders are rare among the elderly. Rather, studies suggest that a large number of substance abusers survive to late life, and a significant number of elderly individuals develop substance use disorders after age 65. Also, many elderly individuals continue to seek treatment for these conditions. For example, after examining treatment records of inpatients treated at Department of Veterans Affairs medical centers in 1987, Moos et al. (1994) reported that 98,000 had substance abuse diagnoses. Of these, 21,139 were 55 years of age and older. While the large majority of these cases had singular diagnoses of alcohol abuse/dependence (58.2%), a second group of 2,887 patients (13.7%) had diagnoses of drug dependence/psychosis. The data provided by Moos and colleagues (1994) suggest that a significant portion of elderly patients treated at Department of Veterans Affairs medical centers carry diagnoses of substance abuse other than alcohol abuse.

However, there are at least two essential issues that have not been adequately addressed in the current treatment literature. These issues include (a) development of treatment strategies that are unique to geriatric patients, and (b) development of programs to address the unique factors that contribute to and/or maintain substance use disorders in elderly individuals.

Potential Obstacles to Successful Treatment

Cognitive Deficits

A number of reports indicate that cognitive deficits are moderately predictive of treatment outcome. Based on these reports, it appears that alcoholics with the highest degree of cognitive impairment have the poorest prognosis for recovery (Parsons, 1994; Parsons, Schaeffer, & Glenn, 1990; Sussman, Rychtarik, Mueser, Glynn, & Prue, 1986). Some authors have suggested that the relation between neuropsychological functioning and prognosis is the direct product of an inability, on the impaired patient's part, to fully utilize treatment opportunities requiring higher order cognitive processes (e.g., verbal abstraction) (Goldman, 1986; Gordon, Kennedy, & McPeake, 1988; Wilkinson & Sanchez-Craig, 1981). However, these conclusions should be tempered by other studies that suggest that neuropsychological functioning, as assessed by standard laboratory measures, has little to do with abstinence following treatment (Eckardt et al., 1988) or that neuropsychological functioning is only a weak predictor of drinking behavior following treatment

(See Donovan, Walker, & Kivlahan, 1987). These conflicting results have led some to suggest that neuropsychological functioning is a moderator of treatment and exerts its effect on treatment efficacy in an indirect rather than direct manner (Goldman, 1990). In either case, it would appear that disruption of normal neuropsychological functioning present in many recently detoxified alcoholics may render them unable to fully use current treatment methods that require higher order cognitive functioning. It is also the case that treatment becomes increasingly difficult as cognitive impairment increases. When cognitive impairment is severe, it affects elderly individuals' abilities to learn and retain new information, impedes application of new problem-solving strategies, and/or causes impaired insight accompanied by executive function deficits which often decrease the awareness of the need for change. Finally, when compared to young substance abusers, elderly substance abusers often exhibit slower recovery of cognitive functioning following cessation of substance use. For alcoholism, this decreased recovery curve has been the most well documented. These findings have implications for timing of treatment. We recommend that in older alcoholics, treatment aimed at ameliorating substance abuse not be initiated for 2 to 4 weeks following abstinence.

Concomitant Psychiatric Disorders

Also, many substance abusers have concomitant psychiatric disorders, particularly major depression, anxiety disorders, and personality disorders. In some cases, substance abuse has served as a major coping mechanism to reduce psychological distress caused by these psychiatric disorders. Similarly, some patients go on to abuse medications initially prescribed for psychiatric conditions and have either developed a tolerance to or become physiologically and psychologically dependent on them (e.g., benzodiazepines). Also, increased risk of relapse in some individuals with alcohol use disorders is associated with depression (Hatsukami & Pickens, 1982). If and when substance use is discontinued, underlying psychiatric disorders contributing to development and maintenance of abuse must be effectively treated in order for patients to maintain abstinence. At least one recent well-controlled study examined the effects of treating coexisting affective disorders on length of sobriety for individuals with a primary diagnosis of alcoholism and a secondary diagnosis of depression (Mason & Kocsis, 1991). Conclusions of this study were somewhat disappointing because it did not appear that treatment of depressed alcoholics with desipramine had a significant effect on length of sobriety following drinking cessation. It may be that amelioration of depression is not a strong enough factor in and of itself to increase length of sobriety in primary alcoholics. However, it may also be that individuals who have primary diagnoses of depression and secondary diagnoses of substance use disorders would benefit significantly more (i.e., exhibit increased length of sobriety) from treatment of their psychiatric conditions. More research is required before these questions can be answered definitively.

Withdrawal Symptoms

Elderly individuals often experience more severe side effects when withdrawn from substances (Brower et al., 1994). Because of this, health care providers must be acutely aware of the possibility that symptoms that follow inadvertent periods of forced abstinence (e.g., hospitalization, etc.) are withdrawal symptoms. Health care professionals will need to keep in mind the possibility of substance abuse and be aware of the typical withdrawal symptoms associated with popular medications, including alcohol and benzodiazepines.

Treatment Implications and Recommendations

Pharmacotherapy

When treating symptoms of anxiety in elderly adults, we encourage practitioners to consider use of antianxiety agents that have demonstrated efficacy in the elderly but have little, if any, effect on cognitive functioning. One such antianxiety agent is buspirone. When compared to lorazepam and placebo, at least one study indicates that a single dose of buspirone does not cause impairment on tests requiring recent verbal memory, vigilance, or attention (Lawlor et al., 1992). Also, antidepressant medications, particularly tricyclics, are effective in treating some specific types of anxiety disorders

(e.g., agoraphobia). Ayd (1994) provides several alternative pharmacotherapies for treatment of anxiety disorders in the elderly.

While clinicians can use medication in conjunction with other forms of treatment to ameliorate psychiatric symptoms that accompany substance abuse, studies examining the effect of psychotropic medications on amelioration of substance use disorders and, in particular, alcohol abuse/dependence suggest that these are not effective treatments. Fluoxetine (Kranzler et al., 1995), tricyclic antidepressants such as desipramine (Mason & Kocsis, 1991), and lithium (Dorus et al., 1989) have not been shown to be effective. Other investigations of disulfiram, a drug which causes a violent adverse reaction to alcohol consumption, are also disappointing (Fuller et al., 1986).

Opioid receptor antagonists are more promising for treatment of alcoholism. The rationale supporting use of opioid receptor antagonists is based on results of behavioral, physiological, and biochemical studies that suggest that alcohol affects the endogenous opioid systems of the cerebrum and that individuals who develop alcohol abuse/dependence have genetically based increases in sensitivity of the endogenous opioid system to the effects of alcohol (De Waele & Gianoulakis, 1992, 1994; Gianoulakis, 1990; Linseman, 1989; Volpicelli, Alterman, Hayashida, & O'Brien, 1992). Because of the role of opioid peptides in reinforcement, reward, and analgesia (Olson, Olson, & Kastin, 1989), this increased sensitivity initiates a behavior pattern of increased and prolonged alcohol consumption.

Naltrexone hydrochloride was recently approved by the Food and Drug Administration as an opioid receptor antagonist for treatment of alcohol abuse and dependence. Results of a recent 12-week study suggested that administration of naltrexone hydrochloride significantly decreased subjective reports of alcohol craving, number of days of alcohol use, and percentage of patients who relapsed; 54% of patients who received placebo relapsed while only 23% of patients receiving active medication relapsed (Volpicelli et al., 1992). Moreover, 95% of subjects taking placebo who had one drink went on to relapse, but only 50% of patients on naltrexone relapsed after taking one drink.

There are at least three factors that may contraindicate treatment with opioid receptor antagonists in elderly patients. First, opioid receptor antagonists significantly decrease the effectiveness of analgesics. Because medical conditions that require treatment with opiate-based analgesics do occur among elderly individuals, thorough evaluation of medication profiles is necessary before initiating treatment with opioid receptor antagonists. Similarly, because acute medical conditions requiring administration of opiates occur more frequently among elderly individuals, medical identification bracelets are necessary for all patients maintained on opioid receptor antagonists. In the event of hospitalization for a medical emergency, information provided on the bracelet will be essential to health care providers. Second, because naltrexone does have the potential for hepatotoxicity, evaluation of liver functioning is required before initiating treatment. This is a particularly important consideration for elderly patients with long histories of alcohol abuse/ dependence because of their increased chances for hepatic dysfunction. Third, there is one report of increased arthritic pain in a patient who was administered naltrexone hydrochloride in a double-blind study (Volpicelli et al., 1992). While this finding has not been consistently demonstrated, it is important to consider the appearance or exacerbation of pain syndromes when opioid receptor antagonists are administered, as these drugs do act on the naturally occurring biochemical systems responsible for decreasing pain.

Treatment Program Development

A renewed emphasis is needed on development of treatment programs specifically for geriatric patients with substance use disorders. These programs could take into account the slower recovery times of these older patients following cessation of substance use as well as address common attitudes that impede recovery. Programs could also provide ancillary treatments for comorbid psychiatric disorders. To date, research confirms the improved efficacy of programs designed specifically for treatment of elders. In one study, treatment of elderly individuals with their same-age peers increased treatment completion fourfold (Kofoed, Tolson, Atkinson, Toth, & Turner, 1987) when compared to elderly individuals who participated in

treatment with younger individuals. Not only does homogeneity in age of group members influence outcome, but also type of treatment is important. At least two studies indicate that the older the individuals with alcohol use disorders become, the more important the treatment modality becomes. Rice, Longabaugh, Beattiem, and Noel (1993) found that while younger patients (18–29 years old) appeared to benefit equally from three types of treatment (extended cognitive behavioral therapy, relationship enhancement, and relationship and vocational enhancement), older patients (50+ years old) treated with extended cognitive behavioral therapy exhibited better outcomes at 3 to 6 months follow-up than older patients treated with either of the other therapies.

Kashner, Rodell, Ogden, Guggenheim, and Karson (1992) also examined differences between alcoholics' responses to different treatments based on age. In their investigation, 137 patients over the age of 45 participated in one of two types of inpatient treatments: (a) traditional confrontational treatment designed to overcome denial and resistance; or (b) an older alcoholics rehabilitation (OAR) program that emphasized developing peer relationships, increasing self-esteem, and achieving short-term goals. Of the 137 subjects, 53% were 60 years of age or older. Compared to the traditional confrontational treatment, patients who participated in the OAR treatment made more outpatient visits following inpatient treatment and were 2.9 times more likely to report abstinence at 6 months ($p < .003$) and 2.1 times more likely to report abstinence at 12 months ($p < .04$). Interestingly, abstinence rates increased with age so that while 50-year-old patients who participated in the OAR program were only .5 times more likely to abstain than those treated in the traditional program, patients treated in the OAR program who were 70 years old were 5.1 times more likely to abstain.

Successful treatment of elderly substance abusers is important for a number of reasons. First and foremost, as with all patients who have substance use disorders, their pattern of substance use has caused negative consequences so that at least one major area of functioning is compromised. Successful treatment increases quality of life by decreasing the negative consequences associated with substance use. Treatment also provides opportunities for them to develop more effective means to cope with life tasks. Second, elderly patients with long histories of substance use disorders who receive outpatient follow-up or after-care exhibit decreased mortality when compared to those who do not receive treatment (Moos et al., 1994). Moreover, it appears that the mortality rate decreases as the number of outpatient visits increases (Moos et al., 1994). In this case, the cause of decreased mortality is unclear but may result from increased periods of abstinence following inpatient treatment or an overall reduction in the amount of substances used following inpatient treatment (Bullock, Reed, & Grant, 1992; Moos et al., 1994). Third, in the near future, health care costs associated with treatment of substance use disorders in the elderly will significantly increase. This is in part due to the aging trend in the United States and the increasing longevity of Americans. Fourth, alcohol abuse may contribute to the rate of decline in Alzheimer's disease, so that individuals with dementia of the Alzheimer's type who are heavy alcohol consumers deteriorate more quickly than those who do not use alcohol (Teri, Hughes, & Larson, 1990). Alcohol abuse may also be one predictor of late-onset dementia of the Alzheimer's type (Fratiglioni, Ahlbom, Viitanen, & Winbald, 1993).

Implications, Recommendations, and Future Directions

Treatment

Much work remains to be done in the area of geriatric substance use disorders. We can draw several tentative conclusions from the available treatment literature. First, it appears that, as with most group treatments, some homogeneity of group members is important. More specifically, elderly patients appear to respond better if treated with their same-age peers. Second, it appears that content of treatment programs is important. Those treatments that provide older individuals with problem-solving strategies (e.g., cognitive behavioral psychotherapy), procedures to build social supports, and methods to set short-term attainable goals appear to be more effective than traditional approaches that emphasize confrontation. Differential treatment response may be more reflective of changes in life tasks as one grows older so that those therapies that emphasize increasing coping abilities, improving social relationships, and setting concrete and attainable goals may be more helpful than therapies that are motivational or confrontational in nature. Also, elderly individuals who eventually present for treatment may be more willing to accept the fact that they have a substance use disorder and, as a result, may not need the typical confrontational approaches designed to break down resistance and denial, even though these techniques are effective with younger patients. In any case, additional research is required in order to determine more specifically those factors that are significant predictors of group outcome (e.g., homogeneity), as well as to elucidate those elements of treatment programs that have the strongest impact on substance use disorders in the elderly. In a similar vein, it is necessary to define more clearly the risk factors for development of substance use disorders in the elderly. Some work in this area has already been conducted, but information is limited.

Finally, Speer, O'Sullivan, and Schonfeld (1991) outlined changes needed in social policy and fund allocation in order to effectively treat elderly individuals who have concurrent substance use disorders and psychiatric diagnoses. One of the most pressing issues in this area is the integration of substance abuse treatment and psychiatric treatment, so that abstinence is maintained for a significant period of time following cessation of treatment. Speer and colleagues point out that this type of integration is often hampered by differing ideologies, certifications, and educational experiences of individuals who provide substance abuse treatment and psychiatric treatment.

Assessment

In the area of assessment, at the most basic level, adequate and valid diagnostic criteria for elderly individuals with substance use disorders are required. Inadequate definitions of geriatric substance abuse and dependence have both clinical and empirical ramifications. From a clinical perspective, adequate diagnostic criteria are necessary so that mental and physical health care providers can readily identify and treat patients with substance use disorders and substance misuse problems. From an empirical standpoint, standard and valid diagnostic criteria are essential if we are to begin to truly understand the prevalence of these disorders in elderly individuals. It is likely that lack of adequate diagnostic criteria is one factor contributing to discrepancies between studies examining prevalence rates of substance abuse by the elderly and to the misconception that substance abuse is not a problem for individuals over the age of 60. In modifying current diagnostic criteria, it will be important to consider how substance use disorders are manifested in late life through impairment of age-appropriate life tasks and increased prevalence of psychiatric and medical disorders. Consideration should also be given to symptoms common to the elderly (such as those that result from the aging process) that may mimic symptoms of substance abuse and dependence in younger individuals. When adequate definitions are developed, they can be used to examine prevalence rates of these disorders in elderly individuals.

When assessing possible substance use disorders in the elderly, it is important for health care providers to clearly differentiate cases of misuse from abuse and dependence. Implications for intervention in the case of drug misuse are significantly different than for drug abuse and dependence. As previously mentioned, individuals who misuse medications because they cannot see the label on the prescription container or the directions on the box may only require that the print be enlarged and extraneous information (e.g., number of refills, phone numbers, possible adverse reactions, etc.) removed. While information about adverse reactions, number of refills, etc., is important and should be included, it is usually not needed in order to take the proper dose of medication and so should not be included on the direction label. Individuals working with the elderly can also modify instructions on labels of medication containers to increase the chances of compliance. Some authors report that associating medication instructions with specific times and/or with common daily events (e.g., meal times) increases medication compliance (Hallworth & Goldberg, 1984). With regard to labeling, it is necessary to clarify the ways in which letter size, spacing, and shading affect medication compliance. Misuse can also be decreased by decreasing the number of medications prescribed and by modifying dosing schedules (Salzman, 1995). We have treated patients who exhibited poor medication compliance simply because they were taking so many medications they could not reasonably keep track of all of them. In one case, we were treating an elderly male who was taking eight medications, most of which were taken more than once a day. Attempting to maintain this medication regime would be a daunting task for anyone. Individuals who misuse medication because of misconceptions about how and when they should be taken may only need brief educational interventions. Some studies indicate that fully informing patients of drug usage decreases incidence of medication misuse (Wiederholt, Clarridge, & Svarstad, 1992). Compliance is also associated with visual perception and visual memory abilities. As these abilities deteriorate, adherence to medication schedules decreases (Isaac, Tamblyn, & McGill-Calgary Drug Research Team, 1993). Because of the increased risk of medication noncompliance and misuse, some investigators have developed techniques to predict elderly patients' abilities to comply (Fitten, Coleman, Siembieda, Yu, & Ganzell, 1995). These techniques appear promising, but further research is required before their utility in, and generality across, clinical settings is fully established. In addition to developing specialized programming for treatment of abuse and dependence, special programs are also needed to identify and address environmental and attitudinal predictors of *misuse*.

We also recommend aggressive assessment of elderly individuals in high-risk populations (e.g., hospitalized patients) to identify elders with substance abuse. Initially, this assessment may take the form of screening with brief self-report instruments, such as the MAST. Further evaluation is indicated for those who answer test items in a manner indicative of the presence of substance abuse. This evaluation most often takes the form of clinical interviewing. However, health care providers may also acquire helpful information from interviews with family members and friends or from review of old medical records. Although a diagnosis of substance abuse or dependence may not be recorded, examination of these records will often assist in establishing a pattern of symptoms that suggests the presence of possible substance use disorders. Finally, clinicians need to be aware of risk signs indicating possible addiction. These include concomitant psychiatric conditions, such as depression; fluctuations in cognitive abilities; and long-term use of high-risk prescription medications, such as benzodiazepines.

In order to understand acute and chronic effects of substance use and dependence on cognition in the elderly, a number of areas require further investigation. First, future studies need to focus on controlling identified factors that can contribute to heterogeneity among chronic alcoholics' performance on cognitive tests (e.g., spontaneous recovery of cognitive functioning following drinking cessation, hepatic encephalopathy, etc.). As the literature develops, the impact of these factors can no longer be ignored. Second, more basic research that examines the long-term effects of cannabis, opiate, and hallucinogen use on cognitive functioning in the elderly is necessary. At this time, there are virtually no studies that examine the effects of these drugs on cognition in elderly individuals. Third, with regard to benzodiazepines, researchers need to replicate and extend results of studies that suggest that cognitive impairment persists after chronic benzodiazepine use is discontinued. Current studies suggest two important areas to explore: (a) differential cognitive effects of chronic benzodiazepine use as a result of age and (b) improvement in cognitive functioning following discontinuation of benzodiazepines in individuals with mild to moderate dementia.

Acknowledgments

The authors would like to thank Stephen G. Huegel, Ph.D., for his helpful comments and assistance in preparation of this manuscript.

References

Abrams, R. C., & Alexopoulos, G. S. (1988). Substance abuse in the elderly: Over-the-counter and illegal drugs. *Hospital and Community Psychiatry, 39,* 822–829.

Adams, P. F., & Benson, V. (1992). *Vital health statistics* (ISSN 0083-1972). Hyattsville, MD: U.S. Department of Health and Human Services.

Adams, K. M., Gilman, S., Koeppe, R. A., Kluin, K. J., Brunberg, J. A., Dede, D., Berent, S., & Kroll, P. D. (1993). Neuropsychological deficits are correlated with frontal hypometabolism in positron emission tomography studies of older alcoholic patients. *Alcoholism: Clinical and Experimental Research, 17,* 205–210.

American Psychiatric Association. (1980). *Diagnostic and statistical manual of mental disorders* (3rd ed.). Washington, DC: Author.

American Psychiatric Association. (1987). *Diagnostic and statistical manual of mental disorders* (3rd ed., rev.). Washington, DC: Author.

American Psychiatric Association. (1990). *Benzodiazepine dependence, toxicity, and abuse. A task force report of the American Psychiatric Association.* Washington, DC: Author.

American Psychiatric Association. (1994). *Diagnostic and statistical manual of mental disorders* (4th ed.). Washington, DC: Author.

Arria, A. M., Tarter, R. E., Starzl, T. E., & VanThiel, D. H. (1991). Improvement in cognitive functioning of alcoholics following orthotopic liver transplantation. *Alcoholism: Clinical and Experimental Research, 15,* 956–962.

Atkinson, R. M., Tolson, R. L., & Turner, J. A. (1990). Late versus early onset problem drinking in older men. *Alcoholism: Clinical and Experimental Research, 14,* 574–579.

Ayd, F. J. (1994). Prescribing anxiolytics and hypnotics for the elderly. *Psychiatric Annals, 24,* 91–97.

Baily, M. B., Haberman, P. W., & Alksne, H. (1964). The epidemiology of alcoholism in an urban residential area. *Quarterly Journal of Studies on Alcohol, 26,* 19–40.

Baum, C., Kennedy, P. L., & Forbes, M. B. (1984). Drug use in the United States in 1981. *Journal of the American Medical Association, 241,* 1293.

Beers, M. H., Ouslander, J. G., Rollingher, I., Reuben, D. B., Brooks, J., & Beck, J. C. (1991). Explicit criteria for determining inappropriate medication use in nursing homes. *Archives of Internal Medicine, 151,* 1825–1832.

Brandt, J., Butters, N., Ryan, C., & Bayog, R. (1983). Cognitive loss and recovery in long-term alcohol abusers. *Archives of General Psychiatry, 40,* 435–442.

Braun, C. M., & Richer, M. (1993). A comparison of functional indexes, derived from screening tests, of chronic alcoholic neurotoxicity in the cerebral cortex, retina and peripheral nervous system. *Journal of Studies on Alcohol, 54,* 11–16.

Brower, K. J., Mudd, S., Blow, F. C., Young, J. P., & Hill, E. M. (1994). Severity and treatment of alcohol withdrawal in elderly individuals versus younger patients. *Alcoholism: Clinical and Experimental Research, 18,* 196–201.

Buchsbaum, D. G., Boling, P., & Groh, M. (1987). Residents underdocumentation in elderly patients' records of prescription of benzodiazepine. *Journal of Medical Education, 62,* 438–440.

Bullock, K. D., Reed, R. J., & Grant, I. (1992). Reduced mortality risk in alcoholics who achieve long-term abstinence. *Journal of the American Medical Association, 267,* 668–672.

Carlen, P. L., McAndrews, M. P., Weiss, R. T., Dongier, M., Hill, J. M., Menzano, E., Farcnik, K., Abarbanel, J., & Eastwood, M. R. (1994). Alcohol related dementia in the institutionalized elderly. *Alcoholism, Clinical and Experimental Research, 18,* 1330–1334.

Closser, M. H. (1991). Benzodiazepines and the elderly. A review of potential problems. *Journal of Substance Abuse Treatment, 8,* 35–41.

Copeland, J. R., Davidson, I. A., Dewey, M. E., Gilmore, C., Larkin, B. A., McWilliam, C., Saunders, P. A., Scott, A., Sharma, V., & Sullivan, C. (1992). Alzheimer's disease, other dementias, depression and pseudodementia: Prevalence, incidence and three-year outcome in Liverpool. *British Journal of Psychiatry, 161,* 230–239.

Crook, F. H. (1979). Psychometric assessment in the elderly. In A. Raskin & L. F. Jarvik (Eds.), *Psychiatric symptoms and cognitive loss in the elderly: Evaluation and assessment techniques* (pp. 207–220). Washington, DC: Hemisphere Publishing Corporation.

Cummings, J. L., & Benson, D. F. (1992). *Dementia: A clinical approach.* Boston: Butterworth's.

Darnell, J. C., Murray, M. D., Martz, B. L., & Weinberger, M. (1986). Medication use by ambulatory elderly. An in-home survey. *Journal of the American Geriatrics Society, 34,* 1–4.

De Waele, J. P., & Gianoulakis, C. (1992). Autoradiographic localization of the u and d receptors in the brain of mice selected for their differences in voluntary ethanol consumption. *Abstracts: Society for Neurosciences, 18,* 269.

De Waele, J. P., & Gianoulakis, C. (1994). Enhanced activity of the brain B-endorphin system by free choice ethanol drinking in C57BL/6 but not in DBA/2 mice. *European Journal of Pharmacology, 258,* 119–129.

Donovan, D. M., Queisser, H. R., & O'Leary, M. R. (1976). Group embedded figures test performance as a predictor of cognitive impairment among alcoholics. *International Journal of the Addictions, 11,* 725–739.

Donovan, D. M., Walker, R. D., & Kivlahan, D. R. (1987). Recovery and remediation of neuropsychological functions: Implications for alcoholism rehabilitation process and outcome. In O. A. Parsons, N. Butters, & P. E. Nathan (Eds.), *Neuropsychology of alcoholism: Implications for diagnosis and treatment* (pp. 339–360). New York: Guilford Press.

Dorus, W., Ostrow, D. G., Anton, R., Cushman, P., Collins, J. F., Schaefer, M., Charles, H. L., Desai, P., Hayashida, M., Malkerneker, U., Willenbring, O., Fiscella, R., & Sather, M. R. (1989). Lithium treatment of depressed and nondepressed alcoholics. *Journal of the American Medical Association, 262,* 1646–1652.

Eckardt, M. J., Rawlings, R. R., Graubard, B. I., Faden, V., Martin, P., & Gottschalk, L. A. (1988). Neuropsychological performance and treatment outcome in male alcoholics. *Alcoholism: Clinical and Experimental Research, 12,* 88–93.

Eckardt, M. J., Stapleton, J. M., Rawlings, R. R., Davis, E. Z., & Grodin, D. M. (1995). Neuropsychological functioning in detoxified alcoholics between 18 and 35 years of age. *American Journal of Psychiatry, 152,* 53–59.

Ellis, R. F., & Oscar-Berman, M. (1989). Alcoholism, aging and functional cerebral asymmetries. *Psychological Bulletin, 106,* 128–147.

Ellor, J. R., & Kurz, D. J. (1982). Misuse and abuse of prescription and nonprescription drugs by the elderly. *Nursing Clinics of North America, 17,* 319–330.

Engstrom, A., Adamsson, C., Allebeck, P., & Rydberg, U. (1991). Mortality in patients with substance abuse: A follow-up in Stockholm County, 1973–1984. *International Journal of the Addictions, 26,* 91–106.

Ewing, J. A. (1984). Detecting alcoholism: The CAGE questionnaire. *Journal of the American Medical Association, 252,* 1905–1907.

Fabian, M. S., & Parsons, O. A. (1983). Differential improvements in cognitive functions in recovering alcoholic women. *Journal of Abnormal Psychology, 92,* 81–95.

Finlayson, R. E., Hurt, R. D., Davis, L. J., & Morse, R. M. (1988). Alcoholism in elderly persons: A study of the psychiatric and psychosocial features of 216 inpatients. *Mayo Clinic Proceedings, 63,* 761–768.

Finney, J. W., & Moos, R. H. (1991). The long-term course of treated alcoholism: I. Mortality, relapse and remission rates and comparisons with community controls. *Journal of Studies on Alcohol, 52,* 44–54.

Fitten, L. J., Coleman, L., Siembieda, D. W., Yu, M., & Ganzell, S. (1995). Assessment of capacity to comply with medication regimens in older patients. *Journal of the American Geriatrics Society, 43,* 361–367.

Fitzhugh, L. C., Fitzhugh, K. B., & Reitan, R. M. (1965). Adaptive abilities and intellectual functioning of hospitalized alcoholics: Further considerations. *Quarterly Journal of Studies on Alcohol, 26,* 402–411.

Fuller, R. K., Branchey, L., Brightwell, D. R., Derman, R. M., Emrick, C. D., Iber, F. L., James, K. E., Lacoursiere, R. B., Lee, K. K., Lowenstam, I., Maany, I., Neiderhiser, D., Nocks, J. J., & Shaw, S. (1986). Disulfiram treatment of alcoholism: A Veterans Administration cooperative study. *Journal of the American Medical Association, 256,* 1449–1455.

Fulop, G., Reinhardt, J., Strain, J. J., Paris, B., Miller, M., & Fillit, H. (1993). Identification of alcoholism and depression in a geriatric medicine outpatient clinic. *Journal of the American Geriatrics Society, 41,* 737–741.

Fratiglioni, L., Ahlbom, A., Viitanen, M., & Winbald, B. (1993). Risk factors for late-onset Alzheimer's disease: A population based, case controlled study. *Annals of Neurology, 33,* 258–266.

Freund, G., & Ballinger, W. E. (1991). Loss of synaptic receptors can precede morphological changes induced by alcoholism. *Alcohol and Alcoholism (Suppl.), 1,* 385–391.

Gianoulakis, C. (1990). Characterization of the effect of acute ethanol administration on the release of B-endorphine peptides by the rat hypothalamus. *European Journal of Pharmacology, 180,* 21–29.

Gilberstadt, S., Gilberstadt, H., Zieve, L., Buegel, B., Collier, R., & McClain, C. (1980). Psychomotor performance deficits in cirrhotic patients without overt encephalopathy. *Archives of Internal Medicine, 140,* 519–521.

Glenn, S., Parsons, O. A., & Sinha, R. (1994). Assessment of recovery of electrophysiological and neuropsychological functions in chronic alcoholics. *Biological Psychiatry, 36,* 443–452.

Goldman, M. S. (1986). Neuropsychological recovery in alcoholics: Endogenous and exogenous processes. *Alcoholism: Clinical and Experimental Research, 10,* 136–144.

Goldman, M. S. (1990). Experience-dependent neuropsychological recovery and the treatment of chronic alcoholism. *Neuropsychology Review, 1,* 75–101.

Goldstein, G. (1985). Dementia associated with alcoholism. In

R. E. Tarter & D. H. VanThiel (Eds.), *Alcohol and the brain: Chronic effects* (pp. 283–294). New York: Plenum Press.

Goldstein, G. (1987a). Recovery, treatment, and rehabilitation in chronic alcoholics. In O. A. Parsons, N. Butters, & P. E. Nathan (Eds.), *Neuropsychology of alcoholism: Implications for diagnosis and treatment* (pp. 361–377). New York: Guilford Press.

Goldstein, G. (1987b). Etiological considerations regarding the neuropsychological consequences of alcoholism. In O. A. Parsons, N. Butters, & P. E. Nathan (Eds.), *Neuropsychology of alcoholism: Implications for diagnosis and treatment* (pp. 227–246). New York: Guilford Press.

Gomberg, E. S. (1995). Older women and alcohol: Use and abuse. *Recent Developments in Alcoholism, 12,* 61–79.

Gordon, S. M., Kennedy, B. P., & McPeake, J. D. (1988). Neuropsychologically impaired alcoholics: Assessment, treatment considerations, and rehabilitation. *Journal of Substance Abuse Treatment, 5,* 99–104.

Grant, I., Adams, K. M., & Reed, R. (1984). Aging, abstinence and medical risk factors in the prediction of neuropsychological deficit amongst chronic alcoholics. *Archives of General Psychiatry, 41,* 710–718.

Hallworth, R. B., & Goldberg, L. A. (1984). Geriatric patients' understanding of labeling of medicines: Part 2. Discussion of the results of a two part study and suggested innovations in the labeling of medicines for geriatric patients. *British Journal of Pharmaceutical Practice, 7,* 42–48.

Hatsukami, D., & Pickens, R. W. (1982). Post treatment depression in an alcoholic and drug abuse population. *American Journal of Psychiatry, 139,* 1563–1566.

Helzer, J. E., & Burnam, A. (1991). Epidemiology of alcohol addiction: United States. In N. S. Miller (Ed.), *Comprehensive handbook of drug and alcohol addiction* (pp. 9–38). New York: Marcel Dekker, Inc.

Helzer, J. E., Burnam, A., & McEvoy, L. T. (1991). Alcoholic abuse and dependence. In L. N. Robins & D. A. Regier (Eds.), *Psychiatric disorders in America: The Epidemiologic Catchment Area study* (pp. 81–115). New York: Free Press.

Hesselbrock, M. N., Meyer, R. E., & Keener, J. J. (1985). Psychopathology in hospitalized alcoholics. *Archives of General Psychiatry, 42,* 1050–1055.

Hesselbrock, M. N., Weidenman, M. A., & Reed, H. B. (1985). Effect of age, sex, drinking history and antisocial personality on neuropsychology of alcoholics. *Journal of Studies on Alcohol, 46,* 313–320.

Higgit, A. (1992). Dependency on prescribed drugs. *Reviews in Clinical Gerontology, 2,* 151–155.

Hinrichs, J. V., & Ghoneim, M. M. (1987). Diazepam, behavior, and aging: Increased sensitivity or lower baseline performance. *Psychopharmacology, 92,* 100–105.

Hommer, D. W. (1991). Benzodiazepines: Cognitive and psychomotor effects. In P. P. Roy-Byrne & D. S. Cowley (Eds.), *Benzodiazepines in clinical practice: Risks and benefits* (pp. 113–129). Washington, DC: American Psychiatric Press, Inc.

Isaac, L. M., Tamblyn, R. M., & McGill-Calgary Drug Research Team. (1993). Compliance and cognitive function: A methodological approach to measuring unintentional errors in medication compliance in the elderly. *The Gerontologist, 33,* 772–781.

Jinks, M. J., & Raschko, R. R. (1990). A profile of alcohol and prescription drug abuse in a high-risk community-based elderly population. *Drug Intelligence and Clinical Pharmacy, 24,* 971–975.

Jones, B. M., & Parsons, O. A. (1972). Specific vs. generalized deficits of abstracting abilities in chronic alcoholics. *Archives of General Psychiatry, 26,* 380–384.

Juergens, S. M. (1993). Benzodiazepines and addiction. *Psychiatric Clinics of North America, 16,* 75–86.

Kashner, T. M., Rodell, D. E., Ogden, S. R., Guggenheim, F. G., & Karson, C. N. (1992). Outcomes and costs of two VA inpatient treatment programs for older alcoholic patients. *Hospital and Community Psychiatry, 43,* 985–989.

King, C. J., VanHasselt, V. B., Segal, D. L., & Hersen, M. (1994). Diagnosis and assessment of substance abuse in older adults: Current strategies and issues. *Addictive Behaviors, 19,* 41–55.

Kofoed, L. L. (1984). Abuse and misuse of over-the-counter drugs by the elderly. In R. M. Atkinson (Ed.), *Alcohol and drug abuse in old age.* Washington DC: American Psychiatric Press.

Kofoed, L. L., Tolson, R. L., Atkinson, R. M., Toth, R. F., & Turner, J. A. (1987) Treatment compliance of older alcoholics: An elder-specific approach is superior to "mainstreaming." *Journal of Studies on Alcohol, 48,* 47–51.

Kranzler, H. R., Burleson, J. A., Korner, P., Del Boca, F. K., Bohn, M. J., Brown, J., & Liebowitz, N. (1995). Placebo-controlled trial of fluoxetine as an adjunct to relapse prevention in alcoholics. *American Journal of Psychiatry, 152,* 391–397.

Kunkel, S. R., & Applebaum, R. A. (1992). Estimating the prevalence of long-term disability for an aging society. *Journals of Gerontology, 47,* S253–S260.

Larson, E., Kukull, W. A., Buchner, D., & Reifler, B. V. (1987). Adverse drug reactions associated with global cognitive impairment in elderly persons. *Annals of Internal Medicine, 107,* 169–173.

La Rue, A. (1992). *Aging and neuropsychological assessment.* New York: Plenum.

Lawlor, B. A., Hill, J. L., Radcliffe, J. L., Minichiello, M., Molchan, S. E., & Sunderland, T. (1992). A single oral dose challenge of buspirone does not affect memory processes in older volunteers. *Biological Psychiatry, 32,* 101–103.

Liberto, J. G., Oslin, D. W., & Ruskin, P. E. (1992). Alcoholism in older persons: A review of the literature. *Hospital and Community Psychiatry, 43,* 975–984.

Linseman, M. A. (1989). Central versus peripheral mediation of opioid effects on ethanol consumption in free-feeding rats. *Pharmacology, Biochemistry and Behavior, 33,* 407–413.

Lishman, W. A. (1990). Alcohol and the brain. *British Journal of Psychiatry, 156,* 635–644.

Martin, P. R., Adinoff, B., Weingartner, H., Mukherjee, A. B., & Eckardt, M. J. (1986). Alcoholic organic brain disease: Nosology and pathophysiologic mechanisms. *Progress in Neuropsychopharmacology and Biological Psychiatry, 10,* 147–164.

Martin, P. R., Adinoff, B., Lane, E., Stapleton, J. M., Bone, G. A., Weingartner, H., Linnoila, M., & Eckardt, M. J. (1995). Fluvoxamine treatment of alcoholic amnestic disorder. *European Neuropsychopharmacology, 5,* 27–33.

Mason, B. J., & Kocsis, J. H. (1991). Desipramine treatment of alcoholism. *Psychopharmacology Bulletin, 27,* 155–161.

Mayfield, D. G., McLeod, G., & Hall, P. (1974). The CAGE questionnaire: Validation of a new alcoholism screening instrument. *American Journal of Psychiatry, 131,* 1121–1123.

McInnes, E., & Powell, J. (1994). Drug and alcohol referrals: Are elderly substance abuse diagnoses and referrals being missed? *British Medical Journal, 308,* 444–446.

Miller, N. S., Belkin, B. M., & Gold, M. S. (1991). Alcohol and drug dependence among the elderly: Epidemiology, diagnosis, and treatment. *Comprehensive Psychiatry, 32,* 153–165.

Moos, R. H., Brennan, P. L., & Mertens, J. R. (1994). Mortality rates and predictors of mortality among late-middle-aged and older substance abuse patients. *Alcohol: Clinical and Experimental Research, 18,* 187–195.

Morgan, K., Dallosso, H., Ebrahim, S., Arie, T. & Fentem, P. H. (1988). Prevalence, frequency, and duration of hypnotic drug use among the elderly living at home. *British Medical Journal Clinical Research Edition, 296,* 601–602.

Moss, H. B., Tarter, R. E., Yao, J. K., & VanThiel, D. H. (1992). Subclinical hepatic encephalopathy: Relationship between neuropsychological deficits and standard laboratory tests assessing hepatic status. *Archives of Clinical Neuropsychology, 7,* 419–429.

Nussbaum, P. D., & Allen, D. N. (in press). Recent developments in neuropsychological assessment of the elderly and individuals with severe dementia. In G. Goldstein & T. Incagnoli (Eds.), *Current approaches to neuropsychological assessment* (2nd ed.). New York: Plenum Press.

Olson, G. A., Olson, R. D., & Kastin, A. B. (1989). Endogenous opiates. *Peptides, 11,* 1277–1304.

O'Mahony, J. F., & Doherty, B. (1993). Patterns of neuropsychological performance among recently abstinent alcohol abusers on the WAIS-R and WMS-R sub-tests. *Archives of Clinical Neuropsychology, 8,* 373–380.

Parsons, O. A. (1994). Neuropsychological measures and event related potentials in alcoholics: Interrelationships, long-term reliabilities, and prediction of resumption of drinking. *Journal of Clinical Psychology, 50,* 37–46.

Parsons, O. A., & Nixon, S. J. (1993). Neurobehavioral sequelae of alcoholism. *Neurologic Clinics, 11,* 205–218.

Parsons, O. A., Schaeffer, K. W., & Glenn, S. W. (1990). Does neuropsychological test performance predict resumption of drinking in posttreatment alcoholics? *Addictive Behaviors, 15,* 297–307.

Patterson, J. F. (1987). Triazolam syndrome in the elderly. *Southern Medical Journal, 80,* 1425–1426.

Petersen, D. M. (1988). Substance abuse, criminal behavior and older people. *Generations, 12,* 63–67.

Pollow, R. L., Stoller, E. P., Forster, L. E., & Duniho, T. S. (1994). Drug combinations and potential for risk of adverse drug reaction among community-dwelling elderly. *Nursing Research, 43,* 44–50.

Pollux, P. M., Wester, A., & De Haan, E. H. (1995). Random generation deficit in alcoholic Korsakoff patients. *Neuropsychologia, 33,* 125–129.

Pomara, N., Stanley, B., Block, R., Berchou, R. C., Stanley, M., Greenblatt, D. J., Newton, R. E., & Gershon, S. (1985). Increased sensitivity of the elderly to the central depressant effects of diazepam. *Journal of Clinical Psychiatry, 46,* 185–187.

Pomara, N., Deptula, D., Rubinstein, S., Stanley, B., & Stanley, M. (1988). The effects of diazepam and aging on intrusions. *Psychopharmacology Bulletin, 24,* 228–231.

Pomara, N., Deptula, D., Medel, M., Block, R. I., & Greenblatt, D. J. (1989). Effects of diazepam on recall memory: Relationship to aging, dose and duration of treatment. *Psychopharmacology Bulletin, 25,* 144–148.

Regier, D. A., Boyd, J. H., Burke, J. D., Jr., Rae, D. S., Myers, J. K., Kramer, M., Robins, L. N., George, L. K., Karno, M., & Locke, B. Z. (1988). One-month prevalence rates of mental disorders in the United States. *Archives of General Psychiatry, 45,* 977–986.

Reitan, R. M., & Wolfson, D. (1985). *Neuroanatomy and neuropathology: A clinical guide for neuropsychologists.* Tucson, AZ: Neuropsychology Press.

Rice, C., Longabaugh, R., Beattiem, M. C., & Noel, N. (1993). Age group differences in response to treatment for problematic alcohol use. *Addiction, 88,* 1369–1375.

Ross, H. E., Glaser, F. B., & Germanson, T. (1988). The prevalence of psychiatric disorders in patients with alcohol and other drug problems. *Archives of General Psychiatry, 45,* 1023–1031.

Ryan, C., & Butters, N. (1986). The neuropsychology of alcoholism. In D. Wedding, A. MacNiell-Horton, Jr., & J. Webster (Eds.), *The neuropsychological handbook: Behavioral and clinical perspectives* (pp. 376–409). New York: Springer.

Salmon, D. P., Butters, N., & Heindel, W. (1993). Alcoholic dementia and related disorders. In R. W. Parks, R. F. Zec, & R. S. Wilson (Eds.), *Neuropsychology of Alzheimer's disease and other dementias* (pp. 186–209). New York: Oxford University Press.

Salzman, C. (1995). Medication compliance in the elderly. *Journal of Clinical Psychiatry, 56,* 18–22.

Schonfeld, L. S., & Dupree, L. W. (1991). Antecedents of drinking for early- and late-life onset elderly alcohol abusers. *Journal of Studies on Alcohol, 52,* 587–592.

Seltzer, B., & Sherwin, I. (1978). Organic brain syndromes: An empirical study and critical review. *American Journal of Psychiatry, 135,* 13–21.

Selzer, M. L. (1971). The Michigan Alcohol Screening Test: The quest for a new diagnostic instrument. *American Journal of Psychiatry, 127,* 1653–1658.

Shear, P. K., Jernigan, T. L., & Butters, N. (1994). Volumetric magnetic resonance imaging quantification of longitudinal brain changes in abstinent alcoholics. *Alcoholism: Clinical and Experimental Research, 18,* 172–176.

Shelly, C., & Goldstein, G. (1976). An empirically derived topology of hospitalized alcoholics. In G. Goldstein & C. Neuringer (Eds.), *Empirical studies of alcoholism.* Cambridge, MA: Ballinger.

Smith, H., & Smith, L. (1977). WAIS functioning in cirrhotic and noncirrhotic alcoholics. *Journal of Clinical Psychology, 33,* 309–313.

Solomon, K., & Stark, S. (1993). Comparison of older and younger alcoholics and prescription drug abusers: History and clinical presentation. *Clinical Gerontologist, 12,* 41–56.

Speer, D. C., O'Sullivan, M., & Schonfeld, L. (1991). Dual diagnosis among older adults: A new array of policy planning problems. *The Journal of Mental Health Administration, 18,* 43–50.

Spencer, G. (1989). *Projections of the population of the United States, by age, sex, and race: 1988 to 2080.* Series P-25, no. 1018. Washington DC: U.S. Department of Commerce.

Spitzer, R. L., Endicott, J., & Robins, E. (1978). Research Diagnostic Criteria: Rationale and reliability. *Archives of General Psychiatry, 35,* 773–782.

Storandt, M. (1994). General principles of assessment of older adults. In M. Storandt & G. R. Van den Bos (Eds.), *Neuropsychological assessment of depression and dementia in older adults: A clinician's guide* (pp. 7–32). Washington, DC: American Psychological Association.

Sussman, S., Rychtarick, R. G., Mueser, K., Glynn, S., & Prue, D. M. (1986). Ecological relevance of memory tests and the prediction of relapse in alcoholics. *Journal of Studies on Alcohol, 47,* 305–310.

Tarter, R. E. (1980). Brain changes in chronic alcoholics: A review of psychological evidence. In O. A. Reichler (Ed.), *Addiction and brain damage* (pp. 267–297). Baltimore: University Park Press.

Tarter, R. E., & Parsons, O. A. (1971). Conceptual shifting in chronic alcoholics. *Journal of Abnormal Psychology, 77,* 71–75.

Tarter, R. E., Ryan, C. M. (1986). Neuropsychology of alcoholism: Etiology, phenomenology, process and outcome. *Recent Developments in Alcoholism, 1,* 449–469.

Tarter, R. E., Moss, H., Arria, A., & VanThiel, D. (1990). Hepatic, nutritional, and genetic influences on cognitive process in alcoholics. *National Institute on Drug Abuse Research Monograph Series: 1990 Research Monograph, 101,* 124–135.

Tarter, R. E., Switala, J., Lu, S., & VanThiel, D. (1995). Abstracting capacity in cirrhotic alcoholics: Negative findings. *Journal of Studies on Alcohol, 56,* 99–103.

Tata, P. R., Rollings, J., Collins, M., Pickering, A., & Jacobson, R. R. (1994). Lack of cognitive recovery following withdrawal from long-term benzodiazepine use. *Psychological Medicine, 24,* 203–213.

Teri, L., Hughes, J. P., & Larson, E. (1990). Cognitive deterioration in Alzheimer's disease: Behavioral and health factors. *Journals of Gerontology, 45,* P58–P63.

Thompson, T. L., Moran, M. G., & Neis, A. S. (1983). Psychotropic drug use in the elderly, Part 1. *New England Journal of Medicine, 308,* 134–138.

Tivis, L. J., Parsons, O. A., Glenn, S. W., & Nixon, S. J. (1993). Differences in cognitive impairment between VA and community treatment center alcoholics. *Psychology of Addictive Behaviors, 7,* 43–51.

Trzepacz, P. T., Tarter, R. E., Shah, A., Tringali, R., Faett, D. G., & VanThiel, D. H. (1994). SPECT scan and cognitive findings in subclinical hepatic encephalopathy. *Journal of Neuropsychiatry and Clinical Neurosciences, 6,* 170–175.

Vestal, R. E., McGuire, E. A., Tobin, J. D., Andres, R., Norris, A. H., & Mezay, E. (1977). Aging and ethanol metabolism. *Clinical Pharmacology and Therapeutics, 21,* 343–354.

Victor, M. (1994). Alcoholic dementia. *Canadian Journal of Neurological Sciences, 21,* 88–99.

Victor, M., Adams, R. D., & Collins, G. H. (1989). *The Wernicke-Korsakoff Syndrome. A clinical and pathological study of 245 patients, 82 with postmortem examinations* (2nd ed.). Philadelphia: F. A. Davis.

Volpicelli, J. R., Alterman, A. I., Hayashida, M., & O'Brien, C. P. (1992). Naltrexone in the treatment of alcohol dependence. *Archives of General Psychiatry, 49,* 876–880.

Whitcup, S. M., & Miller, F. (1987). Unrecognized drug dependence in psychiatrically hospitalized elderly patients. *Journal of the American Geriatrics Society, 35,* 297–301.

Wiederholt, J. B., Clarridge, B. R., & Svarstad, B. L. (1992). Verbal consultation regarding prescription drugs: Findings from a statewide study. *Medical Care, 30,* 159–173.

Wiens, A. N., Menustik, C. E., Miller, S. J., & Schmitz, R. E. (1982–1983). Medical-behavioral treatment of the older alcoholic patient. *American Journal of Drug and Alcohol Abuse, 9,* 461–475.

Wilkinson, D. A., & Sanchez-Craig, M. (1981). Relevance of brain dysfunction to treatment objectives: Should alcohol-related cognitive deficits influence the way we think about treatment? *Addictive Behaviors, 6,* 253–260.

Wilson, B., Kolb, B., Odland, L., & Wishaw, I. (1987). Alcohol, sex, age, and the hippocampus. *Psychobiology, 15,* 300–307.

Winick, C. (1962). Maturing out of narcotic addiction. *Bulletin on Narcotics, 14,* 1–7.

Woods, J. H., & Winger, G. (1995). Current benzodiazepine issues. *Psychopharmacology, 118,* 107–115.

Yohman, J. R., Parsons, O. A., & Leber, W. R. (1985). Lack of recovery in male alcoholics' neuropsychological performance one year after treatment. *Alcoholism: Clinical and Experimental Research 9,* 114–117.

Zarit, S. H., Eiler, J., & Hassinger, M. (1985). Clinical assessment. In J. E. Birren & K. W. Schaie (Eds.), *Handbook of the psychology of aging* (pp. 725–754). New York: Van Nostrand Reinhold.

Zimberg, S. (1979). Alcohol and the elderly. In D. M. Petersen, F. J. Whittington, & B. P. Payne (Eds.), *Drugs and the elderly: Social and pharmacological issues* (pp. 28–41). Springfield, IL: Charles C. Thomas.

III

Neuropsychological Disorders of Late Life

10

The Neuropsychology of Alzheimer's Disease

DAVID P. SALMON AND MARK W. BONDI

Introduction

Alzheimer's disease (AD) is a progressive degenerative brain disorder that results in a profound global dementia characterized by severe amnesia with additional deficits in language, "executive" functions, attention, and visuospatial and constructional abilities (Corkin, Davis, Growdon, Usdin, & Wurtman, 1982; Katzman, 1986). Because dementia is associated with more than 50 different causes of brain dysfunction (Haase, 1977; Katzman, 1986) and because there are no known peripheral markers for AD, the disease can only be definitively diagnosed by histopathological verification of the presence of characteristic neurodegenerative abnormalities (i.e., neuritic plaques and neurofibrillary tangles; Khachaturian, 1985). However, documentation of the presence of dementia and the exclusion of all other known potential causes allows probable or possible AD to be clinically diagnosed during life with some certainty (Galasko et al., 1994; Kawas, 1990; McKhann et al., 1984).

Although the cause of AD remains unknown, a number of risk factors have been identified. Age is considered to be the single most important risk factor for dementia of the Alzheimer's type (DAT), given that the prevalence of the disorder rises in an approximately exponential fashion between the ages of 65 and 85 (Katzman & Kawas, 1994). Women appear to have a slightly greater risk for DAT than men (Bachman et al., 1992; Zhang et al., 1990); however, this may be attributable, at least in part, to differential survival rates after the onset of dementia due to their longer life expectancy (Bachman et al., 1993). A previous head injury that led to loss of consciousness or hospitalization has been identified as a risk factor for DAT (Mortimer et al., 1991), particularly (and perhaps exclusively) in conjunction with a newly discovered genetic risk factor (Mayeux et al., 1995). Recently, studies have shown that lack of education and/or low occupational attainment may be an important risk factor for DAT (for review, see Katzman, 1993), perhaps because these variables are a surrogate for a brain or cognitive reserve that helps to delay the onset of the usual clinical manifestations of AD (Katzman, 1993; Katzman & Kawas, 1994; Mortimer, 1988; Stern, Alexander, Prohovnik, & Mayeux, 1992; Stern et al., 1994; Zhang et al., 1990).

The risk of developing DAT is increased approximately fourfold by a family history of AD in a first-degree relative (i.e., mother, father, brother, or sister; van Duijn, Hofman, & Kay, 1991), and with the recent discovery of specific point mutations on the amyloid precursor protein gene of chromosome 21, as well as linkage studies identifying gene loci on chromosomes 1, 14, and 19, there is now little question that this familial association is genetically based (for review, see Katzman & Kawas, 1994). Furthermore, the type $\epsilon4$ allele of the gene for apolipoprotein E (ApoE), a low-density lipoprotein

DAVID P. SALMON • Department of Neurosciences, School of Medicine, University of California, San Diego, La Jolla, California 92093-0948. MARK W. BONDI • Department of Psychiatry, School of Medicine, University of California, San Diego, La Jolla, California 92093-0948; and San Diego Department of Veterans Affairs Medical Center, San Diego, California 92161.

cholesterol carrier, has very recently been identified as another major risk factor because of its over-representation in patients with AD (Corder et al., 1993; Strittmatter et al., 1993). The ApoE ∈4 allele has been found to be present in 50% to 60% of AD patients (compared to 20% to 25% of healthy older adults), regardless of whether they have a family history of dementia, and is currently the most common known genetic risk factor for AD (for review, see Katzman, 1994; Katzman & Kawas, 1994).

The neurodegenerative changes associated with AD include neocortical atrophy, neuron and synapse loss (Terry, Peck, DeTeresa, Schecter, & Horoupian, 1981; Terry et al., 1991), and the presence of senile plaques and neurofibrillary tangles (Terry & Katzman, 1983). These neurodegenerative changes occur primarily in the hippocampus and entorhinal cortex and in the association cortices of the frontal, temporal, and parietal lobes (Hyman, Van Hoesen, Damasio, & Barnes, 1984; Terry & Katzman, 1983). Although the temporal progression of the neuropathological changes of AD is not fully known, recent studies suggest that the hippocampus and entorhinal cortex are involved in the earliest stage of the disease and that frontal, temporal, and parietal association cortices become increasingly involved as the disease progresses (Arriagada, Growdon, Hedley-Whyte, & Hyman, 1992; Bancher, Braak, Fischer, & Jellinger, 1993; Braak & Braak, 1991; De Lacoste & White, 1993; Hyman et al., 1984; Pearson, Esiri, Hiorns, Wilcock, & Powell, 1985). In addition to these cortical changes, subcortical neuron loss occurs in the nucleus basalis of Meynert and the nucleus locus ceruleus, resulting in a decrement in neocortical levels of cholinergic and noradrenergic markers, respectively (Bondareff, Mountjoy, & Roth, 1982; Mann, Yates, & Marcyniuk, 1984; Whitehouse et al., 1982).

A number of studies have shown that there is a strong relationship between the degree of neuropathological abnormality and the severity of dementia in patients with AD (Blessed, Tomlinson, & Roth, 1968; DeKosky & Scheff, 1990; Mann, Marcyniuk, Yates, Neary, & Snowden, 1988; Neary et al., 1986; Terry et al., 1991). In one of the first of these studies, Blessed and colleagues (1968) found that the number of senile plaques in the neocortex of patients with AD correlated significantly with their performance on the Information-Memory-Concen-

tration (IMC) test, a brief neuropsychological measure of dementia. Neary and colleagues (1986) were unable to replicate this finding, but found that a measure of pyramidal cell neuron loss in the neocortex of AD patients was related to level of cognitive functioning. Indeed, in autopsied patients who had also undergone brain biopsy about 3 to 7 years prior to death, there was a continuing decline in both large neuron counts and cognitive functioning over the intervening years, but no increase in number of senile plaques or neurofibrillary tangles (Mann et al., 1988).

Because a continuing loss of large neocortical pyramidal cells occurs in AD and is related to clinical progression, Terry and colleagues (1991) reasoned that extensive synapse loss might also be expected and that this loss might be highly correlated with severity of dementia prior to death. To examine this hypothesis, Terry and colleagues (1991) quantified synaptic density in the midfrontal, inferior parietal, and superior temporal lobe neocortex of patients with AD and determined the degree of its correlation with their performance on three global mental status examinations, the Blessed IMC test, the Mini-Mental State Examination (MMSE), and the Dementia Rating Scale (DRS). The degree of correlation between the mental status examinations and number of neuritic plaques, neurofibrillary tangles, large neurons (> 90 nm), and choline acetyltransferase (ChAT) levels in the three cortical regions was also examined. The results of this study revealed that performance on the three mental status examinations was more highly correlated with synaptic density in the midfrontal and inferior parietal regions of the neocortex than with other neuropathological measures (see Figure 1). A stepwise multiple regression analysis of neuropathological factors that might contribute to DRS performance, for example, produced a model with midfrontal synaptic density, inferior parietal synaptic density, and inferior parietal neuritic plaques that accounted for 92% of the variance in test performance. These results led Terry and colleagues (1991) to suggest that loss of neocortical synapses may be the primary determinant of dementia in AD and that other neuropathological changes may play a secondary role.

As mentioned above, the dementia associated with AD is usually pervasive and profound, partic-

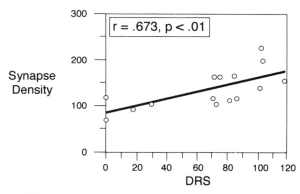

FIGURE 1. The relationship between synaptic density in the midfrontal neocortex and performance on the Dementia Rating Scale (DRS) shortly before death. (Adapted from Terry et al., 1991).

ularly after the disease has progressed beyond its earliest stages. The onset of DAT, however, is insidious and initially is difficult to distinguish from normal cognitive changes that occur with aging. Over the past few decades, extensive research has characterized the neuropsychological features of DAT, particularly with regard to the earliest cognitive changes that are pathognomonic for the disorder and the pattern of cognitive changes that may distinguish DAT from dementia associated with other neurodegenerative diseases (for recent reviews, see Bondi, Salmon, & Butters, 1994; La Rue, 1992; Parks, Zec, & Wilson, 1993). In addition, recent neuropsychological research has focused on newly discovered neuropathological conditions (e.g., the Lewy body variant of AD; Hansen et al., 1990) which may account for at least some heterogeneity in the cognitive manifestations of DAT (Salmon & Galasko, 1996). In this chapter, we briefly review some recent findings in each of these areas of research.

Neuropsychological Detection of Dementia of the Alzheimer's Type

Although DAT involves significant impairments in memory, executive functions, language, and visuospatial and constructional abilities, failure of recent memory is usually the most prominent feature during the early stages of the disease (Hup-

pert & Tym, 1986; Martin, 1987). Accordingly, much of the neuropsychological research concerning early detection of DAT has focused on memory. Numerous studies have shown that measures of the ability to learn new information and retain it over time are quite sensitive in differentiating between mildly demented patients with clinically diagnosed DAT and normal older adults (e.g., Bayles, Boone, Tomoeda, Slauson, & Kaszniak, 1989; Delis et al., 1991; Eslinger, Damasio, Benton, & Van Allen, 1985; Huff et al., 1987; Kaszniak, Wilson, Fox, & Stebbins, 1986; Storandt, Botwinick, Danziger, Berg, & Hughes, 1984).

In one recent study, for example, Welsh and colleagues (Welsh, Butters, Hughes, Mohs, & Heyman, 1991) found that a delayed free recall measure on a verbal memory task was highly effective (i.e., 90% accuracy) in distinguishing between very mildly demented patients with DAT (all with MMSE scores above 24 out of 30) and elderly normal control subjects. In addition, this measure was significantly more effective than measures of learning, confrontation naming, verbal fluency, and constructional ability. Similar results have been obtained in other studies (Flicker, Ferris, & Reisberg, 1991; Knopman & Ryberg, 1989; Morris et al., 1991; Tröster et al., 1993), and in one case (Morris et al., 1991) the effectiveness of memory measures for detecting early DAT was confirmed by histopathologic verification of AD at autopsy.

The primacy and prominence of memory impairment in DAT is consistent with evidence suggesting that neuropathological changes in the hippocampus and entorhinal cortex are the first and most severe to occur in the disease (Braak & Braak, 1991; Hyman et al., 1984). There is now considerable evidence from both human and animal studies that these brain structures are critical for acquisition and retention of new information (for review, see Squire, 1992). It is also possible that early involvement of these structures in AD may lead to decrements in learning and memory during a "preclinical" phase of AD (Katzman, 1994) in which subtle cognitive changes are evident before gradual neural degeneration has spread and reached a level sufficient to produce the full clinical manifestation of the dementia syndrome.

Consistent with this notion, several studies have shown that subtle cognitive decline can be detected in individuals a number of years prior to their meeting established criteria for a clinical diagnosis of DAT (Katzman et al., 1989; La Rue & Jarvik, 1980, 1987), and more recent studies indicate that measures of learning and memory are most effective in this regard (Bayles & Kaszniak, 1987; Bondi et al., 1994; Fuld, Masur, Blau, Crystal, & Aronson, 1990; La Rue, Matsuyama, McPherson, Sherman, & Jarvik, 1992; Linn et al., 1995; Masur, Fuld, Blau, Crystal, & Aronson, 1990; Masur, Sliwinski, Lipton, Blau, & Crystal, 1994). Fuld and colleagues, for example, demonstrated that poor performance on measures of recall from the Fuld Object Memory test (Fuld et al., 1990) or the Selective Reminding Test (Masur et al., 1990) correctly predicted the subsequent development of DAT within the next 5 years. In an extensive follow-up to these studies, Masur and colleagues (1994) found that a logistic regression model containing performance on a delayed recall measure from the Selective Reminding Test, a recall measure from the Fuld Object Memory test, the Digit Symbol Substitution subtest from the Wechsler Adult Intelligence Scale (WAIS), and a measure of verbal fluency was moderately effective in identifying individuals who later developed DAT (32/64; 50%) and provided excellent specificity for identifying individuals who remained free of dementia (238/253; 94%) over a subsequent 11-year period.

A similar result was obtained in a large epidemiological study examining initial neuropsychological test performance of 1,000 nondemented elderly individuals who were followed over the subsequent 13 years (Linn et al., 1995). Fifty-five individuals developed DAT during the study, and development of the disorder was accurately predicted by their initial performance on a delayed recall measure from the Logical Memory subtest of the Wechsler Memory Scale and on the Digit Span subtest from the WAIS. Interestingly, subjects who later developed DAT initially performed worse on the delayed recall measure, but better on the Digit Span subtest, than those who did not. It is also interesting to note that recall and digit span measures predicted subsequent development of dementia even when initial neuropsychological evaluation preceded clinical onset of dementia by 7 years or more.

Another approach to examining potential dec-

rements in learning and memory during a preclinical phase of AD has been to compare the performance of nondemented elderly individuals who have an increased risk for developing the disease due to a positive family history or an ApoE ϵ4 genotype to that of individuals who do not have these risk factors (Bondi et al., 1995; Hom, Turner, Risser, Bonte, & Tintner, 1994; La Rue et al., 1992; Smalley et al., 1992). This approach assumes that nondemented elderly individuals with the risk factor for AD are more likely to be in the preclinical phase of the disease than those who do not have the risk factor, and therefore they are likely to perform worse on sensitive neuropsychological tests.

In one study using this approach, Hom and colleagues (1994) demonstrated that a group of 20 nondemented elderly individuals with a positive family history (FH+) of AD performed significantly worse than 20 age- and education-matched nondemented individuals with a negative family history (FH−) of AD on tests of verbal intelligence and verbal learning and memory. This difference occurred despite the fact that the average performances of both groups on these tests were within normal limits. In a similar study, Bondi and colleagues (1995) longitudinally assessed nondemented FH+ and FH− individuals with quantitative and qualitative indices derived from the California Verbal Learning Test (CVLT; Delis, Kramer, Kaplan, & Ober, 1987). Although the groups were carefully matched in terms of demographic variables and performance on standardized mental status examinations, the FH+ subjects recalled significantly fewer items during learning and delayed recall, produced more intrusion errors, and demonstrated a greater recency effect than the FH− individuals. In addition, five of the nondemented subjects in this study performed on the CVLT in a manner qualitatively similar to that of a group of mildly impaired DAT patients and were subsequently diagnosed with DAT 1 to 2 years following their initial evaluation. Four of these five subjects were FH+, and one had an uninformative family history because no first-degree relative lived long enough to express AD.

With identification of a common and specific genetic risk factor for AD, the ApoE ϵ4 allele, several recent studies have focused on episodic memory changes in nondemented elderly subjects who possess this risk factor. In one study, Reed and colleagues (1994) found that nondemented elderly male individuals with the ϵ4 allele exhibited poorer mean performance on a test of visual memory than their dizygotic twins who did not have the ϵ4 allele. Bondi and colleagues (Bondi et al., 1995) demonstrated that the verbal learning and memory performance of nondemented subjects with the ApoE ϵ4 allele was qualitatively (though not quantitatively) similar to that of patients in the early stages of DAT. Furthermore, nondemented subjects with the ApoE ϵ4 allele recalled fewer items during the learning trials and over delay intervals and used a less effective organizational strategy for learning than carefully matched nondemented subjects without the ApoE ϵ4 allele (see Table 1). Follow-up examinations revealed that 6 of 14 subjects with the ϵ4 allele subsequently developed probable or possible DAT or questionable DAT (i.e., cognitive decline without evidence of significant functional impairment), whereas none of the 26 subjects without an ϵ4 allele demonstrated any cognitive decline.

It is clear from the results of studies reviewed above that decrements in learning and memory are particularly evident in early stages of DAT and are likely to presage the development of the full dementia syndrome. It should be noted, however, that other neuropsychological deficits, such as mildly impaired language, executive functions, and constructional abilities, are often present early in the course of DAT (Salmon, Butters, Thal, & Jeste, in press), and measures of these abilities may also be useful for differentiating between mildly demented patients with DAT and normal elderly individuals. Monsch and colleagues (1992), for example, compared the performances of mild DAT patients and normal elderly control subjects on several types of verbal fluency tasks and found that the semantic category fluency task had greater than 90% sensitivity and specificity for diagnosis of dementia. Similarly high sensitivity (94.3%) and specificity (86.7%) for diagnosis of dementia was demonstrated with the number of categories achieved on a

Table 1. Raw Scores of Apolipoprotein E ϵ4 (n = 17) and Non-ϵ4 (n = 35) Nondemented Elderly Adults on Various Measures from the California Verbal Learning Test (CVLT)[a]

CVLT variables	Apolipoprotein E genotype				Mann-Whitney p value
	ϵ4		Non-ϵ4		
	Mean	(SD)	Mean	(SD)	
Learning					
List A trials 1–5 total	46.0	(13.1)	51.4	(8.5)	0.081
List A trial 1 recall	6.5	(2.3)	6.5	(1.9)	0.449
List A trial 5 recall	10.6	(3.1)	12.4	(2.3)	0.028
List B recall	5.6	(2.0)	6.6	(1.7)	0.030
Retention					
Short delay free recall	8.4	(3.5)	10.5	(2.9)	0.015
Short delay cued recall	9.6	(3.2)	11.3	(3.0)	0.033
Long delay free recall	8.9	(3.9)	11.1	(2.4)	0.019
Long delay cued recall	9.9	(3.3)	11.8	(2.7)	0.022
Long delay savings (%)	80.9	(20.0)	90.3	(14.3)	0.052
Discriminability	91.3	(6.7)	93.7	(6.1)	0.100
Qualitative measures					
Semantic cluster ratio	1.8	(0.7)	2.3	(0.9)	0.027
Recency recall (%)	32.1	(10.7)	27.8	(6.2)	0.041
Learning slope	1.0	(0.5)	1.4	(0.6)	0.021
Cued recall intrusions	3.4	(2.4)	2.7	(2.2)	0.128

[a]Adapted from Bondi et al., 1995.

modified version of the Wisconsin Card Sorting Test in a study that compared the performances of mild DAT patients and normal elderly subjects (Bondi, Monsch, Butters, Salmon, & Paulsen, 1993). These studies in conjunction with those characterizing the memory decrement associated with DAT indicate that considerable progress has been made in identifying early neuropsychological consequences of AD. Continued research in this area is necessary to enhance our ability to clinically detect AD in its earliest stages when potential neuroprotective agents designed to impede progression of the disease might be most effective.

Differentiation of Dementia of the Alzheimer's Type from Other Dementing Disorders

A considerable amount of recent research has been directed at identifying the pattern of cognitive changes that might distinguish DAT from dementia associated with other neurodegenerative diseases. Much of this research has been carried out within the framework of a "cortical–subcortical" distinction (Albert, Feldman, & Willis, 1974; Cummings, 1990; McHugh & Folstein, 1975), which holds that different patterns of primary neuropsychological deficits are associated with neurodegenerative diseases that predominantly involve regions of the cerebral cortex (e.g., Alzheimer's disease, Pick's disease) or that have their primary locus in subcortical brain structures (e.g., Huntington's disease, Parkinson's disease, progressive supranuclear palsy). Studies that address this distinction usually compare and contrast neuropsychological test performance of patients with DAT (a prototypical cortical dementia) with that of patients with Huntington's disease (a prototypical subcortical dementia).

Huntington's disease (HD) is a genetically transmitted neurodegenerative disorder that results in progressive deterioration of the neostriatum (caudate nucleus and putamen; Bruyn, Bots, & Dom, 1979; Vonsattel et al., 1985). Primary clinical manifestations of HD include choreoathetoid movements, a progressive dementia, and emotional or personality changes (Folstein, Brandt, & Folstein, 1990). While DAT is broadly characterized by prominent amnesia with additional deficits in lan-

guage and semantic knowledge (i.e., aphasia), abstract reasoning, other executive functions, and constructional and visuospatial abilities (Bayles & Kaszniak, 1987; Parks et al., 1993), dementia associated with HD involves a moderate memory disturbance, attentional dysfunction, problem-solving deficits, visuoperceptual and constructional deficits, and a deficiency in performing arithmetic (Brandt & Butters, 1986; Butters, Sax, Montgomery, & Tarlow, 1978). Huntington's disease results in little or no aphasia, although patients may be dysarthric due to the motor dysfunction inherent in the disease.

In addition to these differences in the general neuropsychological features of DAT and dementia associated with HD, numerous studies using concepts and experimental procedures of cognitive psychology suggest that there is a fundamental difference in the nature of the memory impairment that occurs in each disorder. Patients with DAT exhibit a severe deficit in episodic memory (i.e., temporally dated autobiographical episodes that depend upon contextual cues for their retrieval) that appears to result from ineffective consolidation (i.e., storage) of new information, whereas the memory disorder of patients with HD is thought to result from a general difficulty in initiating a systematic retrieval strategy when recalling information from either episodic or semantic memory (i.e., overlearned facts and concepts that are not dependent on contextual cues for retrieval).

Evidence for a consolidation deficit in DAT patients includes their showing little improvement in acquiring information over repeated learning trials (Buschke & Fuld, 1974; Masur et al., 1989; Moss, Albert, Butters, & Payne, 1986; Wilson, Bacon, Fox, & Kaszniak, 1983), a tendency to recall only the most recently presented information (i.e., a heightened recency effect) on free recall tasks (Delis et al., 1991; Massman, Delis, & Butters, 1993; Miller, 1971; Pepin & Eslinger, 1989), an inability to benefit normally from effortful or elaborative encoding at the time of acquisition (Knopman & Ryberg, 1989), a failure to demonstrate a normal improvement in performance when memory is tested with a recognition rather than a free recall format (Delis et al., 1991; Miller, 1971; Wilson et al., 1983), and rapid forgetting of information over time (Butters et al., 1988; Moss et al., 1986; Tröster et al., 1993; Welsh et al., 1991).

Although HD patients also exhibit difficulty in learning and recalling information on free recall tasks, evidence of a general retrieval deficit is provided by a marked improvement in their performance when memory is tested with a recognition format (Delis et al., 1991; Moss et al., 1986; but see Brandt, Corwin, & Kraft, 1992) and by their ability to retain information over a delay in near normal fashion (Delis et al., 1991; Moss et al., 1986).

Differences in the nature and pattern of memory impairments associated with cortical and subcortical dementias are highlighted in a recent study by Delis and colleagues (1991). These investigators compared the performances of DAT and HD patient groups on the CVLT, a rigorous test of verbal learning and memory. The CVLT is a standardized memory test that assesses rate of learning, retention after short and long delay intervals, semantic encoding ability, recognition (i.e., discriminability), intrusion and perseverative errors, and response biases. In the test, individuals are verbally presented five presentation/free recall trials of a list of 16 shopping items (four items in each of four categories) and are then administered a single trial using a second, different list of 16 items. Immediately after this final trial, individuals are administered first a free recall and then a cued recall test for items on the first shopping list. Twenty minutes later, free recall and cued recall tests are repeated, followed by a yes-no recognition test consisting of the 16 items on the first shopping list and 28 distractor items.

Delis and colleagues (1991) found that despite comparable immediate and delayed free recall and cued recall deficits, the DAT and HD patients could be differentiated by several other CVLT measures (see Figure 2). A discriminant function analysis revealed that DAT (17 out of 20) and HD (16 out of 19) patients could be effectively distinguished by a model that included two measures derived from the CVLT: (1) the percentage of cued recall intrusions and (2) the difference between recognition discriminability and recall on trial 5 of the initial learning trials. The effectiveness of the first measure reflects the greater susceptibility to proactive interference of DAT patients relative to HD patients (Fuld, Katzman, Davies, & Terry, 1982; Jacobs, Salmon, Tröster, & Butters, 1990; Tröster, Jacobs, Butters, Cullum, & Salmon, 1989). The second measure was effective because it assesses both retention over

time and any potential benefit of a recognition format over free recall, characteristics that should favor HD patients over patients with DAT. Thus, the effectiveness of these particular CVLT measures in discriminating between DAT and HD patients is consistent with the general features of the memory deficits associated with the cortical and subcortical dementias that were described above.

Patients with cortical and subcortical dementia syndromes can also be differentiated by their performances on tests of remote memory. Patients with DAT have a severe retrograde amnesia (i.e., loss of memory for information acquired prior to the onset of their disease) affecting all decades of their lives (Beatty, Salmon, Butters, Heindel, & Granholm, 1988; Hodges, Salmon, & Butters, 1993; Kopelman, 1989; Sagar, Cohen, Sullivan, Corkin, & Growdon, 1988; Wilson, Kaszniak, & Fox, 1981). Several studies indicate that in early stages of DAT, remote memory loss is temporally graded, with memories from the distant past (i.e., childhood and early adulthood) better remembered than memories from the more recent past (i.e., middle and late adulthood) (Beatty & Salmon, 1991; Beatty et al., 1988; Hodges et al., 1993).

In contrast, patients with HD (Albert, Butters, & Brandt, 1981; Beatty et al., 1988) or Parkinson's disease (Freedman, Rivoira, Butters, Sax, & Robert, 1984) suffer only a mild degree of retrograde amnesia that is equally severe across all decades of their

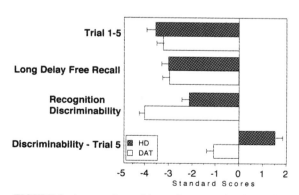

FIGURE 2. A comparison of the performance of patients with dementia of the Alzheimer type (DAT) and Huntington's disease (HD) on several measures from the California Verbal Learning Test (CVLT). The scores are presented in terms of standard scores derived from age- and education-matched normal control subjects. (Adapted from Delis et al., 1991.)

lives. These results suggest that the remote memory deficit of patients with subcortical dementia is another reflection of a general retrieval deficit that equally affects recollection of information from any decade of their lives, whereas the temporally graded remote memory loss of DAT patients is indicative of a failure to adequately consolidate information through repeated processing, rehearsal, or reexposure (see Zola-Morgan & Squire, 1990, for a discussion of the role of consolidation in temporally graded retrograde amnesia).

In addition to their distinct patterns of performance on tests of episodic and remote memory, patients with cortical and subcortical dementia syndromes differ markedly with regard to presence and severity of language deficits. Patients with DAT, for example, are noted for mild anomia and word finding difficulties in spontaneous speech, and some evidence suggests that this deficit is indicative of a loss of semantic knowledge and a breakdown in the organization of semantic memory (for reviews, see Hodges, Salmon, & Butters, 1991; Salmon & Chan, 1994). Consistent with this view, patients with DAT are disproportionately impaired on verbal fluency tasks when they must generate exemplars from a semantic category compared to when they must generate words that begin with a particular letter (Butters, Granholm, Salmon, Grant, & Wolfe, 1987; Monsch et al., 1992); they perform poorly on tests of confrontation naming and tend to produce semantic errors (Bayles & Tomoeda, 1983; Hodges et al., 1991; Huff, Corkin, & Growdon, 1986; Smith, Murdoch, & Chenery, 1989); and they consistently miss the same item across language tests that use different methods and modes of access (Chertkow & Bub, 1990; Hodges, Salmon, & Butters, 1992).

In contrast, patients with HD generally retain their language abilities. For example, HD patients perform at near normal levels on tests of confrontation naming, and the errors they produce are often visuoperceptual rather than semantic (Hodges et al., 1991). Although HD patients perform poorly on tests of verbal fluency, they are equally impaired regardless of the semantic demands of the task (Butters et al., 1987; Monsch et al., 1992), suggesting that their poor fluency is more likely to be related to their general deficiency in initiating an effective retrieval strategy than to a true language deficit.

Chan and colleagues (Chan, Butters, Paulsen, et al., 1993; Chan, Butters, Salmon, & Johnson, 1995; Chan, Butters, Salmon, Johnson, et al., 1995; Chan, Butters, Salmon, & McGuire, 1993) recently initiated a series of studies designed to further investigate the nature of the language and semantic knowledge deficits associated with cortical and subcortical dementia syndromes. These studies used clustering and multidimensional scaling techniques (Romney, Shepard, & Nerlove, 1972; Shepard, Romney, & Nerlove, 1972; Tversky & Hutchinson, 1986) to model the organization of the network of related categories, concepts, and attributes that comprise semantic memory (Collins & Loftus, 1975) in patients with DAT and HD (for review, see Salmon & Chan, 1994). Multidimensional scaling provides a method for generating a spatial representation of the degree of association between concepts in semantic memory. The spatial representation, or cognitive map, generated in this manner clusters concepts along one or more dimensions according to their proximity, or degree of relatedness, in the patient's semantic network. The distance between concepts in the cognitive map reflects the strength of their association.

In a representative study from this series, cognitive maps reflecting the organization of semantic memory were generated for DAT, HD, and normal control subjects (Chan, Butters, Salmon, Johnson, et al., 1995). Maps were generated from proximity data derived from a triadic comparison task in which subjects chose, from among three concepts (i.e., among three animals), two that are most alike. Every possible combination of three animals, from a total sample of twelve animals, was presented to determine the degree of association between each pair of animals in relation to all other animal names.

The results of this analysis revealed that although semantic networks of DAT patients and normal control subjects were best represented by three dimensions (domesticity, predation, and size), they differed significantly in a number of ways. Patients with DAT focused primarily on concrete perceptual information (i.e., size) in categorizing animals, whereas control subjects stressed abstract conceptual knowledge (i.e., domesticity). A number of animals that were highly associated and clustered together for control subjects were not strongly associated for patients with DAT. Also DAT patients were less consistent than normal control subjects in using the various attributes of animals in categorization.

In contrast to DAT patients, semantic networks of HD patients and their age-matched control subjects were best represented by two dimensions (domesticity and size) and were virtually identical. Domesticity was the most salient dimension for categorizing animals for both groups, and HD and normal control subjects did not differ in the importance they applied to various dimensions or in their reliance on a particular dimension for categorization. Thus, organization of semantic memory appears to remain intact in subcortical dementias such as HD, but becomes disorganized in cortical dementias such as DAT.

Another major distinction that can be drawn between patients with cortical and subcortical dementia syndromes is the different patterns of spared and impaired abilities they exhibit on various implicit memory tasks (for reviews, see Bondi et al., 1994; Butters, Salmon, & Heindel, 1995). Implicit memory refers to the unconscious recollection of knowledge that is expressed indirectly through performance of specific operations comprising a task. Classical conditioning, lexical and semantic priming, motor skill learning, and perceptual learning are all considered forms of implicit memory (Squire, 1987). In all of these instances, an individual's performance is facilitated "unconsciously" simply by prior exposure to stimulus material. Implicit memory has been described as being mediated by a distinct memory "system" independent from the conscious, episodic memory system (Schacter, 1987; Schacter & Tulving, 1994; Squire, 1987). Neuropsychological and neurobiological evidence for this distinction is provided by numerous studies that have demonstrated preserved implicit memory in patients with severe amnesia arising from damage to hippocampal formation or to diencephalic brain regions (for review, see Squire, 1987).

Studies comparing patients with cortical or subcortical dementia on various priming tasks have shown that DAT patients, but not HD patients, are significantly impaired on lexical (Bondi & Kaszniak, 1991; Shimamura, Salmon, Squire, & Butters, 1987; Salmon, Shimamura, Butters, & Smith, 1988), semantic (Salmon et al., 1988), and pictorial (Heindel, Salmon, & Butters, 1990) priming tests. For example, Shimamura and colleagues (Salmon et al.,

1988; Shimamura et al., 1987) compared the lexical priming performance of patients with DAT, HD, and alcoholic Korsakoff's syndrome (i.e., circumscribed amnesia) on the word stem completion priming task previously used by Graf and colleagues (Graf, Squire, & Mandler, 1984). In this task, subjects were first exposed to a list of 10 target words (e.g., motel, abstain) and asked to rate each word in terms of "likeability." Following two presentations and ratings of the entire list, subjects were shown three-letter stems (e.g., mot, abs) of words that were and were not on the presentation list and were asked to complete the stems with the "first word that comes to mind." Half of the stems could be completed with previously presented words, while the other half were used to assess baseline guessing rates. Priming is indicated by an increased propensity to complete stems with previously presented words even though previous words are not consciously remembered. The subjects' free recall and recognition abilities (i.e., episodic memory) were assessed with other lists of words.

The results of this study showed that despite equivalent free recall and recognition deficits, amnesic and HD patients exhibited normal levels of stem completion priming, while DAT patients were impaired relative to the other patient groups and normal control subjects.

In contrast to the priming results, HD patients, but not patients with DAT, are impaired on motor skill learning (Eslinger & Damasio, 1986; Heindel, Salmon, Shults, Walicke, & Butters, 1989; Heindel, Butters, & Salmon, 1988), prism adaptation (Paulsen, Butters, Salmon, Heindel, & Swenson, 1993), and weight biasing (Heindel, Salmon, & Butters, 1992), tasks that involve generation and refinement (i.e., learning) of motor programs to guide behavior. In one study, for example, DAT and amnesic patients, as well as normal control subjects, all demonstrated systematic and equivalent improvement across blocks of trials of a rotary pursuit motor skill learning task in which subjects must learn to maintain contact between a stylus held in the preferred hand and a small metallic disk on a rotating turntable (Heindel et al., 1988). In contrast, HD patients were severely impaired in the acquisition of the pursuit rotor motor skill, showing only slight improvement over blocks of trials. This motor skill learning deficit in HD patients was not correlated with their general motor impairment (i.e., chorea) and was confirmed with other tasks that have little, if any, motor component (e.g., weight biasing, prism adaptation).

The double dissociation between AD and HD patients on these various implicit priming and motor skill learning tasks suggests that different forms of implicit memory, all of which are intact in patients with amnesic syndromes, are not mediated by a single neurological substrate. Rather, it appears that there are at least two psychologically and neurologically distinct implicit memory systems. Verbal and pictorial priming may both involve temporary activation of stored representations in semantic memory and may be dependent on the functional integrity of neocortical association areas damaged in AD. Motor skill learning, prism adaptation, and biasing of weight perception, on the other hand, may all involve modification of programmed movement parameters that are likely mediated by a corticostriatal and basal ganglia system that is severely compromised in HD.

The Lewy Body Variant of Alzheimer's Disease

Although the primary manifestation of AD is a profound global dementia, there is considerable heterogeneity in the clinical presentation of the disorder (Katzman, 1986). This heterogeneity may be explained, at least in part, by a recently discovered cliniconeuropathological condition, the Lewy body variant of AD (LBV; for review, see Hansen & Galasko, 1992), which is found in approximately 25% of patients who manifest a syndrome similar to DAT during life. The LBV of AD is characterized by the typical cortical distribution of senile plaques and neurofibrillary tangles associated with AD, the typical subcortical changes of Parkinson's disease (i.e., Lewy bodies and cell loss) in the substantia nigra and other pigmented brain stem nuclei, and the presence of diffusely distributed neocortical Lewy bodies (i.e., abnormal intracytoplasmic eosinophilic neuronal inclusion bodies; for review, see Hansen & Galasko, 1992). Clinically, patients with LBV present with insidious and progressive cognitive decline with no other significant neurologic abnormalities, inexorably progress to severe dementia, and are often diagnosed with probable or possible AD during life (e.g., Hansen et al., 1990).

Despite similarities in the clinical presentation of the two disorders, retrospective studies indicate that patients with LBV may be distinguishable from those with "pure" AD on the basis of specific neurological and neuropsychiatric features. Hansen and colleagues (Galasko, Katzman, Salmon, Thal, & Hansen, 1996; Hansen et al., 1990), for example, found that patients with LBV of AD differed from patients with pure AD in that a greater proportion had mild parkinsonian or extrapyramidal motor findings (e.g., bradykinesia, rigidity, masked facies, gait abnormalities, but no resting tremor). A retrospective study by McKeith and colleagues (McKeith, Perry, Fairbairn, Jabeen, & Perry, 1992) of patients with LBV, or as they refer to it, senile dementia of the Lewy body type, revealed that these patients were significantly more likely than pure AD patients to manifest fluctuating cognitive impairment, visual or auditory hallucinations, unexplained falls, and extrapyramidal features at some point during the course of the disease.

A number of recent retrospective studies have also begun to characterize the nature of the cognitive impairment associated with LBV (Byrne, Lennox, Lowe, & Godwin-Austen, 1989; Forstl, Burns, Luthert, Cairns, & Levy, 1993; Gibb, Esiri, & Lees, 1985; Hansen et al., 1990; McKeith et al., 1992). In one of these studies, Hansen and colleagues (1990) compared the performances of patients with neuropathologically confirmed LBV and those with pure AD on a battery of neuropsychological tests designed to assess memory, attention, language, conceptualization, and visuospatial abilities. Nine patients with LBV were matched one-to-one with nine patients with pure AD on the basis of age, education, overall level of global dementia as assessed by the IMC test of Blessed, and the interval between testing and death. The results of this study indicated that despite equivalent levels of global dementia, patients with LBV performed significantly worse than patients with pure AD on a test of attention (i.e., Digit Span subtest from the WAIS-Revised) and on tests of visuospatial and constructional ability (i.e., Block Design subtest from the Wechsler Intelligence Scale for Children-Revised and Copy-a-Cross test; see Figure 3). In addition, LBV and pure AD patients produced different patterns of impairment on tests of verbal fluency. The LBV group scored significantly lower than the pure AD group on a phoneme-based letter fluency task (i.e., generating words that begin with a particular letter), but the two groups performed similarly on a semantically based category fluency task (i.e., producing words that belong to a particular category). In contrast to these differences, the groups were equivalently impaired on tests of episodic memory, confrontation naming (i.e., Boston Naming Test), and arithmetic.

When results from the Hansen et al. (1990) study were viewed from the perspective of the cortical–subcortical distinction, patients with LBV appeared to exhibit a superimposition of cortical and subcortical neuropsychological impairments. The two groups demonstrated equivalent deficits in cognitive abilities usually affected by AD (e.g., memory, confrontation naming), but LBV patients displayed disproportionately severe deficits in cognitive abilities such as attention, verbal fluency, and visuospatial processing that are prominently affected in subcortical dementia. This pattern of cognitive performance is consistent with the distribution of neuropathological changes in the brains of LBV patients. All patients in the Hansen et al. (1990) study had typical neuropathological changes of AD in the hippocampus and association cortices, as well as subcortical and diffusely distributed neocortical changes associated with Lewy body disease.

Although the Hansen et al. (1990) study suggests that the Lewy body pathology present in LBV contributes importantly to the dementia associated with the disease, the extent of this contribution, and the particular pattern of neuropsychological deficits that may be associated with presence of cortical and subcortical Lewy bodies without concomitant AD, cannot be easily determined by studying these patients. This issue was addressed, however, in a recently completed study of five patients who clinically resembled patients with AD or LBV, but who at autopsy were found to have diffuse Lewy body disease (DLBD) with little or no AD pathology (Salmon et al., 1996). All five patients initially presented with cognitive decline that began insidiously and subsequently developed mild extrapyramidal motor dysfunction, and all were clinically diagnosed with probable or possible AD or one of

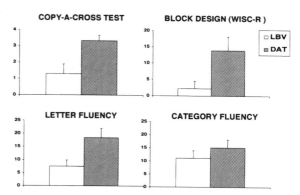

FIGURE 3. A comparison of the performance of patients with autopsy-verified Lewy body variant of Alzheimer's disease (LBV) and autopsy-verified "pure" dementia of the Alzheimer's type (DAT) on the Copy-a-Cross test, the Block Design subtest from the Wechsler Intelligence Scale for Children-Revised (WISC-R), a letter fluency test (FAS), and a category fluency test (animals, fruits and vegetables). (Adapted from Hansen et al., 1990.)

its variants (e.g., LBV, mixed AD and vascular dementia).

Despite the absence of AD pathology, all five DLBD patients exhibited global cognitive decline on neuropsychological testing carried out prior to their death. While deficits were noted in memory, attention, language, executive functions, and visuospatial and visuoconstructional abilities, the pattern and severity of these deficits differed somewhat from that typically observed in patients with DAT. With regard to memory, for example, DLBD patients scored 2 to 3 standard deviations below normal performance on several key measures of the CVLT (i.e., learning on trials 1 through 5, recall on trial 5, short and long delay free recall, recognition discriminability), but they did not exhibit the very poor retention over delay intervals, the increased propensity to produce intrusion errors in the cued recall condition, or the very poor recognition discriminability typical of DAT (Delis et al., 1991). Indeed, when the CVLT scores achieved by DLBD patients were subjected to the previously mentioned discriminant function equations, four of the five patients were classified as "subcortical" and one was classified as "cortical."

When neuropsychological test performance of DLBD patients was directly compared to that of five patients with autopsy-proven pure AD, a number of additional differences were observed. Despite being equated for global severity of dementia and performing similarly on the Digit Span, Boston Naming, Similarities, and Verbal Fluency tests, DLBD patients performed significantly worse than pure AD patients on tests of psychomotor speed and on tests of visuospatial and visuoconstructive abilities. For example, all five DLBD patients exhibited severe psychomotor slowing on parts A and B of the Trail-making test and were significantly slower than pure AD patients in both conditions. In addition, DLBD patients performed significantly worse than pure AD patients on a visuoconstructive task, the Block Design test, with four of the five DLBD patients performing at floor levels and the fifth severely impaired. An additional severe deficit was noted on the copy, but not the command, condition of the Clock Drawing test, and qualitative analysis of the clocks revealed that a significantly greater proportion of DLBD patients (five of five) than pure AD patients (one of five) produced errors related to the spatial layout of the clock (see Figure 4).

The results of the study by Salmon, Galasko, and colleagues (1996) indicate that subcortical and diffusely distributed neocortical Lewy body pathology, without concomitant AD pathology, can produce global cognitive impairment with particularly severe deficits in visuospatial/visuoconstructive abilities and psychomotor speed. In LBV, this pathology is superimposed on neuropathological changes that typically occur in AD, and the resulting neuropsychological impairment appears to reflect the effects of both. For example, patients with LBV, like patients with pure AD, have severe deficits in memory, language, and executive functions, most likely due to severe hippocampal and neocortical damage that occurs in AD (Hansen et al., 1990). In addition, patients with LBV, like patients with DLBD, have particularly severe deficits in visuospatial abilities, attention, and psychomotor processes, which may reflect the additional effects of Lewy body pathology. Thus, both Lewy body pathology and AD pathology appear to contribute importantly to the clinical manifestation of LBV.

The pattern of neuropsychological deficits observed in retrospective studies of patients with autopsy-confirmed LBV have also been observed in recent prospective studies of patients with clinically diagnosed DAT who exhibit mild extrapyramidal motor dysfunction (Girling & Berrios, 1990; Merello et al., 1994; Richards et al., 1993; Soininen et al., 1992), as well as in studies of patients who have been clinically diagnosed with LBV or senile dementia of the Lewy body type on the basis of neurological and neuropsychiatric symptoms (Galloway et al., 1992; Sahgal, Galloway, McKeith, Edwardson, & Lloyd, 1992; Sahgal, Galloway, McKeith, Lloyd, et al., 1992; Sahgal, McKeith, Galloway, Tasker, & Steckler, 1995). The results of these studies indicate that consideration of neuropsychological features associated with LBV may improve the accuracy with which the disorder can be diagnosed during life and thus reduce the apparent heterogeneity in clinical and neuropsychological manifestations of DAT.

Summary

It is evident from the neuropsychological research reviewed in this chapter that considerable progress has been made over the past decade in elucidating the pattern and neuropathological correlates of cognitive deficits associated with AD. In particular, our knowledge has increased greatly with regard to specific neuropsychological deficits that occur in the earliest stages of DAT or that even presage development of dementia. Research has also clearly shown that dementia is not a unitary disorder, but that different patterns of relatively preserved and impaired cognitive abilities can be identified among dementing diseases that have different etiologies and sites of neuropathology. Finally, recent research has shown that the heterogeneity that has been observed in the clinical and cognitive presentation of DAT has a biological basis rooted, at least in part, in the co-occurrence of AD pathology with subcortical and diffusely distributed neocortical Lewy body pathology.

The research reviewed above also has important implications for the study of brain–behavior relationships from a cognitive neuroscience perspective. The study of patients with AD has provided information about the neurological basis of priming and motor skill learning, semantic and episodic memory, and other higher order cognitive processes (e.g., visuospatial skills). As our knowledge of the neuropathology and neuropsychology of

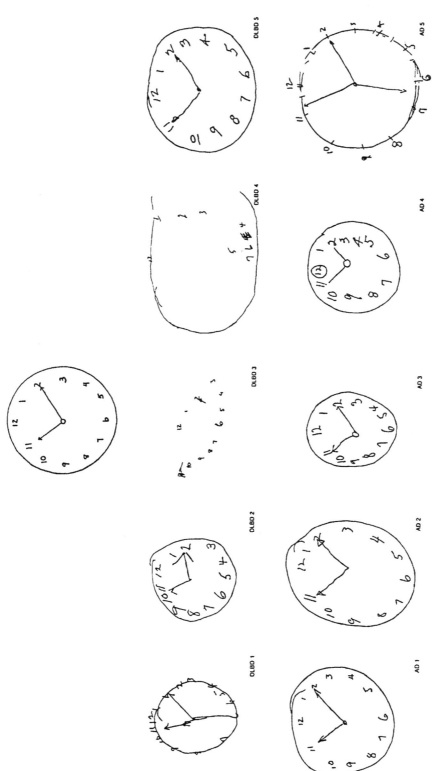

FIGURE 4. Examples of the clocks drawn by patients with diffuse Lewy body disease (DLBD) and Alzheimer's disease (AD) in the copy condition of the Clock Drawing test. The DLBD (cases 1–5) and AD patients (cases 1–5) were matched in terms of overall severity of dementia. The model to be copied is shown at the top. (Adapted from Salmon et al., 1996).

AD grows in coming years, further advances in our understanding of neural mediation of these and other cognitive processes should be possible.

ACKNOWLEDGMENTS

Preparation of this chapter was supported in part by funds from NIA grants AG-05131, AG-12963, and AG-12674; NIMH grant MH-48819; and the Medical Research Service of the Department of Veterans Affairs.

References

Albert, M. L., Feldman, R. G., & Willis, A. L. (1974). The "subcortical dementia" of progressive supranuclear palsy. *Journal of Neurology, Neurosurgery, and Psychiatry, 37,* 121–130.

Albert, M. S., Butters, N., & Brandt, J. (1981). Development of remote memory loss in patients with Huntington's disease. *Journal of Clinical Neuropsychology, 3,* 1–12.

Arriagada, P. V., Growdon, J. H., Hedley-Whyte, E. T., & Hyman, B. T. (1992). Neurofibrillary tangles but not senile plaques parallel duration and severity of Alzheimer's disease. *Neurology, 42,* 631–639.

Bachman, D. L., Wolf, P. A., Linn, R., Knoefel, J. E., Cobb, J., Belanger, A., D'Agostino, R. B., & White, L. R. (1992). Prevalence of dementia and probable senile dementia of the Alzheimer type in the Framingham study. *Neurology, 42,* 115–119.

Bachman, D. L., Wolf, P. A., Linn, R., Knoefel, R. T., Cobb, J. L., Belanger, A. J., White, L. R., & D'Agostino, R. B. (1993). Incidence of dementia and probable Alzheimer's disease in a general population: The Framingham study. *Neurology, 43,* 515–519.

Bancher, C., Braak, H., Fischer, P., & Jellinger, K. A. (1993). Neuropathological staging of Alzheimer lesions and intellectual status in Alzheimer's and Parkinson's disease patients. *Neuroscience Letters, 162,* 179–182.

Bayles, K. A., & Kaszniak, A. W. (1987). *Communication and cognition in normal aging and dementia.* Boston: College-Hill/Little, Brown and Company.

Bayles, K. A., & Tomoeda, C. K. (1983). Confrontation naming impairment in dementia. *Brain and Language, 19,* 98–114.

Bayles, K. A., Boone, D. R., Tomoeda, C. K., Slauson, T. J., & Kaszniak, A. W. (1989). Differentiating Alzheimer's patients from the normal elderly and stroke patients with aphasia. *Journal of Speech and Hearing Disorders, 54,* 74–87.

Beatty, W. W., & Salmon, D. P. (1991). Remote memory for visuospatial information in patients with Alzheimer's disease. *Journal of Geriatric Psychiatry and Neurology, 4,* 14–17.

Beatty, W. W., Salmon, D. P., Butters, N., Heindel, W. C., & Granholm, E. L. (1988). Retrograde amnesia in patients with Alzheimer's disease or Huntington's disease. *Neurobiology of Aging, 9,* 181–186.

Blessed, G., Tomlinson, B. E., & Roth, M. (1968). The association between quantitative measures of dementia and of senile change in the cerebral grey matter of elderly subjects. *British Journal of Psychiatry, 114,* 797–811.

Bondareff, W., Mountjoy, C. Q., & Roth, M. (1982). Loss of neurons of origin of the adrenergic projection to cerebral cortex (nucleus locus ceruleus) in senile dementia. *Neurology, 32,* 164–167.

Bondi, M. W., & Kaszniak, A. W. (1991). Implicit and explicit memory in Alzheimer's disease and Parkinson's disease. *Journal of Clinical and Experimental Neuropsychology, 13,* 339–358.

Bondi, M. W., Monsch, A. U., Butters, N., Salmon, D. P., & Paulsen, J. S. (1993). Utility of a modified version of the Wisconsin Card Sorting test in the detection of dementia of the Alzheimer type. *The Clinical Neuropsychologist, 7,* 161–170.

Bondi, M. W., Monsch, A. U., Galasko, D., Butters, N., Salmon, D. P., & Delis, D. C. (1994). Preclinical cognitive markers of dementia of the Alzheimer type. *Neuropsychology, 8,* 374–384.

Bondi, M. W., Salmon, D. P., & Butters, N. (1994). Neuropsychological features of memory disorders in dementia of the Alzheimer type. In R. D. Terry, R. Katzman, & K. L. Bick (Eds.), *Alzheimer disease* (pp. 41–63). New York: Raven Press.

Bondi, M. W., Salmon, D. P., Monsch, A. U., Galasko, D., Butters, N., Klauber, M. R., Thal, L. J., & Saitoh, T. (1995). Episodic memory changes are associated with the ApoE-ε4 allele in nondemented older adults. *Neurology, 45,* 2203–2206.

Braak, H., & Braak, E. (1991). Neuropathological staging of Alzheimer-related changes. *Acta Neuropathologica, 82,* 239–259.

Brandt, J., & Butters, N. (1986). The neuropsychology of Huntington's disease. *Trends in Neuroscience, 9,* 118–120.

Brandt, J., Corwin, J., & Kraft, L. (1992). Is verbal recognition memory really different in Huntington's and Alzheimer's disease? *Journal of Clinical and Experimental Neuropsychology, 14,* 773–784.

Bruyn, G. W., Bots, G., & Dom, R. (1979). Huntington's chorea: Current neuropathological status. In T. Chase, N. Wexler, & A. Barbeau (Eds.), *Advances in neurology: Vol. 23. Huntington's disease* (pp. 83–94). New York: Raven Press.

Buschke, H., & Fuld, P. A. (1974). Evaluating storage, retention, and retrieval in disordered memory and learning. *Neurology, 24,* 1019–1025.

Butters, N., Sax, D. S., Montgomery, K., & Tarlow, S. (1978). Comparison of the neuropsychological deficits associated with early and advanced Huntington's disease. *Archives of Neurology, 35,* 585–589.

Butters, N., Granholm, E., Salmon, D. P., Grant, I., & Wolfe, J. (1987). Episodic and semantic memory: A comparison of amnesic and demented patients. *Journal of Clinical and Experimental Neuropsychology, 9,* 479–497.

Butters, N., Salmon, D. P., Cullum, C. M., Cairns, P., Tröster, A. I., Jacobs, D., Moss, M. B., & Cermak, L. S. (1988). Differentiation of amnesic and demented patients with the Wechsler Memory Scale-Revised. *The Clinical Neuropsychologist, 2,* 133–144.

Butters, N., Salmon, D. P., & Heindel, W. C. (1995). Specificity of the memory deficits associated with basal ganglia dysfunction. *Revue Neurologique, 150,* 580–587.

Byrne, E. J., Lennox, G., Lowe, J., & Godwin-Austen, R. B. (1989). Diffuse Lewy body disease: Clinical features in 15 cases. *Journal of Neurology, Neurosurgery, and Psychiatry, 52,* 709–717.

Chan, A. S., Butters, N., Paulsen, J. S., Salmon, D. P., Swenson, M. R., & Maloney, L. T. (1993). An assessment of the semantic network in patients with Alzheimer's disease. *Journal of Cognitive Neuroscience, 5,* 254–261.

Chan, A. S., Butters, N., Salmon, D. P., & McGuire, K. A. (1993). Dimensionality and clustering in the semantic network of patients with Alzheimer's disease. *Psychology and Aging, 8,* 411–419.

Chan, A. S., Butters, N., Salmon, D. P., & Johnson, S. A. (1995). Semantic network abnormality predicts rate of cognitive decline in patients with probable Alzheimer's disease. *Journal of the International Neuropsychological Society, 1,* 297–303.

Chan, A. S., Butters, N., Salmon, D. P., Johnson, S. A., Paulsen, J. S., & Swenson, M. R. (1995). Comparison of the semantic networks in patients with dementia and amnesia. *Neuropsychology, 9,* 177–186.

Chertkow, H., & Bub, D. (1990). Semantic memory loss in dementia of Alzheimer's type. *Brain, 118,* 397–417.

Collins, A. M., & Loftus, E. F. (1975). A spreading activation theory of semantic processing. *Psychological Review, 82,* 407–428.

Corder, E. H., Saunders, A. M., Strittmatter, W. J., Schmechel, D. E., Gaskell, P. C., Small, G. W., Roses, A. D., Haines, G. L., & Perick-Vance, M. A. (1993). Gene dose of apolipoprotein E type 4 allele and the risk of Alzheimer's disease in late onset families. *Science, 261,* 921–923.

Corkin, S., Davis, K. L., Growdon, J. H., Usdin, E., & Wurtman, R. J. (1982). *Alzheimer's disease: A report of progress in research. Aging* (Vol. 19). New York: Raven Press.

Cummings, J. L. (1990). *Subcortical dementia.* New York: Oxford University Press.

DeKosky, S. T., & Scheff, S. W. (1990). Synapse loss in frontal cortex biopsies in Alzheimer's disease: Correlation with cognitive severity. *Annals of Neurology, 27,* 457–464.

De Lacoste, M., & White, C. L. (1993). The role of cortical connectivity in Alzheimer's disease pathogenesis: A review and model system. *Neurobiology of Aging, 14,* 1–16.

Delis, D. C., Kramer, J. H., Kaplan, E., & Ober, B. A. (1987). *The California Verbal Learning Test.* New York: Psychological Corporation.

Delis, D. C., Massman, P. J., Butters, N., Salmon, D. P., Kramer, J. H., & Cermak, L. (1991). Profiles of demented and amnesic patients on the California Verbal Learning Test: Implications for the assessment of memory disorders. *Psychological Assessment, 3,* 19–26.

Eslinger, P. J., & Damasio, A. R. (1986). Preserved motor learning in Alzheimer's disease: Implications for anatomy and behavior. *Journal of Neuroscience, 6,* 3006–3009.

Eslinger, P. J., Damasio, A. R., Benton, A. L., & Van Allen, M. (1985). Neuropsychologic detection of abnormal mental decline in older persons. *Journal of the American Medical Association, 253,* 670–674.

Flicker, C., Ferris, S. H., & Reisberg, B. (1991). Mild cognitive impairment in the elderly: Predictors of dementia. *Neurology, 41,* 1006–1009.

Folstein, S. E., Brandt, J., & Folstein, M. F. (1990). Huntington's disease. In J. L. Cummings (Ed.), *Subcortical dementia* (pp. 87–107). New York: Oxford University Press.

Forstl, H., Burns, A., Luthert, P., Cairns, N., & Levy, R. (1993). The Lewy-body variant of Alzheimer's disease: Clinical and pathological findings. *British Journal of Psychiatry, 162,* 385–392.

Freedman, M., Rivoira, P., Butters, N., Sax, D. S., & Robert, G. (1984). Retrograde amnesia in Parkinson's disease. *Canadian Journal of Neurological Sciences, 11,* 297–301.

Fuld, P. A., Katzman, R., Davies, P., & Terry, R. D. (1982). Intrusions as a sign of Alzheimer dementia: Chemical and pathological verification. *Annals of Neurology, 11,* 155–159.

Fuld, P. A., Masur, D. M., Blau, A. D., Crystal, H., & Aronson, M. K. (1990). Object-memory evaluation for prospective detection of dementia in normal functioning elderly: Predictive and normative data. *Journal of Clinical and Experimental Neuropsychology, 12,* 520–528.

Galasko, D., Hansen, L. A., Katzman, R., Wiederholt, W., Masliah, E., Terry, R. D., Hill, L. R., Lessin, P., & Thal, L. J. (1994). Clinical-neuropathological correlations in Alzheimer's disease and related disorders. *Archives of Neurology, 51,* 888–895.

Galasko, D., Katzman, R., Salmon, D. P., Thal, L. J., & Hansen, L. A. (1996). Clinical and neuropathological findings in Lewy body dementias. *Brain and Cognition, 31,* 166–175.

Galloway, P. H., Sahgal, A., McKeith, I. G., Lloyd, S., Cook, J. H., Ferrier, I. N., & Edwardson, J. A. (1992). Visual pattern recognition memory and learning deficits in senile dementias of Alzheimer and Lewy body types. *Dementia, 3,* 101–107.

Gibb, W. R. G., Esiri, M. M. & Lees, A. J. (1985). Clinical and pathological features of diffuse cortical Lewy body disease (Lewy body dementia). *Brain, 110,* 1131–1153.

Girling, D. M., & Berrios, G. E. (1990). Extrapyramidal signs, primitive reflexes and frontal lobe function in senile dementia of the Alzheimer type. *British Journal of Psychiatry, 157,* 888–893.

Graf, P., Squire, L. R., & Mandler, G. (1984). The information that amnesics do not forget. *Journal of Experimental Psychology: Learning, Memory, and Cognition, 10,* 164–178.

Haase, G. R. (1977). Diseases presenting as dementia. In C. E. Wells (Ed.), *Dementia* (2nd ed., pp. 27–67). Philadelphia: F. A. Davis.

Hansen, L. A., & Galasko, D. (1992). Lewy body disease. *Current Opinion in Neurology and Neurosurgery, 5,* 889–894.

Hansen, L., Salmon, D. P., Galasko, D., Masliah, E., Katzman, R., DeTeresa, R., Thal, L. J., Pay, M. M., Hofstetter, R., Klauber, M. R., Rice, V., Butters, N., & Alford, M. (1990). The Lewy body variant of Alzheimer's disease: A clinical and pathologic entity. *Neurology, 40,* 1–8.

Heindel, W. C., Butters, N., & Salmon, D. P. (1988). Impaired learning of a motor skill in patients with Huntington's disease. *Behavioral Neuroscience, 102,* 141–147.

Heindel, W. C., Salmon, D. P., Shults, C., Walicke, P., & Butters,

N. (1989). Neuropsychological evidence for multiple implicit memory systems: A comparison of Alzheimer's, Huntington's and Parkinson's disease patients. *Journal of Neuroscience, 9,* 582–587.

Heindel, W. C., Salmon, D. P., & Butters, N. (1990). Pictorial priming and cued recall in Alzheimer's and Huntington's disease. *Brain and Cognition, 13,* 282–295.

Heindel, W. C., Salmon, D. P., & Butters, N. (1992). The biasing of weight judgments in Alzheimer's and Huntington's disease: A priming or programming phenomenon? *Journal of Clinical and Experimental Neuropsychology, 13,* 189–203.

Hodges, J. R., Salmon, D. P., & Butters, N. (1991). The nature of the naming deficit in Alzheimer's and Huntington's disease. *Brain, 114,* 1547–1558.

Hodges, J. R., Salmon, D. P., & Butters, N. (1992). Semantic memory impairment in Alzheimer's disease: Failure of access or degraded knowledge? *Neuropsychologia, 30,* 301–314.

Hodges, J. R., Salmon, D. P., & Butters, N. (1993). Recognition and naming of famous faces in Alzheimer's disease: A cognitive analysis. *Neuropsychologia, 31,* 775–788.

Hom, J., Turner, M. B., Risser, R., Bonte, F. J., & Tintner, R. (1994). Cognitive deficits in asymptomatic first-degree relatives of Alzheimer's disease patients. *Journal of Clinical and Experimental Neuropsychology, 16,* 568–576.

Huff, F. J., Corkin, S., & Growdon, J. H. (1986). Semantic impairment and anomia in Alzheimer's disease. *Brain and Language, 28,* 235–249.

Huff, F. J., Becker, J. T., Belle, S. H., Nebes, R. D., Holland, A. L., & Boller, F. (1987). Cognitive deficits and clinical diagnosis of Alzheimer's disease. *Neurology, 37,* 1119–1124.

Huppert, F. A., & Tym, E. (1986). Clinical and neuropsychological assessment of dementia. *British Medical Bulletin, 42,* 11–18.

Hyman, B. T., Van Hoesen, G. W., Damasio, A., & Barnes, C. L. (1984). Alzheimer's disease: Cell-specific pathology isolates the hippocampal formation. *Science, 225,* 1168–1170.

Jacobs, D., Salmon, D. P., Tröster, A. I., & Butters, N. (1990). Intrusion errors in the figural memory of patients with Alzheimer's and Huntington's disease. *Archives of Clinical Neuropsychology, 5,* 49–57.

Kaszniak, A. W., Wilson, R. S., Fox, J. H., & Stebbins, G. T. (1986). Cognitive assessment in Alzheimer's disease: Cross-sectional and longitudinal perspectives. *Canadian Journal of Neurological Sciences, 13,* 420–423.

Katzman, R. (1986). Alzheimer's disease. *New England Journal of Medicine, 314,* 964–973.

Katzman, R. (1993). Education and the prevalence of dementia and Alzheimer's disease. *Neurology, 43,* 13–20.

Katzman, R. (1994). Apolipoprotein E and Alzheimer's disease. *Current Opinion in Neurobiology, 4,* 703–707.

Katzman, R., & Kawas, C. (1994). The epidemiology of dementia and Alzheimer disease. In R. D. Terry, R. Katzman, & K. L. Bick (Eds.), *Alzheimer disease* (pp. 105–122). New York: Raven Press.

Katzman, R., Aronson, M., Fuld, P., Kawas, C., Brown, T., Morgenstern, H., Frishman, W., Gidez, L., Eder, H., & Ooi, W. L. (1989). Development of dementing illness in an 80-year-old volunteer cohort. *Annals of Neurology, 25,* 317–324.

Kawas, C. H. (1990). Early clinical diagnosis: Status of

NINCDS-ADRDA criteria. In R. E. Becker & E. Giacobini (Eds.), *Alzheimer disease: Current research in early diagnosis.* New York: Taylor & Francis.

Khachaturian, Z. S. (1985). Diagnosis of Alzheimer's disease. *Archives of Neurology, 42,* 1097–1105.

Knopman, D. S., & Ryberg, S. (1989). A verbal memory test with high predictive accuracy for dementia of the Alzheimer type. *Archives of Neurology, 46,* 141–145.

Kopelman, M. D. (1989). Remote and autobiographical memory, temporal context memory and frontal atrophy in Korsakoff and Alzheimer patients. *Neuropsychologia, 27,* 437–460.

La Rue, A. (1992). *Aging and neuropsychological assessment,* New York: Plenum.

La Rue, A., & Jarvik, L. R. (1980). Reflections of biological changes in the psychological performance of the aged. *Age, 3,* 29–32.

La Rue, A., & Jarvik, L. R. (1987). Cognitive function and prediction of dementia in old age. *International Journal of Aging and Human Development, 25,* 79–89.

La Rue, A., Matsuyama, S. S., McPherson, S., Sherman, J., & Jarvik, L. F. (1992). Cognitive performance in relatives of patients with probable Alzheimer disease: An age at onset effect? *Journal of Clinical and Experimental Neuropsychology, 14,* 533–538.

Linn, R. T., Wolf, P. A., Bachman, D. L., Knoefel, J. E., Cobb, J. L., Belanger, A. J., Kaplan, E. F., & D'Agostino, R. B. (1995). The "preclinical phase" of probable Alzheimer's disease: A 13-year prospective study of the Framingham cohort. *Archives of Neurology, 52,* 485–490.

Mann, D. M. A., Yates, P. O., & Marcyniuk, B. (1984). A comparison of changes in the nucleus basalis and locus ceruleus in Alzheimer's disease. *Journal of Neurology, Neurosurgery, and Psychiatry, 47,* 201–203.

Mann, D. M. A., Marcyniuk, B., Yates, P. O., Neary, D., & Snowden, J. S. (1988). The progression of the pathological changes of Alzheimer's disease in frontal and temporal neocortex examined both at biopsy and at autopsy. *Neuropathology and Applied Neurobiology, 14,* 177–195.

Martin, A. (1987). Representation of semantic and spatial knowledge in Alzheimer's patients: Implications for models of preserved learning in amnesia. *Journal of Clinical and Experimental Neuropsychology, 9,* 191–224.

Massman, P. J., Delis, D. C., & Butters, N. (1993). Does impaired primacy recall equal impaired long-term storage?: Serial position effects in Huntington's disease and Alzheimer's disease. *Developmental Neuropsychology, 9,* 1–15.

Masur, D. M., Fuld, P. A., Blau, A. D., Thal, L. J., Levin, H. S., & Aronson, M. K. (1989). Distinguishing normal and demented elderly with the selective reminding test. *Journal of Clinical and Experimental Neuropsychology, 11,* 615–630.

Masur, D. M., Fuld, P. A., Blau, A. D., Crystal, H., & Aronson, M. K. (1990). Predicting development of dementia in the elderly with the selective reminding test. *Journal of Clinical and Experimental Neuropsychology, 12,* 529–538.

Masur, D. M., Sliwinski, M., Lipton, R. B., Blau, A. D., & Crystal, H. A. (1994). Neuropsychological prediction of dementia and the absence of dementia in healthy elderly persons. *Neurology, 44,* 1427–1432.

Mayeux, R., Ottman, R., Maestre, G., Ngai, C., Tang, M.-X.,

Ginsberg, H., Chun, M., Tycko, B., & Shelanski, M. (1995). Synergistic effects of traumatic head injury and apolipoprotein €4 in patients with Alzheimer's disease. *Neurology, 45,* 555–557.

McHugh, P. R., & Folstein, M. F. (1975). Psychiatric symptoms of Huntington's chorea: A clinical and phenomenologic study. In D. F. Benson & D. Blumer (Eds.), *Psychiatric aspects of neurological disease* (pp. 267–285). New York: Raven Press.

McKeith, I. G., Perry, R. H., Fairbairn, A. F., Jabeen, S., & Perry, E. K. (1992). Operational criteria for senile dementia of Lewy body type (SDLT). *Psychological Medicine, 22,* 911–922.

McKhann, G., Drachman, D., Folstein, M., Katzman, R., Price, D., & Stadlin, E. M. (1984). Clinical diagnosis of Alzheimer's disease: Report of the NINCDS-ADRDA work group under the auspices of the Department of Health and Human Services Task Force on Alzheimer's Disease. *Neurology, 34,* 939–944.

Merello, M., Sabe, L., Teson, A., Migliorelli, R., Petracchi, M., Leiguarda, R., & Starkstein, S. (1994). Extrapyramidalism in Alzheimer's disease: Prevalence, psychiatric, and neuropsychological correlates. *Journal of Neurology, Neurosurgery, and Psychiatry, 57,* 1503–1509.

Miller, E. (1971). On the nature of memory disorder in presenile dementia. *Neuropsychologia, 9,* 75–78.

Monsch, A. U., Bondi, M. W., Butters, N., Salmon, D. P., Katzman, R., & Thal, L. F. (1992). Comparisons of verbal fluency tasks in the detection of dementia of the Alzheimer type. *Archives of Neurology, 49,* 1253–1258.

Morris, J. C., McKeel, D. W., Storandt, M., Rubin, E. H., Price, J. L., Grant, E. A., Ball, M. J., & Berg, L. (1991). Very mild Alzheimer's disease: Informant-based clinical, psychometric, and pathologic distinction from normal aging. *Neurology, 41,* 469–478.

Mortimer, J. A. (1988). Do psychosocial risk factors contribute to Alzheimer's disease? In A. S. Henderson & J. H. Henderson (Eds.), *Etiology of dementia of the Alzheimer's type* (pp. 39–52). New York: John Wiley and Sons.

Mortimer, J. A., van Duijn, C. M., Chandra, V., Fratiglioni, L., Graves, A. B., Heyman, A., Jorm, A. F., Kokem, E., Kondo, K., Rocca, W. A., Shalat, S. L., Soininen, H., & Hofman, A. (1991). Head trauma as a risk factor for Alzheimer's disease: A collaborative re-analysis of case-control studies. *International Journal of Epidemiology, 20*(Suppl. 2), S28–S35.

Moss, M. B., Albert, M. S., Butters, N., & Payne, M. (1986). Differential patterns of memory loss among patients with Alzheimer's disease, Huntington's disease and alcoholic Korsakoff's syndrome. *Archives of Neurology, 43,* 239–246.

Neary, D., Snowden, J. S., Mann, D. M. A., Bowen, D. M., Sims, N. R., Northen, B., Yates, P. O., & Davison, A. N. (1986). Alzheimer's disease: A correlative study. *Journal of Neurology, Neurosurgery, and Psychiatry, 49,* 229–237.

Parks, R. W., Zec, R. F., & Wilson, R. S. (Eds.). (1993). *Neuropsychology of Alzheimer's disease and other dementias.* New York: Oxford University Press.

Paulsen, J. S., Butters, N., Salmon, D. P., Heindel, W. C., & Swenson, M. R. (1993). Prism adaptation in Alzheimer's and Huntington's disease. *Neuropsychology, 7,* 73–81.

Pearson, R. C. A., Esiri, M. M., Hiorns, R. W., Wilcock, G. K., & Powell, T. P. S. (1985). Anatomical correlates of the distribution of the pathological changes in the neocortex in Alzheimer disease. *Proceedings of the National Academy of Sciences, USA, 82,* 4521–4534.

Pepin, E. P., & Eslinger, P. J. (1989). Verbal memory decline in Alzheimer's disease: A multiple-processes deficit. *Neurology, 39,* 1477–1482.

Reed, T., Carmelli, D., Swan, G. E., Breitner, J. C., Welsh, K. A., Jarvik, G. P., Deeb, S., & Auwerx, J. (1994). Lower cognitive performance in normal older adult male twins carrying the apolipoprotein E €4 allele. *Archives of Neurology, 51,* 1189–1192.

Richards, M., Bell, K., Dooneief, G., Marder, K., Sano, M., Mayeux, R., & Stern, Y. (1993). Patterns of neuropsychological performance in Alzheimer's disease patients with and without extrapyramidal signs. *Neurology, 43,* 1708–1711.

Romney, A. K., Shepard, R. N., & Nerlove, S. B. (1972). *Multidimensional scaling: Theory and applications in the behavioral sciences* (Vol. II). New York: Seminar Press.

Sagar, J. J., Cohen, N. J., Sullivan, E. V., Corkin, S., & Growdon, J. H. (1988). Remote memory function in Alzheimer's disease and Parkinson's disease. *Brain, 111,* 525–539.

Sahgal, A., Galloway, P. H., McKeith, I. G., Edwardson, J. A., & Lloyd, S. (1992). A comparative study of attentional deficits in senile dementias of Alzheimer and Lewy body types. *Dementia, 3,* 350–354.

Sahgal, A., Galloway, P. H., McKeith, I. G., Lloyd, S., Cook, J. H., Ferrier, N., & Edwardson, J. A. (1992). Matching-to-sample deficits in patients with senile dementias of the Alzheimer and Lewy body types. *Archives of Neurology, 49,* 1043–1046.

Sahgal, A., McKeith, I. G., Galloway, P. H., Tasker, N., & Steckler, T. (1995). Do differences in visuospatial ability between senile dementias of the Alzheimer and Lewy body types reflect differences solely in mnemonic function? *Journal of Clinical and Experimental Neuropsychology, 17,* 35–43.

Salmon, D. P., Shimamura, A., Butters, N., & Smith, S. (1988). Lexical and semantic priming deficits in patients with Alzheimer's disease. *Journal of Clinical and Experimental Neuropsychology, 10,* 477–494.

Salmon, D. P., & Chan, A. S. (1994). Semantic memory deficits associated with Alzheimer's disease. In L. S. Cermak (Ed.), *Neuropsychological explorations of memory and cognition: Essays in honor of Nelson Butters* (pp. 61–76). New York: Plenum Press.

Salmon, D. P., & Galasko, D. (1996). Neuropsychological aspects of Lewy body dementia. In E. K. Perry, R. H. Perry, & I. McKeith (Eds.), *Lewy body dementia* (pp. 99–113). London: Cambridge University Press.

Salmon, D. P., Galasko, D., Hansen, L. A., Masliah, E., Butters, N., Thal, L. J., & Katzman, R. (1996). Neuropsychological deficits associated with diffuse Lewy body disease. *Brain and Cognition, 31,* 148–165.

Salmon, D. P., Butters, N., Thal, L. J., & Jeste, D. V. (in press). Alzheimer's disease: Analysis for the DSM-IV task force. In T. A. Widiger, A. Frances, & H. Pincus (Eds.), *DSM-IV sourcebook* (Vol. IV). Washington, DC: American Psychiatric Association.

Schacter, D. L. (1987). Implicit memory: History and current status. *Journal of Experimental Psychology: Learning, Memory, and Cognition, 13,* 501–518.

Schacter, D. L., & Tulving, E. (Eds.). (1994). *Memory systems 1994*. Cambridge, MA: MIT Press.

Shepard, R. N., Romney, A. K., & Nerlove, S. B. (1972). *Multidimensional scaling: Theory and applications in the behavioral sciences* (Vol. I). New York: Seminar Press.

Shimamura, A. P., Salmon, D. P., Squire, L. R., & Butters, N. (1987). Memory dysfunction and word priming in dementia and amnesia. *Behavioral Neuroscience, 101*, 347–351.

Smalley, S. L., Wolkenstein, B. H., La Rue, A., Woodward, J. A., Jarvik, L. F., & Matsuyama, S. S. (1992). Comingling analysis of memory performance in offspring of Alzheimer patients. *Genetic Epidemiology, 9*, 333–345.

Smith, S. R., Murdoch, B. E., & Chenery, H. J. (1989). Semantic abilities in dementia of the Alzheimer type: 1. Lexical semantics. *Brain and Language, 36*, 314–324.

Soininen, H., Helkala, E. L., Laulumaa, V., Soikkeli, R., Hartikainen, P., & Riekkinen, P. J. (1992). Cognitive profile of Alzheimer patients with extrapyramidal signs: A longitudinal study. *Journal of Neural Transmission, 4*, 241–254.

Squire, L. R. (1987). *Memory and brain*. New York: Oxford University Press.

Squire, L. R. (1992). Memory and the hippocampus: A synthesis from findings with rats, monkeys and humans. *Psychological Review, 99*, 195–231.

Stern, Y., Alexander, G. E., Prohovnik, I., & Mayeux, R. (1992). Inverse relationship between education and parietotemporal perfusion deficit in Alzheimer's disease. *Neurology, 32*, 371–375.

Stern, Y., Gurland, B., Tatemichi, T. K., Tang, M. X., Wilder, D., & Mayeux, R. (1994). Influence of education and occupation on the incidence of Alzheimer's disease. *Journal of the American Medical Association, 271*, 1004–1010.

Storandt, M., Botwinick, J., Danziger, W. L., Berg, L., & Hughes, C. P. (1984). Psychometric differentiation of mild senile dementia of the Alzheimer type. *Archives of Neurology 41*, 497–499.

Strittmatter, W. J., Saunders, A. M., Schmechel, D., Pericak-Vance, M., Enghild, J., Salvesen, G. S., & Roses, A. D. (1993). Apolipoprotein-E—High-avidity binding to B-amyloid and increased frequency of type 4 allele in late-onset familial Alzheimer disease. *Proceedings of the National Academy of Sciences, USA, 90*, 9649–9653.

Terry, R. D., & Katzman, R. (1983). Senile dementia of the Alzheimer type. *Annals of Neurology, 14*, 497–506.

Terry, R. D., Peck, A., DeTeresa, R., Schecter, R., & Horoupian, D. S. (1981). Some morphometric aspects of the brain in senile dementia of the Alzheimer type. *Annals of Neurology, 10*, 184–192.

Terry, R. D., Masliah, E., Salmon, D. P., Butters, N., DeTeresa, R., Hill, R., Hansen, L. A., & Katzman, R. (1991). Physical basis of cognitive alterations in Alzheimer's disease: Synapse loss is the major correlate of cognitive impairment. *Annals of Neurology, 30*, 572–580.

Tröster, A. I., Jacobs, D., Butters, N., Cullum, C. M., & Salmon, D. P. (1989). Differentiating Alzheimer's disease from Huntington's disease with the Wechsler Memory Scale-Revised. *Clinics in Geriatric Medicine, 5*, 611–632.

Tröster, A. I., Butters, N., Salmon, D. P., Cullum, C. M., Jacobs, D., Brandt, J., & White, R. F. (1993). The diagnostic utility of savings scores: Differentiating Alzheimer's and Huntington's diseases with the logical memory and visual reproduction tests. *Journal of Clinical and Experimental Neuropsychology, 15*, 773–788.

Tversky, A., & Hutchinson, J. W. (1986). Nearest neighbor analysis of psychological spaces. *Psychological Review, 93*, 3–22.

van Duijn, C. M., Hofman, A., & Kay, D. W. (1991). Risk factors for Alzheimer's disease: A collaborative re-analysis of case-control studies. *International Journal of Epidemiology, 20* (Suppl. 2).

Vonsattel, J.-P., Myers, R. H., Stevens, T. J., Ferrante, R. J., Bird, E. D., & Richardson, E. P. (1985). Neuropathological classification of Huntington's disease. *Journal of Neuropathology and Experimental Neurology, 44*, 559–577.

Welsh, K., Butters, N., Hughes, J., Mohs, R., & Heyman, A. (1991). Detection of abnormal memory decline in mild cases of Alzheimer's disease using CERAD neuropsychological measures. *Archives of Neurology, 48*, 278–281.

Whitehouse, P. J., Price, D. L., Struble, R. G., Clark, A. W., Coyle, J. T., & DeLong, M. R. (1982). Alzheimer's disease and senile dementia: Loss of neurons in the basal forebrain. *Science, 215*, 1237–1239.

Wilson, R. S., Kaszniak, A. W., & Fox, J. H. (1981). Remote memory in senile dementia. *Cortex, 17*, 41–48.

Wilson, R. S., Bacon, L. D., Fox, J. H., & Kaszniak, A. W. (1983). Primary and secondary memory in dementia of the Alzheimer type. *Journal of Clinical Neuropsychology, 5*, 337–344.

Zhang, M., Katzman, R., Salmon, D. P., Jin, H., Cai, G., Wang, Z., Qu, G., Grant, I., Yu, E., Levy, P., Kauber, M., & Liu, W. T. (1990). The prevalence of dementia and Alzheimer's disease (AD) in Shanghai, China: Impact on age, gender and education. *Annals of Neurology, 27*, 428–437.

Zola-Morgan, S., & Squire, L. R. (1990). The primate hippocampal formation: Evidence for a time-limited role in memory storage. *Science, 250*, 288–290.

11

Frontotemporal Dementias

MAHMOOD A. USMAN

I hate to say it, but for all practical purposes, my wife is dead. Her body is still healthy, she is beautiful, but her brain damage is such that the woman I love is gone forever. My love is so great that I must care for what remains of her.

—*Michael E. Braun*, whose wife has been diagnosed with a frontotemporal dementia

Introduction

The term frontal lobe dementia or frontotemporal dementia refers to a pathologically heterogeneous group of neurodegenerative disorders that primarily affect the frontal and temporal regions of the brain and produce symptoms characteristic of frontotemporal dysfunction. Of these conditions, Pick's disease has been the most studied and best described, but it is nearly indistinguishable on a clinical basis from a number of similar disorders. These patients typically present with dramatic personality changes, socially inappropriate behavior, apathy, and subtle evidence of impairment in frontal and temporal lobe functions and go on to have more global cognitive dysfunction.

Terminology

Numerous names have been proposed for both the clinical syndromes and the various patterns of neuropathology, making the literature on the subject confusing and often contradictory. Since memory impairment is generally a late finding in these disorders, patients in early stages of the disease

usually do not meet *Diagnostic and Statistical Manual of Mental Disorders*, fourth edition (*DSM-IV*) criteria for a dementia and would instead be considered to have a personality change due to a general medical condition (Frances, Pincus, First, & Widiger, 1994). Because of the semantic ambiguity and pathological heterogeneity of these conditions, descriptive clinical terms like frontotemporal dementia (or degeneration) (FTD) are now used most often in describing these cases, rather than specific pathological terms (e.g., Pick's disease) in the absence of neuropathological data. The term frontotemporal degeneration is more anatomically accurate than the more common term frontal lobe dementia and is being used increasingly in the medical literature (Hooten & Lyketsos, 1996).

History

The first case of frontal lobe dementia to be reported, described by Arnold Pick in 1892, was that of a 71-year-old man with a 3-year history of cognitive deterioration (Pick, 1892/1977). Expressive aphasia was prominent, with anomia and frequent paraphasic errors. A postmortem examination subsequently revealed extensive frontotemporal atrophy. The neuropathological changes of neuronal loss, astrocytic gliosis, and enlarged cells containing argyrophilic intranuclear inclusions (Pick bodies) were described by Alois Alzheimer in 1911, and in 1926 the term Pick's disease was first used to describe the condition (Cummings & Benson, 1988). In the 1960s a number of neuropathological studies reported cases of progressive frontal lobe dysfunction in which neither the microscopic characteristics of Alzheimer's disease nor Pick's disease

MAHMOOD A. USMAN • The Alzheimer Center of Pittsburgh, Pittsburgh, Pennsylvania 15205.

were present at autopsy. The medical literature variously describes these cases as dementia of the frontal lobe type (DFT) (Mann, South, Snowden, & Neary, 1993; Neary, Snowden, Northen, & Goulding, 1988), frontal lobe degeneration of the non-Alzheimer type (FLD) (Brun, 1993; Gustafson, Brun, & Passant, 1992), frontotemporal degeneration (Filley, Kleinschmidt-DeMasters, & Gross, 1994), lobar atrophy (Francis et al., 1993; Neary, Snowden, & Mann, 1993b) and dementia lacking distinct histology (DLDH) (Knopman, Mastri, Frey, Sung, & Rustan, 1990). One proposed solution to this ambiguity was the term "Pick complex" to encompass the spectrum of frontal and temporal lobe diseases (Kertesz, Hudson, Mackenzie, & Munoz, 1994). For consistency throughout this chapter, frontotemporal dementia will be used to refer to the clinical syndrome(s), while dementia of the frontal lobe type will refer to a particular pattern of pathology lacking Pick bodies.

Epidemiology

The frontal lobe dementias represent only a small portion of all dementia cases compared to the leading cause, Alzheimer's disease (AD). However, they make up a significant proportion of cases with an early or "presenile" onset. Although pathologically proven cases of Pick's disease have been reported in people as young as their 20s and as late as their 80s, the FTDs are primarily diseases of middle age. One early study of patients with FTD in Sweden and a more recent large series of patients from Manchester both reported the mean age of onset as 54 years (Neary et al., 1987; Sjögren, Sjögren, & Lindgren, 1952). Less common, familial frontal dementias may have an even earlier onset. In one study of two pedigrees of a familial progressive subcortical gliosis, the average age of onset was 46 years (Lanska et al., 1994), and in a large family with a history of frontal lobe dementia with motor neuron disease (Lynch et al., 1994), the mean age of onset was 45 years.

With the exception of Stockholm, which may have a large genetic pool of Pick's disease and other frontal dementias, these disorders are fairly uncommon. Various estimates put the ratio of AD cases to Pick's cases between 100 to 1 and 10 to 1 (Cummings

& Benson, 1988). Non-Pick's FTD appears to be more common than Pick's disease, outnumbering Pick's cases 4:1 in one series (Brun, 1987). The prevalence of all FTDs, compared to AD, has been estimated to be between 1:5 and 1:11 (Mann et al., 1993). A large autopsy study in Sweden (Gustafson et al., 1992) found non-Pick's FTD to make up 10% of all dementia cases, making it the second most common neurodegenerative dementia after AD. While AD affects more women than men (possibly due to longer life expectancy), a slight male predominance may be seen in Pick's disease (Heston, White, & Mastri, 1987), and no gender differences are seen in non-Pick's FTDs. An early study by Sjögren et al. (1952) of Pick's disease gave a range of 2 to 11 years for duration of illness, with a mean of 5 years, while more recent reports (Mann et al., 1993) document durations of between 1 and 23 years, with a mean of over 8 years. Although the precise etiology of these disorders remains unknown, genetics plays a strong role. Between 43% and 60% of all FTD cases have a positive family history (Gustafson, 1993; Neary et al., 1987). Pick's disease appears to follow an autosomal dominant pattern, possibly with incomplete penetrance (Heston, 1986; Sjögren et al., 1952), while an autosomal recessive pattern has been postulated in non-Pick's FTDs. One group studied a family with FTD and mapped the disease locus to chromosome 3 (Brown et al., 1995) but did not see this linkage in other cases (Ashworth et al., 1995).

Clinical History

The clinical history is critical to the diagnosis of frontal lobe dementias, as it is most likely to distinguish these conditions from other dementias (Lishman, 1978). Frontal dementias typically present with a marked change in personality and behavior, accompanied by primarily expressive aphasia and executive dysfunction. Unlike Alzheimer's disease, memory loss is rarely reported by patients or family members as an early symptom. Behavioral changes and social problems may precede cognitive impairment by several years (Miller et al., 1991). These early changes have been labeled "senile self-neglect" (Orrell & Sahakian, 1991). Patients may begin abusing alcohol, engage in impulsive reckless behavior, be sexually indiscriminate, be socially inappropriate, or commit minor crimes. They are frequently described as both apathetic and disinhibited. Patients with frontal dementias are often mistakenly diagnosed as having primary psychiatric conditions, particularly major depression, bipolar disorder, or schizoaffective disorder.

A 50-year-old right-handed divorced diabetic woman presented with a 2-year history of behavioral changes and impaired judgment. Her personal hygiene had deteriorated and her home became filled with trash. She needed to leave her job due to grossly inappropriate behavior. She ate from trash receptacles and stole food from restaurants, despite having adequate money to buy food. Her frequent "binge eating" made it impossible to control her diabetes. She had at least six psychiatric hospitalizations in a 4-month period for depression, "hypomania," inappropriate behavior, and "compulsive eating." Pharmacologic interventions included fluoxetine, methylphenidate, valproic acid, and resperidone. Noncompliance with treatment, poor judgment, and a need for constant supervision led to placement in a residential facility.

On examination, the woman had hypomimic facies and was aprosodic and perseverative in her speech. Verbal stereotypies were present. She was fully oriented. Concentration and divided attention were impaired but verbal memory and language comprehension were largely intact. Judgment and insight were both grossly impaired. Neurological exam revealed glabellar and snout reflexes.

During formal neuropsychological testing, the patient had trouble sitting still and was impulsive in answering questions. She was intermittently cooperative and often refused to proceed further with a given test. Orientation, language comprehension, and spontaneous recall were relatively intact. She endorsed no symptoms on a subjective depression rating scale. She was unable to perform serial subtractions of 7. She made sequential errors on single and double alternating sequence tasks. Visuospatial construction skills were mildly impaired while performance on a visual organization test was only slightly below average. Memory was mildly impaired, with delayed recall of verbal material more affected than immediate recall. Digit span and visual information span were at the 30th and 35th percentiles, respectively.

Computerized tomography (CT) and magnetic resonance imaging (MRI) scans showed diffuse atrophy and a technetium-99m-hexamethylpropyleneamine (^{99}Tc-HMPAO) SPECT scan showed bifrontal hypoperfusion, more prominent on the right than the left. An electroencephalogram (EEG) was reportedly normal. A diagnosis of frontal lobe dementia was made and confirmed independently at a second facility. The patient was subsequently treated with pergolide with mild improvement in some of her symptoms. She remains in a long-term care facility.

This case illustrates a number of features common in frontal lobe dementias. The patient's symptoms began in middle age, were insidious in onset, and were gradually progressive. Personality

changes, including impulsiveness, disinhibition, and socially inappropriate behavior, were mistakenly attributed to "bipolar disorder versus schizoaffective disorder." Apathy, a flattened affect, and perseveration in speech and behavior were prominent features. She developed symptoms of Klüver-Bucy syndrome (hyperorality, gluttony, ingestion of inedible substances) which were mistaken for a primary eating disorder. In fact, one of this patient's psychiatric hospitalizations was to a specialized eating disorders unit.

Neurobehavioral Symptoms

A broad psychiatric symptomatology has been reported in FTD, including depression and paranoid delusions, although it has been claimed that hallucinations have yet to be reported (Jung & Solomon, 1993). Though some patients are euphoric and show affective lability, most FTD patients have a blunted affect. Irritability or aggressiveness is seen in some patients, especially when they are confronted. Stereotypic behaviors, including clapping, grunting, singing, and repetition of short phrases, are all common (Jung & Solomon, 1993). Several authors have reported complex features of obsessive–compulsive disorder, which may be on a continuum with repetitive behaviors and motor stereotypies (Ames, Cummings, Wirshing, Quinn, & Mahler, 1994; Stip, 1995; Tonkonogy, Smith, & Barreira, 1994). An uncommon symptom in FTD, rarely seen in other conditions, is the "mirror sign" in which a patient faces a mirror and converses with his or her reflection (Jung & Solomon, 1993). Blumer and Benson (1975) described the personality changes seen in frontal lobe dysfunction as falling into two categories: the *pseudopsychopathic* (euphoric and disinhibited) and the *pseudodepressed* (apathetic and indifferent). They note that, while presentations with features of both are more common than pure forms of either type, features of the pseudopsychopathic generally predominate. These patterns of personality change are also referred to as *orbitofrontal* and *dorsolateral* frontal lobe syndromes, respectively, relating to the focal lesions most often associated with these presentations. In frontal lobe dementias, which have fairly diffuse lobar degeneration, both patterns of symptoms typically coexist.

Patients with FTD often tend to be nonspontaneous and disinterested in activities or other people. Most will meet criteria for an *apathetic syndrome* in which goal-directed behaviors, goal-directed cognition, and the emotional concomitants are substantially diminished (Marin, 1991; Marin, Fogel, Hawkins, Duffy, & Krupp, 1995). There is speculation that frontal lobe diseases disrupt "gating" mechanisms that integrate emotional components of thought and behavior (Damasio, 1979), thus disrupting the links between rewards and punishments and associated behaviors.

Klüver-Bucy Syndrome

Elements of Klüver-Bucy syndrome may develop early in the course of FTD, particularly with extensive bitemporal involvement (Cummings & Duchen, 1981). First described in monkeys after bilateral temporal lobectomies, it consists of hyperorality (e.g., placing objects in the mouth), hypersexuality, changes in dietary habits or preferences, hypermetamorphosis (automatic exploration of objects in the environment), emotional blunting, and sensory agnosia. Changes in eating habits are often described in FTD patients, including gluttony, change in the type of foods preferred, and ingestion of inedible substances. Obesity and other sequelae of overeating are common. Excessive consumption of alcohol and tobacco have also been reported. Hypermetamorphosis may be considered a form of environmental dependency, discussed below. Auditory or visual agnosia and prosopagnosia, or an inability to recognize faces, may reflect the disturbance of sensory recognition.

Impairment of Attentional Processes

Most FTD patients have a pattern of mental inflexibility or inability to shift between lines of thought. This is manifest in perseveration in speech, thought, and behavior. While some authors speculate that different mechanisms underlie perseveration in these areas (Sandson & Albert, 1984), others hold a more unitary model (Goldberg, 1986). Perseveration in language may relate to impaired access to semantic memory, while motor perseveration may stem from an inability to disengage attention from a task. Conceptual perseveration may be due

to an inability to associate intentions with actions (Sungaila & Crockett, 1993). Deficits in sustained attention are also frequently seen in FTD patients. One study demonstrated that patients with right frontal damage did poorly counting stimuli that occurred once per second but performed normally with stimuli presented at seven per second (Wilkins, Shallice, & McCarthy, 1987)

Executive Dysfunction

A common feature in FTD patients is the inability to recognize errors and correct one's behavior. Little response to external cues or feedback is seen. Response preparation and the inhibition of inappropriate responses are generally poor and may correlate to some degree with right frontal dysfunction (Verfaellie & Heilman, 1987). Planning of behaviors is disrupted, and patients may be unable to accomplish novel tasks, while the ability to perform routine behaviors is unimpaired. Abstract problem-solving tasks and those requiring estimates of size, speed, or other attributes are particularly difficult (Shallice, 1982). Symptoms of apathy may stem, in part, from an inability to prioritize behavior (Sungaila & Crockett, 1993). Many patients may develop stimulus-bound behavior or environmental dependency (L'hermitte, 1986) in which patients automatically engage in behaviors in response to environmental stimuli. One aspect of this is seen in imitative behaviors such as *echopraxia* and *echolalia* defined as the automatic copying of another's behaviors or speech. Some patients with imitative behaviors also show *utilization behavior*, in which they spontaneously handle or use objects they see, despite instructions or cues not to do so. Environmental dependence has been attributed to a loss of *autonomy* from the environment, in which the boundaries of self outside the world become blurred. The symptoms of impaired sustained attention and confabulation have also been described as manifestations of this loss of autonomy. Similarly, FTD patients often lose insight and self-awareness. In a proposed hierarchy of brain function, self-awareness is considered the "highest" of brain functions and is usually localized to the prefrontal regions (Stuss, 1991; Stuss & Benson, 1986), which are invariably affected by FTDs. Early loss of personal awareness, social awareness, and insight are all included in the proposed clinical criteria for FTD (Lund and Manchester Groups, 1994).

Language Impairment

Language dysfunction in frontal lobe dementias is characterized by anomia, often with dysarthria or verbal stereotypies, but largely without paraphasic errors. Speech is often only tangentially appropriate and may contain both grammatical and syntactic errors. Some patients develop echolalia and most go on to terminal mutism (Strub & Black, 1988), although there have been cases of patients who could communicate by writing or typing after speech was lost (Holland, McBurney, Moossy, & Reinmuth, 1985). As discussed later in this chapter and elsewhere in this volume, language impairment is the predominant feature in progressive aphasias.

Memory Impairment and Confabulation

Although verbal and nonverbal memory tend to spared early in the course of FTD, both are eventually impaired. A longitudinal single-case study of a patient confirmed to have Pick's disease showed an unusual pattern of memory loss (Hodges & Gurd, 1994). While free recall was impaired, there was relative preservation of recognition on tests of anterograde memory. Retrograde memory was relatively spared, but autobiographical events tended to be lost while memory of famous faces and events was differentially preserved. The temporally graded decline in memory seen in Alzheimer's disease was absent in this case. Tests of lexical retrieval revealed word-finding difficulties which worsened as the disease progressed. A majority of the memory deficits seen in these patients may be attributed to disturbances of attention and concentration, a vulnerability to interference, failure to use effective encoding strategies, and an overall inability to organize memories, rather than disturbances of recall and recognition (Mayes, 1988; Shimamura, Janowski, & Squire, 1991). Thus, these memory deficits become more pronounced with increasing complexity of material presented. Confabulation, or expression of memories that did not actually take place, is common in frontal lobe dysfunction. A distinction has been made between *fantastic* confabulation with purely fictional content and *momen-tary* confabulation in which actual events are exaggerated or embellished (Berlyne, 1972). There is speculation that confabulation may represent a form of impaired reality testing, in which the patient cannot distinguish between an internal record of actual perceptions and internally generated events and thoughts (Johnson, 1991).

Visuospatial Dysfunction

As with memory, visuospatial functions are largely preserved in the early stages of FTD when compared with AD. Constructional abilities, map reading, spatial orientation, and other *allocentric* spatial tasks are usually intact while *egocentric* spatial tasks, such as pointing out one's body parts, are impaired (Kolb & Whishaw, 1990). This pattern is reversed in parietal lobe damage and AD, in which egocentric tasks are unimpaired and deficits are seen with allocentric tasks.

Physical Findings

Primitive reflexes or "frontal release signs," including grasp responses, a snout reflex, and a glabellar reflex, are often seen early in the course of FTD. Extrapyramidal symptoms, particularly akinesia and rigidity, are common in later stages of the disease. Prominent resting tremor and cogwheel rigidity early in the disease generally indicate an underlying movement disorder, rather than FTD (Klatka, Schiffer, Powers, & Kazee, 1996; Neary & Snowden, 1991). The remainder of the neurological examination is usually unremarkable, unless bulbar signs (e.g., dysphagia), motor weakness, muscle wasting, fasciculations, and/or hyperreflexia indicate an associated motor neuron disease.

Progressive Aphasias

As is the case with a number of neuropathological conditions, clinical symptomatology may vary with degree of pathological involvement of various brain regions and structures. The best described of these clinical variants is often called primary progressive aphasia (PPA) or Mesulam's syndrome (Mesulam, 1982). These patients present with an insidious onset of nonfluent aphasia with hesitant dysprosodic speech, phonemic paraphasic errors, impairment of syntax, and impaired repetition. Language comprehension and other areas of cognition are relatively intact. One study compared performance on the Western Aphasia Battery and Mattis Dementia Rating Scale in 10 patients with PPA to 10 patients with Alzheimer's disease or dominant hemisphere stroke. Patients with PPA demonstrated disproportionate involvement of the anterior cortical portions of the dominant hemisphere in PPA (Karbe, Kertesz, & Polk, 1993). Clinical criteria for PPA have been proposed which include a 2-year history of progressive impairment of language skills with relative preservation of other cognitive skills and independence in activities of daily living (Weintraub, Rubin, & Mesulam, 1990). Although some feel this syndrome is both clinically and pathologically distinct (Kobayashi et al., 1990; Weintraub et al., 1990), others disagree (Croisile, 1992; Green, Morris, Sandson, McKeel, & Miller, 1990; Kertesz et al., 1994; Kirshner, Webb, & Kelly 1984; Snowden & Neary, 1993; Snowden, Neary, Mann, Goulding, & Testa, 1992). A few neuropathological studies have shown that a number of pathological processes involving the left frontal region, including DFT, Pick's disease, and Alzheimer's disease, may produce this clinical syndrome (Feher, Doody, Whitehead, & Pirozzolo, 1991). The term semantic dementia has been used to describe a clinical syndrome of progressive fluent aphasia, behavioral disturbance, and radiological evidence of temporal lobe atrophy (Hodges, Patterson, Oxbury, & Funnell, 1992). These patients have selective impairment of semantic memory with anomia, loss of single-word comprehension, and a reading disorder suggestive of surface dyslexia. Other areas of language and cognition, including episodic memory, are intact. Other cases have been described in which there is a mixed transcortical pattern of aphasia (Ikejiri et al., 1993; Mehler, 1988). Some cases are clearly familial with an autosomal dominant pattern of inheritance (Morris, Cole, Banker, & Wright, 1984; Snowden & Neary, 1993).

Dementia with Motor Neuron Disease

Dementia associated with motor neuron disease is an increasingly recognized form of frontal

lobe dementia. Some have estimated that it may represent up to 8% of dementia cases (Cooper, Jackson, Lennox, Lowe, & Mann, 1995; James Lowe, personal communication). Recent studies of patients diagnosed with amyotrophic lateral sclerosis (ALS) have revealed evidence of frontotemporal dysfunction and atrophy (Kiernan & Hudson, 1994). Originally described as a dementia-parkinsonism complex that was believed to be restricted to the island of Guam, these cases are now believed to be part of a spectrum of conditions ranging from "pure" ALS without dementia at one extreme to a frontal lobe dementia without pyramidal symptoms but with neuropathological features of ALS at the other extreme. One group has described a "disinhibition-dementia-parkinsonism-amyotrophy complex" (DDPAC) with linkage to chromosome 17q21-22 (Lynch et al., 1994; Wilhelmson, Lynch, Pavlou, Higgins, & Nygaard, 1994). Clinical description of this condition appears to be consistent with what other groups call frontal lobe dementia with motor neuron disease (Caselli et al., 1993; Neary et al., 1990). Onset is generally in middle age (mean 45 years) but has been reported to range from 27 to 77 years of age. Symptoms typically include an insidious personality change with features of the Klüver-Bucy syndrome, depressed mood, stereotyped or inappropriate behaviors, rigidity, and bradykinesia. Many, though not all, of these patients also have clinical features of motor neuron disease, including weakness, muscle wasting, fasciculations, and hyperreflexia. It remains to be seen if this condition shares a common etiology with classic ALS or if new treatments available for motor neuron disease are effective in this condition.

Diagnostic Testing

As noted in the sections above, clinical history, physical and mental status exams and psychometric testing are the most crucial in assessment of the patient with suspected FTD. Some specific diagnostic tests are warranted, although they most often are normal or reveal nonspecific changes. The EEG tends to be normal until late stages of the disease when diffuse slowing is seen. A number of authors have suggested that a lack of slowing on EEG tends to favor a diagnosis of FTD over Alzheimer's disease, but this observation has not been empirically validated. Structural neuroimaging techniques (CT or MRI) often demonstrate focal atrophy, primarily involving anterior frontal lobes and inferior temporal lobes (Tobo, Mitsuyama, Ikari, & Itoi, 1984), but may be normal, particularly early in the disease process (Stip, 1995). Functional neuroimaging studies measure either regional blood flow (single photon emission computed tomography [SPECT] or regional cerebral blood flow [^{133}Xe rCBF]) or regional brain metabolism (positron emission tomography [PET]) and are more helpful in differential diagnosis of frontal lobe dementias. Findings from functional neuroimaging procedures are more likely to correspond to neuropsychological deficits than structural imaging methods (Osimani, Ichise, Chung, Pogue, & Freedman, 1994). Frontal and/or temporal hypoperfusion or hypometabolism is typically found in patients with frontal dementia of varying types of pathology (Figure 1) (Friedland et al., 1993; Namikawa, 1993; Szelies & Karenberg, 1986). A study using ^{99}Tc-HMPAO SPECT showed that FTD patients tended to have more hypoperfusion of the orbital frontal region than of the dorsolateral areas and more anterior temporal flow deficits than dorsal temporal deficits (Starkstein et al., 1994). One study using ^{133}Xe rCBF showed bifrontal deficits in 25 of 26 FTD cases, while the remaining case had primarily right frontal hypoperfusion (Risberg, Passant, Warkentin, & Gustafson, 1993). It has been suggested that patients clinically diagnosed with Alzheimer's disease who display predominant frontal hypoperfusion or hypometabolism may actually have FTD; this has not been validated with pathological studies (Jagust, Reed, Seab, Kramer, & Budinger, 1989; Salmon et al., 1994). These findings are not, however, specific to these conditions. Bifrontal deficits have been reported in schizophrenia and depressive disorders (Holman & Devous, 1992). These deficits are also seen in progressive supranuclear palsy and moderate to severe Alzheimer's disease, though usually not without other findings (Goto et al., 1993; Holman & Devous, 1992; Holman, Johnson, Gerada, Carvalho, & Satlin, 1992). At best, these techniques should be considered as supportive of a clinical diagnosis, rather than diagnostic themselves (Neary et al., 1987). Functional activation studies, where the subject performs a specific cognitive task during tracer uptake, may increase specificity of these techniques. In one study, 13 of 15 FTD patients had a decreased level of frontal activation during the Word Fluency test when compared to a group of 49 normal subjects. Positron emission tomography scanning has revealed loss of sensorimotor pyramidal neurons in ALS (Kew et al., 1994) and may also show frontal

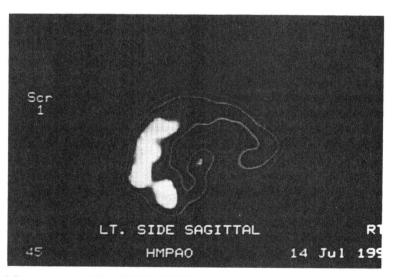

FIGURE 1. A blood flow scan using Tc99m HMPAO SPECT in a 65-year-old woman with frontal lobe dementia and severe dysarthria. In this parasagittal view of the left hemisphere, profound left frontal hypoperfusion is apparent.

hypoperfusion in patients with motor neuron disease with dementia. Electromyography is indicated in patients with pyramidal symptoms. Newer imaging techniques, such as magnetic resonance spectroscopy, may show more promise as diagnostic tools in FTD than other currently used imaging techniques (Shonk et al., 1995; Smith, Gallenstein, Layton, Kryscio, & Markesbery, 1993).

Neuropsychological Assessment

Most commonly used screening tests for dementia, such as the Mini-Mental State Examination (MMSE) (Folstein, Folstein, & McHugh, 1975), contain weak measures of frontal lobe function and are very insensitive to FTD. It is not uncommon for a patient with a moderately advanced clinical diagnosis of FTD to score 29 or 30 on the MMSE (Royall, Mahurin, & Cornell, 1994; Royall, Mahurin, & Plotnick, 1992). Since test-taking behaviors may be profoundly altered, any form of quantitative, norm-based psychometric testing may be of limited value (Sungaila & Crockett, 1993). Since these patients may do fairly well in highly controlled, structured settings, relatively unstructured tasks must be included in the assessment of a patient with suspected frontotemporal dysfunction. Open-ended tasks such as writing a story, drawing pictures, unstructured constructional tasks, carrying on a conversation, or responding to ambiguous stimuli (as in the Thematic Apperception Test) should be included. Measures that combine quantitative measures of performance with description, such as the Boston Process Approach (Milberg, Hebben, & Kaplan, 1986) are useful in these conditions. Quantitative tests sensitive to frontal dysfunction, including the Wisconsin Card Sorting Test (WCST) (Heaton,

1981), Halstead's Category Test (HCT) (Reitan & Wolfson, 1985), Shallice's Cognitive Estimates (Shallice & Evans, 1978), Butters' 20 Questions, EXIT (Royall et al., 1994), Trail-making test (Lezak, 1983), and Verbal Fluency tests are indicated in patients suspected to have FTD (Hodges & Gurd, 1994). One shortcoming of the WCST and the HCT in this population is that the continuous feedback given for each trial may make patients frustrated and angry, which, in turn, negatively affects performance (Sungaila & Crockett, 1993). Simple bedside tests including the "go-no-go" procedure (Weintraub & Mesulam, 1985), alternating hand sequences, or alternating repetitive figures such as the graphomotor pattern, cursive Ms and Ns, or series of loops (Luria, 1980) are particularly useful (Figures 2 and 3). The Trail-making test is a simple and very useful test of mental flexibility in FTD, particularly if there is a marked discrepancy between performance on parts A and B (Sungaila & Crockett, 1993). Simple tests of attention span (backwards digit span), vigilance (Continuous Performance Task), and verbal fluency (Controlled Oral Word Association test) are often helpful (Lezak, 1983). Although recognition and recall tend to be preserved, tests such as the Hopkins Verbal Learning Test (HVLT) (Brandt, 1991) and California Verbal Learning Test (CVLT) (Delis, Kramer, Kaplan, & Ober, 1987) may reveal impairment attributable to attentional deficits or perseveration. Most studies of neuropsychological impairment in FTD have shown little correlation between level of impairment and duration of illness, suggesting wide variation in the course of the disease (Elfgren, Passant, & Risberg, 1993). Behavioral changes may be quantified using structured inventories that use information from family members or clinical staff. These measures include the Neuropsychiatric In-

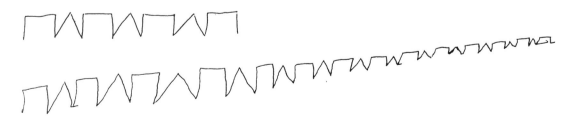

FIGURE 2. This reproduction of the Luria graphomotor pattern by a 49-year-old man with frontal lobe dementia demonstrates progressive micrographia and convergence toward the sample given on the upper line.

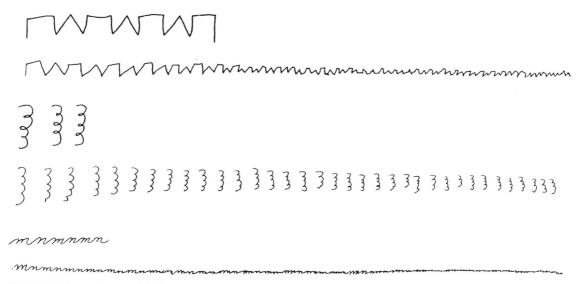

FIGURE 3. Reproductions of the Luria graphomotor pattern, loops, and the cursive letters *m* and *n* by a 46-year-old woman with frontal lobe dementia demonstrate preservative errors and severe micrographia.

ventory (Cummings et al., 1994; Mega, Cummings, Fiorello, & Gornbein, 1996), the Columbia University Scale (Devanand et al., 1992), the Portland Adaptability Inventory (Lezak, 1989), and the Functional Rating Scale (Tuokko & Crockett, 1991).

Clinical Criteria for Frontal Lobe Dementias

A significant portion of the medical literature on frontal dementias has been produced by two groups: one in Lund, Sweden (Drs. Brun, Englund, Gustafson, and Passant), and the other in Manchester, England (Drs. Mann, Neary, and Snowden). Two international conferences on these conditions were held in Lund in 1986 and 1992, leading to a set of clinical and pathological criteria for these disorders. A similar, multiaxial set of diagnostic criteria was also proposed by Baldwin and Förstl in 1993. Clinical criteria from the Lund consensus statement (Lund and Manchester Groups, 1994) are presented in Table 1. They consist of 10 behavioral symptoms, four affective symptoms, four language symptoms, and four physical signs. In addition, spatial orientation and praxis are preserved, EEG is normal, imag-

ing studies show frontotemporal abnormalities, and psychometric testing shows frontal dysfunction. Supportive and exclusionary criteria are also included. This is the first methodical attempt to define diagnostic criteria for these diseases and is, by far, the most complete. By contrast, *DSM-IV* (Frances, Pincus, First, & Widiger, 1994) includes for the first time a diagnostic category for "dementia due to Pick's disease," but the clinical criteria are identical to those of Alzheimer's disease.

The major shortcoming of the Lund–Manchester criteria is that there is no hierarchy to these criteria (e.g., minimum number of symptoms from each category that must be met). No validation studies have been done for these criteria, nor have correlations for individual symptoms been made with clinical diagnosis. Many of the symptoms appear to be nonspecific (e.g., loss of insight), and others are most often seen late in the disease process (e.g., utilization behavior). Similarly, EEG (particularly late in the disease) may have diffuse slowing, and brain imaging studies (particularly early in the course of the illness) may be normal. Despite these shortcomings, the Lund–Manchester criteria remain the most useful and most comprehensive guide to diagnosis of frontal dementias.

Table 1. Proposed Lund and Manchester Clinical Criteria for Frontotemporal Dementia[a]

Core diagnostic features
  Behavioral disorder
    Insidious onset and slow progression
    Early loss of personal awareness (neglect of personal hygiene and grooming)
    Early loss of social awareness (lack of social tact, misdemeanors such as shoplifting)
    Early signs of disinhibition (such as unrestrained sexuality, violent behavior, inappropriate jocularity, restless pacing)
    Mental rigidity and inflexibility
    Hyperorality (oral/dietary changes, overeating, food fads, excessive smoking and alcohol consumption, oral exploration of objects)
    Stereotyped and perseverative behavior (wandering, mannerisms such as clapping, signing, dancing, ritualistic preoccupation such as hoarding, toileting, and dressing)
    Utilization behavior (unrestrained exploration of objects in the environment)
    Distractability, impulsivity, and impersistence
    Early loss of insight into the fact that the altered condition is due to a pathological change of own mental state
  Affective symptoms
    Depression, anxiety, excessive sentimentality, suicidal and fixed ideation, delusion (early and evanescent)
    Hypochondriasis, bizarre somatic preoccupation (early and evanescent)
    Emotional unconcern (emotional indifference and remoteness, lack of empathy and sympathy, apathy)
    Amimia (inertia, aspontaneity)
  Speech disorder
    Progressive reduction of speech (aspontaneity and economy of utterance)
    Stereotypy of speech (repetition of limited repertoire of words, phrases, or themes)
    Echolalia and perseveration
    Late mutism
  Spatial orientation and praxis preserved
  (Intact abilities to negotiate the environment)
  Physical signs
    Early primitive reflexes
    Early incontinence
    Late akinesia, rigidity, tremor
    Low and labile blood pressure
  Assessment findings
    Normal EEG despite clinically evident dementia
    Brain imaging (structural, functional, or both: predominant frontal or anterior temporal abnormality, or both)
    Neuropsychology (profound failure on "frontal lobe" tests in the absence of severe amnesia, aphasia, or perceptual spatial disorder)
Supportive diagnostic features
  Onset before 65
  Positive family history of similar disorder in a first-degree relative
  Bulbar palsy, muscular weakness and wasting, fasciculations (motor neuron disease)
Diagnostic exclusion features
  Abrupt onset with ictal events
  Head trauma related to onset
  Early severe amnesia
  Early spatial disorientation, lost in surroundings, defective localization of objects
  Early severe apraxia
  Logoclonic speech with rapid loss of train of thought
  Myoclonus
  Cortical bulbar and spinal deficits
  Cerebellar ataxia
  Choreoathetosis
  Early, severe, pathological EEG
  Brain imaging (predominant postcentral structural or functional deficit; multifocal cerebral lesions on CT or MRI)
  Laboratory tests indicating brain involvement or inflammatory disorder (e.g., multiple sclerosis, syphilis, AIDS and herpes simplex encephalitis)
Relative diagnostic exclusion features
  Typical history of chronic alcoholism
  Sustained hypertension
  History of vascular disease (e.g., angina, claudication)

[a]Adapted from The Lund and Manchester Groups, 1994.

Clinical Differential Diagnosis

Although disputed (Joynt & Shoulson, 1985), most clinicians agree that in a majority of cases frontotemporal dementias can be reliably differentiated from Alzheimer's disease and other dementias on clinical grounds (Table 2). Unlike Alzheimer's disease, recognition memory, language comprehension, motor praxis, and visuospatial skills are relatively preserved early in the course of FTD. Both diseases may share some clinical features, including apathy and anomia, but clinical history and psychometric testing will usually differentiate between these conditions. Clinicians and nonclinicians may notice the differences at a global qualitative level. For example, one patient's spouse reported that "Alzheimer's disease robs a person of their intellect but this [FTD] robs a person of himself." In a recent study of 170 autopsies of patients clinically diagnosed with probable AD, 21 patients (12%) were found to have an incorrect diagnosis (Klatka et al., 1996). Only five of those patients (2.9% of the total autopsies) were found to have DFT or Pick's disease at autopsy. Two of the five were reported to have a clinical history of "early personality changes." Differentiating between the various pathological processes producing the syndrome of FTD is a more difficult task. While some have proposed that Pick's disease has more features of cortical dysfunction (aphasia, amnesia, agnosia, and acalculia) than the other primarily subcortical diseases, this assumption has never been validated. Since a characteristic feature of the subcortical dementias is disproportionate frontal lobe dysfunction (Cummings & Benson, 1984) and each disease process that produces FTD has both cortical and subcortical pathology, clinical utility of this distinction is doubtful in the case of frontal dementias.

Neuropathology of Pick's Disease

The pathological description of "classic" Pick's disease includes focal atrophy of frontal and anterior temporal lobes, neuronal loss, swollen "balloon-shaped" neurons (Pick cells), and unusual intranuclear inclusions (Pick bodies). The frontotemporal atrophy is often striking, often distinguishing it from AD on macroscopic examination. The gross brain weight may be as little as 700 g, compared to an average brain weight of 1,394 g in normal young males (Adams & Victor, 1989). Affected regions may be sharply demarcated from parietal lobes and the posterior two thirds of the temporal lobes. Cerebral gyri may be so narrowed that the term "knife-blade atrophy" has often been used to describe the morphology. In half of all cases the left frontal lobe is more severely affected, and in only a third is the atrophy symmetric. Parietal lobe involvement is uncommon (Lang, Bergeron, Pollanen, & Ashby, 1994), and involvement of the occipital lobe is exceedingly rare.

The most characteristic microscopic change is presence of rounded or oval-shaped filamentous inclusions in the cytoplasm of remaining neurons (Pick bodies). These inclusions are weakly eosinophilic in routine hematoxylin-eosin preparations but are strongly argyrophilic in the presence of silver stains, such as Bielschowsky's silver impregnation preparations. Electron microscopy suggests that they are composed of neurofilaments, paired helical filaments, and vesiculated endoplasmic reticulum. This is supported by immunohistochemical data showing staining with monoclonal antibody against neurofilament proteins (e.g., tau-1 and Alz-50) and antitubulin antisera (Munoz-Garcia & Ludwin, 1984). A recent study showed that Pick bodies are intensely stained by antibodies directed against complement membrane attack complex (MAC) and one of its three inhibitors, protectin. Of the remaining two inhibitors, vitronectin is weakly stained in

Table 2. Features Distinguishing Frontotemporal Dementia (FTD) from Alzheimer's Disease (AD)[a]

	FTD	AD
Language	Expressive impairment greater than receptive	Receptive impairment greater than expressive
	Stereotypies	Paraphasic errors
Visuospatial skills	Impaired	Relatively spared
Memory	Relatively spared	Impaired
Calculation	Relatively spared	Impaired
Personality	Markedly different Disinhibition	Relatively unchanged
Klüver-Bucy syndrome	Often present	Absent

[a]Adapted from Cummings, 1988; Neary & Snowden, 1991.

Pick bodies, and clusterin is absent from inclusion bodies but is found in nearby neurons, including ballooned cells (Yashura, Aimi, McGeer, & McGeer, 1994). Pick bodies are also labeled by antibodies against the N-terminal and intermediate regions of amyloid precursor protein (APP) and weakly by anti-ubiquitin antibodies (Tranchant, Muller, & Warter, 1992). Some neurons in Pick's disease, including ballooned cells, are stained by antibodies directed against all but the N-terminal segment of APP (Yashura et al., 1994). Regional and laminar distribution of Pick bodies were described in a study based on 16 cases (Hof, Bouras, Perl, & Morrison, 1994). Large concentrations of inclusion bodies were noted in Ammon's horn, subiculum, entorhinal cortex, and the granule cell layer of the dentate gyrus. In frontal and temporal neocortex, the highest densities were noted in layers II and VI.

An extracellular or "ghost" Pick body was recently described as a blurred, weakly argyrophilic mass in the neuropil, composed of 13-nm fibrils and glial filament bundles (Izumiyama, Ikeda, & Oyanagi, 1994). Unlike intraneuronal Pick bodies, they were not labeled by anti-tau or anti-ubiquitin antibodies and are weakly stained by antiglial fibrillary acidic protein. There is speculation that the ghost Pick body is left behind after the death of the neuron, losing its tau and ubiquitin reactivity and inducing a glial reaction in the process.

Neurofibrillary tangles are present in Pick's disease, though in smaller amounts and in a different distribution than in AD. Neuritic plaques and dystrophic neurites are generally absent (Benzing, Mufson, & Armstrong, 1993). As in AD, tangles are intensely stained by antibodies directed against casein kinase II (Baum et al., 1992). They are most common in layers II and III (Hof et al., 1994), in contrast to AD where they are found throughout layers II, III, V, and VI (Arnold, Hymann, & Van-Hoesen, 1994). Neuronal loss in Pick's disease is most prominent in layer III. The finding of neuritic plaques in a few cases has suggested that AD and Pick's disease could coexist in some patients (Hof et al., 1994). Microvascular changes, including decreased microvascular density and presence of atrophic vessels, are most prominent in layers III and VI of the frontotemporal cortex and have been described in Pick's and many other dementing illnesses (Buee et al., 1994). Neuropil threads are also present in both AD and Pick's disease (Davis, Wang, & Markesbery, 1992), but quantitative studies have shown density of neocortical threads to be much less in Pick's disease (Cochran, Fox, & Mufson, 1994).

Another type of intraneuronal inclusion body, the Hirano body, has also been reported in Pick's disease (Hirano, 1994). These inclusions are highly eosinophilic, have a characteristic fine crystalloid structure, and are seen most often in the neuronal processes of the CA1 area in Ammon's horn. They contain epitopes of actin, actin-associated proteins, tau, middle-molecular-weight neurofilament subunits, and a C-terminal fragment of APP. However, these inclusions are by no means specific to Pick's disease and may be found in AD, motor neuron diseases, and in some clinically normal elderly individuals.

Granulovacular or spongiform changes are frequently seen in Pick's disease, and white matter degeneration may be extensive in some cases. A study of microglial cells in Pick's disease, using the monoclonal antibody Ki-M1P, showed that severely affected neocortical areas and underlying white matter had a marked increase in microglial cell density (Paulus, Bancher, & Jellinger, 1993). A neurochemical study which included three cases of autopsy-confirmed Pick's disease (Francis et al., 1993) showed that, unlike the situation in AD, choline acetyltransferase activity was normal. In addition, it was found that serotonin receptors were markedly reduced while measures of presynaptic serotonergic activity were normal or increased. One patient with no history of dementia had neurochemical abnormalities and neuropathology characteristic of Pick's disease, suggesting that these changes may be present prior to onset of clinical symptoms (Sparks et al., 1994).

Based on variations in neuropathological findings, Pick's disease has been divided into "classical" and "generalized" variants (Munoz-Garcia & Ludwin, 1984). The former group had primarily cortical involvement with Pick bodies in neocortex and hippocampus, while the latter group also had extensive involvement of subcortical structures, including degeneration of the caudate. In classical cases, Pick bodies were composed of straight fibrils with a variable diameter, averaging 15 nm. In the generalized group, fibrils were covered by a granular material of presumed ribosomal origin. In one report from a similar generalized case (Yamazaki, Makano, Imazu, Kaieda, & Terashi, 1994), Pick bodies were also seen in astrocytes within subcortical white matter of the temporal lobe.

Neuropathology of Non-Pick's Frontal Dementias

The most common frontal dementia appears to be the condition most often referred to as dementia of the frontal lobe type or DFT. In this condition, frontal and temporal atrophy is seen with microscopic loss of large cortical neurons, spongiform degeneration of superficial neuropil, and only a mild degree of gliosis. Ballooned neurons are uncommon, and inclusion bodies are absent, producing a picture "characteristic of Pick's except [without] either Pick's bodies or Pick's cells" (Hulette & Crain, 1992). The limbic system and striatum may be affected to some degree. Speculation that DFT is actually a prion disease has been abandoned since it has been shown that the host encoded prion protein (PrP) is absent in both DFT and Pick's disease (Collinge & Palmer, 1993; Collinge et al., 1994). The PrP has been found in some cases of familial progressive subcortical gliosis but without mutation of the PrP gene (Petersen et al., 1995).

Pathological descriptions of progressive aphasia have been quite variable, and the pathological distinctiveness of this condition remains controversial. Nearly all studies have reported asymmetric frontal and/or temporal atrophy. Most often, nonspecific pathological changes (e.g., neuronal loss and gliosis) are also seen. Normal choline acetyltransferase with reduced somatostatin-like immunoreactivity has been reported (Mehler, Horoupian, Davies, & Dickson, 1987), as have Alz-50 positive neurons in temporal and parietal cortices without ubiquitin-positive cells, Pick bodies, Lewy bodies, or spongiform changes (Scheltens, Ravid, & Kamphorst, 1994).

Another neuropathological pattern described with the clinical picture of FTD and frontal atrophy was labeled dementia lacking distinctive histologic features (DLDH) (Knopman et al., 1990). Microscopically, these patients had vacuolation of layer II and astrocytosis that was either diffuse or restricted to deep layers. Neuritic plaques, neurofibrillary tangles, inclusion bodies, and ballooned cells were conspicuously absent. Some patients had hippocampal and amygdaloid involvement, and all had some substantia nigra involvement. Thalamic and striatal gliosis were seen in some patients. These changes closely resemble those seen in motor neuron disease (MND) with dementia, and 5 of the 14 patients in the study had hypoglossal degeneration, with at least two developing clinical MND. Unfortunately, immunohistochemical staining for tau and ubiquitin were not done in this study, so it is not known if the inclusion bodies typical of MND with dementia were present. Many cases previously described as progressive subcortical gliosis also appear to be part of the ALS–frontotemporal dementia continuum (Cooper et al., 1995).

Neuropathological Differential Diagnosis

In their consensus statement, the Lund and Manchester groups give three pathological patterns associated with the syndrome they describe as frontotemporal dementia (Lund and Manchester Groups, 1994). These are (1) the frontal lobe degeneration type (equivalent to DFT) with atrophy, neuronal loss, and mild gliosis but without inclusion bodies or balloned cells and without tau or ubiquitin staining of characteristic features; (2) the Pick-type with similar features but also with inflated cells and Pick bodies which are argyrophilic and both tau and ubiquitin immunopositive; and (3) the motor neuron disease type with inclusions that are ubiquitin immunopositive but react to tau or silver stains. Neuropathological features of Alzheimer's disease and prion diseases are given as exclusionary features. This list does not appear to be all-inclusive, omitting, for example, cases with extensive subcortical gliosis or with substantial involvement of the striatum. The most striking feature of the consensus statement categories is that they require immunohistochemical staining for diagnosis. A study of immunohistochemical techniques has shown that anti-tau staining identified corticobasal degeneration, Alzheimer's disease, and Pick's disease while anti-ubiquitin identified the inclusions of MND with dementia and anti-alpha-B-crystallin identified inflated neurons (Cooper et al., 1995). Immuno-histochemical staining for these substances is now essential for the accurate diagnosis of these conditions.

Treatment of Frontal Lobe Dementias

All frontal dementias are incurable and, to a large extent, untreatable. Anecdotal reports have been made and indicate improvement in some cognitive symptoms (e.g., perseveration) with use of dopaminergic agents (Imamura et al., 1994). There may be relatively more improvement with post-synaptic agonists (bromocriptine or pergolide) than other compounds, as is seen in progressive supranuclear palsy (Jackson, Jankovic, & Ford, 1983). Psychiatric manifestations are also treated symptomatically. Depression and psychosis are managed with antidepressants (e.g., selective serotonin reuptake inhibitors or SSRIs) or antipsychotics (e.g., risperidone). Agitated behavior is often managed with trazodone, antipsychotics, benzodiazepines, or valproic acid. In one patient with FTD treated with fluoxetine for pathological affect, intermittent rhythmic myoclonus developed with both fluoxetine and trazodone, suggesting a supersensitivity of serotonin 5HT1A receptors (Lauterbach, 1994). Another group found the combination of lithium and an SSRI to be particularly effective (Anderson, Scott, & Harborne, 1995). Behavioral disturbances may necessitate placement in a facility with a controlled environment (e.g., a locked dementia unit), and a significant number of patients may require long-term psychiatric hospitalization.

Summary

This chapter summarizes the current body of knowledge relating to frontotemporal dementias. Given the multitude of conflicting and often ambiguous terms used to describe these conditions, the existing literature is difficult to interpret. The recently proposed clinical and pathological criteria for these diseases strive to make this material less ambiguous in the future. Although pathologically heterogeneous, these conditions tend to share a common clinical presentation that can generally be distinguished from Alzheimer's disease and other causes of dementia. In the assessment of these cases, clinical history, informal behavioral observations, and open-ended semi-structured tasks are most helpful. Diagnostic testing, including structural and functional neuroimaging and EEGs, often are normal or reveal nonspecific deficits. Until more is known about the neuropathological processes underlying these diseases and better methods are developed for distinguishing between them, direct interventions in the course of these diseases are impossible. At this time, treatment is limited to attempts to ameliorate specific symptoms with psychotropic medications and behavioral and environmental interventions.

References

Adams, R. D., & Victor, M. (1989). *Principles of neurology.* New York: McGraw-Hill, Inc.

Ames, D., Cummings, J. L., Wirshing, W. C., Quinn, B., & Mahler, M. (1994). Repetitive and compulsive behavior in frontal lobe degenerations. *Journal of Neuropsychiatry and Clinical Neurosciences, 6,* 100–113.

Anderson, I. M., Scott, K., & Harborne, G. (1995). Serotonin and depression in frontal lobe dementia. *American Journal of Psychiatry, 152,* 645.

Arnold, S. E., Hymann, B. T., & VanHoesen, G. W. (1994). Neuropathologic changes of the temporal pole in Alzheimer's disease and Pick's disease. *Archives of Neurology, 51,* 145–150.

Ashworth, A., Brown, J., Gydesen, S., Sorensen, S. A., Rossor, M. N., Hardy, J., & Collinge, J. (1995). Frontal lobe or "nonspecific" dementias are genetically heterogeneous. *Neurology, 45,* 1781.

Baldwin, B., & Förstl, H. (1993). "Pick's Disease"—101 years and still there, but in need of reform. *British Journal of Psychiatry, 163,* 100–104.

Baum, L., Masliah, E., Iimoto, D. S., Hansen, L. A., Halliday, W. C., & Saitoh, T. (1992). Casein kinase II is associated with neurofibrillary tangles but is not an intrinsic component of paired helical filaments. *Brain Research, 573,* 126–132.

Benzing, W. C., Mufson, E. J., & Armstrong, D. M. (1993). Alzheimer's disease-like dystrophic neurites characteristically associated with senile plaques are not found within other neurodegenerative diseases unless amyloid beta-protein deposition is present. *Brain Research, 606,* 10–18.

Berlyne, N. (1972). Confabulation. *British Journal of Psychiatry, 120,* 31–39.

Blumer, D., & Benson, D. F. (1975). Personality changes with frontal and temporal lobe lesions. In D. F. Benson & D.

Blumer (Eds.), *Psychiatric aspects of neurologic disease* (pp. 151–170). San Francisco: Grune & Stratton.

Brandt, J. (1991). Hopkins Verbal Learning Test: Development of a new memory test with six equivalent forms. *The Clinical Neuropsychologist, 5,* 125–142.

Brown, J., Ashworth, A., Gydesen, S., Sorensen, A., Rossor, M., Hardy, J., & Collinge, J. (1995). Familial non-specific dementia maps to chromosome 3. *Human Molecular Genetics, 4,* 1625–1628.

Brun, A. (1987). Frontal lobe degeneration of non-Alzheimer type. I. Neuropathology. *Archives of Gerontology and Geriatrics, 6,* 193–208.

Brun, A. (1993). Frontal lobe degeneration of non-Alzheimer type revisited. *Dementia, 4*(3–4), 126–131.

Buee, L., Hof, P. R., Bouras, C., Delacourte, A., Perl, D. P., Morrison, J. H., & Fillit, H. M. (1994). Pathological alterations of the cerebral microvasculature in Alzheimer's disease and related dementing disorders. *Acta Neuropathology (Berlin), 5,* 469–480.

Caselli, R. J., Windebank, A. J., Petersen, R. C., Komori, T., Parisi, J. E., Okazaki, H., Kokmen, E., Iverson, R., Dinapoli, R. P., Graff-Radford, N. R., & Stein, S. D. (1993). Rapidly progressive aphasic dementia and motor neuron disease. *Annals of Neurology, 33*(2), 200–207.

Cochran, E. J., Fox, J. H., & Mufson, E. J. (1994). Severe panencephalic Pick's disease with Alzheimer's disease-like neuropil threads and synaptophysin immunoreactivity. *Acta Neuropathologica, 88*(5), 479–484.

Collinge, J., & Palmer, M. S. (1993). Prion diseases in humans and their relevance to other neurodegenerative diseases. *Dementia, 4,* 178–185.

Collinge, J., Palmer, M. S., Sidle, K. C., Mahal, S. P., Campbell, T., Brown, J., Hardy, J., Brun, A. E., Gustafson, L., & Bakker, E. (1994). Familial Pick's disease and dementia in frontal lobe degeneration of non-Alzheimer type are not variants of prion disease. *Journal of Neurology, Neurosurgery and Psychiatry, 57,* 762.

Cooper, P. N., Jackson, M., Lennox, G., Lowe, J., & Mann, D. M. (1995). Tau, ubiquitin, and alpha B-crystallin immunohistochemistry define the principal causes of degenerative frontotemporal dementia. *Archives of Neurology, 52,* 1011–1015.

Croisile, B. (1992). Progressive cognitive disorders due to focal cortical atrophy. *European Journal of Medicine, 1*(3), 177–182.

Cummings, J. L., & Benson, D. F. (1984). Subcortical dementia. *Archives of Neurology, 41,* 874–879.

Cummings, J. L., & Benson, D. F. (1988). Cortical dementias: Alzheimer's disease and other cortical degenerations. In J. L. Cummings & D. F. Benson (Eds.), *Dementia: A clinical approach* (pp. 45–93). Oxford: Butterworth-Heinemann.

Cummings, J. L., & Duchen, L. W. (1981). The Kluver-Bucy syndrome in Pick disease. *Neurology, 31,* 1415–1422.

Cummings. J. L., Mega, M., Gray, K., Rosenberg-Thompson, S., Carusi, D. A., & Gornbein, J. (1994). The Neuropsychiatric Inventory: Comprehensive assessment of psychopathology in dementia. *Neurology, 44,* 82.

Damasio, A. R. (1979). The frontal lobes. In K. M. Heilman & E. Valenstein (Eds.), *Clinical neuropsychology* (pp. 360–412). New York: Oxford University Press.

Davis, D. G., Wang, H. Z., & Markesbery, W. R. (1992). Image analysis of neuropil threads in Alzheimer's, Pick's, diffuse Lewy body disease and in progressive supranuclear palsy. *Journal of Neuropathology and Experimental Neurology, 51*(6), 594–600.

Delis, D. C., Kramer, J. M., Kaplan, E., & Ober, B. A. (1987). *California Verbal Learning Test, Adult version: Manual.* San Antonio, TX: The Psychological Corporation.

Devanand, D. P., Miller, L., Richards, M., Marder, K., Bell, K., Mayeux, R., & Stern, Y. (1992). The Columbia University Scale for psychopathology in Alzheimer's disease. *Archives of Neurology, 49,* 371–376.

Elfgren, C., Passant, U., & Risberg, J. (1993). Neuropsychological findings in frontal lobe dementia. *Dementia, 4*(3–4), 214–219.

Feher, E. P., Doody, R. S., Whitehead, J., & Pirozzolo, F. J. (1991). Progressive nonfluent aphasia with dementia: A case report. *Journal of Geriatric Psychiatry and Neurology, 4,* 236–240.

Filley, C. M., Kleinschmidt-DeMasters, B. K., & Gross, K. F. (1994). Non-Alzheimer fronto-temporal degenerative dementia. A neurobehavioral and pathologic study. *Clinical Neuropathology, 3,* 109–116.

Folstein, M. F., Folstein, S. E., & McHugh, P. R. (1975). "Mini-Mental State" A practical method for grading the cognitive state of patients for the clinician. *Journal of Psychiatry, 12,* 189–198.

Frances, A., Pincus, H. A., First, M. B., & Widiger, T. A. (1994). *Diagnostic criteria from DSM-IV.* Washington, DC: American Psychiatric Association.

Francis, P. T., Holmes, C., Webster, M. T., Stratmann, G. C., Procter, A. W., & Bowen, D. M. (1993). Preliminary neurochemical findings in non-Alzheimer dementia due to lobar atrophy. *Dementia, 4*(3–4), 172–177.

Friedland, R. P., Koss, E., Lerner, A., Hedera, P., Ellis, W., Dronkers, N., Ober, B. A., & Jagust, W. J. (1993). Functional imaging, the frontal lobes, and dementia. *Dementia, 4*(3–4), 192–203.

Goldberg, E. (1986). Varieties of perseveration: A comparison of two taxonomies. *Journal of Clinical and Experimental Neuropsychology, 8,* 710–726.

Goto, I., Taniwaki, T., Hosokawa, S., Otsuka, M., Ichiya, Y., & Ichimiya, A. (1993). Positron emission tomographic (PET) studies in dementia. *Journal of the Neurological Sciences, 114*(1), 1–6.

Green, J., Morris, J. C., Sandson, J., McKeel, D. W. J., & Miller, T. W. (1990). Progressive aphasia: A precursor of global dementia? *Neurology, 40,* 423–429.

Gustafson, L. (1993). Clinical picture of frontal lobe degeneration of non-Alzheimer type. *Dementia, 4,* 143–148.

Gustafson, L., Brun, A., & Passant, U. (1992). Frontal lobe degeneration of non-Alzheimer type. *Baillieres Clinical Neurology, 3,* 559–582.

Heaton, R. K. (1981). *Wisconsin Card Sorting Test manual.* Odessa, FL: Psychological Assessment Resources.

Heston, L. L. (1986). Clinical genetics of dementing illness. *Neurologic Clinics, 4*(2), 439–445.

Heston, L. L., White, J. A., & Mastri, A. R. (1987). Pick's

disease. Clinical genetics and natural history. *Archives of General Psychiatry*, *44*, 409–411.

Hirano, A. (1994). Hirano bodies and related neuronal inclusions. (Review). *Neuropathology and Applied Neurobiology*, *20*(1), 3–11.

Hodges, J. R., & Gurd, J. M. (1994). Remote memory and lexical retrieval in a case of frontal Pick's disease. *Archives of Neurology*, *51*, 821–827.

Hodges, J. R., Patterson, K., Oxbury, S., & Funnell, E. (1992). Semantic dementia. *Brain*, *115*, 1783–1806.

Hof, P. R., Bouras, C., Perl, D. P., & Morrison, J. H. (1994). Quantitative neuropathologic analysis of Pick's disease cases: Cortical distribution of Pick bodies and coexistence with Alzheimer's disease. *Acta Neuropathology* (Berlin), *2*, 115–124.

Holland, A. L., McBurney, D. H., Moossy, J., & Reinmuth, O. M. (1985). The dissolution of language in Pick's disease with neurofibrillary tangles: A case study. *Brain and Language*, *24*(1), 36–58.

Holman, B. L., & Devous, M. D. (1992). Functional brain SPECT: The emergence of a powerful clinical method. *The Journal of Nuclear Medicine*, *33*(10), 1888–1904.

Holman, B. L., Johnson, K. A., Gerada, B., Carvalho, P., & Satlin, A. (1992). The scintigraphic appearance of Alzheimer's disease: A prospective study using technetium-99m-HMPAO SPECT. *Journal of Nuclear Medicine*, *33*, 181–185.

Hooten, W. M., & Lyketsos, C. G. (1996). Frontotemporal dementia: A clinicopathological review of four postmortem studies. *Journal of Neuropsychiatry and Clinical Neurosciences*, *8*, 10–19.

Hulette, C. M., & Crain, B. J. (1992). Lobar atrophy without Pick bodies. *Clinical Neuropathology*, *11*(3), 151–156.

Ikejiri, U., Tanabe, H., Nakagawa, Y., Kashiwagi, A., Okuda, J., Shiraishi, J., & Nishimura, T. (1993). Two cases of primary progressive non-fluent aphasia. *No To Shinkei—Brain and Nerve*, *45*(4), 370–376.

Imamura, T., Suzuki, K., Yamadori, A., Sahara, M., Nagasawa, H., Itoh, M., & Itoh, H. (1994). Improved perseveration with amantadine. *No To Shinkei*, *46*, 556–562.

Izumiyama, Y., Ikeda, K., & Oyanagi, S. (1994). Extracellular or ghost Pick bodies and their lack of tau immunoreactivity: A histological, immunohistochemical and electron microscopic study. *Acta Neuropathology*, *87*, 277–283.

Jackson, J. A., Jankovic, J., & Ford, J. (1983). Progressive supranuclear palsy: Clinical features and response to treatment in 16 patients. *Annals of Neurology*, *13*, 273–278.

Jagust, W. J., Reed, B. R., Seab, J. P., Kramer, J. H., & Budinger, T. F. (1989). Clinical-physiologic correlates of Alzheimer's disease and frontal lobe dementia. *American Journal of Physiologic Imaging*, *4*(3), 89–96.

Johnson, M. K. (1991). Reality monitoring: Evidence from confabulation in organic brain disease patients. In G. P. Prigatano & D. L. Schacter (Eds.), *Awareness of deficit after brain injury* (pp. 176–197). New York: Oxford University Press.

Joynt, R. J., & Shoulson, I. (1985). Dementia. In K. M. Heilman & E. Valenstein (Eds.), *Clinical neuropsychology* (pp. 453–479). Oxford, England: Oxford University Press.

Jung, R., & Solomon, K. (1993). Clinical practice and service development—psychiatric manifestations of Pick's disease. *International Psychogeriatrics*, *5*(2), 187–202.

Karbe, H., Kertesz, A., & Polk, M. (1993). Profiles of language impairment in primary progressive aphasia. *Archives of Neurology*, *50*(2), 193–201.

Kertesz, A., Hudson, L., Mackenzie, I. R., & Munoz, D. G. (1994). The pathology and nosology of primary progressive aphasia. *Neurology*, *44*(11), 2065–2072.

Kew, J. J. M., Brooks, D. J., Passingham, R. E., Rothwell, J. C., Frackowiak, R. S. J., & Leigh, P. N. (1994). Cortical function in progressive lower motor neuron disorders and amyotrophic lateral sclerosis: A comparative PET study. *Neurology*, *44*, 1101–1110.

Kiernan, J. A., & Hudson, A. J. (1994). Frontal lobe atrophy in motor neuron diseases. *Brain*, *117*, 747–757.

Kirshner, H. S., Webb, W. G., & Kelly, M. P. (1984). Language disturbance: An initial symptom of cortical degenerations and dementia. *Archives of Neurology*, *41*, 491–496.

Klatka, L. A., Schiffer, R. B., Powers, J. M., & Kazee, A. M. (1996). Incorrect diagnosis of Alzheimer's disease. A clinicopathologic study. *Archives of Neurology*, *53*, 35–42.

Knopman, D. S., Mastri, A. R., Frey, W. H., Sung, J. H., & Rustan, T. (1990). Dementia lacking distinctive histologic features: A common non-Alzheimer degenerative dementia. *Neurology*, *40*(2), 251–256.

Kobayashi, K., Kurachi, M., Fukutani, Y., Inao, G., Nakamura, I., & Yamaguchi, N. (1990). Progressive dysphasic dementia with localized cerebral atrophy: Report of an autopsy. *Clinical Neuropathology*, *9*(5), 254–261.

Kolb, B., & Whishaw, I. Q. (1990). Fundamentals of human neuropsychology. In *Fundamentals of human neuropsychology*. New York: Freeman.

Lang, A. E., Bergeron, C., Pollanen, M. S., & Ashby, P. (1994). Parietal Pick's disease mimicking cortical-basal ganglionic degeneration. *Neurology*, *44*(8), 1436–1440.

Lanska, D. J., Currier, R. D., Cohen, M., Gambetti, P., Smith, E. E., Bebin, J., Jackson, J. F., Whitehouse, P. J., & Markesbery, W. R. (1994). Familial progressive subcortical gliosis. *Neurology*, *44*, 1633–1643.

Lauterbach, E. C. (1994). Reversible intermittent rhythmic myoclonus with fluoxetine in presumed Pick's disease. *Movement Disorders*, *9*(3), 343–346.

Lezak, M. D. (1983). *Neuropsychological assessment*. New York: Oxford University Press.

Lezak, M. D. (1989). Assessment of psychosocial dysfunctions resulting from head trauma. In A. R. Liss (Ed.), *Assessment of the behavioral consequences of head trauma* (pp. 113–143). New York: Oxford University Press.

L'hermitte, F. (1986). Human autonomy and the frontal lobes: Part II: Patient behavior in complex and social situations: The "environmental dependency syndrome." *Annals of Neurology*, *19*, 335–343.

Lishman, W. A. (1978). Organic psychiatry. In W. A. Lishman (Ed.), *Organic psychiatry*. London: Blackwell Scientific Publications.

Lund and Manchester Groups. (1994). Clinical and neuropathological criteria for frontotemporal dementia. *Journal of Neurology, Neurosurgery and Psychiatry, 57,* 416–418.

Luria, A. R. (1980). *Higher cortical functions in man.* New York: Basic Books.

Lynch, T., Sano, M., Marder, K. S., Bell, K. L., Foster, N. L., Defendini, R. F., Sima, A. A. F., Keohane, C., Nygaard, T. G., Fahn, S., Mayeux, R., Rowland, L. P., & Wilhelmsen, K. C. (1994). Clinical characteristics of a family with chromosome 17-linked disinhibition-dementia-parkinsonism-amyotrophy complex. *Neurology, 44,* 1878–1884.

Mann, D. M., South, P. W., Snowden, J. S., & Neary, D. (1993). Dementia of frontal lobe type: Neuropathology and immunohistochemistry. *Journal of Neurology, Neurosurgery and Psychiatry, 56*(6), 605–614.

Marin, R. S. (1991). Apathy: A neuropsychiatric syndrome. *Journal of Neuropsychiatry, 3,* 243-254.

Marin, R. S., Fogel, B. S., Hawkins, J., Duffy, J., & Krupp, B. (1995). Apathy: A treatable syndrome. *Journal of Neuropsychiatry and Clinical Neurosciences, 7,* 23–30.

Mayes, A. E. (1988). The memory problems caused by frontal lobe lesions. In *Human organic memory disorders* (pp. 102–123). Cambridge, England: Cambridge University Press.

Mega, M. S., Cummings, J. L., Fiorello, T., & Gornbein, J. (1996). The spectrum of behavioral changes in Alzheimer's disease. *Neurology, 46,* 130–135.

Mehler, M. F. (1988). Mixed transcortical aphasia in nonfamilial dysphasic dementia. *Cortex, 24*(4), 545–554.

Mehler, M. F., Horoupian, D. S., Davies, P., & Dickson, D. W. (1987). Reduced somatostatin-like immunoreactivity in cerebral cortex in nonfamilial dysphasic dementia. *Neurology, 37*(9), 1448–1453.

Mesulam, M. (1982). Slowly progressive aphasia without generalized dementia. *Annals of Neurology, 14,* 592–598.

Milberg, W. P., Hebben, N., & Kaplan, E. (1986). The Boston process approach to neuropsychological assessment. In I. Grant & K. M. Adams (Eds.), *Neuropsychological assessment of neuropsychiatric disorders* (pp. 65–86). New York: Oxford University Press.

Miller, B. L., Cummings, J. L., Villanueve-Meyer, J., Boone, K., Mehringer, C. M., Lesser, I. M., & Mena, I. (1991). Frontal lobe degeneration: Clinical neuropsychological and SPECT characteristics. *Neurology, 41,* 1374–1382.

Morris, J. C., Cole, M., Banker, B. Q., & Wright, D. (1984). Hereditary dysphasic dementia and the Pick-Alzheimer spectrum. *Annals of Neurology, 16*(4), 455–466.

Munoz-Garcia, D., & Ludwin, S. K. (1984). Classic and generalised variants of Pick's disease: A clinicopathological, ultrastructural, and immunocytochemical and comparative study. *Annals of Neurology, 16,* 467–480.

Namikawa, T. (1993). Frontal lobe dementia—two cases diagnosed by SPECT. *Brain and Nerve, 45*(12), 1155–1159.

Neary, D., & Snowden, J. S. (1991). Frontal lobe function and dysfunction. In H. S. Levin, H. M. Eisenberg, & A. L. Benton (Eds.), *Dementia of the frontal lobe type* (pp. 304–317). New York: Oxford University Press.

Neary, D., Snowden, J. S., Shields, R. A., Burjan, A. W., Northen, B., MacDermott, N., Prescott, M. C., & Testa, H. J. (1987). Single photon emission tomography using 99mTc-HMPAO in the investigation of dementia. *Journal of Neurology, Neurosurgery and Psychiatry, 50*(9), 1101–1109.

Neary, D., Snowden, J. S., Northen, B., & Goulding, P. (1988). Dementia of frontal lobe type. *Journal of Neurology, Neurosurgery and Psychiatry, 51,* 353–361.

Neary, D., Snowden, J. S., Mann, D. M., Northen, B., Goulding, P. J., & MacDermott, N. (1990). Frontal lobe dementia and motor neuron disease. *Journal of Neurology, Neurosurgery and Psychiatry, 53,* 23–32.

Neary, D., Snowden, J. S., & Mann, D. M. (1993a). Familial progressive aphasia: its relationship to other forms of lobar atrophy. *Journal of Neurology, Neurosurgery and Psychiatry, 56*(10), 1122–1125.

Orrell, M. W., & Sahakian, B. J. (1991). Dementia of the frontal lobe type. *Psychological Medicine, 21,* 553–556.

Osimani, A., Ichise, M., Chung, D. G., Pogue, J. M., & Freedman, M. (1994). SPECT for differential diagnosis of dementia and correlation of rCBF with cognitive impairment. *Canadian Journal of Neurological Sciences, 21*(2), 104–111.

Paulus, W., Bancher, C., & Jellinger, K. (1993). Microglial reaction in Pick's disease. *Neuroscience Letters, 1,* 89–92.

Petersen, R. B., Tabaton, M., Chen, S. G., Monari, L., Richardson, S. L., Lynch, T., Manetto, V., Lanska, D. J., & Markesbery, W. R. (1995). Familial progressive subcortical gliosis: Presence of prions and linkage to chromosome 17. *Neurology, 45,* 1062–1067.

Pick, A. (1977). On the relation between aphasia and senile atrophy of the brain. In D. A. Rottenberg & F. H. Hochberg (Eds.), *Neurological classics in modern translation* (pp. 35–40). New York: Hafner Press. (Original work published 1892)

Reitan, R. M., & Wolfson, D. (1985). *The Halstead-Reitan neuropsychological test battery: Theory and clinical interpretation.* Tucson, AZ: Neuropsychology Press.

Risberg, J., Passant, U., Warkentin, S., & Gustafson, L. (1993). Regional cerebral blood flow in frontal lobe dementia of non-Alzheimer type. *Dementia, 4*(3–4), 186–187.

Royall, D. R., Mahurin, R. K., & Plotnick, E. (1992). Bedside assessment of executive cognitive impairment: The executive interview. *Journal of the American Geriatric Society, 40,* 1221–1226.

Royall, D. R., Mahurin, R. K., & Cornell, J. (1994). Bedside assessment of frontal degeneration: Distinguishing Alzheimer's disease from non-Alzheimer's cortical dementia. *Experimental Aging Research, 20,* 95–103.

Salmon, E., Sadzot, B., Maquet, P., Degueldre, C., Lemaire, C., Rigo, P., Comar, D., & Franck, G. (1994). Differential diagnosis of Alzheimer's disease with PET. *Journal of Nuclear Medicine, 35*(3), 391–398.

Sandson, J., & Albert, M. (1984). Varieties of perseveration. *Neuropsychologia, 22,* 715–732.

Scheltens, P., Ravid, R., & Kamphorst, W. (1994). Pathologic findings in a case of primary progressive aphasia. *Neurology, 44*(2), 279–282.

Shallice, T. (1982). Specific impairments in planning. *Philosophical Transactions of the Royal Society of London (Series B: Biological Sciences). 298*(1089), 199–209.

Shallice, T., & Evans, M. E. (1978). The involvement of the frontal lobes in cognitive estimation. *Cortex, 4,* 294–303.

Shimamura, A. P., Janowski, J. S., & Squire, L. R. (1991). What is the role of frontal lobe damage in memory disorders? In H. S. Levin, H. M. Eisenberg, & A. L. Benton (Eds.), *Frontal lobe function and dysfunction* (pp. 173–195.). New York: Oxford University Press.

Shonk, T. K., Moats, R. A., Gifford, P., Michaelis, T., Mandigo, J. C., & Izumi, J. (1995). Probable Alzheimer disease: Diagnosis with proton MR spectroscopy. *Radiology, 195*(1), 65–72.

Sjögren, T., Sjögren, H., & Lindgren, A. G. H. (1952). Morbus Alzheimer and morbus Pick. *Acta Psychiatrica et Neurologica Scandinavica, 82,* 1–152.

Smith, C. D., Gallenstein, L. G., Layton, W. J., Kryscio, R. J., & Markesbery, W. R. (1993). 31P magnetic resonance spectroscopy in Alzheimer's and Pick's disease. *Neurobiologic Aging, 14*(1), 85–92.

Snowden, J. S., & Neary, D. (1993). Progressive language dysfunction and lobar atrophy. *Dementia, 4*(3–4), 226–231.

Snowden, J. S., Neary, D., Mann, D. M., Goulding, P. J., & Testa, H. J. (1992). Progressive language disorder due to lobar atrophy. *Annals of Neurology, 31*(2), 174–183.

Sparks, D. L., Danner, F. W., Davis, D. G., Hackney, C., Landers, T., & Coyne, C. M. (1994). Neurochemical and histopathologic alterations characteristic of Pick's disease in a nondemented individual. *Journal of Neuropathology and Experimental Neurology, 53*(1), 37–42.

Starkstein, S. E., Migliorelli, R., Teson, A., Sabe, L., Vazquez, S., Turjanski, M., Robinson, R. G., & Leiguarda, R. (1994). Specificity of changes in cerebral blood flow in patients with frontal lobe dementia. *Journal of Neurology, Neurosurgery and Psychiatry, 57*(7), 790–796.

Stip, E. (1995). Compulsive disorder and acquired antisocial behavior in frontal lobe dementia. *Journal of Neuropsychiatry and Neurosciences, 7,* 116.

Strub, R. L., & Black, F. W. (1988). *Neurobehavioral disorders. A clinical approach.* Philadelphia: F. A. Davis Company.

Stuss, D. T. (1991). Disturbance of self-awareness after frontal system damage. In G. P. Prigatano and D. L. Schacter (Ed.), *Awareness of deficit after brain injury* (pp. 63–83). Oxford, England: Oxford University Press.

Stuss, D. T., & Benson, D. F. (1986). *The frontal lobes.* New York: Raven Press.

Sungaila, P., & Crockett, D. J. (1993). Dementia and the frontal lobes. In R. W. Parks, R. F. Zec, & R. S. Wilson (Eds.), *Neuropsychology of Alzheimer's disease and other dementias* (pp. 235–264). Oxford, England: Oxford University Press.

Szelies, B., & Karenberg, A. (1986). Disorders of glucose metabolism in Pick's disease. *Fortschritte der Neurologie-Psychiatrie, 54*(12), 393–397.

Tobo, M., Mitsuyama, Y., Ikari, K., & Itoi, K. (1984). Familial occurrence of adult-type neuronal ceroid lipofuscinosis. *Archives of Neurology, 41,* 1091–1094.

Tonkonogy, J. M., Smith, T. W., & Barreira, P. J. (1994). Obsessive–compulsive disorders in Pick's disease. *Journal of Neuropsychiatry Clinical Neurosciences, 6*(2), 176–180.

Tranchant, C., Muller, S., & Warter, J. M. (1992). Ubiquitin and degenerative disease of the central nervous system. *Review of Neurology, 12,* 731–735.

Tuokko, H. A., & Crockett, D. (1991). Assessment of everyday functioning in normal and malignant memory disordered elderly. In D. E. Tupper & K. D. Cicerone (Eds.), *The neuropsychology of everyday life: Issues in development and rehabilitation* (pp. 135–182). Boston: Kluwer Academic.

Verfaellie, M., & Heilman, K. M. (1987). Response preparation and response inhibition after lesions of the medial frontal lobe. *Archives of Neurology, 44,* 1265–1271.

Weintraub, S., & Mesulam, M. (1985). Mental state assessment of young and elderly adults in behavioral neurology. In M. Mesulam (Ed.), *Principles of behavioral neurology* (pp. 71–123). Philadelphia: F. A. Davis Company.

Weintraub, S., Rubin, N. P., & Mesulam, M. (1990). Primary progressive aphasia: Longitudinal course, neuropsychological profile and language features. *Archives of Neurology, 47,* 1329–1335.

Wilhelmsen, K. C., Lynch, T., Pavlou, E., Higgins, M., & Nygaard, T. G. (1994). Localization of disinhibition-dementia-parkinsonism-amyotrophy complex to 17q21-22. *American Journal of Human Genetics, 55,* 1159–1165.

Wilkins, A. J., Shallice, T., & McCarthy, R. (1987). Frontal lesions and sustained attention. *Neuropsychologia, 25,* 359–365.

Yamazaki, M., Makano, I., Imazu, O., Kaieda, R., & Terashi, A. (1994). Astrocytic straight tubules in the brain of a patient with Pick's disease. *Acta Neuropathologica, 88*(6), 587–591.

Yashura, O., Aimi, Y., McGeer, E. G., & McGeer, P. L. (1994). Expression of the complement membrane attach complex and its inhibitors in Pick disease brain. *Brain Research, 2,* 346–349.

12

Vascular Dementia

Clinical Assessment, Neuropsychological Features, and Treatment

SUSAN E. McPHERSON AND JEFFREY L. CUMMINGS

Introduction

Vascular dementia (VaD) is the second leading cause of dementia in the elderly, accounting for 15–25% of cognitive decline in aged individuals (Roman, 1991). Despite high prevalence, VaD has not been studied as extensively as other dementias, such as Alzheimer's disease (AD). Worldwide epidemiologic studies have found consistent increases in the prevalence of VaD with advancing age (Rocca et al., 1991; Suzuki, Kutsuzawa, Nakajinia, & Hatano, 1991; Yamaguchi, Ogata, & Yoshida, 1992). Studies reveal that in the United States the prevalence of stroke rises exponentially with age, doubling each decade (Kurtzke, 1985). The estimated prevalence of patients over the age of 60 surviving an ischemic stroke is 1,640,800. Of these patients, approximately 25% develop dementia. It is further estimated that in at least 62% of patients with dementia and ischemic stroke, cognitive impairment dementia is the direct result of cerebrovascular disease (Tatemichi, Desmond, & Mayeux, 1992).

Research on VaD has been limited by the heterogeneity of the disease. Lesions may appear in cortical areas, subcortical regions, strategic locations (e.g., angular gyrus, thalamic), or in combined cortical and subcortical regions. Until recently, clinical studies of patients with infarcts grouped together patients with various types of neuropathologic changes. Recent research definitions developed by an international committee of experts from the National Institute of Neurological Diseases and Stroke (NINDS) and the Association Internationale pour la Recherche et l'Enseignement en Neurosciences (AIREN) resolve this heterogeneity by classifying the disease into distinct subgroups of cerebrovascular lesions (Roman et al., 1993).

This chapter presents the new diagnostic criteria for VaD, reviews available studies that characterize the new subtypes, discusses treatment considerations for patients with VaD, and provides suggestions for future directions in research.

Diagnostic Criteria

The concept of VaD has undergone dramatic changes over the past 20 years. Hachinski, Lassen, and Marshall (1974) introduced the term "multi-infarct dementia" to describe the dementia associated with multiple cerebrovascular infarctions. These investigators ascribed the mental status changes in patients with VaD to tissue destruction and not cerebral hypoperfusion. The terms vascular dementia and multi-infarct dementia are often used interchangeably. In more recent classifications, VaD is used as a more inclusive term encompassing

SUSAN E. McPHERSON • Department of Psychiatry and Biobehavioral Sciences, University of California, Los Angeles, School of Medicine, Los Angeles, California 90024; and Cedars Sinai Alzheimer's Disease Research and Treatment Center, Los Angeles, California 90024. JEFFREY L. CUMMINGS • Department of Neurology, University of California, Los Angeles, School of Medicine, Los Angeles, California 90024; and West Los Angeles Veterans Affairs Medical Center, Los Angeles, California 90095-1769.

several subtypes of dementia including those secondary to stroke, hemorrhagic events, or ischemic changes.

The third edition of the *Diagnostic and Statistical Manual of Mental Disorders* (*DSM-III*; American Psychiatric Association, 1980) adopted the term multi-infarct dementia to describe a condition marked by (1) the presence of dementia, (2) a stepwise deteriorating course with a "patchy" pattern of deficits, (3) evidence of focal neurological signs and symptoms, and (4) evidence from history, physical examination, or laboratory tests of significant cerebrovascular disease judged to be etiologically related to the disturbance. A diagnosis of dementia required a loss of intellectual abilities of sufficient severity to interfere with social or occupational functioning, the presence of memory impairment, and evidence of deficit in at least one additional area of functioning such as abstract reasoning, judgment, language functions (aphasia), recognizing or identifying objects (agnosia), constructional skills, motor activities (apraxia), or personality. A diagnosis of dementia also required that the cognitive disturbance was not solely secondary to a delirium and that there be evidence of a specific organic factor etiologically related to the disturbance. The revision of *DSM-III*, or *DSM-III-R* (American Psychiatric Association, 1987), used identical diagnostic criteria for both dementia and the subclassification of multi-infarct dementia.

The *DSM-IV* (American Psychiatric Association, 1994) has adopted the term vascular dementia to replace the older term multi-infarct dementia. The *DSM-IV* criteria for a diagnosis of VaD include (1) evidence of memory impairment marked by an inability to learn new information or recall previously learned information and one or more of the following cognitive disturbances: aphasia, apraxia, agnosia, or disturbances of executive function; (2) cognitive deficits that cause significant impairment in social or occupational functioning and represent decline from a previous level of functioning; (3) focal neurological signs and symptoms or laboratory evidence of cerebrovascular disease judged to be etiologically related to the disturbance; and (4) deficits not occuring exclusively in the course of the delirium. The *DSM-IV* diagnostic criteria do not specify the physiologic subtypes of VaD.

Recently, new diagnostic criteria for VaD were developed by the NINDS-AIREN international work group. According to these criteria, a diagnosis of probable VaD includes (1) a diagnosis of dementia, (2) evidence of cerebrovascular disease defined by the presence of focal signs on neurologic examination and evidence of relevant cerebrovascular disease by brain imaging, and (3) a relationship of (1) and (2) manifested by the presence of one of the following: (a) onset of dementia within 3 months of a recognized stroke, (b) abrupt deterioration in cognitive functions, or (c) fluctuating, stepwise progression of cognitive deficits (Roman et al., 1993). These criteria define dementia as a decline in memory and intellectual abilities that causes impairment in ability to function in daily living. Impaired functioning in daily living must be due to cognitive impairment and not be secondary to physical handicaps produced by stroke or aphasia. Cognitive decline is manifested by impairment of memory with deficits in at least two of the following additional domains: orientation, attention, language-verbal skills, visuospatial abilities, calculations, executive functions, motor control, praxis, abstraction, and judgment.

Neuropathologically, VaD is defined as dementia resulting from ischemic or hemorrhagic brain lesions or from cerebral ischemic-hypoxic injuries such as those caused by cardiac arrest. This definition excludes those cases due to pure asphyxia, respiratory failure, carbon monoxide poisoning, or cyanide poisoning (Roman et al., 1993).

The following ischemic VaD syndromes have been defined (Table 1): (1) multi-infarct dementia (involving both cortical and subcortical regions), (2) strategic single-infarct dementia, (3) small-vessel disease with dementia, (4) hypoperfusion, (5) hemorrhagic dementia, and (6) combinations of the above lesions and other, yet unknown factors (Roman et al., 1993). The first three conditions have received modest attention in the neuropsychology literature and will be discussed in detail.

Clinical Features of VaD

Epidemiologically, VaD is characterized by an earlier age of onset than is seen in AD and a tendency to affect men more than women (Morimatsu,

Table 1. Classification and Neuropsychological Features of VaD Syndromes

VaD type	Vessels involved	Neuropsychological deficits
Multi-infarct dementia		
Cortical	Anterior middle posterior cerebral	Aphasia, agnosia, amnesia, apraxia
Mixed (cortical and subcortical)	Cortical vessels and subcortical arteriols	Variable pattern of deficits including language and memory
Strategic infarct dementia		
Angular gyrus syndrome	Posterior branch of middle cerebral arteries	Anomia, alexia with agraphia, Gerstmann syndrome, constructional disturbance
Caudate infarction	Lenticulo-striate branch of anterior or middle cerebral arteries	Memory, attention, set shifting, verbal fluency; planning, organizing and sequencing
Globus pallidus infarction	Lenticulo-striate branch of middle cerebral artery	Disorders of memory and set shifting
Thalamic infarction	Thalamo-perforant branches of posterior cerebral arteries	Abnormalities of memory, verbal fluency, mental control, set shifting, sequential reasoning, motor programming
Small-vessel disorders		
Lacunar state	Subcortical arterioles	Set shifting, verbal fluency, attention, abstraction
Binswanger's disease	Subcortical arterioles	Impairment of memory attention, gait disturbance, motor performance, set shifting

Hirai, Muramatsu, & Yoshikawa, 1975; Tomlinson, Blessed, & Roth, 1970). The cardinal clinical features of VaD include an abrupt onset, stepwise deterioration, fluctuating course, nocturnal exacerbation of confusion, previous history of hypertension, and a history of neurological symptoms of transient ischemia (Erkinjuntti, Haltia, Palo, Sulkava, & Paetau, 1988; Hachinski et al., 1975). Vascular dementia can present with a gradually progressive course with periods of partial intellectual recovery or periods of stability (Hershey, Modic, Greenough, & Jaffe, 1987). The absence of typical historical features does not exclude a diagnosis of VaD (Hershey et al., 1987; Meyer, McClintic, Rogers, Sims, & Mortel, 1988).

On clinical examination, patients with VaD exhibit focal neurological signs and symptoms (Bucht, Adolfson, & Winblad, 1984; Hachinski et al., 1975; Ladurner, Iliff, & Lechner, 1982; Loeb & Gandolfo, 1983; Rosen, Terry, Fuld, Katzman, & Peck, 1980). Limb rigidity, psychomotor slowing, incontinence, and gait abnormality are often present (Hershey et al., 1987; Ishii, Nishihara, & Imamura, 1986; Roman, 1987). Pseudobulbar palsy with mild dysarthria is also common (Powell, Cummings, Hill, & Benson, 1988). Patients with VaD are likely to have elevated blood pressure, and heart murmurs, angina, heart failure, and electrocardiographic (ECG) abnormalities are commonly associated with VaD (Bucht et al., 1984; St. Claire & Whalley, 1983; Tresch, Folstein, Rabins, & Hazzard, 1985).

Etiology

Vascular dementia can be caused by a variety of factors or conditions. The most common etiology of VaD is ischemic cerebral injury resulting from occlusion of cerebral blood vessels from thrombotic or embolic disorders (Cummings & Benson, 1992). Anoxic ischemic disorders resulting from cardiopulmonary arrest, recurrent hypotension, anemia, and sleep apnea syndrome can also cause VaD. Mechanical vascular conditions (i.e., " 'pipestem' basilar artery" or a giant cerebral aneurysm) and hemorrhagic disorders also result in VaD. Conditions known to exacerbate VaD include cardiac and renal failure, toxic disorders (secondary to cardiac or antihypertensive agents), and depression (Cummings & Benson, 1992).

Behavioral and Neuropsychological Aspects of Vascular Dementia

Multiple Infarct Dementia

The literature on VaD is limited, and a characteristic pattern of neuropsychologic test outcomes has not been identified. Prior studies of cognitive deficits associated with VaD combined all patients with cerebrovascular pathology into a single group, regardless of the location or severity of lesions. The "patchy" pattern of neuropsychological deficits thought to be characteristic of multi-infarct dementia (MID) may be an artifact of studying patients with a variety of types and locations of neuropathologic changes.

The cerebrovascular lesions associated with the multiple infarct dementia are multiple, large complete infarcts usually involving cortical and subcortical areas (Roman et al., 1993). These criteria, defined by the NINDS-AIREN work group, allow for the possibility that multiple infarcts limited to the cortex cause MID. Cortical infarction most often results from embolic or thrombotic occlusion of large and/or medium-sized vessels. The clinical picture associated with dementia is manifested when multiple, bilateral cortical infarcts are present (Cummings & Benson, 1992).

Multi-infarct dementia is associated with a variable pattern of cognitive deficits. Depending on the cortical territory irrigated by the involved vessel, patients may present with aphasia, apraxia, or deficits in visuospatial and visuomotor performance. Aphasia and apraxia typically appear following occlusion of the middle cerebral artery affecting the left hemisphere (Benson, 1979; Benson & Geschwind, 1975; Geschwind, 1975). Fluent aphasic output is associated with lesions posterior to the central fissure and nonfluent aphasias result from infarctions anterior to the Rolandic fissure (Cummings & Benson, 1992). Infarctions immediately adjacent to the sylvian fissure disrupt repetition. The ability to repeat is preserved when the perisylvian area is spared. Global aphasia is the result of infarction of the entire dominant left cerebral artery territory. Infarction of the right middle cerebral artery may result in abnormalities in language melody, dressing, and visuospatial orientation and visuomotor performance (Hemphill & Klein, 1948; Ross, 1981).

Neuropsychological Studies

Relatively few investigations exist on the neuropsychological aspects of MID. The majority of available studies have relied on relatively small sample sizes and combined all patients with cerebrovascular pathology into a single group, resulting in a heterogeneous or patchy pattern of deficits. Perez and colleagues (1975) compared the neuropsychological performance of three groups of patients: MID, AD, and vertebrobasilar insufficiency (VBI patients). Patients with MID exhibited more subtest scatter on the Wechsler Adult Intelligence Scale (WAIS) than either of the other two groups. These investigators concluded that the lack of homogeneity in test scores reflected the patchy nature of the disease process as well as variation in the "site, location, extent and number of cerebral infarctions." Patchy deficits alone are not diagnostic of MID. Approximately 50% of normal adults exhibit differences of seven or more points between scaled scores on the Wechsler Adult Intelligence Scale-Revised (WAIS-R) subtests (La Rue, 1992).

Investigations of language in patients with MID have suggested that spontaneous output is marked by shorter phrase length, restricted lexical variability, and simplified syntax (Hier, Hagenlocker, & Shindler, 1985). Speech regulation disorders such as perseveration and intrusions (Shindler, Caplan, & Hier, 1984), as well as impairment of mechanical aspects of speech (e.g., pitch, melody, articulation, rate) are also present (Powell et al., 1988). Patients with MID exhibit deficits on tasks of confrontation naming, although less severe than those of comparably demented AD patients (Powell et al., 1988). Verbal fluency has been found to be impaired in MID (Gainotti, Galtagirone, Masullo, & Miceli, 1980), and disorders of word recognition, naming, and repetition have also been reported (Kontiola, Laaksonen, Sulkava, & Erkinjuntti, 1990).

Language differences may not be entirely reliable or helpful in distinguishing MID from AD. At least two studies have found no differences on tests of confrontation naming and verbal fluency between the two disorders (Fischer, Gatterer, Marterer, & Danielczyk, 1988; Loewenstein et al., 1991).

Studies of memory functions in MID have failed to show differences between patients with AD and those with MID when level of severity of dementia was controlled. La Rue (1989) administered a 10-item learning task (Fuld Object Memory Evaluation; Fuld, 1981) to nine inpatients with MID. Three of the patients performed within normal limits, one patient had marked retrieval deficits, one patient had an amnestic-type memory deficit, and four exhibited impaired information storage. Variability in performance was related to the overall severity of dementia and to the presence or absence of depression. However, Loewenstein and colleagues (1991) reported that patients with AD made more intrusion errors on the Fuld Object Memory Evaluation than patients with MID.

Strategic Single-Infarct Dementia

Advanced diagnostic imaging techniques have made it possible to recognize small strategically located infarctions which disrupt multiple cognitive operations. These lesions may be located cortically or subcortically. The majority of neuropsychological studies of strategic infarcts have focused on those to the inferior parietal lobe, caudate nucleus, globus pallidus, and thalamus.

Angular Gyrus Syndrome

Angular gyrus syndrome results from lesions to the inferior parietal lobule and shares several clinical features with AD (Cummings & Benson, 1992). The complete syndrome includes fluent aphasia, alexia with agraphia, Gerstmann syndrome (acalculia, right–left disorientation, dysgraphia, and finger agnosia), and constructional disturbances. Patients also perform poorly on verbal learning tests. The syndrome is difficult to distinguish from AD on neurologic exam and diagnostic imaging because focal motor and/or sensory signs may be absent, and lesions are not always detected by computerized tomography (CT). Clinically, patients with AD are often unaware of language and memory problems. However, patients with angular gyrus syndrome frequently complain of their language disturbance (e.g., inability to remember names) and tend to be frustrated and apologetic about their inability to communicate. Although patients with AD and angular gyrus syndrome both make verbal paraphasias, the paraphasias made by patients with angular gyrus syndrome are closer to the target word. Reading comprehension is impaired in both conditions. Nonverbal memory is preserved in angular gyrus syndrome and impaired in AD.

Caudate Infarction

Neuroanatomical connections between the dorsolateral prefrontal cortex and the caudate nucleus, globus pallidus, and thalamus form the dorsolateral prefrontal-subcortical circuit (Cummings, 1993). The neuropsychological profile of damage to this circuit involves deficits primarily in executive functions and motor programming. There is variability in the profile of neuropsychological and behavioral changes depending upon the extent and location of damage in the circuit, and patients with circuit lesions often meet criteria for dementia.

There are few neuropsychological studies of patients with focal caudate lesions. Mendez, Adams, and Lewandowski (1989) found that patients with dorsal or ventral caudate lesions exhibited deficits in memory, attention, and set shifting. The behavioral changes manifested by patients with dorsal caudate lesions included confusion and disinterest, while patients with ventral caudate lesions exhibited disinhibited, euphoric, and inappropriate behaviors (Mendez et al., 1989). Animals with caudate lesions exhibit impaired performance on tasks involving spatial choice and memory and disruption of responses to reinforcement and conditioning (Oberg & Divac, 1979).

Pallidal Infarcts

Reports of focal damage to the globus pallidus are limited to case studies or multi-case reports, many of which involved patients with damage secondary to carbon monoxide poisoning. Deficits on tests of memory and set shifting were reported in one case study of bilateral globus pallidus hemorrhages (Strub, 1989).

Thalamic Infarcts

In contrast to the limited neuropsychological information on caudate and globus pallidus lesions, there is an extensive body of literature on the neuropsychological sequelae of strategic thalamic infarcts. Reports of cognitive deficits in patients with bilateral paramedian thalamic infarction include poor performance on tasks of memory (Eslinger, Warner, Grattan, & Easton, 1991; Gentilini, De Renzi, & Crisi, 1987; Stuss, Guberman, Nelson, & Larochelle, 1988), reduced verbal fluency, decreased mental control, and intact language (Eslinger et al., 1991). Behaviorally, patients with thalamic infarcts exhibit dysphoria, irritability, disinhibition, apathy, utilization behavior, and distractability (Bogousslavsky et al., 1988; Eslinger et al., 1991; Gentilini et al., 1987).

Case studies have revealed that patients with left medial dorsal thalamic infarction often manifest deficits on tests of "frontal lobe" function, including reduced word list generation and poor executive functions (Sandson, Daffner, Carvalho, & Mesulam, 1991). Apathy and memory impairment have also been observed (Sandson et al., 1991). Other investigators have documented executive deficits including perseveration, inability to shift cognitive set, decreased verbal fluency, and increased susceptibility to interference (Eslinger et al., 1991; Mennemeier, Fennell, Valenstein, & Heilman, 1992; Pepin and Pepin, 1993); poor sequential reasoning; and poor motor programming (Eslinger et al., 1991; Mennemeier et al., 1992).

Damage to each of the structures described above disrupts the dorsolateral prefrontal-subcortical circuit, resulting in a pattern of memory disturbance and deficits of executive functions, meeting criteria for a diagnosis of dementia.

Neuropsychological Aspects of Small-Vessel Disease

Small vessels penetrating from larger arteries irrigate the deep gray matter nuclei (basal ganglia, thalamus) and deep white matter. These small vessels are subject to arteriosclerotic injuries and multiple occlusions resulting in a dementia syndrome. Small-vessel disease with dementia can be divided into two categories: lacunar state and Binswanger's disease.

Lacunar State

Although there exists an extensive literature on lacunar state, very few studies have included neuropsychological evaluations. In the few neuropsychological investigations that exist, a pattern of executive deficits has been identified. Wolfe, Linn, Babikian, and Albert (1990) studied 11 patients with multiple subcortical lacunae, seven of whom had lacunae in both the basal ganglia and periventricular white matter (PVWM). They identified a pattern of deficits similar to that seen in patients with frontal lobe dysfunction, including difficulties in set shifting ability, decreased word list generation, and apathy.

Other investigators have suggested that number of infarcts, extent of periventricular lucency, and severity of ventricular enlargement, but not volume of infarction, were the factors associated with impaired performance on neuropsychological tests, specifically those thought to be dependent on executive function such as phonemic and semantic fluency, simple attention, and abstraction (Corbett, Bennett, & Kos, 1994).

Characterization of the types of deficits associated with small-vessel disease has been advanced by recent progress in understanding frontal-subcortical circuits. Circuits originating in dorsolateral prefrontal cortex mediate executive function and motor programming. Infarcts in subcortical regions such as the basal ganglia and deep white matter disrupt the circuit, resulting in deficits in these functions. The same subcortical structures that, when infarcted, produce a syndrome of strategic infarct dementia (caudate nucleus, globus pallidus, thalamus) are also affected in lacunar state.

Binswanger's Disease

Binswanger's disease (BD) is a gradually progressive syndrome caused by ischemic injury to the deep white matter of the cerebral hemispheres. Clinical risk factors for BD include hypertension, diabetes, cardiovascular disease, and recurrent hypotension. A history of repeated small strokes, usually lacunae, and evidence of discrete neurologic deficits are often present (Babikian & Ropper, 1987; Caplan & Schoene, 1978; Goto, Ishii, & Fukasawa, 1981; Loizou, Kendall, & Marshall, 1981; Nichols & Mohr, 1986; Tomonaga, Yamanouchi, Tohgi, & Kemeyama, 1982). The white matter disease of BD causes direct axon injury as well as disconnection of subcortical structures from an intact cerebral cortex (Roman, 1987).

Clinical manifestations of BD include a slowly progressive dementia marked by pseudobulbar palsy, emotional incontinence, lateralized motor signs, corticospinal or corticobulbar tract dysfunction, and gait disturbance (Aronson & Perl, 1974; Babikian & Ropper, 1987; Biemond, 1970; Burger, Burch, & Kunze, 1976; Caplan & Schoene, 1978; Goto et al., 1981; Loizou et al., 1981; Nichols & Mohr, 1986; Tomonaga et al., 1982). Early in the course of the disease the gait features small steps (marche à petits pas) and there are frequent falls; urinary urgency or incontinence is typically present (Roman, 1987). Changes in mood and behavior are common (Babikian & Ropper, 1987). Frontal lobe-like signs including personality change, loss of initiative, reduced drive, impaired insight, apathy, and abulia typically occur (Ishii et al., 1986; Lotz, Ballinger, & Quisling, 1986). Other frequent manifestations of the disease include mutism, bradykinesia, rigidity, and dysarthria resembling Parkinson's disease or progressive supranuclear palsy (Roman, 1987). Glabellar, snout, rooting, and grasp reflexes and bilateral or unilateral pyramidal tract signs are usually present.

Neuropsychological investigations of BD have focused primarily on the relationship between neuropsychological test performance and evidence of periventricular white matter changes. Rao, Mittenberg, Bernardin, Haughton, and Leo (1989) administered an extensive battery of neuropsychological tests to 50 normotensive, middle-aged, healthy volunteers and found no significant neuropsychological differences between subjects with and without white matter changes. There was no relationship between severity of leukoaraiosis and neuropsychological test performance. However, the sample size was small and only 2 of the 10 subjects with white matter changes had moderately severe white matter alterations. Steingart and colleagues (1987a) administered a brief neuropsychological screening examination to a group of nondemented subjects

with and without evidence of leukoaraiosis on CT. The group with leukoaraiosis exhibited a higher frequency of abnormal gait and focal neurologic signs and performed worse on tests of memory and language. The same investigators found that patients with AD and evidence of leukoaraiosis performed more poorly on cognitive tests than AD patients without leukoaraiosis (Steingart et al., 1987b).

Libon, Scanlon, Swenson, and Coslet (1990) compared the neuropsychological test performance of four groups of patients, including individuals with (1) no evidence of deep white matter disease or dementia, (2) no dementia but evidence of white matter changes on imaging, (3) dementia with no evidence of deep white matter changes, and (4) dementia with evidence of deep white matter changes. As expected, patients with dementia performed more poorly on tests of immediate and delayed recall; significant differences were also found on tests of memory between the two nondemented groups of patients (groups 1 and 2), despite no difference in the frequency of stroke and neurologic signs between groups. Those with white matter changes did more poorly. Although this study does not define a pattern of neuropsychological deficits associated with BD, it does provide evidence that patients who show periventricular hyperintensities on magnetic resonance imaging (MRI) may be at risk for developing a dementing illness.

At least one study has suggested that neuropsychological deficits in small-vessel disease might be associated with volume of infarcted tissue. Boone and coworkers (1992) found that patients with white matter lesion areas of greater than 10 cm^3 performed significantly more poorly on tasks of simple and divided attention and made more perseverative responses and achieved fewer categories on a card sorting task than patients with less extensive ischemic injury. No deficits were found on tests of word list generation or on tests of memory.

In a recent study, patients with AD were compared to those with VaD (small-vessel disease) as defined by evidence of significant white matter hyperintensities on MRI or leukoaraiosis on CT (Kertesz & Clydesdale, 1994). Patients with VaD exhibited greater difficulty on tasks related to executive function including sequential reasoning and analysis, dysgraphia, and motor performance. The AD patients performed more poorly on tasks of paragraph recall and sentence repetition. Subjects with subcortical lacunar infarcts were noted to perform below the level of the control subjects on tasks of response inhibition, set shifting, and semantic clustering. Kertesz and Clydesdale (1994) suggest that new evidence of the existence of frontal subcortical circuits best explains the pattern of deficits found in these patients with damage restricted to subcortical structures.

Recent neuropsychological investigations have suggested that patients with small-vessel disease and ischemic injury to deep hemispheric gray and white matter structures exhibit deficits on tests of frontal functions before the onset of memory or other cognitive disturbances (Boone et al., 1992; Wolfe et al., 1990). These findings indicate that changes in executive function occur well before the onset of memory deficits in subcortical VaD, are a potential key to identifying patients at risk for developing VaD, and may differentiate patients with early VaD from those with AD.

Depression in VaD

In addition to the neuropsychologic complications of stroke discussed above, ischemic brain injury can also result in neuropsychiatric disorders such as depression, psychosis, and anxiety. The reported prevalence of depression occurring after a stroke ranges from as low as 0% to as high as 71%, with a mean of 29% (Cummings & Sultzer, 1993). Depression is most commonly associated with lacunar infarcts and Binswanger's disease, has been variably associated with multiple large strokes, and is rarely observed with thalamic infarcts (Cummings & Sultzer, 1993).

Several possible factors contribute to depression in patients with VaD. Lesion location, particularly those involving the cortical or subcortical structures of the left frontal lobe, have been associated with depressive mood changes (Robinson & Starkstein, 1990). Lesion size has been proposed to contribute to changes in mood (Schwartz et al., 1990), and reduced global hypoperfusion (Rogers, Meyer, Mortel, Mahurin, & Judd, 1986) and neurochemical alterations may be contributory factors

(Bernheimer, Birkmeyer, Hornykiewicz, Jellinger, & Seitelberger, 1973; Wallin et al., 1989). Age, gender, heredity, and personality style may also be associated with susceptibility to depression (Cummings, Miller, Hill, & Neshkes, 1987; Katzman & Terry, 1983; Starkstein et al., 1989).

The differential diagnosis of depression associated with stroke is complex. Two clinical symptoms deserve special recognition: pseudobulbar palsy and the dementia syndrome of depression. Pseudobulbar palsy is a behavioral condition which involves the loss of control of emotional affect, dysarthria, dysphagia, an exaggerated gag reflex, and brisk jaw and facial reflexes (Langworthy & Hesser, 1940). The most common symptom of pseudobulbar affect in elderly patients is forced weeping, an exaggerated display of crying and distress usually brought on by a minor emotional stimulus and out of proportion to the precipitating event. Pseudobulbar affect is accompanied by focal neurological signs (e.g., dysarthria, dysphagia, abnormal reflexes), which help to distinguish it from major depression (Cummings & Sultzer, 1993).

The dementia syndrome of depression is a condition involving cognitive impairment, primarily memory dysfunction, occurring in conjunction with depression. The cognitive impairment resolves with treatment of the mood disorder (Cummings & Sultzer, 1993). There are several factors that distinguish the dementia syndrome of depression from major depression associated with stroke. First, the dementia syndrome of depression generally occurs in the absence of any known cerebral event or degenerative condition or in the presence of a single stroke. The onset of depression in VaD is characteristically associated with several strokes. Second, the onset of depression follows stroke in VaD. However, in the dementia syndrome of depression the onset of cognitive impairment follows the mood disorder. Third, neurologic examination typically reveals no focal signs in the dementia syndrome of depression, but reveals pyramidal or extrapyramidal signs following stroke. Fourth, the cognitive impairment associated with the dementia syndrome of depression resolves following treatment, but does not resolve following treatment in patients with depression associated with stroke. Finally, a family history of mood disorder or past history of depression is more often associated with the dementia syndrome of depression (Cummings & Sultzer, 1993).

Treatment of VaD

Treatment of stroke is primarily pharmacologic and focuses on the prevention of stroke and attempts to decrease the worsening of dementia. Control of hypertension reduces the risk of stroke and is a major goal of therapy. Other means of stroke prevention are also used. Aspirin, a platelet antiaggregant, is the drug most often prescribed for patients with VaD. New platelet antiaggregants, such as ticlopidine, may help to prevent stroke and worsening of dementia in patients who do not respond to or cannot tolerate aspirin. Leukopenia occurs in 2% of patients treated with ticlopidine, requiring patients to have a complete blood count (CBC) every other week for the first 3 months of treatment. Embolic strokes are most often treated with anticoagulant medication, such as coumadin. However, this treatment is warranted only in relatively high-functioning patients who have an identified source of cerebral emboli and do not have a gait disturbance or are at risk for falling.

Treatment of the neuropsychiatric aspects of VaD (depression, psychosis, anxiety) can also reduce patient distress and improve quality of life. There are few systematic studies of the effectiveness of specific agents in the treatment of poststroke depression. Studies of depression in poststroke patients without significant cognitive compromise suggest that the mood symptoms respond to compounds commonly used for treatment of depression. Such studies have focused on nortriptyline (Lipsey, Robinson, Pearlson, Rao, & Price, 1984), trazodone hydrochloride (Reding et al., 1986), methylphenidate (Lingam, Lazarus, Groves, & Oh, 1988), and dextroamphetamine (Masand, Murray, & Pickett, 1991). These studies provide support for the use of a trial of antidepressant medication in patients with VaD and depression.

Nonpharmacologic treatment of VaD includes referrals for psychological counseling, support group participation, community resources, and legal guidance. Psychotherapy support groups help patients and family members cope with physical illness, occupational disability, interpersonal isolation, and dramatic changes in social and family roles associated with stroke and VaD.

Summary

As new, innovative drug therapies are made available for the treatment of VaD, the accurate classification and neuropsychological characterization of patients at risk will be critical in identifying those patients who might benefit. Advances in medical technology have made it possible to improve our understanding of small-vessel disease. The increased sensitivity of MRI has made possible the detection of subcortical white matter lesions, which are invisible on CT. Improved understanding of the neuroanatomical linkages between frontal and subcortical areas allows for new hypotheses regarding the neuropsychological phenomenology of VaD. Improved diagnostic criteria have provided the framework for future research focusing on defining the pattern of neuropsychological deficits associated with each of the subtypes of VaD. Finally, studies focusing on those at risk for developing VaD will be helpful in determining factors which might protect such patients from developing a dementia syndrome.

ACKNOWLEDGMENTS

This project was supported by the Department of Veterans Affairs and a National Institute on Aging Alzheimer's Disease Core Center grant (AG10123).

References

American Psychiatric Association. (1980). *Diagnostic and statistical manual of mental disorders (3rd ed.)*. Washington, DC: Author.

American Psychiatric Association. (1987). *Diagnostic and statistical manual of mental disorders (3rd ed.-rev.)*. Washington, DC: Author.

American Psychiatric Association. (1994). *Diagnostic and statistical manual of mental disorders (4th ed.)*. Washington, DC: Author.

Aronson, S. M., & Perl, D. P. (1974). Clinical neuropathological conference. *Diseases of the Nervous System, 35*, 286–291.

Babikian, V., & Ropper, A. H. (1987). Binswanger's disease: A review. *Stroke, 18*, 2–12.

Benson, D. F. (1979). *Aphasia, alexia, and agraphia*. New York: Churchill Livingstone.

Benson, D. F., & Geschwind, N. (1975). Psychiatric conditions associated with focal lesions of the central nervous system. In S. Arieti & M. Reiser (Eds.), *American handbook of psychiatry* (Vol. 4, pp. 208–243). New York: Basic Books.

Bernheimer, H., Birkmeyer, W., Hornykiewicz, O., Jellinger, K., & Seitelberger, F. (1973). Brain dopamine and the syndromes of Parkinson and Huntington: Clinical, morphological and neurochemical correlations. *Journal of Neurology and Science, 20*, 415–455.

Biemond, A. (1970). Binswanger's subcortical arteriosclerotic encephalopathy and the possibility of its clinical recognition. *Psychiatria, Neurologia, Neurochirugia, 73*, 413–417.

Bogousslavsky, J., Ferrazzini, M., Regli, F., Assal, G., Tanabe, H., & Delaloye-Bischof, A. (1988). Manic delirium and frontal lobe syndrome with paramedian infarction of the right thalamus. *Journal of Neurology, Neurosurgery, and Psychiatry, 51*, 116–119.

Boone, K. B., Miller, B. L., Lesser, I. M., Mehringer, C. M., Hill-Gutierrez, E., Goldberg, M. A., & Berman, N. G. (1992). Neuropsychological correlates of white-matter lesions in healthy elderly subjects: A threshold effect. *Archives of Neurology, 49*, 549–554.

Bucht, G., Adolfson, R., & Winblad, B. (1984). Dementia of the Alzheimer type and multi-infarct dementia: A clinical description and diagnostic problems. *Journal of the American Geriatrics Society, 32*, 491–498.

Burger, P. C., Burch, J. G., & Kunze, U. (1976). Subcortical arteriosclerotic encephalopathy (Binswanger's disease): A vascular etiology of dementia. *Stroke, 7*, 626–631.

Caplan, L. R., & Schoene, W. C. (1978). Clinical features of subcortical arteriosclerotic encephalopathy (Binswanger's disease). *Neurology, 28*, 1206–1215.

Corbett, A. J., Bennett, H., & Kos, S. (1994). Cognitive dysfunction following subcortical infarction. *Archives of Neurology, 51*, 999–1007.

Cummings, J. L. (1993). Frontal-subcortical circuits and human behavior. *Archives of Neurology, 50*, 873–880.

Cummings, J. L., Benson, D. F. (1992). *Dementia: A clinical approach*. Boston: Butterworth-Heinenmann.

Cummings, J. L., & Sultzer, D. L. (1993). Depression in multi-infarct dementia. In S. E. Starkstein & R. G. Robinson (Eds.), *Depression in neurologic disease* (pp. 165–185). Baltimore: Johns Hopkins University Press.

Cummings, J. L., Miller, B., Hill, M. A., & Neshkes, R. (1987). Neuropsychiatric aspects of multi-infarct dementia and dementia of the Alzheimer's type. *Archives of Neurology, 44*, 389–393.

Erkinjuntti, T., Haltia, M., Palo, J., Sulkava, R., & Paetau, A. (1988). Accuracy of the clinical diagnosis of vascular dementia: A prospective clinical and post-mortem neuropathological study. *Journal of Neurology, Neurosurgery, and Psychiatry, 51*, 1037–1044.

Eslinger, P. J., Warner, G. C., Grattan, L. M., & Easton, J. D. (1991). "Frontal lobe" utilization behavior associated with paramedian thalamic infarction. *Neurology, 41*, 450–452.

Fischer, P., Gatterer, G., Marterer, A., & Danielczyk, W. (1988). Nonspecificity of semantic impairment in dementia of the Alzheimer's type. *Archives of Neurology, 45*, 1341–1343.

Fuld, P. A. (1981). *The Fuld Object Memory Evaluation*. Chicago: Stoelting Instruments.

Gainotti, G., Galtagirone, C., Masullo, C., & Miceli, G. (1980). Patterns of neuropsychologic impairment in various diagnostic groups of dementia. In L. Amaducci, A. N. Davidson, & P. Antuono (Eds.), *Aging of the brain and dementia*: Vol. 13. *Aging* (pp. 245–250). New York: Raven Press.

Gentilini, M., De Renzi, E., & Crisi, G. (1987). Bilateral paramedian thalamic artery infarcts: Report of eight cases. *Journal of Neurology, Neurosurgery, and Psychiatry, 50*, 900–909.

Geschwind, M. (1975). The apraxias: Neural mechanisims of disorders of learned movement. *American Scientist, 63*, 188–195.

Goto, K., Ishii, N., & Fukasawa, H. (1981). Diffuse white-matter disease in the geriatric population: A clinical, neuropathological, and CT study. *Radiology, 141*, 687–695.

Hachinski, V. I., Lassen, N. A., & Marshall, J. (1974). Multi-infarct dementia: A cause of mental deterioration in the elderly. *The Lancet, 2*, 207–209.

Hachinski, V. I., Iliff, L. D., Phil, M., Zilhka, E., Du Bolay, G. H., McAllister, V. L., Marshall, J., Ross Russell, R. W., & Symon, L. (1975). Cerebral blood flow in dementia. *Archives of Neurology, 32*, 632–637.

Hemphill, R. E., & Klein, R. (1948). Contribution to the dressing disability as a focal sign and to the imperception phenomena. *Journal of Mental Science, 94*, 611–622.

Hershey, L. A., Modic, M. T., Greenough, G., & Jaffe, D. F. (1987). Magnetic resonance imaging in vascular dementia. *Neurology, 37*, 29–36.

Hier, D. B., Hagenlocker, K., & Shindler, A. G. (1985). Language disintegration in dementia: Effects of etiology and severity. *Brain and Language, 25*, 117–133.

Ishii, N., Nishihara, Y., & Imamura, T. (1986). Why do frontal lobe symptoms predominate in vascular dementia with lacunes? *Neurology, 36*, 340–345.

Katzman, R., & Terry, R. (1983). Normal aging of the nervous system. In R. Katzman & R. Terry (Eds.), *The neurology of aging* (pp. 15–50). Philadelphia: F. A. Davis.

Kertesz, A., & Clydesdale, S. (1994). Neuropsychological deficits in vascular dementia versus Alzheimer's disease. *Archives of Neurology, 51*, 1226–1231.

Kontiola, P., Laaksonen, R., Sulkava, R., & Erkinjuntti, T. (1990). Pattern of language impairment is different in Alzheimer's disease and multi-infarct dementia. *Brain and Language, 38*, 364–383.

Kurtzke, J. F. (1985). Epidemiology of cerebrovascular disease. In F. H. McDowell & L. R. Kaplan (Eds.), *Cerebrovascular survey report for the National Institute of Neurological Disorders and Stroke*. Bethesda, MD: National Institutes of Health.

Ladurner, G., Iliff, L. D., & Lechner, H. (1982). Clinical factors associated with dementia in ischemic stroke. *Journal of Neurology, Neurosurgery, and Psychiatry, 45*, 97–101.

Langworthy, O. R., & Hesser, F. H. (1940). Syndrome of pseudobulbar palsey: An anatomic and physiologic analysis. *Archives of Internal Medicine, 65*, 106–121.

LaRue, A. (1989). Patterns of performance on the Fuld Object

Memory Evaluation in elderly inpatients. *Journal of Clinical and Experimental Neuropsychology, 11,* 409–422.

LaRue, A. (1992). *Aging and neuropsychological assessment.* New York: Plenum.

Libon, D. J., Scanlon, M., Swenson, R., & Coslet, H. B. (1990). Binswanger's disease: Some neuropsychological considerations. *Journal of Geriatric Psychiatry and Neurology, 3,* 31–40.

Lingam, V. R., Lazarus, L. W., Groves, L., & Oh, S. H. (1988). Methylphenidate in treating post-stroke depression. *Journal of Clinical Psychiatry, 49,* 151–153.

Lipsey, J. R., Robinson, R. G., Pearlson, G. D., Rao, K., & Price, T. R. (1984). Nortriptyline treatment of post-stroke depression: A double-blind study. *Lancet, 1,* 297–300.

Loeb, C., & Gandolfo, C. (1983). Diagnostic evaluation of degenerative and vascular dementia. *Stroke, 14,* 399–401.

Loewenstein, D. A., D'Elia, L., Guterman, A., Eisdorfer, C., Wilkie, F., LaRue, A., Mintzer, J., & Duara, R. (1991). The occurrence of different intrusive errors in patients with Alzheimer's disease, multiple cerebral infarctions and major depression. *Brain and Cognition, 16,* 104–117.

Loizou, L. A., Kendall, B. E., & Marshall, J. (1981). Subcortical arteriosclerotic encephalopathy: A clinical and radiological investigation. *Journal of Neurology, Neurosurgery, and Psychiatry, 44,* 294–304.

Lotz, P. R., Ballinger, W. E., Jr., & Quisling, R. G. (1986). Subcortical arteriosclerotic encephalopathy: CT spectrum and pathologic correlation. *American Journal of Roentgenology, 147,* 1209–1214.

Masand, P., Murray, G. B., & Pickett, P. (1991). Psychostimulants in post-stroke depression. *Journal of Neuropsychiatry and Clinical Neuroscience, 3,* 23–27.

Mendez, M. F., Adams, N. L., & Lewandowski, K. S. (1989). Neurobehavioral changes associated with caudate lesions. *Neurology, 39,* 349–354.

Mennemeier, M., Fennell, E., Valenstein, E., & Heilman, K. M. (1992). Contributions of the left intralaminar and medial thalamic nuclei to memory: Comparisons and report of a case. *Archives of Neurology, 49,* 1050–1058.

Meyer, J. S., McClintic, K. L., Rogers, R. L., Sims, P., & Mortel, K. F. (1988). Aetiological considerations and risk factors for multi-infarct dementia. *Journal of Neurology, Neurosurgery, and Psychiatry, 51,* 1489–1497.

Morimatsu, M., Hirai, S., Muramatsu, A., & Yoshikawa, M. (1975). Senile degenerative brain lesions and dementia. *Journal of the American Geriatrics Society, 23,* 390–406.

Nichols, F. T., III, & Mohr, J. P. (1986). Binswanger's subacute arteriosclerotic encephalopathy. In H. J. M. Barnett, J. P. Mohr, B. M. Stein, & F. M. Yatsu (Eds.), *Stroke: Pathophysiology, diagnosis, and management* (pp. 875–885). New York: Churchill Livingstone Inc.

Oberg, R. G. E., & Divac, I. (1979). Cognitive functions of the neostriatum. In I. Divac & R. G. E. Oberg (Eds.), *The neostriatum.* New York: Pergamon.

Pepin, E. P., & Pepin, A. P. (1993). Selective dorsolateral frontal lobe dysfuntion associated with diencephalic amnesia. *Neurology, 43,* 733–741.

Perez, F. I., Rivera, V. M., Meyer, J. S., Gay, J. R. A., Taylor, R.

L., & Mathew, N. T. (1975). Analysis of intellectual and cognitive performance in patients with multi-infarct dementia, vertebrobasilar insufficiency with dementia and Alzheimer's disease. *Journal of Neurology, Neurosurgery, and Psychiatry 38,* 533–540.

Powell, A. L., Cummings, J. L., Hill, M. A., & Benson, D. F. (1988). Speech and language alterations in multi-infarct dementia. *Neurology, 38,* 717–719.

Rao, S. M., Mittenberg, W., Bernardin, L., Haughton, V., & Leo, G. J. (1989). Neuropsychological test findings on subjects with leukoaraiosis. *Archives of Neurology, 46,* 40–47.

Reding, M. J., Orto, L. A., Winter, S. W., Furtuna, I. M., Di Ponte, P., & McDowell, F. H. (1986). Anti-depressant therapy after stroke. A double blind trial. *Archives of Neurology, 43,* 763–765.

Robinson, R. G., & Starkstein, S. E. (1990). Current research in affective disorders following stroke. *Journal of Neuropsychiatry and Clinical Neuroscience, 2,* 1–14.

Rocca, W. A., Hofman, A., Brayne, C., Breteler, M. M. B., Clarke, M., Copeland, J. R. M., Dartigues, J. F., Engedal, K., Hagnell, O., Heeren, T. J., Jonker, C., Lindesay, J., Lobo, A., Mann, A. H., Mölsä, P. K., Morgan, K., O'Connor, D. W., da Silva Droux, A., Sulkava, R., Kay, D. W. K., & Amaducci, L. (1991). The prevalence of vascular dementia in Europe: Facts and fragments from 1980–1990 studies. *Annals of Neurology, 30,* 817–824.

Rogers, R. L., Meyer, J. S., Mortel, K. F., Mahurin, R. K., & Judd, B. W. (1986). Decreased cerebral blood flow precedes multi-infarct dementia, but follows senile dementia of the Alzheimer-type. *Neurology, 36,* 1–6.

Roman, G. C. (1987). Senile dementia of the Binswanger type: A vascular form of dementia in the elderly. *Journal of the American Medical Association, 258,* 1782–1788.

Roman, G. C. (1991). The epidemiology of vascular dementia. In A. Hartmann, W. Kuschinsky, & S. Hoyer (Eds.), *Cerebral ischemia and dementia* (pp. 9–15). Berlin: Springer-Verlag.

Roman, G. C., Tatemichi, T. K., Erkinjuntti, T., Cummings, J. L., Masdeu, J. C., Garcia, J. H., Amaducci, L., Orgogozo, J. M., Brun, A., Hofman, A., Moody, D. M., O'Brien, M. D., Yamaguchi, T., Grafman, J., Drayer, B. P., Bennett, D. A., Fisher, M., Ogata, J., Kokmen, E., Bermejo, F., Wolf, P. A., Gorelick, P. B., Bick, K. L., Pajeau, A. K., Bell, M. A., DeCarli, C., Culebras, A., Korczyn, A. D., Bogousslavsky, J., Hartmann, A., & Scheinberg, P. (1993). Vascular dementia: Diagnostic criteria for research studies. *Neurology, 43,* 250–260.

Rosen, W. G., Terry, R. D., Fuld, P. A., Katzman, R., & Peck, A. (1980). Pathological verification of ischemic score in differentiation of dementias. *Annals of Neurology, 7,* 486–488.

Ross, E. D. (1981). The aprosodias. *Archives of Neurology, 38,* 561–569.

Sandson, T. A., Daffner, K. R., Carvalho, P. A., & Mesulam, M. M. (1991). Frontal lobe dysfunction following infarction of the left-sided medial thalamus. *Archives of Neurology, 48,* 1300–1303.

Schwartz, J. A., Speed, N. M., Mountz, J. M., Gross, M. D., Modell, J. G., & Kuhl, D. E. (1990). ^{99m}Tc-Hexamethyl-propyleneamine oxime single photon emission CT in poststroke depression. *American Journal of Psychiatry, 147,* 242–244.

Shindler, A. G., Caplan, L. R., & Hier, D. B. (1984). Intrusions and perseverations. *Brain and Language, 23,* 148–158.

Starkstein, S. E., Robinson, R. G., Honig, M. A., Parikh, R. M., Joselyn, J., & Price, T. R. (1989). Mood changes after right-hemisphere lesions. *British Journal of Psychiatry, 155,* 79–85.

St. Claire, D., & Whalley, L. J. (1983). Hypertension, multi-infarct dementia and Alzheimer's disease. *British Journal of Psychiatry, 143,* 274–276.

Steingart, A., Hachinski, V., Lau, C., Fox, A. J., Diaz, F., Cape, R., Lee, D., Inzitari, D., & Merskey, H. (1987a). Cognitive and neurological findings in demented patients with diffuse white matter lucencies on CT scan (leuko-araiosis). *Archives of Neurology, 44,* 32–35.

Steingart, A., Hachinski, V., Lau, C., Fox, A. J., Diaz, F., Cape, R., Lee, D., Inzitari, D., & Merskey, H. (1987b). Cognitive and neurological findings in demented patients with diffuse white matter lucencies on CT scan (leuko-araiosis). *Archives of Neurology, 44,* 36–39.

Strub, R. L. (1989). Frontal lobe syndrome in a patient with bilateral globus pallidus lesions. *Archives of Neurology, 46,* 1024–1027.

Stuss, D. T., Guberman, A., Nelson, R., & Larochelle, S. (1988). The neuropsychology of paramedian thalamic infarction. *Brain and Cognition, 8,* 348–378.

Suzuki, K., Kutsuzawa, T., Nakajinia, K., & Hatano, S. (1991). Epidemiology of vascular dementia and stroke in Akita, Japan.

In A. Hartmann, W. Kuschinsky, & S. Hoyer (Eds.), *Cerebral ischemia and dementia* (pp. 16–24). Berlin: Springer-Verlag.

Tatemichi, T. K., Desmond, D. W., & Mayeux, R. (1992). Dementia after stroke: Baseline frequency, risks, and clinical features in a hospitalized cohort. *Neurology, 42,* 1185–1193.

Tomlinson, B. E., Blessed, G., & Roth, M. (1970). Observations on the brains of demented old people. *Journal of Neurological Science, 11,* 205–242.

Tomonaga, M., Yamanouchi, H., Tohgi, H., & Kemeyama, M. (1982). Clinicopathologic study of progressive subcortical vascular encephalopathy (Binswanger type) in the elderly. *Journal of the American Geriatrics Society, 30,* 524–529.

Tresch, D. D., Folstein, M. F., Rabins, P. V., & Hazzard, W. R. (1985). Prevalence and significance of cardiovascular disease and hypertension in elderly patients with dementia and depression. *Journal of the American Geriatrics Society, 33,* 530–537.

Wallin, A., Alafuzoff, I., Carlsson, A., Eckernas, S. A., Gottfries, C. G., Karlsson, I., Svennerholm, L., & Winblad, B. (1989). Neurotransmitter deficits in a non-multi-infarct category of vascular dementia. *Acta Neurologica Scandinavica, 79,* 397–406.

Wolfe, N., Linn, R., Babikian, V. L., & Albert, M. L. (1990). Frontal systems impairment following multiple lacunar infarcts. *Archives of Neurology, 47,* 129–132.

Yamaguchi, T., Ogata, J., & Yoshida, F. (1992). Epidemiology of vascular dementia in Japan. Proceedings of the NINDS-AIREN International Workshop on Vascular Dementia, National Institutes of Health, Bethesda, MD, April 19–21. *New Issues in the Neurosciences, 4.*

13

Neuropsychological Evaluation of Subcortical Dementia

MARK R. LOVELL AND STANLEY S. SMITH

Introduction

Dementia is a condition that often afflicts the elderly, and the assessment of dementing disorders has become the pursuit of many neuropsychologists. The differential diagnosis of dementias of different etiologies through neuropsychological assessment has become a particularly fertile area of research and clinical activity. The term *subcortical dementia* has become increasingly popular as a descriptor of neurobehavioral decline secondary to neuropathological or neurophysiological changes in subcortical brain structures. However, the concept of subcortical dementia has been controversial and has undergone considerable revision and expansion over the past two decades.

This chapter reviews the concept of subcortical dementia with specific reference to neuropsychological evaluation of the geriatric patient.

Historical Perspective

Although neurobehavioral dysfunction has long been linked to subcortical brain structures (Naville, 1922; von Stockert, 1932), the term subcortical dementia was first formally introduced by Albert and colleagues (Albert, Feldman, & Willis, 1974) to describe a pattern of cognitive decline in five cases of progressive supranuclear palsy (PSP). Based on these cases, their past clinical experience, and a review of the literature at that time, Albert et al. (1974) identified four clinical features that distinguished the dementia of PSP from dementias whose primary site of neuropathology was presumed to be the cerebral cortex. These features included (1) slowness of thought processes, (2) forgetfulness, (3) apathy or depression, and (4) impaired ability to manipulate acquired knowledge. Subcortical dementia was further distinguished from cortical dementia syndromes by the relative absence of impairment of *higher cortical functions* (apraxia, amnesia, agnosia, and aphasia) in patients whose dementia involved subcortical brain regions. Albert et al. (1974) asserted that dementia syndromes that were the result of subcortical pathology were highly similar clinically to the dementia syndrome associated with bilateral frontal lobe disease, and that the pathological mechanisms that were at the basis of both of these syndromes involved timing and activation.

The slowness of thought processes that characterized PSP was pervasive and appeared to affect all other cognitive processes. Patients characteristically performed poorly on tasks that required verbal manipulation of information or perceptual motor skills only if held to strict time limitations. Their performance improved significantly if they were afforded extra time to complete the task. The mood changes that characterized PSP were described as falling into two categories: (1) depression or apathy, and (2) irritability and/or euphoria.

Albert et al. (1974) distinguished the "forget-

MARK R. LOVELL • Division of Neuropsychology, Henry Ford Hospital, Detroit, Michigan 48202. STANLEY S. SMITH • Department of Psychiatry, Medical College of Pennsylvania and Hahnemann University–Allegheny Campus, Pittsburgh, Pennsylvania 15212.

fulness" that characterized PSP from the amnesia frequently seen in cortical dementias such as dementia of the Alzheimer's type (DAT) as being related primarily to a disruption of mental processing speed rather than to an inability to form new memories per se. They observed that PSP patients typically performed normally on tests of recent and remote memory if given adequate time and encouragement when they were being tested for recall of the material. This was quite different from the pattern of cortical dementias such as DAT that were characterized by pervasive faulty encoding and retrieval of information.

Finally, Albert and colleagues (1974) identified a deficit in the ability to calculate, think abstractly, or otherwise perform intellectual tasks that involved the manipulation of acquired knowledge. These deficits in *fundamental functions* (i.e., processes related to the maintenance and regulation of level of arousal) were thought to be characteristic of PSP and were contrasted with deficits in *instrumental functions* that involved language, praxis, and gnosis. Fundamental functions were hypothesized to facilitate or modulate instrumental processes.

At approximately the same time that the original paper by Albert et al. (1974) described the subcortical dementia syndrome in PSP patients, McHugh and Folstein (1975) independently described a similar pattern of decline in eight patients with Huntington's disease (HD). They described a dementia syndrome that was characterized by a general loss of efficiency of thinking and memory, and a progressive apathy. Similar to the original description of intellectual decline in PSP described by Albert et al. (1974), McHugh and Folstein (1975) emphasized absence of aphasia, apraxia, alexia, and agnosia in HD patients. Later, Bowen (1976) highlighted the neurobehavioral deficits seen in patients with Parkinson's disease (PD). Although the cognitive difficulties experienced by those with PD had previously been attributed primarily to motor slowness or depression, there was increasing evidence that the neuropsychological decline seen in PD was unrelated to either motor slowness or depression. Bowen (1976) found primary deficits in concept formation, short-term memory, and set shifting without deficits in other domains of cognitive functioning. It is interesting to note that Albert (1978) observed that patients with PD showed a similar but less dramatic pattern of neuropsychological impairment than did normal elderly patients.

Later, Huber, Shuttleworth, Paulson, Bellchambers, and Clapp (1986) compared 14 patients who met diagnostic criteria for DAT with 38 patients with idiopathic PD and 20 normal control subjects on a neuropsychological test battery designed specifically to highlight differences between the groups. The test battery consisted of the Mini-Mental State Examination (MMSE; Folstein, Folstein, & McHugh, 1975), a battery of language tests, a motor sequencing task, Part A of the Trail-making test (Reitan, 1958), a digit span test, a paired-associates memory task, and the Zung Self-Rated Depression Scale (Zung, 1965). All subjects were comparable in age and in years of education. The three groups' performances differed significantly from one another on all but the digit span test and the registration portion of the MMSE, suggesting that any other group differences were not the result of differences in attentiveness. Both the Parkinson's group and the normal sample performed significantly better than the DAT group on word fluency, naming, vocabulary, orientation, motor sequencing and Part A of the Trail-making test. Both the PD and DAT patients performed more poorly than the normal sample on the MMSE, paired associates task, and the visuospatial task, but the degree of impairment was more severe for the DAT patients. Both PD and DAT patients had higher depression scores than the normal sample, and the differences between the two patient groups were not significant. Huber and colleagues (1986) concluded that subcortical and cortical forms of dementia could be differentiated neuropsychologically if specific tasks were used to evaluate cognitive processes across different multiple domains of cognitive functioning.

While the use of the term subcortical dementia was becoming increasingly popular during the late 1970s and early 1980s, the term was by no means universally accepted. Some neuroscientists believed that there was insufficient evidence of a dementia syndrome that was pathologically and clinically distinct from other dementing disorders. Several researchers hypothesized that many subcortical dementia syndromes were actually cases of DAT. For instance, Boller, Mizutoni, Roessmann, and Gambetti (1980) reported that the rate of histologically established brain changes demonstrating

Alzheimer's disease in autopsied patients was over six times (33%) the rate of DAT in an age-matched sample (5.1%). They suggested that the dementia observed in these patients prior to their deaths may have been attributable to DAT rather than to their Parkinson's disease. However, as pointed out by Cummings and Benson (1984), the senile plaques and neurofibrillary tangles that may characterize the neuropathology of DAT also increase with age in the brains of "normal" elderly patients who do not suffer from dementia. Their presence in the brains of PD patients does not mean that the cognitive difficulties demonstrated by this group were attributable to DAT. Mayeux, Stern, Rosen, and Benson (1984) also suggested that there was not sufficient evidence of a distinct syndrome of subcortical dementia. To support this belief, they compared over 100 patients with DAT, HD, and PD at different stages of progression of the diseases and did not find a specific pattern of neuropsychological decline in the HD or PD patients that was significantly different from the DAT patients, although the DAT group generally showed more impairment that did the other two groups. However, it should be pointed out that these researchers did not conduct comprehensive neuropsychological assessments and used only a modified MMSE to assess differences between the groups. Given the brief nature of the MMSE and its limitations as a differential diagnostic tool (Cummings, 1990), the failure of this test to discriminate different dementia syndromes is not surprising. Mayeux et al. (1984) also suggested that the term subcortical dementia was misleading because HD patients may have frontal lobe degeneration and DAT patients may have subcortical degeneration. However, as Cummings and Benson (1984) pointed out, what separates the two dementia syndromes is the *primary* site of neuropathology. For instance, the subcortical brain areas are known to have rich neuronal connections with frontal brain areas. Therefore, a lesion at any point in this frontal subcortical circuit may produce deficits that are consistent with subcortical dysfunction. Cummings and Benson (1984) further stressed the importance of understanding *functional systems* within the brain (i.e., brain areas that work in concert to produce a given behavior) rather than attempting to localize brain lesions on a strictly anatomical basis.

As mentioned at the beginning of this chapter,

the concept of subcortical dementia has been broadened over the past decade. While originally confined to PSP, HD, and PD, the term is currently used to describe a number of degenerative, vascular, metabolic, and demyelinating diseases. Table 1 provides a brief review of disorders that have been described as subcortical dementias.

One of the most intriguing hypotheses to arise from the literature in the last five years has been that depression represents a type of subcortical dementia (see Nussbaum, Chapter 17). This hypothesis has been based on several different lines of research. First of all, a number of researchers have documented similarities in neuropsychological test performance between individuals suffering from depression and those who have subcortical dementia syndromes (Massman, Delis, Butters, DuPont, & Gillin, 1992). Although patients with depression were well known to have difficulty in the area of memory (Danion et al., 1991; King, Caine, Conwell, & Cox, 1991), the memory profiles of these groups were quite different from the performance of DAT patients. In contrast to the performance of patients with DAT who have deficiencies in storage and encoding of new information, patients with depression typically perform much better on recognition memory tasks (King et al., 1991) and retain more information once they learn it. Depressed patients also have been observed to make fewer intrusion errors on verbal learning tasks (Wolfe, Granholm, Butters, Saunders, & Janowsky, 1987).

In addition to reporting similarities on neuropsychological test performance between depressed patients and patients with subcortical dementias, researchers have also pointed to the high incidence of depression in patients with classical subcortical dementia syndromes such as HD, PD, and PSP as evidence of the link between depression and subcortical brain areas (Caine & Shoulson, 1983; Mayeux et al., 1984). This link has also been established through neuroradiological and metabolic studies of individuals suffering from depression. In one such study, Coffey, Figiel, and Djang (1989) found a higher number of periventricular white matter abnormalities on magnetic resonance imaging (MRI) in elderly depressed patients compared to nondepressed patients. Using positron emission tomography (PET) scan data, Baxter et al. (1985) found a reduced rate of metabolic activity in the basal gan-

Table 1. Dementia Syndromes Thought to Reflect Primarily Subcortical Dysfunction

Disease process	Site of pathology	Mechanism
Parkinson's disease	Substantia nigra	Dopamine receptor loss
Huntington's disease	Caudate nuclei	Autosomal dominant gene that leads to progressive cell loss
Progressive supranuclear palsy	Globus pallidus, substantia nigra, subthalamic and red nucleus of thalamus	Neurofibillary tangles, fibrillary gliosis, demyelination
Multiple sclerosis	Multifocal sites throughout cortical and subcortical structures	Demyelination of neurons, thought to be due to defective immunoregulation
Wilson's disease	Lenticular nucleus, putamen, caudate, globus pallidus	Autosomal dominant gene that leads to dysregulation of copper metabolism
HIV dementia	Multifocal sites, basal ganglia	Immunodeficiency virus
Subcortical vascular dementia	Multifocal sites periventricular areas	Cerebrovascular disease

glia of unipolar depressives compared to non-depressed subjects. Similar results were obtained in a study that used single photon emission computed tomography (SPECT) (O'Connell et al., 1989).

Neuropsychological Assessment of Patients with Subcortical Dementia

Although the term subcortical dementia has been applied to a growing number of neurobehavioral disorders, the characteristic deficits that originally described the syndrome have remained the diagnostic cornerstones of this group of disorders. More recent neuropsychological studies have generally provided support for the central role of slowed processing, memory disturbance, executive functioning deficits, and affective changes in subcortical dementia, as well as comparing and contrasting dementia patients across different areas of functioning. This research has also investigated impairment of visuospatial processes in patients with subcortical dementias. Following a brief discussion of general assessment issues in working with geriatric patients, this section will discuss patterns of cognitive impairment in patients with cortical and subcortical dementias and will provide general guidelines for the selection of a neuropsychological test battery.

General Assessment Issues

Given the multitude of neurological disorders that can afflict the elderly and the potential impor-

tance of neuropsychological assessment in the diagnostic process, it is important to structure the neuropsychological evaluation in such a way that yields diagnostic information that is maximally useful in the differential diagnosis process. Assessment of elderly patients with suspected dementia can present a challenge to the neuropsychologist. As is the case with neuropsychological evaluation of all elderly patients, the ability of the dementia patient to participate in the neuropsychological evaluation process may be limited to relatively brief assessment strategies (see Lovell & Nussbaum, 1994, for a more thorough discussion of general issues regarding assessment of the elderly). On a practical level, the neuropsychological evaluation may be limited in time and scope by the patient's frailty or unwillingness to engage in a lengthy evaluation process. It is also important to recognize that dementia syndromes are often progressive in nature, and neuropsychological assessment strategies should be broad enough to allow for the measurement of the patient's cognitive deficits when they are mild, as well as when they become more severe, later in the illness. In addition, behavioral sequelae that typically accompany subcortical dementias (e.g., emotional lability, apathy, agitation) may require the examiner to limit the evaluation to a relatively brief time period. For this reason, most approaches to neuropsychological evaluation of patients suspected of having a subcortical dementia have been relatively brief, focused strategies rather than more comprehensive approaches that use lengthy test batteries. While we emphasize the importance of using relatively brief assessment approaches in this chapter, it is important that the assessment approach not be so brief that specific information regarding different cognitive domains of functioning cannot be gleaned from the evaluation. For instance, although useful as a component of the evaluation process, the MMSE should not be used in the absence of more domain-specific test instruments.

In the interest of both brevity and diagnostic utility, we have used a cognitive screening instrument in combination with individual measures that tap specific cognitive processes.

Although there are a number of screening instruments that are routinely employed in the neuropsychological assessment of the elderly, the Neurobehavioral Cognitive Status Examination (NCSE; Northern California Neurobehavioral Group, Inc., 1988) provides a brief, but broad-based assessment of cognitive functioning in the areas of attention, memory, language, constructional ability, verbal reasoning, and calculational ability. The NCSE is relatively unique among screening instruments in that the most difficult item from each domain of cognitive functioning is presented to the patient first. If this item is completed successfully, that portion of the evaluation is terminated. This screening item allows the examiner to obtain basic information regarding the patient's level of functioning in a very brief period of time. If the patient fails the screening item, the metric items are administered, which allows for a more thorough evaluation. The unimpaired patient can usually complete the NCSE within 10 min by passing all of the screening items. Completion of all of the metric items for an impaired patient usually takes from 20 to 30 min.

Another screening instrument that is useful as a tool for evaluating dementia is the Dementia Rating Scale (DRS; Mattis, 1988). The DRS is an instrument that appears to be particularly well suited for the assessment of subcortical dementia syndromes. The DRS consists of five general scales: attention, initiation/perseveration, construction, conceptualization, and memory. With the exception of the memory scale, more difficult items are presented at the beginning of each scale, which if successfully completed, allow the examiner to skip similar but less difficult items which immediately follow. The DRS is particularly well suited for assessing psychomotor and initiation deficits found in patients with subcortical dementias related to PD and Wilson's disease.

As mentioned earlier, use of screening instruments is not sufficient to provide detailed information that is likely to aid in differential diagnosis of cortical and subcortical dementias. Table 2 provides a listing of neuropsychological test instruments that are likely to be useful in this regard. Since the use of these test instruments in the evaluation of specific subcortical dementia syndromes will be more thoroughly discussed in other chapters in this text, only a brief review will be provided in this chapter. Although this table lists a number of tests which have proven to be useful, most approaches to assessment of subcortical dementias have used a subset of these tests that allows for completion of the evaluation in 1 to 2 hr.

Speed of Information Processing

Impairment of mental processing speed (bradyphrenia) has been described as the hallmark of subcortical dementia syndromes (Cummings & Benson, 1984; Huber & Shuttleworth, 1990). Although mental slowing does occur in patients with cortical dementias, it is usually less prominent than in the subcortical dementia syndromes. Differences between subcortical and cortical dementia patients have been substantiated through neuropsychological studies. For example, Beatty, Goodkin, Monson, and Beatty (1988) found that decreased speed of information processing was the most common finding in patients with multiple sclerosis (MS), as measured by the Symbol-Digit Modalities Test-Revised (Smith, 1982). Along similar lines, investigators have found impaired performance on scanning rate (Wilson, Kaszniak, Klawans, & Garron, 1980) and reaction time (Evarts, Teravainen, & Calne, 1981) in PD patients. More recently, Rao, St. Aubin-Faubert, and Leo (1989) found cognitive scanning rate to be significantly impaired in 36 MS patients. This slowing was independent of slowness secondary to motor involvement.

Neuropsychological assessment of information processing speed is complicated somewhat by the existence of a required motor response in many tests that purport to measure processing speed. For instance, the written portion of the Symbol-Digit Modalities Test-Revised (Smith, 1982) requires the patient to copy a series of numbers under the appropriate symbol, while under time pressure. For this reason, this task is as much a test of motor speed and

Table 2. Neuropsychological Tests that May Be Useful in the Assessment of Subcortical Dementias

Cognitive domain	Neuropsychological test
Information processing	Symbol-Digit Modalities-Revised (Smith, 1982)
	Trail Making Test-Part A (Reitan, 1958)
	Paced Auditory Serial Addition Test (Gronwall, 1977)
Attention and memory	Digit span scale from the WAIS-R (Wechsler, 1981)
	Visual Memory Span subtest from the WMS-R (Wechsler, 1987)
Verbal	California Verbal Learning Test (Delis, Kramer, Kaplan, & Ober, 1987)
	Hopkins Verbal Learning Test (Brandt, 1991)
	Rey Auditory Verbal Learning Test (Rey, 1964)
	Logical Memory subtest from the WMS-R (Wechsler, 1987)
Visual	Visual Reproduction subtest from the WMS-R (Wechsler, 1987)
	Recognition Memory Test (Warrington, 1984)
	Rey Complex Figure test-Recall Condition (Osterrieth, 1944)
Remote	Famous Faces Test (Albert, Butters, & Brandt, 1981)
Language	Controlled Oral Word Association Test (Benton & Hamsher, 1978)
	Boston Naming Test (Kaplan, Goodglass, & Weintraub, 1983)
	Token Test (DeRenzi & Vignolo, 1962)
Visuospatial and	Rey Complex Figure-Copy Condition (Rey, 1964)
constructional processes	Hooper Visual Organization Test (Hopper, 1958)
	Block Design scale from the WAIS-R (Wechsler, 1981)
	Judgment of Line Orientation (Benton, Hamsher, Varney, & Spreen, 1983)
	Clock Drawing test (Freedman et al., 1994)
Executive processes	Trail Making Test-Part B (Reitan, 1958)
	Wisconsin Card Sorting Test (Heaton, 1981)
	Similarities scale from the WAIS-R (Wechsler, 1981)
	Stroop Color Word Test (Golden, 1978)
Bradyphrenia	Symbol-Digit Modalities Test-Revised (Smith, 1982)
	Continuous Performance Test (Loong, 1988)
Depression	Beck Depression Inventory (Beck, Ward, Mendelson, Mock, & Erbaugh, 1961)
	Geriatric Depression Scale (Yesavage, Brink, Rose, & Lum, 1983)
	Zung Self-Rated Depression Scale (Zung, 1965)

coordination as it is of processing speed. Fortunately, the test can be administered so that an oral response is required rather than the copying of the numbers using paper and pencil. This makes this component of the test quite useful for evaluation of patients suspected of suffering from subcortical dementias. The Paced Auditory Serial Addition Test (PASAT) has been used as a test of information processing, particularly with head-injured patients (Gronwall, 1977). Although this test may be useful in younger patients with relatively mild symptoms, it has been our experience that this test is too challenging for elderly patients or for patients with more advanced symptoms. Part A of the Trail-making test (Reitan, 1958) also measures visual scanning and processing but has the disadvantage of requiring a sophisticated motor response, which may limit its

usefulness in patients who have impairment of motor processes.

Memory

Impairment of memory occurs in both dementia and subcortical dementia syndromes, but the severity and pattern of impairment may be quite different. Although there has been great progress in understanding the nature of memory impairment in subcortical dementia and how these conditions differ from the cortical dementias, questions still remain regarding specific similarities and differences between subtypes of subcortical dementia (e.g., PD, HD, PSP), and there is a growing realization that these conditions are not identical with regard to the effect of the disease on memory processes (Massman, Delis, & Butters, 1990).

Despite the need for continued study regarding memory impairment in differing subcortical disease processes, some general conclusions can be drawn from existing research. First of all, research has suggested that immediate memory or attention span is most often not impaired in patients with either cortical dementias such as DAT (Rosen, 1983), subcortical dementias related to HD (Caine, Ebert, & Weingartner, 1977), PD (Huber et al., 1986), or MS (Rao, 1989). Memory impairment has also been found to be more severe in DAT than in PD (Gainotti, Caltagirone, Massullo, & Miceli, 1980; Huber et al., 1986). In addition to differences between cortical and subcortical dementia patients regarding severity of impairment, the pattern of memory dysfunction may also be quite different in subcortical and cortical dementias. For example, subcortical dementia patients may demonstrate deficits in free recall that are similar to DAT patients. However, recognition memory is usually superior to free recall in subcortical dementia patients, and their performance improves if they are provided with cues (Butters et al., 1983; Helkala, Laulumeaa, Soininen, & Riekkinen, 1988; Wilson et al., 1987). In contrast, patients with DAT typically forget rapidly and are not aided significantly by cues (Butters et al., 1983).

In evaluating memory processes in the elderly patient, it is important to sample from as many aspects of mnestic processes as is allowed by the testing situation and the patient's ability to participate in the assessment. List learning procedures such as the California Verbal Learning Test (CVLT; Delis, Kramer, Kaplan, & Ober, 1987), the Rey Auditory Verbal Learning Test (RVLT; Rey, 1964), and the Hopkins Verbal Learning Test (HVLT; Brandt, 1991) are extremely useful and allow for assessment of multiple aspects of memory including immediate recall, learning with repeated trials, delayed free recall, and recognition. The CVLT and the RVLT have the advantage of distractor lists of words that allow for assessment of proactive and retroactive interference, but may be too difficult for more severely demented patients. The HVLT has the advantage of employing a shorter word list and having three rather than five repetitions of the list, but it does not have a distractor list. The HVLT also

has six relatively equivalent forms which allows for assessment of memory across multiple assessments.

Visual memory processes can be evaluated by a number of procedures that require a motor response or are relatively motor-free. The Visual Reproduction subtest of the Wechsler Memory Scale-Revised (Wechsler, 1987) provides an evaluation of visual memory under both immediate and delayed conditions. The stimuli are reproduced by drawing, and therefore the test requires a motor response. This requires that the neuropsychologist use clinical judgment in evaluating the contribution of mnestic and constructional processes in the patient's response. Similarly, the Rey Complex Figure Test (Rey, 1964) also requires the patient to draw the stimuli but is still useful in assessing visual memory. Recognition memory tests such as the Continuous Visual Memory Test (Trahan & Larrabee, 1983) and the Recognition Memory Test (Warrington, 1984) represent motor-free tests which can be used with elderly patients. However, these tests do not allow for the evaluation of free recall and are both somewhat time-consuming.

Although still in need of further investigation, past research into remote memory in patients with subcortical dementia syndromes has suggested that there is often impairment in this area in patients with PD (Huber et al., 1986), MS (Beatty et al., 1988), and HD (Albert, Butters, & Brandt, 1981). Remote memory has typically been assessed through the use of the Famous Faces and Famous Events tests (Albert, 1978), which evaluate the patient's recognition of faces and events associated with decades from the 1920s through the 1970s. Although these procedures are useful at the current time, the material contained within them is now somewhat dated and is in need of revision.

Executive Processes

The concept of executive processes refers to the ability of the individual to formulate goals (volition), plan, engage in purposive action to carry out goals, and effectively perform the goal and monitor the behavior (Lezak, 1995). Executive processes also involve the ability to shift conceptual sets and maintain attention. Impairment of executive processes has been described in patients with a number of presumable subcortical illnesses including PD

(Arnett, Rao, Bernardino, & Grafman, 1994; Beatty, Hames, Blanco, & Paul, 1995; Caltagirone, Carlesimo, Fadda, & Ronracci, 1991; Flowers & Robertson, 1985; Taylor, Saint-Cyr, & Lang, 1986) and MS (Beatty et al., 1988). Although executive functioning deficits are often common in cortical dementias such as DAT, impairment in this area is relatively less severe and is usually not the prominent neuropsychological deficit (Cummings & Benson, 1984). One study that compared patients with DAT, PD, and PSP (Pillon, DuBois, Lhermitte, & Agid, 1986) found that DAT patients performed significantly better on the Wisconsin Card Sorting Test than did samples of PD and PSP patients who were matched to the DAT group with regard to level of severity of the dementia. The high incidence of executive functioning deficits in patients with subcortical dementia is thought to underlie the close association of subcortical nuclei with frontal brain areas (Cummings, 1990).

Executive functions presumably involve multiple aspects of cognitive processes, and, therefore, assessment of executive processes should involve the use of tasks that tap these processes. As mentioned previously, the WCST has proven to be a particularly useful instrument. This test is not timed and therefore does not require motor speed to complete. Minimal motor coordination is also required to sort the cards. Abstract reasoning tasks such as the Similarities subtest of the Wechsler Adult Intelligence Scale-Revised (WAIS-R; Wechsler, 1981) assess verbal abstract reasoning and also provide useful information. The Stroop test (Golden, 1978) is also a useful measure of executive processes and provides further information about speed of information processing.

Language

Performance on formal tests of language is often used to separate subcortical and cortical dementia syndromes. Impairment of language processes can occur with both subcortical and cortical dementias, but the pattern of language impairment is often quite different. First of all, word finding impairment (dysnomia) is one of the hallmarks of DAT (Albert, 1981). Confrontation naming tests such as the Boston Naming Test (Kaplan, Good-

glass, & Weintraub, 1983) have been particularly useful in measuring impairment in this area. Auditory comprehension may also be impaired, particularly in the later stages of the disease. In contrast, dysnomia is rare in patients with subcortical dementias, but verbal fluency as measured by the ability to recite as many words as possible beginning with a given letter of the alphabet is characteristically impaired (Huber & Shuttleworth, 1990; Huber et al., 1986).

Clinical assessment of language processes should involve evaluation of comprehension, repetition, fluency, and naming. Comprehension can be evaluated informally by asking the patient to complete increasingly complex sequences of commands or it can be evaluated formally through the use of the Token Test (De Renzi & Vignolo, 1962). Repetition is evaluated by having the patient repeat increasingly long sentences. As mentioned previously, verbal fluency is often impaired in the subcortical dementias and can be easily evaluated through the use of the Controlled Oral Word Association Test (Benton & Hamsher, 1978). Dysnomia can be formally evaluated through the use of the Boston Naming Test although most screening instruments such as the NCSE or the DRS have visual confrontation naming tasks.

Visuospatial and Constructional Processes

Neuropsychological studies have documented impairment of visuospatial processes in patients with HD (Brouwers, Cox, Martin, Chase, & Fedio, 1984; Josiassen, Curry, & Mancall, 1983), MS (Rao et al., 1984), and PD (Gainotti et al., 1980; Huber et al., 1986). However, studies of subcortical dementia syndromes have been hampered somewhat by the motor requirements of many neuropsychological test instruments that purport to measure visuospatial processes (e.g., the Rey Complex Figure, block design tasks). Given the prominent motor impairment that exists in the subcortical dementias, these tests represent a potential impediment to evaluating visuospatial processes.

Several studies have used motor-free tasks to evaluate visuospatial processes in patients with subcortical dementias. For instance, Peyser, Rao, LaRocca, and Kaplan (1990) have recently suggested a relatively brief test battery (2 hr) that minimizes speed of motor responding as a major factor and uses relatively motor-free procedures such as the Hooper Visual Organization Test (1958) and a modified Block Design subtest from the WAIS-R (Wechsler, 1981). Benton's Line Orientation and Visual Form Discrimination tests (Benton, Hamsher, Varney, & Spreen, 1983) also represent useful and well-researched tests of visuospatial analysis which are motor-free. One method of evaluating constructional processes is through the use of tasks that require the patient to reproduce test stimuli by drawing them. The Rey Complex figure (Rey, 1964) is commonly employed for this purpose and also allows for the assessment of immediate and delayed memory processes. Constructional processes can also be evaluated with the Block Design and Object Assembly subtests of the WAIS-R (Wechsler, 1981). The Clock Drawing test (Freedman et al., 1994) is a relatively new test that requires the patient to draw the face of a clock in a given time. This test takes only a few minutes to administer and provides information on planning as well as on constructional processes.

Depression

Depression has often been associated with subcortical dementia syndromes related to HD (Caine & Shoulson, 1983), PSP (Janati & Appel, 1984), PD (Kostic, Djuric, & Covickovic-Sternic, 1994; Santamaria, Tolosa, & Valles, 1986), and MS (Beatty et al., 1988; Minden & Schiffer, 1990). Although depression is known to occur in cortical dementia syndromes such as DAT (Miller, Chang, Oropilla, & Mena, 1994; Sim & Sussman, 1962), depressive symptoms are generally thought to be less severe in cortical dementia than in subcortical dementia (Cummings & Benson, 1984). In contrast, depression is frequently observed in patients with subcortical dementia syndromes such as MS and PD (Cummings, 1990). The issue of mood disorders in subcortical dementia syndromes is a complex one due to the likely role of both brain-related factors (i.e., changes in brain anatomy or physiology) and environmental factors (i.e., reaction to having a chronic disabling illness) in the genesis of the illness. Currently, the exact contributions of these

factors are unknown and remain a topic of continued research and debate.

Traditional personality measures such as the Minnesota Multiphasic Personality Inventory-2 (MMPI-2; Hathaway & McKinley, 1989) have limited usefulness with elderly patients due to their length and the limited time usually available to complete the assessment. For this reason, brief rating scales have become quite popular in evaluating the elderly.

Depressive symptoms should be evaluated and can be accomplished through several self-rating scales such as the Zung Self-Rating Depression Scale (Zung, 1965) and the Beck Depression Inventory (Beck, Ward, Mendelson, Mock, & Erbaugh, 1961). The Geriatric Depression Scale (Yesavage, Brink, Rose, & Lum, 1983) represents a brief and particularly useful rating scale which has become popular over the last 5 years. The Hamilton Rating Scale for Depression (Hamilton, 1960) also provides a useful assessment tool.

Current Diagnostic Issues

In attempting to better understand subcortical dementia syndromes, it is important to recognize current diagnostic criteria and the limitations of these criteria. The most recent version of the *Diagnostic and Statistical Manual of Mental Disorders* (*DSM-IV*; American Psychiatric Association, 1994) lists the following criteria for a diagnosis of dementia: (1) Impairment must exist of multiple areas of cognitive functioning that include memory impairment and dysfunction in at least one other domain of cognitive functioning (aphasia, apraxia, agnosia, executive functioning); (2) impairment must be severe enough to result in dysfunction of social or occupational functioning (performance of activities of daily living, difficulties at work); (3) impairment must represent a decline from the patient's previous level of functioning; and (4) impairment cannot be secondary to a delirium.

Although *DSM-IV* provides separate diagnostic codes for subtypes of dementing conditions that are generally regarded as subcortical in nature (dementia due to HIV, Parkinson's disease, Huntington's disease), there is currently no diagnostic code for subcortical dementia. The application of current *DSM-IV* dementia criteria to the syndromes of subcortical dementia is problematic for several reasons. First of all, the assessment of whether or not there has been a significant decline in social or occupational functioning is highly subjective and difficult to measure uniformly. Second, unlike cortical dementia syndromes such as DAT and Pick's disease, many patients with diseases of the subcortical region do not develop full dementia syndromes, while they may have cognitive or emotional impairments that are meaningful. Cummings and Benson (1983) have therefore suggested the use of an alternative definition of dementia which does not emphasize a decline in social or occupational functioning. They emphasize objective assessment of the cognitive domains of memory, visuospatial processes, emotional or personality change, language, and cognition (i.e., intellectual processes) through the use of neuropsychological testing. Performance that falls two or more standard deviations below the mean indicates impairment. This is a pragmatic approach to defining dementia syndromes which may reduce confusion in the field.

Summary

This chapter has reviewed the concept of subcortical dementia from a historical perspective. We have also endeavored to provide a framework for neuropsychological assessment of subcortical dementia syndromes and have emphasized the use of neuropsychological assessment results in the differential diagnosis process.

The concept of subcortical dementia has contributed important information to our understanding of brain–behavior relationships in the elderly. To date, there has been much controversy about the neuroanatomical specificity of subcortical dementia syndromes. However, in our opinion, the label has clinical utility in separating patients with dementias of differing etiologies. The concept of subcortical dementia also has heuristic value and has promoted continued research regarding dementing disorders in the elderly. It is hoped that future research will lead to a clarification of diagnostic criteria for subcortical dementia and its continued acceptance as a separate diagnostic category.

References

Albert, M. L. (1978). Subcortical dementia. In R. Katzman & K. L. Bick (Eds.), *Alzheimer's disease: Senile dementia and related disorders* (pp. 173–180). New York: Raven Press.

Albert, M. S. (1981). Geriatric neuropsychology. *Journal of Consulting and Clinical Psychology, 49*, 835–850.

Albert, M. L., Feldman, R. G., & Willis, A. (1974). The "subcortical dementia" of progressive supranuclear palsy. *Journal of Neurology, Neurosurgery, and Psychiatry, 37*, 121–130.

Albert, M. S., Butters, N., & Brandt, J. (1981). Patterns of remote memory in amnesic and demented patients. *Archives of Neurology, 38*, 495–500.

American Psychiatric Association (1994). *Diagnostic and statistical manual of mental disorders* (4th ed.). Washington, DC: Author.

Arnett, P. A., Rao, S. M., Bernardino, I., & Grafman, J. (1994). The relationship between frontal lobe lesions and Wisconsin Card Sorting Test performance in patients with multiple sclerosis. *Neurology, 44*, 420–425.

Baxter, L. R., Phelps, M. E., Mazziotta, J. C., Schwartz, J. M., Gemer, R. H., Selin, C. E., & Sumida, R. M. (1985). Cerebral metabolic rates for glucose in mood disorders: Studies with positron emission tomography and fluorodeoxyglucose F18. *Archives of General Psychiatry, 46*, 243–250.

Beatty, W. W., Goodkin, D. E., Monson, N., & Beatty, P. A. (1988). Anterograde and retrograde amnesia in patients with chronic progressive multiple sclerosis. *Archives of Neurology, 45*, 611–619.

Beatty, W. W., Hames, K. A., Blanco, C. R., & Paul, R. H. (1995). Verbal abstraction deficit in multiple sclerosis. *Neuropsychology, 9*, 198–205.

Beck, A. T., Ward, C. H., Mendelson, M., Mock, J., & Erbaugh, J. (1961). An inventory for measuring depression. *Archives of General Psychiatry, 4*, 561–571.

Benton, A. L., & Hamsher, K. (1978). *Multilingual aphasia examination*. Iowa City, IA: The University of Iowa Press.

Benton, A. L., Hamsher, K., Varney, N. R., & Spreen, O. (1983). *Contributions to neuropsychological assessment*. New York: Oxford University Press.

Boller, F., Mizutoni, T., Roessmann, U., & Gambetti, P. (1980). The dementia of Parkinson's disease: Clinicopathological correlations. *Annals of Neurology, 7*, 329–335.

Bowen, D. F. (1976). Behavioral alterations in patients with basal ganglia lesions. In J. Yahr (Ed.), *The basal ganglia* (pp. 169–177). New York: Raven Press.

Brandt, J. (1991). The Hopkins Verbal Learning Test: Development of a new memory test with six equivalent forms. *The Clinical neuropsychologist, 5*, 125–142.

Brouwers, P., Cox, C., Martin, A., Chase, T., & Fedio, P. (1984). Differential perceptual-spatial impairment in Huntington's and Alzheimer's dementias. *Archives of Neurology, 41*, 485–490.

Butters, N., Albert, M. S., Sax, D. S., Miliotis, P., Nagode, J., & Sterste, A. (1983). The effect of verbal mediators on the pictorial memory of brain-damaged patients. *Neuropsychologia, 21*, 307–322.

Caine, E. D., & Shoulson, I. (1983). Psychiatric syndromes in

Huntington's disease. *American Journal of Psychiatry, 140,* 728–733.

Caine, E. D., Ebert, M. H., & Weingartner, H. (1977). An outline for the analysis of dementia: The memory disorder of Huntington's disease. *Neurology, 27,* 1087–1092.

Caltagirone, C., Carlesimo, G. A., Fadda, L., & Ronracci, S. (1991). Cognitive functioning in multiple sclerosis: A subcortical pattern of neuropsychological impairment. *Behavioral Neurology, 4,* 129–141.

Coffey, C. E., Figiel, G. S., & Djang, W. T. (1989). Subcortical white matter hyperintensity on magnetic resonance imaging: Clinical and neuroanatomic correlates in the elderly depressed. *Journal of Neuropsychiatry and Clinical Neuroscience, 1,* 135–144.

Cummings, J. L. (1990). *Introduction.* In J. L. Cummings (Ed.), *Subcortical dementia* (pp. 1–16). New York: Oxford University Press.

Cummings, J. L., & Benson, D. F. (1983). *Dementia: A clinical approach.* Boston: Butterworths.

Cummings, J. L., & Benson, D. F. (1984). Subcortical dementia: Review of an emerging concept. *Archives of Neurology, 41,* 874–879.

Danion, J. M., Willard-Schroeder, D., Zimmerman, M. A., Grange, D., Schlienger, J. L., & Singer, L. (1991). Explicit memory and repetition priming in depression. *Archives of General Psychiatry, 48,* 707–711.

Delis, D. C., Kramer, J. H., Kaplan, E., & Ober, B. A. (1987). *California Verbal Learning Test: Research edition.* New York: Psychological Corporation.

De Renzi, E., & Vignolo, L. A. (1962). The Token Test: A sensitive test to detect disturbances in aphasics. *Brain, 85,* 665–678.

Evarts, E. V., Teravainen, H., & Calne, D. B. (1981). Reaction time in Parkinson's disease. *Brain, 104,* 167–186.

Flowers, K. A., & Robertson, C. (1985). The effect of Parkinson's disease on the ability to maintain a mental test set. *Journal of Neurology, Neurosurgery, and Psychiatry, 48,* 517–529.

Folstein, M. F., Folstein, S. E., & McHugh, P. R. (1975). Minimental state: A practical guide for grading the mental state of patients for the clinician. *Journal of Psychiatric Research, 12,* 189–198.

Freedman, M., Leach, L., Kaplan, E., Winocur, G., Shulman, K. I., & Delis, D. (1994). *Clock drawing: A neuropsychological analysis.* New York: Oxford University Press.

Gainotti, G., Caltagirone, C., Massullo, C., & Miceli, G. (1980). Patterns of neuropsychological impairment in various diagnostic groups of dementia. In L. Amaducci, A. N. Davison, & P. Antvono (Eds.), *Aging of brain and dementia* (pp. 245–250). New York: Raven Press.

Golden, C. J. (1978). *The Stroop Color and Word Test.* Chicago, IL: Stoelting.

Gronwall, D. (1977). Paced Auditory Serial Addition Test: A measure of recovery from concussion. *Perceptual and Motor Skills, 44,* 367–373.

Hamilton, M. (1960). A rating scale for depression. *Journal of Neurology, Neurosurgery, and Psychiatry, 32,* 51–56.

Hathaway, S. R., & McKinley, J. C. (1989). *Minnesota Multi-phasic Personality Inventory-2.* Minneapolis, MN: University of Minnesota Press.

Heaton, R. K. (1981). *Wisconsin Card Sorting Test.* Odessa, FL: Psychological Assessment Resources.

Helkala, E. V., Laulumeaa, V., Soininen, H., & Riekkinen, P. (1988). Recall and recognition memory in patients with Alzheimer's and Parkinson's diseases. *Annals of Neurology, 24,* 214–217.

Hooper, H. E. (1958). *The Hooper Visual Organization Test.* Los Angeles: Western Psychological Services.

Huber, S. J., & Shuttleworth, E. C. (1990). Neuropsychological assessment of subcortical dementia. In J. L. Cummings (Ed.), *Subcortical dementia* (pp. 71–86). New York: Oxford University Press.

Huber, S. J., Shuttleworth, E. C., Paulson, G. W., Bellchambers, M. J., & Clapp, L. E. (1986). Cortical vs. subcortical dementia. *Archives of Neurology, 43,* 392–394.

Janati, A., & Appel, A. R. (1984). Psychiatric aspects of progressive supranuclear palsy. *Journal of Nervous and Mental Disease, 172,* 85–89.

Josiassen, R., Curry, L., & Mancall, E. (1983). Development of neuropsychological deficits in Huntington's disease. *Neuropsychologia, 40,* 791–796.

Kaplan, E., Goodglass, H., & Weintraub, S. (1983). *Boston Naming Test.* Philadelphia: Lea & Febiger.

King, D. A., Caine, E. D., Conwell, Y., & Cox, C. (1991). The neuropsychology of depression in the elderly: A comparative study of normal aging and Alzheimer's disease. *The Journal of Neuropsychiatry and Clinical Neuroscience, 3,* 163–168.

Kostic, V. S., Djuric, B. M., & Covickovic-Sternic, N. (1994). Depression and Parkinson's disease: Possible role of serotinergic mechanisms. *Journal of Neurology, 12,* 94–96.

Lezak, M. D. (1995). *Neuropsychological assessment* (3rd ed.). New York: Oxford University Press.

Loong, J. W. K. (1988). *The Continuous Performance Test.* San Luis Obispo, CA: Wang Neuropsychological Laboratory.

Lovell, M. R., & Nussbaum, P. D. (1994). Neuropsychological assessment. In C. E. Coffey & J. L. Cummings (Eds.), *Textbook of geriatric neuropsychiatry* (pp. 129–144). Washington, DC: American Psychiatric Press.

Massman, P. J., Delis, D. C., & Butters, N. (1990). Are all subcortical dementias alike?: Verbal learning and memory in Parkinson's and Huntington's disease patients. *Journal of Clinical and Experimental Neuropsychology, 12,* 729–744.

Massman, P. J., Delis, D. C., Butters, N., DuPont, R. M., & Gillin, J. C. (1992). The subcortical dysfunction hypothesis of memory deficits in depression: Neuropsychological validation in a subgroup of patients. *Journal of Clinical and Experimental Neuropsychology, 14,* 687–706.

Mattis, S. (1988). *Dementia Rating Scale (DRS).* Odessa, FL: Psychological Assessment Resources.

Mayeux, R., Stern, Y., Rosen, J., & Benson, D. F. (1984). Is "subcortical dementia" a recognizable clinical entity? *Annals of Neurology, 14,* 278–283.

McHugh, P. R., & Folstein, M. F. (1975). Psychiatric syndromes of Huntington's chorea: A clinical and pharmacologic study. In D. F. Benson & D. Blumer (Eds.), *Psychiatric aspects of neurologic disease.* New York: Grune and Stratton.

Miller, B. L., Chang, L., Oropilla, G., & Mena, I. (1994). Alzheimer's disease and frontal lobe dementia. In C. E. Coffey & J. L. Cummings (Eds.), *Textbook of geriatric neuropsychiatry* (pp. 389–404). Washington, DC: American Psychiatric Press.

Minden, S. L., & Schiffer, R. B. (1990). Affective disorders in multiple sclerosis. *Archives of Neurology, 47*, 98–104.

Naville, F. (1922). Etudes sur les complications et les sequelles mentales de l' encephalic epidemique, La bradyphrenic. *L' Encephale, 17*, 369–375.

Northern California Neurobehavioral Group, Inc. (1988). *The Neurobehavioral Cognitive Status Examination*. Fairfax, CA: Author.

O'Connell, R. A., Van Heertum, R. L., Billick, S. B., Holt, A. R., Gonzalez, A., Notardonato, H., Luck, D., & King, L. N. (1989). Single photon emission computed tomography (SPECT) with (123) IMP in the differential diagnosis of psychiatric disorders. *The Journal of Neuropsychiatry and Clinical Neuroscience, 1*, 145–152.

Osterrieth, P. A. (1944). Le test de copie d'une figure complexe. *Archives de Psycholgie, 30*, 206–356.

Peyser, J. M., Rao, S. M. LaRocca, N. G., & Kaplan, E. (1990). Guidelines for neuropsychological research in multiple sclerosis. *Archives of Neurology, 47*, 94–97.

Pillon, B., Dubois, B., Lhermitte, F., & Agid, Y. (1986). Heterogeneity of cognitive impairment in progressive supranuclear palsy, Parkinson's disease, and Alzheimer's disease. *Neurology, 36*, 1179–1185.

Rao, S. M. (1989). The neuropsychology of multiple sclerosis: A critical review. *Journal of Clinical and Experimental Neuropsychology, 8*, 503–542.

Rao, S. M., Hammeke, T. A., McQuillen, M. P., Khatri, B. O., Rhodes, A. M., & Pollard, S. (1984). Memory disturbance in chronic progressive multiple sclerosis. *Archives of Neurology, 41*, 625–631.

Rao, S. M., St. Aubin-Faubert, P., & Leo, G. T. (1989). Information processing speed in patients with multiple sclerosis. *Journal of Clinical and Experimental Neuropsychology, 11*(4), 471–477.

Reitan, R. M. (1958). Validity of the trail making test as an indicator of organic brain damage. *Perceptual and Motor Skills, 8*, 271–276.

Rey, A. (1964). *L'Examen clinique en psychologie*. Paris: Presses Universitaires de France.

Rosen, W. G. (1983). Neuropsychological investigation of memory, visuoconstructional, visuoperceptual, and language abilities in senile dementia of the Alzheimer's type. In R. Mayeux & W. G. Rosen (Eds.), *The dementias* (pp. 65–73). New York: Raven Press.

Santamaria, J., Tolosa, E., & Valles, A. (1986). Parkinson's disease with depression: A possible subgroup of ideopathic parkinsonism. *Neurology, 36*, 1130–1133.

Sim, M., & Sussman, I. (1962). Alzheimer's disease: Its natural history and differential diagnosis. *Journal of Nervous and Mental Disease, 135*, 489–499.

Smith, A. (1982). *Symbol-Digit Modalities Test-Revised*. Los Angeles: Western Psychological Services.

Taylor, A. E., Saint-Cyr, J. A., & Lang, A. E. (1986). Frontal lobe dysfunction in Parkinson's disease. *Brain, 109*, 845–883.

Trahan, D. E., & Larrabee, G. J. (1983). *Continuous Visual Memory Test*. Odessa, FL: Psychological Assessment Resources.

von Stockert, F. G. (1932). Subcorticale demenz. *Archives of Psychiatry, 97*, 77–100.

Warrington, E. K. (1984). *Recognition Memory Test*. Windsor: Canada: Nfer-Nelson.

Wechsler, D. (1981). *Wechsler Adult Intelligence Scale-Revised*. New York: The Psychological Corporation.

Wechsler, D. (1987). *Wechsler Memory Scale-Revised*. New York: The Psychological Corporation.

Wilson, R. S., Kaszniak, A. W., Klawans, H. L, & Garron, D. C. (1980). High speed memory scanning in parkinsonism. *Cortex, 16*, 67–72.

Wilson, R. S., Como, P. G., Garron, D. C., Klawans, H. L., Barr, A., & Klawans, D. (1987). Memory failure in Huntington's disease. *Journal of Clinical and Experimental Neuropsychology, 9*, 147–154.

Wolfe, J., Granholm, E., Butters, N., Saunders, E., & Janowsky, D. (1987). Verbal memory deficits associated with major affective disorders: A comparison of unipolar and bipolar patients. *Journal of Affective Disorders, 13*, 83–92.

Yesavage, J. A., Brink, T. L., Rose, T. L., & Lum, O. (1983). Development and validation of a geriatric depression screening scale: A preliminary report. *Journal of Psychiatric Research, 17*, 37–49.

Zung, W. W. K. (1965). A self-rating depression scale. *Archives of General Psychiatry, 12*, 63–70.

14

Alcoholic Korsakoff's Syndrome

MARLENE OSCAR-BERMAN AND DENISE L. EVERT

Introduction

Prolonged and heavy alcohol consumption is a well-known cause of brain damage and neuropsychological deficits (Talland & Waugh, 1969). Observations of brain images using techniques such as magnetic resonance imaging (MRi) and computerized tomography (CT) generally provide evidence of a relationship between extensive alcohol consumption and structural brain changes (Pfefferbaum & Rosenbloom, 1993). Similarly, results of neuropsychological tests sensitive to impaired mental processes after damage to particular brain systems have disclosed changes in cognitive abilities in chronic alcoholics (e.g., Walsh, 1994). One of the most tragic of the possible legacies of decades of chronic alcoholism is the severe neuropsychological condition Korsakoff's syndrome. Alcoholic Korsakoff's syndrome is characterized, most dramatically, by amnesia (memory loss), and it often is referred to as *alcohol amnestic disorder*. The amnesia of Korsakoff's syndrome does not encompass all memories equally. Instead, memory loss for recent events—anterograde amnesia—is considerably more severe than loss of memories for information learned prior to the onset of alcoholism—retrograde amnesia. Because patients with Korsakoff's syndrome have a permanent short-term memory impairment, that is, they are unable to remember new information for more than a few seconds, virtually nothing new is learned.

MARLENE OSCAR-BERMAN AND DENISE L. EVERT • Laboratory of Neuropsychology, Division of Psychiatry, and Department of Neurology, Boston University School of Medicine, Boston, Massachusetts 02118; and Psychology Research Service, Department of Veterans Affairs Medical Center, Boston, Massachusetts 02130.

Although amnesia is the most clearly defined and described symptom of Korsakoff's syndrome, Talland (1965) and Meissner (1968) have pointed to the inaccuracy of the classical description of the problem: "The defect can only loosely be said to be a defect in memory. The basic defect extends to much more than simply memory functions, and leaves some memory functions untouched" (Meissner, 1968, p. 6). Indeed, preserved memory capacities was a popular topic during the 1980s and continues to be one. Many investigators have demonstrated that patients with Korsakoff's syndrome are able to remember some things very well, for example, general rules for solving problems (Oscar-Berman & Zola-Morgan, 1980). Recent priming studies have explored the nature and extent of these preserved memories (e.g., see Cermak, Verfaellie, Letourneau, & Jacoby, 1993; Smith & Oscar-Berman, 1990; Verfaellie, Milberg, Cermak, & Letourneau, 1992). Beyond the amnesia in Korsakoff's syndrome, additional domains of cognitive impairments include visuospatial, abstraction, and problem-solving deficits and abnormal perseverative responding, that is, the unwanted repetition of a previous response or inappropriate behavior (see Evert & Oscar-Berman, 1995). Also, Korsakoff patients often are emotionally apathetic and may even appear unaware of their disabilities (Talland, 1965). In effect, they live permanently in the past, and they have few worries about their present difficulties.

Despite impairments in memory and other cognitive functions, overall intelligence, as measured by standardized IQ tests, usually remains intact in Korsakoff patients. This is because memories formed and skills acquired before the onset of prolonged heavy drinking remain preserved compared to those recently acquired. Thus, general intelligence is mostly spared, since the types of information and abilities tapped by IQ tests often rely on general knowledge easily retrieved from memories stored before the alcoholism began.

Alcoholics, whether or not they have Korsakoff's syndrome, may differ in their neuropsychological profiles and brain damage. Lishman (1990) and others (e.g., Arendt, Bigl, Arendt, & Tennestedt, 1983; Butters & Granholm, 1987; Butters & Jernigan, 1995; Wilkinson & Carlen, 1982) suggest distinct subgroups or clinical forms of alcoholics according to differences in the brain's vulnerability to alcoholism. These differences in vulnerability derive from two particular pathological influences which may operate independently in some people and interact in others. The first, characterized on brain scans as shrinkage of the cerebral cortex, as well as possible atrophy of basal forebrain regions (see Figure 1), is thought to result from the direct neurotoxic effects of alcohol. The second, characterized by damage to the diencephalon, is attributed to vitamin B_1 (thiamine) deficiency, which may cause blood vessels to rupture in that region. According to Lishman and colleagues, alcoholics who are susceptible to alcohol toxicity alone may develop transient or permanent cognitive deficits associated with cortical shrinkage (Jacobson, Acker, & Lishman, 1990; Lishman, 1990). Those who are susceptible to thiamine deficiency alone will develop a mild or transient Korsakoff state, with anterograde amnesia as a salient feature. Individuals with dual vulnerability, suffering from a combination of alcohol neurotoxicity and thiamine deficiency, will have widespread damage to large regions of the cerebral cortex, as well as to structures deep within the brain. These people will exhibit severe anterograde amnesia as well as other cognitive impairments, such as visuoperceptual abnormalities and decreased abstracting and problem-solving abilities (Jacobson et al., 1990; Lishman, 1990).

In the present chapter, we first describe Korsakoff's syndrome in the context of normal chronological aging, because the disorder occurs in middle to late adulthood (Talland, 1965; Victor, Adams, & Collins, 1971). Next, we describe etiologies, antecedents, and incidence of Korsakoff's syndrome. We then review the brain systems which have commonly been implicated in Korsakoff's syndrome. In describing the purported sites of damage, we also review evidence of concomitant neuropsychological consequences of damage to these systems. We conclude with a summary which emphasizes the presence of widespread brain damage and an array of neuropsychological deficits in alcoholic Korsakoff patients. We advise that prevention of the disorder be an important goal, because known clinical treatments have no proven efficacy for long-term benefit.

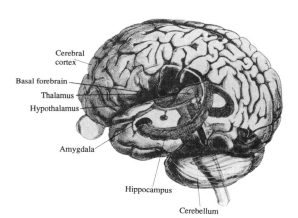

FIGURE 1. The brain structures that have been implicated in the amnesia of alcoholic Korsakoff's syndrome include parts of the limbic system (especially the hippocampus and amygdala), parts of the diencephalon (especially the mammillary bodies of the hypothalamus and the dorsomedial nucleus within the thalamus), and parts of the basal forebrain (especially the nucleus basalis of Meynert). Damage to the cerebral cortex and the limbic system may be responsible for additional abnormalities that have been observed in Korsakoff patients.

Alcoholism and Aging

It is important in considering alcoholic populations (with and without Korsakoff's syndrome) to be able to differentiate, describe, and quantify the separate contributions of aging and alcoholism to cognitive decline and brain changes. Alcoholism among the elderly—although not as prevalent as in other age groups—clearly is a serious problem (National Institute on Alcohol Abuse and Alcoholism, 1993). Wilkinson and Carlen (1982) compared radiological brain scans of non-Korsakoff alcoholics to those of neurological controls across five age decades. A striking characteristic of the brains of the alcoholics was abnormal ventricular enlargement and widening of the cerebral sulci. Of special interest was the fact that the ventricles and sulci became increasingly wider with increasing age both in the alcoholic and control groups. In the 1950s, Courville also described this feature of cerebral atrophy in the brains of alcoholics and likened it to brain shrinkage that occurs with normal chronological aging (see Courville, 1966). That is, alcoholics and normal aging individuals showed fairly uniform cortical atrophy, most prominent in the frontal lobes and extending backwards to the parietal lobes (the top and sides of the brain above the temporal lobes). This finding also has been reported by others (see Wood & Elias, 1982). More recently, Pfefferbaum and colleagues (1992) used MRI techniques and found evidence of increased brain tissue loss in alcoholics, compared with nonalcoholics, even after their age had been taken into account.

From the observed similarities in the brains of alcoholic and aging individuals sprang the search for parallels in functional decline associated with alcoholism and aging. The *premature aging hypothesis* (Parsons & Leber, 1982; Ryan, 1982; Ryan & Butters, 1986) has been put forth in two versions. Both forms of the premature aging hypothesis posit qualitative as well as quantitative parallels between certain neuropsychological changes due to aging and those due to alcoholism. According to the first version, the *accelerated aging* interpretation, alcoholism is accompanied by the precocious onset of neuroanatomical and behavioral changes typically associated with advancing age. Cognitively, or neuropsychologically, alcoholics become old before their time. The second version places the timing of the changes somewhat differently. In this view, which has been labeled the *increased vulnerability* interpretation, the aging brain is more vulnerable to the deleterious influences of toxic substances, including ethanol, than the brain of a younger person. Therefore, the cognitive decline associated with normal chronological aging (beginning at around age 50) receives added momentum from the effect of alcohol abuse. This version predicts that older alcoholics will be impaired compared to age-matched nonalcoholics and younger alcoholics; however, the same will not necessarily be true of younger alcoholics, since they will not have begun to manifest the changes associated with aging.

Does alcoholism cause premature aging, or do the behavioral consequences of aging and alcoholism merely mimic each other? So far, the literature relating the two types of pathological influence suggests that causality is unlikely (e.g., see Ellis & Oscar-Berman, 1989, and Ryan & Butters, 1986). In order to evaluate these hypotheses, we carried out a series of experiments on alcoholic and nonalcoholic men between the ages of 25 and 75 years and studied their perceptual, intellectual, and cognitive abilities (reviewed by Ellis & Oscar-Berman, 1989). Specifically, we looked for the differential effects of aging, alcoholism, and the interaction of aging and alcoholism on visual, auditory, and tactual perception, memory, and cerebral lateralization.

Results of our studies indicate that visual, auditory, and tactual processing and memory functions, as well as cross-modal associative functions, were more severely disrupted by aging than by alcoholism. The compounded effects of aging and alcoholism rarely were observed, and whenever we did find even modest support for the premature aging hypothesis, it was only for the version that posited an increased vulnerability with aging (Oscar-Berman, Hancock, Mildworf, Hutner, & Weber, 1990; Oscar-Berman, Pulaski, Hutner, Weber, & Freedman, 1990). Consequently, the concept of aging as a model for the study of alcoholism may have to serve chiefly as a metaphor.

It should be noted that patients with Korsakoff's syndrome had the most profound deficits on the tasks we gave, their deficits being more severe than those of the oldest of the alcoholics without Korsakoff's syndrome (Oscar-Berman, Hancock, et al., 1990; Oscar-Berman, Pulaski, et al., 1990). Interestingly, Wilkinson and Carlen (1982) indicated that the cortical brain morphology findings from patients with Korsakoff's syndrome were not age-related, as they were in alcoholics without Korsakoff's syndrome. This may be because patients with Korsakoff's syndrome already have suffered maximal alcohol-related brain damage, such that age-related cortical cell loss becomes irrelevant.

Etiologies, Antecedents, and Incidence of Alcoholic Korsakoff's Syndrome

Alcoholism is the most common cause of Korsakoff's syndrome. S. S. Korsakoff was a 19th-century Russian physician who observed amnesic patients with widespread brain damage from alcoholism (Victor & Yakovlev, 1955), but that was not the only cause of the syndrome that bears his name. Korsakoff noted other medical causes as well, including nutritional deficiencies, severe and prolonged gastrointestinal disturbances, and toxemia in pregnancy. Since that time, others also have reported cases of Korsakoff's syndrome in the absence of alcoholism (Ferrari, Baratelli, Colombo, Vitaloni, & Broggini, 1991; Okino, Sakajiri, Fukushima, Ide, & Takamori, 1993; Parkin, Blunden, Rees, & Hunkin, 1991). For example, Parkin et al. (1991) and Okino et al. (1993) described individual nonalcoholic patients who developed amnesia following severe gastrointestinal disease, intravenous feeding, and gastrointestinal surgery which is thought to be an important risk factor for thiamine deficiency. The patterns of the patients' anterograde and retrograde memory impairments were comparable to those observed in patients with alcoholic Korsakoff's syndrome. Similarly, Ferrari et al. (1991) described a nonalcoholic surgical patient who developed Korsakoff's syndrome as a result of thiamine deficiency during a lengthy course of intravenous therapy in the postoperative period. Additional rare causes of Korsakoff's syndrome that have been reported in the absence of alcoholism are intraventricular hemorrhage (Donnet, Balzamo, Royere, Grisoli, & Ali Cherif, 1992), thalamic infarction (Cole, Winkelman, Morris, Simon, & Boyd, 1992), T-cell lymphoma (Engel, Grunnet, & Jacobs, 1991), Creutzfeldt-Jakob disease (Pietrini, 1992), and multiple sclerosis (Vighetto, Charles, Salzmann, Confavreux, & Aimard, 1991). The focus of the present chapter, however, is alcoholic Korsakoff's syndrome.

In the acute phase, Korsakoff's syndrome often occurs together with Wernicke's encephalopathy; the diagnosis at this stage is Wernicke-Korsakoff syndrome. Wernicke's encephalopathy refers to alcohol-related brain disorder characterized behaviorally by general confusion, abnormal gaze and gait, and incoherent speech (Victor et al., 1971).

With abstinence and vitamin supplements (chiefly with thiamine), the encephalopathy clears, but amnesia usually persists. Korsakoff's syndrome does not always occur with Wernicke's encephalopathy. Blansjaar, Vielvoye, van Dijk, and Rijnders (1992) followed 44 patients with alcohol amnestic disorder, prospectively from 1987 to 1990, and found that 33 of the patients did not have the acute symptoms of Wernicke's encephalopathy nor a medical history to suggest its existence. However, because the encephalopathy commonly occurs with Korsakoff's syndrome (Victor et al., 1971), the term Wernicke-Korsakoff syndrome has been used synonymously with Korsakoff's syndrome. In about 75% of patients with acute symptoms of Wernicke-Korsakoff syndrome, anterograde amnesia persists and is irreversible (Victor et al., 1971). In general, Korsakoff's syndrome itself, with anterograde amnesia as the symptom standing in sharp contrast to other cognitive deficits described below, is not a common condition. According to one estimate, only 10 per million (0.001%) of patients admitted for the first time to a psychiatric clinic exhibited characteristics of alcoholic Korsakoff's syndrome (Centerwall & Criqui, 1978). Although statistics on the prevalence of alcoholic Korsakoff's syndrome vary, the incidence of severe alcohol-related brain degeneration, including Korsakoff's syndrome, is approximately 10% of adult dementias in the United States (Martin & Eckardt, 1985; Wells, 1979).

Since not all alcoholics develop Korsakoff's syndrome, some research investigators have suggested a possible genetic component, or inborn predisposition for its occurrence. Evidence in favor of a genetic predisposition for developing Korsakoff's syndrome revolves around the demonstration of an enzyme deficiency in Korsakoff patients, thought to be inherited, such that their bodies cannot use enzymes (e.g., transketolase) to metabolize thiamine efficiently (Blass & Gibson, 1977). In a recent study, Butterworth, Kril, and Harper (1993) found significant reductions of thiamine-dependent enzymes in autopsied cerebellar samples from alcoholic patients with a diagnosis of Wernicke-Korsakoff syndrome. The enzyme activities in brain samples from non-Korsakoff alcoholics were within normal limits and did not differ significantly from controls, thereby implicating abnormal enzyme metabolic processes in the pathogenesis of Wernicke-Korsakoff syndrome. Corroborating evidence comes from findings that thiamine deficiency in animals can lead to brain damage and memory impairments (Markowitsch & Pritzel, 1985; Witt & Goldman-Rakic, 1983).

Taken together, these findings suggest that people with a metabolic disorder that does not permit normal use of thiamine and/or individuals who do not eat enough thiamine-rich foods may be at risk for brain lesions and neuropsychological sequelae associated with Korsakoff's syndrome. However, when Blansjaar, Zwang, and Blijenberg (1991) examined transketolase isoenzyme patterns in Korsakoff patients, their relatives, non-Korsakoff alcoholic controls, and nonalcoholics, they found little evidence to support the hypothesis of an inborn enzyme abnormality in Korsakoff patients. In summary, there is some evidence for the role of thiamine deficiency in amnesia, but the link between abnormal thiamine metabolism and genetic inheritance of a predisposition for developing Korsakoff's syndrome is not decisive.

Brain Damage and Associated Neuropsychological Changes

In striving for a complete neuropsychological profile of alcoholic Korsakoff's syndrome, researchers have attempted to assess the relationship between (a) brain systems in which damage has been observed and (b) cognitive impairments. Associations between brain changes and cognitive deficits have been inferred, in part, from knowledge about the neuropsychological impairments known to occur from damage to specific brain systems. The type and extent of brain damage can be determined by close examination of the nerve cells themselves (neuropathological evidence) and by using MRI and CT scanning techniques that allow the brain to be viewed in vivo inside the skull (neuroradiological evidence). Other evidence can be obtained by using technology that is sensitive to measures of brain function (functional imaging techniques and electrophysiology). Functional brain imaging techniques have the ability to detect variables such as the flow of blood around the brain and brain metabolism. Electrophysiological measures are sensitive to brain electrical activity generated by nerve im-

pulses. Scientists use computers to translate the information obtained from these measures into meaningful pictures which, in turn, make it possible to view the functioning of the brain while an individual is thinking or performing a task. When applied to Korsakoff patients, most of these procedures—neuropathology, neuroradiology, and functional imaging—have shown brain shrinkage in the form of widening of the sulci and/or enlargement of the ventricles, as well as decreased blood flow and cerebral metabolism.

In an attempt to understand the mechanisms underlying the neuropsychological impairments in Korsakoff patients, scientists have considered the brain regions commonly believed to be damaged (see Figure 1). They include portions of the limbic system, especially the hippocampus and amygdala in the temporal lobes; parts of the diencephalon (e.g., the mammillary bodies of the hypothalamus and the dorsomedial thalamic region), a region of the brain nestled within the limbic system directly above the brain stem; neocortical regions; and basal forebrain structures (located just in front of the diencephalon) which are rich sources of neurotransmitters (Arendt et al., 1983; Charness, 1993; Lishman, 1990; Talland & Waugh, 1969; Victor et al., 1971; Walsh, 1994). These brain regions have different functions, and there is increasing evidence that damage to each system is responsible for specific realms of functional impairments in Korsakoff patients. However, there is a vast and complex array of pathways interconnecting different areas of the brain, and complex cognitive abilities can simultaneously involve attention, perception, motivation, memory, and other parallel functions. Therefore, the consequences of damage to one structure or system can involve multiple domains of functional abilities.

The Limbic System

The limbic system is a conglomerate of interconnected structures (including the hippocampus and amygdala) located deep inside the brain. Because the limbic system is a complex structure, its functions are diverse and varied. Memory loss similar to the amnesia in Korsakoff patients has long been associated with surgical lesions of the temporal lobe which include the hippocampus and the amygdala (Petri & Mishkin, 1994). Studies of hippocampal function have refined and broadened our understanding of the important role of the hippocampus in memory (Zola-Morgan & Squire, 1993). The role of the amygdala in memory functioning has not been established so definitively, but the association of stimulus and reward, a key ingredient in learning (Bower & Hilgard, 1975), is thought to converge in the amygdala (Murray & Mishkin, 1985).

In addition to memory impairments, anomalies most probably related to limbic system damage that have been observed in alcoholic Korsakoff patients include emotional changes and a reduced ability to integrate information coming in from more than one sense modality (e.g., cross-modal functions). Because emotional changes and cross-modal deficits in Korsakoff patients have been among the most inadequately researched of their abnormalities, they remain poorly understood.

A recent investigation of emotional functioning examined the ability of Korsakoff and non-Korsakoff alcoholics to identify and recognize emotional states from facial expressions and verbal utterances (Oscar-Berman, Hancock, et al., 1990). The stimulus materials were photographs of faces expressing one of four emotions (happiness, sadness, anger, or neutrality) and auditory recordings of sentences with emotional intonations or semantic meanings expressing the same emotions. The findings revealed significant deficits in visual and auditory emotional perception and memory by the Korsakoff patients, but only minor deficits in non-Korsakoff alcoholics. Thus, whether the emotional materials were pictures or sentences, the Korsakoff patients generally made fewer correct identifications and had poorer memory for the materials than age-matched nonalcoholic and alcoholic controls. The alcoholics and nonalcoholic controls over age 50 also performed poorly on many of the tasks, but well above the levels of the Korsakoff patients. In another study of emotional perception and memory in Korsakoff patients (compared to former heavy drinkers and light drinkers) no group differences in emotional responsiveness were observed (Douglas & Wilkinson, 1993). In one task of that study, the subjects were asked to respond rapidly to audiotaped emotional words by giving the first word that came to mind; then the subjects were asked to re-

member the associated words and rate them for likeability. In another task of the same study, the subjects were shown slides of men's faces paired with descriptor statements about an emotional or neutral activity, and the subjects were asked to imagine the man doing the described activity. In a subsequent recognition test, the subjects were presented with pairs of faces (one new; one not) from which to choose the familiar one; after making a choice, the subjects were asked to rate it for likeability. In both of the tasks, despite severely impaired memory performance by the Korsakoff patients, their patterns of emotional responsiveness were indistinguishable from those of the former heavy drinkers and light drinkers. The investigators suggested, therefore, that the notion of flattening of emotional responsiveness as a central characteristic of Korsakoff's syndrome needs to be reexamined, and that a distinction needs to be made between their expression of affect and their perception/memory of emotional stimuli.

The amygdala is important in integrating information from the senses. It sends and receives nerve fibers to and from brain regions involved in processing sensory information (Murray & Mishkin, 1985). To explore this multimodal aspect of amygdala functioning in Korsakoff patients, we examined cross-modal transfer—the ability to use one sense (such as vision) to learn something in another sense (such as touch) (Oscar-Berman, Pulaski, et al., 1990). Alcoholics with and without Korsakoff's syndrome were taught to choose specific forms or textures that they could see but not touch, or vice versa. These subjects were then asked to recognize the visual cues by touch alone and the tactual cues by sight alone. Patients with Korsakoff's syndrome had significant cross-modal impairments, a finding that is in keeping with possible involvement of the amygdala and functionally related regions of the cerebral cortex. Alcoholics and nonalcoholic controls over age 50 also displayed deficits but their impairments were mild compared to the Korsakoff alcoholics and therefore were attributed to decreased visual and tactual abilities unrelated to cross-modal functions per se. In contrast, another study of cross-modal functions found that patients with Korsakoff's syndrome were poor at identifying circles and arcs from tactile cues alone, but they did not differ from alcoholic controls in their ability to match the tactile feel of an arc with the visual appearance of a circle from which the arc was taken (Shaw, Kentridge, & Aggleton, 1990). However, in this same study, a group of patients with amnesia from encephalitis (which causes limbic system damage unrelated to alcoholism) was impaired only in the cross-modal identification task. The results of both studies (Oscar-Berman, Pulaski, et al., 1990; Shaw et al., 1990) are consistent with the notion that limbic regions in the temporal lobe are important for cross-modal functions. Since Korsakoff patients were impaired in one study (Oscar-Berman, Pulaski, et al., 1990), but not in the other (Shaw et al., 1990), it is possible that (a) the limbic system damage in Korsakoff patients is insufficient to account for all types of cross-modal deficits and/or that (b) cross-modal deficits do not necessarily result from limbic system damage in Korsakoff's syndrome.

The Diencephalon

The diencephalon is a region nestled in the center of the brain. It acts like a way station for nerve signals coming in and going out to many other areas of the brain. Although it is not known what role diencephalic structures play in cognition, including memory functioning, damage to this region has been clearly documented in amnesic patients with and without Korsakoff's syndrome (Butters & Stuss, 1989; Victor et al., 1971; Victor, Adams, & Collins, 1989). The main diencephalic areas that have been implicated in memory functioning are the mammillary bodies of the hypothalamus, the dorsomedial thalamic nucleus (Figure 1), and the nerve fibers connecting these two structures. These regions have been singled out for study because of their anatomical connections with the hippocampus and amygdala (known to be involved in memory functioning) and because structural damage in the diencephalon has been found in many memory-disordered patients (Butters & Stuss, 1989; Victor et al., 1989). For example, patients with acute, alcoholic Wernicke's encephalopathy who do not receive thiamine treatment may show evidence of hemorrhagic lesions within the region around the diencephalon (Butters & Stuss, 1989). In addition, amnesia has been associated with damage to dien-

cephalic structures following trauma, stroke, and brain tumors (Butters & Stuss, 1989).

In one study, Butters and colleagues obtained MRI scans from Korsakoff and non-Korsakoff alcoholics (Butters & Jernigan, 1995; Jernigan, Butters, DiTraglia, & Cermak, 1991; Jernigan, Schafer, Butters, & Cermak, 1991). The Korsakoff patients showed widespread reductions in gray matter volumes in addition to increases in cerebrospinal fluid, with greatest reductions observed in diencephalic structures. Volume losses in anterior portions of the diencephalon, medial temporal lobe structures, and the orbitofrontal cortex were found to differentiate best between the Korsakoff and control groups. (The cortical findings are described in the next section.) These findings were used to support both the commonly held view that damage to diencephalic structures is involved in anterograde amnesia and that other regions, such as the hypothalamus and hippocampus, may contribute to Korsakoff patients' amnesic symptoms as well (Brion, 1969; Petri & Mishkin, 1994). However, in a different study comparing MRI measures of diencephalic damage in alcoholics with and without the amnesia of Korsakoff's syndrome, it was found that diencephalic atrophy was of similar frequency in both groups (Blansjaar et al., 1992). Based on these results, the investigators suggested that diencephalic lesions develop regardless of whether patients acquire the amnesia of Korsakoff's syndrome and are not so much typical of Korsakoff's syndrome as they are of chronic alcoholism and malnutrition.

As noted earlier, several investigators have stressed the idea that diencephalic damage in Korsakoff patients is caused by thiamine deficiency, while cortical abnormalities (described in the next section) are caused by alcohol neurotoxicity or by other conditions associated with alcoholism (e.g., liver disease or head trauma). However, Joyce (1994) has stated that thiamine malnutrition affecting the diencephalon can account for all clinical forms of brain damage in alcoholics whether it is minimal cognitive impairment, amnesia, or dementia. With regard to the role of diencephalic damage in Korsakoff's syndrome, it is important to note that Korsakoff described neuropathology in the cerebral cortex, but he did not specify a subcortical locus of brain damage for the syndrome bearing his name. Rather, he described a set of neuropsychological characteristics in association with various etiologies (Victor & Yakovlev, 1955). The brain regions that have been implicated in the syndrome (mainly diencephalic structures) were described much later by investigators such as Brion (1969) and Victor et al. (1971, 1989) who used different neuropsychological criteria to classify the patients whose brains were later examined at autopsy. To date, controversy still exists with regard to the critical lesion site(s). Therefore, the idea that alcoholic Korsakoff's syndrome can be "neuropathologically confirmed" (e.g., Butterworth et al., 1993; Martin, McCool, & Singleton, 1993) without knowledge of ante mortem neuropsychological symptomatology may be misleading.

The Cerebral Cortex

In patients with alcoholic Korsakoff's syndrome, brain damage is not restricted to limbic and diencephalic regions. Rather, the damage is widespread and is thought to involve large regions of the cerebral cortex as well. In postmortem studies of neuropathology in alcoholics with and without Korsakoff's syndrome, Harper and colleagues have documented reductions in the volume of the cerebral cortex (Harper & Kril, 1993). Most of the tissue loss from the cerebral hemispheres could be explained as reduction of cerebral white matter volume (nerve fibers), but shrinkage of cortical gray matter (cell bodies) in the frontal lobes was especially evident at the microscopic level. Brain imaging procedures also have revealed cortical atrophy, manifested as a widening of the cortical sulci and enlargement of the cerebral ventricles (Adams et al., 1993; Butters & Jernigan, 1995; Cala, Jones, Mastaglia, & Wiley, 1978; Pfefferbaum et al., 1992; Volkow et al., 1992). The investigators who compared Korsakoff and non-Korsakoff alcoholics observed that Korsakoff patients had greater ventricular size, lower gray matter volume in the anterior diencephalon (i.e., hypothalamus) and basal forebrain nuclei (e.g., septal nuclei), and smaller gray matter volumes in mesial temporal and orbitofrontal cortex (e.g., Butters & Jernigan, 1995).

Morphological and structural imaging abnormalities in frontal brain regions of alcoholic Korsakoff patients have been frequently reported (see Pfefferbaum & Rosenbloom, 1993, for a compre-

hensive review). In addition, a study using functional imaging techniques also found evidence for frontal involvement (Hunter et al., 1989). Hunter and colleagues measured regional cerebral blood flow in Korsakoff patients. In comparison to nonalcoholic control subjects, Korsakoff patients showed a trend toward reduced blood flow (hypoperfusion) in frontal areas as well as several significant correlations between the degree of flow reduction in frontal areas and the degree of impairment on memory and orientation tests (less flow corresponded to increased impairments). Hunter et al. (1989) noted that the frontal hypoperfusion could mean that a normal tissue mass has reduced neuronal activity, that a reduced tissue mass has normal activity levels, or some of both. They further noted that since some CT and neuropathological studies point to structural loss of gray and white matter in the frontal lobes of Korsakoff patients, the metabolic impairment in this region probably reflects, at least in part, reduced tissue mass.

In most studies of Korsakoff's syndrome, neuropsychological deficits have been assessed independently of brain changes. As noted earlier, the importance of using both approaches (neuropsychological and structural) is to evaluate ideas about the connection between the locus of the damage and the nature of the decline in cognitive functioning in order to better understand brain–behavior relationships. In studies where both types of measures have been used, results have not revealed consistent convergence between structural damage and functional loss. For example, in the studies by Jernigan and colleagues, although several significant correlations were found between MRI measures and performance on cognitive tests, there was little evidence of a relationship between gray matter measures and cognitive test scores (Butters & Jernigan, 1995; Jernigan, Butters, et al., 1991).

There is abundant neuropsychological evidence of alcoholism-related cortical damage in Korsakoff patients. Examples of such deficits are difficulty with tests of problem-solving (Butters & Granholm, 1987; Oscar-Berman, 1973), spatial memory (Joyce & Robbins, 1991; Oscar-Berman, Hutner, & Bonner, 1992; Verfaellie et al., 1992), visual associations (Oscar-Berman & Zola-Morgan, 1980), and tactual learning (Oscar-Berman, Pulaski, et al., 1990). Butters and colleagues (Butters &

Granholm, 1987; Butters & Jernigan, 1995; Butters & Stuss, 1989) determined that long-term alcoholics with and without Korsakoff's syndrome had more difficulties with conceptualization, problem-solving, and visuospatial tasks than did short-term alcoholics and nonalcoholic controls. Korsakoff patients had the most severe deficits, but even short-term alcoholics performed more poorly than nonalcoholic controls, suggesting a continuum of impairments in these cognitive skills: The greater the lifetime consumption of alcohol, the greater the deficits in performance on the tasks. However, loss of memory skills did not fit the "continuity model," because there were a number of differences between Korsakoff and non-Korsakoff alcoholic groups which reflected qualitative, rather than quantitative, distinctions. For example, Butters and colleagues determined that while the inability of Korsakoff patients to learn new information involved an increased sensitivity to interference, the mild learning deficits in non-Korsakoff alcoholics did not reflect this process. Further, the amnesia in Korsakoff patients was determined to be neither modality-specific nor material-specific, whereas memory impairments in alcoholics were more pronounced with visuospatial information than verbal information. They also found a small group of alcoholics, called borderline Korsakoffs, with amnesic symptoms severe enough for a clinical diagnosis of Korsakoff's syndrome, but not severe enough to interfere with their daily activities. Borderline Korsakoffs did not perform as poorly on anterograde memory tests as did Korsakoff patients, nor did they show a pattern of rapid forgetting and mild retrograde amnesia characteristic of Korsakoff's syndrome. Based on all of these findings, Butters proposed that the continuity model was applicable only to alcoholics' visuoperceptual and conceptual deficits consequent to cortical damage. For these cognitive abilities, the greater the lifetime consumption of alcohol, the greater the deficits in performance. For memory, the continuity model was thought to be invalid. Long-term alcoholism resulted in mild memory problems, but some acute event (e.g., thiamine deficiency and resultant hemorrhagic brain lesions) was needed to produce the Korsakoff amnesia.

Neuropsychological evidence of damage to cortical regions in Korsakoff patients has implicated the frontal lobes more than any other brain area. Korsakoff patients show clinical signs associated with damage to frontal brain systems, for example, disinhibition, reduced attention and susceptibility to interference, poor judgment and planning abilities, and abnormal response perseveration (see Butters, Granholm, Salmon, & Grant, 1987; Evert & Oscar-Berman, 1995; and National Institute on Alcohol Abuse and Alcoholism, in press, for reviews). Delis, Squire, Bihrle, and Massman (1992) compared the performance of Korsakoff patients with that of patients with frontal lobe lesions on a multicomponent sorting task designed to test frontal functioning by isolating and measuring specific components of problem-solving ability. The investigators found that both groups of patients were impaired on eight of the nine components of the task, suggesting that a range of diverse deficits (in abstract thinking, cognitive flexibility, and behavior regulation) contributes to the problem-solving impairments of these patients.

Neuropsychological evidence of frontal system damage in Korsakoff patients has raised the possibility that it may play a role—as yet undefined—in their anterograde amnesia. To test this notion, Joyce and Robbins (1991) tested Korsakoff and non-Korsakoff alcoholics on traditional neuropsychological tests of frontal lobe function and on computerized tests of planning (Tower of London task) and spatial working memory, both of which are also sensitive to frontal damage. The Korsakoff patients demonstrated deficits on the planning task which could not be explained by abnormalities of memory including spatial span, nor by visuoperceptual disturbances. The investigators interpreted their findings as support for the view that in alcoholic Korsakoff's syndrome, in addition to amnesia, there is a specific disturbance of frontal lobe function, characterized by poor strategy organization and abnormal perseveration. Impairments shown by the alcoholic controls, in contrast, did not reflect specific frontal dysfunction. In another study, Shimamura, Janowsky, and Squire (1991) compared Korsakoff patients, non-Korsakoff amnesics, and frontal lobe patients on the Initiation-Perseveration Index of the Dementia Rating Scale (Mattis, 1976). They found that the Korsakoff patients were as impaired as the frontal patients. The Korsakoff and non-Korsakoff amnesic patients were impaired on the Memory Index of the same test, whereas the frontal patients were not, supporting the view that abnormal perseverative responding is dissociable from poor performance on certain tests of memory.

Research using tests that are highly sensitive to frontal lobe damage in monkeys also supports the view of frontal system dysfunction in alcoholic Korsakoff's syndrome (Oscar-Berman et al., 1992; see Oscar-Berman & Hutner, 1993, for review). In our laboratory, for example, we conducted a series of experiments to assess frontal integrity in a simple and direct way; we used classical delayed reaction tasks such as delayed response (DR) and delayed alternation (DA) (reviewed by Oscar-Berman, 1994, and Oscar-Berman, McNamara, & Freedman, 1991). We selected the paradigms precisely because of their special sensitivity to frontal system damage, especially perseverative responding. Abnormal perseverative responding is thought to underlie frontal patients' deficits on many tasks, including DR and DA. Furthermore, successful performance on DR and DA tasks is known to rely upon different underlying neuroanatomical and neuropsychological mechanisms. Specifically, there are at least two subsystems within the frontal lobes: a dorsolateral system and an orbitofrontal system (on the ventral surface). While the dorsolateral system contains intimate connections with other neocortical sites, its connections with limbic sites are less striking than those of the orbitofrontal system. The dorsolateral system, although important for successful performance on both DR and DA, is especially important for DR performance, in which visuospatial, mnemonic, and attentional functions are considered critical. By contrast, functions involved in response inhibition have been linked to the orbitofrontal system. The orbitofrontal system is intimately connected with basal forebrain and limbic structures; its connections with other neocortical regions are not as extensive as those of the dorsolateral system. The orbitofrontal system, like the dorsolateral system, supports successful performance on both DA and DR, but it is especially important for DA. It should be emphasized, however, that the dorsolateral/orbitofrontal dichotomy described here is not all-or-none and is intended only as a useful way of viewing frontal system diversity (Oscar-Berman et al., 1991).

We examined the performance of Korsakoff patients on these tasks to assess possible frontal dysfunction in alcoholic amnesia. We also studied a number of other patient groups. A group of patients with CT-documented bilateral frontal lobe lesions was included to establish baseline levels attributable to known prefrontal pathology; another group of patients with left frontal lesions and Broca's aphasia was included to determine whether intact language was critical for successful performance; a third group with amnesia from anterior communicating artery disease was included to assess the contribution of amnesia unrelated to alcoholism (Freedman & Oscar-Berman, 1986). Results from the bilateral frontal patients supported other findings (Pribram, Ahumada, Hartog, & Roos, 1964) that frontal lobotomies lead to DA deficits. Our bilateral frontal patients had the most severe deficits on DA and DR, but Korsakoff patients also were impaired on both. Deficits on delayed reaction tasks correlated with independent measures of perseverative responding (on the Wisconsin Card Sorting Test; Heaton, 1981), but did not correlate with short-term memory loss (Wechsler Memory Scale scores) or loss of expressive language (Broca's aphasia). This pattern of results suggested not only that perseveration is dissociable from memory and expressive language skills, but also that deficits by Korsakoff patients on DA and DR were due to brain damage separable from that causing amnesia (see also Bowden, 1990). In a later experiment (Oscar-Berman et al., 1992), we presented the DR task in two sensory modalities (vision and audition) to extend the generality of the findings. Korsakoff patients showed impairments in both modalities.

Other Brain Systems

Neurons interact with one another through the release and uptake of neurotransmitters. There are many different types of neurotransmitters which originate in several central systems of the brain. Neurotransmitters play important roles in memory functioning. The major neurotransmitters purported to be involved in memory functioning are those of the cholinergic, catecholaminergic, and serotonergic systems. Although no definitive conclusions have been drawn about relationships between memory loss and abnormalities in these neurotransmitter systems, the research findings have suggested interesting avenues for possible treatment.

A major source of a cholinergic neurotransmitter, acetylcholine, thought to be important for normal memory functioning, is the nucleus basalis of Meynert located in the basal forebrain (in front of the diencephalon; see Figure 1). The nucleus basalis of Meynert connects with other regions of the brain (such as the hippocampus and cerebral cortex) implicated in memory functioning. Acetylcholine deficiency in the nucleus basalis of Meynert has been linked to memory disturbances in alcoholic Korsakoff patients (Arendt, 1993), and damage to the nucleus basalis of Meynert and adjacent sites has been linked to memory disturbances in Alzheimer's patients and in patients with ruptured anterior communicating artery aneurysms (Arendt et al., 1983; Damasio, Graff-Radford, Eslinger, Damasio, & Kassell, 1985; Gade, 1982). Administration of anticholinergic drugs to healthy subjects produces temporary cognitive deficits that resemble Korsakoff's amnesia (Kopelman, 1985). Based on the relationship between cholinergic deficiency and memory impairments, investigators have attempted to improve memory in alcoholic Korsakoff patients using substances that increase cholinergic functioning. For example, in a study using thyrotropin-releasing hormone (TRH) to enhance cholinergic transmission, Khan, Mirolo, Claypoole, and Hughes (1993) gave the hormone to chronic alcoholics who exhibited memory impairments. The researchers found that only patients with a shorter duration of alcohol use (mean of 16 years) performed significantly better with TRH (as compared with a placebo) on a test involving verbal learning and memory. The alcoholics with a more chronic history (mean of 27 years) did not show such a response. In a study of thyrotropin responses to TRH by alcoholics with and without Korsakoff's syndrome, Thakore and Dinan (1993) found that 45% of patients with alcoholic Korsakoff's syndrome and 18% of non-Korsakoff alcoholics had a blunted response to TRH and also to a thyroid-stimulating hormone stimulation test.

Korsakoff patients also have reduced cerebrospinal fluid levels of catecholamine metabolites that correlate with memory loss. Administration of catecholaminergic agents appears to facilitate memory processing in these patients by increasing attention (see Martin & Nimmerrichter, 1993). However, Halliday, Ellis, and Harper (1992) conducted a postmortem analysis of neurons in the brain stem locus ceruleus—a source of catecholamines—in chronic alcoholics with and without a history of memory impairment suggestive of Korsakoff's syndrome, and they found no evidence of significant cellular pathology. Administration of serotonergic agents has facilitated memory processes in some impaired alcoholics, but only with temporary effects (Martin & Nimmerrichter, 1993). Degeneration has been shown in serotonin-rich regions of the brain stem of alcoholics, but the pathology was evident regardless of history of memory impairment (Halliday, Ellis, Heard, Caine, & Harper, 1993). Thus, alcohol-associated damage to serotonergic neuronal populations in the brain may not contribute to memory impairment, or serotonin administration may facilitate memory functioning indirectly (e.g., by increasing attention). Future research on the role of neurotransmitter systems in specific neuropsychological functions will help direct strategies for treating neurological disorders related to alcoholism, as well as for understanding the brain mechanisms involved in normal and abnormal memory processes.

Future Directions for Clinical Research

Clinicians hope that research on the causes, development, and behavioral manifestations of neurological disorders will lay the groundwork for improved diagnosis and treatment (Oscar-Berman, 1988). With regard to Korsakoff's syndrome, some progress has been made toward applying research outcomes directly to treatment of the amnesia. As was discussed, numerous pharmacological treatments have been applied in an attempt to improve memory, with varying results (Martin & Nimmerrichter, 1993; McEntee & Mair, 1990); future research is needed in this area. Clinicians and researchers also have considered strategies for prevention of alcoholic Korsakoff's syndrome (Bond & Homewood, 1991). For example, in Australia, there is controversy regarding whether flour and alcoholic beverages should be fortified with thiamine in an attempt to prevent Wernicke's encephalopathy and Korsakoff's syndrome (Bond & Homewood, 1991; Clark, 1990). The debate mainly centers on two issues: (1) the as-yet unproven relationship between thiamine deficiency and amnesia and (2) the difficulty in establishing cost-effectiveness for implementation of dietary fortification (see Bowden, 1990; Clark, 1990; Dignam, 1991; Wodak, Richmond, & Wilson, 1990; Yellowlees, 1990).

So far, results from studies of treatments to improve memory functioning show no consistent trends. The inconsistencies may be due in part to different criteria used across laboratories for establishing alcohol-related memory impairments, as well as the diversity within the samples of alcoholics studied. Nonetheless, with abstinence some alcoholics show a slow reversal of neuropsychological symptoms (Drake et al., 1995) and brain atrophy (Butters & Jernigan, 1995). For this reason, limited intake of alcohol is strongly recommended to prevent the occurrence of permanent abnormalities.

Summary

Korsakoff's syndrome is characterized primarily by a severe anterograde amnesia, and it occurs more often with prolonged alcoholism than from other etiologies. In alcoholic Korsakoff's syndrome, additional neuropsychological changes occur as well, including emotional abnormalities and cognitive impairments in visuospatial functioning, problem-solving, and other abilities. Alcoholics who do not develop Korsakoff's syndrome may exhibit some of the same nonamnesic symptoms as patients with Korsakoff's syndrome, but not nearly with the same severity. Alcoholism does not seem to accelerate chronological aging, although older non-Korsakoff alcoholics may be more vulnerable to cognitive decline than younger alcoholics. The amnesia in alcoholic Korsakoff patients is thought to be caused mainly by subcortical damage to structures in the limbic system, diencephalon, and/or basal forebrain; the additional neuropsychological changes probably reflect cortical dysfunction (especially in prefrontal brain systems), as well as limbic system damage. Since neuropsychological impairments have not consistently responded to experimental treatments, the best method of prevention of alcohol-related brain damage is the judicious use of alcohol.

ACKNOWLEDGMENTS

Preparation of this article was supported in part by funds from the National Institute on Alcohol Abuse and Alcoholism (R01 AA07112); a training grant from the National Institute on Deafness and Other Communication Disorders (T32 DC00017); and the Medical Research Service of the U.S. Department of Veterans Affairs.

References

Adams, K. M., Gilman, S., Koeppe, R. A., Kluin, K. J., Brunberg, J. A., Dede, D., Berent, S., & Kroll, P. D. (1993). Neuropsychological deficits are correlated with frontal hypometabolism in positron emission tomography studies in older alcoholic patients. *Alcoholism: Clinical and Experimental Research, 17,* 205–210.

Arendt, T. (1993). The cholinergic deafferentation of the cerebral cortex induced by chronic consumption of alcohol: Reversed by cholinergic drugs and transplantation. In W. A. Hunt & S. J. Nixon (Eds.), *Alcohol-induced brain damage.* NIAAA research monograph No. 22 (pp. 431–460). Rockville, MD: USDHHS, NIH Publication No. 93-3549.

Arendt, T., Bigl, V., Arendt, A., & Tennestedt, A. (1983). Loss of neurons in the nucleus basalis of Meynert in Alzheimer's disease, paralysis agitans, and Korsakoff's disease. *Acta Neuropathologica, 61,* 101–108.

Blansjaar, B. A., Zwang, R., & Blijenberg, B. G. (1991). No transketolase abnormalities in Wernicke-Korsakoff patients. *Journal of Neurological Sciences, 106,* 88–90.

Blansjaar, B. A., Vielvoye, G. J., van Dijk, J. G., & Rijnders, R. J. (1992). Similar brain lesions in alcoholics and Korsakoff patients: MRI, psychometric, and clinical findings. *Clinical Neurology and Neurosurgery, 94,* 197–203.

Blass, J. P., & Gibson, G. E. (1977). Abnormality of a thiamin-requiring enzyme in patients with Wernicke-Korsakoff syndrome. *New England Journal of Medicine, 297,* 1367–1370.

Bond, N. W., & Homewood, J. (1991). Wernicke's encephalopathy and Korsakoff's psychosis: To fortify or not to fortify? *Neurotoxicology and Teratology, 13,* 353–355.

Bowden, S. C. (1990). Separating cognitive impairment in neurologically asymptomatic alcoholism from Wernicke-Korsakoff syndrome. Is the neuropsychological distinction justified? *Psychological Bulletin, 107,* 355–366.

Bower, G. H., & Hilgard, E. R. (1975). *Theories of learning.* Englewood Cliffs, NJ: Prentice Hall.

Brion, S. (1969). Korsakoff's syndrome: Clinico-anatomical and physiopathological considerations. In G. A. Talland & N. C. Waugh (Eds.), *The pathology of memory* (pp. 29–39). New York: Academic Press.

Butters, N., & Granholm, E. (1987). The continuity hypothesis: Some conclusions and their implications for the etiology and neuropathology of alcoholic Korsakoff's syndrome. In O. A. Parsons, N. M. Butters, & P. Nathan (Eds.), *Neuropsychology of alcoholism: Implications for diagnosis and treatment* (pp. 176–206). New York: Guilford Press.

Butters, N., & Jernigan. T. (1995, June). *Cognitive and morphometric features of long-term alcoholics with and without Korsakoff's syndrome.* Paper presented at the Annual Scientific Meeting, Research Society on Alcoholism, Steamboat Springs, CO.

Butters, N., & Stuss, D. T. (1989). Diencephalic amnesia. In F. Boller & J. Grafman (Eds.), *Handbook of neuropsychology* (Vol. 3, pp. 107–148). New York: Elsevier Science Publishers.

Butters, N., Granholm, E., Salmon, D. P., & Grant, I. (1987). Episodic and semantic memory: A comparison of amnesic and demented patients. *Journal of Clinical and Experimental Neuropsychology, 5,* 479–497.

Butterworth, R. F., Kril, J. J., & Harper, C. G. (1993). Thiamine-dependent enzyme changes in the brains of alcoholics: Relationship to the Wernicke-Korsakoff syndrome. *Alcoholism: Clinical and Experimental Research, 17,* 1084–1088.

Cala, L. A., Jones, B., Mastaglia, F. L., & Wiley, B. (1978). Brain atrophy and intellectual impairment in heavy drinkers: A clinical, psychometric and computerized tomography study. *Australian/New Zealand Journal of Medicine, 8,* 147–153.

Centerwall, B. S., & Criqui, M. H. (1978). Prevention of the Wernicke-Korsakoff syndrome. A cost-benefit analysis. *New England Journal of Medicine, 299,* 285–289.

Cermak, L. S., Verfaellie, M., Letourneau, L., & Jacoby, L. L. (1993). Episodic effects on picture identification for alcoholic Korsakoff patients. *Brain and Cognition, 22,* 85–97.

Charness, M. E. (1993). Brain lesions in alcoholics. *Alcoholism: Clinical and Experimental Research, 17,* 2–11.

Clark, A. L. (1990). Thiamine in our bread and wine? *Medical Journal of Australia, 153,* 115.

Cole, M., Winkelman, M. D., Morris, J. C., Simon, J. E., & Boyd, T. A. (1992). Thalamic amnesia: Korsakoff syndrome due to left thalamic infarction. *Journal of the Neurological Sciences, 110,* 62–67.

Courville, C. B. (1966). *Effects of alcohol on the nervous system of man.* Los Angeles, CA: San Lucas Press.

Damasio, A. R., Graff-Radford, N. R., Eslinger, P. J., Damasio, H., & Kassell, N. (1985). Amnesia following basal forebrain lesions. *Archives of Neurology, 3,* 263–271.

Delis, D. C., Squire, L. R., Bihrle, A., & Massman, P. (1992). Componential analysis of problem-solving ability: Performance of patients with frontal lobe damage and amnesic patients on a new sorting test. *Neuropsychologia, 30,* 683–697.

Dignam, P. (1991). Thiamine in our bread and wine. *Medical Journal of Australia, 155,* 205–206.

Donnet, A., Balzamo, M., Royere, M. L., Grisoli, F., & Ali Cherif, A. (1992). Transient Korsakoff's syndrome after intraventricular hemorrhage [on-line]. *Neurochirurgie, 38,* 102–104. Abstract from: MEDLINE.

Douglas, J. J., & Wilkinson, D. A. (1993). Evidence of normal emotional responsiveness in alcoholic Korsakoff's syndrome in the presence of profound memory impairment. *Addiction, 88,* 1637–1645.

Drake, A. I., Butters, N., Shear, P. K., Smith, T. L., Bondi, M., Irwin, M., & Schuckit, M. A. (1995). Cognitive recovery with

abstinence and its relationship to family history for alcoholism. *Journal of Studies on Alcohol, 55,* 104–109.

Ellis, R. J., & Oscar-Berman, M. (1989). Alcoholism, aging, and functional cerebral asymmetries. *Psychological Bulletin, 106,* 128–147.

Engel, P. A., Grunnet, M., & Jacobs, B. (1991). Wernicke-Korsakoff syndrome complicating T-cell lymphoma: Unusual or unrecognized? *Southern Medical Journal, 84,* 253–256.

Evert, D. L., & Oscar-Berman, M. (1995). Alcohol-related cognitive impairments—An overview of how alcoholism may affect the workings of the brain. *Alcohol Health and Research World, 19,* 89–96.

Ferrari, V., Baratelli, E., Colombo, C., Vitaloni, L., & Broggini, M. (1991). Wernicke-Korsakoff syndrome caused by prolonged infusion therapy during the postoperative period [on-line] *Recenti Progressi in Medicina, 82,* 672–674. Abstract from: MEDLINE.

Freedman, M., & Oscar-Berman, M. (1986). Bilateral frontal lobe disease and selective delayed respoonse deficits in humans. *Behavioral Neuroscience, 100,* 337–342.

Gade, A. (1982). Amnesia after operations on aneurysms of the anterior communicating artery. *Surgery Neurology, 18,* 46–49.

Halliday, G., Ellis, J., & Harper, C. (1992). The locus coeruleus and memory: A study of chronic alcoholics with and without the memory impairment of Korsakoff's psychosis. *Brain Research, 598,* 33–37.

Halliday, G., Ellis, J., Heard, R., Caine, D., and Harper, C. (1993). Brainstem serotonergic neurons in chronic alcoholics with and without the memory impairment of Korsakoff's psychosis. *Journal of Neuropathology and Experimental Neurology, 52,* 567–579.

Harper, C. G., & Kril, J. J. (1993). Neuropathological changes in alcoholics. In W. A. Hunt & S. J. Nixon (Eds.), *Alcohol-induced brain damage.* NIAAA research monograph No. 22 (pp. 39–69). Rockville, MD: USDHHS, NIH Publication No. 93-3549.

Heaton, R. K. (1981). *A manual for the Wisconsin Card Sorting Test.* Odessa, FL: Psychological Assessment Resources, Inc.

Hunter, R., McLuskie, R., Wyper, D., Patterson, J. ,Christie, J. E., Brooks, D. N., McCulloch, J., Fink, G., & Goodwin, G. M. (1989). The pattern of function-related regional cerebral blood flow investigated by single photon emission tomography with ^{99m}Tc-HMPAO in patients with presenile Alzheimer's disease and Korsakoff's psychosis. *Psychological Medicine, 19,* 847–855.

Jacobson, R. R., Acker, C. F., & Lishman, W. A. (1990). Patterns of neuropsychological deficit in alcoholic Korsakoff's syndrome. *Psychological Medicine, 20,* 321–334.

Jernigan, T. L., Butters, N., DiTraglia, G., & Cermak, L. S. (1991). Reduced cerebral grey matter observed in alcoholics using magnetic resonance imaging. *Alcoholism: Clincal and Experimental Research, 15,* 418–427.

Jernigan, T. L., Schafer, K., Buters, N., & Cermak, L. S. (1991). Magnetic resonance imaging of alcoholic Korsakoff patients. *Neuropsychopharmacology, 4,* 175–186.

Joyce, E. M. (1994). Aetiology of alcoholic brain damage: Alcoholic neurotoxicity or thiamine malnutrition? *British Medical Bulletin, 50,* 99–114.

Joyce, E. M., & Robbins, T. W. (1991). Frontal lobe function in Korsakoff and non-Korsakoff alcoholics. Planning and spatial working memory. *Neuropsychologia, 29,* 709–723.

Khan, A., Mirolo, M. H., Claypoole, K., & Hughes, D. (1993). Low-dose thyrotropin-releasing hormone effects in cognitively impaired alcoholics. *Alcoholism: Clinical and Experimental Research, 17,* 791–796.

Kopelman, M. D. (1985). Rates of forgetting in Alzheimer-type dementia and Korsakoff's sydnrome. *Neuropsychologia, 23,* 623–638.

Lishman, W. A. (1990). Alcohol and the brain. *British Journal of Psychiatry, 156,* 635–644.

Markowitsch, H. J., & Pritzel, M. (1985). The neuropathology of amnesia. *Progress in Neurobiology, 25,* 189–287.

Martin, P. R., & Eckardt, M. J. (1985). Pharmacological interventions in chronic organic brain syndromes associated with alcoholism. In C. A. Naranjo & E. M. Sellers (Eds.), *Research advances in new psychopharmacological treatments for alcoholism* (pp. 257–272). Amsterdam: Elsevier Science Publishers.

Martin, P. R., & Nimmerrichter, A. A. (1993). Pharmacological treatment of alcohol-induced brain damage. In W. A. Hunt & S. J. Nixon (Eds.), *Alcohol-induced brain damage.* NIAAA research monograph No. 22 (pp. 461–477). Rockville, MD: USDHHS, NIH Publication No. 93-3549.

Martin, P. R., McCool, B. A., & Singleton, C. K. (1993). Genetic sensitivity to thiamine deficiency and development of alcoholic organic brain disease. *Alcoholism: Clinical and Experimental Research, 17,* 31–37.

Mattis, S. (1976). Mental status examination of organic mental syndrome in the elderly patient. In L. Bellack & T. B. Karasu (Eds.), *Geriatric psychiatry* (pp. 77–121). New York: Grune & Stratton.

McEntee, W. J., & Mair, R. G. (1990). The Korsakoff syndrome: A neurochemical perspective. *Trends in Neurosciences, 13,* 340–344.

Meissner, W. W. (1968). Learning and memory in the Korsakoff syndrome. *International Journal of Neuropsychiatry, 4,* 6–20.

Murray, E. A., & Mishkin, M. (1985). Amygdalectomy impairs cross-modal associations in monkeys. *Science, 228,* 604–606.

National Institute on Alcohol Abuse and Alcoholism. (1993). *Eighth special report to the U. S. Congress on alcohol and health from the Secretary of Health and Human Services* (DHHS Publication No. ADM-281-91-0003). Alexandria, VA: EEI.

National Institute on Alcohol Abuse and Alcoholism. (in press). *Ninth special report to the U. S. Congress on alcohol and health from the Secretary of Health and Human Services* (DHHS Publication). Alexandria, VA: EEI.

Okino, S., Sakajiri, K. I., Fukushima, I., Ide, Y., & Takamori, M. (1993). A case of Wernicke-Korsakoff syndrome caused by gastrojejunostomy: Specific findings of MRI and SPECT. [online]. *Rinsho Shinkeigaku, 33,* 530–534. Abstract from: MED-LINE.

Oscar-Berman, M. (1973). Hypothesis testing and focusing behavior during concept formation by amnesic Korsakoff patients. *Neuropsychologia, 11,* 191–198.

Oscar-Berman, M. (1988). Links between clinical and experimental neuropsychology. *Journal of Clinical and Experimental Neuropsychology, 11,* 571–588.

Oscar-Berman, M. (1994). Comparative neuropsychology. Brain functions in nonhuman primates and human neurobehavioral disorders. In L. S. Cermak (Ed.), *Neuropsychological explorations of memory and cognition: A tribute to Nelson Butters* (pp. 9–30). New York: Plenum Press.

Oscar-Berman, M., and Hutner, N. (1993). Frontal lobe changes after chronic alcohol ingestion. In W. A. Hunt & S. J. Nixon (Eds.), *Alcohol-induced brain damage.* NIAAA research monograph No. 22 (pp. 121–156). Rockville, MD: USDHHS, NIH Publication No. 93-3549.

Oscar-Berman, M., & Zola-Morgan, S. M. (1980). Comparative neuropsychology and Korsakoff's syndrome. I: Spatial and visual reversal learning. *Neuropsychologia, 18,* 499–512.

Oscar-Berman, M., Hancock, M., Mildworf, B., Hutner, N., & Weber, D. A. (1990). Emotional perception and memory in alcoholism and aging. *Alcoholism: Clinical and Experimental Research, 14,* 383–393.

Oscar-Berman, M., Pulaski, J. L., Hutner, N., Weber, D. A., & Freedman, M. (1990). Cross-modal functions in alcoholism and aging. *Neuropsychologia, 28,* 851–869.

Oscar-Berman, M., McNamara, P., & Freedman, M. (1991). Delayed-response tasks: Parallels between experimental ablation studies and findings in patients with frontal lesions. In H. S. Levin, H. M. Eisenberg, & A. L. Benton (Eds.), *Frontal lobe function and dysfunction* (pp. 230–255). New York: Oxford University Press.

Oscar-Berman, M., Hutner, N., & Bonner, R. T. (1992). Visual and auditory spatial and nonspatial delayed-response performance by Korsakoff and non-Korsakoff alcoholic and aging individuals. *Behavioral Neuroscience, 106,* 613–622.

Parkin, A. J., Blunden, J., Rees, J. E., & Hunkin, N. M. (1991). Wernicke-Korsakoff syndrome of nonalcoholic origin. *Brain and Cognition, 15,* 69–82.

Parsons, O. A., & Leber, W. R. (1982). Premature aging, alcoholism, and recovery. In W. G. Wood and M. F. Elias (Eds.), *Alcoholism and aging: Advances in research* (pp. 79–92). Boca Raton, FL: CRC Press.

Petri, H. L., & Mishkin, M. (1994). Behaviorism, cognitivism and the neuropsychology of memory. *American Scientist, 82,* 30–37.

Pfefferbaum, A., & Rosenbloom, M. J. (1993). In vivo imaging of morphological brain alterations associated with alcoholism. In W. A. Hunt & S. J. Nixon (Eds.), *Alcohol-induced brain damage.* NIAAA research monograph No. 22 (pp. 71–87). Rockville, MD: USDHHS, NIH Publication No. 93-3549.

Pfefferbaum, A., Lim, K. O., Zipursky, R. B., Mathalon, D. H., Rosenbloom, M. J., Lane, B., Ha, C. N., & Sullivan, E. V. (1992). Brain gray and white matter volume loss accelerates with aging in chronic alcoholics: A quantitative MRI study. *Alcoholism: Clinical and Experimental Research, 16,* 1078–1089.

Pietrini, V. (1992). Creutzfeldt-Jakob disease presenting as Wernicke-Korsakoff syndrome. *Journal of the Neurological Sciences, 108,* 149–153.

Pribram, K. H., Ahumada, A., Hartog, J., & Roos, L. (1964). A progress report on the neurological processes disturbed by frontal lesions in primates. In J. M. Warren & K. Akert (Eds.), *The frontal granular cortex and behavior* (pp. 28–55). New York: McGraw-Hill.

Ryan, C. (1982). Alcoholism and premature aging: A neuropsychological perspective. *Alcoholism: Clinical and Experimental Research, 6,* 79–96.

Ryan, C., & Butters, N. (1986). Neuropsychology of alcoholism. In D. Wedding, A. M. Horton, & J. S. Webster (Eds.), *The neuropsychology handbook* (pp. 376–409). New York: Springer.

Shaw, C., Kentridge, R. W., & Aggleton, J. P. (1990). Cross-modal matching by amnesic subjects. *Neuropsychologia, 28,* 665–671.

Shimamura, A. P., Janowsky, J. S., & Squire, L. R. (1991). What is the role of frontal lobe damage in memory disorders? In H. S. Levin, H. M. Eisenberg, & A. L. Benton (Eds.), *Frontal lobe function and dysfunction* (pp. 173–195). New York: Oxford University Press.

Smith, M. E., & Oscar-Berman, M. (1990). Repetition priming of words and pseudowords in divided attention and in amnesia. *Journal of Experimental Psychology: Learning, Memory, and Cognition, 16,* 1033–1042.

Talland, G. A. (1965). *Deranged memory: A psychonomic study of the amnesic syndrome.* New York: Academic Press.

Talland, G. A., & Waugh, N. C. (Eds.). (1969). *The pathology of memory.* New York: Academic Press.

Thakore, J. H., & Dinan, T. G. (1993). Serum thyrotropin responses to thyrotropin-releasing hormone in Korsakoff's syndrome. *Acta Psychiatrica Scandinavica, 88,* 218–220.

Verfaellie, M., Milberg, W. P., Cermak, L. S., & Letourneau, L. L. (1992). Priming of spatial configurations in alcoholic Korsakoff's amnesia. *Brain and Cognition, 18,* 34–45.

Victor, M., & Yakovlev, P. I. (1955). S. S. Korsakoff's psychic disorder in conjunction with peripheral neuritis. A translation of Korsakoff's original article with brief comments on the author and his contribution to clinical medicine. *Neurology, 5,* 394–406.

Victor, M., Adams, R. D., & Collins, G. H. (1971). *The Wernicke-Korsakoff syndrome.* Philadelphia: F. A. Davis.

Victor, M., Adams, R. D., & Collins, G. H. (1989). *The Wernicke-Korsakoff syndrome* (2nd ed.) Philadelphia: F. A. Davis.

Vighetto, A., Charles, N., Salzmann, M., Confavreux, C., & Aimard, G. (1991). Korsakoff's syndrome as the initial presentation of multiple sclerosis. *Journal of Neurology, 238,* 351–354.

Volkow, N. D., Hitzemann, R., Wang, G.-J., Fowler, J. S., Burr, G., Pascani, K., Dewey, S. L., & Wolf, A. P. (1992). Decreased brain metabolism in neurologically intact healthy alcoholics. *American Journal of Psychiatry, 149,* 1016–1022.

Walsh, K. (1994). *Neuropsychology. A clinical approach.* New York: Churchill Livingstone.

Wells, C. E. (1979). Diagnosis of dementia. *Psychosomatics, 20,* 517–522.

Wilkinson, D. A., & Carlen, P. L. (1982). Morphological abnormaliteis in the brains of alcoholics: Relationship to age, psychological test scores and patient type. In W. G. Wood & M. F. Elias (Eds.), *Alcoholism and aging: Advances in research* (pp. 61–77). Boca Raton, FL: CRC Press.

Witt, E. D., & Goldman-Rakic, P. S. (1983). Intermittent thiamin deficiency in the rhesus monkey. II: Evidence for memory loss. *Annals of Neurolgoy, 13,* 396–401.

Wodak, A., Richmond, R., & Wilson, A. (1990). Thiamine fortification and alcohol. *Medical Journal of Australia, 152,* 97–99.

Wood, W. G., & Elias, M. F. (Eds.). *(1982). Alcoholism and aging: Advances in research.* Boca Raton, FL: CRC Press.

Yellowlees, P. (1990). Thiamine in our bread and wine. *Medical Journal of Australia, 153,* 567.

Zola-Morgan, S. M., & Squire, L. (1993). Neuroanatomy of memory. *Annual Review of Neuroscience, 16,* 547–563.

15

Parkinson's Disease

Neurobehavioral Consequences of Basal Ganglia Dysfunction

MARK W. BONDI AND ALEXANDER I. TRÖSTER

Introduction

Parkinson's disease (PD) is the most common disease affecting the basal ganglia. It is a progressive, degenerative neurologic disorder that affects approximately 1 in 100 people over the age of 60 in the United States (Duvoisin, 1984). The neurochemistry and neuropathology of PD arise from changes in the nigrostriatal system and mesolimbic and mesocortical pathways (Bernheimer, Birkmayer, Hornykiewicz, Jellinger, & Seitelberger, 1973; Taylor, Saint-Cyr, & Lang, 1986). The classic motor symptoms of PD include a resting tremor, generally increased muscle tone (rigidity), and difficulty in initiating voluntary movements (bradykinesia). Symptoms of this kind are associated with damage to the basal ganglia and are termed *extrapyramidal* symptoms because of their origins outside of the corticospinal or pyramidal tract; such terminology may be misleading, however, since at least some of the involuntary movements associated with PD are actually effected through the pyramidal tract (Nolte, 1988).

In 1817 James Parkinson originally described the signs and symptoms of several patients he had examined, all of whom shared a similar clinical presentation. In this initial description, he noted

MARK W. BONDI • Department of Psychiatry, School of Medicine, University of California, San Diego, La Jolla, California 92093-0948; and San Diego Department of Veterans Affairs Medical Center, San Diego, California 92161. ALEXANDER I. TRÖSTER • Department of Neurology, University of Kansas Medical Center, Kansas City, Kansas 66160-7314.

changes in motor function and remarked that the senses and intellect remained "uninjured," yet research has demonstrated that PD adversely affects cognitive and other psychologic functions as well (Pollock & Hornabrook, 1966). Motor and cognitive functions are both affected by these neuropathologic changes, with the majority of patients developing some discrete cognitive deficits, and a sizeable percentage further developing dementia (Hietanen & Teravainen, 1986; Lees, 1985; Mayeux & Stern, 1983; Pirozzolo, Hansch, Mortimer, Webster, & Kuskowski, 1982). Affective disturbances commonly appear in PD also; estimates indicate that approximately 40% of PD patients develop a major depression or dysthymic disorder (Mayeux et al., 1986).

As we have witnessed over the preceding decade, significant advances in our knowledge of the pathoanatomic and pathophysiologic mechanisms of PD have also advanced our understanding of the cognitive and affective sequelae of PD. The following sections of this chapter provide an overview of the clinical, pathological, neuropsychological, and affective features associated with Parkinson's disease.

Overview of Clinical Features

Parkinsonism, Parkinson's Disease, and Parkinsonian-Plus Syndromes

Parkinson's disease and parkinsonism are not synonymous. Whereas PD refers to a specific disease entity, parkinsonism refers to a syndrome which PD shares with several other disorders. Specifically, parkinsonism refers to a constellation of four cardinal motor signs (tremor, bradykinesia, rigidity, and postural abnormalities). This parkinsonian syndrome can be a manifestation of not only PD, but also a variety of other neurodegenerative, toxic, metabolic, vascular, traumatic, and infectious conditions (Koller & Megaffin, 1994), as well as psychogenic movement disorders (Marjama, Tröster, & Koller, 1995). Neurodegenerative conditions other than PD giving rise to the parkinsonian syndrome (e.g., progressive supranuclear palsy, striatonigral degeneration, Shy-Drager syndrome, olivopontocerebellar atrophy) have variously been referred to as multiple system atrophies, atypical parkinsonism, and parkinsonian-plus syndromes. The term parkinsonian-plus syndromes appears clinically useful because it captures the concept that such syndromes are differentiated from PD by the presence of additional, non-parkinsonian signs (e.g., prominent dysautonomia in Shy-Drager syndrome; supranuclear gaze palsy in progressive supranuclear palsy).

Diagnosis

The diagnosis of PD is not made until the motor signs (typically two among resting tremor, rigidity, and bradykinesia) are clinically evident. Because the parkinsonian syndrome rarely emerges in its entirety early in the course of the disease, and because some patients first present with nonmotor complaints (e.g., sensory changes such as pain and tingling, loss of smell, depression, signs of autonomic dysfunction such as constipation and orthostatic hypotension, and dementia) (Pahwa & Koller, 1995), differential diagnosis can be difficult during the earliest stages. Indeed, the few studies that have evaluated the accuracy of clinical diagnosis via postmortem neuropathologic verification indicate diagnostic accuracy to be approximately 75% (Hughes, Daniel, Kilford, & Lees, 1992; Rajput, Rozdilsky, & Rajput, 1991). Consequently, additional criteria have been proposed by some (e.g., Gibb, 1989; Koller, 1992) to differentiate PD from other conditions leading to parkinsonism. For example, while PD typically shows responsiveness to levodopa treatment, parkinsonian-plus syndromes show poor response to such treatment. Because PD often has a unilateral onset (i.e., presents as hemiparkinsonism), some consider bilateral disease onset as likely reflecting another disorder. In addition, many clinicians will not make a diagnosis of PD until a clear progression of signs and symptoms is observed. Whether such additional, more rigid diagnostic criteria demonstrate greater specificity without sacrificing sensitivity remains to be verified by prospective clinicopathologic investigations. Given the present lack of agreement on a single set of diagnostic criteria, Calne, Snow, and Lee (1992) have advocated a less rigid system that classifies PD as clinically possible, probable, and definite—much like that of the criteria forwarded by McKhann et al. (1984) for diagnosing Alzheimer's disease (see also Salmon, Chapter 10 of this volume).

Although cognitive and behavioral abnormalities frequently occur early in the course of PD, they do not constitute part of the formal diagnostic criteria for PD. Nonetheless, neuropsychological findings are of considerable importance in the comprehensive work-up of the patient with parkinsonism for several reasons. Baseline evaluations serve to characterize the nature and extent of cognitive changes and thus permit a judgment about whether such changes are consistent or inconsistent with PD. As part of serial neuropsychological evaluation, the baseline provides a standard against which to measure the evolution of a possible dementia, as well as cognitive changes related to comorbid conditions (e.g., depression) and to pharmacologic and surgical treatment. Given that PD likely has an extended latent (or prodromal) period (Pahwa & Koller, 1995), the utility of neuropsychological evaluation in the detection of presymptomatic PD, heretofore neglected, deserves empirical attention.

Generally, when cognitive deficits occur early in PD, such deficits are most often observed in the domains of executive, visuospatial-perceptual, and memory function. In mild PD dementia, the pattern of cognitive deficits, on a global level, corresponds to that characteristic of "subcortical" dementia (see Butters, Granholm, Salmon, Grant, & Wolfe, 1987). More detailed information concerning the effect of PD on different cognitive domains is presented later in the chapter.

Epidemiology

Prevalence and Incidence of Parkinson's Disease

Rough prevalence estimates of PD vary widely by geographic regions, ranging from 10 per 100,000 in Igbo-Ora, Nigeria, to 350 per 100,000 in Limousin, France (Román, Zhang, & Ellenberg, 1995). Whether the variability in prevalence reflects true geographic variation or artifact is unclear. In addition to being complicated by differences among studies in sampling methods, as well as case definition and ascertainment methods, prevalence rates are biased by different population age distributions across regions. Even if age-adjusted prevalence rates are reported, comparisons remain difficult because adjustments are based on different standard populations. Zhang and Román (1993) thus calculated age-adjusted prevalence rates by adjusting to the U.S. population the prevalence rates published in studies also reporting local population age distributions. Although not free of potential artifacts, these more comparable figures indicate a prevalence range from 18 per 100,000 in provincial China to 182 per 100,000 in Iceland. Similar age-adjusted rates for three U.S. studies range from 98 to 175 per 100,000.

Zhang and Román (1993) also provided age-adjusted incidence rates, and these range from 1.9 per 100,000 in provincial China to 22.1 per 100,000 in the earlier Rochester, Minnesota, study (Kurland, 1958). Age-adjusted incidence in the most recent Rochester study (Rajput, Offord, Beard, & Kurland, 1984) was 19.1 per 100,000. Although age-adjusted prevalence and incidence rates of PD vary considerably across countries, two observations have been made more consistently. Specifically, PD is slightly more common among men than women and reaches a peak incidence among individuals ages 70–79 years.

Risk Factors for Parkinson's Disease

The etiology of PD remains unknown and is likely multifactorial (Ellenberg, 1995), but a host of potential risk factors for development of PD, including toxic, genetic, dietary, and demographic factors, have been investigated. Risk factors identi-

fied more consistently include residence in industrial or rural areas with exposure to pesticides, herbicides, and well water (Aquilonius & Hartvig, 1986; Hubble, Cao, Hassanein, Neuberger, & Koller, 1993; Koller et al., 1990; Tanner, 1989), increasing age (see Román et al., 1995, for review), family history of neurologic disease (Hubble et al., 1993), and depression (Hubble et al., 1993).

Genetic factors likely play a more minor role in the development of PD (cf. Golbe, 1995, for a more optimistic view that genetic factors underlie potential PD variants). Although Golbe et al. (1993) reported PD to be transmitted in an apparently autosomal dominant fashion in one large Italian kindred, Koller and Megaffin (1994) suggest that intermarriage in earlier generations of this kindred might underlie a spurious inheritance pattern. Other genetic studies have failed to demonstrate an increased occurrence of PD in monozygotic twins. Ward and colleagues (1983), for example, found only one of 43 monozygotic twin pairs studied to be concordant for PD. However, investigations have also demonstrated that a genetic susceptibility may exist when considering subtypes such as early-onset parkinsonism (Alonso, Otero, D'Regules, & Figueroa, 1986; Barbeau & Poucher, 1982). Others maintain that the concordance of tremor-dominant PD in monozygotic twins suggests that genetic susceptibility is important in this variety of Parkinson's disease (Jankovic & Reches, 1986). Román et al. (1995) also argue that the finding of a higher age-adjusted PD prevalence ratio among blacks in the United States than in Africa favors only a limited genetic role in the etiology of PD. Thus, although a single genetic determinant is unlikely to underlie PD development, genetic factors might nonetheless convey a predisposition to development of PD.

Neuroanatomy, Neurochemistry, and Neuropathology

Morphologic changes in parkinsonism vary according to etiology. Idiopathic PD is the most common form; other forms such as parkinsonism arising from cerebrovascular disease, trauma, toxic substances, tumors, or encephalitis account for less than 20% of cases (see Jellinger, 1986; McPherson & Cummings, 1996, for reviews). Idiopathic PD is characterized neuropathologically by a loss of pigmented cells in the pars compacta (or compact zone) of the substantia nigra and the presence of Lewy bodies (abnormal intracytoplasmic eosinophilic neuronal inclusion bodies) in the substantia nigra, locus ceruleus, dorsal vagal nucleus, and substantia innominata (Hansen & Galasko, 1992; Jellinger, 1987).

Tretiakoff (1919) first discovered the loss of pigmented cells of the substantia nigra upon postmortem examination of a small sample of PD patients. The lesions he observed resulted from a loss of the melanin-containing, dopaminergic cells. More recent work has shown that the threshold for the development of mild motor symptoms associated with PD requires a disproportionately high level of destruction (approximately 80% cell loss) within the substantia nigra (Bernheimer et al., 1973).

The striatum contains more than 80% of the total brain dopamine (Hornykiewicz, 1966) and, in PD, dopamine concentrations are markedly reduced in all structures belonging to the nigrostriatal system (Bernheimer et al., 1973; Hornykiewicz & Kish, 1986). Also, dopamine-synthesizing enzymes such as tyrosine hydroxylase and DOPA decarboxylase, as well as metabolites like homovanillic acid, dihydroxyphenylacetic acid, and 3-methoxytyramine, are all reduced in PD (Hornykiewicz & Kish, 1986). From a historical perspective, PD represented the first documented example of a disease that was consistently correlated with a deficiency in a specific neurotransmitter system (Hornykiewicz, 1966).

However, not all the symptoms of PD are exclusively attributable to the dopaminergic cell loss of the nigrostriatal pathway. Losses occur in the noradrenergic neurons of the locus ceruleus, the nucleus basalis of Meynert, the serotonergic neurons of the raphé nuclei, and the dorsal vagal nucleus (Côté & Crutcher, 1985; Jellinger, 1986). Both the locus ceruleus and the raphé nuclei have widespread projections throughout the brain, including the cerebellum and neocortex. Dopaminergic projections to the limbic system and the frontal neocortex exist also. Thus, because of the widespread and variable morphologic and biochemical changes in PD, the specific loci and synaptic mechanisms that account for all of the parkinsonian symptoms remain uncertain (Côté & Crutcher, 1985).

Cellular inclusions, termed Lewy bodies, are also found in the majority of PD patients, although they are not exclusively pathognomonic of PD (Forno, 1986). Nonetheless, Lewy bodies are a highly characteristic feature of PD, with the greatest concentrations found in the substantia nigra and locus ceruleus (Duffy & Tennyson, 1965; Gibb, 1989; Greenfield & Bosanquet, 1953) and not in the dorsal vagal nucleus or substantia innominata as Lewy himself first thought (Lewy, 1912, 1923). Speculation regarding the predominance of Lewy bodies in the substantia nigra and locus ceruleus centers on the role of neuromelanin in promoting or inducing the formation of these inclusion bodies (Forno, 1986).

Lewy (1912) described these cellular inclusions, with the aid of the Mann stain (a trichrome stain), as red spherical or elongated staining structures within a blue halo of cytoplasm. The electron-dense core contains predominantly protein-rich bundles of fragmented neurofilaments. It is a distinctive neuronal inclusion that appears wherever there is an excessive loss of neurons; thus, it is always found in the substantia nigra upon autopsy in PD patients. Lewy bodies are therefore found in every case of clinically diagnosed PD (except in a few cases with the pathology of an alternative disorder such as postencephalitic parkinsonism; see below), thereby enabling the neuropathologist to diagnose PD (Gibb, 1989).

Variants of Parkinsonism

As stated earlier, a number of syndromes exhibit parkinsonian motor signs, and each has varying degrees of similarity based on neuropathologic comparisons with idiopathic PD and possesses its own classification scheme. A partial list of such movement disorders that have symptom overlap with idiopathic PD includes juvenile-onset parkinsonism, Shy-Drager syndrome, progressive supranuclear palsy, Parkinson-dementia complex of Guam, Steele-Richardson-Olszewski syndrome, Hallervorden-Spatz disease, corticobasal degeneration, drug-induced parkinsonism, and postencephalitic parkinsonism. While discussion of each of these conditions is beyond the scope of this chapter, the last two conditions, drug-induced parkinsonism and postencephalitic parkinsonism, will be given brief mention, and the reader is referred to additional sources for information on at least some of these other parkinsonian disorders (Cummings, 1990; Jankovic and Tolosa, 1993; McPherson & Cummings, 1996).

Postencephalitic Parkinsonism

Individuals who develop parkinsonian motor signs and symptoms secondary to an encephalitis are diagnosed as having postencephalitic parkinsonism under current nomenclature. In 1917, for example, a worldwide epidemic of "sleeping sickness," or encephalitis lethargica, broke out, and many of these individuals further developed parkinsonian symptomatology (Duvoisin, 1984). The acute inflammatory process of encephalitis lethargica was presumed to be caused by a virus, which Von Economo (1931) stated had a predilection for the mesencephalon and diencephalon (Gibb, 1989). Interestingly, Lewy bodies are not part of the pathological findings in postencephalitic parkinsonism (Gibb, 1989). The incidence of postencephalitic parkinsonism rapidly declined after 1926, although rare cases with comparable clinical features continue to appear (Espir & Spalding, 1956; Hunter & Jones, 1966; see also Cummings & Benson, 1992, for discussion). As the mortality rate of those individuals exposed to the encephalitis lethargica epidemic of 1917 continues to increase, the incidence of postencephalitic parkinsonism is decreasing (Klawans & Cohen, 1970). While anticholinergic drugs provide an average of 20% to 25% reduction of symptoms in idiopathic PD, their efficacy in postencephalitic parkinsonism is much greater (Duvoisin, 1984).

Drug-Induced Parkinsonism

Administration of the neurotoxin 1-methyl-4-phenyl-1,2,3,6-tetrahydropyridine (MPTP) to humans and other primates induces persistent parkinsonian symptoms. These symptoms also show palliative responses to classical antiparkinsonian drug therapy (see Jenner & Marsden, 1989, for discussion). Approximately 1 hr following administration of the toxin to primates, animals become increasingly akinetic and exhibit rigidity of the limbs, freezing episodes, postural instabilities, and loss of vocaliza-

tion and blink reflex. There is, however, a low incidence of tremor and, unlike in idiopathic PD, evidence of partial recovery following MPTP administration, probably reflecting the limited pathological foci of MPTP-induced parkinsonism (Jenner & Marsden, 1989). In humans, MPTP-induced parkinsonism is almost exclusively found in a group of intravenous drug users in northern California who inadvertently injected the substance which was derived as a by-product of a laboratory-made "designer drug" (Ballard, Tetrud, & Langston, 1985). A postmortem study of MPTP in man demonstrated that the toxin destroyed the cells of the pars compacta of the substantia nigra, but not cells of the locus ceruleus (Davis et al., 1979). As in postencephalitic parkinsonism, anticholinergic drugs provide a significant reduction of symptoms (Duvoisin, 1984).

The discovery of MPTP as a highly selective neurotoxin that targets the substantia nigra for cell death has not only provided a means of producing an animal model to study PD, but also contributed to the evolution of hypotheses regarding the etiology of PD. The identification of a chemical agent producing PD lends support to the claim (Barbeau, 1984) that PD may be an environmentally based disease, acquired through exposure to unknown neurotoxins that over a lifetime destroy neural tissue with great precision and selectivity.

Dementia in Parkinson's Disease

Description, Prevalence, and Neuropathologic Correlates

Although not included in James Parkinson's original description of the disease, there is a higher prevalence of dementia in patients with PD than in the general population of the same age. However, estimates of the prevalence of dementia in PD vary tremendously. In a recent review, Rajput (1992) indicated that estimates of the prevalence of dementia in PD vary from 8% (Taylor, Saint-Cyr, & Lang, 1985) to 81% (Martin, Loewenson, Resch, & Baker, 1973), but when the sample population, the case ascertainment, and the methodology are all taken into account, the prevalence figures for dementia most widely accepted appear to range from 20% to

40% (Brown & Marsden, 1984; Cummings, 1988; Martilla & Rinne, 1976; Mohr, Mendis, & Grimes, 1995).

As with other dementing illnesses (see Ineichen, 1987; see also Chapter 10 of this volume), estimates of the prevalence of dementia in PD have varied widely due to differences in dementia definitions, sampling techniques, and sensitivity of test instruments used to identify cases. For example, Cummings (1988) demonstrated that studies that used a nonstandardized clinical examination found the lowest prevalence rates of dementia in PD (approximately 30%); studies using a brief structured mental status examination such as the Mini-Mental State Examination (Folstein, Folstein, & McHugh, 1975) found somewhat higher prevalence rates (approximately 40%); and studies using standardized neuropsychological tests found the highest prevalence rates (approximately 70%).

As these findings indicate, different methods of defining dementia have led to widespread variations in the prevalence rates of PD dementia. According to most current definitions, however, the syndrome of dementia involves deterioration in two or more of the following domains of psychological functioning: memory, language, visuospatial skills, judgment or abstract thinking, and emotion or personality (see American Psychiatric Association, 1994; Bayles & Kaszniak, 1987; Cummings & Benson, 1992). In some diagnostic schemes, such as in the fourth edition of the *Diagnostic and Statistical Manual of Mental Disorders* (*DSM-IV*; American Psychiatric Association, 1994), memory impairment and at least one other cognitive deficit must be present and severe enough to significantly interfere with one's usual social or occupational functioning. Furthermore, the cognitive impairment must represent a significant decline from a previous level of intact functioning, and it must not occur exclusively during the course of delirium.

Cummings and Benson (1992), however, differ from the *DSM-IV* diagnostic criteria by defining dementia solely on the basis of an acquired and persistent impairment of intellectual functioning affecting at least three of the above-mentioned domains of psychological functioning. Also, memory impairment is not a necessary feature (e.g., Pick's disease has relatively preserved memory in the early and middle phases of the illness), and verification of

functional decline is not required. Cummings and Benson (1992) have argued that the requirement of social or occupational disability in the *DSM* renders the definition imprecise and relatively unquantifiable. Thus, patients with minimally demanding circumstances in their daily lives would not be considered demented with the same disability that would warrant that diagnosis in an individual with more exacting situations. Parkinson's disease patients with relatively mild but clinically significant cognitive deficits might be expected to fit this latter classification scheme of dementia more easily than that of the *DSM-IV* criteria (McPherson & Cummings, 1996). Furthermore, the application of the criteria for dementia in *DSM-IV* (American Psychiatric Association, 1994) to PD is considered particularly problematic, because in practice it is difficult to establish whether the impairment in social or occupational functioning stems from the cognitive (as required by these criteria) or from the physical impairments associated with PD.

Cummings and Benson (1992) also point out, however, that few, if any, dementias are truly global, equally affecting all spheres of cognitive functioning, although dementia is often mistakenly thought of as a global disorder. Neuropathologically distinct dementing diseases appear to be associated with different patterns of relatively preserved and impaired cognitive abilities. This observation underlies the distinction between *cortical* and *subcortical* dementia (Albert, Feldman, & Willis, 1974; Cummings, 1990; Cummings & Benson, 1992). For example, dementia syndromes associated with neurodegenerative diseases that primarily involve regions of the cerebral cortex (e.g., Alzheimer's disease) are broadly characterized by a prominent amnesia (affecting both recall and recognition abilities) as well as deficits in language and semantic knowledge (i.e., aphasia), "executive" functions, and constructional and visuospatial abilities (see Bayles & Kaszniak, 1987; Cummings & Benson, 1992), whereas those dementing illnesses that have their primary locus in subcortical brain structures (e.g., Parkinson's disease, white matter diseases, subcortical vascular disorders) typically demonstrate a slowing of cognition, moderate memory disturbance (recognition abilities superior to recall abilities), attentional dysfunction, problem-solving deficits, and little or no aphasia, apraxia, or agnosia. A prominent affective disturbance (usually depression) is also commonly associated with subcortical dementias. As expected, many of the parkinsonian motor signs and symptoms are evident in the subcortical dementias as well (Cummings & Benson, 1992).

Thus, the most common pattern of cognitive changes characterizing the dementia of PD is consistent with the pattern of subcortical dementia, although some demented PD patients manifest both cortical and subcortical patterns of intellectual change. Dementia in PD is typically characterized by an inability to develop successful problem-solving strategies, poor concept formation, lowered verbal fluency, impaired set shifting ability, difficulties with initiation, impaired and slowed memory, difficulty with visuospatial skills, and a slowed rate of information processing or bradyphrenia (see Cummings & Benson, 1992; McPherson & Cummings, 1996; Taylor, Saint-Cyr, Lang, & Kenny, 1986). Cortical patterns of intellectual decline such as aphasia, agnosia, or a severe anterograde or retrograde amnesia are not commonly observed in the dementia associated with PD (see Cummings & Benson, 1992; McPherson & Cummings, 1996). However, when these cortical features are present in a PD patient, coexistent Alzheimer's disease may be suspected.

Investigators have speculated that the source of the dementia in PD may be due to the direct effects of subcortical degenerative changes (i.e., dopaminergic depletion of striatal structures secondary to cell losses in the substantia nigra), superimposed Alzheimer's type degenerative changes, or a combination of these two factors (Freedman, 1990; Pirozzolo, Swihart, Rey, Mahurin, & Jankovic, 1993). Furthermore, a number of recent studies have shown that all or very nearly all (i.e., 96%) brains of patients with PD have Lewy bodies in the neocortex (Hughes et al., 1992; Perry et al., 1991; Schmidt et al., 1991).

Some investigators have reported that demented patients with idiopathic PD have cortical lesions indistinguishable from those of AD patients (Boller, Mizutani, Roessmann, & Gambetti, 1980; Hakim & Mathieson, 1979). Variations in subcortical and cortical lesions may explain some of the clinical similarities and differences between the dementias of PD and AD; degeneration of the nucleus basalis of Meynert and locus ceruleus, for example,

are common to both disorders (see Growdon & Corkin, 1986). However, more recent studies (Ball, 1984; Chui et al., 1986; Mann & Yates, 1983) have found little evidence for a systematic association between AD and dementia in PD (see Pirozzolo et al., 1993).

Neurochemical changes also demonstrate similarities and differences between AD and PD dementia. Both diseases show decreased acetylcholine, somatostatin, norepinephrine, and serotonin. Dopamine reductions in AD, however, are smaller and more variable than in PD (see Growdon & Corkin, 1986). Agid, Ruberg, Dubois, and Javoy-Agid (1984) speculate that reductions of choline acetyltransferase activity in nondemented PD patients indicate that the degeneration of subcortical cholinergic neurons precedes the intellectual decline commonly associated with decreased cholinergic activity. Denervation hyperactivity of the remaining cholinergic neurons is proposed to maintain normal intellectual functioning at this stage, but it would no longer be able to do so once neurons are unable to adequately compensate for neuronal loss (see Pirozzolo et al., 1993, for discussion).

Rather than a single syndrome and underlying neuropathology characterizing the dementia of PD, one or more specific intellectual disorders resulting from different lesions appears likely (Pirozzolo et al., 1993). Thus, one might expect to observe specific neurotransmitter deficiencies associated with particular cognitive disorders. This issue would appear to be best explored by clinicopathologic investigations (Pirozzolo et al., 1993).

Risk Factors for Dementia in Parkinson's Disease

As is true for most dementias, increasing age represents one of the most consistently reported risk factors for the development of dementia in PD (e.g., Biggins et al., 1992; Stern, Marder, Tang, & Mayeux, 1993). Other potential risk factors include low socioeconomic status and education (Glatt et al., 1996; Salganik & Korczyn, 1990), older age at disease onset (Biggins et al., 1992; Glatt et al., 1996; Lieberman et al., 1979), more severe extrapyramidal signs (Marder, Tang, Côté, Stern, & Mayeux, 1995), depression (Marder et al., 1995; Stern, Marder, et al., 1993), and the development of confusion or psychosis on levodopa (Stern, Marder, et al., 1993). Individuals with PD and dementia, compared to nondemented individuals with PD, even when matched for age, gender, and severity and duration of illness, have been found to die sooner during a 7-year follow-up study (Piccirilli, D'Alessandro, Finali, & Piccinin, 1994).

Because the apolipoprotein E gene type 4 allele (Apo ε4) is associated with development and age at onset of AD, and because AD and PD share some biologic and clinical features, two recent studies have examined whether the ε4 genotype is a genetic risk factor for dementia in PD. Both studies observed no significant differences in ε4 allele frequency among PD patients with and without dementia and normal control subjects, suggesting that the biologic basis for dementia in PD and AD might differ (Koller et al., 1995; Marder et al., 1994).

Specific Cognitive Functions

Although James Parkinson (1817) originally contended that the "senses and intellect remain uninjured," this conclusion was eventually challenged by a host of other investigators (see Goetz, 1992, for historical review) and today we recognize a number of cognitive changes which are commonly seen in patients with PD. As discussed, a sizeable minority of PD patients develop a frank dementia, and even among those PD patients without dementia, a characteristic pattern of discrete cognitive deficits emerges (see Huber & Cummings, 1992; McPherson & Cummings, 1996, for review). The following section provides an overview of specific cognitive domains and the typical patterns of performance of nondemented PD patients in each of these areas.

Attention/Concentration

Performance on most simple attentional tasks, such as digit span, is not significantly affected in PD (Huber, Freidenberg, Shuttleworth, Paulson, & Christy, 1989; Lees & Smith, 1983; Pillon, Dubois, Lhermitte, & Agid, 1986). More complex aspects of attentional skills, however, may demonstrate some decline in PD, although the evidence is equivocal across studies. Wilson and colleagues (Wilson,

Kaszniak, Klawans, & Garron, 1980), for example, were among the first to demonstrate cognitive slowing (or bradyphrenia) in PD patients on a memory scanning task. However, Rafal et al. (Rafal, Posner, Walker, & Friedrich, 1984) were not able to demonstrate a reduction in the speed of information processing, suggesting that the dopaminergic deficit in PD may not give rise to bradyphrenia (see also Pirozzolo et al., 1993, for discussion). On still other tasks, such as internal allocation of attentional resources, PD patients have demonstrated impairment in the executive control of attention (Girotti et al., 1986; Gotham, Brown, & Marsden, 1988). Thus, as Mahurin, Feher, Nance, Levy, and Pirozzolo (1993) point out, although motor response slowing has been observed in PD, potential interactions of cognitive slowing with symptom presentation and the clinical features of PD have not been fully clarified.

Language

Individuals with PD frequently demonstrate abnormalities related to the motor aspects of speech, such as dysarthria (Cummings, Darkins, Mendez, Hill, & Benson, 1988), and dysarthria might underlie the infrequently reported sentence repetition impairments in PD (Matison, Mayeux, Rosen, & Fahn, 1982). Motoric speech disturbances probably do not account for impairments on generative naming tasks (Gurd & Ward, 1989) and other language tests. Although PD patients are reported to be impaired on some language tests, there is general consensus that frank aphasias are not part of the PD cognitive profile (Cummings et al., 1988; Levin & Katzen, 1995). Perhaps it is for this reason that relatively little empirical attention has been devoted to language in PD. Among studies examining language in PD, phonetics (i.e., appreciation of rules governing language sounds, their combination, and pronunciation) has not been investigated extensively. Instead, the focus has been on syntax (i.e., appreciation of the rules governing the ordering of words in a meaningful manner) and semantics (i.e., knowledge of words and their referents).

Phonetics

Two recent studies suggest the possibility of subtle phonetic impairment in early PD, but these results are best considered tentative because the observed impairments might be of nonlinguistic origin. Grossman, Carvell, Stern, Gollomp, and Hurtig (1992) reported that PD patients had more difficulty than controls in detecting sentence errors involving the phonologic alteration of a closed class word. Although this suggests that PD might subtly compromise phonetic ability, it is equally possible that attentional difficulties account for the observed impairment. Similarly, Brentari, Poizner, and Kegl's (1995) conclusion that two PD patients' disturbances in the temporal organization and coordination (i.e., execution) of American Sign Language's distinctive features reflect a phonetic deficit might be alternatively interpreted as reflecting PD patients' more general difficulties in sequencing (e.g., Beatty & Monson, 1990b).

Syntax

There is increasing agreement that nondemented PD patients demonstrate difficulty in comprehending more complex syntax and that their spontaneous language output is syntactically simplified. Furthermore, syntactic changes are more pronounced in demented PD patients than in nondemented ones (Cummings et al., 1988). What remains at issue is whether the syntactic changes observed in PD reflect true language changes or attentional, executive, and memory dysfunction. Cummings et al. (1988), Illes (1989), Illes, Metter, Hanson, and Iritani (1988), and Lieberman, Friedman, and Feldman (1990) reported that spontaneous speech samples of PD patients are syntactically simplified and that there are more frequent and longer pauses in the flow of speech. Illes et al. (1988) suggested that the decreased syntactic complexity of PD patients' speech might reflect an adaptation to their increasing dysarthria. Although this possibility cannot be excluded, it is unlikely that decreased syntactic complexity represents simply an adaptation to dysarthria. Specifically, several studies have reported alterations in PD patients' comprehension of syntax even when the tasks minimize motoric speech demands (Grossman et al., 1991, 1992; Lieberman et al., 1990, 1992; Natsopoulos et al., 1991). Whether syntactic alterations in the language of PD patients represent attentional and memory dysfunction is less clear. Whereas syntactic comprehension in general emerged unrelated to attentional and memory dysfunction in some studies (Grossman et al., 1992; Lieberman et al., 1990), Grossman et al. (1992) nonetheless proposed that some highly specific aspects of sentence comprehension might be related to attention.

Semantics

With respect to semantic tasks, the majority of studies indicate that nondemented PD patients are impaired on generative naming tasks that use semantic constraints (i.e., category fluency). Impairments on verbal fluency tasks that use lexical constraints (i.e., letter or phonemic fluency) have been less consistently observed and variously characterized by decreased output or increased perseverations and intrusions. In addition, impairments relative to normal control subjects might be evident on only some letters or categories (Auriacombe et al., 1993; Bayles, Trosset, Tomoeda, Montgomery, & Wilson, 1993; Beatty, Monson, & Goodkin, 1989; Cooper, Sagar, Jordan, Harvey, & Sullivan, 1991; Lees & Smith, 1983; Levin, Llabre, & Weiner, 1989). Although PD patients are impaired on alternating fluency tasks (e.g., letter-letter and letter-category) (Cooper et al., 1991; Downes, Sharp, Costall, Sagar, & Howe, 1993) suggesting that attentional impairments might underlie poor performance on some tests of verbal fluency, recent findings indicating that cuing improves verbal fluency performance (Downes et al., 1993; Randolph, Braun, Goldberg, & Chase, 1993) have been interpreted as consonant with a retrieval deficit (Auriacombe et al., 1993; Randolph, Braun, et al., 1993).

It is also possible that category fluency performance in PD, or at least in PD dementia, is impaired due to a degradation or inaccessibility of semantic network contents. Tröster, Heindel, Salmon, and Butters (1989) found that only demented PD patients' category fluency was impaired relative to that of normal controls. Furthermore, the qualitative characteristics of demented PD patients' performance (i.e., a proclivity to generate category labels rather than specific category members, such as "fruit" rather than "apple") resembled that reported for AD patients (Tröster, Salmon, McCullough, & Butters, 1989).

Although verbal fluency impairments have generally been accepted to be more severe in AD than in PD, two recent studies have reported the contrary. Stern, Richards, Sano, and Mayeux (1993) found that both demented and nondemented PD patients perform more poorly on verbal fluency than AD patients, with comparable severity of overall cognitive impairment. Bayles et al. (1993), on the other hand, found that demented PD and AD patients performed similarly on letter and semantic fluency tasks.

It is generally agreed that word knowledge, as assessed with vocabulary tests, is relatively preserved in PD (Huber, Shuttleworth, Paulson, Bellchambers, & Clapp, 1986; Matison et al., 1982; Pirozzolo et al., 1982; Tröster, Fields, Paolo, & Koller, 1996). It is possible, however, that a subset of PD patients with dysnomia perform more poorly also on vocabulary tests (Beatty & Monson, 1989a).

Findings with respect to visual confrontation naming in PD are less uniform. While some have reported mild dysnomia even in early PD (Globus, Mildworf, & Melamed, 1985; Matison et al., 1982), others have not (Freedman, Rivoira, Butters, Sax, & Feldman, 1984; Levin et al., 1989). It is likely that as severity of cognitive impairment in PD increases so does the likelihood of dysnomia (e.g., Cummings et al., 1988; Tröster, Fields, et al., 1996).

Apraxia

Praxis (the ability to carry out purposeful movements in the absence of paralysis or paresis) has not been widely investigated in PD but is generally held to be a feature of cortical rather than subcortical dementias. Although Lees and Smith (1983) did not find evidence of dyspraxia in early PD, two other studies did find evidence of subtle practic deficits in early PD. Goldenberg, Wimmer, Auff, and Schnaberth (1986) reported an impairment of ideomotor praxis involving whole limbs, and Grossman et al. (1991) found PD patients to make "body part-for-object" errors on representational praxis tasks.

Spatial Cognition

There is considerable controversy as to whether PD causes a primary impairment in visu-ospatial function. Passafiume, Boller, and Keefe (1986) strongly suggest that visuospatial impairment is universally present in patients with Parkinson's disease, whereas Brown and Marsden (1986) maintain that neither a review of the literature nor the results of their research give support to the idea of a generalized visuospatial deficit in Parkinson's disease.

Most investigators agree, however, that visuospatial function is not a unitary phenomenon and it includes concepts of spatial perception, space exploration, personal space cognition, topographical memory, constructional ability (De Renzi, 1980), or alternative classifications such as (a) the appreciation of the relative positions of stimulus objects in space, (b) the integration of those objects into a coherent spatial framework, and (c) the execution of mental operations involving spatial concepts (Boller et al., 1982; see also Brown & Marsden, 1986, for review).

Brown and Marsden (1986) suggest that the most basic evidence for a spatial deficit in PD arises from consistent findings of lower performance IQ scores in comparison to verbal IQ scores on such tests as the Wechsler Adult Intelligence Scale (WAIS; Wechsler, 1958). Loranger, Goodell, Lee, and McDowell (1972) found a verbal performance IQ split of more than 20 points in nearly 60% of PD patients, compared with lowered percentage of splits of 20 points or more in normal control (2%) and depressed subjects (20%). Loranger et al. (1972) and other investigators (Meier & Martin, 1970) concluded that these results are indicative of a primary cognitive deficit linked to visuospatial dysfunction. Brown and Marsden (1986), however, contend that a more parsimonious explanation might be that deficits reflect impairments in motor speed and manual dexterity (i.e., most of the performance IQ subtests are timed tasks and require writing or the manipulation of objects); they further state that this issue can only be resolved with experiments designed to separate and analyze individually the different functional components of such tasks.

Early studies designed to specifically examine visuospatial function in PD used a rod and frame apparatus (Proctor, Riklan, Cooper, & Teuber, 1964; Teuber & Proctor, 1964). The procedures required subjects to adjust a line to a vertical position when they were in an upright position as well as when they were blindfolded and tilted in a chair; they were also required to adjust themselves to an upright position while blindfolded and tilted. Patients with PD had no difficulty with the first condition (i.e., adjusting a line to vertical), but demonstrated significant decrements in adjusting the line once tilted and in uprighting themselves.

Bowen and colleagues (Bowen, Burns, Brady, & Yahr, 1976; Bowen, Hoehn, & Yahr, 1972) used other visuospatial tasks with PD patients, such as a route walking task, in which nine spots were laid out on the floor in a 3×3 grid, and subjects were given a paper map with the same floor pattern represented on it. On the map a path was drawn, passing through a number of the dots. Subjects were instructed to use the map to guide them while walking on the grid, following the same path outlined on the map held in their hands. "The crucial instruction was that the subject was not allowed to turn the map around, so that on some occasions the subject would have to turn his body in the opposite direction to that represented literally on the map." (Brown & Marsden, 1986, p. 989). Results demonstrated PD patients to have greater confusion with right and left turns, especially on those occasions when the subject was required to extrapolate the body image to interpret the map correctly (see Brown & Marsden, 1986, for discussion). Bowen et al. (1976) earlier showed subjects a dorsal and ventral representation of a human figure and required them to point out on their own bodies the body parts and locations indicated on the representation. Again, PD patients demonstrated impairment, particularly on those items that required a mental rotation.

Brown and Marsden (1986) contend that such results are not indicative of a primary spatial deficit, but instead reflect an inability in *shifting* mental perspectives from one orientation to another, which has been aptly demonstrated to be impaired in PD patients on tests of both cognitive and motor abilities (Cools, Van Den Berken, Horstink, Van Spaendonk, & Berger, 1984; Lees & Smith, 1983; Taylor, Saint-Cyr, & Lang, 1986):

> The ability to shift a cognitive or motor strategy or "set", is not in itself a spatial function. However, an impairment in "shifting ability" may manifest itself in poor performance on a spatial task where shifting is required. Such poor performance is not a spatial deficit … In no study is there unequivocal evidence for a spatial deficit in Parkinson's disease. (Brown & Marsden, 1986, p. 989)

Because of the complexity involved in many of the tasks used to assess visuospatial function in PD, it has been difficult to delineate the specific influence of visuospatial factors from other cognitive, praxic, and memory factors in completing such tasks. De Renzi, Faglioni, and Scotti (1971) suggest that a more definitive answer might be obtained by employing elementary tasks that tap the basic mechanisms underlying spatial abilities (see also Brown & Marsden, 1986, for discussion). Della Sala, Di Lorenzo, Giordana, and Spinnler (1986), for example, have found no significant differences between PD patients and normal control subjects on tests requiring prediction of line trajectories from line segments. In a study conducted by Mortimer, Pirozzolo, Hansch, and Webster (1982), it was concluded that visuospatial impairment in PD may be a function of deficiencies in spatial memory or the manipulation of spatial information, rather than defects in simple visual discrimination. Brown and Marsden (1986) tested right–left discrimination and the manipulation of those concepts in different spatial perspectives and found that PD patients did not differ from normal subjects in the spatial components of the task. Similar findings were also reported by Taylor, Saint-Cyr, and Lang (1986).

Memory

Explicit Memory

Explicit or declarative memory, which refers to the conscious recollection of previously acquired information, is the type of memory assessed by classic, clinical tests of recall and recognition. One common, dichotomous classification of explicit memory (i.e., the distinction between episodic and semantic memory; Tulving, 1983) is based on the type of information stored in memory. Episodic memory contains context-linked information whose retrieval depends upon spatial and temporal cues. For example, remembering whether one took one's last dose of a medication requires retrieval of an episodic memory (i.e., where and when one took the medicine). Semantic memory, in contrast, refers to information that is context-free and usually overlearned. Thus, recollection that $3 \times 3 = 9$, that Yosemite National Park is in California, and that the colors of the American flag are red, white, and blue can be achieved without recalling the episode (or spatiotemporal context) in which that information was acquired.

Although of general heuristic value in understanding anterograde amnesia (i.e., impaired learning and retention of new information after occurrence of cerebral insult), the application of the episodic–semantic distinction to retrograde amnesia (i.e., impaired recollection of information acquired before cerebral insult) is more problematic (see Heindel, Salmon, & Butters, 1993). For this reason, studies concerning remote memory (or retrograde amnesia) in PD are reviewed briefly before studies of episodic and semantic memory.

Remote Memory

In general, retrograde amnesia is not apparent in PD until a significant decline in overall cognitive functioning is apparent (Freedman et al., 1984; Huber, Shuttleworth, & Paulson, 1986). Using the battery developed by Albert, Butters, and Levin (1979), which requires recall and recognition of information pertaining to famous individuals and events of the 1920s and 1970s and the identification of famous individuals from their photographs, Freedman et al. (1984) and Huber, Shuttleworth, and Paulson (1986) found that cognitively impaired PD patients performed more poorly than controls on all parts of the test. Furthermore, PD patients' impairment was similarly severe across all decades, a feature unlike that observed in AD, which results in a temporally graded retrograde amnesia (with relative sparing of more distant events) (see Beatty, 1994, for review). Although PD patients' remote geographical memory has also been found to be impaired (Beatty & Monson, 1989b), the presence/absence of a temporal gradient for such information has not been investigated.

Although Sagar, Cohen, Sullivan, Corkin, and Growdon (1988) found the recognition of events in remote memory to be relatively intact in PD, PD patients had difficulty dating these events, independent of the overall severity of cognitive impairment. These authors thus suggest that deficient temporal memory or recency discrimination or sequencing,

rather than a retrieval deficit, might underlie the remote memory difficulties observed in PD.

Episodic Memory

Whereas studies of the pattern of performance of PD patients on episodic memory tests have yielded remarkably consistent findings, the anatomic substrate and cognitive mechanisms underlying this memory impairment continue to be debated. The performance of PD patients on clinical memory tests (involving retention of word lists, prose passages, paired associates, and designs) is characterized by impaired recall but relatively intact recognition (Beatty, Staton, Weir, Monson, & Whitaker, 1989; Bondi & Kaszniak, 1991; Breen, 1993; Buytenhuijs et al., 1994; Cohen, Bouchard, Scherzer, & Whitaker, 1994; Helkala, Laulumaa, Soininen, & Reikkinen, 1988; Huber, Shuttleworth, Paulson, Bellchambers, & Clapp, 1986; Levin et al., 1989; Mohr et al., 1990; Pillon, Deweer, Agid, & Dubois, 1993; Tsai, Lu, Hua, Lo, & Lo, 1994). Typically, PD patients without overt dementia demonstrate relatively normal rates of forgetting and tend to commit few intrusion errors (i.e., do not produce material extraneous to the stimuli presented). This pattern is in contrast to that observed in AD: the similar impairment of both recall and recognition, rapid rates of forgetting, and heightened sensitivity to proactive interference as shown by the proclivity for intrusion errors and perseverations (see Bondi, Salmon, & Butters, 1994, for review). Although PD patients with dementia demonstrate poorer recognition memory (with recognition still relatively better than free recall), demonstrate more rapid rates of forgetting, and commit more intrusion errors than PD patients without dementia, these memory abnormalities are still not as pronounced as in AD patients with comparable overall severity of cognitive impairment (Beatty, Monson, & Goodkin, 1989; Kramer, Levin, Brandt, & Delis, 1989; Massman, Delis, Butters, Levin, & Salmon, 1990; Pillon et al., 1993; Stern, Richards, et al., 1993).

The above observations, together with the noted lack of a temporal gradient in the retrograde amnesia of PD patients, have been interpreted as indicating that PD memory deficits reflect these patients' difficulty in retrieval, rather than encoding or storage operations. Taylor, Saint-Cyr, and Lang (1986) also suggested that the episodic memory deficits of PD patients might reflect a deficiency in strategy generation secondary to frontal lobe dysfunction, and that such executive deficits are most pronounced on tasks demanding self-initiated planning.

Taylor, Saint-Cyr, and Lang's (1986) proposal that deficient self-initiated strategic information processing underlies PD cognitive deficits is attractive from both psychological and neuroanatomic standpoints. From a psychological perspective, it is accepted that executive dysfunction is frequently seen even in early PD (Levin & Katzen, 1995). Given the significant demands of many memory tests on executive dysfunction (Levin & Katzen, 1995) one might a priori expect executive dysfunction to affect performance on such memory tests.

From an anatomic standpoint, it is well known that the striatum and frontal cortex are connected via parallel circuits (Alexander, DeLong, & Strick, 1986; Cummings, 1993), and that these frontostriatal circuits have connections to structures important to memory, such as the entorhinal cortex (Mega & Cummings, 1994). Indeed, there are at least two possible pathophysiologic mechanisms by which frontal dysfunction might compromise memory in PD. Thalamic inhibition mediated by increased GABAergic output from basal ganglia to thalamus (Albin, 1995) might in turn decrease the thalamus's glutamine-mediated excitatory influence on the frontal cortex (Albin, 1995; Hallett, 1993), thereby disrupting a circuit integrating executive and memory functions. Such frontal dysfunction might be accentuated by dopaminergic cell loss in the ventral tegmental area adjacent to the substantia nigra (Javoy-Agid et al., 1981) and the consequent lateral prefrontal cortical dopaminergic depletion via mesolimbic-cortical pathway dysfunction (Taylor, Saint-Cyr, & Lang, 1986). However, it is also theoretically plausible that striatal pathophysiology in PD leads to memory disruption independent of frontal dysfunction. That is, basal ganglia dysfunction might inhibit thalamus function, and more particularly the dorsomedial nucleus of the thalamus, which is not only a site of the confluence of basal ganglia and mesial temporal lobe systems, but also itself a structure important to memory. Consequently, striatal pathophysiology observed in PD

might disturb memory relatively directly by disrupting, inter alia, dorsomedial thalamic activity or more indirectly by virtue of disrupting thalamic-mesial temporal circuits.

Despite converging evidence supporting Taylor, Saint-Cyr, and Lang's (1986) frontal dysfunction hypothesis of memory impairment in PD, several uncertainties remain. One major reason for this uncertainty is that there is little agreement about the role of the frontal lobes in memory (see Shimamura, 1994, for review). In their recent review, Tröster and Fields (1995) discussed four broad approaches to evaluate the potential frontal dysfunction contribution to memory impairment in PD: examination of the qualitative characteristics of PD memory impairment and their comparison to those reported in studies of patients with frontal lobe lesions; correlation of memory and executive function test scores; investigation of PD patients' performances on memory tests thought to be sensitive to frontal but not temporal pathology; and neuroimaging studies of cerebral blood flow and metabolism.

Perhaps the most compelling evidence that frontal dysfunction can affect memory comes from studies reporting PD patients to be impaired on memory tasks that are particularly sensitive to frontal dysfunction (e.g., recency discrimination, delayed response and delayed alternation, source memory, and conditional associative learning; for review, see Tröster & Fields, 1995). However, this does not imply that their impairments on clinical memory tests are solely attributable to frontal dysfunction. In some cases, executive dysfunction might be neither sufficient nor necessary for PD patients to demonstrate impairments on traditional clinical memory tests. For example, at least some groups of PD patients have been shown to demonstrate impaired memory but intact executive functions (e.g., Mohr et al., 1990), or intact memory but impaired executive functions (e.g., Owen et al., 1992). Even if executive deficits affect performance on clinical memory tests, the shared variance attributable to the relationship between executive and memory test scores is typically modest (ranging from 4% to 50%, with the preponderance of values falling into the lower end of this range; Tröster & Fields, 1995). With regard to qualitative similarities among PD and frontal lesion patients' memory test performances, much of the support comes from studies interpreting diminished semantic encoding as an executive deficit. However, semantic encoding deficiencies are not ubiquitous in PD, nor are they a necessary consequence of frontal lesions. In summary, although it is likely that frontally mediated executive deficits adversely affect many aspects of memory test performance in PD, executive dysfunction is unlikely to be the sole determinant of memory impairment in PD.

Semantic Memory

Semantic memory is usually assessed with tasks such as the Vocabulary and Information subtests of the Wechsler Adult Intelligence Scale-Revised (WAIS-R; Wechsler, 1981), which require the examinee to orally provide word definitions and answers to general factual knowledge questions; letter and category verbal fluency tests; and visual confrontation naming tests. In addition, some investigators use an examinee's ability to engage in semantic clustering on word list learning tasks and to appreciate category shifts as indices of the integrity of semantic memory.

As discussed in the section on language, early PD patients' performance on vocabulary is typically preserved (Huber, Shuttleworth, Paulson, et al., 1986; Matison et al., 1982; Pirozzolo et al., 1982; Tröster, Fields, et al., 1996) and apparently is not affected by potential retrieval deficits as suggested by the observation that PD patients derive as much benefit as normal controls from the provision of the multiple-choice recognition format relative to the standard free recall format of the WAIS-R as a neuropsychological instrument (Tröster, Fields et al., 1996). Nonetheless, a subset of early, nondemented PD patients with visual confrontation naming impairment scored more poorly on vocabulary than PD patients without dysnomia (Beatty & Monson, 1989a; Beatty, Monson, et al., 1989). Whereas Pirozzolo et al. (1982) observed PD patients to be impaired on the Information subtest, Randolph, Mohr, and Chase (1993) and Tröster, Fields, et al. (1996) did not.

As already mentioned, the findings pertaining to visual confrontation naming in PD are not consistent. It is of interest that the one study examining error types and effects of cuing on PD naming performance (Matison et al., 1982) showed that errors were largely semantic and that PD patients derived significant benefit from the provision of the phonemic cues. This qualitative analysis provides further support for the view that semantic memory deficits in PD involve difficulty in accessing and retrieving semantic representations rather than a degradation of the structure of semantic knowledge.

Implicit Memory

Recent investigations indicate that patients with cortical and subcortical dementia syndromes can be differentiated by their performances on various implicit memory tasks (for reviews, see Bondi et al., 1994; Salmon & Butters, 1995). Implicit memory refers to the unconscious recollection of knowledge that is expressed indirectly through the performance of the specific operations comprising a task. Classical conditioning, lexical and semantic priming, motor skill learning, and cognitive- or perceptual-skill learning are all considered forms of implicit memory (Schacter, 1987; Squire, 1987). In these instances, an individual's performance is facilitated "unconsciously" simply by prior exposure to stimulus material. Implicit memory has been described as a distinct memory "system" independent of the conscious, episodic memory system (Schacter, 1987; Schacter & Tulving, 1994; Squire, 1987). Neuropsychological and neurobiological evidence for this distinction is provided by numerous studies over the past decade that have demonstrated preserved implicit memory in patients with severe amnesia arising from damage to the hippocampal formation or to diencephalic brain regions (for review, see Squire, Knowlton, & Musen, 1993).

Patients with cortical dementias (i.e., AD) have been found to be significantly impaired on lexical (Bondi & Kaszniak, 1991; Shimamura, Salmon, Squire, & Butters, 1987), semantic (Salmon, Shimamura, Butters, & Smith, 1988), and pictorial (Heindel, Salmon, & Butters, 1990) priming tests, whereas subcortical dementia patients (e.g., Huntington's disease [HD] and PD) have demonstrated normal verbal (Bondi & Kaszniak, 1991; Salmon et al., 1988) and pictorial priming ability (Heindel et al., 1990). For example, Bondi and Kaszniak (1991) compared the lexical priming performance of patients with AD and PD on the word stem completion priming task previously used by Graf and colleagues (Graf, Squire, & Mandler, 1984; Salmon et al., 1988). The PD patients exhibited intact stem completion priming. In contrast, the AD patients showed little or no tendency to complete the stems with the previously presented words and demonstrated significantly less priming than normal control subjects and PD patients. The results of this and other studies of priming suggest that this form of implicit memory may be dependent on the association cortices that are damaged in AD but relatively intact in PD patients without overt dementia (Bondi & Kaszniak, 1991).

In contrast to the priming results, subcortical dementia patients such as those with HD are impaired on tests of motor skill learning (Heindel, Butters, & Salmon, 1988; Heindel, Salmon, Shults, Walicke, & Butters, 1989), prism adaptation (Paulsen, Butters, Salmon, Heindel, & Swenson, 1993), and weight biasing (Heindel, Salmon, & Butters, 1992) tasks that are performed normally by most AD patients. All of these tasks involve the generation and refinement (i.e., learning) of motor programs to guide behavior. For example, in one motor skill learning task, rotary pursuit, subjects must learn over repeated trials to maintain contact between a stylus held in the preferred hand and a small metallic disk on a rotating turntable. Heindel and colleagues (1988) tested AD, HD, and amnesic patients on this task over six blocks of trials, with each block consisting of four 20-s trials. The total time on target for each trial was recorded. The results of this study showed that AD and amnesic patients, as well as normal control subjects, all demonstrated systematic and equivalent improvement across blocks of trials. In contrast, the HD patients were severely impaired in the acquisition of the pursuit rotor motor skill, showing only slight improvement over blocks of trials. This motor skill learning deficit in HD patients was not correlated with their general motor impairment (i.e., chorea) and was confirmed with other tasks that have little, if any, motor component (e.g., weight biasing, prism adaptation). These results suggest that motor skill acquisition is dependent on the integrity of the basal ganglia structures damaged in HD and independent of the cortical, hippocampal, and diencephalic brain regions affected in AD and circumscribed amnesia.

Evidence concerning procedural or skill learning in PD, however, has been mixed (see Salmon & Butters, 1995, for review). Nondemented PD patients have shown impairment on some procedural learning tasks such as the Tower of Toronto puzzle (Saint-Cyr, Taylor, & Lang, 1988) and the skill learning component of a fragmented pictures task (Bondi & Kaszniak, 1991; Bondi, Kaszniak, Bayles, & Vance, 1993), but not on other skill learning tasks such as mirror-reversed reading (Bondi & Kaszniak, 1991; Harrington, Haaland, Yeo, & Marder, 1990) and pursuit-rotor tracking (Bondi & Kaszniak, 1991; Heindel et al., 1989). Across different studies, too, conflicting results have also been reported for the same procedural learning task. For example, whereas Bondi and Kaszniak (1991) and Heindel et al. (1989) found nondemented PD patients to show learning curves equivalent to those of controls on pursuit-rotor tracking tasks, Harrington and colleagues (1990) reported PD patients to be impaired in pursuit-rotor tracking. However, in contrast to the other two studies, Harrington et al. studied pursuit-rotor learning across three days rather than a single day. In the Harrington et al. study, the PD patients showed a similar amount of learning as control subjects across trial blocks in the first day, but less learning across days. It may therefore be that differences in the results of these pursuit-rotor learning studies are attributable to the fact that Harrington et al. tested subjects across three consecutive days. Patients with PD may have been more disrupted in their motor procedural learning by other motor activities in which they engaged between each of the days in the Harrington et al. study. This possibility raises the question of whether interference or set shifting requirements may be a critical determinant of whether nondemented PD patients are impaired in motor procedural learning tasks.

In a direct test of this notion, Kaszniak and colleagues (Kaszniak, Trosset, Bondi, & Bayles, 1992) examined nondemented PD patients on a modification of the serial reaction time (SRT) task developed by Nissen and colleagues (Nissen & Bullemer, 1987; Nissen, Willingham, & Hartman, 1989). When given this task, patients with alcoholic Korsakoff's syndrome perform similar to age-matched control subjects, showing the same pattern of SRT improvement with practice on a repeating stimulus sequence (spatial location of visual stimuli) and the same pattern of slowing upon switching to a random sequence. Kaszniak et al. (1992) predicted that PD patients would acquire the procedural learning of the repeating sequence as well as control subjects; however, given the expectation that PD patients would have difficulty in set shifting when going from the random trial block back to the repeating sequence blocks, they further predicted that the PD group would show less of a decrease in SRT latency than the control group. That is, the shift from nonpredictive back to predictive information was expected to be more costly in terms of demands for the PD patients because of their hypothesized deficits in shifting sets.

The pattern of results was as predicted and consistent with the interpretation that nigrostriatal dysfunction in PD does not result in impaired procedural learning for tasks that involve high predictability (e.g., pursuit-rotor learning, mirror-reversed reading, and repeated sequences of SRT tasks) and require no shifting of set. However, when procedural learning tasks do not provide highly predictive information (e.g., fragmented pictures skill learning), or when a shift in the predictive value of information occurs (e.g., repeat to random and back to repeat SRT trials), PD patients are impaired in their task performance. The impairment observed by Kaszniak et al. (1992) was also correlated with performance on the modified Wisconsin Card Sorting Test (Hart, Kwentus, Wade, & Taylor, 1988), consistent with the interpretation that difficulties in set shifting play a role in the SRT results obtained by Kaszniak et al. (1992). Difficulties on both tasks may reflect a common dysfunction of semi-closed neuronal circuitry loops between the basal ganglia and the frontal cortex (DeLong & Georgopoulos, 1981; DeLong, Georgopoulos, & Crutcher, 1983).

Executive Function

The frontal lobes are implicated in a number of higher level functions. These functions include concept formation, abstract reasoning, planning, organization, initiation, feedback utilization, inhibition of irrelevant responses, and cognitive flexibility. Deficits in these abilities are thought to have their greatest impact on tasks of novel problem-solving (see Stuss & Benson, 1986). Previous research on PD patients has consistently demonstrated circumscribed deficits on most tasks thought to be sensitive to the integrity of the frontal lobes (Cools et al., 1984; Lees & Smith, 1983; Taylor, Saint-Cyr, & Lang, 1986).

Lees and Smith (1983) were among the first investigators to observe impaired performance on the Wisconsin Card Sorting Test and verbal fluency in PD patients, including those patients restricted to the earliest, untreated stages of the disease. These deficits were observed within the context of preserved intellectual and recognition memory functions. These authors concluded that the results implied selective dysfunction within the frontal lobes. Similarly, Cools et al. (1984) demonstrated a "diminished shifting aptitude" in PD patients with intact intellectual functions. Patients with PD were impaired on tasks involving the ability to reorganize behavior according to the requirements of a task; diminished shifting aptitude was observed on motor and sorting tasks guided by self-generated information.

In efforts to explain such frontal-like deficits in PD, Taylor and colleagues (1986) adopted a functional/anatomic hypothesis concerning semi-closed neuronal circuitry or "loops" between striatal and frontal cortical areas. DeLong and colleagues (DeLong and Georgopoulos, 1981; DeLong et al., 1983) first proposed the concept of "motor" and "complex" loops existing between the basal ganglia and frontal cortex. The "complex" loop is thought to transmit information through the striatum to granular frontal association areas thought to be involved in more purely cognitive operations. Using this theoretical framework, Taylor, Saint-Cyr, and Lang (1986) predicted that cognitive deficits in PD would occur as a consequence of the disturbed outflow of neuronal activity from the striatum (particularly the caudate nucleus); abilities thought to be dependent on the integrity of the frontal lobes would, therefore, be affected because of subcortical deafferentation of the prefrontal cortex.

Through extensive testing of memory, visuospatial, and executive functions, the degree to which circumscribed deficits were attributable to the integrity of the frontal lobes could be ascertained. Results indicated no evidence of generalized disruption of cognitive processes. Rather, only five tests distinguished PD from the normal control subjects: the Wisconsin Card Sorting Test, free recall of items from the Rey Auditory Verbal Learning Test,

Bead-Tapper, the Delayed Recognition Test spatial list (Albert & Moss, 1984), and immediate recall of the logical passages on the Wechsler Memory Scale. These deficits were taken to reflect an impairment in the ability to spontaneously generate efficient strategies when relying on self-directed, task-specific planning. Since the prefrontal cortex is presumed to play an important role in self-directed behavioral planning, these investigators concluded that the neostriatal outflow model, in predicting the consequences of caudate nucleus dysfunction, was supported. Also, this conclusion is strengthened by the lack of deficits on tests presumably related to other cortical areas, such as recognition memory and most visuospatial tasks (see also Brown & Marsden, 1986; Flowers, Pearce, & Pearce, 1984).

Taylor, Saint-Cyr, and Lang (1986) further argue that the disturbed neostriatal outflow model would have to explain not only the lack of deficits associated with all but the frontal region, but also intact performance on tasks which are also associated with the frontal region. Their investigation demonstrated intact performance on tests of verbal fluency (cf. Lees & Smith, 1983) and design fluency, as well as the ability to maintain an alternating cognitive set on the Trail Making Test (parts A and B). Taylor, Saint-Cyr, and Lang (1986) reasoned that the outflow model, in placing emphasis on activity in the frontal lobes, takes account of the massive corticocortical support this region receives in the processing of familiar, structured and rule-bound behavior. Thus, Taylor and colleagues (1986) highlighted that PD results in a loss of internally guided behavior which is expressed differentially in the diminished planning of motor, cognitive, and emotional behaviors, secondary to disturbed neostriatal outflow to the prefrontal cortical regions which are thought to subserve these abilities.

Recent studies have further implicated frontal system dysfunction in performances of PD patients on other card sorting tasks as well as on tasks of temporal ordering and sequencing (Beatty & Monson, 1990a; Bondi et al., 1993; McFie & Thompson, 1972; Sagar, Sullivan, Gabrieli, Corkin, & Growdon, 1988; Sullivan, Sagar, Gabrieli, Corkin, & Growdon, 1989). Research has demonstrated that the ability to make judgments of temporal order is dissociable from the capacity to recognize previous events (see Squire, 1987; Schacter, 1987, for discus-

sion), suggesting that recognition memory and recency discrimination are served by independent cognitive processes (see Sagar et al., 1988, for discussion). Korsakoff's syndrome patients, for example, exhibit a severe deficit in remembering the temporal order of learned material that is described as being too large to be explained by impaired memory for the material itself (Squire, 1982). Patients with surgical lesions involving the frontal lobes (Milner, 1971, 1974) have demonstrated this dissociation as well, suggesting that the frontal lobes play an important role in this type of cognitive operation.

Temporal ordering and recognition memory have been assessed in PD patients with verbal material. Sagar et al. (1988) administered a continuous recognition memory and recency discrimination paradigm (cf. Hirst & Volpe, 1982). Test questions appeared at various intervals after presentation of target stimuli. The results demonstrated that PD patients were disproportionately impaired in recency discrimination relative to content recognition; they also showed deficits in content recognition only at the shortest stimulus-test intervals. They suggested that recency discrimination deficits and impaired short-term memory processing are specific cognitive deficits in PD and may be linked to subcortical deafferentation of the frontal lobes.

Several teams of investigators have suggested that frontal system dysfunction may be an underlying mechanism accounting for cognitive difficulties of PD patients in other domains such as memory, visuospatial and perceptual skills, and language (Bondi et al., 1993; Bowen et al., 1976; Brown & Marsden, 1984, 1986; Della Salla et al., 1986; Frith, Bloxham, & Carpenter, 1986; Levin, Tomer, & Rey, 1992; Taylor, Saint-Cyr, & Lang, 1986; see also Taylor & Saint-Cyr, 1992, for discussion). Bondi and colleagues (1993), for example, administered three categories of neuropsychological tests to a group of nondemented PD patients: (a) tests sensitive to frontal system dysfunction, (b) tests of learning and memory, and (c) tests of visuospatial and perceptual skills. Results demonstrated that memory and visuospatial test performances in PD patients no longer differed from those of elderly control subjects once scores on the frontal system tasks were statistically covaried. However, the converse was not true. Performances of patients with PD on the frontally related tasks were still significantly poorer than that of control subjects even when memory and visuospatial test performance was covaried. Bondi et al. (1993) concluded that frontal system dysfunction appeared to account for many of the apparent failures in other task domains.

Nonetheless, given the multifactorial nature of many neuropsychological tasks, it remains difficult to establish the precise contributions of so-called frontal system or executive skills to impaired performances in other cognitive domains such as memory. It is clear that there is a complex interaction between frontally mediated executive deficits in PD and performance in other cognitive domains. Furthermore, as some authors have suggested (see Tröster & Fields, 1995), although frontal executive deficits in PD may account for at least some of the difficulties in other task domains, frontal system dysfunction may not adequately account for all cognitive impairments seen in PD patients without overt dementia.

Depression

Incidence and Prevalence

Depression is acknowledged to be a common concomitant of Parkinson's disease and more severe and frequent in PD than in other conditions with chronic physical limitations (Rao, Huber, & Bornstein, 1992; Starkstein & Mayberg, 1993). Although prevalence estimates of depression in PD vary widely (from 20% to 90%) (Rao et al., 1992), the majority of studies estimate it at 40%, with half that number of patients having major depression and the other half minor depression (Starkstein & Mayberg, 1993). As Cummings (1992) has pointed out, several factors likely underlie the discrepant prevalence estimates: patient selection biases, different methods of assessment, different definitions of depression, and different thresholds for identification of depression. In addition, regardless of whether studies of depression in PD use the syndrome model (diagnostic criteria) or the symptom approach (symptom rating scales), they likely overestimate depression in PD because the symptoms of PD and depression overlap (Rao et al., 1992). Because prevalence of depression also is influenced by inci-

dence of new cases, duration, and recurrence of depression, Dooneief et al. (1992) suggest that incidence might provide a more accurate estimate of risk of depression in PD than prevalence. Dooneief et al. (1992) reported an incidence of depression in PD of 1.86% per year, a number considerably higher than incidence of depression reported for the general population 40 years and older.

Depression: Reaction to or Biological Concomitant of Parkinson's Disease?

Considerable attention has been devoted to the debate about whether depression in PD is endogenous or reactive. Concerning biological correlates of depression in PD, there is general agreement that dopaminergic abnormalities are unlikely to be significantly related to depression (Mayeux, 1990). Rather, there is at least tentative, converging evidence that depression in PD relates to serotonergic depletion (for review, see Mayberg & Solomon, 1995).

Some authors suggested that depression in PD is likely a function of both reaction to physical challenges and biological changes evident in PD (e.g., Taylor, Saint-Cyr, Lang, & Kenny, 1986). Brown and Jahanshahi (1995) recently proposed what they call a "crude model" of factors causing and modifying depression in PD. They suggest that proximal causes of depression in PD are related to biochemical changes and handicap. However, they suggest that much empirical attention will have to be devoted to studying how impairment and consequent disability translate into handicap and how individuals' demographic backgrounds (e.g., age), their personal (e.g., coping strategies) and social (e.g., social support) resources, and their specific life circumstances (e.g., nature of work) modify the relationships among impairment, disability, and handicap.

Clinical Correlates of Depression in Parkinson's Disease

There is some suggestion that depressive symptoms may vary as a function of disease progression. Huber, Freidenberg, Paulson, Shuttleworth, and Christy (1990) reported that symptoms related to self-reproach and mood were evident early in the course of the disease and stayed stable. In contrast, somatic symptoms were present early in the disease and increased in severity with disease progression, and vegetative signs were evident only later in the course of the disease. Perhaps this heterogeneity of symptoms over the course of the disease underlies the apparent lack of relationship between depression and age, age at disease onset, and disease duration. Alternatively, Cummings (1992) has suggested that there might be two groups of PD patients, those with and without mood changes, and that membership in these groups remains relatively stable over time. Consequently, when these subgroups are combined, possible relationships among depression and clinical variables might be obscured. The majority of studies have also not found a reliable relationship between mood changes and motor manifestations of PD, but it is possible that depression is more common among those with pronounced gait and postural changes (Cummings, 1992).

Influence of Depression on Cognition in Parkinson's Disease

Cross-sectional studies, with generally smaller sample sizes, have yielded contradictory results concerning the impact of depression on cognition in PD. More recent longitudinal studies, and cross-sectional studies carefully matching patient groups for a host of demographic and disease factors, yield converging evidence that depression exacerbates cognitive (and especially, memory) impairment in PD (Starkstein et al., 1989; Tröster, Paolo, et al., 1995), and that depression might be a risk factor for dementia in PD (Marder et al., 1995; Stern, Marder, Tang, & Mayeux, 1993).

Perhaps the most compelling evidence that depression affects cognition in PD comes from longitudinal studies by Starkstein and colleagues examining the relationship between depression and decline in cognition and activities of daily living (Starkstein, Bolduc, Mayberg, Preziosi, & Robinson, 1990; Starkstein, Mayberg, Leiguarda, Preziosi, & Robinson, 1992; Starkstein, Preziosi, Bolduc, & Robinson, 1990). These authors have reported that Mini-Mental State Examination (MMSE) (Folstein et al., 1975) and activities of daily living (ADL) scores of a depressed PD group declined more rapidly than those of a nondepressed group; that initial depression score predicted extent of cognitive decline; and that extent of cognitive and ADL impairment was greater in PD patients with major depression than in those with mild depression. Because potentially confounding variables were not controlled for simultaneously in these studies, Tröster, Paolo, et al. (1995) examined performance of PD groups with and without depression (matched for age, education, gender, age at disease onset, disease duration, and disease severity) on the Mattis Dementia Rating Scale (DRS) (Mattis, 1988). Relative to matched controls, both depressed and nondepressed PD groups demonstrated impairments on the Conceptualization and Initiation/Perseveration subtests, but only the depressed group demonstrated an impairment on the Construction and Memory subtests.

Because Tröster, Paolo, et al. (1995) used only the DRS, and because the depressed PD group's overall severity of cognitive impairment was more pronounced than that of the nondepressed PD group, these authors were not able to establish whether impairment of the depressed relative to the nondepressed PD group was merely one of quantity or one also of quality. Using a broader neuropsychological test battery, Tröster, Stalp, Paolo, Fields, and Koller (1995) found that, relative to a nondepressed PD group matched for age, education, gender, disease severity, age at disease onset, and disease duration, a depressed PD group had more severe impairments in immediate verbal recall and semantic verbal fluency. In addition, relative to a normal control group, only the depressed PD group demonstrated impairments in visual confrontation naming and letter fluency. However, once the two PD groups were also matched for overall severity of cognitive impairment, differences among their test scores disappeared. This finding suggests that depression exacerbates PD cognitive (and especially memory) impairment, but that it does not appreciably alter its quality.

That depression affects predominantly quantity rather than quality of cognitive impairment in PD is plausible if one considers that at least one subgroup of patients with depression develops a subcortical-type dementia (Massman, Delis, Butters, Dupont, & Gillin, 1992). That is, depression might exacerbate the frontostriatal pathophysiology of PD. The observation that depression can exacerbate memory and language impairments of PD is also consistent with recent findings concerning the pathophysiology of depression in PD. More specifically, Torack and Morris (1988) reported that neuropathology common to depressed PD patients involved the ventral tegmental area, hippocampus, and entorhinal cortex. Ring et al. (1994) found that relative to patients with only PD, depressed PD patients demonstrated regional blood flow abnormalities in the medial frontal and cingulate cortices, an abnormality also found in patients with only depression. Mayberg (1994) too reported that individuals with basal ganglia disease and depression, regardless of the etiology of the basal ganglia dysfunction, demonstrate bilateral glucose metabolism reductions in the inferior prefrontal and anterior temporal regions. Interestingly, the apparent medial and inferior frontal pathophysiology observed in PD with depression appears not to exacerbate executive dysfunction often evident in PD. Neither Starkstein et al. (1989) nor Tröster, Stalp, et al. (1995) found greater executive dysfunction in depressed patients compared to nondepressed PD patients.

Treatment and Management of Parkinson's Disease

Pharmacologic Treatment

Koller and Megaffin (1994) emphasize the importance of education and reassurance in treatment of the newly diagnosed PD patient. The mainstay of pharmacologic treatment in PD continues to be levodopa, which serves to increase brain dopamine levels. The drug (combined with carbidopa to counter the peripheral side effects of dopamine) is decarboxylated to dopamine both in the gut and liver and in the brain after crossing the blood-brain barrier. The most pronounced effects of levodopa-carbidopa combination (Sinemet) are observed on bradykinesia and rigidity, and to a lesser extent on tremor. Postural stability and autonomic dysfunction symptoms typically do not respond to levodopa. Recent studies indicate a controlled-release version of the drug (Sinemet-CR) to be helpful in

reducing "off" time and early morning dystonia. Side effects of levodopa treatment include "on–off" phenomena and dyskinesia. Levodopa and dopamine agonists used in conjunction with levodopa, such as pergolide (Permax) and bromocriptine (Parlodel), have also been related to hallucinations (especially visual), delusions, delirium, mania, and a predisposition to depression.

Although levodopa has generally been held not to affect cognition, recent studies indicate that levodopa treatment has heterogeneous effects on different test performances (i.e., improves, worsens, and leaves unaffected certain cognitive functions). Unfortunately, the literature to date makes it difficult to discern consistent effects of levodopa on cognition. Lange et al. (1992) reported that while performance on three "frontal" tasks (attentional set shifting, spatial working memory, and Tower of London) was superior on than off levodopa, performance on three tasks with predominant memory components (spatial and pattern recognition, associative learning, and delayed matching-to-sample) was unaffected. To complicate matters further, it appears that all executive functions are not uniformly affected by levodopa (Gotham et al., 1988) such that some test performances improve, others worsen, and yet others appear unaffected. Furthermore, even within one test (e.g., Tower of London), different variables might bear a different relationship to levodopa treatment (Owen et al., 1995).

Because monoamine oxidase-B (MAO-B) and catechol-O-methyl transferase (COMT) catalyze the breakdown of dopamine and levodopa, drugs inhibiting these enzymes have been investigated as potential antiparkinsonian agents. The MAO-B inhibitor selegiline (Eldepryl; l-deprenyl) has been widely evaluated and is thought to protect nigral neurons. The exact mechanism by which selegiline might protect nigral neurons is unknown. Nonetheless, because selegiline appears to delay the requirement for symptomatic treatment (Parkinson Study Group, 1989) and has been shown to be effective as an initial treatment in early PD, there is general agreement that selegiline should be the first treatment in PD patients who can tolerate this drug (Koller & Megaffin, 1994). Although clinical studies with COMT inhibitors (e.g., tolcapone and entacapone) have only recently been initiated, there is tentative evidence that such drugs might be useful adjuncts to levodopa treatment (Klockgether, Löschmann, & Wüllner, 1994).

In PD cases where tremor is the predominant problem, treatment with anticholinergics such as benztropine (Cogentin), trihexphenidyl (Artane), and amantadine (Symmetrel) can be beneficial. Although negative side effects on cognition have been only inconsistently reported (Levin & Katzen, 1995), the potential of cognitive as well as physical side effects have led some (e.g., Koller & Megaffin, 1994) to argue against use of anticholinergics in individuals older than 70 years. For similar reasons, use in PD of antidepressants other than cyclic agents (which have more potent anticholinergic properties among antidepressants) has been recommended.

Functional Neurosurgery

One approach to restoring striatal dopaminergic function is cerebral implantation of autologous adrenal medullary tissue or fetal mesencephalic tissue. It is now acknowledged that adrenal medullary tissue does not survive (Goetz, DeLong, Penn, & Bakay, 1993; Klockgether et al., 1994). Although use of fetal mesencephalic tissue appears more promising (Lindvall et al., 1994), immunologic problems and ethical issues are unresolved (Klockgether et al., 1994). There is only one report of neuropsychological consequences of fetal tissue implantation (Sass et al., 1995), best considered preliminary as it is based on four patients. Specifically, Sass et al. (1995) reported that three patients with bilateral caudate and one patient with right caudate mesencephalic tissue implants demonstrated significant improvements from presurgical baseline in verbal memory up to 24 months after surgery. However, these improvements were not maintained 36 months after surgery. In addition, no significant changes in verbal and nonverbal cognitive ability and in information processing speed were observed postoperatively. It is thus possible that mesencephalic tissue implantation at least temporarily slows progression of verbal memory deficits.

Although a report of the surgical treatment of Parkinson's disease was first published in 1941, recent advances in stereotactic neurosurgery have led to renewed interest in thalamotomy and pallidotomy as treatments for PD (see Burchiel, 1995, and Laitinen, 1995, for reviews). Despite numerous reports that pallidotomy can markedly improve rigidity, bradykinesia, tremor, balance, and medication-induced dyskinesia (e.g., Dogali et al., 1995; Laitinen, 1994), neuropsychological consequences are sparsely and inadequately documented. Laitinen (1994) reported that following pallidotomy, patients performed more quickly and accurately on all parts of the Purdue pegboard. In addition, left pallidotomy was associated with significant improvements in speed of performance on the Stroop Color Word Test, whereas right pallidotomy was associated with a nonsignificant improvement on the Stroop test. Although unilateral thalamotomy can effectively control tremor, the few studies including neuropsychological evaluation suggest that adverse cognitive side effects can occur. Vilkki and Laitinen (1974) reported that left thalamotomy was associated with language and speech decrements and that right thalamotomy led to transient visuoperceptual changes (decrements on a facial matching task). Darley, Brown, and Swenson (1975) observed that particularly left thalamotomy or combined thalamotomy/pallidotomy involved risk of postoperative language dysfunction. More than 20% of their sample of 123 PD patients experienced expressive language decrements, but only a much smaller number developed comprehension or naming problems. Rossitch et al. (1988), although using a relatively brief neuropsychological test battery and a group of patients whose movement disorders were of various etiologies, found that significant reductions in language and memory occurred in 7 out of 18 patients (only one of these seven had PD, and this patient had previously undergone a contralateral thalamotomy). Laitinen (1994) reported that left thalamotomy was also associated with slower and more error-prone performance on the Stroop test.

Given the irreversibility and potential cognitive side effects of thalamotomy and pallidotomy, recent efforts have been directed at evaluating the benefits of chronic stimulation of the thalamus and pallidum. Initial studies indicate that chronic stimulation of the ventral intermediate (VIM) nucleus of the thalamus leads to improvements in tremor and medication-induced dyskinesia (Benabid et al., 1991; Blond & Siegfried, 1991; Caparros-Lefebvre et al., 1993). Blond et al. (1992) and Caparros-Lefebvre, Blond, Pécheux, Pasquier, and Petit

(1992) reported that in a small series of patients (10 with PD and 4 with essential tremor, and 9 with PD, respectively), no significant changes were observed pre- to postsurgery on a modified mini-mental state exam, the WCST, and a verbal fluency test. Pallidal stimulation has not yet been adequately evaluated, but Siegfried and Lippitz (1994) reported significant improvements in hypokinesia, on–off fluctuations, and gait and speech disturbances in three PD patients, 1 to 9 months postoperatively.

Summary

Parkinson's disease is one of the most common neurologic diseases afflicting older adults. Although its primary motor symptoms (resting tremor, muscular rigidity, slowness of movement or bradykinesia, stooped posture) were accurately described more than 175 years ago, its cause or causes are still unknown. Neuropathologic features of PD include cell losses in the substantia nigra and other subcortical structures and associated reductions in dopamine levels in the striatum. Pharmacologic treatment of PD continues to center on dopaminergic replacement, although a new generation of functional neurosurgical techniques such as pallidotomies are also available. The use of levodopa and other dopamine agonists provides significant reductions in motor symptoms and substantially reduces the impact of PD on everyday functioning (La Rue, 1992). Their impact on ameliorating cognitive sequelae associated with PD are less clear. With the serendipitous discovery of MPTP-induced parkinsonism, researchers have found renewed interest in potential etiologic factors (i.e., PD-causing neurotoxins) that may prove useful in eventually preventing onset of PD (see Langston & Tanner, 1992).

While severe cognitive decline is not observed in the majority of patients with PD (i.e., dementia prevalence ranges between 20% and 40%), a characteristic pattern of neuropsychological deficits is routinely noted. Depression is also a common concomitant of PD. When cognitive deficits occur early in PD, such deficits are most often observed in domains of executive, visuospatial-perceptual, and memory function. Recognition memory appears to be generally spared, whereas PD patients have greater difficulty with tests of free recall. Across studies, frontal executive skills appear to be among the earliest and most consistently impaired domains of functioning and may also contribute to performance deficits in other cognitive areas such as memory and visuoperceptual skills. In mild PD dementia, the pattern of cognitive deficits, on a global level, corresponds to that characteristic of subcortical dementia (see Butters et al., 1987; Cummings, 1990).

McPherson and Cummings (1996) note that the caudate nucleus, globus pallidus, and thalamus are member structures of frontal-subcortical neuronal circuits that link these subcortical nuclei with specific regions of the frontal lobe, and disruption of the circuits results in cognitive deficits similar to those occurring with frontal lobe dysfunction (see also Cummings, 1993). Thus, many of the neuropsychological changes noted in PD can be ascribed to interruption of frontal-subcortical circuit function (McPherson & Cummings, 1996). However, more detailed studies characterizing the role of frontal system abilities in PD and their contributions to other cognitive tasks are needed (see Tröster & Fields, 1995). Although once relegated solely to aspects of motor control and function, it is clear from the neurobehavioral consequences of PD that the basal ganglia plays a much more important role in both cognitive and affective functions than previously thought.

ACKNOWLEDGMENTS

This work was supported in part by funds from the Medical Research Service of the Department of Veterans Affairs and by National Institute on Aging grants AG12674 (Dr. Bondi) and AG10182 (Dr. Tröster). The authors wish to thank Julie A. Fields for assistance with manuscript preparation.

References

Agid, Y., Ruberg, M., Dubois, B., & Javoy-Agid, F. (1984). Biochemical substrates of mental disturbances in Parkinson's disease. In R. G. Hassier & J. F. Christ (Eds.), *Parkinson-specific motor and mental disorders* (pp. 211–218). New York: Raven Press.

Albert, M. L., & Moss, M. (1984). The assessment of memory disorders in patients with Alzheimer's disease. In L. R. Squire & N. Butters (Eds.), *Neuropsychology of memory* (pp. 236–246). New York: Guilford Press.

Albert, M. L., Feldman, R. G., & Willis, A. L. (1974). The "subcortical dementia" of progressive supranuclear palsy. *Journal of Neurology, Neurosurgery, and Psychiatry, 37,* 121–130.

Albert, M. S., Butters, N., & Levin, J. (1979). Temporal gradients in the retrograde amnesia of patients with alcoholic Korsakoff's disease. *Archives of Neurology, 36,* 211–216.

Albin, R. L. (1995). The pathophysiology of chorea/ballism and parkinsonism. *Parkinsonism and Related Disorders, 1,* 3–11.

Alexander, G. E., DeLong, M. R., & Strick, P. L. (1986). Parallel organization of functionally segregated circuits linking basal ganglia and cortex. *Annual Review of Neuroscience, 9,* 357–381.

Alonso, M. E., Otero, E., D'Regules, R., & Figueroa, H. H. (1986). Parkinson's disease: A genetic study. *Canadian Journal of Neurological Sciences, 13,* 248–251.

American Psychiatric Association. (1994). *Diagnostic and statistical manual of mental disorders* (4th ed.). Washington, DC: Author.

Aquilonius, S. M., & Hartvig, P. (1986). A Swedish country with unexpected high utilization of antiparkinsonian drugs. *Acta Neurologica Scandinavica, 74,* 379–382.

Auriacombe, S., Grossman, M., Carvell, S., Gollomp, S., Stern, M. B., & Hurtig, H. I. (1993). Verbal fluency deficits in Parkinson's disease. *Neuropsychology, 7,* 182–192.

Ball, M. J. (1984). The morphological basis of dementia in Parkinson's disease. *Canadian Journal of Neurological Sciences, 11,* 180–184.

Ballard, P. A., Tetrud, J. W., & Langston, J. W. (1985). Permanent human parkinsonism due to 1-methyl-4-phenyl-1,2,3,6-tetrahydropyridine (MPTP): Seven cases. *Neurology, 35,* 949–956.

Barbeau, A. (1984). Etiology of Parkinson's disease: A research strategy. *Canadian Journal of Neurological Sciences, 11,* 24–28.

Barbeau, A., & Poucher, E. (1982). New data on the genetics of Parkinson's disease. *Canadian Journal of Neurological Sciences, 11,* 151–155.

Bayles, K. A., & Kaszniak, A. W. (1987). *Communication and cognition in normal aging and dementia.* Boston: Little, Brown, & Co./College-Hill Press.

Bayles, K. A., Trosset, M. W., Tomoeda, C. K., Montgomery, E. B., & Wilson, J. (1993). Generative naming in Parkinson's disease patients. *Journal of Clinical and Experimental Neuropsychology, 15,* 547–562.

Beatty, W. W. (1994). Remote memory in retrospect. In L. S. Cermak (Ed.), *Neuropsychological explorations of memory and cognition: Essays in honor of Nelson Butters* (pp. 215–221). New York: Plenum Press.

Beatty, W. W., & Monson, N. (1989a). Lexical processing in Parkinson's disease and multiple sclerosis. *Journal of Geriatric Psychiatry and Neurology, 2,* 145–152.

Beatty, W. W., & Monson, N. (1989b). Geographical knowledge in patients with Parkinson's disease. *Bulletin of the Psychonomic Society, 27,* 473–475.

Beatty, W. W., & Monson, N. (1990a). Problem solving in Parkinson's disease: Comparison of performance on the Wisconsin and California Card Sorting Tests. *Journal of Geriatric Psychiatry & Neurology, 3,* 163–171.

Beatty, W. W., & Monson, N. (1990b). Picture and motor sequencing in Parkinson's disease. *Journal of Geriatric Psychiatry and Neurology, 3,* 192–197.

Beatty, W. W., Monson, N., & Goodkin, D. E. (1989). Access to semantic memory in Parkinson's disease and multiple sclerosis. *Journal of Geriatric Psychiatry and Neurology, 2,* 153–162.

Beatty, W. W., Staton, R. D., Weir, W. S., Monson, N., & Whitaker, H. A. (1989). Cognitive disturbances in Parkinson's disease. *Journal of Geriatric Psychiatry and Neurology, 2,* 22–33.

Benabid, A. L., Pollack, P., Gervason, C., Hoffman, D., Gao, D. M., Hommel, M., Perret, J. E., & deRougemont, J. (1991). Long-term suppression of tremor by chronic stimulation of the ventral intermediate thalamic nucleus. *Lancet, 337,* 403–406.

Bernheimer, H., Birkmayer, W., Hornykiewicz, O., Jellinger, K., & Seitelberger, F. (1973). Brain dopamine and the syndromes of Parkinson and Huntington: Clinical, morphological, and neurochemical correlations. *Journal of Neurological Sciences, 20,* 415–455.

Biggins, C. A., Boyd, J. L., Harrop, F. M., Madeley, P., Mindham, R. H. S., Randall, J. I., & Spokes, E. G. S. (1992). A controlled, longitudinal study of dementia in Parkinson's disease. *Journal of Neurology, Neurosurgery and Psychiatry, 55,* 566–571.

Blond, S., & Siegfried, J. (1991). Thalamic stimulation for the treatment of tremor and other motor movement disorders. *Acta Neurochirurgica, 52* (Suppl.), 109–111.

Blond, S., Caparros-Lefebvre, D., Parker, F., Assaker, R., Petit, H., Guieu, J. D., & Christiaens, J. L. (1992). Control of tremor and involuntary movement disorders by chronic stereotactic stimulation of the ventral intermediate thalamic nucleus. *Journal of Neurosurgery, 77,* 62–68.

Boller, F., Mizutani, T., Roessmann, U., & Gambetti, P. (1980). Parkinson's disease, dementia and Alzheimer's disease: Clinicopathological correlations. *Annals of Neurology, 7,* 329–335.

Boller, F., Passafiume, D., Keefe, M. C., Rogers, K., Morrow, L., & Kim, Y. (1982). Visuospatial impairment in Parkinson disease: Role of perceptual and motor factors. *Archives of Neurology, 41,* 485–490.

Bondi, M. W., & Kaszniak, A. W. (1991). Implicit and explicit memory in Alzheimer's disease and Parkinson's disease. *Journal of Clinical and Experimental Neuropsychology, 13,* 339–358.

Bondi, M. W., Kaszniak, A. W., Bayles, K. A., & Vance, K. T. (1993). Contributions of frontal system dysfunction to memory and perceptual abilities in Parkinson's disease. *Neuropsychology, 7,* 89–102.

Bondi, M. W., Salmon, D. P., & Butters, N. (1994). Neuropsychological features of memory disorders in Alzheimer's disease. In R. D. Terry, R. Katzman, and K. L. Bick (Eds.), *Alzheimer's disease* (pp. 41–63). New York: Raven Press.

Bowen, F. P., Hoehn, M. M., & Yahr, M. D. (1972). Parkinsonism: Alterations in spatial orientation as determined by a route-walking test. *Neuropsychologia, 10,* 355–361.

Bowen, F. P., Burns, M. M., Brady, E., & Yahr, M. D. (1976). A note on alterations of personal orientation in parkinsonism. *Neuropsychologia, 14*, 425–429.

Breen, E. K. (1993). Recall and recognition memory in Parkinson's disease. *Cortex, 29*, 91–102.

Brentari, D., Poizner, H,. & Kegl, J. (1995). Aphasic and parkinsonian signing: Differences in phonological disruption. *Brain and Language, 48*, 69–105.

Brown, R., & Jahanshahi, M. (1995). Depression in Parkinson's disease: A psychosocial viewpoint. In W. J. Weiner & A. E. Lang (Eds.), *Advances in neurology: Vol. 65. Behavioral neurology of movement disorders* (pp. 61–84). New York: Raven Press.

Brown, R. G., & Marsden, C. D. (1984). How common is dementia in Parkinson's disease? *Lancet, 2*, 1262–1265.

Brown, R. G., & Marsden, C. D. (1986). Visuospatial function in Parkinson's disease. *Brain, 109*, 987–1002.

Burchiel, K. J. (1995). Thalamotomy for movement disorders. *Neurosurgery Clinics of North America, 6*, 55–71.

Butters, N., Granholm, E., Salmon, D. P., Grant, I., & Wolfe, J. (1987). Episodic and semantic memory: A comparison of amnesic and demented patients. *Journal of Clinical and Experimental Neuropsychology, 9*, 479–497.

Buytenhuijs, E. L., Berger, H. J. C., Van Spaendonck, K. P. M., Horstink, W. I. M., Borm, G. F., & Cools, A. R. (1994). Memory and learning strategies in patients with Parkinson's disease. *Neuropsychologia, 32*, 335–342.

Calne, D. B., Snow, B. J., & Lee, C. (1992). Criteria for diagnosing Parkinson's disease. *Annals of Neurology, 32* (Suppl.), 125–127.

Caparros-Lefebvre, D., Blond, S., Pécheux, N., Pasquier, F., & Petit, H. (1992). Evaluation neuropsychologique avant et après stimulation thalamique chez 9 parkinsoniens. *Révue Neurologique, 148*, 117–122.

Caparros-Lefebvre, D., Blond, S., Vermersch, P., Pécheux, N., Guieu, J. D., & Petit, H. (1993). Chronic thalamic stimulation improves tremor and levodopa-induced dyskinesias in Parkinson's disease. *Journal of Neurology, Neurosurgery, and Psychiatry, 56*, 268–273.

Chui, H. C., Mortimer, J. A., Slager, V., Zarow, C., Bondneff, W., & Webster, D. D. (1986). Pathologic correlates of dementia. *Archives of Neurology, 43*, 991–995.

Cohen, H., Bouchard, S., Scherzer, P., & Whitaker, H. (1994). Language and verbal reasoning in Parkinson's disease. *Neuropsychiatry, Neuropsychology, and Behavioral Neurology, 7*, 166–175.

Cools, A. R., Van Den Berken, J. H. L., Horstink, M. W. I., Van Spaendonk, K. P. M., & Berger, H. J. C. (1984). Cognitive and motor shifting aptitude disorder in Parkinson's disease. *Journal of Neurology, Neurosurgery, and Psychiatry, 47*, 443–453.

Cooper, J. A., Sagar, H. J., Jordan, N., Harvey, N. S., & Sullivan, E. V. (1991). Cognitive impairment in early, untreated Parkinson's disease and its relationship to motor disability. *Brain, 114*, 2095–2122.

Côté, L., & Crutcher, M. D. (1985). Motor functions of the basal ganglia and disease of transmitter metabolism. In E. R. Kandel & J. H. Schwartz (Eds.), *Principles of neural science* (2nd ed., pp. 525–536). New York: Elsevier Science Publishing Co.

Cummings, J. L. (1988). The dementias of Parkinson's disease: Prevalence, characteristics, neurobiology, and comparison with dementia of the Alzheimer type. *European Neurology, 28* (Suppl. 1), 15–23.

Cummings, J. L. (Ed.). (1990). *Subcortical dementia*. New York: Oxford University Press.

Cummings, J. L. (1992). Depression and Parkinson's disease: A review. *American Journal of Psychiatry, 149*, 443–454.

Cummings, J. L. (1993). Frontal-subcortical circuits and human behavior. *Archives of Neurology, 50*, 873–880.

Cummings, J. L., & Benson, D. F. (Eds.). (1992). *Dementia: A clinical approach* (2nd ed.). Boston: Butterworth-Heinemann.

Cummings, J. L., Darkins, A., Mendez, M., Hill, M. A., & Benson, D. F. (1988). Alzheimer's disease and Parkinson's disease: Comparison of speech and language alterations. *Neurology, 38*, 680–684.

Darley, F. L., Brown, J. R., & Swenson, W. M. (1975). Language changes after neurosurgery for parkinsonism. *Brain and Language, 2*, 65–69.

Davis, G. C., Williams, A. C., Markey, S. P., Ebert, M. H., Calne, E. D., Reichert, C. M., & Kopin, I. J. (1979). Chronic parkinsonism secondary to intravenous injection of meperidine analogues. *Psychiatry Research, 1*, 249–254.

Della Sala, S., Di Lorenzo, G., Giordana, A., & Spinnler, H. (1986). Is there a specific visuo-spatial impairment in parkinsonians? *Journal of Neurology, Neurosurgery, and Psychiatry, 49*, 1258–1265.

DeLong, M. R., & Georgopoulos, A. P. (1981). Motor functions of the basal ganglia. In J. M. Brookhart & V. B. Mountcastle (Eds.), *Handbook of physiology* (Sect. 1, Vol. 2, pp. 1017–1061). Bethesda, MD: American Physiological Society.

DeLong, M. R., & Georgopoulos, A. P., Crutcher, M. D. (1983). Cortico-basal ganglia relations and coding of motor performance. *Experimental Brain Research, 49* (Suppl. 7), 30–40.

De Renzi, E. (1980). *Disorder of space exploration and cognition*. Chichester: Wiley.

De Renzi, E., Faglioni, P., & Scotti, G. (1971). Judgment of spatial orientation in patients with focal brain damage. *Journal of Neurology, Neurosurgery, and Psychiatry, 34*, 489–495.

Dogali, M., Fazzini, E., Kolodny, E., Eidelberg, D., Sterio, D., Devinsky, O., & Beri, A. (1995). Stereotactic ventral pallidotomy for Parkinson's disease. *Neurology, 45*, 753–761.

Dooneief, G., Mirabello, E., Bell, K., Marder, K., Stern, Y., & Mayeux, R. (1992). An estimate of the incidence of depression in idiopathic Parkinson's disease. *Archives of Neurology, 49*, 305–307.

Downes, J. J., Sharp, H. M., Costall, B. M., Sagar, H. J., & Howe, J. (1993). Alternating fluency in Parkinson's disease: An evaluation of the attentional control theory of cognitive impairment. *Brain, 116*, 887–902.

Duffy, P. E., & Tennyson, V. M. (1965). Phase and electron microscopic observations of Lewy bodies and melanin granules in the substantia nigra and locus ceruleus in Parkinson's disease. *Journal of Neuropathology and Experimental Neurology, 24*, 398–414.

Duvoisin, R. C. (1984). *Parkinson's disease: A guide for patient and family*. New York: Raven Press.

Ellenberg, J. H. (1995). Early life and demographic factors predisposing to Parkinson's disease. In J. H. Ellenberg, W. C. Koller, & J. W. Langston (Eds.), *Etiology of Parkinson's disease* (pp. 277–294). New York: Marcel Dekker.

Espir, M. L. E., & Spalding, J. M. K. (1956). Three recent cases of encephalitis lethargica. *British Medical Journal, 1,* 1141–1144.

Flowers, K. A., Pearce, I., & Pearce, J. M. S. (1984). Recognition memory in Parkinson's disease. *Journal of Neurology, Neurosurgery, and Psychiatry, 47,* 1174–1181.

Folstein, M. F., Folstein, S. E., & McHugh, P. R. (1975). "Minimental state": A practical method for grading the cognitive state of patients for the clinician. *Journal of Psychiatry Research, 12,* 189–198.

Forno, L. S. (1986). Lewy body in Parkinson's disease. In M. D. Yahr & K. J. Bergmann (Eds.), *Advances in neurology: Vol. 45. Parkinson's disease* (pp. 35–44). New York: Raven Press.

Freedman, M. (1990). Parkinson's disease. In J. L. Cummings (Ed.), *Subcortical dementia* (pp. 108–122). New York: Oxford University Press.

Freedman, M., Rivoira, P., Butters, N., Sax, D. S., & Feldman, R. S. (1984). Retrograde amnesia in Parkinson's disease. *Canadian Journal of Neurological Sciences, 11,* 297–301.

Frith, C. D., Bloxham, C. A., & Carpenter, K. N. (1986). Impairments in the learning and performance of a new manual skill in patients with Parkinson's disease. *Journal of Neurology, Neurosurgery, and Psychiatry, 49,* 661–668.

Gibb, W. R. G. (1989). The neuropathology of parkinsonian disorders. In J. Jankovic & E. Tolosa (Eds.), *Parkinson's disease and movement disorders* (pp. 205–224). Baltimore: Urban & Schwarzenberg.

Girotti, F., Carella, R., Grassi, M. P., Soliveri, P., Marano, R., & Caroceni, T. (1986). Motor and cognitive performances of parkinsonian patients in the on and off phases of the disease. *Journal of Neurology, Neurosurgery, and Psychiatry, 49,* 657–660.

Glatt, S. L., Hubble, J. P., Lyons, K., Paolo, A., Tröster, A. I., Hassanein, R. E. S., & Koller, W. C. (1996). Risk factors for dementia in Parkinson's disease: Effect of education. *Neuroepidemiology, 15,* 20–25.

Globus, M., Mildworf, B., & Melamed, E. (1985). Cerebral blood flow and cognitive impairment in Parkinson's disease. *Neurology, 35,* 1135–1139.

Goetz, C. G. (1992). The historical background of behavioral studies in Parkinson's disease. In S. J. Huber & J. L. Cummings (Eds.), *Parkinson's disease: Neurobehavioral aspects* (pp. 3–9). New York: Oxford University Press.

Goetz, C. G., DeLong, M. R., Penn, R. D., & Bakay, R. A. E. (1993). Neurosurgical horizons in Parkinson's disease. *Neurology, 43,* 1–7.

Golbe, L. I. (1995). Genetics of Parkinson's disease. In J. H. Ellenberg, W. C. Koller, & J. W. Langston (Eds.), *Etiology of Parkinson's disease* (pp. 115–140). New York: Marcel Dekker.

Golbe, L. I., Lazzarini, A. M., Schwarz, K. O., Mark, M. H., Dickson, D. W., & Duvoisin, R. C. (1993). Autosomal dominant parkinsonism with benign course and typical Lewy-body pathology. *Neurology, 43,* 2222–2227.

Goldenberg, G., Wimmer, A., Auff, E., & Schnaberth, G. (1986). Impairment of motor planning in patients with Parkinson's

disease: Evidence from ideomotor apraxia. *Journal of Neurology, Neurosurgery, and Psychiatry, 49,* 1266–1272.

Gotham, A. M., Brown, R. G., & Marsden, C. D. (1988). "Frontal" cognitive function in patients with Parkinson's disease "on" and "off" levodopa. *Brain, 111,* 299–321.

Graf, P., Squire, L. R., & Mandler, G. (1984). The information that amnesics do not forget. *Journal of Experimental Psychology: Learning, Memory, and Cognition, 10,* 164–178.

Greenfield, J. G., & Bosanquet, F. D. (1953). The brain-stem lesions in parkinsonism. *Journal of Neurology, Neurosurgery, and Psychiatry, 16,* 213–226.

Grossman, M., Carvell, S., Gollomp, S., Stern, M. B., Vernon, G., & Hurtig, H. I. (1991). Sentence comprehension and praxis deficits in Parkinson's disease. *Neurology, 41,* 1620–1628.

Grossman, M., Carvell, S., Stern, M. B., Gollomp, S., & Hurtig, H. I. (1992). Sentence comprehension in Parkinson's disease: The role of attention and memory. *Brain and Language, 42,* 347–384.

Growdon, J. H., & Corkin, S. (1986). Cognitive impairments in Parkinson's disease. In M. D. Yahr & K. J. Bergmann (Eds.), *Advances in neurology: Vol. 45. Parkinson's disease* (pp. 383–392). New York: Raven Press.

Gurd, J. M., & Ward, C. D. (1989). Retrieval from semantic and letter-initial categories in patients with Parkinson's disease. *Neuropsychologia, 27,* 743–746.

Hakim, A. M., & Mathieson, G. (1979). Dementia in Parkinson's disease: A neuropathological study. *Neurology, 29,* 1209–1214.

Hallett, M. (1993). Physiology of basal ganglia disorders: An overview. *Canadian Journal of Neurological Sciences, 20,* 177–183.

Hansen, L. A., & Galasko, D. (1992). Lewy body disease. *Current Opinion in Neurology and Neurosurgery, 5,* 889–894.

Harrington, D. L., Haaland, K. Y., Yeo, R. A., & Marder, E. (1990). Procedural memory in Parkinson's disease: Impaired motor but not visuoperceptual learning. *Journal of Clinical and Experimental Neuropsychology, 12,* 323–339.

Hart, R. P., Kwentus, J. A., Wade, J. B., & Taylor, J. R. (1988). Modified Wisconsin Card Sorting Test in elderly normal, depressed and demented patients. *Clinical Neuropsychologist, 2,* 49–56.

Heindel, W. C., Salmon, D. P., Shults, C. W., Walicke, P. A., & Butters, N. (1989). Neuropsychological evidence for multiple implicit memory systems: A comparison of Alzheimer's, Huntington's and Parkinson's disease patients. *Journal of Neuroscience, 9,* 582–587.

Heindel, W. C., Butters, N., & Salmon, D. P. (1988). Impaired learning of a motor skill in patients with Huntington's disease. *Behavioral Neuroscience, 102,* 141–147.

Heindel, W. C., Salmon, D. P., & Butters, N. (1990). Pictorial priming and cued recall in Alzheimer's and Huntington's disease. *Brain and Cognition, 13,* 282–295.

Heindel, W. C., Salmon, D. P., & Butters, N. (1992). The biasing of weight judgments in Alzheimer's and Huntington's disease: A priming or programming phenomenon? *Journal of Clinical and Experimental Neuropsychology, 13,* 189–203.

Heindel, W. C., Salmon, D. P., & Butters, N. (1993). Cognitive approaches to the memory disorders of demented patients. In

P. B. Sutker & H. E. Adams (Eds.), *Comprehensive handbook of psychopathology* (2nd ed., pp. 735–761). New York: Plenum Press.

Helkala, E.-L., Laulumaa V., Soininen, H., & Reikkinen, P. J. (1988). Recall and recognition memory in patients with Alzheimer's and Parkinson's diseases. *Annals of Neurology, 24,* 214–217.

Hietanen, M., & Teravainen, H. (1986). Cognitive performance in early Parkinson's disease. *Acta Neurologica Scandinavica, 73,* 151–159.

Hirst, W., & Volpe, B. T. (1982). Temporal order judgments with amnesia. *Brain and Cognition, 1,* 294–306.

Hornykiewicz, O. (1966). Dopamine (3-hydroxytyramine) and brain function. *Pharmacology Review, 18,* 377–396.

Hornykiewicz, O., & Kish, S. J. (1986). Biochemical pathophysiology of Parkinson's disease. In M. D. Yahr & K. J. Bergmann (Eds.), *Advances in neurology: Vol. 45. Parkinson's disease* (pp. 19–34). New York: Raven Press.

Hubble, J. P., Cao, T., Hassanein, R. E. S., Neuberger, J. S., & Koller, W. C. (1993). Risk factors for Parkinson's disease. *Neurology, 43,* 1693–1697.

Huber, S. J., & Cummings, J. L. (Eds.). (1992). *Parkinson's disease: Neurobehavioral aspects.* New York: Oxford University Press.

Huber, S. J., Shuttleworth, E. C., & Paulson, G. W. (1986). Dementia in Parkinson's disease. *Archives of Neurology, 43,* 987–990.

Huber, S. J., Shuttleworth, E. C., Paulson, G. W., Bellchambers, M. J. G., & Clapp, L. E. (1986). Cortical vs. subcortical dementia: Neuropsychological differences. *Archives of Neurology, 43,* 392–394.

Huber, S. J., Freidenberg, D. L., Shuttleworth, E. C., Paulson, G. W., & Christy, J. A. (1989). Neuropsychological impairments associated with severity of Parkinson's disease. *Journal of Neuropsychiatry and Clinical Neurosciences, 1,* 155–159.

Huber, S. J., Freidenberg, D. L., Paulson, G. W., Shuttleworth, E. C., & Christy, J. A. (1990). The pattern of depressive symptoms varies with progression of Parkinson's disease. *Journal of Neurology, Neurosurgery, and Psychiatry, 53,* 275–278.

Hughes, A. J., Daniel, S. E., Kilford, L., & Lees, A. J. (1992). Accuracy of the clinical diagnosis of idiopathic Parkinson's disease: A clinicopathological study of 100 cases. *Journal of Neurology, Neurosurgery, and Psychiatry, 55,* 181–184.

Hunter, R., & Jones, M. (1966). Acute lethargica-type encephalitis. *Lancet, 2,* 1023–1024.

Illes, J. (1989). Neurolinguistic features of spontaneous language production dissociate three forms of neurodegenerative disease: Alzheimer's, Huntington's, and Parkinson's. *Brain and Language, 37,* 628–642.

Illes, J., Metter, E. J., Hanson, W. R., & Iritani, S. (1988). Language production in Parkinson's disease: Acoustic and linguistic considerations. *Brain and Language, 33,* 146–160.

Ineichen, B. (1987). Measuring the rising tide. How many dementia cases will there be by 2001? *British Journal of Psychiatry, 150,* 193–200.

Jankovic, J., & Reches, A. (1986). Parkinson's disease in monozygotic twins. *Annals of Neurology, 19,* 405–408.

Jankovic, J. & Tolosa, E. (Eds.). (1993). *Parkinson's disease and movement disorders* (2nd ed.). Baltimore: Williams & Wilkins.

Javoy-Agid, F., Taquet, H., Ploska, A., Cherif-Zahar, C., Ruberg, M., & Agid, Y. (1981). Distribution of catecholamines in the ventral mesencephalon of human brain, with special reference to Parkinson's disease. *Journal of Neurochemistry, 36,* 2101–2105.

Jellinger, K. (1986). Overview of morphological changes in Parkinson's disease. In M. D. Yahr & K. J. Bergmann (Eds.), *Advances in neurology: Vol. 45. Parkinson's disease* (pp. 1–18). New York: Raven Press.

Jellinger, K. (1987). The pathology of parkinsonism. In C. D. Marsden & S. Fahn (Eds.), *Neurology: Vol. 7. Movement disorders 2* (pp. 124–165). London: Butterworths.

Jenner, P., & Marsden, C. D. (1989). MPTP-induced parkinsonism as an experimental model of Parkinson's disease. In J. Jankovic & E. Tolosa (Eds.), *Parkinson's disease and movement disorders* (pp. 37–48). Baltimore: Urban & Schwarzenberg.

Kaszniak, A. W., Trosset, M. W., Bondi, M. W., & Bayles, K. A. (1992). Procedural learning of Parkinson's disease patients in a serial reaction time task. *Journal of Clinical and Experimental Neuropsychology, 14,* 51.

Klawans, H. L., & Cohen, M. M. (1970). Diseases of the extrapyramidal system. In H. F. Dowling (Ed.), *Disease-a-month.* Chicago: Year Book Medical Publishers, Inc.

Klockgether, T., Löschmann, P. A., & Wüllner, U. (1994). New medical and surgical treatments for Parkinson's disease. *Current Opinion in Neurology, 7,* 346–352.

Koller, W., Vetere-Overfield, B., Gray, C., Alexander, C., Chin, T., Dolezal, J., Hassanein, R., & Tanner, C. (1990). Environmental risk factors in Parkinson's disease. *Neurology, 40,* 1218–1221.

Koller, W. C. (1992). How accurately can Parkinson's disease be diagnosed? *Neurology, 42* (Suppl. 1), 6–16.

Koller, W. C., & Megaffin, B. B. (1994). Parkinson's disease and parkinsonism. In C. E. Coffey & J. L. Cummings (Eds.), *Textbook of geriatric neuropsychiatry* (pp. 433–456). Washington, DC: American Psychiatric Press.

Koller, W. C., Glatt, S. L., Hubble, J. P., Paolo, A., Tröster, A. I., Handler, M. S., Horvat, R. T., Martin, C., Schmidt, K., Karst, A., Wijsman, E. M., Yu, C. E., & Schellenberg, G. D. (1995). Apolipoprotein E genotypes in Parkinson's disease with and without dementia. *Annals of Neurology, 37,* 242–245.

Kramer, J. H., Levin, B. E., Brandt, J., & Delis, D. C. (1989). Differentiation of Alzheimer's, Huntington's, and Parkinson's disease patients on the basis of verbal learning characteristics. *Neuropsychology, 3,* 111–120.

Kurland, L. T. (1958). Epidemiology: Incidence, geographic distribution and genetic considerations. In W. S. Field (Ed.), *Pathogenesis and treatment of parkinsonism* (pp. 5–49). Springfield, IL: Charles C. Thomas.

Laitinen, L. V. (1994). Ventroposterolateral pallidotomy. *Stereotactic and Functional Neurosurgery, 62,* 41–52.

Laitinen, L. V. (1995). Pallidotomy for Parkinson's disease. *Neurosurgery Clinics of North America, 6,* 105–112.

Lange, K. W., Robbins, T. W., Marsden, C. D., James, M., Owen,

A. M., & Paul, G. M. (1992). L-Dopa withdrawal in Parkinson's disease selectively impairs cognitive performance on tests sensitive to frontal lobe dysfunction. *Psychopharmacology*, *107*, 394–404.

Langston, J. W., & Tanner, C. M. (1992). Etiology. In W. C. Koller (Ed.), *Handbook of Parkinson's disease* (2nd ed., pp. 369–381). New York: Marcel Dekker, Inc.

La Rue, A. (1992). *Aging and neuropsychological assessment*. New York: Plenum Press.

Lees, A. J. (1985). Parkinson's disease and dementia. *Lancet 2*, 43–44.

Lees, A. J., & Smith, E. (1983). Cognitive deficits in the early stages of Parkinson's disease. *Brain*, *106*, 257–270.

Leverenz, J., & Sumi, S. M. (1986). Parkinson's disease in patients with Alzheimer's disease. *Archives of Neurology*, *43*, 662–664.

Levin, B. E., & Katzen, H. L. (1995). Early cognitive changes and nondementing behavioral abnormalities in Parkinson's disease. In W. J. Weiner & A. E. Lang (Eds.), *Advances in neurology: Vol. 65. Behavioral neurology of movement disorders* (pp. 85–95). New York: Raven Press.

Levin, B. E., Llabre, B. M., & Weiner, W. J. (1989). Cognitive impairments associated with early Parkinson's disease. *Neurology*, *39*, 557–561.

Levin, B. E., Tomer, R., & Rey, G. J. (1992). Cognitive impairments in Parkinson's disease. *Neurologic Clinics*, *10*, 471–485.

Lewy, F. H. (1912). Paralysis agitans. I. Pathologische anatomie. In M. Lewandowsky (Ed.), *Handbuch der Neurologie* (pp. 920–933). Berlin: Springer.

Lewy, F. H. (1923). *Die Hehre vom Tonus und der Bewegung*. Berlin: Springer.

Lieberman, A., Dziatolowski, M., Kupersmith, M., Serby, M., Goodgold, A., Korein, J., & Goldstein, M. (1979). Dementia in Parkinson's disease. *Annals of Neurology*, *6*, 335–359.

Lieberman, P., Friedman, J., & Feldman, L. S. (1990). Syntax comprehension deficits in Parkinson's disease. *Journal of Nervous and Mental Disease*, *178*, 360–365.

Lieberman, P., Kako, E., Friedman, J., Tajchman, G., Feldman, L. S., & Jiminez, E. B. (1992). Speech production, syntax comprehension, and cognitive deficits in Parkinson's disease. *Brain and Language*, *43*, 169–189.

Lindvall, O., Sawle, G., Widner, H., Rothwell, J. C., Bjîrklund, A., Brooks, D., Brundin, P., Frackowiak, R., Marsden, C. D., Odin, P., & Rehncrona, S. (1994). Evidence for long-term survival and function of dopaminergic grafts in progressive Parkinson's disease. *Annals of Neurology*, *35*, 172–180.

Loranger, A. W., Goodell, H., Lee, J. E., & McDowell, F. (1972). Levodopa treatment of Parkinson's syndrome. *Archives of General Psychiatry*, *26*, 163–168.

Mahurin, R. K., Feher, E. P., Nance, M. L., Levy, J. K., & Pirozzolo, F. J. (1993). Cognition in Parkinson's disease and related disorders. In R. W. Parks, R. F. Zec, & R. S. Wilson (Eds.), *Neuropsychology of Alzheimer's disease and other dementias* (pp. 308–349). New York: Oxford University Press.

Mann, D. M. A., & Yates, P. O. (1983). Pathological basis for neurotransmitter changes in Parkinson's disease. *Neuropathology and Applied Neurobiology*, *9*, 3–19.

Marder, K., Maestre, G., Cote, L., Mejia, H., Alfaro, B., Halim, A., Tang, M., Tycko, B., & Mayeux, R. (1994). The apolipoprotein ε4 allele in Parkinson's disease with and without dementia. *Neurology*,. *44*, 1330–1331.

Marder, K., Tang, M. X., Côté, L., Stern, Y., & Mayeux, R. (1995). The frequency and associated risk factors for dementia in patients with Parkinson's disease. *Archives of Neurology*, *52*, 695–701.

Marjama, J., Tröster, A. I., & Koller, W. C. (1995). Psychogenic movement disorders. *Neurologic Clinics*, *13*, 283–297.

Martilla, R. J., & Rinne, U. K. (1976). Dementia in Parkinson's disease. *Acta Neurologica Scandinavica*, *54*, 431–441.

Martin, W. E., Loewenson, R. B., Resch, J. A., & Baker, A. B. (1973). Parkinson's disease: Clinical analysis of 100 patients. *Neurology*, *23*, 783–790.

Massman, P. J., Delis, D. C., Butters, N., Levin, B. E., & Salmon, D. P. (1990). Are all subcortical dementias alike?: Verbal learning and memory in Parkinson's and Huntington's disease patients. *Journal of Clinical and Experimental Neuropsychology*, *12*, 729–744.

Massman, P. J., Delis, D. C., Butters, N., Dupont, R., & Gillin, J. C. (1992). The subcortical dysfunction hypothesis of memory deficits in depression: Neuropsychological validation in a subgroup of patients. *Journal of Clinical and Experimental Neuropsychology*, *14*, 687–706.

Matison, R., Mayeux, R., Rosen, J., & Fahn, S. (1982). "Tip-of-the-tongue" phenomenon in Parkinson's disease. *Neurology*, *32*, 567–570.

Mattis, S. (1988). *Dementia rating scale*. Odessa, FL: Psychological Assessment Resources.

Mayberg, H. S. (1994). Frontal lobe dysfunction in secondary depression. *Journal of Neuropsychiatry and Clinical Neurosciences*, *6*, 428–442.

Mayberg, H. S., & Solomon, D. H. (1995). Depression in Parkinson's disease: A biochemical and organic viewpoint. In W. J. Weiner & A. E. Lang (Eds.), *Advances in neurology: Vol. 65. Behavioral neurology of movement disorders* (pp. 49–60). New York: Raven Press.

Mayeux, R. (1990). Parkinson's disease: A review of cognitive and psychiatric disorders. *Neuropsychiatry, Neuropsychology, and Behavioral Neurology*, *3*, 3–14.

Mayeux, R., & Stern, Y. (1983). Intellectual dysfunction and dementia in Parkinson's disease. In R. Mayeux & W. G. Rosen (Eds.), *The dementias* (pp. 211–228). New York: Raven Press.

Mayeux, R., Stern, Y., Williams, J. B. W., Côté, L., Frantz, A., & Dyrenfurth, I. (1986). Clinical and biochemical features of depression in Parkinson's disease. *American Journal of Psychiatry*, *143*, 756–759.

McFie, J., & Thompson, J. A. (1972). Picture arrangement: A measure of frontal lobe function? *British Journal of Psychiatry*, *121*, 547–552.

McKhann, G., Drachman, D., Folstein, M., Katzman, R., Price, D., & Stadlan, E. M. (1984). Clinical diagnosis of Alzheimer's disease: Report of the NINCDS-ADRDA Work Group under the auspices of the Department of Health and Human Services Task Force on Alzheimer's disease. *Neurology*, *34*, 939–944.

McPherson, S., & Cummings, J. L. (1996). Neuropsychological aspects of Parkinson's disease and parkinsonism. In I. Grant &

K. M. Adams (Eds.), *Neuropsychological assessment of neuropsychiatric disorders* (2nd ed.) (pp. 288–311). New York: Oxford University Press.

Mega, M. S., & Cummings, J. L. (1994). Frontal-subcortical circuits and neuropsychiatric disorders. *Journal of Neuropsychiatry and Clinical Neurosciences, 6,* 358–370.

Meier, M. J., & Martin, W. E. (1970). Intellectual changes associated with levodopa therapy. *Journal of the American Medical Association, 213,* 465–466.

Milner, B. (1971). Interhemispheric differences in the localization of psychological processes in man. *British Medical Bulletin, 27,* 272–277.

Milner, B. (1974). Hemisphere specialization: Scope and limits. In F. O. Schmitt & F. G. Worden (Eds.), *The neurosciences third study program.* Cambridge, MA: Massachusetts Institute of Technology Press.

Mohr, E., Juncos, J., Cox, C., Litvan, I., Fedio, P., & Chase, T. N. (1990). Selective deficits in cognition and memory in high-functioning parkinsonian patients. *Journal of Neurology, Neurosurgery, and Psychiatry, 53,* 603–606.

Mohr, E., Mendis, T., & Grimes, J. D. (1995). Late cognitive changes in Parkinson's disease with an emphasis on dementia. In W. J. Weiner & A. E. Lang (Eds.), *Advances in neurology: Vol. 65. Behavioral neurology of movement disorders* (pp. 97–113). New York: Raven Press.

Mortimer, J. A. Pirozzolo, F. J., Hansch, E. C. & Webster, D. D. (1982). Relationship of motor symptoms to intellectual deficits in Parkinson's disease. *Neurology, 32,* 133–137.

Natsopoulos, D., Katsarou, Z., Bostantzopoulos, G., Grouios, G., Mentemopoulos, G., & Logothetis, J. (1991). Strategies in comprehension of relative clauses in parkinsonian patients. *Cortex, 27,* 255–268.

Nissen, M. J., & Bullemer, P. (1987). Attentional requirements of learning: Evidence from performance measures. *Cognitive Psychology, 19,* 1–32.

Nissen, M. J., Willingham, D., & Hartman M. (1989). Explicit and implicit remembering: When is learning preserved in amnesia? *Neuropsychologia, 27,* 341–352.

Nolte, J. (1988). *The human brain: An introduction to its functional anatomy* (2nd ed.). Washington, DC: C. V. Mosby Co.

Owen, A. M., James, M., Leigh, P. N., Summers, B. A., Marsden, C. D., Quinn, N. P., Lange, K. W., & Robbins, T. W. (1992). Fronto-striatal cognitive deficits at different stages of Parkinson's disease. *Brain, 115,* 1727–1751.

Owen, A. M., Sahakian, B. J., Hodges, J. R., Summers, B. A., Polkey, C. E., & Robbins, T. W. (1995). Dopamine-dependent frontostriatal planning deficits in early Parkinson's disease. *Neuropsychology, 9,* 126–140.

Pahwa, R., & Koller, W. C. (1995). Defining Parkinson's disease and parkinsonism. In J. H. Ellenberg, W. C. Koller, & J. W. Langston (Eds.), *Etiology of Parkinson's disease* (pp. 1–54). New York: Marcel Dekker.

Parkinson, J. (1974). An essay on the shaking palsy. In J. Marks (Ed.), *Treatment of parkinsonism with L-dopa* (pp. 9–17). New York: American Elservier Publishing Co. (Original work published 1817)

Parkinson Study Group. (1989). Effect of deprenyl on the progression of disability in early Parkinson's disease. *New England Journal of Medicine, 321,* 1364–1371.

Passafiume, D., Boller, F., & Keefe, M. C. (1986). Neuropsychological impairment in patients with Parkinson's disease. In I. Grant & K. M. Adams (Eds.), *Neuropsychological assessment of neuropsychiatric disorders* (pp. 374–383). New York: Oxford University Press.

Paulsen, J. S., Butters, N., Salmon, D. P., Heindel, W. C., & Swenson, M. R. (1993). Prism adaptation in Alzheimer's and Huntington's disease. *Neuropsychology, 7,* 73–81.

Perry, E. K., McKeith, I., Thompson, P., Marshall, E., Kerwin, J., Jabeen, S., Edwardson, J. A., Ince, P., Blessed, G., Irving, D., & Perry, R. H. (1991). Topography, extent, and clinical relevance of neurochemical deficits in dementia of Lewy body type, Parkinson's disease, and Alzheimer's disease. *Annals of the New York Academy of Sciences, 640,* 142–152.

Piccirilli, M., D'Alessandro, P., Finali, G., & Piccinin, G. L. (1994). Neuropsychological follow-up of parkinsonian patients with and without cognitive impairment. *Dementia, 5,* 17–22.

Pillon, B., Dubois, B., Lhermitte, F., & Agid, Y. (1986). Heterogeneity of cognitive impairment in progressive supranuclear palsy, Parkinson's disease, and Alzheimer's disease. *Neurology, 36,* 1179–1185.

Pillon, B., Deweer, B., Agid, Y., & Dubois, B. (1993). Explicit memory in Alzheimer's, Huntington's, and Parkinson's diseases. *Archives of Neurology, 50,* 374–379.

Pirozzolo, F. J., Hansch, E. C., Mortimer, J. A., Webster, D. D., & Kuskowski, M. A. (1982). Dementia in Parkinson's disease: A neuropsychological analysis. *Brain and Cognition, 1,* 71–83.

Pirozzolo, F. J., Swihart, A. A., Rey, G., Mahurin, R., & Jankovic, J. (1993). Cognitive impairments associated with Parkinson's disease and other movement disorders. In J. Jankovic & E. Tolosa (Eds.), *Parkinson's disease and movement disorders* (2nd ed., pp. 493–510). Baltimore: Williams & Wilkins.

Pollock, M., & Hornabrook, R. W. (1966). The prevalence, natural history and dementia of Parkinson's disease. *Brain, 89,* 429–448.

Proctor, F., Riklan, M., Cooper, I. S., & Teuber, H. L. (1964). Judgment of visual and postural vertical by parkinsonian patients. *Neurology, 14,* 287–293.

Rafal, R. D., Posner, M. I., Walker, J. A., & Friedrich, F. J. (1984). Cognition and the basal ganglia: Separating mental and motor components of performance in Parkinson's disease. *Brain, 107,* 1083–1094.

Rajput, A. H. (1992). Prevalence of dementia in Parkinson's disease. In S. J. Huber & J. L. Cummings (Eds.), *Parkinson's disease: Neurobehavioral aspects* (pp. 119–131). New York: Oxford University Press.

Rajput, A. H., Offord, K. P., Beard, C. M., & Kurland, L. T. (1984). Epidemiology of parkinsonism: Incidence, classification, and mortality. *Annals of Neurology, 16,* 278–282.

Rajput, A. H., Rozdilsky, B., & Rajput, A. (1991). Accuracy of clinical diagnosis in parkinsonism: A prospective study. *Canadian Journal of Neurological Science, 18,* 275–278.

Randolph, C., Braun, A. R., Goldberg, T. E., & Chase, T. N. (1993). Semantic fluency in Alzheimer's, Parkinson's, and

Huntington's disease: Dissociation of storage and retrieval failures. *Neuropsychology, 7,* 82–88.

Randolph, C., Mohr, E., & Chase, T. N. (1993). Assessment of intellectual functioning in dementing disorders: Validity of WAIS-R short forms for patients with Alzheimer's, Huntington's, and Parkinson's disease. *Journal of Clinical and Experimental Neuropsychology, 15,* 743–753.

Rao, S. M., Huber, S. J., & Bornstein, R. A. (1992). Emotional changes with multiple sclerosis and Parkinson's disease. *Journal of Consulting and Clinical Psychology, 60,* 369–378.

Ring, H. A., Bench, C. J., Trimble, M. R., Brooks, D. J., Frackowiak, R. S. J., & Dolan, R. J. (1994). Depression in Parkinson's disease: A positron emission study. *British Journal of Psychiatry, 165,* 333–339.

Román, G. C., Zhang, Z. X., & Ellenberg, J. H. (1995). The neuroepidemiology of Parkinson's disease. In J. H. Ellenberg, W. C. Koller, & J. W. Langston (Eds.), *Etiology of Parkinson's disease* (pp. 203–243). New York: Marcel Dekker.

Rossitch, E., Zeidman, S. M., Nashold, B. S., Horner, J., Walker, J., Osborne, D., & Bullard, D. E. (1988). Evaluation of memory and language function pre- and post-thalamotomy with an attempt to define those patients at risk for postoperative dysfunction. *Surgical Neurology, 29,* 11–16.

Sagar, H. J., Cohen, N. J., Sullivan, E. V., Corkin, S., & Growdon, J. H. (1988). Remote memory function in Alzheimer's disease and Parkinson's disease. *Brain, 111,* 185–206.

Sagar, H. J., Sullivan, E. V., Gabrieli, J. D. E., Corkin, S., & Growdon, J. (1988). Temporal ordering and short-term memory deficits in Parkinson's disease. *Brain, 111,* 525–539.

Saint-Cyr, J. A., Taylor, A. E., & Lang, A. E. (1988). Procedural learning and neostriatal dysfunction in man. *Brain, 111,* 941–959.

Salganik, I., & Korczyn, A. (1990). Risk factors for dementia in Parkinson's disease. In M. B. Streifler, A. D. Korczyn, E. Melamed, & M. B. H. Youdim (Eds.), *Advances in neurology: Vol. 53. Parkinson's disease: Anatomy, pathology, and therapy* (pp. 343–347). New York: Raven Press.

Salmon, D. P., & Butters, N. (1995). Neurobiology of skill and habit learning. *Current Opinion in Neurobiology, 5,* 184–190.

Salmon, D. P., Shimamura, A. P., Butters, N., & Smith, S. (1988). Lexical and semantic priming in patients with Alzheimer's disease. *Journal of Clinical and Experimental Neuropsychology, 10,* 477–494.

Sass, K. J., Buchanan, C. P., Westerveld, M., Marek, K. L., Farhi, A., Robbins, R. J., Naftolin, F., Vollmer, T. L., Leranth, C., Roth, R. H., Price, L. H., Bunney, B. S., Elsworth J. D., Hoffer, P. B., Redmond, D. E., & Spencer, D. S. (1995). General cognitive ability following unilateral and bilateral fetal ventral mesencephalic tissue transplantation for treatment of Parkinson's disease. *Archives of Neurology, 52,* 680–686.

Schacter, D. L. (1987). Implicit memory: History and current status. *Journal of Experimental Psychology: Learning, Memory, and Cognition, 13,* 501–518.

Schacter, D. L., & Tulving, E. (Eds.). (1994). *Memory systems 1994.* Cambridge, MA: MIT Press.

Schmidt, M. L., Murray, J., Lee, V. M.-Y., Hill, W. D., Wertkin, A., & Trojanowski, J. Q. (1991). Epitote map of neurofilament protein domains in cortical and peripheral nervous system Lewy bodies. *American Journal of Pathology, 139,* 53–65.

Shimamura, A. P. (1994). Memory and frontal lobe function. In M. S. Gazzaniga (Ed.), *The cognitive neurosciences* (pp. 803–813. Cambridge, MA: MIT Press.

Shimamura, A. P., Salmon, D. P., Squire, L. R., & Buttes, N. (1987). Memory dysfunction and word priming in dementia and amnesia. *Behavioral Neuroscience, 101,* 347–351.

Siegfried, J., & Lippitz, B. (1994). Chronic electrical stimulation of the VL-VPL complex and of the pallidum in the treatment of movement disorders: Personal experience since 1982. *Stereotactic and Functional Neurosurgery, 62,* 71–75.

Squire, L. R. (1982). The neuropsychology of human memory. *Annual Review of Neuroscience, 5,* 241–273.

Squire, L. R. (1987). *Memory and brain.* New York: Oxford University Press.

Squire, L. R., Knowlton, B., & Musen, G. (1993). The structure and organization of memory. *Annual Review of Psychology, 44,* 453–495.

Starkstein, S. E., & Mayberg, H. S. (1993). Depression in Parkinson's disease. In S. E. Starkstein & R. G. Robinson (Eds.), *Depression in neurologic disease* (pp. 97–116). Baltimore: Johns Hopkins University Press.

Starkstein, S. E., Rabins, P. V., Berthier, M. L., Cohen, B. J., Folstein, M. F., & Robinson, R.G. (1989). Dementia of depression among patients with neurological disorders and functional depression. *Journal of Neuropsychiatry and Clinical Neurosciences, 1,* 263–268.

Starkstein, S. E., Bolduc, P. L., Mayberg, H. S, Preziosi, T. J., & Robinson, R. G. (1990). Cognitive impairments and depression in Parkinson's disease: A follow-up study. *Journal of Neurology, Neurosurgery, and Psychiatry, 53,* 597–602.

Starkstein, S. E., Preziosi, T. J., Bolduc, P. L., & Robinson, R. G. (1990). Depression in Parkinson's disease. *Journal of Nervous and Mental Disease, 178,* 27–31.

Starkstein, S. E., Mayberg, H. S., Leiguarda, R., Preziosi, T. J., & Robinson, R. G. (1992). A prospective, longitudinal of depression, cognitive decline, and physical impairments in patients with Parkinson's disease. *Journal of Neurology, Neurosurgery, and Psychiatry, 55,* 377–382.

Stern, Y., Marder, K., Tang, M. X., & Mayeux, R. (1993). Antecedent clinical features associated with dementia in Parkinson's disease. *Neurology, 43,* 1690–1692.

Stern, Y., Richards, M., Sano, M., & Mayeux, R. (1993). Comparison of cognitive changes in patients with Alzheimer's and Parkinson's disease. *Archives of Neurology, 50,* 1040–1045.

Stuss, D. T., & Benson, D. F. (1986). *The frontal lobes.* New York: Raven Press.

Sullivan, E. V., Sagar, H. J., Gabrieli, J. D. E., Corkin, S., & Growdon, J. H. (1989). Different cognitive profiles on standard behavioral tests in Parkinson's disease and Alzheimer's disease. *Journal of Clinical and Experimental Neuropsychology, 11,* 799–820.

Tanner, C. M. (1989). The role of environmental toxins in the etiology of Parkinson's disease. *Trends in Neuroscience, 12,* 49–54.

Taylor, A. E., & Saint-Cyr, J. A. (1992). Executive function. In S.

J. Huber & J. L. Cummings (Eds.), *Parkinson's disease: Neurobehavioral aspects* (pp. 74–85). New York: Oxford University Press.

Taylor, A. E., Saint-Cyr, J. A., & Lang, A. E. (1986). Frontal lobe dysfunction in Parkinson's disease: The cortical focus of neostriatal outflow. *Brain, 109*, 845–883.

Taylor, A. E., Saint-Cyr, J. A., & Lang, A. E. (1985). Dementia prevalence in Parkinson's disease. *Lancet, 1* (8436), 1037.

Taylor, A. E., Saint-Cyr, J. A., Lang, A. E., & Kenny, F. T. (1986). Parkinson's disease and depression: A critical re-evaluation. *Brain, 109*, 279–292.

Teuber, H. L., & Proctor, F. (1964). Some effects of basal ganglia lesions in subhuman primates and man. *Neuropsychologia, 2*, 85–93.

Torack, R. M., & Morris, J. C. (1988). The association of ventral tegmental area histopathology with adult dementia. *Archives of Neurology, 45*, 497–501.

Tretiakoff, C. (1919). *Contribution á l'étude de l'anatomia pathologique du locus niger*. Thése: Université de Paris.

Tröster, A. I., & Fields, J. A. (1995). Frontal cognitive function and memory in Parkinson's disease: Toward a distinction between prospective and declarative memory impairments. *Behavioural Neurology, 8*, 59–74.

Tröster, A. I., Heindel, W. C., Salmon, D. P., & Buttes, N. (1989). Category fluency performance in Parkinson's disease with and without dementia. *The Clinical Neuropsychologist, 3*, 284.

Tröster, A. I., Salmon, D. P., McCullough, D., & Butters, N. (1989). A comparison of the category fluency deficits associated with Alzheimer's and Huntington's disease. *Brain and Language, 37*, 500–513.

Tröster, A. I., Paolo, A. M., Lyons, K. E., Glatt, S. L., Hubble, J. P., & Koller, W. C. (1995). The influence of depression on cognition in Parkinson's disease: A pattern of impairment distinguishable from Alzheimer's disease. *Neurology, 45*, 672–676.

Tröster, A. I., Stalp, L. D., Paolo, A. M., Fields, J. A., & Koller, W. C. (1995). Neuropsychological impairment in Parkinson's disease with and without depression. *Archives of Neurology, 52*, 1164–1169.

Tröster, A. I., Fields, J. A., Paolo, A. M., & Koller, W. C. (1996). Performance of individuals with Parkinson's disease on the Vocabulary and Information subtests of the WAIS-R as a neuropsychological instruments. *Journal of Clinical Geropsychology, 2*, 215–223.

Tsai, C.-H., Lu, C.-S., Hua, M.-S., Lo, W.-L., & Lo, S.-K. (1994). Cognitive dysfunction in early onset parkinsonism. *Acta Neurologica Scandinavica, 89*, 9–14.

Tulving, E. (1983). *Elements of episodic memory*. London: Oxford University Press.

Vilkki, J., & Laitinen, L. V. (1974). Differential effects of left and right ventrolateral thalamotomy on receptive and expressive verbal performances and face-matching. *Neuropsychologia, 12*, 11–19.

Von Economo, E. (1931). *Encephalitis lethargica. Its sequelae and treatment* (K. O. Newman, Trans.). London: Oxford University Press.

Ward, C. D., Duvoisin, R. C., Ince, S. E., Nutt, J. D., Eldridge, R., & Calne, D. B. (1983). Parkinson's disease in 65 pairs of twins and in a set of quadruplets. *Neurology, 33*, 815–824.

Wechsler, D. (1958). *The measurement and appraisal of adult intelligence*. Baltimore: Williams & Wilkins.

Wechsler, D. (1981). *Wechsler Adult Intelligence Scale-Revised*. New York: The Psychological Corporation.

Wilson, R. S., Kaszniak, A. W., Klawans, H. L., & Garron, D. C. (1980). High-speed memory scanning in parkinsonism. *Cortex, 16*, 67–72.

Zhang, Z. X., & Román, G. C. (1993). Worldwide occurrence of Parkinson's disease: An updated review. *Neuroepidemiology, 12*, 195–208.

16

Huntington's Disease

FREDERICK W. BYLSMA

Introduction

The major clinical features of Huntington's disease (HD) were first eloquently described by George Huntington, a Long Island physician, in a concise report to a medical society (Huntington, 1872). Huntington reported on three notable features that distinguish this disease from "common" (Sydenham's) chorea: (1) It tended to be passed from generation to generation within families; (2) the disease usually was not evident until adulthood; and (3) of special note for psychologists and psychiatrists, those suffering from the disease tended to also display symptoms of "insanity," usually depression and suicidal tendencies. Huntington, describing the dementia of HD, observed that "the mind becomes more or less impaired" as the disease progresses. For most patients "mind and body both gradually fail until death." He noted that no treatment was available at that time and relegated the disease into the class of the "incurables."

Clinical Features and Neuropathology

Huntington's disease is a neurodegenerative genetic disorder that is inherited as an autosomal dominant trait with full lifetime penetrance. As such, offspring of affected individuals have a 50% chance of inheriting the genetic mutation from their affected parent. If they have, they will go on to develop the disease during their lifetime, provided

FREDERICK W. BYLSMA • Department of Psychiatry and Behavioral Sciences, Division of Medical Psychology, The Johns Hopkins University School of Medicine, Baltimore, Maryland 21287.

they do not die of competing causes prior to disease onset. The prevalence of HD is estimated to range between 0.005% and 0.01%, or 5 to 10 cases per 100,000 individuals (Bryois, 1989; Conneally, 1984; Folstein, 1989). In the United States, there are approximately 25,000 affected individuals.

Onset of disease, most often defined by the onset of involuntary movements (chorea), is insidious and typically occurs between 35 and 45 years of age. Onset age ranges from childhood (5 years of age) to the eighth decade of life, and duration of disease averages 15 to 17 years. Disease duration appears to be related to age of onset; those with earlier age of onset show a more malignant course with the most rapid decline (Myers et al., 1991; Young et al., 1986; but see Roos, Hermans, Vegtervan der Vlis, van Ommen, & Bruyn, 1993, and Feigin et al., 1995).

The progressive motor disorder of HD comprises both the defining involuntary component (i.e., chorea and dystonia) and a voluntary component (i.e., bradykinesia, rigidity, gait disorder, motor impersistence). Oculomotor impairments are also prominent. Patients with HD display an inability to smoothly track slowly moving targets with their eyes, and their saccadic eye movements are of increased latency and decreased velocity and are often hypometric (Lasker, Zee, Hain, Folstein, & Singer, 1987, 1988; Leigh, Newman, Folstein, Lasker, & Jensen, 1983). Chorea and oculomotor impairments are prominent early in the disease, but chorea plateaus in the middle stages of illness and may decline substantially in the late stages. Voluntary motor impairment tends to increase steadily throughout the course of illness, culminating in an akinetic rigidity in the later stages of disease (Folstein, 1989).

As Huntington noted in his initial description, cognitive and psychiatric symptoms are prominent features of HD. Indeed, because of the prominence of the cognitive disorder and relative restriction of neuropathological changes in HD to the basal ganglia, Huntington's disease has been described as the prototypic "subcortical dementia" (McHugh & Folstein, 1973, 1975). Subcortical dementias are characterized by slowed thinking; memory impairments in the form of inefficient learning of new information with poor recall in the face of relatively retained recognition memory; and difficulty in mentally manipulating acquired information. The aphasia, apraxia, and agnosia typical of cortical dementias such as Alzheimer's disease are not prominent in HD (Cummings & Benson, 1984; Folstein, Brandt, & Folstein, 1991). The dementia of HD is discussed in greater detail in later sections of this chapter.

In addition to the cognitive and neurological impairments, psychiatric and emotional disturbances frequently occur in HD. Many HD patients experience profound depression, and a few become manic or suffer a bipolar disorder (Folstein, Abbott, Chase, Jensen, & Folstein, 1983; Shoulson, 1990). While depression might not be considered an unlikely outcome for someone suffering an incurable disease, in many cases depression antedates the onset of motor symptoms (and therefore diagnosis) by many years. This suggests that these affective symptoms are part of the neuropsychiatric symptom complex of HD and are not an understandable reaction to knowledge of disease status (McHugh, 1989). Other emotional symptoms, such as irritability, aggression, apathy, sexual disorders, alcohol or drug abuse, schizophreniform thought disorder, and conduct disorder are also prominent (Bylsma et al., 1996; Folstein et al., 1991; Folstein, Franz, Jensen, Chase, & Folstein, 1983; Pflanz, Besson, Ebmeier, & Simpson, 1991; Shiwach, 1994; Shoulson, 1990).

Postmortem examination of brains of HD patients reveals striking atrophy of the head of the caudate nucleus even at the earliest stages of disease, while the putamen is less affected (e.g., Dom, Malfroid, & Baro, 1976; Vonsattel et al., 1985). Microscopic examination reveals a relatively selective loss of small, spiny neurons in the dorsomedial aspects of the head of the caudate nucleus in the early stages of disease. As the disease progresses, both the head and body of the caudate, as well as the putamen, become involved (Vonsattel et al., 1985). The globus pallidus appears to lose relatively few neurons.

Atrophy of the cerebral cortex has also been observed in the autopsied brains of HD patients (De la Monte, Vonsattel, & Richardson, 1988; Forno & Jose, 1973). Comparisons of neuron counts in the dorsolateral prefrontal cortex in brains of HD patients and neurologically normal control subjects have shown neuronal loss in layers III, V, and VI of the cortex (Hedreen, Peyser, Folstein, & Ross, 1991; Sotrel et al., 1991), demonstrating clear neuroanatomical abnormalities in the frontal lobes of HD patients. It remains unclear whether loss of frontal cortical cells is part of the primary neuropathology of HD or occurs as a reaction to loss of connections with striatal neurons in the frontal striatal loops (Alexander, DeLong, & Strick, 1986). These frontal cortex abnormalities fit well with descriptions of HD patients' cognitive performance as appearing similar to that of patients with frontal lobe lesions and may prove important for explaining the full clinical syndrome of HD.

Currently, it is believed that the most likely pathophysiological mechanism of cell death in HD is depicted by the "excitotoxin hypothesis." This hypothesis proposes that glutamate and its analogs have a toxic effect on striatal neurons due to a defect in the N-methyl-D-aspartate (NMDA) subtype of glutamate receptors on striatal neurons (Coyle & Schwarz, 1976; McGeer & McGeer, 1976; Young et al., 1988). The defect results in prolonged and/or excessive excitation of those neurons, which ultimately results in their death (Albin et al., 1990). The hypothesis is supported by animal research showing that glutamatergic analogs, such as quinolinic, ibotenic, or kainic acid, create a pattern of striatal lesions that is similar to that observed in the brains of HD patients (Coyle & Schwarz, 1976; Hantraye, Riche, Maziere, & Isacson, 1990; McGeer & McGeer, 1976). This hypothesis has served as the theoretical basis for recent clinical treatment trials of putative therapeutic agents in HD (described below).

Genetics

Only recently has there been a systematic search for the genetic mutation responsible for

Huntington's disease. A national registry for Huntington's disease patients was instituted in 1979. The National Institutes of Health funded two Huntington's disease research centers in 1980. The goals of the centers were to determine the cause of HD, to better understand the natural history of the disease, and to develop better treatments and management plans for affected patients.

The first important genetic finding was the chromosomal locus of the HD gene. Gusella and colleagues (1983), using genetic linkage analysis, reported the tip of the short arm of chromosome 4 as the location. The genetic defect itself was not identified. A number of associated genetic markers were identified, making possible presymptomatic genetic linkage testing for HD in asymptomatic at-risk individuals. The test was not definitive, but for most at-risk individuals it afforded an estimate of the certainty of developing or not developing the disease in the range of 95% to 99%.

A decade later, the genetic defect that causes Huntington's disease was identified. An unstable expansion of trinucleotide repeats (cytosine-adenine-guanine; CAG) in the IT15 gene located on the tip of chromosome 4 was identified as the genetic abnormality responsible for Huntington's disease (Huntington's Disease Collaborative Research Group, 1993). In normal individuals, the number of CAG repeats ranges between 7 and 31, while in individuals affected with Huntington's disease there are greater than 37 repeats. There is a relationship between age at onset of disease and repeat length, with earlier onset associated with a larger number of repeats. This is particularly true for repeat lengths over 50, but the relationship is less clear for shorter repeat lengths (Stine et al., 1993). The discovery of the genetic mutation led to hope that a cure or treatment might be quickly discovered, however this is not likely. The gene is unlike any other known gene, and its function remains unclear.

One hypothesis to explain the selective vulnerability of striatal tissues in HD has been a selective overrepresentation of the genetic mutation in striatal tissues, particularly the caudate nucleus. This hypothesis has proven to be false. Both the HD gene messenger ribonucleic acid and its protein product, called *huntingtin*, are widely expressed throughout the brain and in non-neural tissues (Li et al., 1993; Sharp et al., 1995; Strong et al., 1993). The gene is expressed at its highest level in neuronal tissue, but there is considerable expression in tissues throughout the body (Huntington's Disease Collaborative Research Group, 1993; Li et al., 1993; Strong et al., 1993). Within the central nervous system, the highest concentrations are in the cortex and cerebellum, with only moderate gene expression in the striatum (Sharp et al., 1995). The regional distribution of the HD gene expression does not match the regional distribution of HD neuropathology, effectively ruling out regional gene distribution as a viable substrate for the regional neuropathological changes of HD.

An alternate explanation for the pattern of neuropathology in HD is a selective vulnerability of striatal neurons to an aberrant function of the mutated HD gene product. Recent research has shown that the HD gene product is located in the cytoplasm of neurons (DiFiglia et al., 1995; Sharp et al., 1995; Trottier et al., 1995). DiFiglia et al. (1995) report that huntingtin is located in cell bodies and dendrites, in the matrix of the cytoplasm, and near, but outside, vesicles. These authors propose that huntingtin may be involved in vesicle transport within cells. Trottier et al. (1995) report that huntingtin appears to be located in cell bodies of cerebellar Purkinje cells and some dopaminergic cells of the substantia nigra, but not in the majority of striatal cell bodies. Punctate staining of cortical cells suggested that huntingtin is also located in nerve endings, and subcellular fractionation studies revealed huntingtin in the fraction associated with synaptic vesicles. Sharp et al. (1995) report similar findings, but importantly, they also found huntingtin in the nerve terminals of caudate and putamen neurons. None of these studies found the HD gene messenger RNA or huntingtin in neuronal nuclei or mitochondria, and each independently concludes that the HD gene is, therefore, not involved in transcription. In summary, huntingtin is found in nerve terminals and appears to be associated with some aspect of synaptic vesicle function, although the precise role remains unknown. The regional distribution of huntingtin is intriguing but does not speak directly to the regional neuropathology in HD. Sharp et al. (1995) speculate that other, yet uncharacterized proteins might interact with huntingtin to produce the selective damage.

One such protein, huntingtin-associated protein-1 (HAP-1), has recently been discovered (Li et al., 1995). As huntingtin is not like any known gene, HAP-1 is unlike any other known protein, and its function is unknown. This protein shows a specific interactive affinity for huntingtin, and the strength of the binding is related to the length of the trinucleotide repeat in the huntingtin gene product; longer repeat lengths yield stronger binding. Importantly, HAP-1 protein, unlike the huntingtin gene, is found only in brain tissue and not peripheral tissues. It is detected in its highest concentrations in areas of the brain that are most vulnerable in HD—the caudate and cortex—and therefore holds promise as a substrate for the selective brain pathology of HD.

The role of huntingtin remains poorly understood, although there is evidence that it is necessary for normal fetal development. Mouse embryonic models have been developed that have one or no copies of huntingtin in their chromosomes (Duyao et al., 1995; Nasir et al., 1995). In one study, those that were homozygous for the deletion did not survive gestation past the 8th day at a stage preceding the development of neural tissue (Duyao et al., 1995). Heterozygous embryos survived to adulthood but developed motor and cognitive abnormalities. Neuropathological examination of the adult heterozygotic mice revealed cell loss in the subthalamic nucleus (Nasir et al., 1995). These data indicate that huntingtin is necessary for normal embryonic growth and that this gene is important for normal basal ganglia development. In addition, these authors suggest that the abnormal huntingtin gene responsible for the development of HD results in an abnormal "gain of function" rather than "loss of function." Li et al. (1995) interpret their finding of a stronger HAP-1 association with expanded polyglutamine repeat lengths than with shorter ones as supportive of that hypothesis.

The discovery of the HD gene, the huntingtin protein, and the HAP-1 protein are very important steps in understanding the neuropathological mechanism of HD. If the interaction of huntingtin and HAP-1 are shown to be involved in the neuropathological process in HD, then they could be the target of future therapeutic interventions. That is, if blocking the natural interaction of HAP-1 and huntingtin blocks or slows the neuropathological process, this might be a very powerful method of slowing or arresting the progress of disease.

The Cognitive Disorder of Huntington's Disease

Very early in the course of HD, patients and family members report a decline in cognitive performance. Patients describe difficulty in planning and organizing their daily routines. Family members report the patient to be less flexible in thinking and less adaptable in behavior. Formal testing of early-stage HD patients clearly documents significant declines that are consistent with these reports. Attention, memory, visuomotor and visuographic abilities, and executive functions such as planning and monitoring activities, mental flexibility, and set shifting are all impaired in early HD patients (Brandt & Bylsma, 1993). In many respects, this pattern of impairment is reminiscent of that observed in patients with prefrontal cortex lesions. This resemblance is not unexpected, given the extensive reciprocal connections between basal ganglia structures and many areas of frontal cortex (Alexander et al., 1986). Of the five anatomically discrete and functionally specific circuits described, three involve caudate projections and are thought to be involved in aspects of cognitive performance. The other two circuits involve the putamen and are thought to be involved in the motor disorder of HD.

Given the coincident onset of motor and cognitive abnormalities in HD, the relationship between the two has been a topic of investigation. In general, studies have shown no relationship between cognitive performance and severity of chorea (Girotti, Marano, Soliveri, Geminiani, & Scigliano, 1988; Heindel, Butters, & Salmon, 1988). This is consistent with Alexander et al.'s (1986) delineation of the distinct reciprocal frontal striatal circuits involved in motor versus cognitive functions.

Functional impairments are also prominent in early HD and become worse over time. Indices measuring functional abilities, such as the Total Functional Capacity (TFC; Shoulson & Fahn, 1979) and the Huntington's Disease Activities of Daily Living (HD-ADL) scales (Bylsma, Rothlind, Hall, Folstein, & Brandt, 1993; Folstein, 1989), consistently show stronger relationships with cognitive decline than motor impairments in HD (Bamford, Caine, Kido, Plassche, & Shoulson, 1989; Mayeux, Stern, Herman, Greenbaum, & Fahn, 1986; Rothlind, Bylsma, Brandt, Peyser, & Folstein, 1993).

Rothlind et al. (1993) reported chorea to be the aspect of the motor disorder least predictive of functional performance in HD. So, although chorea is the defining feature of the disease, it is the cognitive disorder that contributes most to functional impairments in HD.

Specific Cognitive Functions

Attention and Concentration

As indicated above, attentional difficulties are an early problem for HD patients. Of the Wechsler Adult Intelligence Scale-Revised (WAIS-R; Wechsler, 1981) subtests, HD patients perform worst on those that involve the "freedom from distraction" factor (Arithmetic, Digit Span, Digit Symbol) (Josiassen, Curry, & Mancall, 1983; Strauss & Brandt, 1986). Attentional impairments are thought to be the basis for HD patients' difficulties with mental arithmetic (Brandt, Folstein, & Folstein, 1988; Caine, Bamford, Schiffer, Shoulson, & Levy, 1986). Performance on the Stroop Color Word Test (Stroop, 1935) and the Brief Test of Attention (Schretlen, Bobholz, & Brandt, 1996) and other such complex attentional tasks is also impaired in mildly affected patients (Paulsen et al., 1996; Schretlen, Brandt, & Bobholz, 1996) and becomes worse as the disease progresses.

Language

In contrast to cortical dementias such as Alzheimer's disease (AD), aphasia is not a prominent feature of the dementia of HD (Folstein et al., 1991). However, motor speech impairments such as dysarthria and dysprosodia are common, affecting nearly half of patients early in the disease and progressing such that all patients produce essentially unintelligible speech in the late stages of disease (Gordon & Illes, 1987; Illes, 1989; Podoll, Caspary, Lange, & Noth, 1988). The syntactic complexity of oral and written communication becomes reduced, culminating in incomplete sentence phrases or single word utterances in the late stages. Despite this, syntactic structure remains correct and speech content appropriate until very advanced disease (Gordon & Illes, 1987; Illes, 1989; Podoll et al., 1988).

Other aspects of language are also affected. Patients with HD are impaired on tests of confronta-

tion naming, although their errors are more often due to perceptual impairments than semantic network abnormalities (Hodges, Salmon, & Butters, 1990; Podoll et al., 1988). Repetition and narrative language tend to be disrupted due to speech timing impairments. Responses are delayed, leaving conversation with long pauses between sentences or words in a sentence (Podoll et al., 1988). On verbal fluency tasks, HD patients generate fewer words than normal, a deficit attributed to a breakdown in retrieval processes, not disruption of semantic networks. Patients with HD are equally impaired on phonemic and semantic fluency tasks, unlike AD patients, who suffer a breakdown of semantic networks (Martin & Fedio, 1983) and who are more impaired on semantic than phonemic fluency tasks (Monsch et al., 1994). Also, AD patients fail to benefit from retrieval cues during semantic fluency tasks, but HD patients generate significantly more words when cues are given (Randolf, Braun, Goldberg, & Chase, 1993).

Spatial Cognition

Performance on visuospatial tasks is impaired early in the disease process. Patients with HD are slow and inaccurate in copying geometric designs (Brouwers, Cox, Martin, Chase, & Fedio, 1984) and are impaired on the Block Design and Object Assembly subtests of the WAIS-R. Deficits are also observed on the Mosaic Comparisons Test, which is untimed and requires no motor response (Fedio, Cox, Neophytides, Canal-Frederick, & Chase, 1979), indicating that these impairments are not completely attributable to patients' motor disorders.

A major component of the visuospatial impairment of HD involves mental manipulation of self or objects in space. Potegal (1971) showed HD patients to be unable to accurately locate a previously visualized target after taking one step to the left or right, suggesting that HD patients are unable to adjust cognitive representations of position in space after a self-initiated movement. Mohr et al. (1991) found HD patients to be impaired on tasks of general visuospatial processing as well as on tasks requiring imagined movement of objects in space. Brouwers et al. (1984) found HD patients to be impaired on one such test, the Standardized Road Map Test of Directional Sense (Money, 1976). Similarly, Bylsma, Brandt, and Strauss (1992) found that HD patients were impaired on a version of the Semmes Route Walking Test (Semmes, Weinstein, Ghent, & Teuber, 1955, 1963). Patients with HD were particularly impaired on trials that required mental rotation of the route maps to adjust for their actual movements along the route. Together, these findings suggest that HD patients suffer a defect in egocentric, or personal, orientation of self in space.

Memory

Also appearing early in the course of HD are difficulties with explicit memory, manifesting as deficits in learning and retaining new information (Caine, Ebert & Weingartner, 1977; Moses, Golden, Berger, & Wisniewski, 1981) and recalling previously learned material (Beatty, Salmon, Butters, Heindel, & Granholm, 1988; Brandt, 1985). Early studies attributed deficits in learning new information to inefficient encoding (Weingartner, Caine, & Ebert, 1979). However, demonstrations of significantly better recognition (often approaching that of healthy controls) than on-demand recall on verbal memory tests indicate that HD patients do encode and retain the material to be learned (Butters, Wolfe, Granholm, & Martone, 1986; Butters, Wolfe, Martone, Granholm, & Cermak, 1985; Delis et al., 1991; Moss, Albert, Butters, & Payne, 1986; see Brandt, Corwin, & Krafft, 1992). These findings have lead to the hypothesis that HD patients' verbal memory deficits result more from inefficient retrieval strategies than encoding problems (Brandt, 1985; Butters, 1984; Butters, Salmon, & Heindel, 1990).

Memory for nonverbal material has been less well studied in HD. Patients with HD performed normally on a visual delayed response task, but were significantly impaired on a similar task requiring delayed spatial alternation (Oscar-Berman & Zola-Morgan, 1980; Oscar-Berman, Zola-Morgan, Öberg, & Bonner, 1982). Immediate memory for visual material is only mildly affected in HD patients, as indexed by normal recall and reproduction of line drawings on the Visual Reproduction subtest of the Wechsler Memory Scale-Revised (WMS-R; Wechsler, 1987) (Jacobs, Salmon, Tröster, & Butters, 1990; Jacobs, Tröster, Buttes, Salmon, & Cermak, 1990). Yet, in contrast to demonstrated near-normal recognition of verbal material, recognition of spatial locations, colors, patterns, and faces is impaired in HD (Moss et al., 1986).

Two important features of HD patients' memory performance on anterograde memory tests distinguish these patients from amnesic patients and AD patients. First, on both verbal and nonverbal memory tasks, HD patients make few intrusion errors on recall tasks (Butters, Granholm, Salmon, Grant, & Wolfe, 1987; Delis et al., 1991; Jacobs, Salmon, et al., 1990; Jacobs, Tröster, et al., 1990), and they tend to retain what they learn over at least a brief (30-min) period of time (Butters, Salmon, & Cullum, 1988; Delis et al., 1991).

Performance of HD patients on retrograde memory tests also distinguishes them from other memory-disordered patients, such as those with amnestic Korsakoff's syndrome (KS). On tests assessing memory for past public events, KS patients show a distinct temporal gradient, with more recent events being recalled less well than more distant events (Albert, Butters, & Brandt, 1981a). However, HD patients show a "flat" retrograde amnesia profile with equal recall of events across all time periods (Albert, Butters, & Brandt, 1981b; Beatty et al., 1988). This pattern is taken to support the hypothesis that a general retrieval deficit is the basis of HD patients' memory impairment.

There is a complicated and growing literature concerning the performance of HD patients on tests of implicit memory. Implicit memory refers to a class of improved performances that reflect the influence of prior learning episodes, but (unlike explicit recall and recognition memory measures) do not require conscious recollection of those episodes (Schacter, 1987). Implicit memory measures are of interest and importance for neuropsychology because it has been demonstrated that patients with severe explicit memory disorders such as AD and KS can nonetheless demonstrate preserved learning on implicit memory tasks. These findings indicate that this type of memory is not reliant on the limbic/diencephalic memory system, and there has been an increasing effort to discern the neural substrate of implicit learning. Studies have contrasted memory-disordered patients known to have lesions in the diencephalic/limbic system, such as AD and KS patients, to memory-disordered patients with no such lesions, such as HD patients.

In general such studies have demonstrated that AD and KS patients are impaired on most tests of lexical, semantic, and pictorial priming, but HD patients' performances on these tests are most often unimpaired (Bylsma, Rebok, & Brandt, 1992; Heindel, Salmon, Shults, Walicke, & Butters, 1989). In contrast, on implicit tests assessing acquisition of motor, visuomotor, perceptual, or cognitive skills, HD patients are typically impaired while AD and KS patients perform relatively better. Specifically, HD patients demonstrate impaired performance acquiring mirror-reading skills, despite normal explicit recognition of test stimuli (Martone, Butters, Payne, Becker, & Sax, 1984); an inability to improve performance on pursuit rotor task with practice (Heindel et al., 1988, 1989); lack of a weight biasing effect (Heindel, Salmon, & Butters, 1991); failure to show adaptation effects to prism lens distortion (Paulsen, Butters, Salmon, Heindel, & Swenson, 1993); failure to improve performance on the Tower of Hanoi task with practice (Butters et al., 1985; Saint-Cyr, Taylor, & Lang, 1988); failure to generalize task skills and no beneficial effect of route predictability on a maze learning task (Bylsma, Brandt, & Strauss, 1990); and impaired performance on the Serial Reaction Time task, assessing motor sequence learning (Knopman & Nissen, 1991; Willingham & Koroshetz, 1993). Importantly, in these studies there was little correlation between the severity of motor impairment and performance; more often severity of dementia was the best predictor.

These findings support the hypothesis that the basal ganglia are important for acquisition of skill-based knowledge. The basal ganglia appear to be crucial for generalizing across stimulus situations and for allowing use of across-situation regularity, patterning, and organization of stimuli to improve performance. A likely basis of impairment is the inability to generate and retain central motor programs or expectancies that are required for skill learning.

Longitudinal Studies of Cognition in Huntington's Disease

There have been surprisingly few studies of the progression of clinical symptoms in HD and even fewer documenting cognitive decline over time. Penney, Young, and Shoulson (1990) report that the rate of decline in functional abilities is more rapid in patients with early onset (particularly juvenile onset) when compared to those with later onset. A

similar relationship between onset age and rate of decline was reported by Myers et al. (1991). Kieburtz et al. (1994) found the rate of functional decline to correlate with age of onset but not with length of the CAG expansion at IT15. However, Feigin et al. (1995) found no relationship between functional decline and onset age.

In the cognitive domain, Hodges et al. (1990) contrasted the performance of equally demented HD and AD patients on tests of semantic and episodic memory on two occasions separated by 1 year. Patients with AD showed greater declines than HD patients on several tests assessing semantic knowledge (Boston Naming Test, Number Information Test, Similarities subtest of the WAIS-R, category fluency). In contrast, HD patients showed greater declines than AD patients on the Controlled Oral Word Association Test, a test of letter-cued verbal fluency.

Recently, we assessed clinical and cognitive progression in a group of 46 early HD patients with measures of neurological impairment (QNE; Quantitated Neurological Examination) and a detailed neuropsychological examination on three occasions each separated by 1 year (Brandt et al., 1996). The test battery consisted of tests known to be sensitive to mild "subcortical" dementia of HD, focusing on attention, memory, and executive functions. Performance measures from the battery were subjected to principal components factor analysis (with orthogonal rotation) to reduce the number of variables for statistical analyses. The factor solution yielded three factors accounting for 69.4% of the variance in the intercorrelation matrix. The first factor (51.5% of the variance) was a general cognitive factor (WAIS-R Vocabulary and Block Design; Controlled Oral Word Association Test; Developmental Test of Visual-Motor Integration). Factor 2 (9.4% of the variance) comprised tests of memory and attention (Hopkins Verbal Learning Test; Brief Test of Attention; Stroop Color Word Test; Trail Making Test). Factor 3 (8.4% of the variance) assessed categorization (cards/sort and perseverative errors from the Wisconsin Card Sorting Test).

The patients were divided by median split into those with short CAG repeat lengths (< 47 repeats; n = 25) and those with long repeat lengths (≥ 47 repeats; n = 21). These groups were contrasted for baseline characteristics and for rate of decline on clinical indices of disease severity and cognitive performance. At baseline, the groups were equal for years of education and duration of disease. However, the short repeat group was significantly older and had a later disease onset than the long repeat group. This was not unexpected, given the previous demonstrations of an inverse relationship between CAG repeat length and age at onset. The groups were not different on the QNE indices of disease severity or any cognitive measure, although the short repeat group was more functionally impaired than the long repeat group at baseline.

Contrasting the groups over the three annual visits revealed groups to differ in their rate of progression of neurological impairment, with the long repeat group showing more rapid progression as indexed by total QNE score and Motor Impairment Scale (MIS) subscale, which measures voluntary motor impairment. Similarly, on Cognitive Factor 1 (general cognitive abilities), the short repeat group performed at a similar level over three visits while the long repeat group showed significantly more rapid decline. Together, these findings indicate that a longer CAG repeat length is associated with an earlier onset of disease and a more malignant disease course, although the mechanism for these effects is unknown. Such studies of the natural course of HD are important for future clinical trials. It is necessary to know how quickly each aspect of the disease declines in untreated patients so that the beneficial effects of putative therapeutic agents can be demonstrated. Our longitudinal study is continuing.

Treatment

Presymptomatic Testing of At-Risk Individuals

Disease onset is most often delayed past the childbearing years, so many individuals with HD genetic mutation have passed it on to their children before they themselves show any signs of disease. The recent advent of presymptomatic testing programs, initially using genetic linkage (Gusella et al., 1983) and now by direct genetic testing (Huntington's Disease Collaborative Research Group, 1993), has allowed neurologically normal individ-

uals who are at risk for the disease (i.e., have an affected parent) to obtain information about their own genetic status before disease starts.

Funding was obtained for a presymptomatic testing program at the Johns Hopkins University School of Medicine to provide genetic information to individuals at risk for HD in the context of a research study. There was justifiable concern that informing individuals that they will, with high probability, develop a fatal neurodegenerative disease might result in negative psychological consequences. A rigorous protocol was implemented to decrease the likelihood of such events. Participants in the study are required to have a confidant who accompanies them for all study visits, to be deemed psychiatrically and neurologically normal at the time the genetic test was requested, and to come to at least four genetic and psychological counseling sessions prior to being informed of their genetic status. The experience of the program at Johns Hopkins University is that, regardless of whether individuals received news that they would/would not develop the disease, the vast majority of participants experienced no short-term or long-lasting detrimental consequences (Brandt et al., 1989; Codori & Brandt, 1994).

Also in the context of the program, efforts have been directed toward determining whether there are clinical, cognitive, or neuropsychiatric characteristics that can predict onset of disease. Each participant in the program undergoes a baseline neurological, cognitive, and psychiatric assessment. These assessments are repeated annually for a minimum of 3 years after disclosure of genetic status, and many participants are followed annually for longer periods. The goal is to document clinical correlates of conversion from unaffected status to active disease. Once active disease has been discovered, data from the pre-onset visits can be examined for changes in cognitive performance, neurological status, and psychiatric or emotional state, which are predictive of the transition. With this information in hand from a sufficient number of people, it may be possible to determine when someone is about to become affected. Such information could be used to counsel individuals who remain at risk for the disease. To date, there have been few such status conversions, so the utility of this strategy remains to be determined.

Presymptomatic determination of genetic status is an important aspect of the treatment of HD. Such knowledge allows individuals at risk for the disease to make informed family planning (i.e., whether to have children or not), financial, employment, and health care decisions. In addition, prenatal testing of at-risk fetuses can determine whether the gene has been passed, and this information can be used in decisions about whether to terminate a pregnancy. Use of genetic information for such decisions, whether by individuals at risk for HD or other genetic conditions, will most likely increase in the future as genetic testing becomes more readily available through commercial testing centers. Knowing the circumstances under which providing such information is likely to result in negative consequences for the individual is of vital importance.

Treatment of Clinically Affected Patients

There are no known treatments for Huntington's disease. That is, there are no known ways to prevent someone who has the HD genetic mutation from developing the disease, and there are no treatments which slow the progressive neuropathological changes once they commence. There are, however, effective methods for treating some of the *symptoms* of Huntington's disease—motor disorder and psychiatric symptoms in particular.

There have been several attempts to affect the rate of decline in HD patients. Early studies took the approach attempting to modulate levels of neurotransmitters that are altered in the brains of HD patients due to striatal neuron death. Replacement of gamma-aminobutyric acid (GABA) with muscimal, a GABA agonist, resulted in no amelioration of symptoms (Shoulson, Goldblatt, Charlton, & Joynt, 1978; Foster, Chase, Denaro, Hare, & Taminga, 1983). A similar approach to reduce increased striatal dopamine in HD (Sanberg & Coyle, 1984) by administering dopamine antagonists resulted in a reduction of involuntary movements, but no slowing of disease progression (Folstein, 1989).

A recent strategy has been to prevent or slow striatal cell death. Based upon the theory of glutamate-mediated excitotoxicity as the mechanism of cell death in HD, blocking this effect by administering glutamate antagonists was attempted.

In a 3-year double-blind placebo-controlled study, no benefit of baclofen was found (Shoulson et al., 1989). A hypothesis was generated from the excitotoxin theory that the proximal cause of cell death was the generation of excessive neurotoxic oxygen free radicals, resulting in damage to cell membranes, intracellular proteins, and nuclear DNA (Coyle & Puttfarken, 1993). In in vitro and in vivo studies, the administration of free radical scavengers—substances which quickly bind to and neutralize oxygen free radicals—reduced or prevented the excitotoxic effects of glutamine agonists (Miyamoto & Coyle, 1990; Miyamoto, Murphy, Schnaar, & Coyle, 1989). Clinical trials of known oxygen free radical scavengers were instituted in HD patients. A double-blind placebo-controlled trial of D-α-tocopherol (vitamin E) revealed no effect on disease progression in the group as a whole, but did reveal suggestive findings for patients who were early in the course of disease (Peyser et al., 1995). A similar study of idebenone, a more potent free radical scavenger, found no effect on disease progression, even those in the early stages of disease (Ranen et al., 1996). While the outcomes of these latter studies have been disappointing, the laboratory studies continue to show such a strategy to be a viable one. A strategy for future clinical trials may be administering combinations of glutamine antagonists and oxygen free radical scavengers.

Although no treatments to slow the progression of disease have yet been discovered, greater success has been achieved in treating some of the motor symptoms and most of the psychiatric symptoms that HD patients experience. Treatment of the motor disorder of HD can be problematic, however, because of the two components. Typically, treatment is sought for involuntary movements, and pharmacotherapy for that aspect can exacerbate the voluntary motor disorder (Folstein, 1989). Therefore, the first line of treatment for difficulties with chorea should be environmental or behavioral. Special chairs which keep the patient in a semi-reclining position, padding around chairs and beds, and use of ankle or wrist weights have been shown to be beneficial in some cases. Stress and anxiety exacerbate chorea, so keeping the patient's environment quiet and consistent can help reduce chorea. As a last resort, pharmacotherapy, typically with neuroleptic medications (i.e., haldol, fluphenazine, thioridazine), should be considered if the chorea is very debilitating and if behavioral and environmental manipulations have proven ineffective. Careful patient monitoring for side effects is necessary, particularly for parkinsonism and increased voluntary motor impairment (Ranen, Peyser, & Folstein, 1993). For management of other aspects of the motor disorder such as dysphagia, dysarthria, rigidity, and gait disorders, pharmacotherapy is rarely beneficial. Environmental manipulations, reducing anxiety, and education of the patient and caregivers through consultation with occupational therapists, physical therapists, or speech pathologists can be helpful (Ranen et al., 1993).

Psychiatric disorders, although quite common, are often undertreated in Huntington's disease patients. Symptoms and disorders include irritability, aggression, apathy, depression, and occasionally, bipolar disorder or frank mania. Delusions, hallucinations, schizophreniform disorders, obsessions, and sexual disorders are also frequent. Ranen et al. (1993) review in detail therapeutic strategies to treat each of these symptoms, drawing on the expertise gained from many years of treating HD patients in the clinic of the Baltimore Huntington's Disease Project at the Johns Hopkins Hospital. The reader is referred to their handbook, *A Physician's Guide to the Management of Huntington's Disease*, available through the Huntington's Disease Society of America or the Huntington Society of Canada, for a more detailed discussion of therapeutic strategies. The basic thrust of their recommendations will be reviewed here.

In general, psychiatric symptoms in HD patients can be treated pharmacologically as easily and effectively as in other psychiatric patients, and clinicians should not be reluctant to attempt to do so. The medications which are effective for general psychiatric patients are also effective for HD patients and typically do not adversely affect the motor disorder of HD. In some cases, reduction of psychiatric symptoms and the coincident stress and anxiety may lead to improvements in motor symptoms, particularly chorea.

Ranen et al. (1993) suggest that psychiatric symptoms be treated aggressively, but carefully, starting with lower than normal doses and increasing medications in small steps. Because patients with brain damage due to trauma or degenerative disease are typically more sensitive to medications than persons with uncompromised brain function, patients need to be closely monitored for side effects, particularly medication-induced delirium and increased motor disorders. Adequate therapeutic response may be achieved on lower than normal doses of medication. Likewise, a delirium may be induced by a "typical" dose of medication.

Summary

These are exciting times in the study of Huntington's disease. The recent discovery of the genetic mutation responsible for the disease, its protein product (huntingtin), and an associated protein (HAP-1) provide the underpinnings for further research to understand the pathophysiological basis of striatal cell death in HD. In addition, these findings will serve to focus the search for potential therapeutic agents to slow or arrest decline in affected patients and delay the onset of disease in unaffected gene carriers. Our longitudinal studies of the natural history of cognitive, neurological, and functional change and of frontal-striatal atrophy in HD continue. These studies will provide essential information about rate of change in untreated HD patients to compare to measures in treatment trials. As we await viable treatments for the disease itself, our efforts to find better palliative treatments for the symptoms that accompany the disease are ongoing. The next decade holds the promise of exciting discoveries in the treatment of this tragic illness.

ACKNOWLEDGMENTS

The author is indebted to many colleagues and collaborators who have assisted greatly in my understanding of this disease—particularly Jason Brandt, Ph.D., and Susan Folstein, M.D. The ongoing support of the Research Center Without Walls for Huntington's Disease, the Baltimore Huntington's Disease Project (Christopher A. Ross, M.D., Principal Investigator) is also acknowledged. This work was supported in part by grants NS16375 and NS24841 from the National Institute of Neurological Disorders and Stroke.

References

Albert, M. S., Butters, N., & Brandt, J. (1981a). Patterns of remote memory in amnesic and demented patients. *Archives of Neurology*, 38, 495–500.

Albert, M. S., Butters, N., & Brandt, J. (1981b). Development of remote memory loss in patients with Huntington's disease. *Journal of Clinical Neuropsychology*, 3, 1–12.

Albin, R. L., Young, A. B., Penney, J. B., Handelin, B., Balfour, R., Anderson, K. D., Markel, D. S., Tourtellotte, W. W., & Reiner, A. (1990). Abnormalities of striatal projection neurons and N-methyl-D-aspartate receptors in presymptomatic Huntington's disease. *New England Journal of Medicine*, 322, 1293–1298.

Alexander, G. E., DeLong, M. R., & Strick, P. L. (1986). Parallel organization of functionally segregated circuits linking basal ganglia and cortex. *Annual Review of Neuroscience*, 9, 357–381.

Bamford, K. A., Caine, E. D., Kido, D. K., Plassche, W. M., & Shoulson, I. (1989). Clinical-pathological correlation in Huntington's disease: A neuropsychological and computed tomography study. *Neurology*, 39, 796–801.

Beatty, W. W., Salmon, D. P., Butters, N., Heindel, W. C., & Granholm, E. (1988). Retrograde amnesia in patients with Alzheimer's disease and Huntington's disease. *Neurobiology of Aging*, 9, 181–186.

Brandt, J. (1985). Access to knowledge in the dementia of Huntington's disease. *Developmental Neuropsychology*, 1, 335–348.

Brandt, Folstein, S. E., & Folstein, M. F. (1988). Differential cognitive impairment in Alzheimer's disease and Huntington's disease. *Annals of Neurology*, 23, 555–561.

Brandt, J., Quaid, K. A., Folstein, S. E., Garber, P., Maestri, N. E., Abbott, M. H., Slavney, P. R., Franz, M. L., Kasch, L., & Kazazian, H. H. (1989). Presymptomatic diagnosis of delayed-onset disease with linked DNA markers: The experience in Huntington's disease. *Journal of the American Medical Association*, 26, 3108–3114.

Brandt, J., Corwin, J. & Krafft, L. (1992). Is verbal recognition memory really different in Huntington's and Alzheimer's disease? *Journal of Clinical and Experimental Neuropsychology*, 14, 773–784.

Brandt, J., Bylsma, F. W., Gross, R., Stine, O. C., Ranen, N., & Ross, C. A. (1996). Trinucleotide repeat length and clinical progression in Huntington's disease. *Neurology*, 46, 527–531.

Brouwers, P., Cox, C., Martin, A., Chase, T., & Fedio, P. (1984). Differential perceptual-spatial impairment in Huntington's and Alzheimer's dementias. *Archives of Neurology*, 41, 1073–1076.

Bryois, C. (1989). [The length of survival and cause of death in Huntington chorea]. *Schweizer Archiv für Neurologie und Psychiatrie*, 140, 101–115.

Butters, N. (1984). The clinical aspects of memory disorders: Contributions from experimental studies of amnesia and dementia. *Journal of Clinical Neuropsychology*, 6, 17–36.

Butters, N., Wolfe, J., Martone, M., Granholm, E., & Cermak, L. S. (1985). Memory disorders associated with Huntington's disease: Verbal recall, verbal recognition, and procedural memory. *Neuropsychologia*, 23, 729–743.

Butters, N., Wolfe, J., Granholm, E., & Martone, M. (1986). An assessment of verbal recall, recognition and fluency abilities in patients with Huntington's disease. *Cortex*, 22, 11–32.

Butters, N., Granholm, E., Salmon, D. P., Grant, I., & Wolfe, J., (1987). Episodic and semantic memory: A comparison of amnesic and demented patients. *Journal of Clinical and Experimental Neuropsychology*, 9, 479–497.

Butters, N., Salmon, D. P., & Cullum, C. M. (1988). Differentiation of amnesic and demented patients with the Wechsler Memory Scale-Revised. *The Clinical Neuropsychologist*, 2, 133–148.

Butters, N., Salmon, D. P., & Heindel, W. C. (1990). Processes underlying the memory impairments of demented patients. In E. Goldberg (Ed.), *Contemporary neuropsychology and the legacy of Luria* (pp. 99–126). Hillsdale, NJ: Lawrence Erlbaum.

Bylsma, F. W., Brandt, J., & Strauss, M. E. (1990). Aspects of procedural memory are differentially impaired in Huntington's disease. *Archives of Clinical Neuropsychology*, 5, 287–297.

Bylsma, F. W., Brandt, J., & Strauss, M. E. (1992). Personal and extrapersonal orientation in Huntington's disease patients and those at risk. *Cortex*, 28, 113–122.

Bylsma, F. W., Rebok, G., & Brandt, J. (1992). Long-term retention of implicit learning in Huntington's disease. *Neuropsychologia*, 29, 1213–1221.

Bylsma, F. W., Rothlind, J., Hall, M. H., Folstein, S. E., & Brandt, J. (1993). Assessment of adaptive functioning in Huntington's disease. *Movement Disorders*, 8, 183–190.

Bylsma, F. W., Como, P., Paulsen, J., Jones, R., Rey, G., Saint-Cyr, J., & Stebbins, G., and the Huntington's Study Group. (1996). Noncognitive symptoms in Huntington's disease [Abstract]. *Journal of the International Neuropsychological Society*, 2, 35.

Caine, E. D., Ebert, M. H., & Weingartner, H. (1977). An outline for the analysis of dementia. *Neurology*, 27, 1087–1092.

Caine, E. D., Bamford, K. A., Schiffer, R. B., Shoulson, I., & Levy, S. (1986). A controlled neuropsychological comparison of Huntington's disease and multiple sclerosis. *Archives of Neurology*, 43, 249–254.

Codori, A. M., & Brandt, J. (1994). Psychological costs and benefits of predictive testing for Huntington's disease. *American Journal of Medical Genetics (Neuropsychiatric Genetics)*, 54, 174–184.

Conneally, P. M. (1984). Huntington's disease: Genetics and epidemiology. *American Journal of Human Genetics*, 36, 506–526.

Coyle, J. T., & Puttfarken, P. (1993). Oxidative stress, glutamate and neurodegenerative disorders. *Science*, 262, 689–695.

Coyle, J. T., & Schwarz, R. (1976). Lesions of striatal neurons with kainic acid provides a model for Huntington's disease. *Nature*, 263, 244–246.

Cummings, J. L., & Benson, D. F. (1984). Subcortical dementia: Review of an emerging concept. *Archives of Neurology*, 41, 874–879.

De la Monte, S. M., Vonsattel, J.-P., & Richardson, E. P., Jr.

(1988). Morphometric demonstration of atrophic changes in the cerebral cortex, white matter, and neostriatum in Huntington's disease. *Journal of Neuropathology and Experimental Neurology*, 47, 516–525.

Delis, D. C., Massman, P. J., Butters, N., Salmon, D. P., Cermak, L. S., & Kramer, J. H. (1991). Profiles of demented and amnesic patients on the California Verbal Learning Test: Implications for the assessment of memory disorders. *Psychological Assessment: A Journal of Consulting and Clinical Psychology*, 3, 19–26.

DiFiglia, M., Saap, E., Chase, K., Schwarz, C., Meloni, A., Young, C., Martin, E., Vonsattel, J.-P., Carraway, R., Reeves, S. A., Boyce, F. M., & Aronin, N. (1995). Huntingtin is a cytoplasmic protein associated with vesicles in human and rat brains neurons. *Neuron*, 14, 1075–1081.

Dom, R., Malfroid, M., & Baro, F. (1976). Neuropathology of Huntington's disease. *Neurology*, 26, 64–68.

Duyao, M. P., Auerbach, A. B., Ryan, A., Persichetti, F. I., Barnes, G. T., McNeil, S. M., Ge, P., Vonsattel, J. P., Gusella, J. F., Joyner, A. L., & MacDonald, M. E. (1995). Trinucleotide repeat length instability and age of onset in Huntington's disease. *Science*, 269, 407–410.

Fedio, P., Cox, C. S., Neophytides, A., Canal-Frederick, G., & Chase, T. N. (1979). Neuropsychological profile of Huntington's disease. *Advances in Neurology*, 23, 239–255.

Feigin, A., Kieburtz, K., Bordwell, K., Como, P., Steinberg, K., Sotack, J., Zimmerman, C., Hickey, C., Orme, C., & Shoulson, I. (1995). Functional decline in Huntington's disease. *Movement Disorders*, 10, 211–214.

Folstein, S. E. (1989). *Huntington's disease. A disorder of families.* Baltimore: The Johns Hopkins University Press.

Folstein, S. E., Abbott, M. H., Chase, G. A., Jensen, B. A., & Folstein, M. F. (1983). Association of affective disorder with Huntington's disease in a case series and in families. *Psychological Medicine*, 13, 537–542.

Folstein, S. E., Franz, M. L., Jensen, B., Chase, G. A., & Folstein, M. F. (1983). Conduct disorder and affective disorder among the offspring of patients with Huntington's disease. In S. B. Guze, F. L. Earls, & J. E. Barrett (Eds.), *Childhood psychopathology and development* (pp. 231–245). New York: Raven Press.

Folstein, S. E., Brandt, J., & Folstein, M. F. (1991). Huntington's disease. In J. L. Cummings (Ed.), *Subcortical dementia* (pp. 87–107). New York: Oxford University Press.

Forno, L. S., & Jose, C. (1973). Huntington's chorea: A pathological study. In A. Barbeau, T. N. Chase, & G. W. Paulson (Eds.), *Advances in neurology: Vol. 1. Huntington's disease.* New York: Raven Press.

Foster, N. L., Chase, T. N., Denaro, A., Hare, T. A., & Taminga, C. A. (1983). THIP treatment of Huntington's disease. *Neurology*, 33, 637–639.

Girotti, F., Marano, R., Soliveri, P., Geminiani, G., & Scigliano, G. (1988). Relationship between motor and cognitive disorders in Huntington's disease. *Journal of Neurology*, 235, 454–457.

Gordon, W. P., & Illes, J. (1987). Neurolinguistic characteristics of language production in Huntington's disease: A preliminary report. *Brain and Language*, 31, 1–10.

Gusella, J. F., Wexler, N. S., Conneally, P. M., Naylor, S. L., Anderson, M. A., Tanzi, R. E., Watkins, P. C., Ottina, K., Wallace, M. R., Sakaguchi, A. Y., Young, A. B., Shoulson, I., Bonnilla, E., & Martin, J. B. (1983). A polymorphic DNA marker linked to Huntington's disease. *Nature*, 306, 234–238.

Hantraye, P., Riche, D., Maziere, M., & Isacson, O. (1990). A primate model of Huntington's disease: Behavioral and anatomical studies of unilateral excitotoxic lesions of the caudate-putamen in the baboon. *Experimental Neurology*, 108, 91–104.

Hedreen, J. C., Peyser, C. E., Folstein, S. E., & Ross, C. A. (1991). Neuronal loss in layers V and VI of the cerebral cortex in Huntington's disease. *Neuroscience Letters*, 133, 257–261.

Heindel, W. C., Butters, N., & Salmon, D. P. (1988). Impaired learning of motor skill in patients with Huntington's disease. *Behavioral Neuroscience*, 102, 141–147.

Heindel, W. C., Salmon, D. P., Shults, C. W., Walicke, P. A., & Butters, N. (1989). Neuropsychological evidence for multiple implicit memory systems: A comparison of Alzheimer's, Huntington's, and Parkinson's disease patients. *Journal of Neuroscience*, 9, 582–587.

Heindel, W. C., Salmon, D. P., & Butters, N. (1991). The biasing of weight judgments in Alzheimer's and Huntington's disease: A priming or programming phenomenon? *Journal of Clinical and Experimental Neuropsychology*, 13, 189–203.

Hodges, J. R., Salmon, D. P., & Butters, N. (1990). Differential impairment of semantic and episodic memory in Alzheimer's and Huntington's diseases: A controlled prospective study. *Journal of Neurology, Neurosurgery, and Psychiatry*, 53, 1089–1095.

Huntington, G. (1872). On chorea. *Advances in Neurology*, 1, 33–35.

Huntington's Disease Collaborative Research Group. (1993). A novel gene containing a trinucleotide repeat that is expanded and unstable on Huntington's disease chromosomes. *Cell*, 71, 971–983.

Illes, J. (1989). Neurolinguistic features of spontaneous language production dissociate three forms of neurodegenerative disease: Alzheimer's, Huntington's, and Parkinson's. *Brain and Language*, 37, 628–642.

Jacobs, D., Salmon, D. P., Tröster, A. I., & Butters, N. (1990). Intrusion errors in the figural memory of patients with Alzheimer's and Huntington's disease. *Archives of Clinical Neuropsychology*, 5, 49–57.

Jacobs, D., Tröster, A. I., Butters, N., Salmon, D. P., & Cermak, L. S. (1990). Intrusion errors on the visual reproduction test of the Wechsler Memory Scale and the Wechsler Memory Scale-Revised: An analysis of demented and amnesic patients. *The Clinical Neuropsychologist*, 4, 177–191.

Josiassen, R. C., Curry, L. M., & Mancall, E. L. (1983). Development of neuropsychological deficits in Huntington's disease. *Archives of Neurology*, 40, 791–796.

Kieburtz, K., MacDonald, M., Shih, C., Feigin, A., Steinberg, K., Bordwell, K., Zimmerman, C., Srinidhi, J., Sotack, J., Gusella, J., & Shoulson, I. (1994). Trinucleotide repeat length and progression of illness in Huntington's disease. *Journal of Medical Genetics*, 31, 872–874.

Knopman, D. S., & Nissen, M. J. (1991). Procedural learning is impaired in Huntington's disease: Evidence from the serial reaction time task. *Neuropsychologia, 29,* 245–254.

Lasker, A. G., Zee, D. S., Hain, T. C., Folstein, S. E., & Singer, H. S. (1987). Saccades in Huntington's disease: Initiation defects and distractibility. *Neurology, 37,* 427–431.

Lasker, A. G., Zee, D. S., Hain, T. C., Folstein, S. E., & Singer, H. S. (1988). Saccades in Huntington's disease: Slowing and dysmetria. *Neurology, 38,* 364–370.

Leigh, R. J., Newman, S. A., Folstein, S. E., Lasker, A. G., & Jensen, B. A. (1983). Abnormal ocular motor control in Huntington's disease. *Neurology (Cleveland), 33,* 1268–1275.

Li, S.-H., Schilling, G., Young, W. S., III, Li, X.-J., Margolis, R. L., Stine, O. C., Wagster, M. V., Abbott, M. H., Franz, M. L., Ranen, N. G., Folstein, S. E., Hedreen, J. C., & Ross, C. A. (1993). Huntington's disease gene (IT15) is widely expressed in human and rat tissues. *Neuron, 11,* 985–993.

Li, X.-J., Li, S.-H., Sharp, A. H., Nuclfora, F. C., Jr., Schilling, G., Lanahan, A., Worley, P., Snyder, S. H., & Ross, C. A. (1995). A huntingtin-associated protein enriched in brain with implications for pathology. *Nature, 378*(6555), 398–402.

Martin, A., & Fedio, P. (1983). Word production and comprehension in Alzheimer's disease: The breakdown of semantic knowledge. *Brain and Language, 19,* 124–141.

Martone, M., Butters, N., Payne, M., Becker, J., & Sax, D. S. (1984). Dissociations between skill learning and verbal recognition in amnesia and dementia. *Archives of Neurology, 41,* 965–970.

Mayeux, R., Stern, Y., Herman, A., Greenbaum, L., & Fahn, S. (1986). Correlates of early disability in Huntington's disease. *Annals of Neurology, 20,* 727–731.

McGeer, E. G., & McGeer, P. L. (1976). Duplication of biochemical changes of Huntington's chorea. In A. Barbeau & T. R. Brunette (Eds.), *Progress in neurogenetics.* (pp. 645–650). Amsterdam: Excerpta Medic Foundation.

McHugh, P. R. (1989). The neuropsychiatry of basal ganglia disorders: A triadic syndrome and its explanation. *Neuropsychiatry, Neuropsychology, and Behavioral Neurology, 2,* 239–246.

McHugh, P. R., & Folstein, M. F. (1973). Subcortical dementia. Address to the American Academy of Neurology, Boston, MA.

McHugh, P. R., & Folstein, M. F. (1975). Psychiatric symptoms of Huntington's chorea: A clinical and phenomenological study. In D. F. Benson & D. Blumer (Eds.), *Psychiatric aspects of neurological disease* (pp. 267–285). New York: Raven Press.

Miyamoto, M., & Coyle, J. T. (1990). Idebenone attenuates neuronal degeneration induced by intrastriatal injection of excitotoxins. *Experimental Neurology, 108,* 38–45.

Miyamoto, M., Murphy, T. H., Schnaar, R. L., & Coyle, J. T. (1989). Antioxidants protect against glutamate cytotoxicity in a neuronal cell line. *Journal of Pharmacology and Experimental Therapeutics, 250,* 1132–1140.

Mohr, E., Brouwers, P., Claus, J. J., Mann, U. M., Fedio, P., & Chase, T. N. (1991). Visuospatial cognition in Huntington's disease. *Movement Disorders, 6,* 127–132.

Money, J. (1976). *A Standardized Road Map Test of Directional Sense.* San Rafael, CA: Academic Therapy Publications.

Monsch, A. U., Bondi, M. W., Butters, N., Paulsen, J. S., Salmon, D. P., Brugger, P., & Swenson, M. R. (1994). A comparison of category and letter fluency in Alzheimer's and Huntington's disease. *Neuropsychology, 8,* 25–30.

Moses, J. A., Jr., Golden, C. J., Berger, P. A., & Wisniewski, A. M. (1981). Neuropsychological deficits in early, middle, and late stages of Huntington's disease as measured by the Luria-Nebraska Neuropsychological Battery. *International Journal of Neuroscience, 14,* 95–100.

Moss, M. B., Albert, M. S., Butters, N., & Payne, M. (1986). Differential patterns of memory loss among patients with Alzheimer's disease, Huntington's disease, and alcoholic Korsakoff's syndrome. *Archives of Neurology, 43,* 239–246.

Myers, R. H., Sax, D. S., Koroshetz, W. J., Mastromauro, C., Cupples, L. A., Kiely, D. K., Pettengill, F. K., & Bird, E. D. (1991). Factors associated with slow progression in Huntington's disease. *Archives of Neurology, 48,* 800–804.

Nasir, J., Floresco, S. B., O'Kusky, J. R., Diewert, V. M., Richman, J. M., Zeisler, J., Borowski, A., Marth, J. D., Phillips, A. G., & Hayden, M. R. (1995). Targeted disruption of the Huntington's disease gene results in embryonic lethality and behavioral and morphological changes in heterozygotes. *Cell, 81,* 811–812.

Oscar-Berman, M., & Zola-Morgan, S. (1980). Comparative neuropsychology and Korsakoff's syndrome. I. Spatial and visual reversal learning. *Neuropsychologia, 18,* 499–512.

Oscar-Berman, M., Zola-Morgan, S. M., Öberg, R. G. E., & Bonner, R. T. (1982). Comparative neuropsychology and Korsakoff's syndrome. III. Delayed response, delayed alternation, and DRL performance. *Neuropsychologia, 20,* 187–202.

Paulsen, J. S., Butters, N., Salmon, D. P., Heindel, W. C., & Swenson, M. R. (1993). Prism adaptation in Alzheimer's and Huntington's disease. *Neuropsychology, 7,* 73–81.

Paulsen, J. S., Como, P., Rey, G., Bylsma, F., Jones, R., Saint-Cyr, J., Stebbins, G., & The Huntington Study Group. (1996). The clinical utility of the Stroop Test in a multicenter study of Huntington's disease [Abstract]. *Journal of the International Neuropsychological Society, 2,* 35.

Penney, J. B., Young, A. B., & Shoulson, I. (1990). Huntington's disease in Venezuela: 7 years of follow-up on symptomatic and asymptomatic individuals. *Movement Disorders, 5,* 93–99.

Peyser, C. E., Folstein, M. F., Chase, G. A., Starkstein, S. E., Brandt, J., Cockrell, J. R., Bylsma, F., Coyle, J. T., McHugh, P. R., & Folstein, S. E. (1995). A trial of D-α-tocopherol in Huntington's disease. *American Journal of Psychiatry, 152,* 1771–1775.

Pflanz, S., Besson, J. A. O., Ebmeier, K. P., & Simpson, S. (1991). The clinical manifestations of mental disorder in Huntington's disease: A retrospective case record study of disease progression. *Acta Psychiatrica Scandinavica, 83,* 53–60.

Podoll, K., Caspary, P., Lange, H. W., & Noth, J. (1988). Language functions in Huntington's disease. *Brain, 111,* 1475–1503.

Potegal, M. (1971). A note on spatial motor deficits in patients with Huntington's disease: A test of a hypothesis. *Neuropsychologia, 9,* 233–235.

Randolf, C., Braun, A. R., Goldberg, T. E., & Chase, T. E. (1993). Semantic fluency in Alzheimer's, Parkinson's, and Huntington's disease: Dissociation of storage and retrieval. *Neuropsychology, 7*, 82–88.

Randolph, C. (1991). Implicit, explicit, and semantic memory functions in Alzheimer's disease and Huntington's disease. *Journal of Clinical and Experimental Neuropsychology, 13*, 479–494.

Ranen, N. G., Peyser, C. E., & Folstein, S. E. (1993). *A physician's guide to the management of Huntington's disease: Pharmacologic and non-pharmacologic interventions.* New York: The Huntington's Disease Society of America.

Ranen, N. G., Peyser, C. E., Coyle, J., Bylsma, F. W., Sherr, M., Day, L., Folstein, M. F., Brandt, J., Ross, C. A., & Folstein, S. E. (1996). A controlled trial of idebenone in Huntington's disease. *Movement Disorders, 11*, 549–554.

Roos, R. A. C., Hermans, J., Vegter-van der Vlis, M., van Ommen, G. J. B., & Bruyn, G. W. (1993). Duration of illness in Huntington's disease is not related to age at onset. *Journal of Neurology, Neurosurgery, and Psychiatry, 56*, 98–100.

Rothlind, J. C., Bylsma, F. W., Brandt, J., Peyser, C., & Folstein, S. E. (1993). Cognitive and motor correlates of everyday functioning in early Huntington's disease. *Journal of Nervous and Mental Disease, 181*, 194–199.

Saint-Cyr, J. A., Taylor, A. E., & Lang, A. E. (1988). Procedural learning and neostriatal learning in man. *Brain, 111*, 941–959.

Sanberg, J. H., & Coyle, J. T. (1984). Scientific approaches to Huntington's disease. *Critical Reviews in Clinical Neurobiology, 1*, 1–44.

Schacter, D. (1987). Implicit memory: History and current status. *Journal of Experimental Psychology: Learning, Memory and Cognition, 13*, 501–518.

Schretlen, D., Brandt, J., & Bobholz, J. H. (1996). Validation of the Brief Test of Attention in patients with Huntington's disease and amnesia. *The Clinical Neuropsychologist, 10*, 90–95.

Schretlen, D., Bobholz, J. H., & Brandt, J. (1996). Development and psychometric properties of the Brief Test of Attention. *The Clinical Neuropsychologist, 10*, 80–89.

Semmes, J., Weinstein, S., Ghent, L., & Teuber, H.-L. (1955). Spatial orientation in man after cerebral injury: I. Analyses by locus of lesion. *The Journal of Psychology, 39*, 227–244.

Semmes, J., Weinstein, S., Ghent, L., & Teuber, H.-L. (1963). Correlates of impaired orientation in personal and extrapersonal space. *Brain, 86*, 742–772.

Sharp, A. H., Loev, S. J., Schilling, G., Li, S.-H., Li, X-J., Bao, J., Wagster, M., Kotzuk, J. A., Steiner, J. P., Lo, A., Hedreen, J., Sisodia, S., Snyder, S. H., Dawson, T. M., Byugo, D. K., & Ross, C. A. (1995). Widespread expression of Huntington's disease gene (IT15) protein product. *Neuron, 14*, 1065–1074.

Shiwach, R. (1994). Psychopathology in Huntington's disease patients. *Acta Psychiatrica Scandinavica, 90*, 241–246.

Shoulson, I. (1990). Huntington's disease: Cognitive and psychiatric features. *Neuropsychiatry, Neuropsychology, and Behavioral Neurology, 3*, 15–22.

Shoulson, I., & Fahn, S. (1979). Huntington's disease: Clinical care and evaluation. *Neurology, 29*, 1–3.

Shoulson, I., Goldblatt, D., Charlton, M., & Joynt, R. J. (1978). Huntington's disease: Treatment with muscimal, a GABA-mimetic drug. *Annals of Neurology, 4*, 279–284.

Shoulson, I., Odoroff, C., Oakes, D., Behr, J., Goldblatt, D., Caine, E., Kennedy, J., Miller, C., Bamford, K., Rubin, A., Plumb, S., & Kurlan, R. (1989). A controlled clinical trial of baclofen as protective therapy in early Huntington's disease. *Annals of Neurology, 25*, 252–259.

Sotrel, A., Paskevich, P. A., Kiely, D. K., Bird, E. D., Williams, R. S., & Myers, R. H. (1991). Morphometric analysis of the prefrontal cortex in Huntington's disease. *Neurology, 41*, 1117–1123.

Stine, O. C., Pleasant, N., Franz, M. L., Abbott, M. H., Folstein, S. E., & Ross, C. A. (1993). Correlation between the onset age of Huntington's disease and length of the trinucleotide repeat in IT-15. *Human Molecular Genetics, 2*, 1547–1549.

Strauss, M. E., & Brandt, J. (1986). An attempt at presymptomatic identification of Huntington's disease with the WAIS. *Journal of Clinical and Experimental Neuropsychology, 8*, 210–218.

Strong, T. V., Tagle, D. A., Valdes, J. M., Elmer, L. M., Boehm, K., Swaroop, M., Kaatz, K. W., Collins, F. S., & Albin, R. L. (1993). Widespread expression of the human and rat Huntington's disease gene in brain and nonneuronal tissues. *Nature Genetics, 5*, 259–265.

Stroop, J. R. (1935). Studies of interference in serial verbal reactions. *Journal of Experimental Psychology, 18*, 643–662.

Trottier, Y., Devys, D., Imbert, G., Saudou, F., An, I., Lutz, Y., Weber, C., Agid, Y., Hirsch, E. C., & Mandel, J.-L. (1995). Cellular localization of the Huntington's protein and discrimination of the normal and mutated form. *Nature Genetics, 10*, 104–110.

Vonsattel, J. P., Myers, R. H., Stevens, T. J., Ferrante, F. J., Bird, E. D., & Richardson, E. P., Jr. (1985). Neuropathological classification of Huntington's disease. *Journal of Neuropathology and Experimental Neurology, 44*, 559–577.

Wechsler, D. (1987). *The Wechsler Memory Scale-Revised* (Manual). New York: The Psychological Corporation.

Wechsler, D. (1981). *The Wechsler Adult Intelligence Scales-Revised* (Manual). New York: The Psychological Corporation.

Weingartner, H., Caine, E. D., & Ebert, M. H. (1979). Encoding processes, learning, and recall in Huntington's disease. In T. N. Chase, N. S. Wexler, & A. Barbeau (Eds.), *Advances in neurology* (Vol. 23, pp. 215–226). New York: Raven Press.

Willingham, D. B., & Koroshetz, W. J. (1993). Evidence for dissociable motor skills in Huntington's disease patients. *Psychobiology, 21*, 173–182.

Young, A. B., Shoulson, I., Penney, J. B., Starosta-Rubinstein, S., Gomez, F., Travers, H., Ramos-Arroyo, M. A., Snodgrass, S. R., Bonilla, E., Moreno, H., & Wexler, N. (1986). Huntington's disease in Venezuela: Neurological features and functional decline. *Neurology, 36*, 244–249.

Young, A. B., Greenamyre, J. T., Hollingsworth, Z., Albin, R., D'Amato, C., Shoulson, I., & Penney, J. (1988). NMDA receptor losses in putamen from patients with Huntington's disease (HD). *Science, 241*, 981–983.

17

Late-Life Depression

A Neuropsychological Perspective

PAUL DAVID NUSSBAUM

Introduction

This chapter reviews the literature on late-life depression. Support for a neuroanatomical substrate underlying depression in late life will be articulated using findings from the neuropsychological, neuroimaging, and medical literature. This chapter does not cover treatment issues for depression in late life, but the reader is referred to Chapter 3, *Mood Disorders*, in this text. The purpose of this chapter is to integrate findings from diverse literature and to review evidence suggesting that depression in late life is a unique disorder, different from depression in young adulthood, and related to dysfunction of particular regions of the brain.

Concept of Late-Life Depression

According to the National Institutes of Health (NIH) Consensus Development Conference Statement (1993), depression is broadly defined as a syndrome that encompasses physiological, affective, and cognitive manifestations. Relying on criteria detailed in the revised third edition of the *Diagnostic and Statistical Manual of Mental Disorders* (*DSM-III-R*) (American Psychiatric Association [APA], 1987) for the diagnosis of depression, the NIH panel underscored the classic symptoms of appetite and weight change, disturbed sleep, motor

agitation or retardation, fatigue and loss of energy, depressed or irritable mood, loss of interest or pleasure in previously pleasurable activities, feelings of worthlessness, self-reproach, excessive guilt, suicidal thinking or attempts, and difficulty with concentration.

The panel reported the difficulty in recognizing depression in late life compared to early life because of clinician bias that depression is normal for advanced age, older adults' predisposition to report somatic complaints that may mask depression, medical comorbidity, and concomitant presence of dementia. Although there is an argument made for the differences of early versus late-onset depression, the same criteria for diagnosing depression (APA, 1987) are typically used. This leads to some uncertainty about the appropriateness of considering late-life depression as a separate disorder that requires different assessment and treatment approaches than depression in young adulthood.

Indeed, a recent review of the literature pertaining to depression in late life points out several limitations with regard to studies on the differences between early and late-life depression (Caine, Lyness, & King, 1993). These authors argue that relevant literature contains studies that include primarily psychiatric and community-based subjects, employ inconsistent diagnostic and inclusionary criteria, and overly control for increased medical comorbidity with advanced age. It is problematic to separate coexisting disorders in older hospitalized or institutionalized individuals. Examples of coexisting disorders—mood disorder and medical illness—include arthritis, hypertension, diabetes, vi-

PAUL DAVID NUSSBAUM • Aging Research and Education Center, Lutheran Affiliated Services, Mars, Pennsylvania 16046; and Department of Neurology, University of Pittsburgh School of Medicine, Pittsburgh, Pennsylvania 15261.

sion and hearing deficits, stroke, and progressive dementias. Indeed, Caine and colleagues (1993) note that there is no valid methodology for identifying primary versus secondary psychiatric conditions. As a result, research findings pertaining to late life depression are generally based on limited, if not skewed, samples and may not reflect the reality of depression in the aged. Caine and colleagues further assert that medical illness accounts for much of the observed heterogeneity in presentation and outcome in late-life depression. However, in a recent, thorough study investigating the neuropsychological effects of depression and age in an older sample, King, Cox, Lyness, and Caine (1995) found that medical illness had minimal influence on neuropsychological test performance in same-age depressed and nondepressed elderly. Clearly the influence of medical illness and age on depression in late life is an area that requires additional investigation.

Caine and colleagues (1993), therefore, recommend caution in attempts to describe different samples (young vs. old) as similar or different with regard to clinical depression. They argue that some clinical studies impose rigid inclusion criteria that typically bias results. Further, these authors argue that the literature of late-life depression inappropriately defines age at onset as a dichotomous variable. At present, it remains unclear if age-associated clinical variability can be dichotomized. The validity of late-life depression as a separate clinical phenomena is further challenged by the fact that existing research studies have not employed consistent age cutoffs for "elderly": ages range from 45 to 65 years. Indeed, King and colleagues (1995) report no significant relationships between age of onset of first depressive episode and neuropsychological performance. Caine and colleagues (1993) argue for treating age and age at onset as continuous variables to assess significant trends.

Risk factors for depression in young adulthood and late life are similar. According to the NIH Consensus Development Conference Statement (1993), the major social and demographic risk factors include female gender, unmarried and particularly widowed marital statuses, experience of stressful life events, and lack of a supportive social network. For the older adult, the coexistence of medical illness with depression has been a reliable research finding.

There is little doubt that the clinical research methodology for the study of late-life depression is problematic. Within this context, however, Caine and colleagues (1993) in their review of the literature suggest some tentative conclusions with regard to differences between early-life and late-life depression. First, a positive family history of affective disorder is associated with onset of depression early in life but not necessarily in late life. Older depressed subjects may suffer less guilt or suicidal ideation, but more weight loss, psychomotor abnormalities, and suicidal behavior. Research findings on psychotic behavior across the life span are mixed, and no conclusions can yet be made. Intellectual impairment can occur among both the young depressed and elderly depressed, but with advanced age there is an increase in variability of neuropsychological performance. Cognitive impairment in the depressed older adult may represent an early marker of progressive dementia (Nussbaum, Kaszniak, Allender, & Rapcsak, 1995). This finding suggests a changing and perhaps unique neurophysiological substrate for depression in late life (Folstein & Rabins, 1991; Nussbaum, 1994). Indeed, a significant increase in brain abnormalities as measured by magnetic resonance imaging (MRI) for older depressed subjects compared to young depressed and compared to same-age nondepressed controls has been consistently reported (Coffey, Figiel, Djang, & Saunders, 1989; Coffey, Figiel, Djang, & Weiner, 1990). It remains unclear if the MRI-measured cortical and subcortical changes in older depressed patients are related to dysphoric mood and cognitive dysfunction.

A recently published study assessed the risk factors for first onset of depression in middle age (defined as age 40 to 64) and late life (defined as 65 years of age and older) (Gallo, Royall, & Anthony, 1993). Major depression was diagnosed using the Diagnostic Interview Schedule (Eaton et al., 1989) and the *Diagnostic Statistical Manual for Mental Disorders*, third edition (*DSM-III*) (APA, 1980). For those middle-aged subjects, risk factors for onset of major depression included female gender, low education achievement (less than 12 years, particularly for women), nonminority status (i.e., being white but not Hispanic), being separated or divorced, and currently not working for pay. For subjects 65 years and older, risk factors for onset of first episode of major depression included low education achievement (particularly for women), female gender, and nonminority status. The finding of increased risk for less educated females compared to females and males who complete 12 years of school is of interest particularly because females with 12 years of school have no difference in risk for depression compared to similarly educated males. Data from other studies on depression and risk factors indicate that education level needs to be understood in relation to physical illness, disability, and social network characteristics (Phifer & Murrell, 1986).

Late-life depression remains an ill-defined concept, one that appears to lack convincing empirical support at present. The literature is difficult to integrate because some studies define late-life depression as a first episode of depression after a given age cutoff—variable as this "age" may be—and other studies simply use the label "late-life depression" to describe a mood disorder in older age, first onset or not. The emergence of a syndrome called late-life depression will need to be supported by empirical findings with replication. The study of depression across the life span, employing age as a continuous rather than dichotomous variable, might better identify unique clinical and behavioral markers that emerge with advanced age (Caine et al., 1993).

Prevalence of Late-Life Depression

Among individuals 65 years of age and older, approximately 1 million people suffer from major depression (NIH Consensus Development Conference Statement, 1993). An estimated 5 million more older adults suffer symptoms of depression severe enough to require treatment (NIH Consensus Development Conference Statement, 1993). These estimates do not provide a breakdown, however, of the number of individuals who experience depression for the first time after age 65 versus those who have depression late in life as part of a lifelong pattern. Blazer (1993) reviewed the epidemiological literature on depression in late life. For older adults who reside in the community, the prevalence of reported depressive symptoms ranged from 10% to 25%, and the prevalence of clinically diagnosed major depression was approximately 1% to 5%. The

prevalence of depressive symptoms reported by older adults in acute care settings is 25%, while the prevalence range for major depression is 5% to 10%. For long-term care facilities, prevalence of depressive symptoms is 30% and major depression prevalence is 5% to 15%.

The prevalence of both current and lifetime major depression has been found to be higher in young and middle-aged adults than in older adults (Blazer, 1994), and age has not been found to be a significant predictor of depression, while medical illness and situational factors have (Blazer, 1994). In contrast, one theory attempts to explain the epidemiological data of depression by asserting that aging may act as a protective agent against onset of depression (Henderson, 1994).

Thus, although older adults suffer less from major depression than younger and middle-aged adults, a significant number experience depressive symptoms (Blazer, 1993). Of particular concern is the fact that while the elderly comprise but 12% of the total population, they account for 25% of suicides (Blazer, 1993). Additionally, it is known that depression imposes substantial economic and emotional costs on society. Indeed, the annual costs of depression in the United States is approximately $43.7 billion (Greenberg, Stiglin, Finkelstein, & Berndt, 1993). This has raised particular concerns and has prompted strategies for educating primary care physicians to better recognize depression in all age groups and to implement immediate treatment (Santiago, 1993).

Neuropsychological Aspects of Late-Life Depression

There is a relatively extensive literature on cognitive functioning and the older depressed patient. Much of the literature highlights the presence of cognitive impairment particularly with effort-demanding tasks that deplete the limited attentional capacity system (Weingartner, 1986). Older depressed individuals tend to demonstrate at least mild deficits on tasks measuring secondary memory, verbal fluency, visuospatial skill, novel problem-solving, and sustained attention (Caine, 1986; Folstein & McHugh, 1978; Kaszniak & Christenson, 1994; King et al., 1995). The presence of cognitive impairment in older depressed patients, however, does not necessarily indicate whether the depression is causing the cognitive dysfunction. Some have argued that depression entails a continuum of cognitive dysfunction from mild attentional deficits to severe dementia (Cassens, Wolfe, & Zola, 1990).

The issue of dementia related to depression, or *pseudodementia*, has generated much debate and controversy (Nussbaum, 1994). The term pseudodementia was proposed for clinical use in 1961 to depict clinical conditions in which symptoms consistent with dementia (at that time, dementia was considered irreversible) later resolved (Kiloh, 1961). Further, Kiloh noted that endogenous depression most often presented similar to the clinical picture of irreversible dementia. According to Kiloh, the term pseudodementia was purely descriptive, was not nosologically based, and carried no diagnostic weight.

Symptoms thought to characterize pseudodementia include memory impairment, bradyphrenia, bradykinesia, distractability, inattention, reduced concentration, confusion, and diminished conceptual abilities in the context of depressed mood (Haggerty, Golden, Evans, & Janowski, 1988). In an effort to counter growing confusion with the concept pseudodementia and to underscore the validity of the cognitive impairment evinced by some elderly depressed, new clinical terms were introduced. These included "dementia syndrome of depression" (Folstein & McHugh, 1978), "depression induced organic mental disorder" (McAllister, 1983), "four ideal types of depression and dementia syndromes" (Feinberg & Goodman, 1984), and "depression related cognitive dysfunction" (Stoudemire, Hill, Gulley, & Morris, 1989). Unfortunately, while conceptually interesting, the reliance on clinical description did not clarify issues of etiology.

Recent literature on pseudodementia has focused more on understanding the potential neuroanatomical substrate underlying the symptom cluster of mood disturbance, motor dysfunction, and cognitive impairment frequently associated with depression in late life. Indeed, Folstein and Rabins (1991) introduced the term SOTAN, an acronym for "syndrome of the aminergic nuclei," to replace the label pseudodementia because it initiated a relationship between observed behavior and neuroanatomy.

From their review of the neurochemical changes that occur in the brains of older patients with depression, Parkinson's disease, Huntington's disease, and Alzheimer's disease, Folstein and Rabins (1991) posited that each of these conditions represented diseases of brain pathways that carry aminergic fibers from the brain stem to higher cortical regions. They proposed, therefore, the existence of a common neural mechanism that underlies changes in mood, motor functioning, and cognitive capacity. By focusing on the neuropathological mechanisms that might underlie the presenting symptoms of pseudodementia, Folstein and Rabins attempted to redirect investigative efforts away from a clinical labeling approach. Interestingly, the theory that depression, dementia, and other symptom clusters may represent common central nervous system pathways for many different neurological disorders had previously been advanced (Caine, 1981; Post, 1975).

To further explore the presence of a neuroanatomical substrate underlying the symptom cluster in elderly depressed, two major avenues of research have been developed. One involves the longitudinal investigation of cognitive status in elderly depressed patients, and the second pertains to the application of neuroimaging technology with older depressed individuals.

Longitudinal Investigation

Longitudinal cognitive assessment of elderly depressed might provide evidence for a profile of neuropsychological impairment that can then be related to particular neuroanatomical regions. Further, longitudinal cognitive assessment may produce support for the idea that depression in some older adults presents as the first sign of a later developing progressive dementia.

Five studies have followed older depressed patients to document the frequency of later cognitive deterioration (King, Caine, Conwell, & Cox, 1991; Kral, 1983; Kral & Emery, 1989; Nussbaum, Kaszniak, Allender, & Rapcsak, 1995; Reding, Haycox, & Blass, 1985). For 4 to 18 years (mean of 8 years) Kral (1983) semiannually followed 22 older patients (mean age = 76.5) "diagnosed" with pseudodementia. Twenty of the 22 patients (91%) developed Alzheimer's disease (AD) by the end of the research period. The diagnosis of AD was supported by postmortem neuropathologic evidence obtained on three brains (Kral & Emery, 1989). Of the 22 patients followed, 11 were alive at the end of the study, 9 of whom were demented and living either in hospitals or in nursing homes. Two women were alive and well at the end of the study. The interpretation of the study is made difficult because Kral used the term pseudodementia as a diagnosis and because there was inadequate description of the subjects and of how diagnoses were made. However, the study illuminated the need for investigation of the relationship between depression with cognitive impairment and the aging brain.

In a subsequent anecdotal report (Kral & Emery, 1989), a combination of data from the original Kral (1983) study and clinical data provided by Dr. Emery were analyzed. Forty-four elderly patients described as suffering from "depressive pseudodementia" were included. At the end of the follow-up period (average of 8 years), 39 out of the original 44 (89%) developed AD. Original electroencephalogram (EEG) and computerized tomography (CT) scans conducted on some of the patients were normal. However, by the end of the study, these patients demonstrated intellectual deterioration, abnormal EEG, and abnormal CT characterized by dilation of the ventricles and cortical atrophy. Further, for cases where postmortem autopsies were available, the neuropathology was consistent with AD. The authors speculated that depression might predispose an AD process, particularly when positive heredity for dementia is present. Importantly, the findings of this anecdotal report should be interpreted with caution because no control group was employed, and base rates for intellectual deterioration and neuroanatomical changes in otherwise healthy older adults were not considered.

Reding et al. (1985) followed 28 older patients diagnosed as having a nondementing depression per *DSM-III* (APA, 1980) criteria and neurological and psychiatric evaluations. The study covered 3 years and resulted in 16 of 28 (57%) developing "frank dementia." Thirteen of these 16 patients demonstrated some sign, often subtle, of neurological disease. Variables that identified those depressed patients who developed dementia included evidence of cerebrovascular, extrapyramidal, or spinocerebellar disease; an elevated Modified Hachinski Ischemic Scale (Rosen, Terry, & Fuld, 1980) score; a low mental status score; an elevated dementia behavior score; and confusion in response to low doses of tricyclic antidepressants. The neurological and Modified Hachinski Ischemic Scale score proved most beneficial in predicting later development of dementia. Reding and colleagues (1985) also speculated that depression may initially present as the first sign of a later developing progressive dementia.

Nussbaum et al. (1995) followed 35 older adults (70 years and older) diagnosed (per *DSM-III-R*) (APA, 1987) with either major depression or dysthymia, both without cognitive impairment. Diagnoses were made independently from a review of all medical and neuropsychological data by two board-certified specialists expert in differential diagnosis with the older adult. Repeat neuropsychological examinations were administered at the end of the study period (approximately 2 years), and 8 patients (22%) demonstrated progressive dementia consistent with AD. Predictors of later cognitive decline included the presence of deep white matter and subcortical lesions as measured by brain CT/MRI and abnormal electrocardiogram (EKG) conducted at the initial evaluation. These authors asserted that for older depressed patients, an abnormal brain CT/MRI in the presence of a normal cognitive profile may represent a neurobiological marker for development of progressive dementia. This study lacked sophisticated analysis of neuroimaging data, relying instead on a dichotomous normal–abnormal scale.

Finally, poor confrontation naming was found to be predictive of depression severity at 6 months discharge in a small sample of inpatient elderly diagnosed with major depression without cognitive impairment (King et al., 1991). Poor naming was thought to reflect subtle cerebral changes that might influence the course of depression in the elderly. This represents one of the only studies to document neuropsychological markers predictive of outcome for elderly depressed. Although Nussbaum et al. (1995) used multiple neuropsychological measures in their study, none were found to be predictive of later cognitive decline in elderly depressed.

In contrast to the findings of the studies described above, a recent longitudinal study (Sachdev, Smith, Lepan, & Rodriguez, 1990) found no substantial decline in a sample of 19 middle-aged adults "diagnosed" with pseudodementia. No decline was found across a 12-year time period, which may not be significant given the fact that the mean age of the sample at the start of the investigation was 53. Nonetheless, Sachdev and colleagues (1990) asserted that pseudodementia may be established by a diagnosis of non-organic psychiatric illness, past history of psychiatric illness, and thorough exclusion of organic factors.

Overall, the longitudinal studies reviewed above suggest that depression in some older adults might represent an early marker for a later developing progressive dementia. Potential neurobiological markers that identify depressed patients who are likely to decline cognitively include signs of spinocerebellar, extrapyramidal, and cerebrovascular disease and abnormal CT/MRI scans (subcortical and white matter abnormalities). Potential neuropsychological markers of later cognitive decline in elderly depressed include general impaired mental status and confrontation naming deficit. Future longitudinal investigations of elderly depressed will need to address the methodological concerns raised by the studies above.

Neuroimaging and Late-Life Depression

Neuroimaging technology has provided important preliminary findings regarding changes in brain structure of elderly depressed. For example, one clinical marker that appears to be promising for differentiating depression in late life from AD is the presence of leukoaraiosis, defined as a diminution in the density of brain white matter as visualized either by CT or MRI (Hachinski, Potter, & Merskey, 1987). Coffey and Figiel (1991) encouraged use of the term "subcortical encephalomalacia" (malacia means morbid softening or thinning) to describe brain changes in elderly depressed because it includes subcortical gray matter and brain stem lesions in addition to changes in deep white matter. As such, this chapter shall use the term subcortical encephalomalacia to describe brain changes measured by neuroimaging procedures in elderly depressed.

Prior to a review of the literature on MRI-measured brain changes in elderly depressed, it is important to understand the base rate of similar changes in normotensive, nondepressed, healthy young and healthy elderly. For the healthy young, defined as those under the age of 60, subcortical encephalomalacia occurs in approximately 20% of the population (Rao, Mittenberg, Bernardin, Haughton, & Leo, 1989). In contrast, 80% of the young subjects demonstrate normal MRI scans. Estimates of the occurrence of MRI-measured subcortical encephalomalacia in non-neurologically impaired healthy elderly subjects have ranged from 18% to over 60% (Coffey & Figiel, 1991). The MRI-measured brain changes in healthy elderly, however, tend to be mild in severity (Coffey & Figiel, 1991).

Studies that have employed MRI technology with elderly depressed (Coffey et al., 1989; Coffey et al., 1990; Figiel et al., 1991; Krishnan et al., 1988; Robinson, Morris, & Federoff, 1990) have reported a higher percentage of deep white matter lesions (85–100%), periventricular hyperintensity (86%), cortical atrophy (96%), changes in subcortical gray matter nuclei (51%), and subcortical lesions than that reported for presumably healthy elderly.

One prospective study (Coffey et al., 1989) of elderly depressed patients (mean age = 71.3) referred for electroconvulsive therapy (ECT) demonstrated subcortical white matter hyperintensity in all 51 of the patients (100%) administered MRI. Subsequent analyses revealed that all of the patients (100%) had periventricular hyperintensity, 44 of 51 (86%) had deep white matter hyperintensity, 49 of 51 (96%) had cortical atrophy, and 26 of 51 (51%) had changes in subcortical gray matter nuclei. The authors reported that the majority (80%) of the patients had late-onset depression.

Likewise, Krishnan and colleagues (1988) found a higher percentage (85%) of deep white matter lesions in older depressed patients than healthy elderly, as reported in the literature. They posited a relationship between white matter lesions and depressed mood in older adults. Further, the authors reported a relationship between white matter lesions and advanced age. Since no control group was employed in this study, caution is warranted with interpretation of the results.

Age, again, was found to be an important variable with regard to incidence of white matter lesions in elderly depressed (Figiel et al., 1991). These authors reported a higher incidence of caudate (60%

vs. 11%) and large deep white matter hyperintensities (60% vs. 11%) in late-onset (>60) compared to early-onset depressed subjects (<60). These authors speculated that late-onset depression might be mediated by caudate and white matter structural changes.

In an attempt to understand the clinical significance of MRI-measured subcortical hyperintensity in patients with depression, Coffey and colleagues (1990) compared the prevalence and severity of subcortical hyperintensity in elderly patients (over age 60) to an age- and gender-matched healthy control group. All healthy normal controls evinced mild changes in subcortical hyperintensity, and elderly depressed patients referred for ECT had significantly more severe white matter changes and a higher number of lesions in the subcortical gray nuclei. For both the controls and depressed sample, severity of subcortical hyperintensity was related to the presence of risk factors for vascular disease.

The literature on brain MRI-measured changes in elderly depressed provides preliminary evidence for a relationship between age, white matter and gray matter changes, and depression. However, caution is warranted with interpretation of the studies due to methodological concerns: Some studies did not use a control group such as healthy, nondepressed elderly; standard neuropsychological measures were routinely excluded; and although diagnoses were applied using standard criteria (i.e., *DSM-III-R*), some of the studies used mixed samples such as major depression and bipolar disorder or depression and dementia cases.

Subcortical Encephalomalacia and Cognitive Functions

The literature reviewed above highlights the relationship between MRI subcortical encephalomalacia and depression in late life. In contrast, there is little evidence for a relationship between subcortical encephalomalacia and cognitive impairment in elderly depressed (Coffey & Figiel, 1991). Coffey and colleagues (1989) demonstrated a relationship between severity of MRI-measured white matter changes and presence of verbal and figural memory impairments as measured by the Wechsler Memory Scale (Russell, 1975). Nussbaum and colleagues (1995) reported that abnormal brain MRI

scans predicted cognitive decline in 23% of a sample of initially nondemented elderly depressed. Other research has identified extrapyramidal signs, spinocerebellar disease, cerebrovascular disease, an elevated Modified Hachinski Ischemic Scale score (Rosen et al., 1980), and impaired mental status as predictors of later cognitive decline in a sample of elderly depressed without dementia. In a recent investigation of the relationship between subcortical lesions and cognitive functioning (Wolfe, Linn, Babikian, Knoefel, & Albert, 1990), older subjects (mean age = 64.6) with multiple subcortical lacunae displayed greater neuropsychological impairment and a higher incidence of depression than same-age medical inpatient controls. The pattern of cognitive impairment demonstrated by the subjects (shifting sets, response inhibition, and other executive functions) was consistent with frontal system dysfunction. The finding of cognitive impairment and depressed mood related to frontal system dysfunction in elderly inpatients supports the idea that depressed mood (Figiel et al., 1991) and cognitive impairment (Coffey et al., 1989; Nussbaum et al., 1995) might result from a common neuroanatomical substrate (King & Caine, 1990).

The relationship between presence of deep white matter and subcortical lesions and cognitive impairment/decline in older patients diagnosed as depressed is consistent with studies that reflect an association between subcortical encephalomalacia and dementia severity in AD (Steingart et al., 1987), but contrasts with studies documenting no relation between subcortical encephalomalacia and neuropsychological status in middle-aged normotensive subjects (Rao et al., 1989) or healthy elderly with deep white matter changes on MRI (Tupler, Coffey, Logue, Djang, & Fagan, 1992). Longitudinal research is one approach promoted by Rao and colleagues (1989) to determine whether MRI-measured subcortical encephalomalacia has any predictive value of later cognitive decline in elderly depressed.

Depression: The Subcortical Syndrome Debate

From the literature reviewed above, there is emerging evidence for a subcortical-frontal neuroanatomical substrate underlying depressed mood and cognitive impairment in some elderly depressed (Cummings, 1993; Folstein & Rabins, 1991; Nussbaum, 1994). Indeed, two recent articles (Krishnan, 1993; Sano, 1991) underscored the importance of the prefrontal cortex, subcortex, and in particular, the basal ganglia to the manifestation of depression in late life. The contribution of subcortical neural systems to depressed mood is also supported by the poststroke depression literature that suggests a relationship between depressed mood and lesions of the left basal ganglia and left frontal lobe (Robinson, 1987; Robinson & Starkstein, 1991; Starkstein et al., 1991). A subcortical dysfunction underlying the cognitive impairment in depressed patients also has corroboration from a recent study (Massman, Delis, Butters, Dupont, & Gillin, 1992) that found memory and new learning deficits of some depressed patients (approximately 30%) to be identical to patients suffering from Huntington's disease, a subcortical-based process (caudate nucleus), but different from that of AD patients, primarily a cortical-based process. Indeed, the pattern of cognitive impairment related to depression has been described as a subcortical dementia (King & Caine, 1990).

Despite the emerging evidence of a relationship between subcortical regions, dysphoric mood, and cognitive impairment in elderly depressed, the exact nature of this relationship remains unknown. One hypothesis regarding this relationship is that subcortical encephalomalacia, as measured by MRI, might disconnect or disrupt pathways that bridge subcortical regions to the frontal cortex.

One recent study (King et al., 1995) directly refutes the theory of a subcortical pattern of mood and cognitive dysfunction in elderly depressed. Compared to age- and education-matched controls, a sample of older unipolar depressed inpatients demonstrated neuropsychological deficits in naming, mental slowing, attentional and retrieval difficulties, visuospatial processing, and constructional praxis. These deficits were thought to represent a pattern of neuropsychological dysfunction distinct from that of younger depressed. Further, King and colleagues (1995) argued that the pattern of neuropsychological dysfunction could not be characterized by a subcortical dementia and instead more accurately reflected a pattern of diffuse cortical im-

pairment. Further, they speculated that the neuropsychological impairment and perhaps mood disorder associated with depression might reflect covert disease processes that significantly affect brain integrity.

Conclusion

Several broad conclusions can be generated from the literature reviewed in the present chapter. Older adults experience less clinical major depression than young adults, although they report substantially more depressive symptoms. Those elders who reside in nursing homes or are hospitalized with medical illness suffer rates of major depression significantly higher than community dwelling elderly. Unfortunately, late-life depression is not well defined nor operationalized in a consistent manner across the literature. It is unclear if late-life depression implies first onset of depression or recurrence of a lifelong pattern of mood disorder in the later years of one's life. Late life is defined as 45 years and over in several studies, while 65 and over represents the age threshold for late life in other studies. The use of age as a dichotomous variable has been challenged as inappropriate, and an argument for using age as a continuous variable was made (Caine et al., 1993). Blazer (1993) pointed out that age is not related to onset of depression, a finding that is directly counterintuitive to the concept of late-life depression. The existing research on late-life depression suffers methodological problems sufficient to prevent definitive conclusions regarding its clinical nosology or identification as a clinical entity separate from depression in young adults. Indeed it remains unclear if late-life depression should be considered a clinical entity with a unique physiological, neuroanatomical, and psychosocial profile, separate from depression that recurs in individuals over the age of 65.

Risk factors for late-life depression are quite similar to those for depression in young adults, even for those older adults with first-onset depression after the age of 60. This finding again raises concern regarding the appropriateness of considering late-life depression as a separate entity from depression at other ages. Of interest is the finding that educational achievement is a primary risk factor for both early and late-onset depression. Indeed, females who complete less than 12 years of school experience the greatest risk for depression. This finding warrants caution since physical illness, disability, and extent of social network are three variables that typically correlate with level of education and therefore may confound the import of education as a risk factor for depression in females. Family history of depression appears to be a stronger correlate of early-onset depression, but this finding is not conclusive. There is a suggestion, therefore, that genetics may be more critical for depression in young adults than for depression in the elderly.

Relatively new research on the changes in both structural and functional neuroimaging may provide the most compelling evidence that late-life depression, defined as first onset after age 60, carries unique clinical markers compared to depression in young adults. Specifically, changes in both gray and white brain matter compared to nondepressed, same-age controls indicate that mood disorder—depression—in late life is related to specific neuroanatomical changes, a finding that is at present not well documented in young adults. The anterior cortex and subcortical regions appear to be most vulnerable in late-life depression. This is of interest given the review on neuropsychological functioning in elderly depressed which suggests greater cognitive deficits related to anterior and subcortical pathology. Indeed, there is an argument that the cognitive profiles of older depressed persons are most similar to profiles of individuals with known diseases of the subcortex (i.e., Huntington's disease) and is most accurately described as a subcortical dementia (Caine, 1986). This argument, however, is challenged by recent neuropsychological data that indicates a diffuse cortical pathology in elderly depressed (King et al., 1995).

More research is needed that compares structural and functional neuroimaging data of young and older depressed individuals (first onset and recurrence) in order to better understand the relationship of depression in late life and the brain changes noted above. Indeed, age and medical illness may account more significantly for the changes in brain structure and physiology than presence of depression in late life. Further, cognitive impairment is not isolated to late-onset depression and occurs in similar patterns in young depressed.

Future clinical research might benefit from focus on the following major areas of investigation:

1. There is a clear need to develop standard definitions, operationalization, and perhaps diagnostic criteria of late-life depression. This would not only assist in reducing the confusion that presently exists in the literature on late-life depression, but would also promote more valid methodology for research. Information is needed to determine if late-life depression can only occur as a first-onset depressive disorder, to establish the standard age threshold for use of the term late-life depression, and to determine whether those who experience depression across the life span into advanced years are different from those who suffer first onset of depression after the standard age threshold.

2. Continued longitudinal research is needed to better understand the neuroimaging and neuropsychological findings of first-onset depression in late life. This will promote better understanding of the neuroanatomical substrates that underlie the mood disorder, cognitive impairment, and motor slowing that typically occur with depression in late life. Further, the assertion that first-onset depression in late life may represent an early marker to Alzheimer's disease may be properly assessed using longitudinal research methodology as described above.

3. Risk factors for depression in late life represents another important area of research that deserves continued study. In order to best delineate the differences between depression in young adults versus first-onset, late-life depression, risk factors such as genetic predisposition need to be demonstrated and replicated. As noted above, this area of study has demonstrated more similarities than differences in risk factors between young and older first-onset depressed persons.

4. Although treatment of depression was not presented in the current chapter, this area of investigation remains vital to our understanding of the clinical phenomenology of depression in late life and might assist in better delineating differences between early and late-onset depression. Clearly, as with all research, po-

tential confounding variables such as physical and emotional status, psychosocial stressors, and health disability need to be controlled. Treatment interventions such as psychopharmacology, psychotherapy, and electroconvulsive therapy can be compared for efficacy across the life span and related to changes in functional and structural neuroimaging data and neuropsychological performance.

5. The argument by Caine et al. (1993) that age might best be used as a continuous rather than dichotomous variable should be considered as an appropriate research methodology. This is supported by the finding that age does not correlate with presence of depression (Blazer, 1993), and indeed, no convincing evidence exists for an age threshold to make dichotomous comparisons. This is exemplified most clearly in the literature where age thresholds for operationalization of late-life depression range from age 45 to over age 65.

6. Finally, the idea that aging itself protects against the onset of depression (Henderson, 1994) requires further investigation. This theory is based on the finding that older adults have lower rates of major depression than young adults. Interpretation of this finding includes the following possibilities: Older individuals simply do not report enough symptoms to meet strict diagnostic criteria for major depression; a higher mortality rate among depressed persons may lead to a reduced prevalence of major depression; older adults experience episodes of major depression that are shorter in duration; the biological basis of depression changes across the lifespan, becoming reduced with advanced years; and perhaps with aging there develops a psychological immunization that protects against onset of depression.

These are but a few of the challenges and suggested approaches for clinical researchers interested in advancing our understanding of late-life depression. With the demographic revolution that is taking place in the United States and the economic and emotional burden created by major depression, late-life depression represents a vital area of clinical research for the 21st century.

References

American Psychiatric Association. (1987). *Diagnostic and statistical manual of mental disorders* (3rd ed., rev.). Washington, DC: Author.

Blazer, D. G. (1993). *Depression in late life* (2nd ed.) St. Louis, MO: Mosby.

Blazer, D. G. (1994). Is depression more frequent in late life? *The American Journal of Geriatric Psychiatry, 2,* 193–199.

Caine, E. D. (1981). Pseudodementia: Current concepts and future directions. *Archives of General Psychiatry, 38,* 1359–1364.

Caine, E. D. (1986). The neuropsychology of depression: The pseudodementia syndrome. In I. Grant & K. M. Adams (Eds.), *Neuropsychological assessment of neuropsychiatric disorders* (pp. 221–243). New York: Oxford.

Caine, E. D., Lyness, J. M., & King, D. A. (1993). Reconsidering depression in the elderly. *The American Journal of Geriatric Psychiatry, 1,* 4–20.

Cassens, G., Wolfe, L., & Zola, M. (1990). The neuropsychology of depressions. *The Journal of Neuropsychiatry and Clinical Neurosciences, 2,* 202–213.

Coffey, C. E., & Figiel, G. S. (1991). Neuropsychiatric significance of subcortical encephalomalacia. In B. J. Carroll & J. E. Barrett (Eds.), *Psychopathology and the brain* (pp. 243–264). New York: Raven Press.

Coffey, C. E., Figiel, G. S., Djang, W. T., & Saunders, W. B. (1989). White matter hyperintensity on magnetic resonance imaging: Clinical and neuroanatomic correlates in the depressed elderly. *Journal of Neuropsychiatry and Clinical Neurosciences, 1,* 135–144.

Coffey, C. E., Figiel, G. S., Djang, W. T., & Weiner, R. D. (1990). Subcortical hyperintensity on magnetic resonance imaging: A comparison of normal and depressed elderly subjects. *American Journal of Psychiatry, 147,* 187–189.

Cummings, J. (1993). Frontal-subcortical circuits and human behavior. *Archives of Neurology, 50,* 873–880.

Eaton, W., Kramer, M., Anthony, J. C., Dryman, A., Shapiro, S., & Locke, B. Z. (1989). The incidence of specific DIS/DSM-III mental disorders: Data from the NIMH Epidemiologic Catchment Area Program. *Acta Psychiatrica Scandinavica, 79,* 163–178.

Feinberg, T., & Goodman, B. (1984). Affective illness, dementia, and pseudodementia. *Journal of Clinical Psychiatry, 45,* 99–103.

Figiel, G. S., Krishnan, K. R. R., Doraiswamy, P. M., Rao, V. P., Nemeroff, C. B., & Boyko, O. B. (1991). Subcortical hyperintensities on brain resonance imaging: A comparison between late age onset and early onset depressed subjects. *Neurobiology of Aging, 26,* 245–247.

Folstein, M. F., & McHugh, P. R. (1978). Dementia syndrome of depression. In R. Katzman, R. D. Terry, & K. L. Bick (Eds.), *Alzheimer's disease, senile dementia and related disorders* (pp. 281–289). New York: Raven Press.

Folstein, M. F., & Rabins, P. V. (1991). Replacing pseudodementia. *Neuropsychiatry, Neuropsychology, and Behavioral Neurology, 4,* 36–40.

Gallo, J. J., Royall, D. R., & Anthony, J. C. (1993). Risk factors for the onset of depression in middle age and later life. *Social Psychiatry and Psychiatric Epidemiology, 28,* 101–108.

Greenberg, P. E., Stiglin, L. E., Finkelstein, S. N., & Berndt, E. R. (1993). The economic burden of depression in 1990. *Journal of Clinical Psychiatry, 54,* 405–418.

Hachinski, V. C., Potter, P., & Merskey, H. (1987). Leuko-araiosis. *Archives of Neurology, 44,* 21–23.

Haggerty, J. J., Golden, R. N., Evans, D. L., & Janowski, D. S. (1988). Differential diagnosis of pseudodementia in the elderly. *Geriatrics, 43,* 61–74.

Henderson, A. S. (1994). Does aging protect against depression? *Social Psychiatry and Epidemiology, 29,* 107–109.

Kaszniak, A. W., & Christenson, G. T. (1994). Differential diagnosis of dementia and depression. In M. Storandt & G. R. VandenBos (Eds.), *Neuropsychological assessment of dementia and depression in older adults: A clinician's guide* (pp. 81–118). Washington, DC: American Psychological Association.

Kiloh, L. G. (1961). Pseudodementia. *Acta Psychiatrica Scandinavica, 37,* 336–351.

King, D. A., & Caine, E. P. (1990). Depression. In J. L. Cummings (Ed.), *Subcortical dementia* (pp. 218–230). New York: Oxford.

King, D. A., Caine, E. P., Conwell, Y., & Cox, C. (1991). Predicting severity of depression in the elderly at six month follow-up: A neuropsychological study. *The Journal of Neuropsychiatry and Clinical Neurosciences, 3,* 64–66.

King, D. A., Cox, C., Lyness, J. M., & Caine, E. D. (1995). Neuropsychological effects of depression and age in an elderly sample: A confirmatory study. *Neuropsychology, 9,* 399–408.

Kral, V. A. (1983). The relationship between senile dementia (DAT) and depression. *Canadian Journal of Psychiatry, 28,* 304–306.

Kral, V. A., & Emery, O. B. (1989). Long-term follow-up of depressive pseudodementia of the aged. *Canadian Journal of Psychiatry, 28,* 445–446.

Krishnan, K. R. (1993). Neuroanatomic substrates of depression in the elderly. *Journal of Geriatric Psychiatry and Neurology, 6,* 39–58.

Krishnan, K. R., Goli, V., Ellinwood, E., France, R. D., Blazer, D. G., & Nemeroff, C. B. (1988). Leukoencephalopathy in patients diagnosed as major depressive. *Biological Psychiatry, 23,* 519–522.

Massman, P. J., Delis, D. C., Butters, N., Dupont, R. M., & Gillin, C. (1992). The subcortical dysfunction hypothesis of memory deficits in depression: Neuropsychological validation in a subgroup of patients. *Journal of Clinical and Experimental Neuropsychology, 14,* 687–706.

McAllister, T. W. (1983). Pseudodementia. *American Journal of Psychiatry, 140,* 528–533.

National Institute of Health Consensus Development Conference Statement (1993). Diagnosis and treatment of depression in late life. *Psychopharmacology Bulletin, 29,* 87–95.

Nussbaum, P. D. (1994). Pseudodementia: A slow death. *Neuropsychology Review, 4,* 71–90.

Nussbaum, P. D., Kaszniak, A. W., Allender, J., & Rapcsak, S. (1995). Cognitive decline in elderly depressed: A follow-up study. *The Clinical Neuropsychologist, 9,* 101–111.

Phifer, J. F., & Murrell, S. A. (1986). Etiologic factors in the onset

of depressive symptoms in older adults. *Journal of Abnormal Psychology, 95,* 282–291.

Post, F. (1975). Dementia, depression, and pseudodementia. In D. F. Benson & D. Blumer (Eds.), *Psychiatric aspects of neurological disease* (pp. 99–120). New York: Grune & Stratton.

Rao, S. M., Mittenberg, W., Bernardin, L., Haughton, V., & Leo, G. J. (1989). Neuropsychological test findings in subjects with leukoaraiosis. *Archives of Neurology, 46,* 40–44.

Reding, M., Haycox, J., & Blass, J. (1985). Depression in patients referred to a dementia clinic. *Archives of Neurology, 42,* 894–896.

Robinson, R. G. (1987). Depression and stroke. *Psychiatric Annals, 17,* 731–740.

Robinson, R. G., & Starkstein, S. E. (1991). Heterogeneity in clinical presentation following stroke: Neuropathological correlates. *Neuropsychiatry, Neuropsychology, and Behavioral Neurology, 4,* 1–3.

Robinson, R. G., Morris, P. L., & Federoff, J. P. (1990). Depression and cerebrovascular disease. *Journal of Clinical Psychiatry, 51,* 26–33.

Rosen, W., Terry, R., & Fuld, M. (1980). Pathological verification of ischemic score in differentiation of dementias. *Annals of Neurology, 7,* 486–488.

Russell, E. W. (1975). A multiple scoring method for the assessment of complex memory functions. *Journal of Consulting and Clinical Psychology, 43,* 800–809.

Sachdev, P. S., Smith, J. S., Lepan, H. A., & Rodriguez, P. (1990). Pseudodementia twelve years on. *Journal of Neurology, Neurosurgery, and Psychiatry, 53,* 254–259.

Sano, M. (1991). Basal ganglia diseases and depression. *Neuropsychiatry, Neuropsychology, and Behavioral Neurology, 4,* 41–48.

Santiago, J. M. (1993). The costs of treating depression. *Journal of Clinical Psychiatry, 54,* 425–426.

Starkstein, S. E., Bryer, J. B., Berthier, M. L., Cohen, B., Price, T. R., & Robinson, T. G. (1991). Depression after stroke: The importance of cerebral hemispheric asymmetries. *The Journal of Neuropsychiatry and Clinical Neurosciences, 3,* 276–285.

Steingart, A., Hachinski, V. C., Lau, C., Fox, A. J., Fox, H., Lee, D., Inzitari, D., & Merskey, H. (1987). Cognitive and neurologic findings in demented patients with diffuse white matter lucencies on computed tomographic scan. *Archives of Neurology, 44,* 36–39.

Stoudemire, A., Hill, C., Gulley, L. R., & Morris, R. (1989). Neuropsychological and biomedical assessment of depression-dementia syndromes. *Journal of Neuropsychiatry and Clinical Neurosciences, 1,* 347–361.

Tupler, L. A., Coffey, C. E., Logue, P. E., Djang, W. T., & Fagan, S. M. (1992). Neuropsychological importance of subcortical white matter hyperintensity. *Archives of Neurology, 49,* 1248–1252.

Weingartner, H. (1986). Automatic and effortful demanding cognitive processes in depression. In L. W. Poon (Ed.), *Clinical memory assessment of older adults* (pp. 218–235). Washington, DC: American Psychological Association.

Wolfe, N., Linn, R., Babikian, V. L., Knoefel, J. E., & Albert, M. L. (1990). Frontal system impairment following multiple lacunar infarcts. *Archives of Neurology, 47,* 129–132.

18

Neuropsychological Aspects of Epilepsy in the Elderly

PETER J. SNYDER AND HARRY W. McCONNELL

Introduction

Epilepsy is a common neurological disorder characterized by sudden brief attacks that may alter motor activity, consciousness, and sensory experiences. Convulsive seizures are the most common type of paroxysmal event, but any recurrent seizure pattern is considered "epileptic." Many forms of epilepsy have been linked to viral, fungal, and parasitic infections of the central nervous system, known metabolic disturbances, the ingestion of toxic agents, brain lesions, tumors or congenital defects, or cerebral trauma. Although the direct causes are not always readily observable, with the advent of sophisticated histological, neuroimaging, and biochemical methods, it is now possible to diagnose the causes of seizure disorders that have, in the past, been difficult to identify. Because it can result from many different types of insults to the central nervous system, epilepsy is best thought of as a class of syndromes rather than a disease per se.

Epilepsy is typically thought of as a disorder or syndrome of younger age, and in fact it is true that a large percentage of patients who present to epilepsy clinics and surgical programs develop seizure disorders prior to middle age. Nonetheless, although there is an initial peak early in life and a relatively stable rate throughout middle age, the incidence and prevalence of epilepsy sharply increases after age 60. Few realize that the incidence of epilepsy in those over age 60 exceeds that in children (Hauser, 1992; Hauser, Annegers, & Kurland, 1993; Scheuer & Cohen, 1993) and that seizures in general, and epilepsy in particular, are among the most common neurologic disorders in the elderly (Scheuer & Cohen, 1993). This is stressed in a recent British study in which almost 25% of all newly identified seizures, although not necessarily epilepsy per se, were accounted for by those age 60 and over (Sander, Hart, Johnson, & Shorvon, 1990). After controlling for known risk factors (discussed below), aging alone seems to be associated with an elevation of risk of about 0.3 for each decade of life after the age of 20. In those age 75 and over, the prevalence of active epilepsy is 1.5% (Hauser, Annegers, & Kurland, 1991).

The prevalence of epilepsy is even higher in some select populations. For example, surveys in chronic care facilities suggest that at least 5% of residents have a diagnosis of epilepsy and that 7% are taking anticonvulsant medications (Hauser et al., 1991). This high prevalence is not surprising given that the major reasons for admission to such facilities are, for the most part, neurologic conditions that are also risk factors for seizures and epilepsy. The incidence of newly diagnosed epilepsy cases in such facilities is over 1% per year (Hauser et al., 1991).

These demographic facts are quite frequently overlooked among epileptologists, and yet we will be forced to pay increasing attention to the pathogenesis, diagnosis, and treatment of seizure disorders of the elderly in the decades to come. The

PETER J. SNYDER • Department of Neurology, Medical College of Pennsylvania and Hahnemann University–Allegheny Campus, Pittsburgh, Pennsylvania 15212. HARRY W. McCONNELL • Institute of Epileptology, Maudsley Hospital, London SE5 8AZ, England.

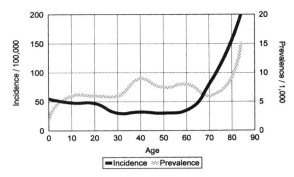

FIGURE 1. Age-specific prevalence for epilepsy and annual incidence (1975–1984) in Rochester, Minnesota. (Reprinted with permission from Hauser et al., 1991, 1993.)

principal reason for this is that the 20th century has seen an unprecedented increase in the absolute number and relative proportion of older persons. We have witnessed not only a dramatic increase in the 65-plus age group, but an extraordinary increase in the 85-plus age cohort (Butler, 1991).

Risk Factors for Seizures and Epilepsy in the Elderly

There exists a broad range of risk factors which predispose elderly individuals to developing seizures and epilepsy. The incidence of conditions that are associated with acute symptomatic seizures (i.e., seizures secondary to other predisposing neurologic conditions) are particularly high in the elderly. Stroke, head injury, and infections of the central nervous system all have relative or absolute peaks in incidence in the oldest age groups (Hauser, 1992; Shorvon, 1988). Metabolic disturbances associated with an increased risk for seizures are also frequent in this age group (Luhdorf, Jensen, & Plesner, 1986). Seizures are often associated with and complicate the management of acute neurologic disease in the elderly and also occur as a symptom of a number of systemic disturbances.

Of the 25,000 or so Americans over the age of 60 who will experience a first acute symptomatic seizure each year, the highest proportion of these individuals, about 35%, will have seizures attributable to an acute cerebrovascular insult (Hauser, 1994). Next in frequency will be seizures with sys-

temic metabolic disturbances, about 15%. About 10% of the cases will be attributable respectively to acute brain trauma, drug and alcohol withdrawal, central nervous system infection, or toxic insults (Hauser, 1994). Additionally, unprovoked seizures or epilepsy, that is, seizure disorders which are not directly attributable to the onset of an acute neurologic condition, are a frequent long-term complication of static neurologic conditions such as stroke and of progressive disorders such as Alzheimer's disease, and they may also occur in the absence of such conditions. The incidence of unprovoked seizures in those over age 60 is about 105 per 100,000 in the population. This translates to between 45,000 and 50,000 new cases each year (Hauser, 1994). As with acute symptomatic seizures, the incidence increases with advancing age.

Despite the impressive array of etiologic factors mentioned above, all of which are particularly common in the elderly, the single largest group, accounting for more than 40% of newly diagnosed cases of epilepsy, are classified as "idiopathic" because they are likely secondary to pathological processes of unknown etiology and are indiscernible by current neurodiagnostic techniques (Hauser, 1994). Finally, epidemiologic studies have suggested that a history of asthma, hypertension, illicit drug use, depression, and/or the use of psychotropic agents all have been demonstrated to increase the risk for epilepsy (Lannon, 1993)

Epileptogenesis and the Aging Brain

In very few of the specific elderly patient groups for which new-onset seizure disorders are common (e.g., post-cerebrovascular accident patients) are the etiological mechanisms for the seizure and epilepsy well understood. Clearly, the field is ripe for investigation. A variety of studies have investigated the relationship between maturational age of experimental animals, most typically rodents, and their propensity to develop seizures in a number of experimental paradigms such as kindling (e.g., Cavazos, Golarai, & Sutula, 1991), the application of kainic acid (e.g., Dawson & Wallace, 1992; Wozniak, Stewart, Miller, & Olney, 1991), and exposure to anoxia (e.g., Jensen, Holmes, Lombroso, Blume, & Firkusny, 1992). These studies, among many others, suggest that there are differences in seizure susceptibility, as well as responses to insults such as hypoxia, between immature and aged animals. Furthermore, recent studies focusing on synaptic reorganization in human hippocampal tissue have supported this general assertion (Babb, Kupfer, Pretorius, Crandall, & Levesque, 1991; Dichter & Weinberger, 1994; McKee, Kowall, & Kosik, 1989).

A number of investigators have studied changes in human brain structure that occur with aging that may have ramifications for the development of seizures. These changes include small, clinically silent infarcts; generalized and focal cortical atrophy; and amyloid deposits in cerebral microvessels. Senile dementia of the Alzheimer's type (SDAT) is associated with prominent derangements of cerebrocortical and hippocampal synaptic density, physiologic activity, and neurochemistry, all of which may be relevant to the increased risk of seizures in patients with this disease (Geddes, Ulas, Brunner, Choe, & Cotman, 1992; Hyman, Penney, Blackstone, & Young, 1994; Scheff, Sparks, & Price, 1993).

Other investigators have examined the potential for increased seizure susceptibility and epileptogenesis in aged rats. Preliminary evidence suggests that aged rats may be more susceptible to kainic acid-induced seizures than younger animals (Wozniak et al., 1991). However, much more work needs to be done in this area. Future research will need to address a range of important issues including (1) the possibility of age-related changes in the susceptibility to develop seizure disorders following similar brain insults, and (2) whether there is a subset of patients with late-onset epilepsy who have an "idiopathic" genetic predisposition for late onset seizures, or whether all such cases are the result of remote symptomatic injury that may or may not be identifiable by currently available diagnostic techniques.

Systemic Disorders Associated with Aging that May Precipitate Seizures

As our bodies age they undergo a whole host of homeostatic metabolic changes, some of which are known to raise the risk of acute symptomatic seizures and possibly epilepsy. Many systemic disorders, various other metabolic disturbances (e.g., electrolyte disturbances), and toxic mechanisms (e.g., abrupt discontinuation of sedative and/or anxiolytic drugs) may lead to acute symptomatic seizures or epilepsy (Loiseau, 1994). To offer one example, changes in the morphology and function of the kidney, as well as changes in the hormonal systems involved in water and sodium regulation, may predispose elderly individuals to a higher incidence of late-onset seizures (e.g., Goyal, 1982; Lindeman, Tobin, & Shock, 1985).

Other examples of age-related changes in systemic functions which lead to a heightened risk of acute symptomatic seizures or epilepsy include changes in drug metabolism and action, a wide variety of endocrinological changes in the elderly, and age-related changes in vision, vestibular functioning, gait, and musculoskeletal functions (all of which predispose elderly to suffer an increased risk of falls and concussive head injuries, with secondary onset of seizure disorders). These are but a few examples of the wide range of physical organ system changes that may contribute to the development of seizures and epilepsy in the elderly (Loiseau, 1994).

Special Diagnostic Considerations

Neurophysiologic Changes Associated with Aging

Most aspects of the clinical evaluation of elderly epilepsy patients do not differ substantially from those afforded to younger patients. There are, however, a few important differences to bear in mind. For example, although the use of EEG in evaluating elderly patients with seizures or epilepsy does not differ substantially from its application in younger patients, it is important to recognize characteristic EEG changes that occur normally with aging or that are seen commonly with either occult or symptomatic disease of the aging brain.

In a large unselected population of young adults, the mean alpha rhythm frequency is 10 to 10.5 Hz. This mean frequency declines in older persons, averaging 9 to 9.5 Hz at age 70 (Katz & Horowitz, 1982) and 8.5 to 9.0 Hz after 80 years of age (Hubbard, Sunde, & Goldensohn, 1976; Wang & Busse, 1969). In patients with frank dementia or with neuropsychological changes indicating impaired memory or cognition, these reductions are much more marked (Pedley & Miller, 1983). The vast majority of these patients show alpha rhythms less than 8.5 Hz. Many considerations other than neurologic disease, however, impinge on these and other measurements. These include cardiopulmonary status, drug use, and metabolic factors (cf. Holmes, 1980).

Certain EEG changes associated with the aging process may easily lead to "false-positive" diagnoses of epileptiform activity. For example, in individuals over 50 years of age, alpha-like activity may be seen over the temporal regions. This electrical activity may be asymmetric and, at times, more conspicuous than the occipital alpha rhythm. Fragments of this temporal alpha-like activity, especially when sharply contoured, may appear as "wicket spikes" or be misinterpreted as epileptiform activity (Pedley, 1994).

These examples of changes in electrophysiologic activity that are associated with aging are offered in order to point out some of the special considerations which must be made as part of the electrophysiologic evaluation of elderly patients. A second type of special consideration relates to the clinical presentation of the seizures themselves.

Behavioral Presentation during Ictal Events

Because such a wide range of age-related changes in the human brain are known to occur, even identical cerebral insults are likely to produce differing seizure types and epileptic syndromes according to the different ages at which they occur. In early adulthood, epilepsy presents most frequently with generalized onset seizures. In the elderly, however, the incidence of partial attacks rises significantly (Dam, Fuglsang-Frederiksen, Svarre-Olsen, & Dam, 1985). This may be explained only in part by the higher frequency, at this age, of identifiable etiologies (such as strokes) that account for about one third of all cases. Nonetheless, as was mentioned above, approximately 40% of cases have no identifiable antecedents. This fact reminds us that aging per se may have an epileptogenic effect on the central nervous system.

Many studies consider partial epileptic seizures with onset in the elderly, but few have focused on the semiological aspects of these seizures (i.e., behavioral and motoric presentation during ictal events). The scrupulous observation and description of ictal semiology, the recognition of consistent stereotyped behaviors during seizures in the same patient, a careful history, identification of likely risk factors, and video-EEG telemetry all contribute to an accurate diagnosis. Unfortunately, video-EEG monitoring, so frequently used in younger epilepsy patients for neurosurgical evaluation, is not commonly used in older patients. In the absence of careful observation and study of ictal semiology during seizures that are documented by EEG or video-EEG telemetry, there is an increased risk that some seizure types will be misdiagnosed as other neurological disorders in the elderly. For instance, periods of prolonged confusion in an elderly patient may sometimes be viewed as related to a dementia (possibly secondary to a progressive organic process, such as SDAT or drug toxicity), whereas such events might actually herald the onset of prolonged ictal states (cf. Ellis & Lee, 1978).

Neuropsychological Evaluation of Elderly Seizure Disorder Patients

In the same way that there is a general paucity of data regarding the clinical manifestation of seizure activity as observed and reviewed via video-EEG telemetry in elderly patients, there is a general lack of information on the neuropsychological presentation of elderly epilepsy patients. In fact, cognitive consequences of seizure and anticonvulsant medications in the elderly may be one of the more widely neglected areas of research within the field of neuropsychology. The primary reason for this appears to be that these patients are infrequently referred for neuropsychological evaluations. This is especially true if the patients have epilepsy only as an accompaniment to other ongoing neurological disorders. A recent informal survey across several major epilepsy centers throughout North America by Dodrill (1994) revealed a general consensus among the attending neuropsychologists in those programs that very few elderly patients with epilepsy are referred to surgical epilepsy programs for evaluation. Systematic neuropsychological evaluations of this population are, for obvious reasons, most likely to occur in such programs. The lack of information on the neuropsychological profile of geriatric epilepsy patients stands in marked contrast to the availability of clinical data on all other age groups.

Nonetheless, one recent preliminary study by Dodrill (1994) at the University of Washington in Seattle reviewed 18 cases of confirmed epilepsy in patients over the age of 60 who had been seen for neuropsychological evaluation in over 23 years of practice. These 18 cases were culled from a larger sample population of approximately 2,700 patients with epilepsy who were referred to his clinic for evaluation. A very preliminary analysis of this data on such an admittedly small sample led to a few tentative conclusions. First, when compared to age-matched healthy normal controls, the group with epilepsy was not markedly below average intellectually, and in fact their IQ scores were slightly higher than those reported in many studies of younger patients with epilepsy (with much earlier ages of onset of seizure disorders).

A second general conclusion from Dodrill's data is that the cognitive deficits found were by no means peculiar to epilepsy. On the contrary, whenever the group with epilepsy performed statistically worse than the normal controls on a number of tests that comprise the Halstead-Reitan Neuropsychological Test battery, a matched sample of elderly patients with other mixed (non-seizure-related) neurological illnesses also had similar performances. In no instance did the epilepsy group perform reliably better or worse than Dodrill's comparison group of neurologically impaired elderly patients without epilepsy.

Additionally, Dodrill (1994) concluded that by their mid-60s the age-matched normal control group showed significant aging effects (i.e., age-related memory impairment) across a variety of neuropsychological tests employed. Even though IQ scores may remain stable because they are age-corrected, the younger normal control subjects' scores on other neuropsychological tests (i.e., memory tests) were found to be substantially higher than those of the elderly persons in good health who were examined in his study (Dodrill, 1994). One possible explanation for this last finding may be related to a measurable amount of hippocampal atrophy that is probably present in one third of normal elderly adults (Golomb et al., 1993). Thus, memory deficits

which are markedly apparent in younger persons with epilepsy relative to their age-matched peers may not be as obvious in older adults.

This last tentative finding has obvious clinical importance for neuropsychologists who are charged with the evaluation, diagnosis, and treatment planning for elderly epilepsy patients. Stated again, the possibility is raised that elderly persons with epilepsy may not be as neuropsychologically impaired, relative to their peers, as younger persons with epilepsy. Elderly patients typically present with a much later age of onset of seizures; they develop seizures for different reasons than do younger persons with epilepsy; and in most cases "one gains the impression that the primary problem is not the seizures at all but instead the underlying neurological difficulty" which gave rise to the seizures (Dodrill, 1994).

Behavioral Syndromes Related to Epilepsy in the Elderly

A survey of the recent literature shows that the prevalence of behavioral and/or psychiatric syndromes in patients with a primary diagnosis of epilepsy is between 35% and 55%, depending on the epidemiologic study (for review, see Smith & Darlington, 1997). There is no evidence at this time to suggest that this is not also true in elderly patients. Tables 1 and 2 list behavioral, psychiatric, and psychosocial symptoms that are often seen comorbidly in patients with seizure disorders of varying types and neuropathological substrates.

Behavioral complications associated with epilepsy include (1) primarily psychosocial problems, such as low self-esteem, dependency, fear of loss of control, stigmatization, loss of independence, and associated marital, transportation, and related problems; (2) neuropsychological disorders which are secondary to the seizures themselves or are secondary to underlying central nervous system (CNS) lesions, neurologic disease, or side effects of certain anticonvulsant medications; (3) psychiatric disorders with a primarily ictal onset, which include ictal dysphoria, psychotic episodes related to the seizures, ictal or postictal intermixed behaviors, and postictal confusional states; and (4) interictal disturbances which include chronic interictal psychosis,

Table 1. Differential Diagnosis of Behavioral Disturbances in Patients with Epilepsy

Behavior changes attributed to anticonvulsant medications
  Direct effect—toxic encephalopathy
  Indirect effects (anemia, hepatotoxicity, drug interactions, folate deficiency, electrolyte imbalance)
Behavioral alterations determined by the personal and social reactions to the epileptic condition

depression, and heightened risk of suicide or self-harm.

Although the investigation of behavioral aspects of epilepsy (with a recent explosion of research and clinical attention paid to quality-of-life aspects of epilepsy in particular) has been occurring over the past few years (cf. McConnell & Snyder, 1997), very few studies have looked at these issues with a specific focus on the particular life events and stressors which are experienced by geriatric patients. Nonetheless, there are a variety of psycho-

Table 2. Behavioral Changes Determined by Existence and Location of the Epileptogenic Focus

Ictal behavioral alterations
  Hallucinations (visual, auditory, somatosensory, olfactory, gustatory, vertiginous-vestibular)
  Autonomic manifestations
  Motor (focal clonus, speech arrest)
  Psychic/cognitive (fear; anxiety; depression; anger, déjà-vu; derealization; depersonalization; dissociatioin; distortion of time, space, and body image; euphoria)
Postictal disturbances
  Depression
  Psychosis
  Aggression
  Confusional states
Interictal psychiatric disorders
  Personality changes
  Schizophrenia-like psychoses
  Affective disturbances
  Dissociative disturbances
  Fugue states, poriomania
  Aggression
  Altered sexual behavior
  Multiple personality
  Depersonalization

social stressors associated with the diagnosis of epilepsy, such as an altered sense of locus of control. The perception of one's loss of control over his or her body along with an associated loss of independence (e.g., loss of a driver's license) usually leads to increased stress and anxiety (Ferrari, Verbanac, & Kane, 1997). Such loss of control may be particularly disturbing to elderly patients, whose perception of increasing physical limitations as a result of normal senescence may be compounded. Collings (1990) noted that individuals diagnosed with epilepsy who perceive that their condition would have little effect on their lives tended to report a greater sense of well-being than those who anticipated obvious and noticeable life changes. Collings believes that this latter phenomenon is due directly to the widely held negative stigma associated with epilepsy.

Anticonvulsant Use and the Elderly

The use and potential behavioral toxicity of anticonvulsants are affected by a number of age-related changes in the elderly. Physiological changes of aging cause changes in the absorption, distribution, metabolism, and excretion of most drugs, which all serve to alter the pharmacokinetics of drug metabolism. Altered pharmacodynamics, compliance, concomitant physical illness, the increased number of prescriptions used, the use of over-the-counter preparations, and other environmental factors may also account for changes in drug distribution in this population (McConnell & Duffy, 1994). Age-related alterations in neuronal cell numbers, neurotransmitter production, the proliferation of receptor sites, second messenger systems, decreased total body water, lean body mass, serum albumin, and cardiac output all affect the pharmacodynamics and distribution of anticonvulsants. Metabolism is directly affected by decreases in hepatic mass and enzyme activity, and absorption is affected by age-related changes affecting the absorptive surface and decreased splanchnic blood flow. The decreased glomerular filtration rate and renal blood flow associated with aging also affect excretion. All these factors must be taken into account when prescribing anticonvulsants for the elderly.

The most commonly prescribed anticonvulsant for the elderly is phenytoin. Phenytoin clearance may be markedly increased in the elderly, and as protein binding is decreased concomitantly, it is important to follow both free and total phenytoin levels. The elderly may also be susceptible to falls with the use of phenytoin and should be monitored closely for phenytoin toxicity, which may result in ataxia and subsequent falls. Patients wearing dentures may also be at increased risk of gingival hyperplasia, and the wearing of dentures may make this side effect particularly difficult and should be considered in choosing an anticonvulsant (Lannon, 1993). Carbamazepine clearance may be up to 40% lower in the elderly, and although there appears to be no significant changes in carbamazepine-10,11-epoxide concentrations, the elderly may be more sensitive to epoxide levels at lower concentrations. As a result, patients should be clinically monitored and should also be watched closely for the development of hyponatremia which may present with lethargy or behavioral alterations. Phenobarbital and primodone are still widely prescribed in the elderly although they appear to cause sedation and cognitive dysfunction at a much higher frequency in the elderly than in younger patients. Depression is also a common side effect with phenobarbital, and given the high incidence of behavioral side effects with this drug, it should not be used as a first-choice therapy in this population. The elderly are, similarly, much more sensitive to the effects of benzodiazepines which may cause delirium, dementia, depression, or increased falls in the elderly. Valproic acid is used with increasing frequency in the elderly for various indications, and there are some theoretical advantages to its use in this population because it has generally fewer effects on the liver's metabolism of concurrently administered drugs. As with phenytoin, one must, however, monitor the free valproate concentrations closely in this population (Scheuer & Cohen, 1993). Of the newer drugs, gabapentin seems to have some promise in this population given that it has very few known drug interactions. The use of lamotrogine, vigabatrin, gabapentin, and other newer anticonvulsants has not been systematically examined in this population.

With the use of all anticonvulsants in the elderly, the clinician must be aware of the greater sensitivity to dose-related neurotoxic side effects.

Often these may develop insidiously and may include ataxia, increased falls, cognitive dulling, memory disturbances, agitation, visual disturbances, and depression. Use of phenytoin, phenobarbital, and benzodiazepines are important risk factors for falls in the elderly, which may result in hip fractures. Free drug concentrations of valproate and phenytoin in particular should be monitored, particularly if the patient is taking other relatively highly protein-bound drugs. Anticonvulsants may also accelerate osteomalacia and osteoporosis, and this may be an important risk factor in the development of hip fractures. The elderly may also be sensitive to cardiac effects of phenytoin and carbamazepine. Baseline electrocardiograms (EKGs) should be obtained before initiation of carbamazepine therapy (Scheuer & Cohen, 1993). With the increased use of other concomitant prescription and nonprescription medications one must always be aware of the possibility of drug interactions to which the elderly may also be particularly susceptible. The use of over-the-counter medications and other concurrent medical illnesses may predispose the elderly to behavioral or cognitive effects of anticonvulsants. The use of aspirin, for example, may result in an increase in levels of phenytoin and valproate, resulting in behavioral toxicity from these drugs without concomitant changes in total drug levels or dosages. The use of antacids may also cause absorption of anticonvulsants. The use of psychotropics may affect seizure threshold and antiepileptic drug (AED) levels, and their levels may also be concomitantly influenced by AEDs. Carbamazepine, phenobarbital, and phenytoin may, for example, decrease haloperidol concentrations, and chlorpromazine may increase phenytoin and valproate concentrations.

Conclusions and Research Directions

In this brief chapter, we have attempted to convey two basic points. First, seizures and epilepsy commonly occur in the elderly. The incidence of epilepsy increases substantially in those over 60 years of age. Overall, epilepsy has an incidence of 48 per 100,000 in the population, but in those over age 60 the rate is 82 per 100,000 per year. As such, this clinical condition is frequently encountered by specialists across neuropsychology, neurology, geriatrics, and psychiatry who care for elderly patients. Second, we have hoped to convey how little we currently understand about the neuropathology, etiologic substrates, neuropsychological presentation, diagnosis, and treatment of epilepsy within the geriatric population. There are several extremely interesting research questions which we hope will be addressed by epileptologists in the coming years. For example, are there differences in the propensity to develop epilepsy following similar brain insults between elderly and young adult individuals? What differences, if any, exist between elderly and young adult individuals in their response to insults, such as hypoxia or trauma? Does the sheer number of neurologic insults accumulating with aging explain the subsequent development of epilepsy? One last research question we find especially intriguing: Do the changes in hippocampal structure associated with Alzheimer's disease lead to patterns of synaptic reorganization that are similar to those seen in younger epilepsy patients with mesial temporal sclerosis?

It will be these questions and many others that we have not or cannot think of that will drive research over the remainder of this "decade of the brain" and in future decades to come. The goal is to produce a knowledge base on geriatric aspects of epilepsy that will eventually complement the vast amount of information obtained thus far on the development, diagnosis, and treatment of seizure disorders within all other younger age groups.

References

Babb, T. L., Kupfer, W. R., Pretorius, J. K., Crandall, P. H., & Levesque, M. F. (1991). Synaptic reorganization by mossy fibers in human epileptic fascia dentata. *Neuroscience, 42*, 351–363.

Butler, R. N. (1991). The challenge of geriatric medicine. In J. D. Wilson, E. Braunwald, K. J. Isselbacher, R. G. Petersdorf, J. B. Martin, A. S. Fauci, & R. K. Root (Eds.), *Harrison's principles of internal medicine* (12th ed., pp. 16–19). New York: McGraw-Hill, Inc.

Cavazos, J. E., Golarai, G., & Sutula, T. P. (1991). Mossy fiber reorganization induced by kindling: Time course of development, progression, and permanence. *Journal of Neuroscience, 11*, 2795–2803.

Collings, J. A. (1990). Epilepsy and well-being. *Social Sciences Medicine, 31*, 165–170.

Dam, A. M., Fuglsang-Frederiksen, A., Svarre-Olsen, U., & Dam, M. (1985). Late-onset epilepsy: Etiologies, types of seizures, and value of clinical investigation, EEG, and computerized tomography scan. *Epilepsia, 26*, 227–231.

Dawson, R., Jr., & Wallace, D. R. (1992). Kainic acid-induced seizures in aged rats: Neurochemical correlates. *Brain Research Bulletin, 29*, 459–468.

Dichter, M. A., & Weinberger, L. M. (1994, March). Epileptogenesis and the aging brain (Platform Presentation). Presented at the Seizures and the Elderly Symposium, Miami, FL.

Dodrill, C. B. (1994, March). Cognitive consequences of seizures and antiepileptic drugs in the elderly (Platform Presentation). Presented at the Seizures and the Elderly Symposium, Miami, FL.

Ellis, J. M., & Lee, S. I. (1978). Acute prolonged confusion in later life as an ictal state. *Epilepsia, 19*, 119–128.

Ferrari, M., Verbanac, A., & Kane, V. (1997). Family systems therapy: An approach to therapy for families with epilepsy. In H. McConnell, & P. J. Snyder, (Eds.), *Psychiatric comorbidity in epilepsy: Basic mechanisms, diagnosis, and treatment.* Washington, DC: American Psychiatric Press.

Geddes, J. W., Ulas, J., Brunner, L. C., Choe, W., & Cotman, C. W. (1992). Hippocampal excitatory amino acid receptors in elderly, normal individuals and those with Alzheimer's disease: Non-N-methyl-D-aspartate receptors. *Neuroscience, 50*, 23–34.

Golomb, J., de Leon, M. J., Kluger, A., George, A. E., Tarshish, C., & Ferris, S. H. (1993). Hippocampal atrophy in normal aging: An association with recent memory impairment. *Archives of Neurology, 50*, 967–973.

Goyal, V. K. (1982). Changes with age in the human kidney. *Experimental Gerontology, 17*, 321–331.

Hauser, W. A. (1992). Seizure disorders: The changes with age. *Epilepsia, 33* (Suppl. 4), S6–S14.

Hauser, W. A. (1994, March). Epidemiology of seizures in the elderly (Platform Presentation). Presented at the Seizures and the Elderly Symposium, Miami, FL.

Hauser, W. A., Annegers, J. F., & Kurland, L. T. (1991). Prevalence of epilepsy in Rochester, Minnesota: 1940–1980. *Epilepsia, 32*, 428–445.

Hauser, W. A., Annegers, J. F., & Kurland, L. T. (1993). Incidence of epilepsy and unprovoked seizures in Rochester, Minnesota: 1935–1984. *Epilepsia, 34*, 453–468.

Holmes, G. H. (1980). The electroencephalogram as a predictor of seizures following cerebral infarction. *Clinical Electroencephalography, 11*, 83–86.

Hubbard, O., Sunde, D., & Goldensohn, E. S. (1976). The EEG in centenarians. *Electroencephalography and Clinical Neurophysiology, 40*, 407–417.

Hyman, B. T., Penney, J. B., Blackstone, C. D., & Young, A. B. (1994). Localization of non-N-methyl-D-aspartate glutamate receptors in normal and Alzheimer hippocampal formation. *Annals of Neurology, 35*, 31–37.

Jensen, F. E., Holmes, G. L., Lombroso, C. T., Blume, H. K., & Firkusny, I. R. (1992). Age-dependent changes in long-term seizure susceptibility and behavior after hypoxia in rats. *Epilepsia, 33*, 971–980.

Katz, R. I., & Horowitz, G. R. (1982). The septuagenarian EEG:

Studies in a selected normal geriatric population. *Journal of the American Geriatrics Society, 3*, 273–275.

Lannon, S. L. (1993). Epilepsy in the elderly. *Journal of Neuroscience Nursing, 25*, 273–282.

Lindeman, R. D., Tobin, J. D., & Shock, N. W. (1985). Longitudinal studies on the rate of decline in renal function with age. *Journal of the American Geriatrics Society, 33*, 278–285.

Loiseau, P. (1994, March). Pathological processes in the elderly and their association with seizures (Platform Presentation). Presented at the Seizures and the Elderly Symposium, Miami, FL.

Luhdorf, K., Jensen, L. D., & Plesner, A. M. (1986). Etiology of seizures in the elderly. *Epilepsia, 27*, 458.

McConnell, H., & Duffy, J. (1994). Neuropsychiatric aspects of medical therapies. In E. Coffey & J. Cummings (Eds.), *American psychiatric press textbook of geriatric psychiatry* (pp. 550–574). Washington, DC: American Psychiatric Press.

McConnell, H., & Snyder, P. J. (Eds.). (1997). *Psychiatric comorbidity in epilepsy: Basic mechanisms, diagnosis, and treatment*. Washington, DC: American Psychiatric Press.

McKee, A. C., Kowall, N. W., & Kosik, K. S. (1989). Microtubular reorganization and dendritic growth response in Alzheimer's disease. *Annals of Neurology, 26*, 652–659.

Pedley, T. A. (1994, March). Electrophysiological studies: Neurophysiology of aging and seizures in the elderly. (Platform Presentation). Presented at the Seizures and the Elderly Symposium, Miami, FL.

Pedley, T. A., & Miller, J. A. (1983). Clinical neurophysiology of aging and dementia. In R. Mayeux & W. G. Rosen (Eds.), *The dementias* (pp. 31–49). New York: Raven Press.

Sander, J. W. A. S., Hart, Y. M., Johnson, A. L., & Shorvon, S. D. (1990). National general practice study of epilepsy: Newly diagnosed epileptic seizures in general population. *Lancet, 336*, 1267–1271.

Scheff, S. W., Sparks, D. L., & Price, D. A. (1993). Quantitative assessment of synaptic density in the entorhinal cortex in Alzheimer's disease. *Annals of Neurology, 34*, 356–361.

Scheuer, M. L., & Cohen, J. (1993). Seizures and epilepsy in the elderly. In O. Dovinsky (Ed.), *Neurologic clinics, epilepsy 1, diagnosis and treatment, 11*, (pp. 787–804). Philadelphia: W. B. Saunders.

Shorvon, S. D. (1988). Late onset seizures and dementia: A review of epidemiology and aetiology. In M. R. Trimble & E. H. Reynolds (Eds.), *Epilepsy, behavior and cognitive function* (pp. 189–207). New York: John Wiley and Sons.

Smith, P. F., & Darlington, C. L. (1997). Neural mechanisms of psychiatric disturbances in epilepsy. In H. McConnell, & P. J. Snyder, (Eds.), *Psychiatric comorbidity in epilepsy: Basic mechanisms, diagnosis, and treatment*. Washington, DC: American Psychiatric Press.

Wang, H. S., & Busse, E. W. (1969). EEG of healthy old persons—a longitudinal study. I. Dominant background activity and occipital rhythm. *Journal of Gerontology, 24*, 419–426.

Wozniak, D. F., Stewart, G. R., Miller, J. P., & Olney, J. W. (1991). Age-related sensitivity to kainate neurotoxicity. *Experimental Neurology, 114*, 250–253.

19

Geriatric Head Injury

ROBERT B. FIELDS

Introduction

Until recently, the topic of traumatic brain injury (TBI) in the elderly, or geriatric head injury (GHI), had received relatively little attention from the neuropsychological community. In fact, there are only a handful of studies which describe the syndrome of GHI in neuropsychological terms (e.g., Fields, 1994; Goldstein et al., in press; Goldstein et al., 1994) or specifically address the neurobehavioral impact of a TBI on an elderly individual (e.g., Deaton, 1990; Fields & Coffey, 1994; Fields, Taylor, & Starratt, 1993; Levin, 1995).

In the absence of neurobehavioral data, most predictions about outcome following GHI have been based on the neurosurgery and trauma literature. Studies in these areas have consistently demonstrated that older patients are at greater risk for negative outcome following a TBI than are younger adults (Annegers, Grabow, Kurland, & Laws, 1980; Carlsson, vonEssen, & Lofgren, 1968; Cartlidge & Shaw, 1981; Fife, Faich, Hollinshead, & Boynton, 1986; Kotwica & Jakubowski, 1992; Luerssen, Klauber, & Marshall, 1988; Pentland, Jones, Roy, & Miller, 1986; Rakier, Guilburd, Soustiel, Zaaroor, & Feinsod, 1995; Vollmer et al., 1991). Support for an age-based vulnerability hypothesis has also been provided by animal studies (Hamm, Jenkins, Lyeth, White-Gbadebo, & Hayes, 1991; Hamm, White-Gbadebo, Lyeth, Jenkins, & Hayes, 1992), the literature on general trauma in humans (Dries & Gamelli, 1992), and clinical observations. For example, most neuropsychologists have evaluated older

patients who were reported to be doing reasonably well prior to a relatively mild TBI, but who never fully recovered from their injury.

Thus, while it has been well established that age is an important general factor in predicting outcome following TBI, the specific role that age plays in outcome is less clear. Specifically, we do not yet know whether all elderly are at risk for negative outcome following TBI, or whether the risk of negative outcome is limited to a subset of vulnerable elderly, while the majority of elderly recover in a manner similar to younger adults. Similarly, we still have a great deal to learn about the mechanisms through which aging makes the brain more susceptible to a traumatic injury and through which a traumatic injury may provoke, or exacerbate, a neurodegenerative process in an aging brain.

The recent interest in GHI appears to come from at least three fronts. First, because the population is aging, cases of GHI now account for a greater percentage of patients treated in emergency rooms and on trauma units, making findings such as increased mortality and longer hospital stays more relevant to clinicians, hospital administrators, and insurance companies. Second, the increased referral of patients for neuropsychological evaluation following GHI has led to the need for practical guidelines for the differentiation of the syndrome of GHI from other conditions, such as dementia. The question of whether postinjury deficits are due to the injury, a preexisting condition, the effects of advanced age, or some combination of these factors is often a difficult one. In addition to clinical and academic interest, the answer to this question for individual patients can have legal implications as well. Finally, the third front is the rapidly growing body of literature on the epidemiological and patho-

ROBERT B. FIELDS • Department of Psychiatry, Allegheny General Hospital, and Allegheny University of the Health Sciences, Pittsburgh, Pennsylvania 15212.

genetic association between head injury in adulthood and risk for Alzheimer's disease.

This chapter begins with an overview of the fairly well established literature on the epidemiology and unique characteristics of geriatric head injuries. From this review, the case will be made that GHI is a unique phenomenon. The second section focuses on neurological sequelae and indices of general outcome following TBI and concludes that despite methodological problems in the literature, advanced age is a significant risk factor for negative outcome. Next, the limited research on the neurobehavioral consequences of brain injury in the elderly will be discussed. The preliminary data in this area suggest that the syndrome of GHI can be differentiated from normal aging and from dementia based on neuropsychological test performance and that neuropsychiatric recovery may differ with age following TBI. Finally, the proposed relationship between TBI in adulthood and Alzheimer's disease will be discussed within the context of current conceptualizations about the central role that amyloid deposition plays in the pathogenesis of Alzheimer's disease and the apparent role that head injury plays in contributing to early amyloid deposition.

Epidemiology and Unique Characteristics of Traumatic Brain Injury in the Elderly

Epidemiology

The incidence of TBI in the general population is approximately 200 per 100,000 (Kraus et al., 1984; Naugle, 1990; Sorenson & Kraus, 1991). However, risk for TBI is clearly age-related. Traumatic brain injury is most common among young adult males, for whom the incidence is approximately 400 per 100,000. Typically, these injuries occur in motor vehicle accidents, and alcohol is often involved. Children are a second risk group and often sustain injuries from falls or other accidents. The elderly comprise a third "at-risk" group. As can be seen in Figure 1, after a period of relatively low risk in middle adulthood, the risk for TBI steadily increases after age 65. What is also noteworthy about these data is that unlike young adults, there is no gender difference among older adults in the

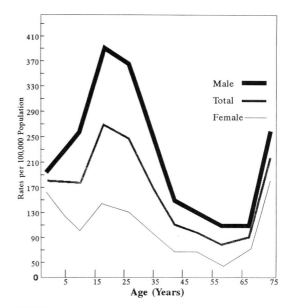

FIGURE 1. Incidence rates of traumatic brain injury by age and sex. (Adapted with permission from Kraus et al., 1984.)

occurrence of these injuries. By comparison, young adult males are approximately three times more likely than young adult females to sustain a TBI, whereas for older adults, men and women are at equal risk.

Mechanism of Injury

Another factor that differs with age is the manner in which the TBI is sustained. With age, there is an increase in the percentage of TBIs that are caused by falls and pedestrian accidents and a decrease in the percentage that are the result of motor vehicle accidents (Naugle, 1990). Among younger adults, motor vehicle accidents are the most common cause of the injury. Among older adults, falls are the most common cause of the injury, and motor vehicle accidents are the second most common cause.

As can be seen in Figure 2, data from our sample of 2,328 patients admitted to the trauma service of a large urban hospital (Fields, 1991) support the findings of others in this regard. In addition to pointing out the unique characteristics of geriatric head injuries, these data have two important implications for the interpretation of age-related differences in outcome. First, the data raise the question

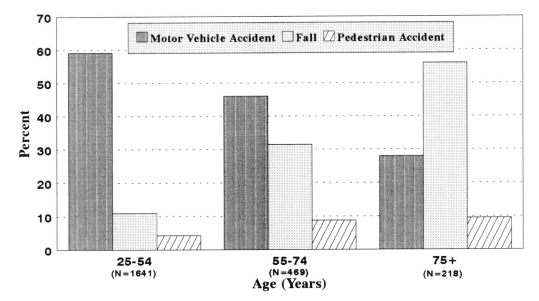

FIGURE 2. Causes of traumatic brain injury by age. p < .0001.

of whether the mechanism of injury must be accounted for when comparing samples of differing age groups. That is, does the variable of mechanism of injury contribute independent variance to outcome? This question has rarely been addressed in the literature. Our own data suggest that while less important than age, general outcome does differ based on mechanism of injury. For example, in one sample of older adults (ages 75–90, n = 121) who sustained a mild TBI, the in-hospital mortality rate was significantly higher when the injury was sustained in a motor vehicle accident (10%) than when it occurred as the result of a fall (2.8%) (Fields & Ackerman, 1991).

The second related implication is that different brain (and nonbrain) injuries are associated with different mechanisms of injury. For example, thoracic injuries (e.g., rib fracture, heart contusion) are more common in motor vehicle accidents whereas subdural bleeds are more common following falls (Fields & Ackerman, 1991). More recently, it has been shown that the deposition of amyloid in the brain is more likely following a TBI sustained in a fall than a TBI sustained via some other mechanism (Roberts et al., 1994). Unfortunately, few studies have taken these factors into account, and as a result, their contribution to age differences in general outcome are unknown.

Prior Head Injury

Among young adults, previous TBI is a known risk factor for future head injury (Annegers et al., 1980; Edna, 1987; Sims, 1985). Documentation of prior TBIs is somewhat difficult because it is typically based on self-report, memory, and subjective interpretation. With these limitations in mind, preliminary data collected in one large trauma database (M. Lovell and S. Smith, personal communication, September 1994) suggest that the frequency of patients who are hospitalized following a TBI reporting a previous TBI is higher among younger adults than older adults. Specifically, in this sample, prior TBI was reported by 32% of a young to middle-age sample (ages 20–50, n = 535), but by only 20% of an older adult sample (ages 60–90, n = 97).

Substance Abuse

Alcohol is another factor that is significantly related to the etiology of, and outcome following, TBI in young adults (Desai et al., 1983; Edna, 1987; Frankowski, 1986; Parkinson, Stephenson, & Phillips, 1985; Ruff et al., 1990). It is also another factor that has not been adequately addressed in the literature on GHI and one for which our data suggest that the assumptions based on young adults may not apply to older adults. As expected, among a sample of over 3,500 patients hospitalized following a TBI at Allegheny General Hospital in Pittsburgh, the frequency of young adults having blood alcohol levels at or above the legal definition of intoxication when brought to the emergency room was relatively high (15- to 24-year-olds = 44%; 35- to 54-year-olds = 39%). Somewhat surprisingly, alcohol was associated with the TBI much less often among the older sample (i.e., 65- to 95-year-olds with legally intoxicated blood alcohol levels = 11%).

Another unique characteristic of the geriatric population is the age difference in the circumstances in which alcohol is involved in the TBI. In our database, legally intoxicated blood alcohol levels were found among young and middle-aged adults whose TBIs occurred in motor vehicle accidents (39%) at approximately the same rate as among those whose TBI occurred because of a fall (35%). In contrast, in the older adult group, among whom alcohol use was less prevalent overall, a legally intoxicated blood alcohol level was significantly more likely when the injury occurred during a fall (17.3%) than when the injury occurred during a motor vehicle accident (6.1%). These data suggest that drinking and driving is less of a problem for the elderly than for younger adults, and that our understanding of the outcome following TBIs that occur as the result of a fall in the elderly must take into account the role of alcohol.

Severity of TBI and Overall Injuries

Finally, we note two more subtle methodological points that are relevant to the investigation of why older adults do not fare as well following TBI as do young and middle-aged adults. First, because outcome following TBI is correlated to the severity of the head injury, if older adults suffer more severe injuries, then age differences in outcome may be due to severity of injury rather than age. In our examination of the natural occurrence of head injuries in a sample of over 3,500 patients, based on Glasgow Coma Scale (GCS; Teasdale & Jennett, 1974) scores in the emergency room, older adults suffered slightly but not dramatically more severe injuries than younger adults (Fields, 1994).

Similarly, the severity of overall injuries was slightly greater in our older sample than in the younger sample. For this analysis, severity of total

body injury was rated with the Injury Severity Scale (ISS; Baker, O'Neil, Haddon, & Long, 1974), which assigns a score based on the severity of injuries in six regions of the body including the head. Severity of total body injury was also noted to be slightly but not dramatically greater with age. These data underscore the importance of controlling for factors such as severity of head injury and severity of other injuries when examining the role that age plays in outcome following TBI.

Summary of Unique Characteristics of Geriatric TBI

To summarize, there is ample evidence to consider geriatric TBI a unique phenomenon. First, TBI is relatively common among the elderly. Second, in contrast to young adults, there is no gender difference in the incidence of TBI among older adults. Third, there are age-related differences in the manner in which TBIs are sustained. That is, with age, there is an increase in falls and pedestrian accidents and a decrease in motor vehicle accidents. Fourth, preliminary data suggest that prior TBI is somewhat less common, or at least reported less, among older adults. Fifth, alcohol is involved in the TBI much less often among older adults than among young and middle-aged adults. However, when alcohol is involved, it is more frequently associated with a fall than a motor vehicle accident. Finally, when looking at the natural occurrence of TBI in the population, older adults seem to suffer slightly but not dramatically more severe head injuries and more severe total body injuries than younger adults, suggesting that these factors need to be taken into account when analyzing outcome data to ensure that age differences in outcome are in fact due to age and not to factors unrelated to age.

Neurological Sequelae and Indices of General Outcome following TBI in the Elderly

Overview of Terminology

Comprehensive reviews of the pathophysiology and natural history of TBI can be found elsewhere (e.g., Alexander, 1995; Bigler, 1991; Gennarelli, 1993; Parker, 1990; Richardson, 1990). To summarize briefly, there is a tremendous amount of variability in the manner in which TBIs occur. In classifying these injuries, the distinctions of focal injuries versus diffuse injuries and primary versus secondary injuries are often useful ones (Gennarelli, 1993). Primary brain injuries typically involve neural or vascular aspects of the brain (Gennarelli, 1993). Damage from the initial trauma of a focal brain injury generally occurs as the result of contact with an external object. Such contact can cause skull fractures, contusions, lacerations, "contrecoup" injuries, and hemorrhage leading to the formation of extradural, subarachnoid, subdural, or intracerebral hematomas (Gennarelli, 1993; Katz, 1992; Richardson, 1990). Diffuse brain injuries, which can produce concussions or prolonged posttraumatic coma, often involve linear acceleration/deceleration or rotational/twisting movements of the brain within the cranial vault. These injuries can produce diffuse axonal shearing as well as lacerations or contusions when the moving brain comes into contact with the more stationary protuberances of the base of the skull (typically in the orbital, frontal, or temporal areas) (Bigler, 1990, 1991; Gennarelli, 1993; Ommaya, Grubb, & Naumann, 1971; Richardson, 1990).

Secondary brain injuries (i.e., those that occur following the initial trauma) can include edema, increased intracranial pressure, ischemia, seizures, and the consequences of the "neurotoxic cascade" (e.g., release of free radicals and excitotoxic neurotransmitters such as glutamate) that occur in response to central nervous system (CNS) trauma (Becker, Verity, Povlishock, & Cheung, 1988; Faden, Demediuk, Panter, & Vink, 1989; Gennarelli, 1993; Katayama, Becker, Tamura, & Hovda, 1990).

Severity of initial injury is the most important factor in predicting postinjury sequelae as well as eventual outcome. Despite its limitations (Sorenson & Kraus, 1991), the GCS (Teasdale & Jennett, 1974) remains the most frequently used method of assessing the severity of a TBI. The GCS is a 15-point global index of consciousness that assesses functions in three domains (i.e., eye opening, verbal response, and motor response). As noted above, the severity of the other injuries which co-occur with the head injury often provides useful prognostic information and can be assessed with scales such as the ISS (Baker et al., 1974). Compared to severity of injury, age is a less powerful predictor of outcome, but it has been associated with increased risk for some, but not all, postinjury problems.

Postinjury Neurological Sequelae

Advanced age is a risk factor for subdural hematomas, intracranial hemorrhages, and posttraumatic infections following TBI (Amacher & Bybee, 1987; Dries & Gamelli, 1992; Fogel & Duffy, 1994; Miller & Pentland, 1989). Postinjury bleeds are more common and more problematic in the elderly for a number of reasons. First, the incidence of nontraumatic intracerebral hemorrhage in the general population increases exponentially with age, making the elderly an "at-risk" population in general (Broderick, Brott, Tomsick, Miller, & Huster, 1993). Second, because brain atrophy increases the distance from the brain surface to the venous sinuses, bridging veins are more vulnerable to rupture with even minor trauma, which increases the risk of subdural hematomas (Cummings & Benson, 1992). Third, because falls are the most common cause of TBI in the elderly, and because subdural hematomas are common consequences of falls, the elderly are particularly vulnerable to subdural bleeds. Finally, these types of injuries may develop in a delayed fashion over time and may go unrecognized in the presence of other injuries (Fogel & Duffy, 1994). For example, in one study of older patients admitted to a hospital because of a fractured bone, 10% were found to have a subdural hematoma as well (Oster, 1977).

The age-related increased risk of posttraumatic intracranial hematomas is particularly problematic after injuries that are classified as being in the mild to moderate range of severity. For example, in their comparison of older (> 65 years, n = 449) and younger (< 65, n = 1,571) patients following TBI of all severities, Pentland et al. (1986) reported a threefold increase in intracranial hematomas among the older sample. However, there was no age difference in the patients whose injuries were severe, among whom intracranial bleeds were common at all ages. In contrast, following TBIs of mild to moderate severity, the frequency of intracranial hematoma was six times greater in the older group. In our study (Fields, Ackerman, & Diamond, unpublished data), of patients who sustained a mild TBI as the result of a fall or a motor vehicle accident, the incidence of intracranial bleeds was related to age and type of injury. As noted in Table 1, intracranial bleeds were significantly more common in the elderly sample in general, but were also more common among those whose injury was sustained in a fall than among those whose injury occurred during a motor vehicle accident.

For other neurological sequelae, there are no age differences, or the effects of age are not well known. Despite the logical prediction that an older skull might be more vulnerable to fracture than a younger skull during a TBI, there is no consistent evidence that this is the case. For example, in one large study of patients with TBI of all severities (Pentland et al., 1986), no age differences were found in the frequency of skull fracture, and in another study of patients with severe TBIs, (Vollmer et al., 1991) only a slight increase with age was found. In our study of the effects of mild TBI (see Table 1), the developing skulls of children were found to be more vulnerable to fracture than the aging skulls of the adult and elderly samples, and no significant increase in the frequency of skull fracture was found with advancing age.

With regard to other neurological sequelae, older adults are not at increased risk to develop brain swelling or a posttraumatic seizure disorder following a TBI (Richardson, 1990). Similar to the data on skull fractures, posttraumatic seizures are in fact more common following TBI in children than in adults (Dalmady-Israel & Zasler, 1993; Fields et al., unpublished data; see Table 1). While it has been postulated that axonal shearing and damage from the release of excitotoxic neurotransmitters is greater among the elderly (Hamm et al., 1991, 1992), this prediction has not yet been proven.

Indices of General Outcome

There are several ways in which general outcome in the initial postinjury period has been assessed. These include survival rates, length of hospital stay, discharge destination, and ability to return to preinjury activities. As is the case with neurological sequelae, initial outcome is influenced most by the severity of the injury, although a number of other factors contribute to outcome.

Following severe TBIs, death, permanent disability, and inability to return to work are more common at all ages. However, age appears to play an independent and significant role in increasing the risk of negative outcome. In the most comprehensive study of age differences in outcome following severe TBI to date, Vollmer et al. (1991) found dramatic age-related differences in outcome at 6 months. Using the Glasgow Outcome Scale (Jennett & Bond, 1975), which measures global outcome on a 5-point scale ranging from good recovery to vegetative survival and death, the mortality rate at 6 months was 28% for the 26- to 35-year-old group and 80% for the over 55-year-old group. In addition, 28% of the younger group were rated as having made a good recovery after 6 months, whereas among the older group, none had made a good recovery. One of the advantages of this study was that the role of age in influencing outcome was assessed by systematically ruling out the effect of other variables. The authors concluded that the variable of age clearly made an independent contribution to outcome in their sample.

Mortality

With regard to the specific question of survival rate following TBI, in keeping with the Vollmer et al. (1991) study, a fairly robust finding in the literature is that older adults are at greater risk for death

Table 1. Differences in Neurological Sequelae following Mild Traumatic Brain Injury Due to Age and Type of Injury[a]

| Age group | Type of injury | n | Percentage of patients with | | |
			Skull fracture	Intracranial bleed	Seizures
0–10	Fall	63	29	6	6
	MVA[b]	42	12	9	0
15–24	Fall	82	15	18	5
	MVA	795	10	4	1
35–54	Fall	169	17	19	5
	MVA	545	11	2	2
65–95	Fall	248	16	40	1
	MVA	229	13	15	0

[a]From Fields et al., unpublished data.
[b]MVA, motor vehicle accident.

following head injury than are young adults or children (e.g., Amacher & Bybee, 1987; Annegers et al., 1980; Fields, 1991; Fife et al., 1986; Pentland et al., 1986; Rakier et al., 1995). However, as noted above, most studies of this outcome measure did not control for factors such as severity of brain injury or severity of other nonbrain injuries. In our attempts to do so (see Table 2), an age by severity of injury interaction was found. As can be seen in Figure 3, when all patients were included regardless of severity of injury, mortality rate was relatively stable through middle adulthood, but increased significantly beginning at age 55 and continued to increase with advancing age. In follow-up analyses (see Table 2), among patients whose injuries were severe, mortality was greater for patients at all ages, but again was highest among the oldest group.

Among patients whose head injuries were considered to be mild, but whose total injuries were not accounted for in the analysis, the mortality rate among the oldest group was approximately eight times greater than the middle age group and 24 times greater than the young adult group. However, when severity of head injury (i.e., mild, GCS = 13–15) and severity of total body injury (i.e., mild, ISS < 10) were controlled, mortality was extremely low for all age groups (see Table 2). These data suggest that while age increases the risk for in-hospital mortality following a head injury at any level of severity, other factors (e.g., severity of other injuries) play a role in the apparent age difference in outcome.

Table 2. Age Differences in Mortality Rates following Traumatic Brain Injuries of Different Severity[a]

Severity of injury	Age			
	0–10	15–24	35–54	65–95
Severe TBI (GCS = 3–8)[b]	24% (n = 42)	19% (n = 289)	21% (n = 196)	54% (n = 162)
Mild TBI (GCS = 13–15)	0% (n = 189)	0.3% (n = 1139)	1% (n = 952)	8% (n = 545)
Mild overall (GCS = 13–15) (ISS <10)[c]	0% (n = 125)	0% (n = 628)	0% (n = 458)	0.5% (n = 187)

[a]*Source*: Fields, 1994; Fields et al., unpublished data.
[b]GCS, Glasgow Coma Scale.
[c]ISS, Injury Severity Scale.

Length of Hospital Stay and Discharge Destination

Several outcome studies have documented that following TBIs of similar severity, older adults stay in a hospital longer and are more likely to be discharged to a nursing home and less likely to be discharged to their home (e.g., Fields, 1991; Fife et al., 1986; Roy, Pentland, & Miller, 1986). Given changes in reimbursement for health care services, these age-related differences have enormous practical and economic significance. Although length of hospital stay increases with age, this increase appears to be a reflection of the interaction between length of stay and discharge destination. In our sample, the mean length of stay for patients discharged to home or to a nursing home did not differ significantly by age (Fields, 1991). That is, patients of any age who are discharged to nursing homes stay in a hospital much longer than patients who return home. Because more older adults are discharged to nursing homes and fewer older adults are discharged home, the overall increase in length of hospital stay for the elderly is due to the fact that a larger percentage of elderly are discharged to nursing homes, not because it takes all older adults longer to recover from their injuries.

Return to Preinjury Functioning

Finally, the literature on young and middle-aged adults suggests that advanced age is a relevant factor in the prediction of return to previous level of functioning. One frequently used index of outcome among young adults is return to school or work. Although this indicator is not meaningful for many older adults (who are retired), and despite the fact that the majority of the studies in this area do not include patients above age 65, it is worth noting that conclusions about the effect of age are, nevertheless, often made. For example, in three recent studies (Ip, Dornan, & Schentag, 1995; Ponsford, Olver, Curran, & Ng, 1995; Ruff et al., 1993), age was found to be a small, but significant, predictor of eventual outcome following severe TBI (among young and middle-aged adults). In the few studies that have assessed this variable among older adults (Alberico, Ward, Choi, Marmarou, & Young, 1987; Davis & Acton, 1988; Pentland et al., 1986), ad-

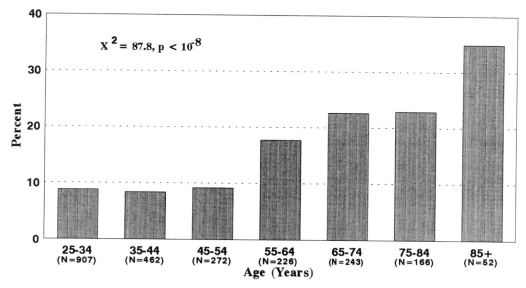

FIGURE 3. Age differences in mortality rate following TBI, all levels of severity.

vanced age has also been found to predict increased difficulty with activities of daily living, increased general disability, and decreased likelihood of returning to work (among those who were working prior to their injury).

Summary

To summarize, the elderly are at risk for some, but not all, neurological sequelae. Of particular concern in this population are intracranial bleeds, which are more common in the elderly in general and more common following falls which are a primary cause of GHI. While many studies fail to account for several factors that influence outcome, advanced age clearly appears to be a risk factor for increased in-hospital mortality, longer hospital stay, and increased likelihood of nursing home placement. However, the available data suggest that while elderly as a group represent an at-risk population, it may be the case that more elderly are at risk, rather than that all elderly take longer to recover. Finally, while it appears that return to preinjury functioning becomes less likely with age, this variable is not well defined for the elderly, and only a handful of studies have addressed it.

Neurobehavioral Consequences of GHI

While limited, the available data on the neurobehavioral consequences of GHI have begun to shed light on some of the central questions that must be addressed in order to define the syndrome of GHI. These questions include: (1) Can the effects of GHI be differentiated from the effects of normal aging? (2) Do the neuropsychological effects of TBI differ with age? (3) Can the syndrome of GHI be differentiated from the syndrome of dementia on the basis of neuropsychological test performance? (4) Do the neuropsychiatric and psychosocial consequences of TBI differ with age?

Can GHI Be Differentiated from Normal Aging?

Indirect support for the hypothesis that the neuropsychological effects of TBI in the elderly can be differentiated from the effects of normal aging comes from the extensive literature on the effects of TBI among young adults (e.g., Levin, Benton, & Grossman, 1982; Levin, Gary, et al., 1990; Levin, Hamilton, & Grossman, 1990) as well as one study (Mazzucchi et al., 1992) which found a high rate of generalized cognitive impairment (i.e., approximately 50%) among a sample of older adults (50–75 years of age) who had recently suffered a TBI.

Two recent studies have directly tested and supported this hypothesis. In the first, Goldstein et al. (1994) compared the performance of older (50 years of age and older) patients who had sustained a TBI of mild (n = 6) or moderate (n = 16) severity with the performance of an older adult control group (n = 16) on selected measures in four cognitive domains: attention (e.g., reciting alphabet, serial 3s, reciting months forward and backward), language (e.g., visual naming, controlled oral word association), memory (e.g., California Verbal Learning Test [CVLT], Continuous Visual Recognition Test), and executive functioning (Wechsler Adult Intelligence Scale-Revised [WAIS-R] Similarities, modified card sorting). Nineteen of the 22 GHI patients were tested within 3 months of their injury. Consistent with the literature on TBI among young adults, significant between-group differences were found in three of the four domains (i.e., language, memory, and executive functioning). The authors concluded that "mild to moderate closed head injury in older adults produces cognitive deficits involving the same neurobehavioral areas affected in young survivors" (p. 964).

In a second study (Goldstein et al., 1996), the performance of 15 GHI patients was compared with the performance of 15 normal elderly controls (and 15 patients with AD, see below) on measures of memory (i.e., dementia version of the CVLT) and language processing (i.e., naming and verbal fluency). Consistent with the findings of their previous study, the GHI group in this study performed significantly worse than the elderly control group on measures of memory and language.

Do the Neuropsychological Effects of TBI Differ with Age?

To provide conclusive support for the contention that TBI produces similar deficits among young and older survivors, a large-scale study of young and older adult TBI patients is needed which takes into account factors such as premorbid level of functioning, role of substance abuse, history of prior head injury, type of injury, severity of injury, type and severity of other nonbrain injuries, and availability of rehabilitation and psychosocial support resources. No such study has been done to date.

In an attempt to address one aspect of this question, Fields (1994) compared the neuropsychological test performance of young (n = 472) and older (n = 96) adults who suffered a mild TBI (i.e., GCS = 13–15) and recovered sufficiently within the first week following their injury to complete a neuropsychological evaluation. A limitation of this study was that it did not address the issue of whether more elderly than young adults were too impaired to be tested (i.e., had more severe initial outcome). However, this design ensured the comparability of the two groups by requiring that all patients met the same inclusion criteria.

As can be seen in Table 3, while the raw scores of the older adults were significantly worse on seven of the eight measures chosen, when the effects of age were controlled by converting raw scores to age-based percentile scores, the groups differed on only one of the eight measures (i.e., Digit Span Backwards; see Table 3). These preliminary data support the conclusion of Goldstein et al. (1994) and suggest that the acute neuropsychological effects of

Table 3. Comparison of Neuropsychological Test Performance of Geriatric Patients (n = 96) versus Young Adult Patients (n = 472) following Mild TBI[a]

Test	Results	
	Raw score	Percentile score
Digit Span Forward	n.s.[b]	n.s.
Digit Span Backward	p < .01	p < .05
Trails A	p < .001	n.s.
Trails B	p < .001	n.s.
Wechsler Memory Scale-Revised		
Logical Memory-I	p < .05	n.s.
Logical Memory-II	p < .01	n.s.
Visual Reproduction-I	p < .001	n.s.
Visual Reproduction-II	p < .001	n.s.

[a]Source: Fields, 1994.
[b]n.s., not significant.

mild TBI among patients whose initial recovery is relatively uncomplicated is not significantly different with age. However, whether there are age differences in the long-term neuropsychological effects of TBI or the course of neuropsychological recovery over time is not yet known.

Can GHI Be Differentiated from Dementia?

The ability to differentiate the syndrome of GHI from dementia is important for clinical as well as legal reasons. Two studies have provided preliminary guidelines in this area. Goldstein et al. (1996) compared the performance of 15 GHI patients following mild to moderate TBI (GCS = 9–15) with the performance of 15 patients with probable Alzheimer's disease (all of whom were considered to be in the early stages of the disease) and 15 elderly controls. The GHI patients were tested approximately 6 weeks postinjury. The test battery chosen for this study specifically included two areas that are impaired in early AD, memory (via the dementia version of the CVLT) and language processing (via tests of object naming and verbal fluency). Not surprisingly, the normal elderly control subjects performed better on the language and memory tasks than both of the patient groups. Of relevance to the current discussion, the patients with AD displayed poorer recall on the dementia version of the CVLT and did not show the normal facilitation of verbal fluency when asked to generate words in specific semantic categories (fruits/vegetables) as opposed to the generation of word lists in more specific phonemic categories (i.e., words beginning with specific letters).

In a second study, Young, Fields, and Lovell (1995) compared the test performance of 33 patients who had sustained a recent GHI (i.e., in the past week) with 35 patients who met criteria for mild dementia on measures of attention (i.e., Digit Span, Trails A), memory (Hopkins Verbal Learning Test), and executive functioning (Trails B). In keeping with the findings of Goldstein et al. (1996), Young et al. found that while the GHI group performed better than the AD group overall, the only significant between-group differences were on measures of memory and executive functioning (see Table 4).

Table 4. Comparison of Neuropsychological Test Performance of GHI Patients (n = 33) versus Patients with Mild Dementia (n = 35)[a]

Test	GHI patients	Dementia patients	p value
Digit Span Forward	7.8	6.9	
Digit Span Backward	5.0	4.5	
Trails A	69.1	97.6	
Trails B	193.8	266.4	p < .01
Hopkins Verbal Learning Test			
Learning Score	6.7	4.8	p < .001
Delayed Recall	5.2	1.8	p < .001

[a]Source: Young, Fields, & Lovell, 1995.

Does Neurobehavioral Functioning Differ with Age following TBI?

Among young adults, neurobehavioral complaints are frequent in the month following a TBI and can include physical changes (e.g., headache, dizziness, sensitivity to light and noise), cognitive difficulties (e.g., concentration, memory), as well as alterations in mood (e.g., depression, posttraumatic anxiety) and behavior (e.g., impulsivity, irritability) (Binder, 1986; Bohnen & Jolles, 1992; Bohnen, Jolles, & Twijnstra, 1992). For most patients, these symptoms resolve in 3 to 6 months. Among the elderly, there is preliminary evidence that neurobehavioral recovery may be different and slightly more complicated.

Levin (1995) reported on a preliminary study using the Neurobehavioral Rating Scale to assess the functioning of GHI, AD, and normal elderly controls across time. One month following their injury, GHI patients reported difficulties in the areas of cognition, meta-cognition, and language. When a subsample of this group was reassessed 6 months following their injury, no significant change in overall symptomatology was reported.

Similar results were found in another study of the natural history of post-TBI complaints in which the self-reports of older patients (ages 50–95, n = 49) were compared with the self-reports of younger patients (ages 18–45, n = 139) 1 and 4 months following their injury (Fields et al., 1993). For this study, a 29-item questionnaire (Post-Traumatic Neurobehavioral Screening Inventory, PTNSI) that assesses symptoms commonly reported following TBI was used (Taylor, Fields, Starratt, Russo, & Diamond, 1993). The two age groups were comparable in terms of severity of head injury and severity of other nonbrain injuries. One month following the injury, neurobehavioral complaints were common among both younger and older patients, and the overall symptom profiles were quite similar, although symptoms of posttraumatic stress disorder were more common among the younger group and fatigue was reported more often in the older group. At the 4-month follow-up, however, age-related differences began to emerge. The older patients endorsed fatigue, difficulty processing information, dysphoric mood, dizziness, and sensitivity to noise significantly more than the younger patients. In addition, there was an age by time interaction found on three of the six subscales of the test (i.e., cognitive, behavior, posttraumatic stress) such that the older patients reported similar, or greater, distress in these areas at 4 months compared to 3 months earlier, whereas the younger patients reported improvement in all of these areas across the same time period. Thus, while preliminary, these findings suggest that the course of neurobehavioral recovery following TBI in the elderly may be different, and somewhat worse, than in younger patients.

Summary

To summarize, while extremely limited, the available data on neurobehavioral outcome suggest that GHI produces neuropsychological effects that are similar to the effects of TBI in young adults and that are distinguishable from the effects of normal aging and dementia. One important implication of these data is that if elderly are evaluated with age-appropriate tests and norms, a significant percentage (perhaps a majority) perform in a manner that is not significantly worse than younger adults, suggesting that not all elderly are at greater risk for negative outcome. With regard to the differentiation of GHI from dementia, the available data suggest that learning, delayed recall, semantic processing, and executive functioning are cognitive domains that should be included in a test battery designed to differentiate these two syndromes. With regard to neurobehavioral outcome, in addition to the general finding that older adults are less likely to return to their preinjury level of functioning, there is now preliminary evidence that the course of recovery for older patients following a TBI may be different, and somewhat worse, than the course for younger patients.

TBI and Alzheimer's Disease

Findings from Dementia Pugilistica

A potential link between TBI and Alzheimer's disease was suggested by the relatively high prevalence of dementia among former boxers who experienced repeated head injuries earlier in life (Corsellis, Bruton, & Freeman-Browne, 1973; Roberts, 1969; Roberts, Allsop, & Bruton, 1990). Dementia pugilistica (DP) or "punch-drunk" syndrome can develop late in a boxer's career or several years after retirement. Typically, DP includes parkinsonian symptoms such as dysarthria and bradykinesia as well as general cognitive deterioration and personality change (Roberts, 1969). Neuroanatomically, abnormalities of the septum pellucidum, cerebellar scarring, and degeneration of the substantia nigra have been reported (Corsellis et al., 1973). Histopathologically, DP was initially described as including neurofibrillary tangles in the absence of senile neuritic plaques (Corsellis et al., 1973). However, recent studies (Allsop, Haga, Bruton, Ishii, & Roberts, 1990; Roberts et al., 1990) have documented that patients with DP have beta-amyloid deposits (i.e., plaques) that are comparable to those seen in AD, suggesting that AD and DP may result from similar pathogenetic processes.

Epidemiological Studies

The question of whether a single significant head injury in adulthood increases the risk of developing dementia in later life has been posed for some time (e.g., Corsellis & Brierly, 1959), but has received increased attention over the past decade with somewhat conflicting results. In the majority of studies comparing AD patients with matched elderly controls, head injury was found to be significantly more common in the histories of the AD patients (Graves et al., 1990; Henderson et al., 1992; Heyman et al., 1984; Mayeux, Ottman, et al., 1993; Mortimer, French, Hutton, & Schuman, 1985; Rasmusson, Brandt, Martin, & Folstein, 1995). Despite methodological differences between studies in areas, such as the definition of "head injury," the odds ratio (OR), or estimate of relative risk for AD in patients with a history of head injury, was fairly comparable in several studies (e.g., Graves et al., 1990, OR = 3.5; Mayeux, Ottman, et al, 1993, OR = 3.7; Mortimer et al, 1985, OR = 4.4). Not surprisingly, other studies have reported greater variability in risk for AD (e.g., Van Duijn et al., 1992, OR = 1.6; Rasmusson et al., 1995, OR = 13.75), and a minority of studies did not find a significant association between a history of TBI and AD (Broe et al., 1990; Chandra, Philipose, Bell, Lazaroff, & Schoenberg, 1987; Williams, Annegers, Kokmen, O'Brien, & Kurland, 1991). In their meta-analysis of the literature in this area, Mortimer et al. (1991) pooled data from several studies and concluded that a history of TBI with loss of consciousness was significantly more common in patients with AD than in controls; also, it appeared to be more of a risk factor for men than women and for sporadic cases of AD than for familial cases.

The issue of sporadic versus familial remains an unresolved one. In one recent study, Rasmusson et al. (1995) found that while a history of head injury was reported in 29% of their AD cases and only 3% of their controls, the OR was higher for the sporadic cases (25.4) than the familial cases (8.25). These authors concluded that "head trauma is involved in the pathogenesis of AD to a greater extent among individuals who do not have a genetic vulnerability to the disease. In contrast, those having the genotype for AD will express it, with or without cranial trauma, if they live long enough" (p. 217). A somewhat different view was expressed by Mayeux et al. (1995), who found that a history of TBI was associated with increased risk for AD only in the presence of a genetic allele that has been associated with an increased risk for AD (i.e., apolipoprotein E ε-4 allele; see below). The OR for AD associated with a history of head injury alone in their sample was 1.5, whereas the OR for AD associated with a history of head injury and at least one ε-4 allele was 10.5. These authors conclude that "the biological effects of head injury may increase the risk of AD, but only through a synergistic relationship with apolipoprotein ε-4" (p. 555). Needless to say, additional prospective studies in this area would be welcome.

General Vulnerability Model

Two explanatory models have been suggested to account for the proposed association between TBI and AD. The first is a general vulnerability hypothesis. In this model, an injury, or injuries, to the brain produce a lasting and possibly cumulative effect on an individual's vulnerability to AD. Possible mechanisms for this vulnerability include neuronal death via axonal shearing or weakening of the blood–brain barrier during the injury, thereby exposing the central nervous system to toxic substances (Nandy, 1981). A comprehensive description of this type of vulnerability model was provided by Satz (1991). In his "threshold theory" model, Satz proposed that vulnerability factors (e.g., low IQ, limited education, head injury) and protective factors (e.g., advanced education, higher IQ) interact to determine an individual's "brain reserve capacity" and "threshold for impairment." Among individuals with a lowered threshold for impairment, a subsequent mild insult will be sufficient for the expression of neuropsychological and/or functional deficits. The appeal of this model is its ability to take multiple factors into account and to provide a general framework for establishing vulnerability. The limitation of this model is its lack of specificity. As Brandt (1995) pointed out, general vulnerability models do not explain why brain surgery, epilepsy, and stroke do not increase the risk for AD or why TBI increases risk specifically for AD and not for other neurodegenerative disorders.

Amyloid Hypothesis: Beta-Amyloid Protein Deposition

A second explanatory model that is receiving more support is based on our current understanding of the pathogenesis of AD. To summarize briefly, this model is based on the role of amyloid deposition in AD and the apparent provocative effects of a TBI on the mechanism of amyloid production and deposition. Support for this model comes from two areas of research: (1) genetic and environmental factors affecting the deposition of the beta-amyloid protein in the brain, and (2) the identification of a possible genetic marker for Alzheimer's disease (i.e., apolipoprotein E ε-4 allele) that appears to have a role in mediating amyloid deposition.

There is now a great deal of evidence that the deposition of beta-amyloid is the central (if not causative) pathological event in the neuronal degeneration that occurs in AD (Hardy, 1994; Hardy & Allsop, 1991). Beta-amyloid protein (bAP) deposits are found at the core of the senile plaques which are common in AD and selected other neurodegenerative disorders, and abnormalities in the processing and deposition of beta-amyloid have been linked to increased risk for AD (Hardy, 1994). Beta-amyloid protein is part of a large transmembrane beta-amyloid precursor protein (bAPP) that is encoded by a gene on chromosome 21 (Kang et al., 1987). Beta-amyloid originates in the metabolism of bAPP, and soluble bAP accumulates in the brains of AD patients until it polymerizes into amyloid fibers (Tabaton, 1994). Deposition of bAP as a result of this "amyloid cascade" (Hardy & Higgins, 1992; Selkoe, 1993) produces neuronal degeneration.

The high prevalence of AD and diffuse deposition of bAP in the brains of patients with Down's syndrome (trisomy 21) (Giaccone et al., 1989) and patients with mutations of the bAPP gene on chromosome 21 (Murrell, Farlow, Ghetti, & Benson, 1991) provides strong evidence of the critical role that bAPP plays in the development of early-onset AD (Hardy, 1994). It also provides a genetic model of how the apparently lifelong overexpression and metabolism of bAPP to bAP may cause AD.

An environmental model of how this process occurs has been proposed based on the findings from patients with DP and young adults who die following severe TBIs. As noted above, the findings of beta-amyloid deposits in patients with DP (Roberts et al., 1990) suggest a causative role of repeated brain injuries in producing a dementia that resembles AD neuropathologically. Furthermore, in a recent study of patients across the age span who died following a severe head injury, beta-amyloid deposits were found in 30% of the patients and bAPP immunoreactivity was increased in all of the patients examined (Roberts, Gentleman, Lynch, & Graham, 1991; Roberts et al., 1994). While more common in older adults, bAP deposition in this study was found in young adults and children as young as 10 years of age. Of relevance to the elderly was the finding that in addition to increased likelihood of bAP deposition with advancing age, there was also increased likelihood of bAP deposition following an injury sustained in a fall than in any other type of injury.

These findings extended the conclusions based on the DP patients and suggested that even one significant brain injury can have a significant effect on the process of amyloid deposition and that this process occurs quite rapidly following CNS injury. While the mechanism by which this process occurs is not yet clear, Roberts et al. (1994) hypothesized that increased expression of bAPP may be part of an acute phase response to neuronal injury in the human brain designed to stabilize damaged synaptic membranes, promote synaptic plasticity, and facilitate repair and regeneration. They suggest further that induction of bAPP in the brain may be a normal, and possibly protective, response to neuronal injury which, in susceptible individuals, might initiate a disease process.

Amyloid Hypothesis: Role of Apolipoprotein E ε-4 Allele

The second key component of the amyloid hypothesis is based on the recent finding that AD has been linked to a specific allele for apolipoprotein E (ApoE) on chromosome 19 (Saunders et al., 1993; Strittmatter et al., 1993). Apolipoprotein E was previously identified as having a role in cholesterol metabolism and, as a result, related to risk for coronary artery disease and stroke (Mahley, 1988). Of relevance to AD, ApoE also has been found to bind with high affinity to beta-amyloid in the cerebrospinal fluid (CSF) and to be present in the senile plaques and tangles that are the hallmark of AD (Saunders et al., 1993). It has been postulated that ApoE contributes to the risk of AD by mediating amyloid deposition (Rebeck, Reiter, Strickland, & Hyman, 1993; Schmechel et al., 1993) via genetic variability of the ApoE allele which has three common variants; ε-2, ε-3, and ε-4. The ε-3 allele is most common and accounts for approximately 78% of the ApoE alleles in American and European whites (vs. 15% for the ε-4 allele and 7% for the ε-2 allele) (Utermann, Langenbeck, Beisiegel, & Weber, 1980). It now appears that the presence of the ε-4 allele increases the risk for AD (Brousseau et al., 1994; Corder et al., 1993; Mayeux, Stern, et al., 1993; Poirier et al., 1993; Saunders et al., 1993; Strittmatter et al., 1993), whereas the presence of ε-2 may be protective against AD (Corder et al., 1994; Talbot et al., 1994). In one study (Mayeux, Stern, et al., 1993), for example, the OR for AD for older adults who were homozygous for the ε-4 allele (i.e., two ε-4 alleles) was 17.9 and the OR for those who were heterozygous (i.e., one ε-4 allele and one other allele) was 4.2 compared to older adults with other ApoE alleles.

The role that ApoE plays following CNS injury is not well understood. Following peripheral nervous system injury, it has been reported that ApoE levels increase 250-fold (Boyles, Notterpek, & Anderson, 1990), possibly to increase cholesterol acquisition by the regenerating nerve (Rubinsztein, 1995). A similar process has been postulated for CNS injury (Mahley, 1988), via a role in cholesterol metabolism, nerve growth, or immunoregulation, but further research in this area is needed. Of relevance to this hypothesis is the aforementioned study by Mayeux et al. (1995) in which a history of head injury was found to be a risk factor for AD only among patients with at least one ε-4 allele. This finding suggests that ApoE may play a role in the process of neuronal repair following TBI, or that the development of AD following TBI results from the interaction between a genetic predisposition (i.e., ApoE ε-4 genotype) and an environmental event (i.e., the TBI).

Further work in this area will need to elucidate the role of ApoE following CNS injury and to determine the specificity of ApoE ε-4 for AD. There is, for example, preliminary evidence that the ε-4 allele is more common in vascular dementia (Shimano et al., 1989) (which is consistent with its role in cholesterol metabolism) and that it may also increase risk for some neurodegenerative disorders, such as Pick's disease, corticobasilar degeneration; and progressive supranuclear palsy (Schneider, Gearing, Robbins, de l'Aune, & Mirra, 1995), but not others (e.g., Parkinson's disease, multiple sclerosis; Rubinsztein et al., 1994). In addition, there is also preliminary evidence that the presence of the ApoE ε-4 allele may play a crucial role in the development of neurofibrillary tangles via its role in the phosphorylation of tau (Strittmatter et al., 1994). Tau is a microtubule associated protein which binds strongly with ApoE ε-3, but not with ApoE ε-4. It has been suggested that the presence of ApoE ε-4 (or the absence of ApoE ε-3) leads to more rapid phosphorylation of tau which in turn leads to instability of the microtubule system in neurons and ultimately the formation of paired helical filaments and neurofibrillary tangles, thereby increasing the risk of AD (Strittmatter et al., 1994). As a result, much more research is needed before it is clear that ApoE plays a critical role in amyloid deposition, that it is a specific marker for AD, and that it is a specific risk factor following TBI. As of now, however, the amyloid hypothesis remains an intriguing one and worthy of the tremendous amount of research activity that it has generated.

Summary

Recent studies have suggested a link between TBI in adulthood and the development of AD. While more prospective longitudinal studies of this proposed association are needed, the available data at the time of this writing are intriguing and provide a conceptual basis for considering head injury as one piece of the pathogenetic puzzle of AD. The notion of reduced brain capacity in AD is a good explanatory model for dementia in general. However, recent data suggest that a more parsimonious explanation can be based on the amyloid hypothesis, which contends that a TBI at any age (but more so in an older brain) can set into motion a response that is protective at the time of the injury but which, for some patients, may lay the foundation for AD. It remains to be seen whether this occurs in a manner in which the TBI per se is an environmental risk factor for AD and therefore is more common in sporadic cases (as suggested by Rasmusson et al., 1995), interacts synergistically with a genetic predisposition and therefore is more common in genetically vulnerable individuals (as suggested by Mayeux et al., 1995), or both. Regardless of the final answer, further research in this area is clearly warranted.

Conclusion

Epidemiological studies consistently document that GHI is a relatively common phenomenon with many unique features. Compared to TBI among young adults, TBI among the elderly differs with respect to gender distribution, mechanism of injury, history of TBI, role of alcohol use, and severity of injury. Outcome following TBI in general is worse among the elderly, although the extent to which variables such as type of injury and severity of other injuries mediate the effects of age is not well known. The limited data on the neuropsychological effects of TBI in the elderly suggest that these effects are similar to the effects of TBI among young adults and can be differentiated from normal aging and dementia; however, studies of the long-term effects of TBI in the elderly do not exist. There is some preliminary evidence that the neuropsychiatric consequences of TBI may be more severe in the elderly, but long-term studies are needed in this area as well. Finally, the proposed link between TBI and AD has led to a greater understanding of the pathogenesis of both. At this point, the hypothesis that TBI increases the risk for AD via early deposition of amyloid is generating increased support, however, additional work is needed to determine if this or some other hypothesis will provide the most convincing explanation of the data.

References

Alberico, A. M., Ward, J. D., Choi, S. C., Marmarou, A., & Young, H. F. (1987). Outcome after severe head injury: Relationship to mass lesions, diffuse injury, and ICP course in pediatric and adult patients. *Journal of Neurosurgery, 67*, 648–656.

Alexander, M. P. (1995). Mild traumatic brain injury: Pathophysiology, natural history, and clinical management. *Neurology, 45*, 1253–1260.

Allsop, D., Haga, S., Bruton, C., Ishii, T., & Roberts, G. W. (1990). Neurofibrillary tangles in some cases of dementia pugilistica share antigens with amyloid B-protein of Alzheimer's disease. *American Journal of Pathology, 136*, 255–260.

Amacher, A. L., & Bybee, D. E. (1987). Toleration of head injury by the elderly. *Neurosurgery, 20*(6), 954–958.

Annegers, J. F., Grabow, J. D., Kurland, L. T., & Laws, E. R. (1980). The incidence, causes, and secular trends of head trauma in Olmsted County, Minnesota, 1935–1974. *Neurology, 30*, 912–919.

Baker, S. P., O'Neil, B., Haddon, W., Jr., & Long, W. B. (1974). The injury severity score: A method of describing patients with multiple injuries and evaluating emergency care. *Journal of Trauma, 14*, 187–196.

Becker, D. P., Verity, M. A., Povlishock, J., & Cheung, M. (1988). Brain cellular injury and recovery: Horizons for improving medical therapies in stroke and trauma. *Western Journal of Medicine, 148*, 670–684.

Bigler, E. D. (1990). *Traumatic brain injury*. Austin, TX: Pro-Ed.

Bigler, E. D. (1991). *Diagnostic clinical neuropsychology*. Austin, TX: University of Texas Press.

Binder, L. M. (1986). Persisting symptoms after mild head injury: A review of the postconcussive syndrome. *Journal of Clinical and Experimental Neuropsychology, 8*, 323–346.

Bohnen, N., & Jolles, J. (1992). Neurobehavioral aspects of postconcussive symptoms after mild head injury. *Journal of Nervous and Mental Disease, 180*, 683–692.

Bohnen, N., Jolles, J., & Twijnstra, A. (1992). Neuropsychological deficits in patients with persistent symptoms six months after mild head injury. *Neurosurgery, 30*, 692–696.

Boyles, J. K., Notterpek, L. M., & Anderson, L. J. (1990). Accumulation of apolipoproteins in the regenerating and remyelinating mammalian peripheral nerve. *Journal of Biological Chemistry, 265*, 17805–17815.

Brandt, J. (1995, February). *Concluding comments (in symposium: Closed head injury and Alzheimer's disease: Epidemiologic, neurobehavioral, and neuropathologic links*. Paper presented at the annual meeting of the International Society of Neuropsychology, Seattle, WA.

Broderick, J. P., Brott, T., Tomsick, T., Miller, R., & Huster, G. (1993). Intracerebral hemorrhage more than twice as common as subarachnoid hemorrhage. *Journal of Neurosurgery, 78*, 188–191.

Broe, G. A., Henderson, A. S., Creasey, H., McCusker, E., Korten, A. S., Jorm, A. F., Longley, W., & Anthony, J. C. (1990). A case-control study of Alzheimer's disease in Australia. *Neurology, 40*, 1698–1701.

Brousseau, T., Legrain, S., Berr, C., Gourlet, V., Vidal, O., & Amouyel, P. (1994). Confirmation of the e4 allele of the apolipoprotein E gene as a risk factor for late-onset Alzheimer's disease. *Neurology, 44*, 342–344.

Carlsson, C. A., vonEssen, C., & Lofgren, J. (1968). Factors affecting the clinical course of patients with severe head injuries. *Journal of Neurosurgery, 29*, 242–251.

Cartlidge, N. E. F., & Shaw, D. A. (1981). *Head injury*. London: W. B. Saunders.

Chandra, V., Philipose, V., Bell, P. A., Lazaroff, A., & Schoenberg, B. S. (1987). Case-control study of late onset "probable Alzheimer's disease." *Neurology, 37*, 1295–1300.

Corder, E. H., Saunders, A. M., Strittmatter, W. J., Schmechel, D. E., Gaskell, P. C., Small, G. W., Roses, A. D., Haines, J. L., & Pericak-Vance, M. A. (1993). Gene dose of apolipoprotein E type 4 allele and the risk of Alzheimer's disease in late onset families. *Science, 261*, 921–923.

Corder, E. H., Saunders, A. M., Risch, N. J., Strittmatter, W. J., Schmechel, D. E., Gaskell, P. C., Jr., Rimmler, J. B., Locke, P. A., Conneally, P. M., Schmader, K. E., Small, G. W., Roses, A. D., Haines, J. L., & Pericak-Vance, M. A. (1994). Protective effect of apolipoprotein E type 2 late onset Alzheimer's disease. *Nature Genetics, 7*, 180–184.

Corsellis, J. A. N., & Brierly, J. B. (1959). Observations on the pathology of insidious dementia following head injury. *Journal of Mental Science, 105*, 714–724.

Corsellis, J. A. N., Bruton, C. J., & Freeman-Browne, D. (1973). The aftermath of boxing. *Psychological Medicine, 3*, 270–273.

Cummings, J. L., & Benson, D. F. (1992). *Dementia: A clinical approach* (2nd ed.). Stoneham, MA: Butterworth-Heinemann.

Dalmady-Israel, C., & Zasler, N. D. (1993). Post-traumatic seizures: A critical review. *Brain Injury, 7*, 263–273.

Davis, C. S., & Acton, P. (1988). Treatment of the elderly brain-injured patient: Experience in a traumatic brain injury unit. *Journal of the American Geriatrics Society, 36*, 225–229.

Deaton, A. Y. (1990, August). *Brain injuries in persons over 50: Different issues, different goals*. Paper presented at the annual meeting of the American Psychological Association, Boston, MA.

Desai, B. T., Whitman, S., Coonley-Hoganson, R., Coleman, T. E., Gabriel, G., & Dell, J. (1983). Urban head injury: A clinical series. *Journal of the National Medical Association, 75*, 875–881.

Dries, D. J., & Gamelli, R. L. (1992). Issues in geriatric trauma. *Medical Intelligence Unit-Trauma 2000*, 191–197.

Edna, T. H. (1987). Head injuries admitted to hospital: Epidemiology, risk factors and long-term outcome. *Journal of Oslo City Hospitals, 37*, 101–116.

Faden, A. I., Demediuk, P., Panter, S. S., & Vink, R. (1989). The role of excitatory amino acids and NMDA receptors in traumatic brain injury. *Science, 244*, 798–800.

Fields, R. (1991). The effects of head injuries in older adults [Abstract]. *Clinical Neuropsychologist, 5*, 252.

Fields, R. (1994, November). *Traumatic brain injury in the elderly*. Paper presented at the annual meeting of the National Academy of Neuropsychology, Orlando, FL.

Fields, R. B., & Ackerman, M. (1991, October). *Differential outcome following mild head injury due to age and type of injury*. Paper presented at the National Academy of Neuropsychology, Dallas, TX.

Fields, R., & Coffey, C. (1994). Traumatic brain injury. In C. E. Coffey & J. L. Cummings (Eds.), *Textbook of geriatric neuropsychiatry* (pp. 470–507). Washington DC: American Psychiatric Press.

Fields, R. B., Taylor, C., & Starratt, G. (1993). Neuropsychiatric complaints following geriatric head injury [abstract]. *Archives of Clinical Neuropsychology, 8*, 223–224.

Fife, D., Faich, G., Hollinshead, W., & Boynton, W. (1986). Incidence and outcome of hospital-treated head injury in Rhode Island. *American Journal of Public Health, 76*, 773–778.

Fogel, B., & Duffy, J. (1994). Elderly patients. In J. M. Silver, S. C. Yudofsky, & R. E. Hales (Eds.), *Neuropsychiatry of traumatic brain injury* (pp. 412–441). Washington DC: American Psychiatric Press.

Frankowski, R. F. (1986). Descriptive epidemiological studies of head injury in the United States: 1974–1984. *Advances in Psychosomatic Medicine, 16*, 153–172.

Gennarelli, T. A. (1993). Mechanisms of brain injury. *Journal of Emergency Medicine, 11*, 5–11.

Giaccone, G., Tagliavani, F., Linoli, G., Bouras, C., Frigerio, L., Frangione, B., & Bugiani, O. (1989). Down's patients: Extracellular preamyloid deposits precede neuritic degeneration and senile plaques. *Neuroscience Letters, 97*, 232–238.

Goldstein, F. C., Levin, H. S., Presley, R. M., Searcy, J., Colohan, A. R. T., Eisenberg, H. M., Jann, B., & Bertolino-Kusnerik, L. (1994). Neurobehavioral consequences of closed head injury in older adults. *Journal of Neurology, Neurosurgery, and Psychiatry, 57*, 961–966.

Goldstein, F. C., Levin, H. S., Roberts, V. J., Goldman, W. P., Kalechstein, A. S., Winslow, M., & Goldstein, S. A. (1996). Neuropsychological effects of closed head injury in older adults: A comparison with Alzheimer's disease. *Neuropsychology, 7*, 147–154.

Graves, A. B., White, E., Koepsell, T. D., Reifler, B. V., van Belle, G., Larson, E., & Raskind, M. (1990). The association between head trauma and Alzheimer's disease. *American Journal of Epidemiology, 131*, 491–501.

Hamm, R. J., Jenkins, L. W., Lyeth, B. G., White-Gbadebo, D. M., & Hayes, R. L. (1991). The effect of age on outcome following traumatic brain injury in rats. *Journal of Neurosurgery, 75*, 916–921.

Hamm, R. J., White-Gbadebo, D. M., Lyeth, B. G., Jenkins, L. W., & Hayes, R. L. (1992). The effect of age on motor and cognitive deficits after traumatic brain injury in rats. *Neurosurgery, 31*, 1072–1078.

Hardy, J. (1994). Alzheimer's disease: Clinical molecular genetics. *Alzheimer's Disease Update, 10*, 239–247.

Hardy, J., & Allsop, D. (1991). Amyloid deposition as the central event in the aetiology of Alzheimer's disease. *Trends in Pharmacological Science, 12*, 383–388.

Hardy, J. A., & Higgins, G. A. (1992). Alzheimer's disease: The amyloid cascade hypothesis. *Science, 256*, 184–185.

Henderson, A. S., Jorm, A. F., Kortem, B. S., Creasey, H., McCusker, E., Broe, G. A., Longley, W., & Anthony, J. C. (1992). Environmental risk factors for Alzheimer's disease: Their relationship to age of onset and to familial or sporadic types. *Psychological Medicine, 22*, 429–436.

Heyman, A., Wilkinson, W. E., Stafford, J. A., Helms, M. J., Sigmon, A. H., & Weinberg, T. (1984). Alzheimer's disease: A study of epidemiological aspects. *Annals of Neurology, 15*, 335–341.

Ip, R. Y., Dornan, J., & Schentag, C. (1995). Traumatic brain injury: Factors predicting return to work or school. *Brain Injury, 9*, 517–532.

Jennett, B., & Bond, M. R. (1975). Assessment of outcome after severe brain injury: A practical scale. *Lancet, 1*, 480–484.

Kang, J., Lemaire, H.-G., Unterbeck, A., Salbaum, J. M., Masters, C. L., Grzeschik, K.-H., Multhaup, G., Beyreuther, K., & Muller-Hill, B. (1987). The precursor of Alzheimer's disease amyloid A4 protein resembles a cell-surface receptor. *Nature, 325*, 733–736.

Katayama, Y., Becker, D. P., Tamura, T., & Hovda, D. A. (1990). Massive increases in extracellular potassium and the indiscriminate release of glutamate following concussive brain injury. *Journal of Neurosurgery, 73*, 889–900.

Katz, D. I. (1992). Neuropathology and neurobehavioral recovery from closed head injury. *Journal of Head Trauma Rehabilitation, 7*, 1–15.

Kotwica, Z., & Jakubowski, J. K. (1992). Acute head injuries in the elderly: An analysis of 136 consecutive patients. *Acta Neurochirurgica, 118*, 98–102.

Kraus, J. F., Black, M. A., Hessol, N., Ley, P., Rokaw, W., Sullivan, C., Bowers, S., Knowlton, S., & Marshall, L. (1984). The incidence of acute brain injury and serious impairment in a defined population. *American Journal of Epidemiology, 119,* 186–201.

Levin, H. (1995, February). *Closed head injury in older adults: Assessment by the neurobehavioral rating scale.* Paper presented at the annual meeting of the International Neuropsychological Society, Seattle, WA.

Levin, H. S., Benton, A. L., & Grossman, R. G. (1982). *Neurobehavioral consequences of closed head injury.* New York: Oxford University Press.

Levin, H. S., Gary, H. E., Eisenberg, H. M., Ruff, R. M., Barth, J. T., Kreutzer, J., High, W. M., Portman, S., Foulkes, M. A., Jane, J. A., Marmarou, A., & Marshall, L. F. (1990). Neurobehavioral outcome 1 year after severe head injury. *Journal of Neurosurgery, 73,* 699–709.

Levin, H. S., Hamilton, W. J., & Grossman, R. G. (1990). Outcome after head injury. In R. Braakman (Ed.), *Handbook of clinical neurology* (Vol. 13, pp. 367–395). New York: Elsevier Science Publishers.

Luerssen, T. G., Klauber, M. R., & Marshall, L. F. (1988). Outcome from head injury related to patient's age: A longitudinal study of adult and pediatric head injury. *Journal of Neurosurgery, 69,* 409–416.

Mahley, R. W. (1988). Apolipoprotein E: Cholesterol transport protein with expanding role in cell biology. *Science, 240,* 622–630.

Mayeux, R., Ottman, R., Tang, M., Noboa-Bauza, L., Marder, K., Gurland, B., & Stern, Y. (1993). Genetic susceptibility and head injury as risk factors for Alzheimer's disease among community-dwelling elderly persons and their first-degree relative. *Annals of Neurology, 33,* 494–501.

Mayeux, R., Stern, Y., Ottman, R., Tatemichi, T. K., Tang, M., Maestre, G., Ngai, C., Tycko, B., & Ginsberg, G. (1993). The apolipoprotein E4 allele in patients with Alzheimer's disease. *Annals of Neurology, 34,* 752–754.

Mayeux, R., Ottman, R., Maestre, G., Ngai, C., Tang, M.-X., Ginsberg, H., Chun, M., Tycko, B., & Shelanski, M. (1995). Synergistic effects of traumatic head injury and apolipoprotein-e4 in patients with Alzheimer's disease. *Neurology, 45,* 555–557.

Mazzucchi, A., Cattelani, R., Missale, G., Gugliotta, M., Brianti, R., & Parma, M. (1992). Head-injured subjects aged over 50 years: Correlations between variables of trauma and neuropsychological follow-up. *Journal of Neurology, 239,* 256–260.

Miller, J. D., & Pentland, B. (1989). The factors of age, alcohol, and multiple injury in patients with mild and moderate head injury. In J. T. Hoff, T. E. Anderson, & T. M. Cole, (Eds.), *Mild to moderate head injury* (pp. 125–133). Boston: Blackwell Scientific.

Mortimer, J. A., French, L. R., Hutton, J. T., & Schuman, L. M. (1985). Head injury as a risk for Alzheimer's disease. *Neurology, 35,* 264–267.

Mortimer, J. A., Van Duijn, C. M., Chandra, V. V., Fratiglioni, L., Graves, A. B., Heyman, A., Jorm, A. F., Kokmen, E., Kondo, K., Rocca, W. A., Shalat, S. L., Soininen, H., & Hofman, A. (1991). Head trauma as a risk factor for Alzheimer's disease: A

collaborative reanalysis of case control studies. *International Journal of Epidemiology, 20,* S28–S35.

Murrell, J., Farlow, M., Ghetti, B., & Benson, M. (1991). A mutation in the amyloid protein associated with hereditary Alzheimer's disease. *Science, 254,* 97–99.

Nandy, K. (1981). Senile dementia: A possible immune hypothesis. In J. A. Mortimer & L. M. Schuman (Eds.), *The epidemiology of dementia* (pp. 87–100). New York: Oxford University Press.

Naugle, R. I. (1990). Epidemiology of traumatic brain injury in adults. In E. D. Bigler (Ed.), *Traumatic brain injury* (pp. 69–103). Austin, TX: Pro-Ed.

Ommaya, A. K., Grubb, R. L., & Naumann, R. A. (1971). Coup and contrecoup injury: Observations on the mechanics of visible brain injuries in the rhesus monkey. *Journal of Neurosurgery, 35,* 368–370.

Oster, C. (1977). Signs of sensory deprivation versus cerebral injury in post-hip fracture patients. *Journal of the American Geriatrics Society, 25,* 368–370.

Parker, R. S. (1990). *Traumatic brain injury and neuropsychological impairment.* New York: Springer-Verlag.

Parkinson, D., Stephenson, S., & Phillips, S. (1985). Head injuries: A prospective, computerized study. *Canadian Journal of Surgery, 28,* 79–83.

Pentland, B., Jones, P. A., Roy, C. W., & Miller, J. D. (1986). Head injury in the elderly. *Age and Ageing, 15,* 193–202.

Poirier, J., Davignon, J., Bouthellier, D., Kogan, S., Bertand, P., & Gauthier, S. (1993). Apolipoprotein E polymorphism in Alzheimer's disease. *Lancet, 342,* 697–699.

Ponsford, J. L., Olver, J. H., Curran, C., & Ng, K. (1995). Prediction of employment status 2 years after traumatic brain injury. *Brain Injury, 9,* 11–20.

Rakier, A., Guilburd, J. N., Soustiel, J. F., Zaaroor, M., & Feinsod, M. (1995). Head injuries in the elderly. *Brain Injury 9,* 187–193.

Rasmusson, D. X., Brandt, J., Martin, D. B., & Folstein, M. F. (1995). Head injury as a risk factor in Alzheimer's disease. *Brain Injury, 9,* 213–219.

Rebeck, G. W., Reiter, J. S., Strickland, D. K., & Hyman, B. T. (1993). Apolipoprotein E in sporadic Alzheimer's disease: Allelic variation and receptor interactions. *Neuron, 11,* 575–580.

Richardson, J. T. E. (1990). *Clinical and neuropsychological aspects of closed head injury.* London: Taylor & Francis.

Roberts, A. J. (1969). *Brain damage in boxers.* London: Pitman.

Roberts, G. W., Allsop, D., & Bruton, C. (1990). The occult aftermath of boxing. *Journal of Neurology, Neurosurgery, and Psychiatry, 53,* 373–378.

Roberts, G. W., Gentleman, S. M., Lynch, A., & Graham, D. I. (1991). BA4 amyloid protein deposition in brain after head trauma. *Lancet, 338,* 1422–1423.

Roberts, G. W., Gentleman, S. M., Lynch, A., Murray, L., Landon, M., & Graham, D. I. (1994). Beta amyloid protein deposition in the brain after severe head injury: Implications for the pathogenesis of Alzheimer's disease. *Journal of Neurology, Neurosurgery, and Psychiatry, 57,* 419–425.

Roy, C. W., Pentland, B., & Miller, J. D. (1986). The causes and consequences of minor head injury in the elderly. *Injury, 17,* 220–223.

Rubinsztein, D. C. (1995). Apolipoprotein E: A review of its roles in lipoprotein metabolism, neuronal growth and repair and as a risk factor for Alzheimer's disease. *Psychological Medicine, 25,* 223–229.

Rubinsztein, D. C., Hanlon, C. S., Irving, R. M., Goodburn, S., Evans, D. G., Kellar-Wood, H., Xuereb, J. H., Bandmann, O., & Harding, A. E. (1994). Apo E genotypes in multiple sclerosis, Parkinson's disease, schwannomas and late-onset Alzheimer's disease. *Molecular and Cellular Probes, 8,* 519–526.

Ruff, R. M., Marshall, L. F., Klauber, M. R., Blunt, B. A., Grant, I., Foulkes, M. A., Eisenberg, H., Jane, J., & Marmarou, A. (1990). Alcohol abuse and neurological outcome of the severely head injured. *Journal of Head Trauma Rehabilitation, 5,* 21–31.

Ruff, R. M., Marshall, L. F., Crouch, J., Klauber, M. R., Levin, H. S., Barth, J., Kreutzer, J., Blunt, B. A., Foulkes, M. A., Eisenberg, H. M., Jane, J. A., & Marmarou, A. (1993). Predictors of outcome following severe head trauma: Follow-up data from the traumatic coma data bank. *Brain Injury, 7,* 101–111.

Satz, P. (1991, August). *Threshold theory: Brain reserve capacity on symptom onset after brain injury: A formulation and review of evidence.* Paper presented at the annual meeting of the American Psychological Association, San Francisco, CA.

Saunders, A. M., Strittmatter, W. J., Schmechel, D., St. George-Hyslop, P. H., Perical-Vance, M. A., Joo, S. H., Rosi, B. L., Gusella, J. F., Crapper-Maclachlan, M. D., Alberts, M. J., Hulette, C., Crain, B., Goldgaber, D., & Roses, A. D. (1993). Association of apolipoprotein E allele (e4) with late onset familial and sporadic Alzheimer's disease. *Neurology, 43,* 1467–1472.

Schmechel, D. E., Saunders, A. M., Strittmatter, W. J., Crain, B. J., Hulette, C. M., Joo, S. H., Pericak-Vance, M. A., Goldgaber, D., & Roses, A. D. (1993). Increased amyloid B-peptide deposition in cerebral cortex as a consequence of apolipoprotein E genotype in late-onset Alzheimer disease. *Proceedings of the National Academy of Sciences, USA, 90,* 9649–9653.

Schneider, J. A., Gearing, M., Robbins, R. S., de l'Aune, W., & Mirra, S. S. (1995). Apolipoprotein E genotype in diverse neurodegenerative disorders. *Annals of Neurology, 38,* 131–135.

Selkoe, D. J. (1993). Physiological production of the amyloid B-protein and the mechanism of Alzheimer's disease. *Trends in Neuroscience, 16,* 403–409.

Shimano, H., Ishibashi, S., Murase, T., Gotohda, T., Yamada, N., Takaku, F., & Ohtomo, E. (1989). Plasma apolipoproteins in patients with multi-infarct dementia. *Atherosclerosis, 79,* 257–260.

Sims, A. C. P. (1985). Head injury, neurosis and accident proneness. *Advances in Psychosomatic Medicine, 13,* 49–70.

Sorenson, S. B., & Kraus, J. F. (1991). Occurrence, severity, and outcomes of brain injury. *Journal of Head Trauma Rehabilitation, 6,* 1–10.

Strittmatter, W. J., Saunders, A. M., Smechel, D., Pericak-Vance, M., Enghild, J., Salvesen, G. S., & Roses, A. D. (1993). Apolipoprotein E: High avidity binding to B-amyloid and increased frequency of type 4 allele in late-onset familial Alzheimer's disease. *Proceedings of the National Academy of Sciences, USA, 90,* 1977–1981.

Strittmatter, W. J., Weisgraber, K. H., Goedert, M., Saunders, A. M., Huang, D., Corder, E. H., Dong, L. M., Jakes, R., Alberts, M. J., Gilbert, J. R., Han, S. H., Hulette, C., Einstein, G., Schmechel, D. E., Pericak-Vance, M. A., & Roses, A. D. (1994). Hypothesis: Microtubule instability and paired helical filament formation in the Alzheimer disease brain are related to apolipoprotein E genotype. *Experimental Neurology, 125,* 163–171.

Tabaton, M. (1994). Research advances in the biology of Alzheimer's disease. *Alzheimer's Disease Update, 10,* 249–255.

Talbot, C., Lendon, C., Craddock, N., Shears, S., Morris, J. C., & Goate, A. (1994). Protection against Alzheimer's disease with apoE-e2. *Lancet, 343,* 1432–1433.

Taylor, C., Fields, R. B., Starratt, G., Russo, B., & Diamond, D. (1993, March). *Neuropsychiatric complaints following traumatic injury: Head injured vs. non-head injured trauma patients.* Paper presented at the annual meeting of the American Neuropsychiatric Association, San Antonio, TX.

Teasdale, G., & Jennett, B. (1974). Assessment of coma and impaired consciousness: A practical scale. *Lancet, 2,* 81–84.

Utermann, G., Langenbeck, U., Beisiegel, U., & Weber, W. (1980). Genetics of the apolipoprotein E system in man. *American Journal of Human Genetics, 32,* 339–347.

Van Duijn, C. M., Tanja, T. A., Haaxma, R., Schulte, W., Saan, R. J., Lameris, A. J., Antonides-Hendriks, G., & Hofman, A. (1992). Head trauma and the risk of Alzheimer's disease. *American Journal of Epidemiology, 135,* 775–781.

Vollmer, D. G., Torner, J. C., Jane, J. A., Sadovnic, B., Charlebois, D., Eisenberg, H. M., Foulkes, M. A., Marmarou, A., & Marshall, L. F. (1991). Age and outcome following traumatic coma: Why do older patients fare worse? *Journal of Neurosurgery, 75,* S37–S49.

Williams, D. B., Annegers, J. F., Kokmen, E., O'Brien, P. C., & Kurland, L. T. (1991). Brain injury and neurologic sequelae: A cohort study of dementia, parkinsonism and amyotrophic lateral sclerosis. *Neurology, 41,* 1554–1557.

Young, L., Fields, R. B., & Lovell, M. (1995). Neuropsychological differentiation of geriatric head injury from dementia (abstract). *Journal of Neuropsychiatry, 7,* 414.

20

Aphasia

PELAGIE M. BEESON AND KATHRYN A. BAYLES

Introduction

Aphasia is an acquired language impairment that results from brain damage to the language dominant hemisphere, typically the left. This clinical entity holds a prominent place in the history of neurology and psychology, as it inspired much of the theoretical development of the anatomical basis of language (Benton & Joynt, 1960; Geschwind, 1963; Joynt & Benson, 1984). In 1836, Marc Dax, a French military surgeon, made the clinical observation that damage to the left side of the brain often resulted in "a loss of memory for words" (Dax, 1865/1984). Dax's work went unpublished for almost 30 years, and it was Paul Broca who engendered interest in the study of aphasia in the 1860s with his case presentations to the Anthropological Society in Paris. In 1861 he described two patients whose aphasia followed lesions to the left frontal lobe, and in 1863, he described eight more cases. After two more years of clinical study, Broca stated, "the loss of speech without the paralysis of the organs of articulation and without the destruction of the intellect, is linked to lesions of the third frontal convolution" (as cited in Berker, Berker, & Smith, 1986, p. 1066).

Several years later, Carl Wernicke (1874) identified a different lesion location associated with an aphasia profile unlike the cases presented by Broca. More importantly, Wernicke set forth an anatomical association model that accounted for aphasia within the context of existing knowledge about the brain (Geschwind, 1963; Wernicke, 1874). The ensuing

four decades was a vigorous epoch in the study of aphasia, language, and brain–behavior relations. Wernicke's model was elaborated by Lichtheim (1885), with significant contributions made by Dejerine (1892), Liepmann (1895), and others. By the turn of the 19th century, several relatively distinct patterns of language impairment had been identified, from which current aphasia classification systems had their beginnings.

The Wernicke-Lichtheim model of aphasia evolved to its modern form through the contributions of Geschwind, Benson, Goodglass, and their Boston colleagues in the 1960s and thus became known to North Americans as the Boston classification system. Other classification systems were developed over the past century (Goldstein, 1948; Luria & Hutton, 1977; Weisenberg & McBride, 1935), but there has been general consistency in the identification of key features of several aphasia syndromes.

The neuroanatomical bases of aphasia classification derive from the relatively invariant location of primary motor and sensory regions in the brain and their adjacent association areas. Lesions anterior to the central fissure are likely to affect motor control and motor planning and thus, the fluency of verbal expression. Similarly, lesions close to the primary auditory region (the posterior, superior temporal lobe) are likely to interfere with auditory comprehension. Because repetition requires relatively intact auditory processing and verbal expression, significant damage anywhere adjacent to the sylvian fissure (i.e., the perisylvian region) may cause disruption; in contrast, preservation of the region leaves repetition relatively intact even though significant language impairment can result from extraperisylvian lesions. Despite these estab-

PELAGIE M. BEESON and KATHRYN A. BAYLES
• National Center for Neurogenic Communication Disorders, University of Arizona, Tucson, Arizona 85721.

298

lished brain–behavior relations, prediction of lesion location from a language profile is only moderately successful because the complex processes underlying language use are widely distributed and vary across individuals.

Classical aphasia syndromes have been criticized as grossly oversimplifying the psycholinguistic and cognitive profiles of affected individuals (Caplan, 1992; Caramazza, 1984). Caramazza, in particular, has been critical of the experimental grouping of subjects by aphasia type with the expectation of homogeneity in lesion location and language deficits within groups. He argues that "brain damage rarely affects a single processing component totally while completely sparing other processing components" (p. 14) and that an "exhaustive" analysis is necessary in order to isolate and examine each processing component that is critical for language in a given individual. Caplan (1992) was similarly critical, noting that the correlation between aphasia syndromes and lesion location should not be taken as evidence that aphasia syndromes reflect disturbances of specific language processors.

We agree that classical aphasia syndromes permit prediction of lesion locations only in a general sense and that aphasia classification does not provide specific information about the nature of language impairment in a given individual. Thus, clinical and research endeavors often demand careful psycholinguistic analysis of language processing, rather than designation of aphasia type. Given that caveat, we believe the relations among aphasia type and lesion location are sufficiently predictable to be clinically useful. More importantly, aphasia taxonomies provide clinicians with an efficient way to designate the cluster of signs observed in a given individual. As such, they are worthy of review.

Aphasia Assessment for Classification

Benton and Joynt (1960) traced the term *aphasia* to its derivation from a Greek word *aphasis* used by the Greek Skeptics in the second century to refer to a philosophy of "nonassertion." The term had no relation to the concept of disordered language; rather it referred to "a condition of mind, according to which we can say that we neither affirm nor deny

anything" (Benton & Joynt, 1960, p. 111/207). In effect, the term captures the essence of the problem faced by a severely aphasic individual: the inability to communicate verbally. The language impairment is rarely complete, however, so *dysphasia* is a more accurate descriptor than aphasia, but the latter has become preferable by convention. Although impaired verbal expression is the most salient feature of aphasia, in most cases, all input and output language modalities are affected: speech, auditory comprehension, reading, and writing.

At present, aphasia syndromes typically are differentiated on the basis of the fluency of spontaneous speech and the adequacy of auditory comprehension, spoken repetition, and confrontation naming. Informal assessment of aphasia can yield fairly reliable aphasia classification for those individuals who exhibit a prototypical aphasia type; our clinical impression is that some 30% to 40% of acutely aphasic individuals can be classified accurately using a decision process such as that depicted in Figure 1.

A more precise and reliable determination of aphasia type is accomplished by means of standardized aphasia tests, such as the Boston Diagnostic Aphasia Examination (Goodglass & Kaplan, 1983), the Western Aphasia Battery (Kertesz, 1982), and the Aphasia Diagnostic Profiles (Helm-Estabrooks, 1992). Such tests use a systematic sampling of language behaviors and criteria for aphasia classification and provide an indication of severity across language domains. With formal assessment, Wertz et al. (1981) found that 76% of 92 aphasic individuals studied were classifiable by aphasia type.

Fluency

Speech and language fluency typically are examined during conversation and descriptive discourse (as in a picture description task). Nonfluent aphasias are characterized by effortful, hesitant speech that may be poorly articulated, and the prosodic melody of spontaneous speech is disrupted. Language is nonfluent because of a reduction in the length and syntactic complexity of utterances. As a rule of thumb, individuals with nonfluent aphasia rarely produce sentences longer than four words and these sentences often lack "little words" such as articles and prepositions, termed "functors." Table

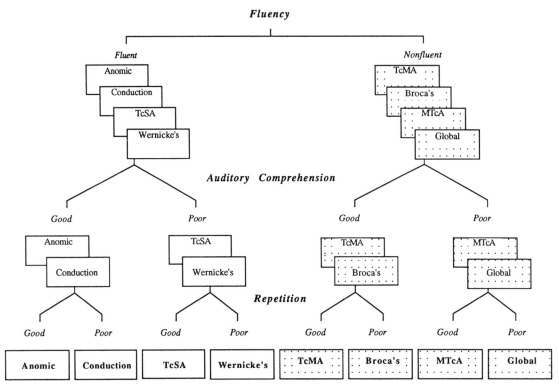

FIGURE 1. Decision tree to guide the classification of aphasia type based upon fluency of spontaneous speech, auditory comprehension, and verbal repetition. TcSA, transcortical sensory aphasia; TcMA, transcortical motor aphasia; MTcA, mixed transcortical aphasia.

1 indicates four nonfluent aphasia types and four fluent aphasia types.

Fluent aphasias are characterized by well-articulated utterances of normal length and prosodic variation. However, utterances often are marred by errors in word choice (i.e., semantic or verbal paraphasias) or sound substitution errors (i.e., phonemic or literal paraphasias), which make them difficult to understand. Nonwords, or neologisms, are produced when sounds are completely off target, so that some utterances are strings of nonwords constituting neologistic jargon.

Auditory Comprehension

Auditory comprehension typically is assessed using tasks of increasing complexity: from the comprehension of single words, to following simple and complex commands, to understanding sentences or paragraphs. Single-word comprehension may be influenced by word frequency, grammatical class (e.g., noun vs. verb), or semantic category (e.g., colors vs. body parts). Even in severely aphasic individuals, comprehension often is preserved for some natural requests, such as "close your eyes" or

Table 1. Aphasia Syndromes Based upon the Boston Classification System

Fluency		
Nonfluent	Fluent	Lesion location
Broca's	Wernicke's	Perisylvian
Global	Conduction	
Transcortical motor	Transcortical sensory	Extraperisylvian
Mixed transcortical	Anomic	

"sit down." The ability to follow commands often deteriorates as requests become complex or place demands on auditory short-term memory. Tasks that require comprehension of connected sentences are most akin to listening in the real world, and frequently there is impairment to some extent even with mild aphasia. However, language in its natural context is often syntactically simple and rich with nonverbal cues so that comprehension of conversation may be surprisingly good. This paradox can give a false impression of intact auditory comprehension, thus validating the need for structured assessment of auditory comprehension.

Repetition

The ability to repeat spoken utterances is of clinical importance because successful verbal repetition appears to depend on an intact perisylvian region. Therefore, aphasia-producing lesions outside of the region surrounding the sylvian fissure (i.e., extraperisylvian) typically preserve the ability to repeat. Repetition is assessed using single words (typically nouns), short phrases, and sentences of increasing length. This progression allows the examiner to observe the point at which repetition breaks down. In the case of perisylvian lesions, repeated utterances tend to be qualitatively similar to spontaneous speech; in contrast, individuals with extraperisylvian lesions may show strikingly superior repetition in comparison to spontaneous output.

Naming

The ability to name objects or pictured items and events is impaired to some extent in all types of aphasia; therefore, impairment of naming ability offers little information specific to lesion localization or aphasia type. In the case of anomic aphasia, naming difficulty may be the *only* language deficit. It is important to examine naming across a variety of word classes and semantic categories. Individuals with aphasia are sensitive to word frequency; more frequently used words tend to be more accessible than those less frequently used. The retrieval of substantive words may be better in running speech than in confrontation naming tasks, and word sub-

stitutions or circumlocutions may mask some instances of anomia.

Reading and Writing

Reading and writing often are impaired in aphasic individuals similar to auditory-verbal deficits. Reading and writing impairments do not determine aphasia classification and are sometimes referred to as "aphasic alexia" and "aphasic dysgraphia," respectively (Friedman & Albert, 1985). However, a careful analysis of reading and writing may reveal impairment of component processes suggestive of specific dyslexic or dysgraphic syndromes. Psycholinguistic analysis of reading and writing disorders is an active area of research, and the reader is referred to recent reviews (Coultheart, Patterson, & Marshall, 1987; Friedman, Ween, & Albert, 1993; Roeltgen, 1993).

Aphasia Syndromes

Aphasias Associated with Perisylvian Lesions

Broca's Aphasia

Broca's aphasia is characterized by nonfluent verbal expression and slow, hesitant, telegraphic speech. Utterances are of reduced length and grammatical complexity, consisting predominantly of nouns with some verbs and descriptive adjectives. They notably lack articles, prepositions, other function words, and grammatical endings of words, such as -ing or -es. This reduction or lack of grammatical structure and morphological markers is referred to as agrammatism and is a relatively common feature of Broca's aphasia. Verbal repetition usually is commensurate with expressive language ability and therefore is restricted to single words or short phrases. Auditory comprehension often is a relative strength and should be adequate for simple conversational interaction. However, auditory comprehension of syntax and morphological markers is frequently impaired. Naming performance is variable.

In the following excerpt from a transcript of an

individual with Broca's aphasia who is describing the picnic scene* from the Western Aphasia Battery (WAB; Kertesz, 1981), the hesitant, telegraphic nature of the verbal output is apparent.

> Is family, um, picnic. And fish, and man is, um, oh, um, reading, and, and, um … Lady is pouring … and sit, um. Son is, is *ha* … is, um, is, um, flying kite. And neighbor is fishing. And neighbor is, um, sailing. And boy is, um, playing in water. And man and lady in … listen to radio … And *daughter*, I mean, dog, oh, *s* …, oh, *s* …, is lady … is man … is *stave, stave* … oh *stay* … I don't know.

Some reading ability may be present, particularly for content words, although semantic errors are not uncommon. Those with severe Broca's aphasia are likely to recognize only highly familiar words. Often there is difficulty associating the correct sound with a given letter so that reading nonwords is not possible, a condition referred to as phonological dyslexia (Marshall & Newcombe, 1973; Patterson, 1981). Writing abilities vary but typically are commensurate with spoken language, yielding somewhat telegraphic, meaningful sentences. Spelling errors are common.

Lesion Characteristics.   Persistent Broca's aphasia is associated with large lesions that not only include Broca's area, but extend superiorly and posteriorly into the Rolandic regions and the anterior parietal lobe. The insula and basal ganglia structures frequently are damaged as well (Mohr, 1976). A small cortical lesion to Broca's area proper does not result in classic Broca's aphasia, but rather in a relatively transient aphasia characterized by mutism, which resolves to apraxia of speech, with no agrammatism or comprehension impairment (Mohr, 1976).

Accompanying Deficits.   Right hemiparesis and hemisensory loss are common in Broca's aphasia, and handwriting often is switched to the nondominant hand. An impairment of motor planning may be exhibited by the left hand and arm (i..e., limb apraxia). The motor speech disorders of dys-

---

*The picture includes a man and a woman having a picnic: the man is reading a book; the woman is pouring a drink; a boy nearby is flying a kite; there is a lake in the distance where people are sailing, fishing, and playing in the sand. Italics are used in the transcriptions to indicate false starts and phonemic and semantic paraphasias.

arthria and apraxia frequently reduce speech intelligibility. Dysarthria, an impairment of speech production due to muscle weakness, slowness, or incoordination, results in imprecise consonant production (Darley, Aronson, & Brown, 1975). An impairment of volitional speech movements, referred to by some as apraxia of speech, results in inconsistent articulatory errors and is thought to reflect an impairment in motor planning for speech (Darley et al., 1975; Square-Storer, 1989). Although there is disagreement as to whether apraxia of speech is an entity apart from aphasia, there is consensus that individuals with Broca's aphasia often have a disorder of phonetic realization (Goodglass, 1993).

Wernicke's Aphasia

Wernicke's aphasia is characterized by fluent speech that may be difficult to comprehend because of the presence of phonemic and semantic paraphasias and neologistic jargon. Utterances often are paragrammatic, that is, they violate the rules of syntax and grammar. Verbal repetition is impaired, typically regardless of the length of the utterance. Auditory comprehension is poor, and the ability to name objects is often quite poor. Individuals with Wernicke's aphasia may be overly talkative, as demonstrated by the WAB picture description given by one of our patients:

> Well here's a, here's a, uh, a man and a *kusbit, kus, kus*, I don't know, a *wuzman*. What's a husband. Yea, a husband. A wife and a husband. And he had a *mack*. And, something to read, read a *cupture*. This was his wife with a napkin and looking at food. And then there was their napkin sitting on this thing. Uh, a child with a little girl on a *map*. I guess she was a little girl, a child, a maybe young person. On the, on the *rip, rip*, oo, I can't say that, anyway. And here with the man, and a bird. I guess there were several people on this *swail*, on this *swait*. Here was another bird. This is a child I guess. Oh, *sanding*. They were *sanding*. Did I say this, here was a girl on a bird. *Swai*. Here was a child with a tree. A card here. Handkerchiefs. Uh, a *tr*, I think that's … oh, and that *map* on the thing, more or less.

Reading ability usually parallels auditory comprehension and may be limited to recognition of some content words; however, reading ability can be relatively preserved in some (Heilman, Rothi,

Campanella, & Wolfson, 1979). Oral reading may contain paraphasias similar to spontaneous speech. Writing typically mirrors spontaneous speech. Less severely impaired individuals may exhibit paragrammatic writing that parallels spoken output, characterized by misuse of functors and morphological endings. Individuals with more severe Wernicke's aphasia may produce writing that is unintelligible or limited to partial lexical knowledge of content words (i.e., ability to write only part of a word).

Lesion Characteristics. Lesions associated with Wernicke's aphasia are in the posterior superior temporal lobe, often extending posteriorly and superiorly into the angular gyrus. Selnes, Knopman, Niccum, and Rubens (1985) found that damage to Wernicke's area was consistently associated with persistent repetition deficits. Restoration of patients' auditory comprehension deficits is thought to be dependent upon sparing of the supramarginal and angular gyri (Kertesz, Lau, & Polk, 1993).

Accompanying Deficits. Wernicke's aphasia may exist in the absence of any other notable neurological deficit, but a visual field defect affecting the upper right quadrant or a complete right hemianopia can coexist. Right hemisensory loss may exist as well.

Conduction Aphasia

Conduction aphasia is characterized by fluent verbal expression and relatively intact auditory comprehension, but verbal repetition is markedly impaired. Paraphasias are prevalent in naming and in repetition, particularly phonemic paraphasias. Patients are often aware of their paraphasic errors and may attempt self-correction repeatedly, a phenomenon referred to as *conduit d'approche*. The speech of individuals with conduction aphasia tends to be well articulated, and grammatical morphemes (such as -ing and -ed) and syntactic constructions can be preserved. The WAB picture description of one of our patients exemplifies the paraphasic output of conduction aphasia and the characteristic *conduit d'approche* as he tried to say the word "picnic" and in another episode with an unknown target for "kank":

About the car, you mean, and the … and a dog and they're in the … and one of the kids, I guess it is in the … I don't know what you'd call … I guess that's a *late*, lake … *Sa … san* … I can't think what it is. And this one's fishing. *Kank*, no. I don't know what she's doin'. And they're having a *pinick, pinick, pick*, picnic *picnickick*, picnic. Is that right? And that's what they're here about, I guess. And what else would a … I can't what the … and a *kank*. *Kank, kank, kank*, no it isn't either … *Sink, kank, kant*, I can't say it, *kank, kant, kink, kink, sank, sink*. I can't say it.

Reading comprehension may be near normal in conduction aphasia. Oral reading is remarkably spared in some individuals, whereas others produce frequent phonemic errors (phonemic paralexias) that mirror their spontaneous speech (Goodglass, 1992; Palumbo, Alexander, & Naeser, 1992). Individuals with conduction aphasia have writing and spelling that are impaired to varying degrees.

Lesion Characteristics. Wernicke (1874) proposed a disconnection theory of conduction aphasia, suggesting that it results from an interruption of the pathways connecting the auditory language and motor speech centers. Although Wernicke had not yet seen such a clinical case, he postulated that the critical connections were located in the insula. Later, Lichtheim (1885) pointed out that such a disconnection would lead to disordered repetition, and in 1901, Dejerine proposed that the arcuate fasciculus was the essential posterior-anterior pathway. This white matter bundle originates in the superior temporal gyrus, runs deep to the supramarginal gyrus, and then projects anteriorly to the dorsolateral frontal lobe. Researchers have elaborated upon the disconnection model and have found that lesions to the supramarginal gyrus and subjacent white matter are most common in conduction aphasia and that the arcuate fasciculus, as well as a shorter pathway deep to the insula, are critical (Damasio & Damasio, 1980; Geschwind, 1965; Petrides & Pandya, 1988). However, conduction aphasia also follows lesions in other portions of the temporoparietal region, so that "disconnection" hypothesis does not apply in all cases (Damasio & Damasio, 1980; Green & Howes, 1977; Palumbo et al., 1992). Conduction aphasia results from left posterior perisylvian lesions that are typically smaller and have lesser extension into the superior temporal gyrus than those that result in Wernicke's aphasia (Goodglass, 1992; Kertesz, Lesk, & McCabe, 1977).

Accompanying Deficits. Conduction aphasia may be accompanied by right hemiparesis, right hemisensory loss, and right hemianopia. Limb apraxia also is seen with conduction aphasia and is severe in some cases.

Global Aphasia

Global aphasia refers to a severe language impairment in all domains. Verbal output is extremely limited and does not improve with repetition. Auditory comprehension also is severely impaired. Many individuals with global aphasia are limited to stereotypic perseverative words (e.g., "fine, fine"), short phrases (e.g., "I can see, I can see") or neologisms (e.g., "nokeydoe, nokeydoe"). Some individuals with global aphasia produce jargon; others have little verbal output.

Reading and writing are severely impaired in global aphasia. There may be recognition of a few concrete nouns. Writing of one's name and of serial numbers up to about 10 may be preserved.

Lesion Characteristics. Global aphasia typically results from extensive lesions encompassing large portions of the perisylvian region. Large lesions that spare the posterior temporoparietal region may evolve to Broca's aphasia (Mohr, 1976), but lesions that affect the entire perisylvian zone are likely to result in persistent global aphasia.

Accompanying Deficits. Global aphasia is often accompanied by right hemiparesis, right hemisensory loss, right homonymous hemianopia, limb apraxia, dysarthria, and apraxia of speech.

Aphasias Associated with Extraperisylvian Lesions

Anomic Aphasia

Individuals with anomic aphasia are fluent, have good auditory comprehension, and have good ability to repeat. Their verbal output usually is well articulated and does not contain phonemic paraphasias, but may include semantic paraphasias. The most prominent feature of this syndrome is the difficulty in word retrieval, particularly of high-content words—nouns, verbs, and adjectives. Word-finding difficulty may result in circumlocutions or the production of relatively empty utterances.

Lesion Characteristics. Anomic aphasia results from lesions in various locations including the angular gyrus and the inferior temporal gyrus (Goodglass, 1993). Whereas the acute presentation of anomic aphasia is often associated with lesions outside the perisylvian zone, anomic aphasia also is the common evolutionary endpoint of patients with all types of aphasia who make good recoveries.

Accompanying Deficits. Anomic aphasia may exist without other significant concomitant neurological deficits, but mild right-sided weakness is not uncommon.

Transcortical Motor Aphasia

Transcortical motor aphasia (TcMA) is a relatively uncommon aphasia syndrome that results from lesions outside the perisylvian zone. It is characterized by the ability to repeat but not produce spontaneous speech. Auditory comprehension is relatively preserved; ability to name is variable (Goodglass, 1993). In its acute presentation, an aphasic individual may be mute or hypophonic, and echolalia is not uncommon (Jonas, 1987). Following an initial period of speech suppression, individuals with TcMA may respond with one- or two-word utterances in a somewhat reactive manner, but propositional utterances are markedly limited. Transcortical motor aphasia resolves relatively quickly, but in some instances, residual speech dysfluency has been reported (Freedman, Alexander, & Naeser, 1984). Reading and writing may be relatively unaffected.

One of our patients, recalling his acute transcortical motor aphasia, described the odd realization that volitional, propositional speech was unavailable to him:

> I realized I couldn't talk ... I thought maybe my vocal cords were paralyzed, so I tried to make other sounds, and I could do that. I could hum, or I could make sounds, but I couldn't make a word. It was like when I tried before to move something with my mind: tele-

kinesis. It was the same feeling that I had trying to make a word ... In the hospital I couldn't talk and the nurse would come in and ask me to say what she said, and I could say it. But I couldn't think of anything to say on my own.

Lesion Characteristics. Transcortical motor aphasia was first described by Lichtheim (1885) and then elaborated upon by Wernicke (1886, 1906). Lichtheim (1885) postulated a disconnection between the "center for the elaboration of concepts" and the "center of motor images." Lesions associated with TcMA are typically anterior or superior to Broca's area, served by the vascular "watershed" zone at the periphery of the anterior branch of the middle cerebral artery. This aphasia also is observed following lesions in the medial frontal region, including the supplementary motor area and the cingulate gyrus of the language dominant hemisphere (Benson, 1993). Lesions causing TcMA are usually smaller than those resulting in Broca's or Wernicke's aphasia.

Accompanying Deficits. Right-sided weakness may result from a lesion producing TcMA, with the right leg more affected than the right arm (Alexander & Schmidt, 1980). There is no associated hemisensory loss or visual impairment.

Transcortical Sensory Aphasia

Transcortical sensory aphasia (TcSA) is characterized by fluent, paraphasic verbal expression, but remarkably preserved verbal repetition. Like individuals with TcMA, those with TcSA may be echolalic, as well as somewhat perseverative. Auditory comprehension is notably impaired. Verbal output is similar to that of Wernicke's aphasia, but is less voluble. Reading and writing often are impaired.

Lesion Characteristics. Typically TcSA results from deep lesions posterior to the perisylvian region in the temporal and parietal lobes in the watershed region between the middle and posterior cerebral arteries, or entirely in the left posterior cerebral artery distribution. A language profile consistent with TcSA is also observed in some individ-

uals with dementia, particularly of the Alzheimer's type (Appel, Kertesz, & Fisman, 1982).

Accompanying Deficits. Transcortical sensory aphasia may be accompanied by right hemianopia. In some cases, right hemisensory loss occurs, and right hemiparesis can be present because of posterior cerebral artery infarction affecting the left cerebral peduncles (Hommel et al., 1990).

Mixed Transcortical Aphasia

Mixed transcortical aphasia (MTcA) has been called isolation aphasia (Geschwind, Quadfasal, & Segarra, 1968) because the perisylvian zone is essentially isolated from the extrasylvian regions. It has the features of global aphasia, with the exception of preserved ability to repeat. Verbal output is seldom meaningful and is often characterized by stereotyped perseverative utterances (Rapcsak & Rubens, 1994). Auditory comprehension is very poor, and naming is severely limited. The preservation of repetition is found during testing, and echolalia is not uncommon (Geschwind et al., 1968). Reading and writing are also severely impaired.

Lesion Characteristics. Mixed transcortical aphasia occurs very infrequently and can follow stroke, affecting both anterior and posterior perisylvian border zones, which includes TcMA and TcSA lesion sites (Rapcsak & Rubens, 1994). Left internal carotid stenosis may result in an arc-shaped area of infarction across the vascular watershed areas of the cerebral arteries (Speedie, Coslett, & Heilman, 1984). Mixed transcortical aphasia may also result from carbon monoxide poisoning, anoxia, or generalized cortical atrophy associated with late-stage dementia (Appel et al., 1982; Whitaker, 1976).

Accompanying Deficits. In some cases MTcA may be accompanied by right hemisensory loss, right-sided weakness, or right hemianopia, but these deficits are inconsistent.

Subcortical Aphasia Syndromes

Aphasia can result from lesions that spare the cerebral cortex. Such lesions may affect the subcortical gray matter, the deep white matter connections in the language dominant hemisphere, or both. Currently the role of subcortical structures in language functions is not well understood; however, research over the past decade has confirmed the importance of the cortical-subcortical loops in language and memory functions (Alexander, Naeser, & Palumbo, 1987; Crosson, 1992; Robin & Schienberg, 1990; Wallesch, 1985). Small lesions of the thalamus, basal ganglia, or subcortical white matter usually do not result in aphasia; however, larger subcortical lesions frequently have been associated with aphasia (Alexander et al., 1987; Crosson, 1992). Significant recovery following subcortical lesions is often reported, however, persistent language impairments also have been documented (Robin & Schienberg, 1990; Wallesch, 1985). There is no single subcortical aphasia profile, but there are some consistent findings relative to lesion location and type of stroke.

Thalamic Aphasia

Crosson (1984) reviewed 37 cases of aphasia resulting from thalamic hemorrhage that were reported in the literature. He reported that hemorrhagic lesions of the dominant thalamus tend to result in a fluent aphasia characterized by semantic paraphasias which sometimes deteriorates to a jargon aphasia; auditory comprehension and verbal repetition are relatively well preserved. In contrast, a review of reported cases of thalamic lesions from infarction by Crosson (1992) indicated that "aphasia after thalamic infarction does not cohere as a syndrome like cases of aphasia after dominant thalamic hemorrhage" (p. 99). These cases included nonfluent output, with greater phonemic than semantic paraphasias, and impaired auditory comprehension together with preserved repetition. The relative preservation of repetition following hemorrhagic and nonhemorrhagic thalamic lesions produces profiles that have been likened to the transcortical aphasias (Helm-Estabrooks & Albert, 1991).

Although it is not clear which thalamic nuclei are important for language, aphasia has been associated with hemorrhage in the region of the pulvinar (i.e., posterior thalamus) and infarctions of the tuberothalamic artery, which serves the ventral anterior nuclei and portions of the anterior, ventral lateral, and dorsomedial nuclei (Crosson, 1992).

Nonthalamic Subcortical Aphasia

Nonthalamic subcortical lesions affecting the basal ganglia and deep white matter may result in several different aphasia profiles. Alexander and colleagues (1987) emphasized the importance of white matter pathways rather than striatal structures in producing language disorders. Hemorrhagic lesions to the basal ganglia have been associated with dysfluent speech (i.e., impaired speech initiation and melodic line) in the presence of fluent language (i.e., relatively normal phrase length and syntax); auditory comprehension may or may not be compromised (Alexander et al., 1987). Naeser and colleagues (1982) reported that auditory comprehension was impaired in cases where basal ganglia lesions extended into the posterior white matter, but not in cases of anterior, superior extension. The aphasia profile associated with lesions of the anterior striatum and anterior white matter may be similar to that of TcMA. The more posterior nonthalamic lesions present a fluent profile that resembles Wernicke's aphasia in some cases (Alexander et al., 1987). Global aphasia with stereotyped utterances has been reported with subcortical lesions that damage both the medial subcallosal fasciculus and the periventricular white matter (Alexander et al., 1987).

Natural Evolution of Aphasia

Some individuals have a transient aphasia because of ischemia that does not result in cell death. In most cases, however, aphasia is a persistent disorder. This does not mean that it is static. In fact, barring further neurological impairments or complications, a positive course of language recovery always ensues, but it is limited by the extent and location of lesions and the integrity of the remaining brain tissue. Improvement of language abilities is variable across modalities, and a progression through various aphasia syndromes is not uncommon (Holland & Bartlett, 1985; Kertesz & McCabe, 1977). Wertz and colleagues (1981) found that almost half of the 96 patients followed from 2 weeks to 6 months after onset of aphasia had changes in symptoms that resulted in reclassification of their aphasia type. Some of the more commonly observed changes are shown in Table 2. It should be noted as well that some individuals who are unclassifiable as to type of aphasia in the acute stage later present one of the classic types of aphasia. Improvement of auditory comprehension is most common, and typical evolutionary endpoints are anomic, Broca's, and conduction aphasias. It is important to keep in mind that there may be little correlation between lesion location and an "evolved" aphasia syndrome. These chronic aphasia syndromes result when a damaged brain continues to process language despite residual impairments and uses biological and behavioral compensations.

Some globally aphasic individuals eventually evolve to Broca's aphasia because of their improved auditory comprehension and verbal output (Mohr, 1976). In contrast, individuals with acute Broca's aphasia, particularly those with cortical lesions that do not extend deep into white matter, can resolve relatively quickly to anomic aphasia. Even some individuals with marked Broca's aphasia during the first several months can eventually recover to anomic aphasia, although it is not uncommon for them to have hesitations and pauses in their speech. Wernicke's aphasia evolves to conduction aphasia if the dense comprehension difficulties and prominent jargon aphasia recede (Goodglass, 1992). Kertesz and Benson (1970) found that neologistic jargon often resolves toward semantic paraphasias and semantic jargon in some individuals, but toward phonemic paraphasias in others. Conduction aphasia that resolves to anomic aphasia is characterized by fluent, grammatical utterances marred by significant anomia and the persistence of phonemic paraphasias in substantive words (Goodglass, 1992). TcMA and TcSA resulting from stroke tend to resolve toward anomia over time (Rapcsak & Rubens,

1994), but recovery from MTcA is highly variable (Kertesz & McCabe, 1977).

Epidemiology

Aphasia is a significant, life-changing sequel of brain damage affecting 1 million Americans (American Heart Association, 1994). The yearly incidence of new cases is estimated at 80,000 by the National Aphasia Association (Klein, 1995). Although individuals of any age can acquire aphasia, it is predominantly a disorder of the aging population; the mean age of the aphasic population in the NINDS Stroke Data Bank from 1983 to 1986 was 67.7 years (Hier, Yoon, Mohr, Price, & Wolf, 1994).

Most aphasias result from stroke (embolic, thrombolic, or hemorrhagic), but some result from trauma, neoplasms, infection or inflammatory processes, or tissue damage during surgery. Aphasia occurs in about 20% of all strokes (American Heart Association, 1994): 58% of left cortical lesions, and 22% of left deep lesions (Hier et al., 1994). It also occurs more frequently following some types of strokes than others; Hier and colleagues (1994) found 40% following cardiac emboli, 24% following atherosclerotic infarction, and about 16% following intracerebral hemorrhage.

Handedness affects the incidence of aphasia as well. Following left hemisphere lesions, left-handed individuals have a lower incidence of aphasia than right-handed individuals (32% compared to 60%, respectively); but following right hemisphere lesions, left-handed individuals have a higher incidence of aphasia (24% compared to 2%) (Benson, 1985).

Although the incidence of stroke is higher in men than women (D'Agostino, Wolf, Belanger, & Kannel, 1994), gender has little, if any, influence on the incidence of aphasia in the stroke population (Hier et al., 1994). Lesions in the same anatomical location produce similar speech and language deficits in males and females (Tranel & Damasio, 1987). Kertesz and Benke (1989) found no significant gender differences with regard to the incidence of anterior versus central versus posterior lesions in aphasic individuals; however, Hier et al. (1994) found that ischemic lesions producing aphasia were more anteriorly situated in women than in men. Also,

Table 2. Some Common Changes in Aphasia Classification over Time

Acute presentation		Chronic presentation
Global	→	Broca's
Broca's	→	Anomic
Wernicke's	→	Conduction
Conduction	→	Anomic
Transcortical sensory	→	Anomic
Transcortical motor	→	Anomic

when stroke type was examined, aphasia was more frequent in women with infarcts (as opposed to hemorrhages) than in men (Hier et al., 1994).

Findings of the relation of gender to aphasia type and severity are mixed. Some studies show that gender does not affect aphasia type or severity (Basso, Spinnler, Vallar, & Zanobio, 1982; Kertesz & Benke, 1989; Wertz et al., 1981), but others report that more women than men exhibit global, Wernicke's, and anomic aphasia (Hier et al., 1994; Schechter, Schejter, Abarbanel, Groswasser, & Solzi, 1985; Sundet, 1986) and that Broca's aphasia is somewhat more common in men (Hier et al., 1994).

The Effect of Age on Aphasia

Age and Aphasia Severity

Several researchers have reported that older individuals who acquire aphasia are likely to have more severe aphasia (Holland & Bartlett, 1985; Smith, 1971); however, others have found no relationship between age at onset and aphasia severity (Wertz et al., 1981; Wertz & Dronkers, 1990). In a study of 94 aphasic individuals who were 75 years or younger, Wertz and colleagues (1981) found no significant correlations between age and severity of aphasia. When comparing aphasic individuals younger than 60 with individuals older than 70, Holland and Bartlett (1985) found that older aphasic persons were more severely impaired and showed less spontaneous recovery than the younger group.

Age and Aphasia Type

It is well documented that individuals with Broca's aphasia are about a decade younger than those with Wernicke's and global aphasia (Basso, Bracchi, Capitani, Laiacona, & Zanobio, 1987; Eslinger & Damasio, 1981; Obler, Albert, Goodglass, & Benson, 1978; Wertz et al., 1981). The reason for this relationship is not known (Eslinger & Damasio, 1981), but Brown and Jaffe (1975) suggested that it may reflect changes in hemispheric lateralization that occur with age. If language lateralization to the dominant hemisphere increases throughout adulthood, then the right hemisphere's contribution to language may be greater in younger individuals. The right hemisphere language profile reflects rela-

tively rich lexical semantics, with impoverished syntax and phonology (Joannette, Goulet, & Hannequin, 1990; Zaidel, 1985), a profile that parallels that of Broca's aphasia (Beeson & Rapcsak, 1995; Rapcsak & Beeson, 1995). This hypothesis would also predict that global aphasia is more likely to result from large lesions in older than younger individuals, because of more complete language lateralization and decreased right hemisphere contributions to language. Several researchers have reported that individuals with global aphasia tend to be older than those having other types of aphasia (Hier et al., 1994; Holland, 1980; Obler & Albert, 1981). Individuals with conduction aphasia were found to be younger than those with Wernicke's and global aphasia by Eslinger and Damasio (1981), but Wertz et al. (1981) did not find this association in subjects tested 7 weeks after onset.

Age and Aphasia Recovery

Although the database is small, several researchers have indicated that age may not be a strong predictor of spontaneous recovery from aphasia (i.e., improvement without treatment) (Basso, Capitani, & Vignolo, 1979; Kertesz & McCabe, 1977; Wertz et al., 1981). In their large group study of aphasic individuals who were 75 years of age or younger, Wertz et al. (1981) found no significant differences in the amount of spontaneous recovery observed during a no-treatment phase among different age groups. They also found that older aphasic individuals (65- to 75-year-olds) were as likely to evolve to another aphasia type as those who were younger (45- to 55-year-olds). Culton (1969) and Kertesz and McCabe (1977) also found no significant relationship between age and language improvement. However, Holland and Bartlett (1985) found that age may limit the spontaneous recovery in individuals who are older than 75. With regard to improvement during aphasia therapy, Sarno (1980) and Wertz and Dronkers (1990) found that older adults benefited as much as younger individuals when equated along relevant variables.

Age-Related Decline in Chronic Aphasia

There has been little research on the effects of aging on individuals with chronic aphasia. It is obvious that normal aging processes interact with a compromised language system. We have observed a subgroup of individuals in our clinic who, after years of language improvement, exhibited a downturn in language abilities without any known change in physical/neurological status. Although such changes tend to occur gradually rather than abruptly, it is possible that a lesioned brain loses compensatory abilities as a function of aging.

Treatment of Aphasia

For clinical aphasiologists, the primary goal of assessment is to formulate a plan for therapeutic intervention and rehabilitation. Although determination of aphasia type and severity is of value, a finer grain analysis of language skills and weaknesses is necessary to plan language therapy adequately. Albert and Helm-Estabrooks (1988) noted that "successful treatments are based on detailed knowledge of the individual patient's cognitive and linguistic assets and deficits and on the identification of the spared and impaired brain regions and pathways that subserve these functions" (p. 1207). The goals of treatment are to (1) maximize the recovery of language, (2) assist in the development of compensatory strategies, and (3) assist aphasic individuals in their adjustment to the difference between their prior and residual language abilities (Rosenbek, LaPointe, & Wertz, 1989).

Efforts to maximize recovery of language include stimulation techniques (Duffy, 1994; Jenkins, Pabón-Jiménez, Shaw, & Sefer, 1975), programmed treatment approaches (Helm-Estabrooks & Albert, 1991), psycholinguistic approaches (Shewan & Bandur, 1994), and treatments derived from cognitive processing models (Caramazza & Hillis, 1990; Hillis, 1994; Mitchum, 1994). Treatment procedures for specific language deficits are described in sources such as *The Manual for Aphasia Therapy* (Helm-Estabrooks & Albert, 1991), *Language Intervention Strategies in Adults* (Chapey, 1994), and *Aphasia Treatment: World Perspectives* (Holland & Forbes, 1993). Clinical aphasiology has benefited from advances in cognitive psychology and psycholinguistics. Models of normal cognition and language processing have inspired the examination and treatment of component processes that can be differentially impaired by brain damage (Mitchum, 1994; Seron & Deloche, 1989). Advances in neuroradiology also have provided additional prognostic information (Knopman et al., 1983; Naeser, Palumbo, Helm-Estabrooks, Stiassny-Eder, & Albert, 1989).

The efficacy of aphasia treatment has been studied by a variety of researchers using group designs of different degrees of experimental rigor, with mixed results (for reviews, see Holland & Beeson, 1995; Rosenbek, et al., 1989; Wertz, 1987). Rosenbek et al. (1989) suggested that this body of research can be understood best if one asks the question: "Whom does aphasia treatment help?" (p. 113). Their review of aphasia efficacy research revealed that treatment helps moderately to mildly aphasic individuals who experienced single occlusive infarcts and who received treatment within 6 months of onset (Basso et al., 1979; Hagen, 1973; Shewan & Kertesz, 1984; Wertz et al., 1981, 1986). Treatment was more effective when it was provided at least 3 hours a week for 5 months or 8 to 10 hours a week for 3 months. Treatment outcomes were poor for individuals who had multiple or bilateral strokes, those who were severely aphasic and received treatment long after onset, and those who received less intense therapy (Lincoln et al., 1984; Sarno, Silverman, & Sands, 1970).

Single-subject research can document the effectiveness of specific clinical approaches for individuals with well-defined aphasic disorders (e.g., Byng, 1988; Wambaugh & Thompson, 1989). Using these designs, researchers have documented clinically significant improvements in individuals who received treatment long after 6 months postonset (Saffran, Schwartz, Fink, Myers, & Martin, 1993; Thompson, Shapiro, & Roberts, 1992).

Instruction in the use of compensatory strategies to capitalize on preserved functions can also be an important part of aphasia treatment. For example, the use of gestures, melodic intonation, drawing, and assistive devices (including "low-tech" communication books and "high-tech" computers) typically requires systematic training to be highly effective (Helm-Estabrooks & Albert, 1991). It is unlikely that the use of compensatory strategies will improve performance on most standardized aphasia tests, except for those that measure functional communication abilities, such as the Communicative

Abilities in Daily Living test (Holland, 1980) or the American Speech-Language-Hearing Association Functional Assessment of Communication Skills for Adults (ASHA FACS; Frattali, Thompson, Holland, & Ferketic, 1995). More importantly, improved communication with the use of compensatory strategies may be powerfully significant in the lives of aphasic individuals and their families.

Living with Aphasia

Reactive and biologically based depression are common during the first 2 years following stroke (Cullum & Bigler, 1991; Robinson & Benson, 1981; Robinson, Lipsey, & Price, 1985). In particular, individuals with anterior left hemisphere lesions are at high risk for depression (Robinson, Kubos, Starr, Rao, & Price, 1983, 1984). Poststroke depression results in symptoms similar to functional depression, including "sadness, anxiety/restlessness, loss of energy, decreased appetite and weight loss, insomnia, social withdrawal, and irritability" (Swindell & Hammons, 1991, p. 332). Without treatment, depression may last 7 to 8 months (Robinson & Price, 1982).

Aphasia interferes with basic human functions of self-expression through verbal communication. Persistent aphasia, even in its mildest form, is a lifelong disability with significant psychosocial impact. Individuals with moderate to severe aphasia experience frustration from recurrent communication failures. Skelley (1975) surveyed 50 individuals who had recovered sufficiently from severe aphasia to comment on their experience. Many indicated that they felt that their ability to comprehend was better than people thought, but that often the verbal input of their communication partners was too much and too fast. Many indicated that they were depressed by the impatience of listeners.

Maximizing Communication with Aphasic Individuals

Understanding the verbal output from individuals with significant residual aphasia requires the active participation of listeners. It is most likely to be successful in an environment with minimal distractions. Eye contact should be maintained so that the listener can perceive the visual aspects of communication and can avoid interrupting the aphasic speaker. It is helpful to become familiar with an individual's aphasia profile and to adopt a listening strategy that is suited to that individual. For example, because nonfluent aphasia results in slow, effortful productions of short utterances lacking functors, the listener should (1) be patient, allowing the aphasic speaker adequate time to formulate and produce his or her utterance; (2) mentally "fill in" the missing words; and (3) try to construct the big picture the speaker is trying to communicate. Because individuals with fluent aphasia can be overly talkative with utterances that include empty comments and paraphasic utterances, the following listening strategies should be kept in mind: (1) Ignore meaningless words, particularly perseverative utterances; (b) listen to vocal pitch and intonation for clues to meaning; and (c) try to abstract the gist while waiting for the meaning to emerge.

Independent of syndrome, when speaking with aphasic individuals, the listener should readily accept communication attempts in all modalities: speech, gestures, drawing, and writing. Written responses can be helpful even if only part of a word is written correctly, such as the initial letter. Confirming messages periodically with the aphasic speaker is useful, especially in the event of communication breakdown. Information can be clarified using brief, syntactically simple questions. In some cases, a listener may need to ask the aphasic speaker to provide information in another modality, such as gesturing or drawing.

Even individuals who recover sufficiently to write about their stroke and aphasia stress the significant impact of aphasia and the need to eliminate distractions in order to handle language tasks. Moore (1994) wrote, "I had a mild stroke, I know … but I cannot today do any two things simultaneously. If you ask me a question, I have to turn off the television, figuratively speaking at least" (p. 102). Moore goes on to say, "If there is a group of people in a room, if there are two or more conversations at the same time, and if people talk loud, that event is cruel torture" (p. 102).

In closing, it should be noted that aphasia can result in a loss of one's "sense of self" and in grieving for one's lost identity (Brumfitt, 1993; Holland & Beeson, 1993). Professionals who provide service to individuals with aphasia are well advised to move beyond the role of the "unveiler of deficits" and to assist these individuals and their families in coping with the distress of aphasia. Successful recovery requires maximizing language ability and compensatory strategies, but also developing a healthy new sense of self.

ACKNOWLEDGMENTS

This work was supported in part by National Multipurpose Research and Training Center Grant DC-01409 from the National Institute on Deafness and Other Communication Disorders. The authors would like to thank Audrey Holland, Steven Rapcsak, and Richard Curlee for their helpful comments and Pam Eshelman for her secretarial assistance.

References

Albert, M. L., & Helm-Estabrooks, N. (1988). Diagnosis and treatment of aphasia, part II. *Journal of the American Medical Association, 259,* 1205–1210.

Alexander, M. P., & Schmidt, M. A. (1980). The aphasia syndrome of stroke in the left anterior cerebral artery territory. *Archives of Neurology, 37,* 97–100.

Alexander, M. P., Naeser, M. A. & Palumbo, C. L. (1987). Correlations of subcortical CT lesion sites and aphasia profiles. *Brain, 110,* 961–991.

American Heart Association. (1994). *Caring for a person with aphasia.* Publication no. 50-1127. Dallas, TX: Author.

Appel, J., Kertesz, A., & Fisman, M. (1982). A study of language functioning in Alzheimer patients. *Brain and Language, 17,* 73–91.

Basso, A., Capitani, E., & Vignolo, L. A. (1979). Influence of rehabilitation on language skills in aphasic patients. *Archives of Neurology, 36,* 190–196.

Basso, A., Spinnler, H., Vallar, G., & Zanobio, M. E. (1982). Left hemisphere damage and selective impairment of auditory verbal short-term memory. A case study. *Neuropsychologia, 20,* 263–274.

Basso, A., Bracchi, M., Capitani, E., Laiacona, M., & Zanobio, M. E. (1987). Age and evolution of language area functions: A study on adult stroke patients. *Cortex, 23,* 475–483.

Beeson, P. M., & Rapcsak, S. Z. (1995, February). *Chronic Broca's aphasia: Evidence for right hemisphere language.* Telerounds Program, National Center for Neurogenic Communication Disorders, Tucson, AZ.

Benson, D. F. (1985). Language in the left hemisphere. In D. F. Benson & E. Zaidel (Eds.), *The dual brain* (pp. 193–203). New York: Guilford Press.

Benson, D. F. (1993). Aphasia. In K. M. Heilman & E. Valenstein (Eds.), *Clinical neuropsychology* (3rd ed.). New York: Oxford University Press.

Benton, A. L., & Joynt, R. L. (1960). Early descriptions of aphasia. *Archives of Neurology, 3,* 109/205–126/222.

Berker, E. A., Berker, A. H., & Smith, A., 1986. Translation of Broca's 1865 report: Localization of speech in the third left frontal convolution. *Archives of Neurology, 43,* 1065–1072.

Brown, J. W., & Jaffe, J. (1975). Hypothesis on cerebral dominance. *Neuropsychologia, 13,* 107–110.

Brumfitt, S. (1993). Losing your sense of self: What aphasia can do. *Aphasiology, 7,* 569–591.

Byng, S. (1988). Sentence processing deficits: Theory and therapy. *Cognitive Neuropsychology, 5,* 629–676.

Caplan, D. (1992). *Language: Structure, processing and disorders.* Cambridge, MA: MIT Press.

Caramazza, A. (1984). The logic of neuropsychological research and the problem of patient classification in aphasia. *Brain and Language, 21,* 9–20.

Caramazza, A., & Hillis, A. E. (1990). Where do semantic errors come from? *Cortex, 26,* 95–122.

Chapey, R. Ed.). (1994). *Language intervention strategies in adult aphasia.* Baltimore: William & Wilkins.

Coultheart, M., Patterson, K., & Marshall, J. C. (Eds.). (1987). *Deep dyslexia* (2nd ed.). New York: Routledge & Kegan Paul.

Crosson, B. (1984). Role of the dominant thalamus in language: A review. *Psychological Bulletin, 96,* 491–517.

Crosson, B. (1992). *Subcortical functions in language and memory.* New York: Guilford Press.

Cullum, C., & Bigler, E. (1991). Short- and long-term psychological status following stroke: Short form MMPI results. *Journal of Nervous and Mental Disease, 179,* 274–278.

Culton, G. L. (1969). Spontaneous recovery from aphasia. *Journal of Speech and Hearing Research, 12,* 825–833.

D'Agostino, R. B., Wolf, P. A., Belanger, A. J., & Kannel, W. B. (1994). Stroke risk profile: The Framingham study. *Stroke, 25,* 40–43.

Damasio, H., & Damasio A. (1980). The anatomical basis of conduction aphasia. *Brain, 103,* 337–350.

Darley, F. L., Aronson, A. E., & Brown, J. E. (1975). *Motor speech disorders.* Philadelphia: W. B. Saunders Company.

Dax, M. (1984). Lesions de la moitie gauche de l'encephale coincident avec l'oublie des signes de la pensée (R. J. Joynt & A. L. Benton, Trans.). The memoir of Marc Dax on aphasia. *Neurology, 14,* 851–854 (Original work published 1865).

Dejerine, J. (1892). Contribution à l'étude anatomoclinique et clinique des differentes variétés de cécité verbale. *Memoires Société Biologique, 4,* 61–90.

Dejerine, J. (1901). *Anatomie des centres nerveux.* Paris: Rueff.

Duffy, J. R. (1994). Schuell's stimulation approach to rehabilitation. In R. Chapey (Ed.), *Language intervention strategies in adult aphasia* (3rd ed., pp. 146–174). Baltimore: Williams & Wilkins.

Eslinger, P. J., & Damasio, A. R. (1981). Age and type of aphasia in patients with stroke. *Journal of Neurology, Neurosurgery, and Psychiatry, 44,* 377–381.

Frattali, C. M., Thompson, C. K., Holland, A. L., & Ferketic, M. M. (1995). American Speech-Language-Hearing Association Functional Assessment of Communication Skills for Adults.

Rockville, MD: American Speech-Language-Hearing Association.

Freedman, M., Alexander, M. P., & Naeser, M. A. (1984). Anatomic basis of transcortical motor aphasia. *Neurology, 34,* 409–417.

Friedman, R., & Albert, M. L. (1985). Alexia. In K. M. Heilman & E. Valenstein (Eds.), *Clinical neuropsychology* (2nd ed.). New York: Oxford University Press.

Friedman, R., Ween, J. E., & Albert, M. L. (1993). Alexia. In K. M. Heilman & E. Valenstein (Eds.), *Clinical neuropsychology* (3rd ed.). New York: Oxford University Press.

Geschwind, N. (1963). Carl Wernicke, The Breslau School, and the history of aphasia. In E. C. Carterette (Ed.), In *Brain function: Speech, language and communication* (Vol. 3, pp. 1–16). Berkeley, CA: University of California Press.

Geschwind, N. (1965). Disconnection syndromes in animals and man. *Brain, 88,* 237–294.

Geschwind, N., Quadfasal, F. A., & Segarra, J. M. (1968). Isolation of the speech area. *Neuropsychologia, 6,* 327–340.

Goldstein, K. (1948). *Language and language disturbances.* New York: Grune & Stratton.

Goodglass, H. (1992). Diagnosis of conduction aphasia. In S. Kohn (Ed.), *Conduction aphasia.* Hillsdale, NJ: Lawrence Erlbaum Associates.

Goodglass, H. (1993). *Understanding aphasia.* San Diego, CA: Academic Press, Inc.

Goodglass, H., & Kaplan, E. (1983a). *Boston diagnostic examination for aphasia.* Philadelphia: Lea & Febiger.

Green, E., & Howes, D. H. (1977). The nature of conduction aphasia: A study of anatomic and clinical features and underlying mechanisms. In H. Whitaker & H. A. Whitaker (Eds.), *Studies in neurolinguistics* (Vol. 3, pp. 123–156).

Hagen, C. (1973). Communication abilities in hemiplegia: Effect of speech therapy. *Archives of Physical Medicine and Rehabilitation, 54,* 454–463.

Heilman, K. M., Rothi, L., Campanella, D., & Wolfson, S. (1979). Wernicke's and global aphasia without alexia. *Archives of Neurology, 36,* 129–133.

Helm-Estabrooks, N. (1992). *Manual of aphasia diagnostic profiles.* Chicago, IL: The Riverside Publishing Company.

Helm-Estabrooks, N., & Albert, M. L. (1991). *Manual of aphasia therapy.* Austin, TX: Pro-Ed.

Hier, D. B., Yoon, W. B., Mohr, J. P., Price, T. R., & Wolf, P. A. (1994). Gender and aphasia in the stroke data bank. *Brain and Language, 47,* 155–167.

Hillis, A. E. (1994). Contributions from cognitive analyses. In R. Chapey (Ed.), *Language intervention strategies in adult aphasia* (3rd ed., pp. 207–219). Baltimore: Williams & Wilkins.

Holland, A. L. (1980). *CADL: Communicative abilities in daily living.* Austin, TX: Pro-Ed.

Holland, A. L., & Bartlett, C. L. (1985). Some differential effects of age on stroke-produced aphasia. In H. K. Ulatowska (Ed.), *The aging brain: Communication in the elderly* (pp. 141–155). San Diego, CA: College-Hill.

Holland, A. L., & Beeson, P. M. (1993). Finding a new sense of self: What the clinician can do to help. A reply to Brumfitt's, Losing one's sense of self following stroke. *Aphasiology, 7,* 569–591.

Holland, A. L., & Beeson, P. M. (1995). Aphasia therapy. In H. S. Kirshner (Ed.), *Handbook of neurological speech and language disorders.* New York: Marcel Dekker, Inc.

Holland, A. L., & Forbes, M. (Eds.). (1993). *Aphasia treatment: World perspectives.* San Diego, CA: Singular.

Hommel, M., Besson, G., Pollak, P., Kahane, P., LeBas, J. F., & Perret, J. (1990). Hemiplegia in posterior cerebral artery occlusion. *Neurology, 40,* 1496–1499.

Jenkins, J. J., Pabón-Jiménez, E., Shaw, R. E., & Williams Sefer, J. (1975). *Schuell's aphasia in adults: Diagnosis, prognosis and treatment* (2nd ed.). Hagerstown, MD: Harper & Row.

Joannette, Y., Goulet, P., & Hannequin, D. (1990). *Right hemisphere and verbal communication.* New York: Springer-Verlag.

Jonas, S. (1987). The supplementary motor region and speech. In E. Perecman (Ed.), *The frontal lobes revisited* (pp. 241–250). Hillsdale, NJ: Lawrence Erlbaum Associates.

Joynt, R. J., & Benson, A. L. (1984). The memoir of Marc Dax on aphasia. *Neurology, 14,* 851–854.

Kertesz, A. (1982). *Western aphasia battery.* New York: Grune & Stratton.

Kertesz, A., & Benke, T. (1989). Sex equality in intrahemispheric language organization. *Brain and Language, 37,* 401–408.

Kertesz, A., & Benson, D. F. (1970). Neologistic jargon: A clinicopathological study. *Cortex, 6,* 362–387.

Kertesz, A., & McCabe, P. (1977). Recovery patterns and prognosis in aphasia. *Brain, 100,* 1–18.

Kertesz, A., Lau, W. K., & Polk, M. (1993). The structural determinants of recovery in Wernicke's aphasia. *Brain and Language, 44,* 153–164.

Kertesz, A., Lesk, D., & McCabe, P. (1977). Isotope localization of infarcts in aphasia. *Archives of Neurology, 34,* 590–601.

Klein, K. (Ed.). (1995). *Aphasia community group manual.* New York: National Aphasia Association.

Knopman, D. S., Selnes, O. A., Niccum, N., Rubens, A. B., Yock, D., & Larson, D. (1983). A longitudinal study of speech fluency in aphasia: CT correlates of recovery and persistent nonfluency. *Neurology, 33,* 1170–1178.

Lichtheim, L. (1885). On aphasia. *Brain, 7,* 434–484.

Liepmann, H. (1895). Über die delirien der alkoholisten und über künstlich beiihnen hervorgerufene Visionen. *Archiv für Psychiatrie und Nervenkrankheiten, 27,* 172–232.

Lincoln, N. B., McGuirk, E., Mulley, G. P., Lendrem, W., Jones, A. C., & Mitchell, J. R. A. (1984). Effectiveness of speech therapy for aphasic stroke patients: A randomized controlled trial. *Lancet, 1,* 1197–1200.

Luria, A. R., & Hutton, J. T. (1977). A modern assessment of the basic forms of aphasia. *Brain and Language, 4,* 129–151.

Marshall, J. C., & Newcombe, F. (1973). Patterns of paralexia: A psycholinguistic approach. *Journal of Psycholinguistic Research, 2,* 175–199.

Mitchum, C. C. (1994). Traditional and contemporary views of aphasia: Implications for clinical management. In E. J. Roth & D. A. Olson (Eds.), *Topics in stroke rehabilitation* (pp. 14–36). Frederick, MD: Aspen Publishers, Inc.

Mohr, J. P. (1976). Broca's area and Broca's aphasia. In H. Whitaker & H. Whitaker (Eds.), *Studies in neurolinguistics* (Vol. 1, pp. 201–235). New York: Academic Press.

Moore, D. (1994). A second start. *Topics in Stroke Rehabilitation, 1*, 100–103.

Naeser, M. A., Alexander, M. P., Helm-Estabrooks, N., Levine, H. L., Laughlin, S. A., & Geschwind, N. (1982). Aphasia with predominantly subcortical lesion sites. Description of three capsular/putaminal aphasia syndromes. *Archives of Neurology, 39*, 2–14.

Naeser, M. A., Palumbo, C. L., Helm-Estabrooks, N., Stiassny-Eder, D., & Albert, M. L. (1989). Severe non-fluency in aphasia: Role of the medial subcallosal fasciculus plus other white matter pathways in recovery of spontaneous speech. *Brain, 112*, 1–38.

Obler, L. K., & Albert, M. L. (1981). Language in the elderly aphasic and in the dementing patient. In M. T. Sarno (Ed.), *Acquired aphasia* (pp. 385–398). New York: Academic Press.

Obler, L. K., Albert, M. L., Goodglass, H., & Benson, D. F. (1978). Aphasia type and aging. *Brain and Language, 6*, 318–322.

Palumbo, C. L., Alexander, M. P., & Naeser, M. A. (1992). CT scan lesion sites associated with conduction aphasia. In S. Kohn (Ed.), *Conduction aphasia*. Hillsdale, NJ: Lawrence Erlbaum Associates.

Patterson, K. E. (1981). Neuropsychological approaches to the study of reading. *British Journal of Psychiatry, 72*, 151–174.

Petrides, M., & Pandya, D. N. (1988). Association fiber pathways to the frontal cortex from the superior temporal region in the rhesus monkey. *The Journal of Comparative Neurology, 273*, 52–66.

Rapcsak, S. Z., & Beeson, P. M. (1995). Broca's aphasia: A right hemisphere hypothesis [Abstract]. *Journal of the International Neuropsychological Society, 1*, 181.

Rapcsak, S. Z., & Rubens, A. B. (1994). Localization of lesions in transcortical aphasia. In A. Kertesz (Ed.), *Localization and neuroimaging in neuropsychology* (pp. 297–329). San Diego, CA: Academic Press, Inc.

Robin, D. A., & Schienberg, S. (1990). Subcortical lesions and aphasia. *Journal of Speech and Hearing Disorders, 55*, 90–100.

Robinson, R. G., & Benson, D. F. (1981). Depression in aphasic patients: Frequency, severity, and clinicopathological correlations. *Brain and Language, 14*, 282–291.

Robinson, R. G., & Price, T. R. (1982). Post-stroke depressive disorders: A follow-up study of 103 patients. *Stroke, 13*, 635–641.

Robinson, R. G., Kubos, K. L., Starr, L. B., Rao, K., & Price, T. R. (1983). Mood changes in stroke patients: Relationship to lesion location. *Comprehensive Psychiatry, 24*, 555–566.

Robinson, R. G., Kubos, K. L., Starr, L. B., Rao, K., & Price, T. R. (1984). Mood disorders in stroke patients: Importance of location of lesion. *Brain, 107*, 81–93.

Robinson, R. G., Lipsey, J. R., & Price, T. R. (1985). Diagnosis and clinical management of post-stroke depression. *Psychosomatics, 26*, 769–778.

Roeltgen, D. P. (1993). Agraphia. In K. M. Heilman & E. Valenstein (Eds.), *Clinical neuropsychology* (3rd ed.). New York: Oxford University Press.

Rosenbek, J., LaPointe, L. L., & Wertz, R. T. (1989). *Aphasia: A clinical approach*. Boston, MA: College Hill.

Saffran, E., Schwartz, M., Fink, R., Myers, J., & Martin, N. (1993). Mapping therapy: An approach to remediating agrammatic sentence comprehension and production. In J. Cooper (Ed.), *Aphasia treatment: Current approaches and research opportunities*. NIDCD monograph 2. Bethesda, MD: National Institutes of Health.

Sarno, M. T. (1980). Language rehabilitation outcome in the elderly aphasic patient. In L. Obler & M. Albert (Eds.), *Language and communication in the elderly aphasic* (pp. 191–204). Lexington, MA: D.C. Health.

Sarno, M. T., Silverman, M., & Sands, E. (1970). Speech therapy and language recovery in severe aphasia. *Journal of Speech and Hearing Research, 13*, 595–606.

Schechter, I., Schejter, J., Abarbanel, M., Groswasser, Z., & Solzi, P. (1985). Age and aphasic syndromes. *Scandinavian Journal of Rehabilitation Medicine* (Suppl. 12), 60–63.

Selnes, O. A., Knopman, D. S., Niccum, N., & Rubens, A. B. (1985). The critical role of Wernicke's area in sentence repetition. *Annals of Neurology, 17*, 549–557.

Seron, X., & Deloche, G. (Eds.). (1989). *Cognitive approaches in neuropsychological rehabilitation*. Hillsdale, NJ: Lawrence Erlbaum Associates.

Shewan, C. M., & Bandur, D. L. (1994). Language-oriented treatment: A psycholinguistic approach to aphasia. In R. Chapey (Ed.), *Language intervention strategies in adult aphasia* (3rd ed., pp. 184–206). Baltimore: Williams & Wilkins.

Shewan, C. M., & Kertesz, A. (1984). Effects of speech and language treatment on recovery from aphasia. *Brain and Language, 23*, 272–299.

Skelley, M. (1975). Rethinking stroke: Aphasic patients talk back. *American Journal of Nursing, 75*, 1140–1142.

Smith, A. (1971). Objective indices of severity of chronic aphasia in stroke patient. *Journal of Speech and Hearing Disorders, 36*, 167–207.

Speedie, L. J., Coslett, H. B., & Heilman, K. M. (1984). Repetition of affective prosody in mixed transcortical aphasia. *Archives of Neurology, 41*, 268–270.

Square-Storer, P. (Ed.). (1989). *Acquired apraxia of speech in aphasic adults*. Hillsdale, NJ: Lawrence Erlbaum Associates.

Sundet, K. (1986). Sex differences in cognitive impairment following unilateral brain damage. *Journal of Clinical and Experimental Neuropsychology, 8*, 51–61.

Swindell, C. S., & Hammons, J. (1991). Poststroke depression: Neurologic, physiologic, diagnostic, and treatment implications. *Journal of Speech and Hearing Research, 34*, 325–333.

Thompson, C. D., Shapiro, L. P., & Roberts, M. et al. (1992). Treatment of sentence production deficits in aphasia: A linguistic-specific approach to *wh*-interrogative training and generalization. *Aphasiology, 7*, 111–133.

Tranel, D., & Damasio, H. (1987, October). *The role of gender in aphasia following focal cerebral lesions*. Paper presented at Academy of Aphasia, Phoenix, AZ.

Wallesch, C. W. (1985). Two syndromes of aphasia occurring with ischemic lesions involving the left basal ganglia. *Brain and Language, 25*, 357–361.

Wambaugh, J. L., & Thompson, C. K. (1989). Training and generalization of agrammatic aphasic adults' *wh*-interrogative productions. *Journal of Speech and Hearing Disorders, 54*, 514.

Weisenberg, T., & McBride, K. E. (1935). *Aphasia: A clinical and psychological study*. New York: Commonwealth Fund.

Wernicke, C. (1874). *Der aphasiche Symptomenkomplex* [The symptom complex of aphasia]. Breslau: Cohen & Weigert.

Wernicke, C. (1886). Einige neuere Arbeiten über Aphasie. *Fortschritte der Medizin, 4*, 377–463.

Wernicke, C. (1906). Der aphasische symptomencomplex. *Deutsche Klinik am Eingange des 20 Jahrhunderts, 6*, 487–556.

Wertz, R. T. (1987). Language treatment for aphasia is efficacious, but for whom? *Topics in Language Disorders, 8*, 1–10.

Wertz, R. T., & Dronkers, N. (1990). Effects of age on aphasia. In E. Cherow (Ed.), *Proceedings of the research symposium on communication sciences and disorders of aging* (pp. 88–98). Rockville, MD: ASHA.

Wertz, R. T., Collins, M. J., Weiss, D., Kurtzke, J. F., Friden, T., Brookshire, R. H., Pierce, J., Holtzapple, P., Hubbard, D. J., Proch, B. E., West, H. A., Davis, L., Matovitch, V., Morley, G. K., & Resurreccion, E. (1981). Veteran's Administration cooperative study on aphasia: A comparison of individual and group treatment. *Journal of Speech and Hearing Research, 24*, 580–594.

Wertz, R. T., Weiss, D. G., Aten, J. L., Brookshire, R. H., Garcia-Buñuel, L., Holland, A. L., Kurtzke, J. F., LaPointe, L. L., Milianti, F. J., Brannegan, R., Greenbaum, H., Marshall, R. C., Vogel, D., Carter, J., Barnes, N. S., & Goodman, R. (1986). Comparison of clinic, home, and deferred language treatment for aphasia. *Archives of Neurology, 43*, 653–658.

Whitaker, H. (1976). A case of the isolation of the language function. In H. Whitaker & H. A. Whitaker (Eds.), *Studies in neurolinguistics* (Vol. 1, pp. 1–58). New York: Academic Press.

Zaidel, E. (1985). Language in the right hemisphere. In D. F. Benson & E. Zaidel (Eds.), *The dual brain* (pp. 205–231). New York: Guilford Press.

21

The Neuropsychology of Stroke

RICHARD C. DELANEY AND LISA D. RAVDIN

Introduction

The study of cerebrovascular disease is of central interest to neuropsychologists involved in both clinical care and research. In clinical settings, the incidence and prevalence of stroke are high in comparison to other neurological disorders. Over a half-million strokes are estimated to occur yearly in the United States alone, and there are over 3 million Americans who have survived a cerebrovascular accident (Dobkin, 1995). For an aging population these statistics are especially pressing, with the incidence of stroke more than doubling with each decade after age 55. Although stroke mortality has been declining, especially from 1960 to 1980, cerebrovascular disease remains the third leading cause of death in the United States. The decline in mortality may relate to better supportive care, more accurate identification of mild strokes, or changes in risk factor management and the natural history of stroke (Shahar et al., 1995). Tremendous resources are allocated to the problems of stroke prevention, acute stroke treatment, poststroke management, and rehabilitation. Neuropsychologists contribute to each of these areas in direct clinical service and outcome research.

Stroke is a primary avenue of neuroscience research because of the heuristic opportunities afforded by relatively focal disruptions of cerebral activity. Benton (1991) provided a historical review of the contributions of stroke research to our models for the aphasias, apraxias, and agnosias, in which he regards the ischemic infarct as "the most valuable experiment of nature available for the clinical study of brain–behavior relationships." As our imaging technology improves, the hypotheses regarding brain–behavior models become increasingly refined, as does our understanding of functional neuroanatomy and neuropsychology.

Therefore, it is essential for neuropsychologists to have an understanding of cerebral blood flow, cerebrovascular disease, and the presentation of stroke syndromes. The present chapter will review these topics with attention to current methods of assessment, intervention, and research on cerebrovascular disease. Where the coverage is necessarily skeletal due to the breadth of topics, the interested reader is provided with references to gain greater depth.

Neurovascular Anatomy and Cerebral Blood Flow

The central nervous system places large demands (approximately one fifth of total) on cardiac output. The brain has a relatively high and stable metabolic rate for oxygen and glucose. Two anterior channels (the carotid system) and two posterior channels (vertebrobasilar system) conduct blood to specific regions of the brain.

The Carotid System

The common carotid arteries arise from the aortic arch (on the right side of the body coming off an initial branch, the innominate artery) and proceed through the neck to the angle of the jaw where they bifurcate to form the internal and external

RICHARD C. DELANEY • Neuropsychology Section, Psychology Service, Veterans Affairs Medical Center, West Haven, Connecticut 06516.   LISA D. RAVDIN • Department of Neurology and Neuroscience, The New York Hospital-Cornell Medical Center, New York, New York 10021.

carotid arteries. The external carotid is primarily responsible for the blood supply to the face, skull, and meninges. By means of anastomotic connections through the retina, and to a lesser extent the meninges, the external carotid arteries can assist in supplying blood to the brain when the internal carotid system is challenged.

Coursing into the skull, the first branch from the internal carotid is the ophthalmic artery which further bifurcates to form the retinal artery. Continuing to the base of the brain the internal carotids yield (1) the posterior communicating arteries, the major anastomotic connection between anterior and posterior flow; and (2) the anterior choroidal arteries, which supply portions of the basal ganglia, anterior hippocampus, and amygdala. The carotid arteries terminate in their bifurcation to form the anterior cerebral and middle cerebral arteries.

The anterior cerebral arteries (ACA) travel forward in rough parallel through the interhemispheric fissure and are typically connected by a small vessel, the anterior communicating artery (ACoA). The ACA are responsible for the perfusion of the medial and polar surfaces of the frontal and parietal lobes, for the anterior 80% of the corpus callosum, and for portions of the basal ganglia through its penetrating branches.

The middle cerebral arteries (MCA) course laterally through the sylvian fissure, sending deep penetrating branches (lenticulostriate arteries) to the medial portions of the basal ganglia, thalamus, and internal capsule. Branching on the surface of the brain, the MCA is responsible for the blood supply to much of the lateral convexity, including frontal, temporal, and parietal cortical regions.

The Vertebrobasilar System

The vertebral arteries arise from the subclavian arteries at the base of the neck and course through the vertebral canal, surrounded by neck vertebrae, entering the skull through the foramen magnum. They join at the rostral end of the medulla to form the basilar artery which runs up the length of the pons to the midbrain. Small branches from this system supply the brain stem and cerebellum. The basilar artery terminates in a bifurcation forming the posterior cerebral arteries (PCA). The PCA provide a blood supply to the inferior medial surfaces and polar regions of the temporal and occipital lobes and to the splenium of the corpus callosum.

Anastomoses

A critical concept to understanding blood flow and the variable effects of vessel blockage is *anastomotic connections*. These are the connections between blood vessels, such that an occluded vessel can be compensated for by increased flow from another vessel at a level above the occlusion. These alternative flow channels vary in effectiveness. Anastomotic connections tend to be less efficacious in the event of sudden blockage than in situations that take years to develop, such as atherosclerosis. The major anastomoses include (in decreasing significance) the Circle of Willis, connections between the internal and external carotid arteries via the ophthalmic artery, and the corticomeningeal anastomoses. The latter include the end arteries of the ACA, MCA, and PCA, which interconnect in their distal territories. Poirier, Gray, and Escourolle (1990) provide an excellent presentation of blood flow dynamics and its relationship to vascular pathology.

Cerebrovascular Disease: Risk Factors and Pathology

Stroke or cerebrovascular accident is defined as a sudden, nonconvulsive, focal, neurologic deficit of vascular origin (Adams & Victor, 1985). The origin may be either ischemic or hemorrhagic, yet the majority of events are typically the former (80%) and associated with atherosclerosis (Millikan, McDowell, & Easton, 1987). Less common causes of stroke include vascular abnormalities of large (e.g., moyamoya, fibromuscular dysplasia) and small (e.g., vasculitis, arteritis, angiopathies) blood vessels. Cerebrovascular events can be classified based on the duration and extent of behavioral dysfunction. As the name implies, the clinical symptoms of transient ischemic attacks (TIA) are not permanent deficits, with resolution within 24 hr. Symptoms of a reversible ischemic neurologic deficit (RIND) last longer but are clinically indiscernible 3 weeks after the onset. An episode of increasing deficit across a period of clinical observation is referred to as stroke in evolution. The most severe and persistent impairments result from completed stroke. Although the event itself is usually sudden, occurring over minutes to hours, the pathological processes responsible are quite gradual and relate to an interplay of risk factors.

Risk Factors

There are several well-established risk factors for stroke that are obviously not treatable. Such factors include age, gender (greater for men), genetic predispositions, and race (e.g., greater for blacks than for whites). The mechanisms by which these operate are complex and interactive (see Gorelick, 1993), relating to the deposition, placement, and progression of atherosclerotic plaques. There are also risk factors that can be treated or altered, though with varying success. Hypertension, cardiac disease (especially atrial fibrillation), diabetes mellitus, high blood lipid levels and hypercholesterolemia, cigarette smoking, alcohol abuse, elevated blood factors (fibrinogen and hematocrit), and physical inactivity are modifiable risk factors (Dyken, 1987; Gorelick, 1995; Sacco, 1995). These factors interact in a complex fashion over time, and recent research suggests some interesting contradictions. For example, the relationship between stroke incidence and such factors as cholesterol levels and cigarette smoking may be weaker in elderly subjects (Fabris et al., 1994). Other studies have found that risk factors, such as diabetes and hypertension, are associated with subtle neuropsychological deficits even prior to an identifiable cerebrovascular event (Bornstein & Kelly, 1991; Waldstein, Manuck, Ryan, & Muldoon, 1991). The elucidation of how these factors contribute to and interact in the development of stroke pathology is an area for future research and can lead to more effective intervention and prevention.

Pathology

The chief pathological process involved in cerebrovascular disease is atherosclerosis. Atherogenesis proceeds through a series of stages, beginning in childhood, and is one of the most common diseases of adult humans (Millikan et al., 1987). The process can be identified as early as the first decade in the aorta, by the second decade in the coronary arteries, and in the 20s in cerebral vessels. In late life, all three regions often show involvement. With respect to cerebral vessels the process is clearly nonrandom, occurring more severely in regions of bifurcation and curvature of vessels. In the initial phase, fatty streaks develop in the arterial wall, and the intima thickens as smooth muscle cells accumulate in the vessel wall. A lipid plaque gradually forms, eventually followed by scarring or fibrosis. The center of fibrous plaques may contain varying amounts of cholesterol crystals, calcium deposits, and lipid particles. The plaques themselves may become thick enough to seriously narrow the lumen of the vessel. The process is exacerbated by high blood pressure and blood platelet/clotting factors. Increased turbulence in the region of vessel damage can sometimes be detected through audition (bruit). As the plaque advances from a "softer" to a "harder" state, hemorrhage, ulceration, thrombosis, or calcification may occur. If the plaque ulcerates there is the opportunity for the release of debris as emboli. A similar process occurs in the smaller penetrating arteries of the brain (sometimes referred to as arteriosclerosis) in which hypertension plays an even more prominent role. Evidence suggests that risk factor management through diet and drug regimens can reverse or delay atherosclerosis (Hennerici, 1991).

Ischemic stroke can occur either through thrombosis, the extensive narrowing of a vessel wall through atherosclerosis, or through embolus, the release of plaque into the system which can suddenly block a smaller vessel "downstream." Both strokes and TIA can result from emboli released either from a developing cerebrovascular thrombus or through pathological processes in the heart (e.g., secondary to the valvular deformations of rheumatic heart disease or myocardial infarction). In the absence of such events, an individual with a developing thrombus is very often symptom-free until considerable narrowing of the vessel has occurred (e.g., 80–90%). It is possible for complete closure of a major vessel to occur without clinical concomitant, since the process occurs over long periods allowing anastomotic connections to become increasingly effective. However, there is emerging evidence that even in the absence of completed strokes, patients with asymptomatic carotid bruit (Naugle, Bridgers, & Delaney, 1986), TIA

(Delaney, Wallace, & Egelko, 1980), or other "reversible ischemia" (Dull et al., 1982) have subtle but identifiable deficits on neuropsychological examination. These findings are consistent with the animal literature which reports that chronic reductions in cerebral blood flow (up to 50%) in the absence of other identifiable abnormalities impair neuronal function (Sekhon, Morgan, Spence, & Weber, 1994).

The ischemic stroke results in a region of tissue damage referred to as an infarct. The actual process that leads to infarction and necrosis is complex, involving both the sudden reduction of glucose and oxygen resources and the termination of venous drainage. The latter leads to a build-up of lactic acid and other cellular metabolites which contribute to acidosis, a release of neurotransmitters, and a loss of autoregulation of blood flow (Welch & Levine, 1991). A central zone of maximal ischemia is surrounded by regions of fluctuating flow, referred to as the "penumbra" (Astrup, Symon, & Siesjo, 1981). The dysregulation of blood flow can extend the infarct by shunting blood away from a border zone. The result is a "luxury perfusion" (hyperemia) of adjacent tissue at the expense of tissue on the edge of viability. Recent research has suggested that the duration for potential recovery of the penumbra also depends on the preservation of energy metabolism, and peri-infarct depolarizations reduce that viability (Hossman, 1994). The physiological and biochemical chain of events defining the extent of infarction provides a basis for research on medical interventions for acute stroke, referred to as neuroprotection.

Hemorrhagic cerebrovascular events include subdural and extradural hematoma, subarachnoid hemorrhage, and intracerebral hemorrhage. Hemorrhage most often results secondary to vessel abnormalities such as arterio-venous malformations and aneurysm but can also occur following traumatic brain injury. A thorough discussion of these disorders is beyond the scope of this chapter (see Millikan et al., 1987). Table 1 provides the major clinical and pathological distinctions between ischemic and hemorrhagic events. Primary intracerebral hemorrhage has as its most typical source the small penetrating arteries of the major vessels, especially the striate arteries of the middle cerebral artery distribution supplying the basal ganglia and internal cap-

Table 1. Clinical Presentation of Infarct versus Intracerebral Hemorrhage[a]

Infarct	Intracerebral hemorrhage
Often history of TIA	No history of TIA
Often onset at rest	Onset frequent during activity
Minimal cranial discomfort	Headache (often severe)
Focal neurologic deficit increasing in stepwise fashion with intact consciousness early	Rapidly advancing neurologic deficit (1–5 hr) with consciousness declining to coma
Normotensive to moderate hypertension	Moderate to severe hypertension
Clear CSF	Blood in CSF
Early CT scan often normal	CT scan shows hemorrhage

[a]From Millikan et al., 1987; TIA, transient ischemic attack; CSF, cerebrospinal fluid; CT, computerized tomography.

sule. The thalamus, brain stem, pons, cerebellum, and cerebral white matter are also at risk. A hemorrhage can act as a space-occupying lesion and can dissect tissue, frequently along fiber tracts. There is a question of whether the etiology of such bleeds relates primarily to microaneurysms or to multiple types of vessel pathologies, but hypertension is clearly a prominent risk factor. A second relatively common source of hemorrhagic stroke is saccular aneurysm, especially in the region of the Circle of Willis. An especially striking syndrome can occur with rupture or clipping of an aneurysm in the anterior communicating artery; the clinical presentation is described below.

Although recent findings have suggested that infarction and hemorrhage share most risk factors, diabetes, ischemic heart disease, and elevated total cholesterol are most frequently associated with infarction. Intracerebral hemorrhage tends to be associated with a poorer prognosis; however, extent of the injury (defining severity of stroke) is the major contributing factor in prognosis (Jorgensen, Nakayama, Raaschou, & Olsen, 1995).

Stroke Syndromes

The behavioral deficits resulting from a single stroke clearly relate to the size and location of the event. There is, of course, additional variability between individuals (e.g., that related to such factors as handedness, gender, and past experience) which make absolute description based simply on topography of the lesions impossible. Nonetheless, there are patterns of impairment which present with sufficient regularity to be described as stroke syndromes relating to specific vascular regions. Their presentation may be partial or both complete and severe. The descriptions below focus on major stroke syndromes and exclude discussion of the multi-infarct states discussed elsewhere in this volume. The syndromes are also more extensively outlined by Adams and Victor (1985).

Anterior Cerebral Artery Syndrome

The basic motor and sensory deficits observed with ACA events are greater for the contralateral foot and leg, with a lesser degree of cortical sensory loss and paresis in the arm. There are often numerous features which are associated with anterior and prefrontal damage, including the "frontal release signs" of reinstated reflexes (e.g., grasp and sucking), the reduction in the modulation of behavior (including disinhibition, perseveration, and/or reduced spontaneity), and emotional dyscontrol. The cluster of symptoms that includes pronounced apathy, lack of insight, inability to complete tasks, and delays in responding is referred to as abulia. Damage to the anterior section of the corpus callosum may result in disconnection syndromes, such as dyspraxia of the left limbs and the inability to name objects placed in the left hand out of view (Bogen, 1985).

Middle Cerebral Artery Syndrome

This syndrome is characterized by sensory and motor impairments, including the loss of fine sensation (discrimination, stereognosis) and paralysis of the contralateral side of the body. The face and arm are typically more severely affected than the leg or foot. Visual impairments often include contralateral homonymous hemianopia or upper quadrantanopia. Infarction in the MCA distribution also produces many of the classical deficit patterns in neuropsychology, with the typical dominant/nondominant hemisphere distinctions. Dominant hemisphere MCA strokes are often associated with language impairments (fluent and nonfluent dysphasias) and

may also result in ideomotor dyspraxia, right–left confusion, and finger agnosia. As described by Albert, Goodglass, Helm, Rubens, and Alexander (1981), MCA strokes produce the classical presentations of global aphasia (with extensive infarct), Broca's aphasia (lesion limited to the superior division of the MCA territory), Wernicke's aphasia (associated with posterior temporal artery infarct), and conduction aphasia (posterior parietal branch). Nondominant hemisphere strokes in the MCA distribution can lead to a syndrome of apractagnosia, the complex of perceptual, spatial, and constructional deficits typically observed following right hemisphere parietal lobe damage. Although unawareness of deficit (anosognosia) and neglect of body (asomatognosia) or contralateral space (hemispatial neglect) are more common with nondominant lesions, these impairments have been reported following both left and right MCA infarct.

Posterior Cerebral Artery Syndrome

Homonymous hemianopia is a prominent feature of posterior cerebral artery stroke. Cortical blindness may present without the patient's awareness of that defect (Anton's syndrome). When visual loss is incomplete, deficits in visual processing may include failures in facial discrimination/recognition (prosopagnosia), visual illusions/hallucinations, achromatopsia, and the inability to identify or focus upon multiple percepts in a complicated visual array (simultanagnosia). Reductions in the ability to learn can be anticipated with most significant strokes, but prominent memory impairments are more often associated with posterior circulation blockage.

Watershed and Hemodynamic Stroke

In the event of marked reductions in global cerebral blood flow, infarction can occur in the border zones between vascular systems. Border zones include cerebral tissue supplied by the most distal branches of the anterior, middle, and posterior cerebral arteries. Such hypoperfusion can result from cardiac arrest, episodes of severe hypotension, perioperative hypoperfusion, and possibly through microemboli (Torvik, 1984). Brain regions at particular risk for such events include the posterior parietal areas (especially the corona radiata), the frontal and occipital poles, the medial temporal lobes (including the hippocampus), and the basal ganglia. Although the tissue changes caused by watershed infarction are not different from other ischemic events, the clinical presentations differ because a different mosaic of damage results. Amnesia secondary to bilateral medial temporal damage could be anticipated. Infarction in the watershed zone is the most common etiology of the transcortical aphasias (see Albert et al., 1981). Hemodynamic stroke has been estimated to represent as many as 10% of stroke unit admissions (Bladin & Chambers, 1994). This type of stroke is especially prevalent in the elderly, since it is so often associated with other systemic medical disorders.

Vertebrobasilar Syndromes

Large strokes in the vertebrobasilar distribution can easily be fatal. Small events in this distribution lead to exquisitely defined patterns of sensory and motor dysfunction, with both contralateral and ipsilateral deficits secondary to damage to neural pathways and to cranial nerves. Thus, multiple medullary and pontine syndromes (medial, lateral, superior, inferior, etc.) can be defined through careful neurological examination. Dizziness, dysphagia, dysarthria, diplopia, and nausea are prime initial symptoms of vertebrobasilar events. Deficits in higher cortical functions are less prominent, though dementia has been linked to chronic vertebrobasilar insufficiency (Perez et al., 1975), perhaps through hypoperfusion or a multi-infarct process.

Anterior Communicating Artery Syndrome

There are numerous subcategories of the major stroke syndromes described above, depending on blockage or hemorrhage of specific branches of major vessels. One that has been of particular interest to neuropsychologists has been referred to as the syndrome of the anterior communicating artery (Alexander & Freedman, 1984). The deficits associated with ACoA hemorrhage typically include a pronounced amnestic syndrome, often with confabulation, and personality changes. The latter may include leucotomy-like effects of apathy, lowered reactivity, and poor insight (Storey, 1970). Cogni-

tive deficits, such as impairments in self-regulatory activities and executive functions have also been reported, implicating basal forebrain dysfunction (Damasio, Graff-Radford, Eslinger, Damasio, & Kassel, 1985; DeLuca, 1992). As in all of the syndromes described above, there is variability in the presentation and persistence of the ACoA syndrome. DeLuca (1993) has provided evidence that cognitive impairments may be the most pervasive finding with ACoA aneurysm hemorrhage. The personality changes and confabulation occur primarily in conjunction with amnesia.

Neuropsychological Assessment and Research with Stroke

Clinical Assessment of Stroke

The types and levels of behavioral dysfunction that occur following cerebrovascular accident are exceedingly broad and varied. Several discussions have been presented which delineate the advantages and utility of objective neuropsychological assessment following stroke (Hom, 1991; Meier, 1970; Reitan, 1970; Reitan & Wolfson, 1993). In addition to basic sensory motor testing, neuropsychological evaluations include challenging tests of higher level processing to identify subtle deficits which often go undetected on clinical neurologic exam (Delaney et al., 1980; Dull et al., 1982; Naugle et al., 1986). Quantitative approaches and instruments with alternate forms also provide the opportunity for objective follow-up to consider change over time or across interventions.

Clinicians who work with stroke patients need to adapt their assessment approaches in order to effectively engage individuals who may have limitations in perceptual processing (i.e., visual field loss and spatial neglect), language skills, or response output capabilities. Formal assessment can be especially challenging in the patient with comprehension deficits, as in Wernicke's aphasia, where intentions and directions must be nonverbally presented. Recognition or matching tasks, especially those that have relatively easy preliminary items (e.g., Ravens Colored Matrices, Benton Visual Form Discrimination Test), may prove useful in engaging the patient. In addition to the standard quantitative analysis, a qualitative approach to assessment can help determine factors underlying success/failure, which will be useful for individualized treatment (e.g., Milberg, Hebben, & Kaplan, 1986). A thorough neuropsychological evaluation will identify the functional areas to target for remediation as well as serve as the baseline for posttreatment comparisons.

The reader is referred to Chapter 24 of this volume for coverage of the broader issues of neuropsychological evaluation of aging patients. With regard to the assessment of stroke patients, the following considerations are also raised:

1. It is important not to become too focused on the most obvious or severe aspects of an impaired presentation, for example, the dysphasia and right hemiparesis of the left hemisphere stroke or the neglect syndrome with left hemiparesis of the right hemisphere stroke. The identification of residual strengths and more subtle deficits also need to be adequately described.

2. Clinicians need to be aware of the dynamic processes involved in neurological insult and recovery. Although stroke produces a resolving lesion with most pronounced dysfunction in the acute phase, even a remarkably "focal" injury can have effects on functions presumed to be subserved by distant neural systems. Von Monakow (1911) is credited with introducing the concept of "diaschisis," which for cerebrovascular disease can be the result of the dysregulation of cerebral blood flow, the release of neurotransmitters, cerebral edema, or neural disconnection.

3. Clinicians should also assess the presence of additional risk factors for neuropsychological impairment (including coexisting medical illness, chronic diabetes/hypertension, etc.), comorbid neurodegenerative disease (including prior TIA, clinically "silent stroke," or other primary dementing illness), and affective distress which might contribute to the obtained profile.

Each of these factors argues for a broad and thorough evaluation. The examiner is cautioned against too many presumptions based upon an expected profile of abilities and deficits in a given patient. Finally, clinical practice has provided numerous examples of differences in the assessment and conclusions reached by professionals of different disciplines, reflecting differences in approach, criteria, and nature of involvement with the patient. Integration of information from neurologists, neuropsychologists, rehabilitation therapists, and nursing is critical to providing the most accurate predictive evaluation.

Overview of Neuropsychological Research with Stroke

Patients with cerebrovascular disease have contributed vastly to our ideas regarding the relationships between regional brain functioning and behavioral abilities. To attempt to cover that literature is beyond the scope of any chapter. The purpose of this section is to present a sampling of important findings relevant to the understanding of cerebrovascular disease and to provide directions for future neuropsychological research.

Sensory Perception and Motor Integration

The important research by Reitan and associates (Reitan & Fitzhugh, 1971) has been previously summarized by Brown, Baird, and Shatz (1986) and by Hom (1991). Not surprisingly, studies indicate that the most marked sensorimotor impairments are contralateral and result from lateralized cerebrovascular lesions in a manner reflecting the classic neural pathways. Recent reports suggest that somatosensory, visual half field, and motor deficits contralateral to a hemispheric stroke may be more common following right than left hemisphere events (Sterzi et al., 1993). However, careful comparisons of subject performances have demonstrated the need to consider within-subject comparisons as well. That is, ipsilateral declines in motor integration or fine discrimination also occur, particularly on more complex tasks. Although ipsilateral sensorimotor deficits may be more common or significant following right hemisphere lesions (Hom & Reitan, 1982), dysfunction of either "normal" hand (i.e., the hand ipsilateral to the infarct) has been well recognized in patients with stroke in either hemisphere (Jebsen, Griffith, Long, & Fowler, 1971). Classical (ideomotor) apraxia, the inability to complete previously learned motor actions to command, is clearly associated with dominant hemisphere lesions (Heilman & Gonzalez Rothi, 1985).

Hemispatial neglect is recognized to occur with much greater frequency following right than left hemisphere infarct (Weinstein & Friedland, 1977), with the perceptual disturbance and inattention expressed more predominantly in contralateral space. However, the presentation of the neglect syndrome is quite variable. Its subcomponents can dissociate depending on the nature of the task (Kinsella, Olver, Ng, Packer, & Stark, 1993) or the cortical and subcortical distribution of the lesion (Heilman, Watson, & Valenstein, 1985; Mesulam, 1982).

It has been argued that the term "left visuospatial neglect" should be regarded as no more than a descriptive shorthand, such as "aphasia," since so many variants exist (Halligan & Marshall, 1992). A goal for neuropsychology is to identify the component processes involved in complex functions and to relate them to specific neural systems. For example, Laeng (1994) used the component process approach to show that different types of spatial dysfunction are observed following lesions to each hemisphere. Right hemisphere stroke affected coordinate spatial functions, which specify exact spatial position of objects. Left hemisphere stroke was associated with reduced categorical spatial skills, defined as the ability to identify broader spatial relationships such as "to the left of."

Language

Historically, the neuropsychological study of stroke-related language dysfunction has represented the most concerted effort to consider component subsystems that contribute to complex behavior (Albert et al., 1981; see also Chapter 20, this volume, for a discussion of language functions in aging patients).

Cognitive and Executive Control Functioning

Lateralized infarct can lead to greater impairment of verbal skills following left hemisphere stroke or of nonverbal skills following right hemisphere stroke, as measured traditionally with the Wechsler Adult Intelligence Scale-Revised (WAIS-R). This is most easily demonstrable acutely and in the presence of dysphasia or apractagnosia. However, stroke also significantly impairs intellectual functions in a more generalized manner involving complex adaptive abilities (Hom & Reitan, 1990). Smaller strokes which involve subcortical systems or white matter, frequently associated with the frontal lobe, are increasingly being linked to subtle declines in executive control (Breteler et al., 1994; Godefroy et al., 1992). Glosser and Goodglass (1990) provide evidence that anterior strokes lead to executive dyscontrol and that such deficits are relatively independent of the linguistic or visual-spatial disorders which may also be present in larger strokes. Significant cognitive impairment following stroke is associated with decreased long-term survival, independent of age, physical disability, and many other usual predictors (Tatemichi et al., 1994).

Memory

Amnestic syndromes have been reported following occlusion of the posterior cerebral artery (Benson, Marsden, & Meadows, 1974), thalamic infarct (von Cramon, Hebel, & Schuri, 1985; Winocur, Oxbury, Roberts, Agnetti, & Davis, 1984), as well as in the ACoA syndrome. Amnestic disturbances associated with vascular syndromes are similar to other mesial temporal/diencephalic amnesias, including bilateral temporal lobe damage and Korsakoff's syndrome. Other research suggests that transient global amnesia, a process of presumably vascular origin, may result in lasting impairment that can go undetected without careful assessment (Hodges & Oxbury, 1990).

Unilateral cortical strokes in the middle cerebral artery distribution do not characteristically present with memory impairment as a primary symptom. However, considerable research has demonstrated that deficits in short-term span, registration, and the initial processing of information occur with lateralized lesions and that this can have material-specific or modality-specific qualities (Barbizet & Cany, 1969; Butters, Samuels, Goodglass, & Brody, 1970). Recently it has been shown that left hemisphere stroke patients can have deficits in both short-term memory (associated with posterior lesions) and long-term memory (associated with anterior lesions) (Beeson, Bayles, Rubens, & Kaszniak, 1993). Neither of these types of deficits was adequately accounted for by dysphasia, but the anterior, long-term memory impairment may be related to executive dyscontrol.

Emotion

The affective consequences of stroke are critical to quality of life and rehabilitation efforts. Recently, considerable research has been directed toward this complex area. In addition to the emotional reactions that result from loss of function or independence, cerebrovascular events produce neuropathological changes that can have a profound effect on emotionality. Emotional sequelae of stroke include anxiety (Castillo, Starkstein, Federoff, Price, & Robinson, 1993), apathy (Starkstein, Federoff, Price, Leiguarda, & Robinson, 1993a), catastrophic reaction (Castillo et al., 1993), lability (Morris, Robinson, & Raphael, 1993), and clinical depression. This section will focus on poststroke depression (PSD), the most commonly observed emotional change, with estimates ranging as high as 50% (Shima, Kitagaw, Kitamura, Fujinawa, & Watanabe, 1994).

Classic descriptions of emotional asymmetries following unilateral lesions involve the dominant hemisphere "catastrophic reaction" (Goldstein, 1939), which includes anxiety and depression, in contrast to the right hemisphere "indifference" reaction which manifests primarily as apathy (Gainotti, 1972, 1989). Consistent with these descriptions, the findings of Robinson, Kubos, Starr, Rao, and Price (1984) suggest that the major determinant of PSD is a left hemisphere cerebrovascular event. The association between laterality of lesion and emotional change is independent of handedness (Robinson et al., 1985) and cortical–subcortical distinctions (Starkstein, Robinson, Berthier, Parikh, & Price, 1988; Starkstein, Robinson, & Price, 1987). Depression has been associated with anterior lesions, with increased severity following lesions that are closer to the frontal pole (Robinson et al., 1984). Anterior-posterior distinctions have also been ob-

served in patients with bilateral lesions (Lipsey, Robinson, Pearlson, Rao, & Price, 1984). After a series of investigations, Starkstein et al. (1987) further conclude that lesion location correlates only with the presence of major, not minor, depression.

Contradictory findings also exist. For example, Schwartz and colleagues (1993) reported a greater incidence of depression following right hemisphere stroke in their sample. These authors suggest that the contradictory findings may be explained by other variables hypothesized to influence PSD, such as lesion size and the time poststroke. The majority of patients in the study by Schwartz et al. (1993a,b) were evaluated 2 months poststroke. Robinson and colleagues (1984) evaluated patients 1 to 3 weeks following the event, and lesions were probably smaller since about 25% had negative computerized tomography (CT) findings. Nelson et al. (1993) failed to find any laterality differences in the acute presentation of depression, but follow-up studies revealed differential recovery rates of poststroke emotional changes associated with lesion laterality (Nelson, Cicchetti, Satz, Sowa, & Mitrushina, 1994). At 2 months poststroke, left hemisphere patients evidenced slower emotional recovery than patients with right hemisphere stroke. Demographic variables such as age and socioeconomic status (income) (Schulz, Tompkins, & Rau, 1988) and history of depression (family or self) (Dam, Pederson, & Ahlgren, 1989) also affect the likelihood of poststroke emotional changes. Recent discussions of "state versus trait" models of depression are valuable in considering how each hemisphere might contribute to the emergence of a depressive episode, with the left hemisphere exerting a regulatory control of affect and with abnormal organization of the right hemisphere predisposing to depression (Boone et al., 1995).

The presence of depression has a direct effect on clinical presentation, functional recovery, and outcome. Poststroke depression may exacerbate cognitive dysfunction. There is an extensive literature which identifies psychomotor skills, attentional control, learning, and memory as the neuropsychological functions most vulnerable to the effects of depression (Boone et al., 1995; Brand, Jolles, & Gipsen-de Wied, 1992; Cassens, Wolfe, & Zola, 1990; Gray, Dean, Rattan, & Cramer, 1987; Sweet,

Newman, & Bell, 1992). Cognitive impairment attributable to PSD varies as a function of degree of affective disturbance as well as lesion size, with deficits most evident in patients with major depression (Bolla-Wilson, Robinson, Starkstein, Boston, & Price, 1989) and more extensive lesions (Robinson, Bolla-Wilson, Kaplan, Lipsey, & Price, 1986).

Late-life depression is one of the most common psychiatric disturbances. Therefore, the elderly may have an increased vulnerability to emotional disturbance following neurologic illness. The presence of depression has been associated with increased mortality in medically ill patients, particularly in the elderly population. Evidence suggests that this holds true for patients with cerebrovascular disease. A 10-year follow-up study of stroke patients demonstrated an increased risk of mortality in depressed versus nondepressed patients (Morris, Robinson, Andrzejewski, Samuels, & Price, 1993).

Fortunately, PSD is responsive to pharmacotherapy. Lazarus and colleagues (1992) reported 80% full or partial alleviation of depressive signs and symptoms, as measured by the Hamilton Rating Scale for Depression, after a 3-week trial of methylphenidate. Other studies demonstrate successful alleviation of depression with traditional antidepressants (i.e., MAO inhibitors, tricyclic antidepressants) (Federoff & Robinson, 1989; Lauritzen et al., 1994; Tiller, 1992) as well as electroconvulsive shock therapy (Currier, Murray, & Welch, 1992). Early identification and a variety of treatment options for PSD may ultimately result in improved functional outcome in a proportion of stroke patients. Cognitive dysfunction attributable to PSD can be considered reversible, since elevations in mood should to some extent improve functional abilities. At the very least, elevated mood will likely have a positive influence on rehabilitation as a result of improved motivation and attention.

Treatment of Cerebrovascular Disease

Current treatment of cerebrovascular disease can be divided into categories of prevention and acute poststroke intervention. One well-established prevention effort is the reduction of stroke risk factors as discussed previously. However, both medical and surgical procedures have also been applied.

Stroke Prevention

The most common and widely employed surgical intervention to prevent stroke is carotid endarterectomy. Not without risk, this procedure continues to be carefully studied for efficacy, leading to changing guidelines for its use (Moore et al., 1995). Because of difficulty with access, vertebral endarterectomy is much less commonly attempted. Other revascularization efforts include surgery to establish new anastomotic connections through bypass graft. The most common of these has been the superficial temporal artery to middle cerebral artery bypass (STA-MCA). This essentially creates an alternate path from an external carotid branch to an internal carotid branch to improve cerebral blood flow. The question as to whether cerebral revascularization is associated with improvements in neuropsychological functioning was reviewed by Baird (1991). Results vary across studies; where gains have been observed they have generally been small, and alternative explanations can be posited. In addition, small declines can occur in some patients, and the prediction of risk has been difficult. Since surgical guidelines, procedures, and expertise are becoming more refined and specific, there is a clear need for continued neuropsychological study in this area.

Medical interventions to minimize the likelihood of stroke have included anticoagulation with warfarin and antiplatelet treatment with aspirin or ticlopidine (Raps & Galetta, 1995). Ticlopidine has been associated with more serious side effects than has aspirin. A promising new antiplatelet agent, clopidogrel, is now under large-scale investigation (van Gijn & Algra, 1994).

Similar to earlier research findings on the effects of vasodilators, it does not appear that stroke prevention efforts routinely lead to improvement or recovery of neuropsychological functioning. However, better control of risk factors (which may result in deferment of the atherosclerotic process), medical interventions, and surgery may lead to a significant reduction not only in completed stroke (for which the benefit is obvious), but also transient events (TIA and RIND). Since there has been limited long-term follow-up research on possible cumulative effects of TIA, it would be of particular interest to study individuals across time to consider functional changes and frequency of recurring TIA.

Acute Stroke Treatment

Another very exciting opportunity for neuropsychological investigation is the emerging field of neuroprotection. This includes hypertensive therapy, hypervolemia, vasodilation, hemodilution, hyperosmolarity, and various agents for the pharmacological attenuation of cellular excitation in the acute phase (Marangos & Lal, 1992; Weinstein & Faden, 1990). The primary scientific rationale for these efforts is salvaging tissue which is marginally viable (the penumbra). Animal model investigations have been promising (Smith & Meldrum, 1995; Wiard, Dickerson, Beek, Norton, & Cooper, 1995). The Working Group on Emergency Brain Resuscitation (1995) has presented an argument for improving the acute implementation of experimentally promising interventions. A list of experimental stroke therapies is provided in Table 2. To date, most experimental treatment protocols have used broad outcome measures of activities of daily living and quality of life. Neuropsychological research can add greater specificity to our understanding of improved outcome.

Recovery and Rehabilitation

As reviewed by Meier and Strauman (1991), there are a number of factors that are believed to contribute to neuropsychological recovery from stroke. These include processes such as the dissipation of diaschisis, regeneration of neural elements (which may have positive or negative effects), redundancy within neural networks, and behavioral substitution. In most studies, increasing age and size of lesion are factors that lead to poorer prognosis for recovery of function.

Neuropsychology has a primary role in the development and application of rehabilitation and remediation strategies following brain damage. The term rehabilitation has been used variously in the literature, but many (e.g., Diller, 1988) employ a broad definition which refers to that phase of care

Table 2. Experimental Therapies for Stroke[a]

Reperfusion
   Thrombolytic agents: intravenous, intra-arterial
   Angioplasty
   Embolectomy
   Acute endarterectomy
Neuroprotective agents
   N-methy-D-aspartate blockers
   Calcium channel blockers
   Glutamate release inhibitors
   21-amino steroids
Surgical decompression
   Lobectomy or hemispherectomy
   Stereotactic aspiration or surgical removal of
     hemorrhage

[a]From the Working Group on Emergency Brain Resuscitation, 1995.

designed to optimize functioning in the physical, psychological, vocational, and social areas for patients with impairments due to disease or trauma. Remediation is a subset of rehabilitation that involves overcoming specific types of failures or learning alternative methods to arrive at a given response.

In their investigations of unilateral stroke patients, Diller and colleagues pioneered many of the remediation techniques that are now standard practice. Some of their earlier studies targeted assessment and retraining of primary disturbances that can interfere with higher order functioning, including ability to profit from cues (Ben-Yishay, Diller, Gerstman, & Gordon, 1970), task persistence (Ben-Yishay, Diller, Gerstman, & Haas, 1968), sensory awareness (Weinberg et al., 1979), and visual scanning and hemi-inattention (Diller & Weinberg, 1977; Weinberg et al., 1977). These investigations served as the groundwork for the development of remediation strategies currently in use, such as perceptual retraining (Diller & Weinberg, 1993), memory training paradigms (Chute & Bliss, 1994), and attention training programs (Sohlberg & Mateer, 1987).

Stroke rehabilitation uses methods similar to those employed with other etiologies (see Sohlberg and Mateer, 1989, for a discussion of theoretical and practical applications). This section focuses briefly on issues relevant to therapy with an elderly stroke population, including premorbid status, targets of intervention, and treatment goals.

To begin with, therapies need to be sensitive to age-related changes in sensory (visual and auditory), motor, and cognitive functions. For example, cognitive decline associated with normal aging, including decreased problem-solving and cognitive flexibility, can be an impediment to the demands of cognitive rehabilitation strategies. Premorbid functional levels determine the complexity of the cognitive exercises and serve to establish treatment goals. Due to the focal nature of stroke-induced deficits, specific impairments are targeted for rehabilitation. Rehabilitation goals for the elderly are focused on increased independence rather than the vocationally driven goals used with younger patients. The goals need to be individualized and directed at improved quality of life, however "quality of life" may be defined differently for each individual.

Dobkin (1991) argues for the initiation of physical and cognitive therapy within days of an acute cerebrovascular event. Prompt intervention is likely to have a positive influence on motivation. So-called spontaneous recovery (dissipation of diaschisis, improved functioning of marginal tissue, etc.) can be expected to occur most rapidly in the first 3 months following the stroke. If therapies begin within this time period, the patient is likely to experience the greatest gains within the rehabilitation setting, serving as a motivating force for continued therapy. Counseling and education about relevant issues such as rate and potential for recovery is essential.

Unawareness of deficits and emotional changes following stroke can be primary obstacles to rehabilitation efforts. Each of these can have a neuropathological (i.e., anosognosia) or psychological (i.e., reactive depression) basis. A patient in denial or one who lacks recognition of impairment will be less likely to actively cooperate with therapies. Although some degree of denial can be adaptive in the acute stage of illness where control is minimal (Levine et al., 1987), extended failure to appreciate or accept one's deficits becomes a deterrent to progress in therapies and in self-initiation of compensatory strategies. Depression also has a negative impact on rehabilitation in terms of participation. Depression-induced dementia may lead to an overestimation of cognitive decline secondary to stroke. Mood-related changes in cognitive abilities need to be identified because they can be responsive to treatment (pharmacotherapy or counseling). Clearly the most beneficial approach to rehabilitation consists of a multidisciplinary team approach which uses input from the patient and supportive family members to address all aspects of functional status. Interventions must be directed toward increasing independence and promoting return to the community in a way that is meaningful to that individual.

Future Research

This chapter has emphasized some of the complexities and variability presented by stroke and cerebrovascular disease. Although stroke can occur in neonates and children, it is of relatively low incidence until the fifth decade of life. Thus, a thorough understanding of cerebrovascular disease is essential to the neuropsychology of aging. Stroke patients will continue to play a major role in neuropsychological research in helping us to further develop models of brain functioning. Additional neuropsychological investigations are essential to continued understanding of the disease process and its effects on brain functioning, particularly in the areas of prevention (risk factor management) and treatment (pharmacological, surgical, and rehabilitation). The following are suggested as salient and timely topics for investigation:

1. The long-term and cumulative effects of TIA; the natural history of TIA from a neuropsychological perspective
2. Risk factor reduction and associated neuropsychological outcome
3. The sensitivity of neuropsychological measurement to neuroprotection and preventive interventions; this research can be accomplished in conjunction with blood flow studies to consider both generalized and specific effects of treatment.
4. Cognitive remediation outcome studies evaluating treatments targeted at specific functional impairments; clinical research must demonstrate generalizability in terms of

meaningful functional gains, such as increased independence or return to the community.

References

Adams, R. D., & Victor, M. (1985). *Principles of neurology*. New York: McGraw-Hill.

Albert, M. L., Goodglass, H., Helm, N. A., Rubens, A. B., & Alexander, M. P. (1981). *Clinical aspects of dysphasia*. New York: Springer-Verlag.

Alexander, M. P., & Freedman, M. (1984). Amnesia after anterior communicating artery aneurysm rupture. *Neurology, 34*, 752–757.

Astrup, J., Symon, L., & Siesjo, B. K. (1981). Thresholds in cerebral ischemia—the ischemic penumbra. *Stroke, 12*, 723–725.

Baird, A. D. (1991). Behavioral correlates of cerebral revascularization. In R. A. Bornstein & G. Brown (Eds.), *Neurobehavioral aspects of cerebrovascular disease* (pp. 297–313). New York: Oxford University Press.

Barbizet, J., & Cany, E. (1969). A psychometric study of various memory deficits associated with cerebral lesions. In G. A. Talland & N. C. Waugh (Eds.), *The pathology of memory* (pp. 49–65). New York: Academic Press.

Beeson, P. M., Bayles, K. A., Rubens, A. B., & Kaszniak, A. W. (1993). Memory impairment and executive control in individuals with stroke-induced aphasia. *Brain and Language, 45*, 253–275.

Benson, D. F., Marsden, C. D., & Meadows, J. C. (1974). The amnesic syndrome of posterior artery occlusion. *Acta Neurologica Scandinavica, 50*, 133–145.

Benton, A. L. (1991). Cerebrovascular disease in the history of neuropsychology. In R. A. Bornstein & G. Brown (Eds.), *Neurobehavioral aspects of cerebrovascular disease* (pp. 1–13). New York: Oxford University Press.

Ben-Yishay, Y., Diller, L., Gerstman, L., & Haas, A. (1968). The relationship between impersistence, intellectual function and outcome of rehabilitation in patients with left hemiplegia. *Neurology, 18*, 852–861.

Ben-Yishay, Y., Diller, L., Gerstman, L., & Gordon, W. (1970). Relationship between initial competence and ability to profit from cues in brain-damaged individuals. *Journal of Abnormal Psychology, 75*(3), 248–259.

Bladin, C. F., & Chambers, B. R. (1994). Frequency and pathogenesis of hemodynamic stroke. *Stroke, 25*, 2179–2182.

Bogen, J. C. (1985). The callosal syndromes. In K. M. Heilman & E. Valenstein (Eds.), *Clinical neuropsychology* (pp. 295–338). New York: Oxford University Press.

Bolla-Wilson, K., Robinson, R. G., Starkstein, S. E., Boston, J., & Price, T. R. (1989). Lateralization of dementia of depression in stroke patients. *American Journal of Psychiatry, 146*, 627–634.

Boone, K. B., Lesser, I. M., Miller, B. L., Wohl, M., Berman, N., Lee, A., Palmer, B., & Back, C. (1995). Cognitive functioning in older depressed outpatients: Relationship of presence and severity of depression to neuropsychological test scores. *Neuropsychology, 9*, 390–398.

Bornstein, R. A., & Kelly, M. (1991). Risk factors for stroke and neuropsychological performance. In R. A. Bornstein & G. Brown (Eds.), *Neurobehavioral aspects of cerebrovascular disease* (pp. 1–13). New York: Oxford University Press.

Brand, A. N., Jolles, J., & Gipsen-de Wied, C. (1992). Recall and recognition memory deficits in depression. *Journal of Affective Disorders, 25*, 77–86.

Breteler, M. M. B., Amerongen, N. M., van Swieten, J. C., Claus, J. J., Grobbee, D. E., van Gijn, J., Hofman, A., & van Harskamp, F. (1994). Cognitive correlates of ventricular enlargement and cerebral white matter lesions on magnetic resonance imaging. *Stroke, 25*, 1109–1115.

Brown, G. G., Baird, A. D., & Shatz, M. W. (1986). The effects of cerebral vascular disease and its treatment on higher cortical functioning. In I. Grant & K. M. Adams (Eds.), *Neuropsychological assessment of neurospsychiatric disorders* (pp. 384–414). New York: Oxford Press.

Butters, N., Samuels, I., Goodglass, H., & Brody, B. (1970). Short term visual and auditory memory disorders after parietal and frontal lobe damage. *Cortex, 6*, 44–59.

Cassens, G., Wolfe, L., & Zola, M. (1990). The neuropsychology of depression. *Journal of Neuropsychiatry and Clinical Neurosciences, 2*, 202–213.

Castillo, C. S., Starkstein, S. E., Federoff, J. P., Price, T. R., & Robinson, R. G. (1993). Generalized anxiety disorder after stroke. *Journal of Nervous and Mental Disease, 181*(2), 100–106.

Chute, D. L., & Bliss, M. E. (1994). ProsthesisWare: Concepts and caveats for microcomputer-based aids to everyday living. *Experimental Aging Research, 20*(3), 229–238.

Currier, M. B., Murray, G. B., & Welch, C. C. (1992). Electroconvulsive therapy for post-stroke depressed geriatric patients. *Journal of Neuropsychiatry and Clinical Neurosciences, 4*(2), 140–144.

Dam, H., Pederson, H. E., & Ahlgren, P. (1989). Depression among patients with stroke. *Acta Psychiatrica Scandinavica, 80*(2), 118–124.

Damasio, A. R., Graff-Radford, N. R., Eslinger, P. J., Damasio, H., & Kassel, N. (1985). Amnesia following basal forebrain lesions. *Archives of Neurology, 42*, 263–271.

Delaney, R. C., Wallace, J. D., & Egelko, S. (1980). Transient cerebral ischemic attacks and neuropsychological deficit. *Journal of Clinical Neuropsychology, 2*, 107–115.

DeLuca, J. (1992). Cognitive dysfunction after aneurysm of the anterior communicating artery. *Journal of Clinical and Experimental Neuropsychology, 14*, 924–934.

DeLuca, J. (1993). Predicting neurobehavioral patterns following anterior communicating artery aneurysm. *Cortex, 29*, 639–647.

Diller, L. (1988). Rehabilitation in traumatic brain injury: Observations on the current U.S. scene. In A. L. Christensen & B. Uzzell (Eds.), *Neuropsychological rehabilitation*. Boston: Kluwer Academic.

Diller, L., & Weinberg, J. (1977). Hemi-inattention in rehabilitation: The evolution of a rational remediation program. *Advances in Neurology, 18*, 63–82.

Diller, L., & Weinberg, J. (1993). Response styles in perceptual retraining. In W. A. Gordon (Ed.), *Advances in stroke reha-bilitation*. Boston: Andover Medical Publishers.

Dobkin, B. (1991). The rehabilitation of elderly stroke patients. *Clinics in Geriatric Medicine, 7*, 507–523.

Dobkin, B. (1995). The economic impact of stroke. *Neurology, 45*(Suppl. 1), S6–S9.

Dull, R. B., Brown, G., Adams, K. M., Shatz, M. W., Diaz, F. G., & Ausman, J. I. (1982). *The Journal of Clinical Neuropsychology, 4*, 151–166.

Dyken, M. L. (1987). Symptoms, epidemiology, and risk factors. In R. E. Dunkle & J. W. Schmidley (Eds.), *Stroke in the elderly* (pp. 3–18). New York: Springer Publishing Company.

Fabris, F. Zanocchi, M., Bo, M., Fonte, G., Poli, L., Bergoglio, I., Farrario, E., & Pernigotti, L. (1994). Carotid plaque, aging, and risk factors. *Stroke, 25*, 1133–1140.

Federoff, J. P., & Robinson, R. G. (1989). Tricyclic antidepressants in the treatment of post-stroke depression. Symposium: Clinical challenges of depression: Timely perspectives in antidepressants. *Journal of Clinical Psychiatry, 50* (Suppl.), 18–23.

Gainotti, G. (1972). Emotional behavior and hemispheric side of the lesion. *Cortex, 8*, 41–55.

Gainotti, G. (1989). The meaning of emotional disturbances resulting from unilateral brain injury. In G. Gainotti & C. Caltagirone (Eds.), *Emotions and the dual brain*. Berlin/Heidelberg: Springer-Verlag.

Glosser, G., & Goodglass, H. (1990). Disorders in executive control functions among aphasic and other brain damaged patients. *Journal of Clinical and Experimental Neuropsychology, 12*, 485–501.

Godefroy, O., Rousseau, M., Leys, D., Destee, A., Scheltens, P., & Pruvo, J. P. (1992). Frontal lobe dysfunction in unilateral lenticulostriate infarcts. *Archives of Neurology, 49*, 1285–1289.

Goldstein, K. (1939). *The organism*. New York: American Book Company.

Gorelick, P. (1993). Distribution of atherosclerotic cerebrovascular lesions: Effects of age, race, and sex. *Stroke, 24*, 116–119.

Gorelick, P. (1995). Stroke prevention. *Archives of Neurology, 52*, 347–355.

Gray, J. W., Dean, R. S., Rattan, G., & Cramer, K. M. (1987). Neuropsychological aspects of primary affective depression. *International Journal of Neuroscience, 32*(3–4), 911–918.

Halligan, P. W., & Marshall, J. C. (1992). Left visuo-spatial neglect: A meaningless entity? *Cortex 28*, 525–535.

Heilman, K. M., & Gonzalez Rothi, L. J. (1985). Apraxia. In K. M. Heilman & E. Valenstein (Eds.), *Clinical neuropsychology* (pp. 131–150). New York: Oxford University Press.

Heilman, K. M., Watson, R. T., & Valenstein, E. (1985). Neglect and related disorders. In K. M. Heilman & E. Valenstein, E. (Eds.), *Clinical neuropsychology* (pp. 243–294). New York: Oxford University Press.

Hennerici, M. G. (1991). Regression of atherosclerosis. In J. W. Norris & V. C. Hachinski (Eds.), *Prevention of stroke* (pp. 49–60). New York: Springer-Verlag.

Hodges, J. R., & Oxbury, S. M. (1990). Persistent memory impairment following transient global amnesia. *Journal of Clinical and Experimental Neuropsychology, 12*, 904–920.

Hom, J. (1991). Contributions of the Halstead-Reitan Battery in the neuropsychological investigation of stroke. In R. A. Bornstein & G. Brown (Eds.), *Neurobehavioral aspects of cerebrovascular disease* (pp. 182–201). New York: Oxford University Press.

Hom, J., & Reitan, R. M. (1982). Effects of lateralized cerebral damage upon contralateral and ipsilateral sensorimotor performances. *Journal of Clinical Neuropsychology, 4*, 249–268.

Hom, J., & Reitan, R. M. (1990). Generalized cognitive function in stroke. *Journal of Clinical and Experimental Neuropsychology, 12*, 644–654.

Hossman, K. A. (1994). Viability thresholds and the penumbra of focal ischemia. *Annals of Neurology, 36*(4), 557–565.

Jebsen, R. H., Griffith, E. R., Long, E. W., & Fowler, R. (1971). Function of the "normal" hand in stroke patients. *Archives of Physical Medicine and Rehabilitation, 52*, 171–175.

Jorgensen, H. S., Nakayama, H., Raaschou, H. O., & Olsen, T. S. (1995). Intracerebral hemorrhage versus infarction: Stroke severity, risk factors, and prognosis. *Annals of Neurology, 38*, 45–50.

Kinsella, G., Olver, J., Ng, K., Packer, S., & Stark, R. (1993). Analysis of the syndrome of unilateral neglect. *Cortex, 29*, 135–140.

Laeng, B. (1994). Lateralization of categorical and coordinate spatial functions: A study of unilateral stroke patients. *Journal of Cognitive Neuroscience, 6*, 189–203.

Lauritzen, L., Bendsen, B. B., Vilmar, T., Bendsen, E. B., Lunde, M., & Bech, P. (1994). Post-stroke depression: Combined treatment with imipramine or desipramine and mianserin: A controlled clinical study. *Psychopharmacology, 114*(1), 119–122.

Lazarus, L. W., Winemiller, D. R., Lingam, V. R., & Neyman, I., Hartmen, C., Abassian, M., Kartan, U., Groves, L. & Fawcett, J. (1992). Efficacy and side effects of methylphenidate for post-stroke depression. *Journal of Clinical Psychiatry, 56*, 447–449.

Levine, J., Warrenburg, S., Kerns, R., Schwartz, G., Delaney, R. C., Fontana, A., Gradman, A., Smith, S., Allen, S., & Cascione, R. (1987). The role of denial in the recovery from coronary heart disease. *Psychosomatic Medicine, 49*, 109–117.

Lipsey, J. R., Robinson, R. G., Pearlson, G. D., Rao, K., & Price, T. R. (1984). Nortriptyline treatment of post-stroke depression: A double-blind study. *Lancet, 1*, 297–300.

Marangos, P. J., & Lal, H. (Eds.). (1992). *Emerging strategies in neuroprotection*. Boston: Birkhauser.

Meier, M. (1970). Objective behavioral assessment in diagnosis and prediction: Presentation 14. In A. L. Benton (Ed.), *Behavioral changes in cerebrovascular disease* (pp. 119–154). New York: Harper and Row.

Meier, M., & Strauman, S. (1991). Neuropsychological recovery after cerebral infarction. In R. A. Bornstein & G. Brown (Eds.), *Neurobehavioral aspects of cerebrovascular disease* (pp. 271–296). New York: Oxford University Press.

Mesulam, M. (1982). A cortical network for directed attention and unilateral neglect. *Annals of Neurology, 10*, 309–325.

Milberg, W. P., Hebben, N., & Kaplan, E. (1986). The Boston process approach to neuropsychological assessment. In I.

Grant & K. M. Adams (Eds.), *Neuropsychological aspects of neuropsychiatric disorders* (pp. 65–86). New York: Oxford University Press.

Millikan, C. H., McDowell, F., & Easton, J. D. (1987). *Stroke*. Philadelphia: Lea and Fibiger.

Moore, W. S., Barnett, H. J. M., Beebe, H. G., Bernstein, E. F., Brener, B. T., Brott, T. Caplan, L. R., Day, A., Goldstone, J., Hobson, R. W., Kempczinski, R. F., Matchar, D. B., Mayburg, M. R., Niolaides, A. N., Norris, J. W., Ricotta, A. J., Robertson, J. T., Rutherford, R. B., Thomas, D., Toole, J. F., Trout, H. H., & Wiebers, D. O. (1995). Guidelines for carotid endarterectomy. *Stroke, 26,* 188–201.

Morris, P. L., Robinson, R. G., Andrzejewski, P., Samuels, J., & Price, T. R. (1993). Association of depression with 10-year post-stroke mortality. *American Journal of Psychiatry, 151*(1), 124–129.

Morris, P. L., Robinson, R. G., & Raphael, B. (1993). Emotional lability after stroke. *Australian and New Zealand Journal of Psychiatry, 27*(4), 601–605.

Naugle, R., Bridgers, S. L., & Delaney, R. C. (1986). Neuropsychological signs of asymptomatic stenosis. *Archives of Clinical Neuropsychology, 1,* 25–30.

Nelson, L. D., Cicchetti, D., Satz, P., Stern, S., Sowa, M., Cohen, S., Mitrushina, M., & van Gorp, W. (1993). Emotional sequelae of stroke. *Neuropsychology, 7*(4), 553–560.

Nelson, L. D., Cicchetti, D., Satz, P., Sowa, M., & Mitrushina, M. (1994). *Journal of Clinical and Experimental Neuropsychology, 16,* 796–806.

Perez, F. I., Rivera, V. M., Meyer, J. S., Gay, J. R. A., Taylor, R. L., & Matthew, N. T. (1975). Analysis of intellectual and cognitive performance in patients with multi-infarct dementia, vertebro-basilar insufficiency with dementia, and Alzheimer's disease. *Journal of Neurology, Neurosurgery, and Psychiatry, 38,* 533–540.

Poirier, J., Gray, F., & Escourolle, R. (1990). *Manual of basic neuropathology* (L. J. Rubenstein, Trans.). Philadelphia: Saunders.

Raps, E. C., & Galetta, S. L. (1995). Stroke prevention therapies and management of patient subgroups. *Neurology, 45* (Suppl. 1), S19–S24.

Reitan, R. M. (1970). Objective behavioral assessment in diagnosis and prediction: Presentation 15. In A. L. Benton (Ed.), *Behavioral changes in cerebrovascular disease* (pp. 155–165). New York: Harper and Row.

Reitan, R. M., & Fitzhugh, K. B. (1971). Behavioral deficits in groups with cerebral vascular lesions. *Journal of Consulting and Clinical Psychology, 37,* 215–223.

Reitan, R. M., & Wolfson, D. (1993). *The Halstead-Reitan Neuropsychological Battery.* Tucson, AZ: Neuropsychology Press.

Robinson, R., Kubos, K., Starr, L., Rao, K., & Price, T. R. (1984). Mood disorders in stroke patients: Importance of location of lesion. *Brain, 107,* 81–93.

Robinson, R. G., Lipsey, J. R., Bolla-Wilson, K., Bolduc, P. L., Pearlson, G. D., Rao, K., & Price, T. R. (1985). Mood disorders in left-handed stroke patients. *American Journal of Psychiatry, 142,* 1424–1429.

Robinson, R. G., Bolla-Wilson, K., Kaplan, E., Lipsey, J. R., & Price, T. R. (1986). Depression influences intellectual impairment in stroke patients. *British Journal of Psychiatry, 148,* 541–547.

Sacco, R. L. (1995). Risk factors and outcomes for ischemic stroke. *Neurology, 45*(Suppl. 1), S10–S13.

Schulz, R., Tompkins, C. A., & Rau, M. T. (1988). A longitudinal study of the psychosocial impact of stroke on primary support persons. *Psychological Aging, 3,* 131–141.

Schwartz, J. A., Speed, N. M., Brunberg, J. A., Brewer, T. L., Brown, M., & Greden, J. F. (1993). *Biological Psychiatry, 33,* 694–699.

Sekhon, L. H. S., Morgan, M. K., Spence, I., & Weber, N. C. (1994). Chronic cerebral hypoperfusion and impaired neuronal function in rats. *Stroke, 25,* 1022–1027.

Shahar, E., McGovern, P. G., Sprafka, J. M., Pankow, J. S., Doliszny, K. M., Luepker, R. V., & Blackburn, H. (1995). Improved survival of stroke patients during the 1980s. *Stroke, 26,* 1–6.

Shima, S., Kitagawa, Y., Kitamura, T., Fujinawa, A., & Watanabe, Y. (1994). Post stroke depression. *General Hospital Psychiatry, 16,* 286–289.

Smith, S. E., & Meldrum, B. S. (1995). Cerebroprotective effects of lamotrigine after focal ischemia in rats. *Stroke, 26,* 117–122.

Sohlberg, M. M., & Mateer, C. A. (1987). Effectiveness of an attention-training program. *Journal of Clinical and Experimental Neuropsychology, 9*(2), 117–130.

Sohlberg, M. M., & Mateer, C. A. (1989). *Introduction to cognitive rehabilitation: Theory and practice.* New York: Guilford Press.

Starkstein, S., Robinson, R., & Price, T. (1987). Comparison of cortical and subcortical lesions in the production of post-stroke disorders. *Brain, 111,* 1045–1059.

Starkstein, S. E., Robinson, R. G., Berthier, L., Parikh, R. M., & Price, T. R. (1988). Differential mood changes following basal ganglia vs. thalamic lesions. *Archives of Neurology, 45,* 725–730.

Starkstein, S. E., Federoff, J. P., Price, T. R., Leiguarda, R., & Robinson, R. G. (1993a). Apathy following cerebrovascular lesions. *Stroke, 24,* 1625–1630.

Starkstein, S. E., Federoff, J. P., Price, T. R., Leiguarda, R., & Robinson, R. G. (1993b). Catastrophic reaction after cerebrovascular lesions: Frequency, correlates and validation of a scale. *Journal of Neuropsychiatry and Clinical Neurosciences, 5*(2), 189–194.

Sterzi, R., Bottini, G., Celani, M. G., Righetti, E., Lamassa, M., Ricci, S., & Vallar, G. (1993). Hemianopia, hemianaesthesia, and hemiplegia after left and right hemisphere damage. A hemisphere difference. *Journal of Neurology, Neurosurgery, and Psychiatry, 56,* 308–310.

Storey, P. B. (1970). Brain damage and personality change after subarachnoid hemorrhage. *British Journal of Psychiatry, 117,* 129–142.

Sweet, J. J., Newman, P., & Bell, B. (1992). Significance of depression in clinical neuropsychological assessment. *Clinical Psychology Review, 12,* 21–45.

Tatemichi, T. K., Paik, M., Bagiella, E., Desmond, D. W., Pirro, M., & Hanzawa, L. K. (1994). Dementia after stroke is a predictor of long term survival. *Stroke, 25,* 1915–1919.

Tiller, J. W. (1992). Post-stroke depression. Second International

Symposium on Moclobemide: RIMA (reversible inhibitor of monoamine oxidase type A): A new concept in the treatment of depression. *Psychopharmacology, 106* (Suppl.), 130–133.

Torvik, A. (1984). The pathogenesis of watershed infarcts in the brain. *Stroke, 15*, 221–223.

van Gijn, J., & Algra, A. (1994). Ticlopidine, trials and torture. *Stroke, 25*, 1097–1098.

von Cramon, D. Y., Hebel, N., & Schuri, U. (1985). A contribution to the anatomical basis of thalamic amnesia. *Brain, 108*, 993–1008.

Von Monakow, C. (1911). Lokalisation der Hirnfunktionen. *Journal für Psychologie und Neurologie, 17*, 185–200.

Waldstein, S. R., Manuck, S. B., Ryan, C. M., & Muldoon, M. F. (1991). Neuropsychological correlates of hypertension: Review and methodologic considerations. *Psychological Bulletin, 110*(3), 451–468.

Weinberg, J., Diller, L., Gordon, W., Gerstman, L., Lieberman, A., Lakin, P., Hodges, G., & Ezrachi, O. (1977). Visual scanning training effect on reading-related tasks in acquired right brain damage. *Archives of Physical Medicine and Rehabilitation, 58*(11), 479–486.

Weinberg, J., Diller, L., Gordon, W., Gerstman, L., Lieberman, A., Lakin, P., Hodges, G., & Ezrachi, O. (1979). Training sensory awareness and spatial organization in people with right brain damage. *Archives of Physical Medicine and Rehabilitation, 60*(11), 491–496.

Weinstein, E. A., & Friedland, R. P. (1977). Hemi-inattention and hemispheric specialization: Introduction and historical review. *Advances in Neurology, 18*, 1–31.

Weinstein, P. R., & Faden, A. I. (Eds.). (1990). *Protection of the brain from ischemia.* Baltimore: Williams and Wilkins.

Welch, K. M. A., & Levine, S. R. (1991). In R. A. Bornstein & G. Brown (Eds.), *Neurobehavioral aspects of cerebrovascular disease* (pp. 1–13). New York: Oxford University Press.

Wiard, R. P., Dickerson, M. C., Beek, O., Norton, R., & Cooper, B. R. (1995). Neuroprotective properties of the novel antiepileptic lamotrigine in a gerbil model of global cerebral ischemia. *Stroke, 26*, 466–472.

Winocur, G., Oxbury, S., Roberts, R., Agnetti, V., & Davis, C. (1984). Amnesia in a patient with bilateral lesions to the thalamus. *Neuropsychologia, 22*, 123–143.

Working Group on Emergency Brain Resuscitation. (1995). Emergency brain resuscitation. *Annals of Internal Medicine, 122*, 622–627.

22

Aging and Mental Retardation

GREGORY T. SLOMKA AND JULIE BERKEY

Introduction

Historically, research efforts have been lacking in the investigation of age-related changes in the physical, psychosocial, and cognitive adaptation of mentally retarded adults. Much remains unknown about how the central nervous system (CNS) ages in this population (Wisniewski & Merz, 1985). While nearly 25 years of effort have been directed at elucidating aspects of cognitive development in mentally retarded children (Hodapp & Zigler, 1995), research on the effects of aging has been limited to the last 10 years.

In terms of accountability, debate among policy-makers in both aging and mental retardation service networks revolves around how best to meet specific needs of an aging mentally retarded citizenry within the context of support systems designed for the aged versus specialized programs dedicated to meet the needs of mentally retarded individuals (Ansello & Rose, 1989; Janicki, 1994). Accordingly, among these agencies is competition for allocation of limited resources (Hogg, 1990). A number of vexing questions remain unresolved. For example, should existing mental retardation (MR) services be expanded to accommodate the needs of seniors, or would this population be best served via inclusion in programs for the aged within the general population?

In terms of eligibility for services no consistent definition of "aged" in mentally retarded populations has been operationalized. This has obvious implications in terms of eligibility for senior services, program planning, and compensatory services. The chronological age at which mentally retarded individuals are considered aged is variably defined, although 60 is the age specified by the 1987 reauthorization of the Older Americans Act (Janicki, 1994). This is particularly pertinent to older persons with Down's syndrome. Increased longevity is documented in this population secondary to improved health care practices, but with this comes a higher incidence of age-related health complications, Alzheimer's-type dementia, and premature aging effects that limit life adaptation in segments of this population. Therefore, eligibility for medical gerontology and social services may be required earlier in this population than for the population at large (Janicki, 1994). It must be recognized that aging within developmentally disabled populations may occur as early as the mid-40s to early 50s (Janicki, Otis, Puccio, Rettig, & Jacobson, 1985). Where premature aging occurs, special guidelines are required to provide appropriate supervision of life activities, programmatic adjustments, and geriatric medical services (Janicki et al., 1985). To meet the overall needs of this special population, appropriate multidisciplinary assessment methodologies are required to ensure the comprehensive delineation of needs. From a service and policy point of view, the impact of the aging process on developmentally disabled persons requires recognition that chronological age should not be the only determinant of need, since the time at which atypical aging may make its impact is variable (Lippman & Loberg, 1985). Because physical and cognitive aging effects manifest differently in this heterogeneous population, the availability of comprehen-

GREGORY T. SLOMKA • Western Psychiatric Institute and Clinic, Pittsburgh, Pennsylvania 15213. JULIE BERKEY • Allegheny General Hospital/Allegheny Neuropsychiatric Institute, Pittsburgh, Pennsylvania 15212.

sive, longitudinal assessment methodologies will be required for purposes of screening. Additionally, improved estimates of life expectancy and specialized needs among homogeneous subgroups within this population are needed in order to identify risk factors that predict morbidity and mortality, as well as to determine service planning (Eyman & Borthwich-Duffy, 1994). As will be discussed, research beyond the parameters of aging within Down's syndrome remains relatively limited. In order to plan for the special needs and supports of an elderly developmentally disabled population expressing risks for dementia and related complications, a broader base of research is needed. In this regard, clinical neuropsychology has much to offer. In the discussion which follows, a review of aging effects in Down's syndrome is summarized. Implications derived from these findings are subsequently generalized to future research directions.

Aging and Mental Retardation

Early studies have not suggested major variations from normal patterns of aging for the population of mentally retarded individuals (Bell & Zubek, 1960; Demaine & Silverstein, 1978; Goodman, 1976). Fisher and Zeaman (1970), in their longitudinal study of intellectual development, indicated that mental age in mentally retarded children increased in linear fashion from age 2 to 16. Higher functioning individuals exhibited a continued pattern of growth into early adulthood. Over the course of adulthood, stability in general intellectual functioning was noted, with a tendency to decline after age 60. Fenner, Hewitt, and Torpy (1987) obtained evidence of a similar pattern of stability of general cognitive ability throughout adulthood, with declines evident in the mid 60s. When one transcends these epidemiological studies, the number of investigations of age-related cognitive risk factors in mentally retarded adults is minimal. Much of our understanding of age-related change and dementia vulnerability in ideopathic forms of mental retardation is inferred from studies of premature aging effects in Down's syndrome. The consensus opinion emerging from this limited database has been that with the exception of Down's syndrome individuals, mentally retarded adults are at the same risk

for pathological aging effects as the population at large. With over 300 etiologies identified as contributory to mental retardation, it remains presumptive that Down's syndrome represents the only condition in which abnormal aging is observed.

There is additional evidence, however, that etiology, level of mental retardation, as well as moderating psychosocial influences predict mortality risk in the elderly mentally retarded population. Wisniewski and Hill (1985) distinguish static etiologies (i.e., posttraumatic, infection, anoxia, etc.) from progressive syndromes (i.e., congenital conditions involving inborn errors of metabolism or neurodegenerative processes). Individuals whose etiologies clustered within the static conditions were presumed to be vulnerable to similar risks as the general population in later life. Progressive CNS processes, among them a number of genetically linked conditions, would be predicted to result in potential dementing effects earlier in life.

Additionally, individuals with moderate to profound mental retardation have been found to be at greatest risk for shorter life expectancies than nonhandicapped controls due to effects of secondary handicapping factors and problems associated with health risks (Eyman & Borthwich-Duffy, 1994). Risk factors associated with type of residency, availability of health care supports, as well as other lifestyle factors have also been correlated with expected life span (Krauss & Seltzer, 1994).

Aging and Down's Syndrome

As was highlighted above, Down's syndrome in comparison to other congenital syndromes or forms of mental retardation has associated with it vulnerability to accelerated neurological aging. Neuropathological aging effects, including loss of acetylcholine, neuronal loss, senile plaques, and neurofibrillary tangle formation, as well as evidence of reduced cerebral metabolism, are virtually ubiquitous in this population with advanced age. While these neuropathological features are characteristic of Alzheimer's dementia in the population at large, specific to Down's syndrome is the temporal course of neuropathological changes to which these individuals are vulnerable, as well as the variable expression of actual dementia.

Thus, individuals with Down's syndrome provide clinicians with a unique opportunity to study the evolution of neuropathological correlates of dementia. As will be discussed, neuropathologically and neurochemically there are sufficient similarities to Alzheimer's dementia to suggest that the abnormal aging seen in Down's syndrome represents a viable model for understanding dementia progression.

It must be emphasized that the unique characteristics distinguishing the lifetime history of the Down's syndrome subject would naturally predispose differences in phenotypic expression of abnormal aging. Aging changes are superimposed upon anomalous brain development, a lifetime history of intellectual retardation, and a divergent path in terms of psychosocial opportunities and attainment of adult life role responsibilities. In addition, confounds associated with specific physical-medical complications are frequently exhibited in this population. Despite these inherent differences, multiple studies have suggested reasonable parsimony between dementia in Down's syndrome and Alzheimer's dementia (Dalton, 1992; Evenhuis, 1990; Lai, 1992; Lai & Williams, 1989).

The increased prevalence of dementia risk in Down's syndrome makes this population ideal for studying risk factors associated with Alzheimer's-type dementia (Wisniewski, Wisniewski, & Wen, 1985). Further, to the degree to which lifetime vulnerabilities to dementia can be understood in a population in which the full range of mental deficiency is expressed, Down's syndrome should serve as a prototype for development of diagnostic, assessment, treatment, and support services across the spectrum of the aged population of mentally retarded individuals.

Down's Syndrome

Down's syndrome is the most common cause of mental retardation in developed countries. One in 600 live births, or approximately 7,000 children per year, are born with Down's syndrome in the United States (Wishart, 1988). Varying levels of mental retardation are expressed within this population. Impaired brain growth and maturation, vulnerability to cardiac abnormalities, dermatoglyphic

changes, immune complications, as well as early age-related pathogenic changes in the central nervous system have been associated with this condition. Table 1 highlights a number of the physical and medical complications expressed in this population and addresses their functional significance for adaption.

Kemper (1988) has delineated specific neurodevelopmental risks leading to atypical brain development. He suggests essentially normal neuronal development up until birth, with progressive curtailment during the first year of postnatal life. Courchesne (1988) offers further substantiation for a model of early developmental arrest. Abnormal progression in brain development, especially atypical neurogenesis and synaptogenesis (Wisniewski, Miezejeski, & Hill, 1988) are thought to contribute to abnormalities expressed in brain morphology. Reduced brain weight, frontocaudal shortening, variable expression of hypoplasia of the frontal lobe, atrophy of the temporal gyrus, decreased size of the cerebellum, and abnormal neurodensity in the hippocampus, neocortex, and varied subcortical structures characterize the atypical brain development in the Down's syndrome phenotype. Thus, these developmental vulnerabilities are important to bear in mind when any attempts at comparative neuropathological examination with Alzheimer's dementia are considered.

Specific medical conditions identified in the Down's syndrome population (see Table 1) tend to occur in higher proportions relative to life span developmental stages. Health-related complications require substantial treatment supports and monitoring (Pueschel, 1990). Access to quality health care within the community is related to quality of life and life expectancy in this population (Krauss & Seltzer, 1994). For the adult with Down's syndrome who is residing in supervised living arrangements, medical care is usually readily available. However, for those individuals outside such systems, these health-related problems may go unrecognized or adequate support systems may not be available to provide treatment. Edgerton (1994) identified four factors that limit the delivery of adequate preventative medical care in developmentally disabled populations: (1) ineffectiveness of such individuals in articulating their health concerns to professional staff secondary to limited verbal skills;

Table 1. Down's Syndrome: Conditions, Treatment, and Sequelae

Frequently occurring Down's syndrome conditions	Programming treatment recommendations	Behavioral/neuropsychological sequelae
Immunology Premature aging	Assessment and skill-matched programming throughout life span	Cognitive, physical, language, sensory adaptive declines

Cardiovascular disease
  Congenital heart disease
  Mitral valve prolapse
  Increased blood pressure
  Obesity
	Pediatric cardiologist involvement for management; ongoing nutrition, fitness, and activity program	Reduced brain oxygenation with possible effects on higher mental functions and psychological processes

Endocrine disease
  Thyroid dysfunction
  Hypothyroidism
	Annual assessment/monitoring for thyroid dysfunction	Growth delays, behavior changes, confusion, lethargy, motivation, depression

Sensory losses
  Vision
    Congenital cataracts
    Acquired cataracts
    Refractive errors
    Strabismus
  Hearing
    High frequency loss
    Conductive loss
    middle ear
	Specialized assessment/monitoring; corrective lenses; hearing aids; environmental accommodations; communicate expectations clearly, slowly; reduce visual confusions; provide socialization opportunities to offset withdrawal	Confusion without reliance on visual or auditory cues; receptive language comprehension decline; decreased ability to follow task demands; decreased interest in socialization participation; inattention; general functional declines

Muscular/skeletal
  Muscular skeletal abnormalities
  Changes in motor skills, coordination, flexibility
	Radiograph spines; exercise to reduce mobility deterioration and muscle atrophy; physical therapy; environmental accommodations in daily activity	Deterioration in ambulation, mobility; fractures; falls; decrease in independent, basic self-help skills such as toileting, feeding; respiratory infections

Dental Periodontal disease	Maintain preventive oral hygiene program; monitor for medication/medical side effects	Reduced feeding abilities, nutrition effects, communication disturbances
Sleep apnea Increases with age	Provide appropriate medical treatment	Lethargy in daytime, behavior problems, developmental growth delays

(2) problems in understanding staff questions and medical instructions; (3) inadequate compliance with therapy or interventive health care maintenance, and (4) failure to monitor or recognize early warning signs and seek appropriate medical care. The range of appropriately trained health professionals, programs, and services in the area of health needs for older mentally retarded citizens are not nearly as comprehensive as pediatric services (Seltzer & Essex, 1993). The better the access to health care and the availability of appropriate lifestyle modifications and supports, the greater the likelihood of maintaining physical condition and a healthier aging process. The health-related complications, sensory losses, and physical limitations that may accompany premature aging in Down's syndrome creates a challenge for management and requires specialized service planning.

Table 1 highlights a number of conditions that hold special implications for the neuropsychologist attempting to conduct comprehensive assessments with this population. For example, chronic effects of long-term sensory deprivation from auditory or visual impairment could affect reality contact. High incidence of hearing loss (more than two thirds of this population with advancing age) could affect communicative effectiveness. Poor muscle tone, atrophy, or skeletal abnormalities secondary to limited stimulation and inactivity could mimic subtle extrapyramidal signs. Further, in the realm of metabolic inefficiencies, expression of thyroid dysfunction would be expected to be variably expressed as a function of age, that is, delayed growth in early childhood with a greater likelihood of cognitive impairment expressed in later adulthood.

Haverman, Maaskant, and Sturman (1989), in contrasting a sample of Down's syndrome and nonspecific etiology subjects with mental retardation in an institutional setting, identified a more substantial vulnerability to auditory and visual handicaps, arthritis, osteoporosis, and epilepsy, in addition to dementia, in a Down's syndrome sample. Effects of quality of life notwithstanding, there appears to be a differential expression of health risks in the Down's syndrome population which must be considered. Thus, Wisniewski and Merz (1985), in conceptualizing aging as a "loss of reserve" (p. 177) phenomenon, emphasize the importance of preventing or otherwise mollifying the expression of medical complications that could potentially burden the central nervous system.

Incidence of Dementia in Down's Syndrome

The introduction of antibiotic treatment for respiratory infections, one of the complications associated with Down's syndrome, has vastly increased life span. Whereas in the 1950s only approximately 50% of those with Down's syndrome survived infancy, the current average life expectancy is approximately 50 years with a substantial number now surviving to the 60s. With increased longevity, however, has come morbidity secondary to both a vulnerability to leukemia as well as dementia. Thase (1982) estimated the mortality rate of Down's syndrome subjects after age 50 as comparable to individuals in the normal population over age 80. Prevalence of dementia increases in an exponential fashion past age 50. Lai and Williams (1989) noted an approximate 8% expression of dementia in young adults with Down's syndrome ages 35 to 49. In the age range 50–59 the prevalence was 55%. For those past age 60 the prevalence rate was 75%. When generalizations are extended to the population at large, Thase (1988) estimated the incidence of dementia to be approximately 30% As Down's syndrome represents approximately 15% of the overall incidence of mental retardation expressed in the population at large, extrapolating from existing demographic data, Steffelaar and Evenhuis (1989) estimated that the proportion of those individuals with Down's syndrome between the years 1990 and 2010 would increase by 75% among those over 40, and by 200% among those over 50. Thus, the impact in terms of an increase in number of individuals at risk for dementia-related complications can be considered substantial.

Genetics

It is hypothesized that the major predisposing factor for early Alzheimer's symptom development in Down's syndrome is an extra copy of the gene that encodes the precursor of amyloid protein

(Goldgaber, Lerman, McBride, Saffiotti, & Gajdusek, 1987; Tanzi et al., 1987). This is presumed to lead to an excessive accumulation of beta-amyloid. The excessive extracellular deposition of amyloid and the accumulation of abnormal neurofibrillary filaments has been linked to this protein. An additional risk factor for developing Alzheimer's dementia neuropathology is inheritance of the apolipoprotein (ApoE) $\epsilon4$ allele. The risk for inheritance of this allele in Down's syndrome does not differ from that in the population at large. The presence of this allele is associated with an earlier onset of dementia and increased senile plaque formation, hence, an earlier and more virulent expression of dementia characteristics. Of further significance is the fact that risk of Down's syndrome is increased 2 to 2.5 times in relatives of subjects identified with dementia of the Alzheimer's type. It is emphasized that a genetic association is not attributed to the majority of individuals with Alzheimer's disease. Thus, any future genetic treatment for the presumed neuropathogenetic effect of Alzheimer's disease and dementia in Down's syndrome would be aimed at reducing the expression of beta-amyloid or its neurotoxic effects; Down's syndrome can be used as a model for understanding these early neurocognitive/neuropathological effects.

Neuropathological Correlates

Structural and Functional Brain Imaging

Imaging studies offer one means to examine patterns of change associated with the course of dementia. As noted earlier, any such studies are complicated by the fact that there are significant developmental differences in the Down's syndrome brain unrelated to acquired cerebral atrophy. Morphometric analysis of Down's syndrome neuropathology has been plagued by problems related to use of inappropriate control groups. Therefore, it has been recommended that comparisons should be made to other nondemented Down's syndrome subjects, and not aging normals (Lott, 1992). Studies using computerized tomography (CT) and magnetic resonance imaging (MRI) have generally demonstrated considerable variability in age-related structural changes. Progressive cortical atrophy and

increases in third ventricle size have been inconsistently reported in older Down's syndrome subjects, but cross-sectional and longitudinal studies using quantitative imaging suggest that significant volume loss tends to occur only in Down's syndrome subjects with clinically identified dementia (Dalton & Crapper, 1977; Lott & Lai, 1982; Schapiro, Azari, Grady, Haxby, & Horowitz, 1992). Further investigation of regional variations associated with onset and progression of Alzheimer's disease is necessary (Schapiro, 1993). The temporal lobes, particularly the hippocampal formation, are identified as areas for close examination (Pearlson et al., 1990).

Functional brain imaging has offered further support for declines in cerebral metabolism paralleling the regional changes seen in dementia of the Alzheimer's type (Schapiro et al., 1988). Johanson et al. (1991), in a longitudinal follow-up with two groups of younger (mean age 33 ± 4 years) and older (mean age 50 ± 8 years) Down's syndrome subjects, documented mean reductions in cerebral blood flow only for older subjects.

Clinicopathological Correlates

An atypical pattern of aging associated with Down's syndrome has been recognized for well over a century. While the association between Alzheimer's disease and Down's syndrome has been recognized for 60 years, the ultimate events leading to this association remain incompletely understood. Lott (1992) provides a historical perspective of the neurobiology of Down's syndrome. Premature CNS aging effects in Down's syndrome are hypothesized to represent premature and exaggerated expression of senile plaque and neurofibrillary tangle formation as well as other neuropathological changes. Khachaturian (1985) established the mean density of senile plaque and neurofibrillary tangle proliferation within the neocortex of individuals under 50 at no more than two to five per 200× microscopic field. In individuals over 75 the density increases to approximately 15 per field. Wisnewski et al. (1985) noted plaque formation in postmortem examinations of Down's syndrome subjects at densities comparable to those of individuals in the normal population over age 75. Their analysis suggested that all individuals with Down's syndrome express significant enough amyloid deposition by age 40 to meet criteria for a differential diagnosis of Alzheimer's disease.

While Kemper's (1988) investigation of this population suggests that similar but distinct abnormalities in both amyloid deposition and atrophic changes occur as early as the first and second decades of life, necropsy examinations in Down's syndrome subjects consistently show the most substantial neuropathological changes (atrophy, neuronal loss, and amyloid deposits) occurring after age 35. Thus, cross-sectional studies of neuropsychological performance prior to and after age 35–40 delineate distinct changes in cognitive ability that appear to be linked to underlying neuropathological processes.

Despite the evidence of neuropathological changes in the brains of individuals with Down's syndrome who come to autopsy over age 40, less than one third had overt indications of dementia. This suggests that it is not the presence of abnormal amyloid deposits alone which marks the onset of dementia. Multiple lines of inquiry have subsequently attempted to define threshold effects which herald onset of dementia. These factors are not completely understood, but recent research has offered a number of insights.

One obvious area of investigation is the expression of senile plaque formation due to the genetic predisposition of Down's syndrome subjects to overproduction of the amyloid protein. Hyman's (1992) review suggests that senile plaque and neurofibrillary tangle development in Down's syndrome is immunohistochemically similar to the neuropathology of Alzheimer's disease. The fact that high densities of senile plaques can be seen in intellectually normal subjects suggests that senile plaque formation alone may be insufficient for the expression of dementia in Alzheimer's disease. Further, senile plaque density has not been found to be a consistently reliable index of dementia severity or onset. Thus, Hof et al. (1995) conclude that early amyloid deposition alone does not account for dementia in Down's syndrome subjects over age 50.

Other investigators have focused on the distribution pattern of senile plaques and neurofibrillary tangles. Hyman (1992) reviewed the regional or topographical proliferation of senile plaques and neurofibrillary tangles. Neurofibrillary tangles were found to be most prominent in the cytoarchitectonic

fields of the hippocampal formation and the association cortices. In contrast, primary sensory and motor cortices were spared. Senile plaque formation was significant in hierarchial distributions within the hippocampus. Hof et al. (1995) replicated earlier findings of Hyman and others. Significant in his study was the fact that plaques were ubiquitous in this population, but that virtually no neurofibrillary tangles were observed in subjects younger than age 40. Hof et al. (1995) and Hyman, West, Rebeck, Lai, and Mann (1995) have proposed that the number of neurofibrillary tangles progressively accumulates in Down's syndrome subjects from age 35 onwards, obeying a hierarchial scheme similar to that seen in dementia of the Alzheimer's type. It appears that 10 to 20 years elapse between the development of initial neurofibrillary tangles in entorhinal cortex and the onset of dementia. After age 50 prominent hippocampal involvement is evident. It is suspected that dementia tends not to proceed unless the neocortex is affected. The earliest dementia indices correlate with hippocampal *and* neurofibrillary tangle development in the inferior temporal regions. Hence, the involvement of the association cortex appears to be a critical and necessary step in dementia onset. In this model dementia may not present until neurofibrillary tangle formation occurs outside the hippocampus and entorhinal cortex. Thus, not only widespread amyloid deposition, but also disruption in cortical circuitry, may be required before dementia is exhibited in Down's syndrome. Understanding of the shared mechanisms of clinical, genetic, and neuropathological mechanisms, however, awaits further confirmation of such hypotheses.

Course of Dementia in Down's Syndrome

Mean age of onset of dementia in Down's syndrome subjects varies between 51 years and 54.2 years (Evenhuis, 1990; Lai & Williams, 1989; Wisniewski et al., 1985). Whereas cross-sectional data suggest mild intellectual changes at approximately age 35, followed by more severe deterioration as neuropathological changes progress, Fenner et al. (1987), as well as Hewitt, Carter, and Jancar (1985), suggest that substantial intellectual deterioration does not occur until late in the fourth decade or early fifth decade, and then in less than 50% of this population. Although Down's syndrome subjects over age 35 exhibit neuropathological changes similar to those seen in non-mentally retarded elderly with Alzheimer's dementia, many do not exhibit definitive dementia characteristics. A protracted prodromal period associated with neuropathological changes is thought to occur prior to the expression of overt dementia. Evidence for such a prolonged prodrome may also exist for a subset of premorbidly normal adults in whom Alzheimer's neuropathological changes, but no manifestations of overt dementia, are apparent (refer to Haxby and Schapiro, 1992, for discussion).

Thus, the course of dementia can clearly be dissociated from that of Alzheimer's disease (Dalton, Crapper, & Schlotterer, 1974; Miniszek, 1983; Oliver & Holland, 1986; Wisniewski et al., 1985; Wisniewski & Rabe, 1986). As previously noted, expression of dementia in Down's syndrome subjects occurs at an earlier age than in normal controls. Preliminary evidence further suggests that progression is more rapid, with mortality 4.9 years to 5.2 years following initial diagnosis (Evenhuis, 1990).

Although differences in the pathogenic expression of dementia in Down's remains difficult to reconcile, a number of models have been proposed which describe the typical course. Schapiro et al. (1988) advanced a two-stage model linked to the progressive evolution of underlying neuropathological changes. An initial stage involving incipient progressive decline in cognitive abilities correlates with abnormal plaque accumulation and early neuronal degeneration. A second stage involving actual loss of overlearned behaviors and subsequent declines in social and adaptive skill competencies with more severe cognitive decline marks a phase of accelerated neurodegeneration and neurofibrillary tangle formation.

Lai and Williams (1989) proposed an alternative three-stage model of deterioration. In the first stage, predominantly cognitive impairment is manifest, consisting of memory impairment, temporal disorientation, reduced motor output (seen in higher functioning individuals), attentional dysfunction, and apathy/reduced social interest. The second stage is marked by losses in instrumental skill func-

tions. Declines in previously established self-care routines become more prominent and extrapyramidal motor signs emerge. Seizures develop at this stage and are distinctly more prevalent than in Alzheimer's dementia of the general population. In the third stage, progressive motor involvement is noted. Loss of ambulatory capacity and incontinence develop. A flexed posture evolves. Eventually, pathological reflexes emerge. Thus, there are a number of similarities between the progression of dementia in Down's syndrome and dementia of the Alzheimer's type, but the former occurs more rapidly.

The reader is cautioned that the staging models advanced by Schapiro et al. (1988) and Lai and Williams (1989) for Down's syndrome, like the stage models of Alzheimer's dementia, do not imply discrete, readily discerned characteristics which correlate with definitive neuropathological markers. Just as differentiation of predementia from dementia in the normal population is a challenge, multiple limitations inherent in assessment of a premorbid intellectually impaired population further confound both differential diagnosis and clinical research.

Emotional–Behavioral Correlates of Aging in Down's Syndrome

Only in the last two decades have there been rigorous efforts to explain the comorbidity of mental retardation and other emotional-behavioral disorders. This research has identified a broad range of psychopathological conditions to which individuals with mental retardation may be vulnerable. Estimates of affective disorder characteristics vary mainly as a function of the heterogeneity of samples studied and the challenge of adequate differential diagnosis in lower functioning individuals. Limited verbal competencies make traditional methods of standardized diagnostic assessment tenuous at best. Therefore, in many instances, diagnosis of affective disorder is based upon a third party informant's description of mood and behavior.

Reiss's (1994) review of dual diagnosis, that is, comorbidity of mental retardation and emotional-behavioral disorders, across 33 studies reflected prevalence rates of 15% to 35%. As such, up to one third of this population may be at risk for a wide range of emotional and behavioral problems. While disproportionate vulnerability to psychopathology has been substantiated for this population, a comprehensive appreciation of life span effects upon the expression of maladaptive behavior and emotional adjustment remains extant. Overall, appreciation of aging effects upon psychosocial adaptation remains quite limited.

Changes in affect have been identified in a number of studies as one marker of dementia onset in Down's syndrome populations. Burt, Loveland, and Lewis (1992) addressed the challenges associated with differential diagnosis of depression versus dementia with comorbid depressive symptomatology. Their review of multiple studies indicated a number of similarities between affective disorder and dementia. Anecdotal data accrued in case studies have consistently suggested that deficits in cognitive ability, memory, and adaptive skill competencies are sequelae of depression in this population (Warren, Holroyd, & Folstein, 1989). Moving beyond case study methodologies, Burt et al. (1995) contrasted age-matched Down's syndrome subjects with individuals whose mental retardation was attributed to other causes. Results were significant in validating the association of affective symptomatology in Down's subjects with dementia. Although it was established, using the Depression Status Inventory, that depressive symptomatology was identifiable in both groups, the non-Down's syndrome subjects who were identified with depressive symptomatology did not exhibit declines on cognitive, memory, or adaptive competency measures. Further, qualitative differences were expressed in the depressive symptomatology of the two groups. Thus, for Down's syndrome subjects in particular, it is difficult to distinguish the effects of primary depression from the comorbid presentation of dementia-depression.

Clearly, characteristics associated with depressive disorder symptomatology merit further investigation. Burt et al. (1992) found severity indices to be important potential predictors of outcome. Cooper and Collacott (1993) found that age of onset of first depressive episode was yet another potential determinant of outcome. It is also necessary to examine the effect of level of premorbid mental retardation and the ultimate expression of affective disorder. For example, clinicians familiar with the differential diagnosis of affective disorder in more severely impaired populations do not anticipate the expression of overt mood-related symptomatology. Rather, the clinical evaluation focuses on elucidating evidence of apathy, social withdrawal, irritability, and increased somatization. Refinement of diagnostic assessment strategies is an important step in any advancement of our understanding of these risk factors.

From yet another perspective, Nelson, Lott, Touchette, Satz, and D'Elia (1995) found distinguishing characteristics in a comparison study of Down's syndrome subjects, Alzheimer's dementia patients, and normal controls based on an evaluation of five emotional factors. While clinical depressive features of dementia were identifiable in the Alzheimer's dementia sample, the Down's syndrome subjects exhibited a greater vulnerability to apathy and indifference. Thus, the investigation of affective changes in aging Down's syndrome subjects must involve determining markers relevant to traditional assessment of affective disorder, as well as indices that permit a determination of possible organic apathy syndrome.

At this time, the relationship of depression and dementia in Down's syndrome remains ambiguous. It must be further recognized that changes in affect have not been a distinguishing hallmark of onset of dementia across studies (Wisniewski et al., 1985). Although attempts have been made to offer algorithms for features which distinguish depression from dementia (Warren et al., 1989), such efforts remain conjectural at best. Burt et al. (1992) conclude that any adult with Down's syndrome suspected of manifesting dementia should first be evaluated for any possible treatable psychiatric disorder, especially depression.

Neuropsychological Assessment

Morris (1994) has emphasized that while dementia is ultimately an acquired, global impairment of higher cognitive functioning and memory, it must be recognized that early deterioration is characteristically selective, insidious, and associated with progressive neuropathological changes at the level of the cerebral substrate. Although the general level of functioning of Down's syndrome subjects is obviously substantially lower than that of the general population, similar specificity in terms of loss of functioning correlated with neuropathological changes can be expected.

Indeed, despite the fact that neurocognitive vulnerability may be masked by severity of associated intellectual impairment, multiple studies using cross-sectional designs have delineated substantial differences in neuropsychological functioning between older and younger subjects. Thus, development of appropriate probes of cognitive functioning within this population is one of the main challenges of any longitudinal research. Toward this end, remarkable heterogeneity has been expressed across methodologies used in the assessment of aging Down's syndrome subjects.

Just as neuropsychological measures have proven sensitive to the detection of effects of cognitive and memory changes in Alzheimer's dementia within the general population, such methodologies distinguish the abnormal aging effects to which individuals with Down's syndrome are vulnerable. As will be discussed, while a number of methodologies used with the general population have proven applicable in the assessment of segments of the Down's syndrome population, attributes specific to this group necessitate a number of adaptations of more traditional forms of neuropsychological assessment.

Intellectual Assessment

When dealing with subjects whose premorbid levels of functioning fall in the mild or borderline ranges of functioning, repetition of any previous standardized ability measure (Wechsler scales, Stanford-Binet, Leiter International Performance Scale, etc.) offers an opportunity to reliably contrast performances on multiple baseline measures over time and document regression (Albert, 1992; Fenner et al., 1987; Haxby, 1989). When confronted with lower functioning subjects (high-moderate or severe to profound levels of mental retardation), floor effects inherent within the instrumentation tend to mitigate any contrast. Thus, intellectual measures

may offer limited utility when applied to longitudinal evaluation of more significantly impaired subjects. As an alternative, neuropsychological tests offer substantially greater sensitivity and specificity.

Neuropsychological Batteries

A review of the literature indicates substantial diversity associated with the tests used in the investigation of dementia in Down's syndrome. Haxby (1989) and Haxby and Schapiro (1992) used the Stanford-Binet L-M combined with a specially designed Down's syndrome Mental Status Examination. Brugge et al. (1994) used the Wechsler Adult Intelligence Scale-Revised (WAIS-R) combined with a diverse battery of neuropsychological measures of attention, memory, language, conceptual ability, as well as motor proficiency based primarily on developmentally less challenging tests standardized for use with children. Vicari, Nocentini, and Caltagirone (1994) similarly used a diverse battery of tests comprising measures, the majority of which might be found in any standardized dementia battery used with the general population. Other batteries have included components based upon nontraditional or experimental test methodologies. For example, Das and Mishra (1995), as a means to more specifically reconcile linguistic and cognitive functioning from a more theory-driven perspective, used the PASS test system (Planning, Attention, Simultaneous, and Successive processing).

While a number of these standardized measures may be sensitive to declines in select cognitive domains within the early phases of dementiform processes in higher functioning individuals, the assessment of more severely impaired populations and those individuals who require longitudinal follow-up over the course of their dementia requires alternative strategies. Based on Dalton's (1992) caveat that no single test of functional impairment will be useful throughout the course of dementia and that every test will eventually succumb to "floor effects," a special emphasis has been placed on development of brief cognitive measures of more elemental functions. As such, in addition to development of a computerized delayed matching to sample test of memory developed by Dalton and

Crapper (1984) to meet demands for longitudinal testing, methodologies applied in cognitive research with nonhuman primates have been modified for use with this population. Dalton's laboratory has, for example, developed the Visual Recognition Span test, the Table Top Spatial Location Test, as well as a series of dyspraxia measures for assessment of more severely impaired populations.

Behavioral Adaptation

Concerns about the utility of a number of cognitive assessment methodologies has led to exploration of alternative methodologies of measurement based on changes in instrumental skill functions or capacity to maintain age-appropriate expectations in areas involving adaptive skill competencies. As such, a variety of standardized rating scales typically used to aid in diagnosis of mental retardation have been applied (Collacott, 1992; Miniszek, 1983; Rasmussen & Sobsey, 1994). While a number of investigators have clearly demonstrated age-related declines in Down's syndrome populations disproportional to matched comparison groups, all such questionnaire-based strategies have not yielded discriminating findings (Silverstein, Herbs, Miller, Nasuta, & Williams, 1986). Concerns have been raised that because individuals with Down's syndrome lead comparatively structured, routinized, and supported lifestyles, impact in terms of declines in day-to-day functioning may be negligible. Further, in the assessment of emotional characteristics, a burden is placed on third party descriptions of behavior.

Neuropsychological Investigations of Down's Syndrome

Course

Crayton and Oliver (1993) provide a succinct review of multiple neuropsychological investigations of this population. These studies, primarily cross-sectional in design, have clearly established a linkage between the expression of abnormal CNS changes in Down's syndrome and Alzheimer's dementia, as well as provided information regarding incidence, course, and pattern of expressed vulnerability in younger versus older Down's syndrome subjects. It has been recognized via postmortem studies that premature expression of senile plaques and neurofibrillary tangles are prevalent in the aging process in Down's syndrome. These neuropathological changes reach proportions which in the normal population correlate with the Alzheimer's phenotype. Although studies have consistently reflected premature aging effects in older compared to younger Down's syndrome subjects relative to control subjects with mental retardation of varied etiologies, it is reiterated that the majority of these individuals do not express frank dementia features for a decade or more past the age of apparent neuropathologic risk (Thase, 1988).

Although a premature disposition to aging was clearly established as a result of early research, it is difficult to derive generalizations from these data.

Widaman, Borthwich-Duffy, and Powers (1994) discuss the methodological constraints on the investigation of aging effects in mentally retarded populations. Advances in assessment methodologies, recognition of public health benefits to be derived from understanding dementia vulnerability in developmentally disabled populations, and corollary improved understanding of the neuropathological changes in the aging central nervous system of Down's syndrome subjects have led more

Table 2. Limitations Associated with Early Research

Predominant use of institutionalized versus community-based populations

Disproportionate representation of very low level functioning subjects

Inadequate description of premorbid functioning levels

Matching for IQ to control for level of mental retardation without eliminating recent dementia effects in the controlled population

Lack of screening for conditions that could be expressed as "pseudodementia"

Baseline data not adjusted for variance attributable to heterogeneity of IQ test measures

Small sample sizes

Lack of age-matched controls

Few studies including subjects in the fifth decade of life or later

Limited sensitivity of cognitive measures used (i.e., floor effects)

recently to studies with longitudinal designs. As such, a number of prospective longitudinal studies are now available for review (Burt et al., 1995; Dalton, 1992; Devenny, Hill, Paxtot, Silverman, & Wisniewski, 1992; Lai, 1992; Lai & Williams, 1989). Haxby and Schapiro's (1992) longitudinal investigation was significant in that it suggested a parallel between aging effects in the normal population and pathological changes in the aging of Down's syndrome individuals. He found that relative to younger subjects, older non-Down's syndrome subjects performed more poorly on measures of general cognitive ability, recent memory, and spatial and constructional abilities. Further, these subjects did not display any select impairment in language or immediate memory span. It was suggested that this pattern of impairment paralleled the age-related changes seen in the population at large. This contrast between predementia cognitive changes in contrast to rapid and progressive neuropsychological changes led to Haxby's two-stage model of the progression of abnormal aging in this population.

In the predementia stage, selective mild cognitive impairment is likely to be expressed. Global deficits in independent activities of daily living during this time are not anticipated. More subtle ramifications upon daily functioning may not be recognized by caregivers, again, relative to the buffers such individuals are provided within many supervised living arrangements. Neuropsychological measures have, however, documented coexisting decrements in cognitive ability. At this stage, brain imaging studies tend not to reflect significant atrophic changes (Schapiro et al., 1989). Cognitive and adaptive deficits within this prodromal phase may be expressed rather benignly for up to 20 years.

Haxby would argue that rather than being reflective of any continuous process of progressive, insidious degeneration, onset of dementia in Down's syndrome represents a fundamental change in the neuropathological processes underlying aging. He suggests that longitudinal data reflect more the triggering of a cascade of related degenerative processes, the clinical manifestations of which result in a relatively rapid and progressive decline in cognitive and adaptive functioning. These more malignant changes are accompanied by neuronal degen-erative changes as exemplified by atrophy and significantly reduced cerebral metabolic rate.

Specific Deficits

Converging evidence from diverse sources suggests that heterogeneous expression of dementiform effects across the boundaries of sensorimotor and higher cognitive functioning must be anticipated. Within this context, there are a number of idiosyncratic vulnerabilities within this population that merit close scrutiny.

Language

Semantic dissolution is a hallmark of Alzheimer's dementia along with a progressive decline in verbal conceptual abilities. This is typically indicated by naming difficulties, literal and semantic paraphasias, as well as comprehension inefficiencies. Syntax and phonology remain relatively preserved. A number of early studies of Down's syndrome subjects (Hewett et al., 1985; Schapiro et al., 1989; Thase, 1982; Thase, Tigner, Smeltzer, & Liss, 1984) included measures of the nominative functions of language. Aging Down's syndrome subjects consistently expressed deficits on such measures. Studies by Haxby (1989) as well as Young and Kramer (1991) were further significant for the demonstration of receptive language deficits. It must be recognized, however, that congenital as well as early acquired risk factors may result in disproportionate vulnerability to premorbid language comprehension and communication deficits in this population (Das & Mishra, 1995; Wisniewski et al., 1988). Vulnerabilities to early expressive language problems and risk factors for hearing loss remain substantial over the life span. Young and Kramer (1991) investigated receptive language in adults with Down's syndrome and identified no hearing impairment. Vulnerabilities to comprehension deficits were identified on the Sequenced Inventory for Communication Development. Therefore, appropriate caution must be taken in examining language-related changes across the life span in Down's syndrome subjects. Traditional language measures may not be sensitive enough to reflect subtle change in a population at risk for significant premorbid vulnerabilities in language development (Brugge et al., 1994).

Memory

A hallmark of dementia is memory impairment. Early studies of Down's syndrome subjects clearly implicated vulnerabilities in this domain (Kolata, 1985; Lott & Lai, 1982; Wisniewski et al., 1985). A number of cross-sectional studies have established age-related decrements in performance across a variety of measures of new learning proficiency (Haxby, 1989; Lai & Williams, 1989; Schapiro et al., 1988). These deficits generalize across measures of both verbal and nonverbal information processing. Also, incremental deficits in new learning have been described in longitudinal investigations (Haxby & Schapiro, 1992). It must be recognized that the majority of these studies have primarily addressed new learning paradigms. Memory consolidation, retention and retrieval strategy utilization, and consequences of impaired memory on daily living skill competencies remain essentially unexplored.

Spatial and Constructional Abilities

Although deficits in visuospatial and visuomotor integration skills represent vulnerabilities in neuropsychological performance which are of particular relevance as Alzheimer's dementia progresses in the general population, these abilities remain only minimally investigated in Down's syndrome populations. Low-level general functioning as well as attentional and motivational factors make it difficult to obtain consistently valid measures of such faculties. Expression of any temporal gradient associated with specific loss of complex, nonverbal, or spatial processing abilities remains elusive.

Dyspraxia

Although dyspraxia is explicit in midstage- to advanced Alzheimer's dementia, this neuropsychological domain remains minimally investigated in Down's syndrome. Recognizing inherent limitations of standardized tests of these abilities, Dalton (1992) has experimented with a video-recorded structured performance test of dyspraxia, but this has not translated into widespread clinical application.

Adaptive Functioning

Elderly adults with Down's syndrome are more likely to lose adaptive skill competencies. This is particularly conspicuous in individuals over age 50 (Zigman, Seltzer, & Silverman, 1994). Rasmussen and Sobsey (1994) have suggested that specific deficits associated with self-care, increased irritability, fear of leaving familiar surroundings, difficulties coping with previously well-ensconced daily routines, and comprehension deficits may herald the onset of dementia. The variety of methodologies used for objectifying adaptive skill competencies as well as the varied life circumstances associated with the support of this population (community-supervised residential and institutional care environments) makes generalizations from such data difficult.

Summary

As has been highlighted above, research on the aging process in mentally retarded populations has focused on Alzheimer's-type dementia associated with Down's syndrome. This focus is in itself not limiting in that knowledge derived from this research can be generalized to aid an expanding citizenry of aging mentally retarded persons. However, it will be necessary in the near future to expand the breadth of these studies. The investigation of CNS development within this population has essentially been polarized. Hodapp and Zigler (1995) provide a review of research on early cognitive development in mentally retarded children. On the opposite end of the age spectrum, a growing body of knowledge has emerged regarding characteristics associated with pathogenesis and course of Alzheimer's-type dementia in Down's syndrome. However, many aspects of normal and pathological aging remain unknown. Hodapp and Zigler (1995) have argued that a substantial portion of the research with children has been conducted "through the lens of normal development" (p. 299). Recognition of congenital syndromes that involve atypical pathways of cognitive development or an alternative structure or modularity of cognitive functioning offers a means to probe both cognitive development and the aging process from an alternative prospective. For example, varied rates of development have been identified in mentally retarded children (see Hodapp and Zigler, 1995, for review). Fragile X syndrome has been associated with a substantial decline in IQ as males proceed through adolescence. While most fragile X male children have mild to moderate mental retardation, the majority of adults with this syndrome function at substantially lower levels (Maes, Fryns, Van Walleghem, & Van den Berghe, 1994). Investigations of the progress of these individuals through adulthood are limited. Similarly, specific neurogenetic syndromes are known to exert very specific influences upon the modularity of cognitive development. For example, Turner's syndrome results in specific deficits in spatial processing abilities, while Klinefelter's syndrome results in relative sparing of spatial abilities, but significant impairment of language. In Turner's syndrome there are medical conditions which may develop, prominent among them Hashimoto's thyroiditis, which could result in development of treatable pseudodementia characteristics. Although neither Turner's syndrome nor Klinefelter's syndrome have associated with them any known increased risk for dementia, they remain nonetheless important paradigms for understanding mechanisms of atypical cognitive development, and hence, potentially abnormal aging. For example, could individuals with presumptive right cerebral hemisphere information processing inefficiencies be more susceptible to adaptational burden with advancing age?

Williams syndrome represents yet another condition in which striking dissociations are seen in cognitive development. It is a rare genetic condition which results in mental retardation and specific dysmorphic as well as organ anomalies. In addition, a unique pattern of neurocognitive strengths and weaknesses is expressed. These individuals possess linguistic skills which rival the deficits they express in general cognitive ability and select aspects of spatial and constructional processing. Belugi, Wang, and Jernigan (1994) have undertaken a probe of cognitive processing differences in a matched Williams syndrome and Down's syndrome sample.

While both groups exhibit similar general cognitive inefficiencies, striking contrasts have bene delineated in terms of information processing abilities. What remains to be discerned are longitudinal ramifications of such atypical cognitive development upon aging and adaptation. Thus, longitudinal examination of diverse congenital conditions such as Turner's syndrome, Klinefelter's syndrome, Williams syndrome, and other conditions may offer unique insights into vulnerability of specific neural systems to aging.

Thus, in addition to risk factors associated with Down's syndrome, there are a number of "neurodevelopmental" disorders which affect CNS development in a specific manner. These syndromes offer a unique scaffold from which aspects of cognitive development can be understood. Examination of such conditions offers an opportunity to foster development of not only more complete models of brain–behavior relationships, but at the same time the delineation from a broad-based neurodevelopmental perspective of influences on adaptation over the life span. As such, continued elucidation of cognitive and adaptive risk factors in this population from a neuropsychological perspective is integral to issues such as programmatic development and resource allocation. From a theoretical perspective, unique insights can also be afforded through the understanding of the aging process in its normal and pathological forms.

References

Albert, M. S. (1992). Parallels between Down syndrome, dementia, and Alzheimer's disease. In L. Nadel & C. J. Epstein (Eds.), *Progress in clinical and biological research: Vol. 379. Down syndrome and Alzheimer disease* (pp. 77–102). New York: Wiley-Liss.

Ansello, E. F., & Rose, T. (1989). *Aging and lifelong disabilities: Partnership for the twenty-first century.* College Park, MD: University of Maryland, Center on Aging.

Bell, A., & Zubek, J. P. (1960). The effect of age on the intellectual performance of defectives. *Journal of Gerontology, 15,* 285–295.

Belugi, V., Wang, P. P., & Jernigan, T. L. (1994). Williams syndrome: An unusual neuropsychological profile. In S. H. Broman & J. Grafman (Eds.), *Atypical cognitive deficits in developmental disorders: Implications for brain function.* Hillsdale, NJ: Lawrence Erlbaum Associates.

Brugge, K. L., Nichols, S. L., Salmon, D. P., Hill, L. R., Delis, D. C., Aaron, L., & Trauner, D. A. (1994). Cognitive impairment in adults with Down's syndrome: Similarities to early cognitive changes in Alzheimer's disease. *Neurology, 44*, 232–238.

Burt, D., Loveland, K., & Lewis, R. (1992). Depression and the onset of dementia in adults with mental retardation. *American Journal on Mental Retardation, 96*, 502–511.

Burt, D. B., Loveland, K. A., Chen, Y. W., Chuang, A., Lewis, K. R., & Cherry, L. (1995). Aging in adults with Down's syndrome: Report from a longitudinal study. *American Journal on Mental Retardation, 100*(3), 262–270.

Collacott, R. A. (1992). The effect of age and residual placement on adaptive behavior of adults with Down's syndrome. *British Journal of Psychiatry, 161*, 675–679.

Cooper, R. A., & Collacott, S. A. (1993). Prognosis of depression in Down syndrome. *Journal of Nervous and Mental Disease, 181*, 1–6.

Courchesne, E. (1988). Physioanatomical considerations in Down's syndrome. In L. Nadel (Ed.), *The psychobiology of Down syndrome* (pp. 291–313). Cambridge, MA: MIT Press.

Crayton, L., & Oliver, C. (1993). Assessment of cognitive functioning in persons with Down syndrome who develop Alzheimer disease. In J. M. Berg, H. Karlinsky, & A. J. Holland (Eds.), *Alzheimer disease, Down syndrome and their relationship*. Oxford, England: Oxford University Press.

Dalton, A. J. (1992), Dementia in Down syndrome: Methods of evaluation. In L. Nadel & C. J. Epstein (Eds.), *Progress in clinical and biological research. Down syndrome and Alzheimer disease* (Vol. 379, pp. 51–76). New York: Wiley-Liss.

Dalton, A. J., & Crapper, D. R. (1977). Down's syndrome and aging of the brain. In P. Mitter (Ed.), *Research to practice in mental retardation* (pp. 391–400). Baltimore: University Park Press.

Dalton, A. J., & Crapper, D. R. (1984). Incidence of memory deterioration in aging persons with Down's syndrome. In J. M. Berg (Ed.), *Perspectives and progress in mental retardation biomedical aspects* (Vol. 2, pp. 55–62). Baltimore: University Press.

Dalton, A. J., Crapper, D. R., & Schlotterer, G. R. (1974). Alzheimer's disease in Down's syndrome: Visual retention deficits. *Cortex, 10*(4), 366–377.

Das, P., & Mishra, R. K. (1995). Assessment of cognitive decline associated with aging: A comparison of individuals with Down syndrome and other etiologies. *Research in Developmental Disabilities, 16*(1), 11–25.

Demaine, G. C., & Silverstein, A. B. (1978). Mental age changes in institutionalized Down's syndrome persons: Semi-longitudinal approach. *American Journal of Mental Deficiency, 82*, 429–432.

Devenny, D., Hill, A. L., Paxtot, O., Silverman, W. P., & Wisniewski, K. E. (1992). Ageing in higher functioning adults with Down's syndrome: An interim report in a longitudinal study. *Journal of Intellectual Disability Research, 36*, 241–250.

Edgerton, R. B., (1994). Quality of life issues: Some people know how to be old. In M. M. Seltzer, M. W. Krauss, & M. P. Janicki (Eds.), *Life course perspectives on adulthood and old age* (pp. 53–66). Washington, DC: American Association on Mental Retardation.

Evenhuis, H. M., (1990). The natural history of dementia in Down's syndrome. *Archives of Neurology, 47*(3), 263–267.

Eyman, R. K., & Borthwick-Duffy, S. A. (1994). Trends in mortality rates on predictions of mortality. In M. M. Seltzer, M. W. Krauss, & M. P. Janicki (Eds.), *Life course perspectives on adulthood and old age* (pp. 93–108). Washington, DC: American Association on Mental Retardation.

Fenner, M. E., Hewitt, K. E., & Torpy, D. M. (1987). Down's syndrome: Intellectual and behavioral functioning during adulthood. *Mental Deficiency Research, 31*, 241–249.

Fisher, M. A., & Zeaman, D. (1970). Growth and decline of retardate intelligence. In N. R. Ellis (Ed.), *International review of research in mental retardation* (Vol. 4, pp. 151–191). New York: Academic Press.

Goldgaber, D., Lerman, M. I., McBride, O. W., Saffiotti, U., & Gajdusek, D. C. (1987). Characterization and chromosomal localization of a cDNA encoding brain amyloid of Alzheimer's disease. *Science, 235*, 877–880.

Goodman, J. F. (1976). Aging and IQ change in institutionalized mentally retarded. *Psychological Reports, 39*, 999–1006.

Haverman, N., Maaskant, M. A., & Sturman, F. (1989). Older Dutch residents of institutions with and without Down syndrome: Comparisons of mortality and morbidity trends and motor/social functioning. *Australia and New Zealand Journal of Developmental Disabilities, 15*(3–4), 241–255.

Haxby, J. V. (1989). Neuropsychological evaluation of adults with Down's syndrome: Patterns of selective impairment in non-demented old adults. *Journal of Mental Deficiency Research, 33*, 193–210.

Haxby, J. V., & Schapiro, M. D. (1992). Longitudinal study of neuropsychological function in older adults with Down syndrome. In L. Nadel & C. J. Epstein (Eds.), *Progress in clinical and biological research: Down's syndrome and Alzheimer disease* (pp. 35–50). New York: Wiley-Liss, Inc.

Hewitt, K. E., Carter, G., & Jancar, J. (1985), Ageing in Down's syndrome. *British Journal of Psychiatry, 147*, 58–62.

Hodapp, R. M., & Zigler, E. (1995). Past, present, and future issues in the developmental approach to mental retardation and developmental disabilities. In D. Cicchetti & D. Cohen (Eds.), *Developmental psychopathology: Risk, disorder, and adaptation* (Vol. 2, pp. 299–331). New York: John Wiley and Sons, Inc.

Hof, P. R., Bouras, C., Perl, D. P., Sparks, D. L., Mehta, N., & Morrison, J. H. (1995). Age-related distribution of neuropathologic changes in the cerebral cortex of patients with Down's syndrome. *Archives of Neurology, 52*, 379–391.

Hogg, J. (1990). International sources and directions in the study of ageing and severe intellectual impairment (mental handicap). Paper presented at the symposium Growing Up and Growing Older, Institute for Research on Mental Retardation and Brain Aging, Troina, Italy.

Hyman, B. T. (1992). Down syndrome and Alzheimer disease. In L. Nadel & C. J. Epstein (Eds.), *Down syndrome and Alzheimer disease* (pp. 123–142). New York: Wiley-Liss.

Hyman, B. T., West, H. L., Rebeck, G. W., Lai, F., & Mann, D. A. (1995). Neuropathological changes in Down's syndrome hippocampal formation. *Archives of Neurology, 52*, 373–378.

Janicki, M. P. (1994). Policies and supports for older persons with mental retardation. In M. M. Seltzer, M. W. Krauss, & M. P. Janicki (Eds.), *Life course perspectives on adulthood and old age* (pp. 213–220). Washington, DC: American Association on Mental Retardation.

Janicki, M. P., Otis, J. P., Puccio, P. S., Rettig, J. H., & Jacobson, J. W. (1985). Service needs among older developmentally disabled persons. In M. P. Janicki & H. M. Wisniewski (Eds.), *Aging and developmental disabilities: Issues and approaches* (pp. 289–304). Baltimore, MD: Brookes.

Johanson, A., Gustafson, L., Brun, A., Risberg, J., Rosen, I., & Tideman, E. (1991). A longitudinal study of dementia of Alzheimer's type in Down's syndrome. *Dementia, 2,* 159–168.

Kemper, T. L. (1988). Neuropathology of Down syndrome. In L. Nadel (Ed.), *The psychobiology of Down syndrome* (pp. 269–289). Cambridge, MA: MIT Press.

Khachaturian, Z. (1985). Diagnosis of Alzheimer's disease. *Archives of Neurology, 42,* 1097–1105.

Kolata, G. (1985). Down syndrome-Alzheimer's linked. *Science, 230,* 1152–1153.

Krauss, M. W., & Seltzer, M. M. (1994). Taking stock: Expected gains from a life-span perspective on mental retardation. In M. M. Seltzer, M. W. Krauss, & M. P. Janicki (Eds.), *Life course perspectives on adulthood and old age* (pp. 213–226). Washington, DC: American Association on Mental Retardation.

Lai, F. (1992). Clinicopathologic features of Alzheimer disease in Down syndrome. In L. Nadel & C. J. Epstein (Eds.), *Down syndrome and Alzheimer disease* (pp. 15–34). New York: Wiley-Liss.

Lai, F., & Williams, R. S. (1989). A prospective study of Alzheimer disease in Down syndrome. *Archives of Neurology, 46,* 849–853.

Lippman, L., & Loberg, D. E. (1985). An overview of developmental disabilities. In M. P. Janicki & H. M Wisniewski (Eds.), *Aging and developmental disabilities: Issues and approaches* (pp. 41–60). Baltimore: Brookes.

Lott, I. T. (1992). The neurology of Alzheimer disease in Down syndrome. In L. Nadel & C. J. Epstein (Eds.), *Down syndrome and Alzheimer disease* (pp. 1–14). New York: Wiley-Liss.

Lott, I. T., & Lai, F. (1982). Dementia in Down syndrome. *Annals of Neurology, 12,* 210.

Maes, B., Fryns, J. P., Van Walleghem, M., & Van den Berghe, H. (1994). Cognitive functioning and information processing of adult mentally retarded men with fragile-X syndrome. *American Journal of Medical Genetics, 50,* 190–200.

Miniszek, N. A. (1983). Development of Alzheimer disease in Down syndrome individuals. *American Journal of Mental Deficiency, 87,* 377–385.

Morris, R. G. (1994). Recent developments in the neuropsychology of dementia. *International Review of Psychiatry, 6,* 85–107.

Nelson, L., Lott, I., Touchette, P., Satz, P., & D'Elia, L. (1995). Detection of Alzheimer disease in individuals with Down syndrome. *American Journal on Mental Retardation, 99*(6), 616–622.

Oliver, C., & Holland, A. J. (1986). Down's syndrome and Alzheimer's disease: A review. *Psychological Medicine, 16,* 307–322.

Pearlson, G. D., Warren, A. C., Starkstein, S. E., Aylward, E. H., Kumar, A. J., Chase, G. A., & Folstein, M. F. (1990). Brain atrophy in 18 patients with Down syndrome: A CT study. *American Journal of Neuroradiology, 11,* 811–816.

Pueschel, S. M. (1990). Clinical aspects of Down's syndrome from infancy to adulthood. *American Journal of Medical Genetics Supplement, 7,* 52–56.

Rasmussen, D. E., & Sobsey, D. (1994). Age, adaptive behavior, and Alzheimer disease in Down syndrome: Cross-sectional and longitudinal analyses. *American Journal on Mental Retardation, 99*(2), 151–165.

Reiss, S. (1994). *Handbook of challenging behavior: Mental health aspects of mental retardation.* Worthington, OH: IDS Publishing Corporation.

Schapiro, M. B. (1993). Neuroimaging in adults with Down's syndrome. In J. M. Berg, H. Karlinsky, & A. J. Holland (Eds.), *Alzheimer disease, Down's syndrome, and their relationship* (pp. 173–197). Oxford, England: Oxford University Press.

Schapiro, M. B., Ball, M. J., Grady, C. L., Haxby, J. V., Kaye, J. A., & Rapoport, S. I. (1988). Dementia in Down's syndrome. *Neurology, 38*(14), 938–942.

Schapiro, M. B., Luxenber, J. S., Kaye, J. A., Haxby, J. V., Friedland, R. P., & Rapoport, S. I. (1989). Serial quantitative CT analysis of brain morphometrics in adult Down's syndrome at different ages. *Neurology, 39,* 1349–1353.

Schapiro, M. B., Azari, N. P., Grady, C. L., Haxby, J. V., & Horowitz, B. (1992). Down's syndrome: Differentiating mental retardation and dementia with brain imaging techniques. In L. Nadel & C. J. Epstein (Eds.), *Down syndrome and Alzheimer disease* (Vol. 379, pp. 103–122). New York: Wiley-Liss.

Seltzer, G. B., & Essex, E. L. (1993). Service needs of persons with mental retardation and developmental disabilities (Robert Wood Johnson Foundation Report). Providence, RI: Brown University, Center for Gerontology and Health Care Research.

Silverstein, A. B., Herbs, D., Miller, T. J., Nasuta, R., & Williams, D. L. (1986). Effects of age on the adaptive behavior of institutionalized individuals with Down syndrome. *American Journal of Mental Deficiency, 90*(6), 659–662.

Steffelaar, J. W., & Evenhuis, H. M. (1989). Life expectancy, Down syndrome, and dementia. *The Lancet, 4*(1), 492–493.

Tanzi, R. E., Gusella, J. F., Watkins, P. C., Bruns, G. A. P., St. George-Hyslop, P., Van Keuren, M. L., Patterson, D., Pagan, S., Kurnit, D. M., & Neve, R. L. (1987). Amyloid B protein gene: cDNA, mRNA distribution, and genetic linkage near the Alzheimer locus. *Science, 235,* 880–884.

Thase, M. E. (1982). Longevity and mortality in Down's syndrome. *Journal of Mental Deficiency Research, 26,* 177–192.

Thase, M. E. (1988). The relationship between Down syndrome and Alzheimer's disease. In L. Nadel (Ed.), *The psychology of Down syndrome* (pp. 345–368). Cambridge, MA: MIT Press.

Thase, M. E., Tigner, R., Smeltzer, D. J., & Liss, L. (1984). Age-related neuropsychological deficits in Down's syndrome. *Biological Psychiatry, 19*(4), 571–585.

Vicari, S., Nocentini, U., & Caltagirone, C. (1994). Neuropsychological diagnosis of aging in adults with Down syndrome. *Developmental Brain Dysfunction, 7,* 340–348.

Warren, A. C., Holroyd, S., & Folstein, M. F. (1989). Major depression in Down's syndrome. *British Journal of Psychiatry, 155,* 202–205.

Widaman, K. F., Borthwich-Duffy, S. A., & Powers, J. C. (1994). Methodological challenges in the study of life-span development of persons with mental retardation. In M. M. Seltzer, M. W. Krauss, & M. P. Janicki (Eds.), *Life course perspectives on adulthood and old age* (pp. 187–212). Washington, DC: American Association on Mental Retardation.

Wishart, J. G. (1988). Early learning in infants and young children with Down syndrome. In L. Nadel (Ed.), *The psychobiology of Down's syndrome* (pp. 7–50). Cambridge, MA: MIT Press.

Wisniewski, H. M., & Merz, G. S. (1985). Aging, Alzheimer's disease, and developmental disabilities. In M. P. Janicki & H. M. Wisniewski (Eds.), *Aging and developmental disabilities: Issues and approaches* (pp. 177–184). Baltimore: Brookes.

Wisniewski, K. E., & Hill, L. (1985). Clinical aspects of dementia in mental retardation and developmental disabilities. In M. P. Janicki & H. M. Wisniewski (Eds.), *Aging and developmental disabilities: Issues and approaches* (pp. 195–210). Baltimore: Brookes.

Wisniewski, K. E., & Rabe, A. (1986). Discrepancy between Alzheimer-type neuropathology and dementia in persons with Down's syndrome. *Annals of the New York Academy of Sciences, 477,* 247–259.

Wisniewski, K. E., Wisniewski, H. M., & Wen, G. Y. (1985). Occurrence of neuropathological changes and dementia of Alzheimer's disease in Down syndrome. *Annals of Neurology, 17,* 278–282.

Wisniewski, K. E., Miezejeski, C. M. & Hill, L. A. (1988). Neurological and psychological status of individual with Down syndrome. In L. Nadel (Ed.), *The psychobiology of Down syndrome* (pp. 315–344). Cambridge, MA: MIT Press.

Young, E. C., & Kramer, B. M. (1991). Characteristics of age related language decline in adults with Down syndrome. *Mental Retardation, 29,* 75–79.

Zigman, W. B., Seltzer, G., & Silverman, W. P. (1994). Behavioral and mental health changes associated with aging in adults with mental retardation. In M. M. Seltzer, M. W, Krauss, & M. P. Janicki (Eds.), *Life course perspectives on adulthood and old age* (pp. 67–92). Washington, DC: American Association on Mental Retardation.

IV

Assessment Procedures and the Older Patient

23

Neurological Evaluation in the Elderly

JON BRILLMAN

Introduction

Various expressions of neurological impairment usually have a direct relationship to advancing age. If one has the good fortune to defer systemic illness, there usually is, to a varying degree, an inexorable decline in coordination, motor function, and intellectual prowess with advancing years. Advanced dementia, parkinsonism, and disorders of praxis are easily recognizable by non-neurologists. More subtle declines in function, such as benign forgetfulness, minor alterations in tone and balance, and early parkinsonism often require the assistance of a neurologist for further definition (Kral, 1962). This chapter demonstrates how the standard neurologic examination may be applied to patients of advanced years and how it may assist the examiner in the differential diagnosis of neurological conditions common to the elderly (Wolfson & Katzman, 1983).

History

History taking, as in all of medicine, is the most important part of the examination, and alert competent clinicians can often make the diagnosis after 2 or 3 minutes of the interview. Nowhere is history taking more crucial than in the examination of the aged individual. In this particular population it is extremely important that a spouse or family member accompany the patient for an objective

JON BRILLMAN • Allegheny General Hospital, Pittsburgh, Pennsylvania 15212.

analysis and for verification of details. The general demeanor of the patient, whether he or she appears happy or depressed, suspicious or sullen, neat or unkempt, cooperative or obstreperous, provides valuable clues as to the nature of his or her physical and mental functioning at home (Cummings & Benson, 1983). If the patient immediately looks to his or her spouse or child for assistance in responding, this is often a clue to cognitive decline. The examiner must observe whether or not the patient is easily distracted, is evasive in answering, or has a tendency to minimize deficits. One common but important difficulty that clinicians may have is distinguishing between confusion and disturbances of language. Confusion, which represents a global cerebral dysfunction resulting from medication, endogenous metabolic factors, or structural dementias, generally manifests as deficits in orientation and memory, but patients are usually able to comprehend, repeat, and name objects. Conversely, patients with aphasias demonstrate difficulties primarily with language and have difficulty repeating, following simple commands, and naming common objects. Aphasias, although part of a cognitive disorder such as Alzheimer's disease, generally indicate a more specific dysfunction in the dominant hemisphere with a more focal structural lesion such as an infarction or tumor (Brown, 1972). Questions to the patient should deal principally with items that affect his or her daily life, such as employment, day-to-day activities in retirement, hobbies, and interests, with careful attention paid to the degree of specificity with which he or she is able to discuss these activities. All neurologists and psychiatrists must familiarize themselves with the Mini-Mental State Examination, which can be carried out in short order in the office setting or by the bedside and can often serve as an objective reference for future decline or improvement (Kahn, Goldfarb, Pollack, & Peck, 1960). In the aging population, it is particularly important for the clinician to ask questions about drinking habits and medications—specifically medications with sedative or mood-altering properties that may have an exaggerated adverse effect on cognition. Here, family members may provide extremely important details about the quantity of drugs that are taken and the effect they have on the patient's functioning.

Although older people are generally not as physically mobile as their younger counterparts, it is important to assess the degree of patient activity. Questions about physical hobbies, such as golf, tennis, and walking, will provide invaluable clues to the overall functioning of the nervous system. Assessment of sleep patterns is also important. Although it is recognized that sleep requirements may decline with advancing years, queries about the regularity of sleep habits, requirements for sleep aids, naps, and tendency to doze off are frequently windows to information about the patient's physical and mental functioning (Weitzman, 1981). In the female population questions about hobbies and other activities should be included with inquiries about the patient's interest in her children and grandchildren. I have found questions about grandchildren, in particular, their health and activity, generally allows for a comfortable interaction with the patient. Once a detailed history has been obtained, ordinarily taking no more than 20 min, the physician should be able to broadly categorize the neurological problem as a movement disorder or cognitive disorder, which are two of the broadest groups of neurologic dysfunction in the elderly.

Neurologic Examination

The standard neurological examination in elderly individuals is somewhat different than in younger patients. Examination of cardiovascular status is of particular importance. This includes auscultation of the heart and the carotid arteries for bruits. In addition, measurement of blood pressure in the lying and standing positions is paramount in order to detect postural hypotension, one of the most common causes of lightheadedness or "dizziness" in aged individuals. The mental state, arguably the most essential part of the neurologic examination in the elderly, is dealt with in detail elsewhere in this book, and the principles of the mental status examination have been previously outlined in the history section. We now review the other components of the standard neurologic examination: cranial nerves; motor, sensory, and cerebellar functions; gait; and the special case of examining the comatose patient, with particular emphasis on elderly patients.

Cranial Nerves

Certain features in the examination of the cranial nerves in older people are distinctive. A good example of this are the pupils and eye movements. In the elderly, the pupils are 2 to 3 mm in diameter and react somewhat sluggishly as compared to a younger person's (Glaser, 1978). In addition, one must be aware that older people commonly use pilocarpine eye drops, thus, small pupils often reflect the popular administration of this medication. Upgaze is also limited in elderly individuals because of fibrosis of the superior rectus muscle (Glaser, 1978). This is important to recognize since disorders of the extrapyramidal systems, such as Parkinson's disease, are associated with limited upgaze as well. Facial expression and mimicry diminish with advancing years. This is of course much more pronounced in patients with parkinsonism as is the inability to inhibit the blink reflex (Myerson's sign). Patients with cerebral degenerative diseases and microvascular ischemic changes may have signs of pseudobulbar palsy which is frequently characterized by dysarthria, poor tongue stimulation, impaired swallowing reflexes with increased gag reflex and an active jaw jerk and snout reflex. The snout reflex is particularly important in cerebral degenerative disorders associated with dementia and is carried out by tapping the upper lip along the sides and observing an immediate pout. This reflex as well as the sucking reflex and the exaggerated jaw reflex, commonly reflect bilateral pyramidal tract dysfunction in the white matter of the brain, releasing the so-called "primitive reflexes" from supersegmental control. Similarly, spontaneous crying and exaggerated emoting to minimal stimuli characterize the pseudobulbar state. Again, this reflects the widespread observations of disinhibition in elderly individuals from frontal lobe control.

Motor Functions

Examination of the extremities should begin with resting tone. The examiner generally observes the way the patient moves his or her limbs, and passive movements will generally show a slight increase in tone in elderly individuals. This is commonly referred to as paratonia. Spasticity due to damage to the pyramidal system is generally characterized by increased flexor tone in the upper extremities and increased extensor tone in the lower extremities. Usually there is a "clasped-knife" phenomenon when the limb is moved rapidly. In contrast, rigidity, the hallmark of Parkinson's disease, will be detected independent of the rate of movement of an extremity. Cogwheeling or ratchet-type rigidity is characteristic of idiopathic Parkinson's disease, and it is difficult to make the diagnosis without this finding. The examiner must look for atrophy, asymmetries, and spastic posture, as described above. Range of motion and alterations in tone, as well as hemiparesis, are most traditionally elicited by having the patients hold their arms straight out with palms up and looking for drift of the affected extremity (Barré's sign). Deep tendon reflexes are checked by tapping on the supinator reflex, biceps, triceps, patellar, and Achilles tendons. The plantar responses detected are observed by stroking the outside of the foot from the heel toward the ball with the patient lying down in an attempt to observe a Babinski reflex. This, of course, when present, is an invariable sign of pyramidal tract disease.

Sensory Functions

In the aging nervous system there is a gradual decline in sensory functions due to receptor degeneration. Occasional polyneuropathies (peripheral nerve damage) can be found in elderly individuals who will complain of paresthesias both in the hands and feet without clear-cut etiology. Normally, vibratory sensation is reduced particularly at the toes, and a mild reduction of joint position sense may also

be present which to some degree accounts for defects in gait. The presence of distal hypalgesia (loss of sensation to pain) and temperature, both in the hands and feet, is characteristic of a symmetrical polyneuropathy often attributable to diabetes mellitus but can be seen in otherwise healthy aged individuals (Dyck, Thomas, Asbury, Winegrad, & Porte, 1987; Harati, 1987). The aging process renders the peripheral nervous system more susceptible to traumatic nerve injury, and compressive neuropathies such as carpal tunnel syndrome, cubital tunnel syndrome, and peroneal palsies are commonly seen in individuals of advanced years who sit and cross their legs for prolonged periods of time or who may be bedridden due to chronic illnesses (Schaumberg, Spencer, & Thomas, 1983). The loss of the protective layer of fat in individuals who lose weight in advanced years also contributes to trauma that may involve exposed nerves next to bony prominences. The special senses, including hearing, taste, and sense of smell, have a reduction in acuity.

Cerebellar Functions

A certain degree of cerebellar atrophy can accompany mild cortical atrophy attributable to aging, varying from patient to patient (Gilman, Bloedel, & Lechtenberg, 1981). This manifests primarily as imbalance and the need to broaden one's gait. Under normal circumstances, however, cerebellar dysfunction is only seen following structural lesions of the cerebellum, which include infarction, cerebellar metastases, cerebellar degeneration due to paraneoplastic disorders, and alcohol- or drug-related cerebellar degeneration. Ordinarily, lesions of the cerebellar hemispheres produce appendicular ataxia or dysmetria demonstrated by finger-to-nose testing or heel-to-knee-to-shin testing. Midline cerebellar lesions will primarily affect gait.

Gait and Station

Most experienced neurologists are able to identify a neurological disturbance simply by observing the gait pattern. A complete neurological examination must include an observation of the patient walking, preferably down a reasonably long corridor, with close attention to associated arm motions, posture, and the fluidity of the turn. Observation of the patient's posture will frequently provide clues to disturbances in motor function and, in particular, extrapyramidal disturbances. "Universal flexion," that is, flexion of the neck, trunk, knees, and upper extremities, is very characteristic of Parkinson's disease. Although there is a tendency for retropulsion (falling backwards) if the patient is jostled backward, usually the patient will pitch forward. Other forms of extrapyramidal disturbances, such as progressive supranuclear palsy, will frequently show a dystonia, and although there is impoverished movement, the tendency may be for the head, neck, and trunk to be arched backwards and frequently to the side as though the patient were looking up at the ceiling (Duvoisin, Golbe, & Lepore, 1987). In all parkinsonian syndromes, postural instability is an extremely important observation, and the examiner can push the patient off balance with relative ease. Midline cerebellar disturbances such as those seen in phenytoin intoxication, alcoholism, or demyelinating disorders can frequently by identified by titubation or a tendency for the head and body to bob up and down or oscillate while standing in a fixed position. The Romberg test is performed by having the patient stand with the feet together and the eyes closed. Under these circumstances the patient uses visual input to maintain his or her balance with the feet close together; however, when the eyes are closed swaying of the trunk begins due to deficient proprioceptive input from the feet. It is frequently a sign of dorsal column dysfunction or large fiber peripheral neuropathy in the legs. Often this is seen in combination with nutritional deficiencies, alcoholism, or subacute combined degeneration due to Vitamin B_{12} deficiency.

Types of Gait Disturbance

Senescent Gait

In advancing years the steps become less sure and smaller. The normal spring to the step, which is seen in youth and is associated with good health and enthusiasm, diminishes in advancing years. There are many causes for a senescent gait, including decreased mobility of the joints, tightness of the hamstrings, decreased proprioceptive input due to

mild peripheral neuropathy, and some degree of cerebral atrophy. All of these factors have been demonstrated to be associated with gait disturbances, and although elderly patients may be otherwise physiologically "well," the gait is almost universally affected with advanced years (Murray, Kory, & Clarkson, 1969). However, in circumstances of advanced dementing illnesses, including Alzheimer's disease, severe cerebral atrophy, communicating hydrocephalus, as well as subcortical arteriosclerotic encephalopathy (Binswanger's disease), the gait may become severely apractic. Under these circumstances the steps are very small and uncertain, and frequently patients cannot take even the smallest step; the feet seem to be magnetized to the floor. Patients are easily tipped over backward or forward, and when asked to stand or get out of bed to walk, they have a great deal of difficulty assuming a balanced posture. The patients frequently position and reposition their feet or oscillate their body vertically in an attempt to maintain balance. Most patients with advanced gait apraxias are unable to walk at all (Sudarsky, 1990).

Parkinson's Disease and Parkinsonism

Parkinsonian gait is marked by flexion of all limbs including the trunk and a tendency to lean forward and pick up speed as one goes on—a gait disturbance referred to as "festination" (Yahr & Bergmann, 1986).

Patients with progressive supranuclear palsy more commonly have axial dystonia with a tendency for the body to be arched slightly backward and an astonished facial appearance rather than a true parkinsonian appearance, which is a relative poverty of expression. Other extrapyramidal disorders, including Shy-Drager syndrome, olivopontocerebellar degeneration, or striatonigral degeneration, are more typically parkinsonian but may also have features of apraxia. It is not always possible to distinguish the gait characteristics of these various disorders from each other.

Hemiparetic Gait

Patients with hemiparesis, most commonly due to cerebral infarction, have arm flexion in the

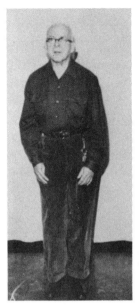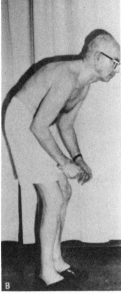

FIGURE 1. Typical (A) appearance and (B) posture in Parkinson's disease.

upper extremity with adduction of the arm held closely to the body and flexion of the fingers but hyperextension of the foot with an equinovarus deformity. The leg is commonly stiff or spastic, and in order to avoid tripping over the toes on the floor, the leg is swung out in a so-called circumducting fashion. This type of gait is most commonly seen with spastic hemiparesis.

Ataxic Gait

Ataxia refers to a disordered balance that is nonspecific with respect to neuroanatomical localization. Patients with cerebellar damage (infarction, hemorrhage, or metastases) will have either appendicular ataxia or vermian ataxia which causes a broad-based gait and a tendency for oscillation of the trunk and head, previously described as titubation. Gait ataxia may also be present in dorsal column dysfunction such as vitamin B_{12} deficiency in which case Rombergism is present (the patient sways with the eyes closed). If there is a severe peripheral neuropathy involving the large fibers in the legs, then gait ataxia may also be present, particularly in the dark where visual input is diminished.

Spastic Gait

Patients with bilateral lower extremity spasticity, commonly seen in cervical spine disease (cervical spondylotic myelopathy), will have a stiff leg or "wooden-legged" gait where there is minimal flexion of the knees while walking. Should this become exaggerated, the adductors of the thighs become particularly tight, and "scissoring" is commonly noted. This is particularly evident in patients who have congenital abnormalities, such as cerebral palsy, due to birth trauma.

Hysterical Gait

This is often the most difficult gait to distinguish, as is the case with many other psychogenic disorders (Keane, 1989). Hysterical gait is a gait disturbance which cannot be satisfactorily explained by any clear-cut neuroanatomical localization. As is often the case with psychogenic disorders, associated features of emotional disturbance should be vigorously sought in a nonthreatening fashion by the examiner. Gait may be bizarre, pitching and starting to one side or the other, wavering suddenly from left to right, or including twirling motions with the arms outstretched and flopping about (astasia-basia). Other patients who are neurologically unsophisticated may take a step with one leg and then drag the other leg behind (puller's), while others may take a step and push the fellow leg (pusher's). The experienced examiner has little difficulty, in general, distinguishing gait disturbances that are non-organic.

Tremor

The classification of tremor in the elderly can be based on whether it occurs during movement or at rest. Resting tremor, usually observed with the hands on the lap, is typical of Parkinson's disease. Usually this is an alternating 3- to 5-Hz flexion extension tremor of the fingers ("pill-rolling"). Essential tremor in the elderly, referred to as "senile tremor" (Haerer, Anderson, & Schoenberg, 1982), is a dominantly inherited disorder most often observed with the hands in posture, either with the arms outstretched or holding an object such as a cup or pencil. Generally the frequency is more rapid (8–10 Hz) than the frequency of parkinsonian tremor and, unlike parkinsonism, the head and voice are often tremulous (Larsen & Calne, 1983). Cerebellar tremor (intention tremor) is demonstrated when the patient reaches to touch an object. Under this circumstance, the finger will be seen to oscillate at a rate of about 5 Hz on attempting to touch the goal.

Headache and Facial Pain in the Elderly

Headache of new onset in older people should be thoroughly evaluated. Although migraine and tension (or muscle contraction) headaches are most often seen in younger patients, they may occur in advancing years, particularly manifested as pain which may appear in the back of the head associated with cervical osteoarthritis (Friedman, 1978). A sedimentation rate should always be obtained in elderly patients with new onset headache to exclude giant cell (or temporal) arteritis, a condition which is potentially remediable with corticosteroids (Bengtsson & Malmvall, 1976). An image of the brain, obtained through computed tomography (CT) or magnetic resonance imaging (MRI), may also exclude an intracerebral process, and it is often wise to consider this in the absence of a ready explanation for recent headache or face pain. Spinal fluid analysis may also be considered to exclude a meningeal process in headache of uncertain etiology.

Facial pain in the elderly may be due to trigeminal neuralgia (tic-doloreaux) disease of the facial structures or to muscle spasms. In trigeminal neuralgia, pain is in the distribution of the trigeminal nerve (usually cranial nerve VII or VIII), unilateral, lancinating, or sudden, and it frequently can be triggered by touching the affected region (Fromm, Terrence, & Maroon, 1984). Pain due to dental, osseous, or sinus disease is more chronic, aching in character, and may extend outside the distribution of the fifth cranial nerve. This also includes the myofacial pain syndrome, often attributable to dysfunction of the temporomandibular joint or spasm of muscles of mastication due to ill-fitting dentures, bruxisms, or tension.

Examination of the Comatose Patient

The examination of a patient in coma is a special circumstance. Patients with decreased responsiveness may appear to the examiner as awake or asleep.

Patients Who Appear to Be Awake

Abulia or Apathy

These patients appear to be awake but are extremely slow in their responses. They frequently appear to be stunned and slowly turn to the examiner when asked to respond to a specific question or to follow an instruction. The mental status examination may be within normal limits, however, it takes an undue length of time to extract a history or to converse with the patient. These patients are those who have bilateral prefrontal disorders due to atrophy, trauma, infarction, or lobotomies.

Psychogenic Unresponsiveness

These patients have psychiatric disorders but appear to be awake, and if they do not respond, they either have hysterical mutism or conversion hysteria. These patients frequently will speak in a whispered voice. Others may have more serious psychiatric disturbances, such as catatonia, which will require relatively acute psychiatric intervention.

Locked-in State

These are patients whose nervous systems have been bisected, usually by an infarction in the pons. Under these circumstances the patient is quadriplegic and usually only can move his or her eyes in a vertical fashion. Nevertheless, the patient is awake and can feel pain. Patients with excellent nursing care can be kept alive for quite some time in this unfortunate condition.

Persistent Vegetative State

These patients are increasingly seen due to incomplete resuscitation after cardiac arrest or hypoxia. Diffuse cerebral ischemia renders both hemispheres damaged. However, since the brain stem is functioning, the patient may appear to be awake, have normal wake–sleep cycles, dart or turn his or her head to the sound of a noise, and have swallowing movements. Nevertheless, the patient does not respond appropriately or interact with the environment. It is required that a month elapse before the diagnosis of persistent vegetative state be made, implying irreversibility (Hansotia, 1985).

Patients Who Appear to Be Asleep

These patients are those who we commonly associate with stupor and coma. Three categories are generally used by the neurologist and have specific meanings: (1) *Drowsiness* is a state in which a patient appears to be asleep but can be easily aroused by voice; (2) *Stupor* is a condition in which a patient is in a deeper state of unresponsiveness and cannot be aroused by voice but can be aroused with painful stimuli; (3) *Coma* is a state where neither voice nor painful stimuli will arouse the patient.

Despite the fact that they are unresponsive, patients in coma require a detailed history. This must be obtained from family members, paramedics, police, or significant others who may be familiar with the patient's prior mental state, medical history, and medication use. The rate of onset of the coma is equally important. Obviously the history of an elderly person who bumped his or her head and became progressively drowsy over 2 weeks until he or she could no longer be awakened implies a subdural hematoma, whereas an elderly patient who suddenly collapses at the dinner table may have had a cardiac arrest and cerebral hypoxia. The rate of onset suggests different disorders.

Neurologic examination of a comatose patient requires knowledge of the pathophysiology of coma (Plum & Posner, 1980). Comatose states may be produced by widespread diffuse bilateral hemisphere disease or brain stem disease affecting the ascending reticular activating system from the mid pons rostrally. The goal, therefore, in examining a comatose patient, is to determine whether or not the coma is due to bilateral hemisphere disease or to brain stem disease, as the correct localization of the lesion will help determine not only the cause of the coma, but the prognosis as well. In order to do this, the clinician needs to understand the different patterns of respiration, pupillary reactions and eye movements, and postures associated with various levels of coma.

Respiration

Simple observation of respiratory patterns is extremely important in examining comatose individuals. If the patient has normal respiration or Cheyne-Stokes respiration (hyperventilation and hypoventilation with interposed periods of apnea), then a lesion is either at the level of the diencephalon or rostral to this. Central neurogenic hyperventilation with respiratory rates of 30 or greater are commonly seen in brain stem lesions, particularly high ones. Apneustic respirations, or prolonged inspiratory cramp with a prolonged expiratory phase, are commonly seen after failure of the pons. Ataxic or agonal respirations, which are irregular ineffective respirations of about four to six per minute, are seen with failure of the medulla oblongata, and this commonly precedes apnea, which requires intubation.

Pupillary Reactions

A bright light is required to identify the state of the pupils in a comatose individual. Pupils that are widely dilated in comatose individuals generally imply cerebral hypoxia, particularly if they are non-reactive. Pinpoint pupils with minimal reactivity imply pontine infarction or hemorrhage but they may also result from narcotic overdose. Mid-positioned to dilated pupils of about 5 to 6 mm that do not respond to light imply infarction or damage to the midbrain. The most important pupillary abnormality, however, is asymmetrical pupils or "anisocoria." Under these circumstances one pupil is dilated and unresponsive. Frequently this implies a shift of supertentorial structures, usually the uncus of the temporal lobe which is herniated through the tentorial incisura and has compressed the midbrain. Under these circumstances patients should be at least drowsy and are frequently stuporous or in coma. An awake patient with anisocoria has less emergent significance, and one must be certain that a mydriatic was not used in the eye.

Of those bedside tests that are performed on comatose patients, tests of eye movements have the most significance. If ocular movements are present, this strongly suggests that the brain stem is functioning, particularly if pupils work normally. If the eyes do not move, however, on first inspection, the examiner should then try to make them move either by head rotation (doll's head maneuver) or ice water calorics. The doll's head maneuver should not be done on a comatose patient where history is incomplete. Under these circumstances there may have been cervical trauma, and turning the head from side to side may dislocate the cervical spine. It is therefore advised that ice water calorics be performed by using a 50-ml syringe, drawing ice water 7 degrees colder than body temperature, and, through a number 18 catheter, inserting the water into the ear rapidly with the eyes held open. Inspection to assure integrity of the tympanic membrane should be carried out first. Under physiologic circumstances the eyes should slowly deviate to the side of the ice water and then jerk back with nystagmus to the midline. The initial deviation of the eyes is due to brain stem function (opposite side), and the nystagmus of the eyes back to the midline is a hemisphere function. If patients have bihemisphere coma, therefore, eyes will move slowly to the side of the ice water and drift slowly back in a smooth fashion to the midline. This test should be done bilaterally. If the eyes do not move after injection of ice water on either side, the brain stem is not functioning and the coma is due to brain stem damage. Occasionally one will encounter a patient with hysterical coma. Under these circumstances painful stimulation will generally not arouse the patient, but insertion of ice water into the ear will cause deviation of the eyes to the side of the ice water and a jerking back of the eyes to the midline. If this reaction is present bilaterally, the implication is that both the brain stem and the hemispheres are working and the coma is non-organic. This is an extraordinarily uncomfortable test and will make most patients violently ill. Curiously, patients with hysterical coma do not seem to respond to this stimulation.

Body Movements

Patients in coma should be stimulated vigorously to test their responsiveness to pain. A satisfactory way of accomplishing this is to put pressure on the supraorbital ridge with one's thumb. This rarely leaves trauma marks and does not cause any intra-ocular trauma if done carefully. If the patient's level of coma is light, then the patient will be aroused and use avoidance measures by pushing the examiner's hand away. If the patient has a lesion at the midbrain level or caudal to this level, decerebrate posturing is likely with adduction and internal rotation of the upper extremity and hyperextension and internal rotation of the lower extremity. This may be bilateral or unilateral. No response to painful stimuli or slight flexion of the knees implies medullary damage and heralds a very poor prognosis. In addition to determining if the coma is attributable to bilateral hemisphere disease or to brain stem disease, it is important to detect whether the brain stem may be failing secondary to transtentorial herniation. Again, patients who have transtentorial herniation due to a rapidly expanding hemisphere or temporal lobe mass will have a progressively deepening coma associated frequently with an enlarged light fixed pupil ipsilateral to the lesion and decerebrate posturing on the opposite side of the body.

Clearly, examination of a comatose patient presents a special challenge to the examiner, however, if the aforementioned principles are followed, the more important questions as to the pathogenesis of the coma and the prognosis may be resolved.

Summary

The special challenge to the examiner in performing a neurologic evaluation in elderly patients is the ability to identify what is "normal aging" and what represents disease. The emphasis of the examination should be on special functions, particularly those vulnerable to advanced years, such as cognition and memory, as well as gait and posture.

The neurologic evaluation of elderly patients requires clinical experience with this age group and a knowledge of those disorders peculiar to them. This will become increasingly important in the coming years as the percentage of our population over age 65 increases.

References

Bengtsson, B. A., & Malmvall, B. E. (1976). Alternate-day corticosteroid regimen in maintenance therapy of giant cell arteritis. *Survey of Ophthalmology, 20*, 247–260.

Brown, J. W. (1972). *Aphasia, apraxia, and agnosia.* Springfield, IL: Charles C. Thomas.

Cummings, J. L., & Benson, D. B. (1983). *Dementia: A clinical approach.* London: Butterworths.

Duvoisin, R. C., Golbe, L. I., & Lepore, F. E. (1987). Progressive supranuclear palsy. *Canadian Journal of Neurologic Science, 14,* 547–554.

Dyck, P. J., Thomas, P. K., Asbury, A. K., Winegrad, A. I., & Porte, D., Jr. (1987). *Diabetic neuropathy.* Philadelphia: W. B. Saunders.

Friedman, A. P. (Ed.). (1978). Headache and related pain syndromes. *Medical Clinics of North America, 62,* 427–623.

Fromm, G. H., Terrence, C. F., & Maroon, J. C. (1984). Trigeminal neuralgia. Current concepts regarding etiology and pathogenesis. *Archives of Neurology, 41,* 1204–1207.

Gilman, S., Bloedel, J., & Lechtenberg, R. (1981). *Disorders of the cerebellum.* Philadelphia: F. A. Davis.

Glaser, J. S. (1978). *Neuro-ophthalmology.* Hagerstown, MD: Harper and Row.

Haerer, A. F., Anderson, D. N., & Schoenberg, B. S. (1982). Prevalence of essential tremor. *Archives of Neurology, 39,* 750.

Hansotia, P. L. (1985). Persistent vegetative state. Review and report of electrodiagnostic studies in eight cases. *Archives of Neurology, 42,* 1048–1052.

Harati, Y. (1987). Diabetic peripheral neuropathies. *Annals of Internal Medicine, 107,* 546–559.

Kahn, R. L., Goldfarb, A. I., Pollack, M., & Peck, A. (1960). Brief objective measures for the determination of mental status in the aged. *American Journal of Psychiatry, 117,* 326–328.

Keane, J. R. (1989). Hysterical gait disorders. *Neurology, 39,* 586.

Kral, V. A. (1962). Senescent forgetfulness: Benign and malignant. *Canadian Medical Association Journal, 86,* 257–260.

Larsen, T. A., & Calne, D. B. (1983). Essential tremor. *Clinical Neuropharmacology, 6,* 185–206.

Murray, M. P., Kory, R. C., & Clarkson, B. H. (1969). Walking patterns in healthy old men. *Journal of Gerontology, 24,* 169.

Plum, F., & Posner, J. B. (1980). *The diagnosis of stupor and coma* (3rd ed.). Philadelphia: F. A. Davis.

Schaumberg, H. H., Spencer, P. S., & Thomas, P. K. (1983). *Disorders of peripheral nerves.* Philadelphia: F. A. Davis.

Sudarsky, L. (1990). Geriatrics: Gait disorders in the elderly. *New England Journal of Medicine, 322,* 1441.

Weitzman, E. D. (1981). Sleep and its disorders. *Annual Review of Neuroscience, 4,* 381–417.

Wolfson, L. W., & Katzman, R. (1983). Neurological consultation at age 80. In R. Katzman & R. D. Terry (Eds.), *Neurology of aging.* Philadelphia: F. A. Davis.

Yahr, M. D., & Bergmann, K. J. (Eds.). (1986). *Advances in Neurology. Vol. 45. Parkinson's disease.* New York: Raven Press.

24

Neuropsychological Assessment

ASENATH LA RUE AND REX SWANDA

Increasing numbers of older adults and the high prevalence of medical, psychiatric, and neurological disorders in later life present a challenge of unprecedented proportions to the health care system. In response, psychologists are becoming better informed about the need for neuropsychological and psychodiagnostic assessment of older persons and better acquainted with tools appropriate for conducting these assessments (Brown & Wiggins, 1994).

This chapter provides an overview and update of methods for addressing the most common referral questions in geriatric neuropsychology. These include (1) screening for possible cognitive impairment, (2) differential diagnosis of neurological and neuropsychiatric disorders in older clients, (3) monitoring change in neuropsychological functions, and (4) formulating treatment and management recommendations based on assessment outcomes. General guidelines for assessment are presented first, followed by discussion of procedures relevant to each referral issue. Special issues in multicultural assessment are discussed in a final section.

The Assessment Process: General Considerations

The assessment process typically relies on at least three sources of data: review of the pertinent

ASENATH LA RUE • Department of Psychiatry, University of New Mexico, Albuquerque, New Mexico 87131; and Department of Psychiatry and Biobehavioral Sciences, University of California, Los Angeles, Los Angeles, California 90024-1759. REX SWANDA • Veterans Affairs Medical Center, Albuquerque, New Mexico 87108.

medical and psychosocial history, clinical interview with the patient and appropriate family or caregivers, and use of formal quantitative or qualitative assessment techniques. Review of the history provides the best opportunity for identifying factors common to older adults that might alter the selection of procedures. These same factors might also be expected to affect the eventual interpretation of the assessment data. Some of these examples include sensory problems in vision and hearing, multiple medical problems and physical discomfort, limited mobility, and sensitivity to medications (La Rue, 1992; Storandt, 1994).

The clinical interview supplements the history by offering an opportunity to collect information and impressions from the patient, as well as family members and caregivers who are close to the patient. The interview provides the structure for the first interaction between the clinician and the patient and, in effect, offers a preview of the behavior that will be encountered in formal assessment procedures. It is an important time for the examiner to clarify the nature and purpose of examination, to establish rapport, and to set the stage for motivated effort in the examination procedures. This initial interaction is invaluable in refining the selection of assessment instruments.

Selection of specific assessment procedures should be based on consideration of the referral issues and should reflect the best match between individual patient characteristics and characteristics of the procedures themselves. Assessing competence of a severely incapacitated, lethargic stroke patient may require only a 10- to 20-min screening, whereas a longer set of procedures, requiring 1 to 4 hr, might be needed with a higher functioning patient to differentiate between dementia and depression, or to establish a baseline for follow-up comparisons.

Most assessment procedures emphasize particular modalities of stimulus presentation and response, which obviously must match the sensory and motor capabilities of the patient. As stated above, the history and interview should alert the examiner to any special needs of the patient. However, the examiner should also consider more subtle patient characteristics which might affect his or her participation in the assessment and thus contribute to the outcome of the examination. Many of these characteristics lie in the arena of personality and emotion. For instance, evidence of lowered frustration tolerance or tenuous cooperation early in the session might lead the examiner to omit a potentially frustrating task (e.g., Wisconsin Card Sorting Test or Paced Auditory Serial Addition Test) or at least delay such procedures until the end of the protocol. Some patients exert greater cooperation and effort on tasks that are perceived as more ecologically valid. Poor stamina, fatigue, or very limited education might justifiably lead the examiner to select less taxing techniques for assessing similar areas of functioning (e.g., the Fuld Object Memory Evaluation rather than the California Verbal Learning Test). On the other hand, obvious indications of psychological contributors, such as depression, illness behavior, or stress may suggest a need for more elaborate assessment of personality and emotional factors.

Aside from more general considerations for test selection (see Lezak, 1995), care should be taken to ensure that the standardization sample on which a given test is based is representative and appropriate for use with a given patient. There has been considerable progress toward this end in recent years, but many well known assessment procedures still do not offer appropriate norms for certain types of older adults (La Rue, 1992). Erickson, Eimon, and Hebben (as cited in Storandt & VandenBos, 1994) have compiled a listing of references on normative studies with older samples, and Spreen and Strauss (1991), La Rue (1992), and Lezak (1995) provide normative data on selected tests.

Interpretation of assessment outcomes for older persons must take into account not only age, education, and medical history, but also genera-

tional and cultural factors. The quality and focus of educational, dietary, exercise, and recreational preferences, as well as language patterns and problem-solving styles, are likely to change over successive generations, and as a result, normative data collected 20 years ago may no longer be applicable to contemporary old persons. Similarly, although concerns regarding cultural bias have received increasing attention in recent years, there is a continuing need to refine interpretation to account for subtle cross-cultural differences in comprehension of terms or approaches to tasks. Older adults who have been less influenced by the English language and customs than their younger relatives may be particularly likely to demonstrate such differences. Each of these influences on interpretation are discussed in more detail below.

Screening for Cognitive Impairment

Mental Status Examinations

Current and projected health needs of the aging population have increased demands for brief evaluations to screen for common cognitive disorders such as dementia. Several cognitive mental status examinations have been developed, ranging from very brief scales of only a few items to lengthier instruments that tap a variety of skills in an abbreviated manner (see Table 1). The general aim of these instruments is to maximize sensitivity to impairment, so that few true cases will be overlooked; then, depending on clinical needs, positive findings on screening can be followed up with more detailed procedures to reduce the incidence of false-positive errors.

Mini-Mental State Examination (MMSE)

The MMSE (Folstein, Folstein, & McHugh, 1975) is the best known cognitive mental status examination. It is a bedside procedure that is easy to administer and has acceptable test–retest reliability and validity relative to the Wechsler Adult Intelligence Scale (Folstein et al., 1975). Extensive norms for age (18 to 85 years and older) and education (no formal schooling to one or more college degrees) have been reported for the MMSE based

Table 1. Comparison of Mental Status Screening Procedures

Test	Time	Test structure	Strengths	Weaknesses
Mental Status Questionnaire	5–10 min	10 mental status items: orientation, personal and general information	Very brief; adequate reliability; rough screening	Relatively insensitive to mild dysfunction
Short Portable Mental Status Questionnaire	5–10 min	10 mental status items: orientation, personal, general information, serial 3s	Very brief; adequate reliability; criteria correct for age, education, race (Scherr et al., 1988)	Relatively insensitive to mild dysfunction
Blessed Information-Memory-Concentration Test	5–10 min	26 mental status items (Katzman et al., 1983): assesses personal information; memory for personal/general information	Very brief; correlates significantly with senile plaque counts	Relatively insensitive to mild dysfunction
Orientation-Memory-Concentration Test	5–10 min	6 mental status items: time of day, month, year, count 20–1, memory phrase, months backward	Very brief; correlates with senile plaque counts	Relatively insensitive to mild dysfunction
Mini-Mental State Examination	5–10 min	Mental status items assess orientation (time, place), registration, attention, calculation, recall, naming, repetition, comprehension, writing, visual construction	Brief; widely used with many populations; many normative studies indicate reliability and sensitivity for screening purposes; has been used cross-culturally	Total cut-off score (23/30) may obscure focal deficits; cautious use with low education
Neurobehavioral Cognitive Status Examination	10–30 min	"Screening" items with "metric" follow-up assess five domains (language, memory, construction, reasoning, calculations) plus attention, orientation, and level of consciousness	Discriminates both psychiatric/neurologic populations; characterizes patterns of dysfunction in profile across domains	Ceiling effects; profile may mischaracterize diagnostic conclusion
Mattis Dementia Rating Scale	10–45 min	Items hierarchically arranged in "screening" format; assesses attention, initiation/perseveration, construction, conceptualization, memory	Designed to differentiate and follow dementia patients; relatively sensitive to mild dysfunction; acceptable validity and reliability	"Total" score may obscure cautious interpretation of subscale performances

on a probability sampling of more than 18,000 adults (Crum, Anthony, Bassett, & Folstein, 1993). The performances of several different cultural and racial groups have been documented on this examination (e.g., Anthony, La Resche, Niaz, Von Korff, & Folstein, 1982; Escobar et al., 1986; Salmon et al., 1989; see section on Culturally Diverse Assessment below), and a modified version has been developed for hearing-impaired adults (Uhlmann, Larson, Rees, Koepsell, & Duckert, 1989).

Crum and colleagues (1993) reported an inverse relationship between MMSE scores and age, ranging from a median score of 29 for ages 18 to 24 years to a median of 25 for 80 years and older. Across the adult age span, a relatively strong association with education was documented, with median scores ranging from 22 for persons with less than 4 years of school to 29 for those with 9 years or more of education.

As part of the trade-off for brevity, clinicians should bear in mind that the MMSE may be relatively insensitive to certain aspects of cognitive functioning, especially in well-educated persons or those with focal impairment. Kupke, Revis, and Gantner (1993) found that the MMSE was sensitive to deficits associated with left hemisphere stroke or dementia, but not to deficits resulting from right hemisphere stroke. In older patients with mild Alzheimer's disease who are otherwise healthy and have a high school education or more, as many as one in three can be expected to score 24 or higher on the MMSE (Galasko et al., 1990), and in this type of population, MMSE performance may be relatively independent of activity-of-daily-living ratings (Reed, Jagust, & Seab, 1989).

Cullum, Thompson, and Smernoff (1993) examined correlations between performances of older adults on the California Verbal Learning Test and their recall of two versions of a three-word recall task, the memory item used on the MMSE. They found only modest correlations between three-word recall and CVLT performance and concluded that the potential risk of false-positive errors based on this brief memory test was unacceptably high. They also noted that the specific words used on the three-time lists had a great impact on recall performance.

In a 3-year longitudinal study of an aging community sample, Mitrushina and Satz (1991) found that a decline of five points or more over a 2-year period was associated with the strong possibility of neurological disorder. In contrast, when Haxby, Raffaele, Gillette, Schapiro, and Rapoport (1992) used the MMSE to examine individual trajectories of cognitive decline among patients with Alzheimer's-type dementia, they found it to be less effective as a measure of longitudinal change than the Wechsler Adult Intelligence Scale or Mattis Dementia Rating Scale and ineffective in predicting the rate of future decline.

Widespread use of the MMSE, by many different types of health professionals, is likely to ensure its continued popularity, despite limitations noted above. However, it is important to be aware of the limitations and to have realistic expectations for the information that can be learned from this gross screening instrument. Suggestions for supplementing the MMSE with other brief procedures in order to increase sensitivity or specificity have been offered by several groups. Galasko and colleagues (1990) found that inclusion of a verbal fluency procedure enhanced sensitivity of the MMSE to patients in a mild Alzheimer's dementia group while reducing the error rate. Teng and Chui (1987) developed a revised version of the MMSE, modifying some items and increasing the scoring range to a total of 100 points, which may enhance the sensitivity and specificity of the instrument.

Neurobehavioral Cognitive Status Examination (NCSE)

The NCSE (Kiernan, Mueller, Langston, & Van Dyke, 1987) quantitatively assesses cognitive performance across several domains of ability, including orientation, attention, language, visual construction, memory, calculations, and reasoning. Screening items at a level passed by most normal persons are presented first; these are followed by simpler items if necessary. Normative data are provided in the manual for older adult volunteers (70 to 92 years) as well as for younger age groups. A preliminary validation study with a neurosurgical population (Schwamm, Van Dyke, Kiernan, Merrin, & Mueller, 1987) found a lower false-negative rate for the NCSE relative to the MMSE and the Cognitive Capacity Screening Examination (7%, 43%, and 53%, respectively).

The heightened sensitivity and profile summary of the NCSE are attractive features, and the availability of age norms makes it relevant for geriatric applications; however there are still relatively few independent validation studies of this instrument. Elderly psychiatric inpatients with either organic mental disorders or depressive disorders were examined by Osato, Yang, and La Rue (1993) using both the NCSE and MMSE. They reported high sensitivity (100%) but low specificity (28%) for the NCSE and the opposite pattern for MMSE, with low sensitivity (46%) but high specificity (89%). Osato et al. (1993) suggested that the optimal method for maximizing sensitivity rates while minimizing false-negative errors in this population would be to identify as impaired those subjects who fall below age cutoffs on two or more scales of the NCSE.

Logue, Tupler, D'Amico, and Schmitt (1993) examined 866 psychiatric inpatients using the NCSE and concluded that the instrument is both practical and well tolerated, but noted substantial differences between the performances of their psychiatric sample in comparison to the original standardization sample. Among other observations, very high percentages of their sample failed the initial screening item for several of the subtest areas (repetition, 56.9%; naming, 54.5%; construction, 89.5%; similarities, 95%; judgment, 85.9%). However, their analyses did support construct validity for the NCSE, and they found predicted age-related decline across the various subtests that reinforced the original assumptions of the NCSE. They suggested that, since the construction item (recall of a geometric configuration) was highly correlated with the (verbal) memory subtest, an alternate measure of constructional ability would be useful. They also expressed concern that the NCSE provides only weak information regarding attention and information-processing speed, and that there is no alternate form for follow-up.

The Mattis Dementia Rating Scale (MDRS)

The MDRS (Mattis, 1988) is composed of five subscales that evaluate attention, perseveration and initiation, construction, memory, and conceptualization. It offers an efficient administration format by presenting items within most domains of ability in the reverse order of difficulty, so that relatively easier items can be omitted if those more difficult

screening items in the range of normal ability are passed. Acceptable concurrent validity and split-half reliability have been found, so this instrument has achieved wide use as a screening procedure for assessing impaired cognitive functioning among older adults (Kaszniak, 1986). Although factor analyses of the scale have not fully supported its original subscale structure (e.g., Smith, Petersen, & Ivnik, 1991), a recent study by Nadler, Richardson, Malloy, Marran, and Brinson (1993) found significant predictive relationships between the subscales of the MDRS and domains of everyday functioning for self-care, safety, money management, cooking, medication administration, and community utilization. The lengthiest of commonly used cognitive mental status exams, the MDRS may be the best candidate for brief geriatric testing when dementia is suspected and when full neuropsychological assessment is not feasible. The inclusion of items that may be sensitive to frontal lobe impairments (e.g., initiation and perseveration) may increase the sensitivity of the MDRS to subcortically mediated dementia syndromes relative to other briefer mental status exams.

Dementia Screening Batteries

Another approach to screening of cognitive functioning among older adults has been to assemble small sets of standardized tests that have been shown to be sensitive to brain impairment. In developing the Iowa Battery for Mental Decline, discriminant analysis was used by Eslinger, Damasio, Benton, and Van Allen (1985) to identify and cross-validate a sensitive combination of standardized procedures (Visual Retention Test, Controlled Oral Word Association, and Temporal Orientation) that correctly classified 89% of dementia cases. A similar method of discriminant analysis was used by Storandt, Botwinick, Danziger, Berg, and Hughes (1984) to develop the Washington University Screening Battery composed of Logical Memory and Mental Control from the Wechsler Memory Scale, Trail-making Part A, and Word Fluency (S and P). This battery effectively discriminated 98% of patients with mild dementia of the Alzheimer's type from age-, sex-, and SES-matched healthy older adults in the initial study. These findings were successfully replicated by Tierney, Snow, Reid,

Zorzitto, and Fisher (1987). However, this latter study reported that this battery did not discriminate among various types of dementias. In a direct comparison of the Iowa and Washington University approaches, Ryan, Paolo, and Oehlert (1989) found greater support for the battery selected by Storandt and colleagues. Equivalent sensitivity was observed for both brief batteries (each correctly identified 79% of demented patients), but there was higher specificity for the Storandt battery (77%) than for the Iowa battery (53%). Harper, Chacko, Kotik-Harper, and Kirby (1992) compared the relative efficacy of the MMSE and the Iowa Battery for Mental Decline in distinguishing depressed older patients with and without dementia. The MMSE and Iowa battery each had an overall accuracy for detecting dementia of about 70%. The visual retention test and verbal fluency measures from the Iowa battery produced substantially fewer false-negative errors compared to the MMSE, but this was at the expense of a much higher rate of false-positive errors.

The Consortium to Establish a Registry for Alzheimer's Disease (CERAD) has developed a brief examination for detection and tracking of cognitive symptoms of dementia of the Alzheimer's type (DAT). The CERAD battery consists of the MMSE, abbreviated tests of verbal fluency, confrontation naming, and constructional praxis and a 10-item word list memory test. Findings published to date are based on DAT patients and healthy control subjects recruited at 23 participating medical centers in the United States. The battery effectively distinguishes between patients with mild DAT and healthy controls (Welsh, Butters, Hughes, Mohs, & Heyman, 1991), and inter-rater agreement, test–retest reliability, and longitudinal validity are in acceptable ranges (Morris et al., 1989; cf. Welsh et al., 1994). Preliminary normative data have recently been published for the CERAD measures based on a sample of 413 healthy controls (Welsh et al., 1994). The normative sample consists of white, predominantly well-educated (only 11% have less than a high school education), and relatively young (mean age = 68 years) adults. Normative data for African-American elderly are anticipated in light of increased enrollment of this group at CERAD study sites in recent years (Ballard, Nash, Raiford, & Harrell, 1993). At present, the utility of the preliminary norms is limited by the broad age spans for which means and standard deviations are reported (50–69 years vs. 70–89 years). Also, data are lacking on the utility of the battery for distinguishing dementia of the Alzheimer's type from other common disorders affecting cognitive performance (e.g., vascular dementia and psychiatric disorders).

Clock Drawing

Clock drawing is a convenient and diagnostically useful neuropsychological test that is seeing increasing use as a dementia screening instrument. While simple to administer, the task requires the patient to integrate many different cognitive mechanisms, including attention, graphomotor, visual perceptual, and constructional functions, as well as executive planning and organizational abilities. Memory and comprehension are also required if the instruction is in the form of a complex command (e.g., "draw a clock, place all the numbers, and set the hands to 10 after 11"), as is the procedure of most clinicians (Freedman et al., 1994). Clock drawing is particularly sensitive to problems of neglect, poor planning and organization, perseveration, and concrete thinking.

Although many clinicians rely on subjective examination of the patient's drawing effort, several scoring systems have been devised (e.g., Freedman et al., 1994) that have demonstrated utility in screening for dementia, differentiating Alzheimer's patients from normal controls (Sunderland et al., 1989; Tuokko, Hadjistavropoulos, Miller, & Beattie, 1992) and, possibly, from patients with vascular dementia (Libon, Swenson, Barnoski, & Sands, 1993).

Differential Diagnosis

A wide range of neurological and psychiatric disorders are observed among older patients. Common presentations include normally aging persons who have concerns about failing capacity; persons with dementing disorders of either the cortical or subcortical type; persons with focal brain deficits related to stroke; and persons with psychiatric disorder accompanied by cognitive complaints or impairments. Other chapters in this volume provide detailed discussions of normal aging and specific disorders. This discussion provides a brief synopsis of neuropsychological tools that can assist in distinguishing among these conditions.

Fixed Batteries

Many clinical laboratories have utilized consistent sets of neuropsychological tasks and instruments over the years to good effect. This approach has generated systematic sets of standardization data and experience with both clinical populations and research groups. The Halstead-Reitan Neuropsychological Battery (HRNB) (Reitan & Wolfson, 1993) represents one of the most widely used and broadly researched batteries, based in large part on procedures that were originally developed or used by Ward Halstead. Since this battery is clearly sensitive to the declines in cognitive ability that can be expected as a function of age (Bak & Greene, 1980), appropriate norms are obviously important to consider for using this battery as well as any other. The work of Heaton, Grant, and Matthews (1991) has provided a clinically useful resource for examining patient performances on an extended Halstead-Reitan battery, stratified by age and education. However, a key drawback to the use of this battery with many older adults is the relatively lengthy sets of procedures that may exceed energy and effort resources and may be relatively insensitive to subtle changes in performance in the lower ranges of performance.

The Luria-Nebraska Neuropsychological Battery (LNNB; Golden, Hammeke, & Purisch, 1980) is a more recently developed battery that includes some of the tasks developed by Luria (e.g., Luria & Majovski, 1977), presented with standardized procedures. A profile format summarizes performance across several scales, and individual scores are interpreted relative to an age- and education-adjusted baseline. Healthy aged individuals score slightly lower than younger adults on a majority of LNNB scales, but clearly outperform brain-damaged patients on all scales (McInnes et al., 1983). Associations of modest strength have been documented between LNNB scales and several measures of everyday functional abilities (McCue, Rogers, & Goldstein, 1990), and a short form of the LNNB, comprising 141 as opposed to 269 items,

has been developed for use with impaired older persons who may not be able to complete the standard examination (McCue, Goldstein, & Shelly, 1989).

Flexible Batteries

A majority of neuropsychologists who work extensively with older adults use flexible batteries composed of a brief core of tests given to all or nearly all patients and additional measures used for specific referral questions or in response to special characteristics of a given patient. Typically, one or more tests are selected to tap each functional area (e.g., attention, language, learning and memory, visuospatial abilities, reasoning, executive functions, and motor functions). Within each area, there are several options for test selection that may serve equally well for basic differential diagnostic tasks. This flexible approach requires experience with a diverse set of assessment tools and knowledge of normative data for each of these instruments.

Table 2 contrasts outcomes for patients with mild Alzheimer's disease, subcortical dementia, and major depression on several tests commonly used in diagnostic assessment. Within this table, "mild deficit" corresponds to performance 1–1.5 standard deviations below an appropriate normative mean (approximately 6th to 16th percentile), "moderate deficit" corresponds to impairments of approximately 1.66 to 3 standard deviations below the normative mean (0.1 to 5th percentile), and "severe deficit" refers to impairments that are more than 3 standard deviations below average, if scorable, or to gross inability to perform the task. Qualitative features of performance are noted in some cases, based on the Boston Process Approach to neuropsychological assessment (e.g., Milberg, Hebben, & Kaplan, 1986) and other investigations (see La Rue, 1992).

The distinction between Alzheimer's disease (a "cortical dementia") and subcortical dementing disorders (e.g., Cummings & Benson, 1984) is arbitrary to a degree (Whitehouse, 1986). There is cell loss or dysfunction in subcortical brain regions in Alzheimer's disease, particularly the basal forebrain, and disorders such as Parkinson's disease, where the primary pathology is in subcortical structures, also produce cortical dysfunction, most notably in the frontal lobes. However, the cortical/subcortical distinction may be useful in alerting a clinician to differences in the relative prominence of neuropsychological impairments for different conditions.

Alzheimer's Disease

Expected performances in Alzheimer's disease (AD), as summarized in Table 2, are for patients with mild disease with a functional level roughly equivalent to a Clinical Dementia Rating score of 1 (Berg, 1988). Persons at this level of impairment have mild but definite impairment in complex independent living skills and are no longer able to meaningfully contribute to community affairs; however, they can perform basic self-care activities, and in casual observation, appear normal in speech and behavior.

Neuropsychological performance in mild Alzheimer's disease has been characterized by Storandt and colleagues (Storandt et al., 1984; Storandt & Hill, 1989), Welsh and colleagues (1991), and many others (for reviews, see Kaszniak, 1986; La Rue, 1992). The most predictable and severe impairments are in the realm of learning and memory. Tests of secondary memory routinely yield large effect sizes in separating patients with mild dementia of the Alzheimer's type from matched controls (see Christensen, Hadzi-Pavlovic, & Jacomb, 1991, for a review). Deficits are noted in immediate recall of supraspan information (e.g., word lists of 10 or more items) and in rate of acquisition of such information with repeated presentation. After delays of 5 min or more, there is a marked reduction in the amount of information that can be spontaneously recalled, and often, benefit from semantic cues is absent or reduced. Recognition testing yields a higher estimate of learning than recall testing, but the amount of information correctly recognized is below expectations for age. Some, but not all, persons with mild Alzheimer's disease make repeated errors of intrusion on verbal learning tasks, and others perseverate in their attempts to reproduce elements of pictures or designs.

The memory tests noted in Table 2 have been normed for geriatric populations and are well represented in studies comparing Alzheimer's patients and normal older adults. For the Logical Memory and Visual Reproduction subtests from the Wechsler Memory Scale (WMS), much of the published outcomes are for the original scale, but similar outcomes are obtained clinically with the Wechsler Memory Scale-Revised (WMS-R). List learning tests such as the Auditory Verbal Learning Test (AVLT; Rey, 1964), California Verbal Learning Test (CVLT; Delis, Kramer, Kaplan, & Ober, 1987), and Object Memory Evaluation (Fuld, 1981) are among the best tests available for detection of mild AD (Christensen et al., 1991). New normative data for ages 56 to 97 are available for the AVLT from Mayo's Older Americans Normative Study (MOANS; Ivnik et al., 1992), and the CVLT was initially normed for ages 17 to 80. For older persons with low education or limited stamina, the Fuld Object Memory Evaluation provides a useful alternative list-learning test. The Visual Reproduction subtest from the WMS-R and the Benton Visual Retention Test (BVRT) have been the most widely used nonverbal memory tests in geriatric clinical research, although both have the disadvantage of confounding visuoconstructive and memory skills. The BVRT is effective in identifying mild dementia relative to normal aging and is the most important component of the Iowa Battery for Mental Decline (Eslinger et al., 1985).

Alzheimer's disease severe enough to meet diagnostic criteria as specified in the fourth edition of the *Diagnostic and Statistical Manual of Mental Disorders* (*DSM-IV*) (American Psychiatric Association, 1994) almost always involves additional neuropsychological deficits along with memory impairment. Huff and colleagues (1987) noted neuropsychological impairment (scores at the 5th percentile or lower) among 95% of patients clinically diagnosed with AD; 12% had only a single area of deficit, 15% had two areas of deficit, and 68% were impaired in three or more abilities. Memory and language impairments were most commonly observed, affecting 87% and 72% of patients, respectively; visuoconstructive or attentional deficits were noted for 44% to 49% of cases. Qualitative features of performance that are relatively distinctive to Alzheimer's disease have been identified for visuospatial tasks (Brantjes & Bouma, 1991), verbal and nonverbal memory tasks (e.g., Butters et al., 1988; Jacobs, Troster, Butters, Salmon, & Cermak, 1990), and semantic memory and language tasks (e.g.,

Table 2. Neuropsychological Findings in Selected Disorders Relative to Normal Aging

Function/test[a]	Alzheimer's disease	Subcortical dementia	Depression
Attention			
Digit Span Forward	Deficit absent or mild	Mild deficit	Mild deficit
Digit Span Backward	Mild to moderate deficit	Moderate deficit	Mild to moderate deficit
WMS-R Mental Control	Deficit absent or mild	Mild deficit	Mild deficit
WMS-R Attention/Concentration Index	Mild deficit	Moderate deficit	Mild to moderate deficit
Language			
Boston Naming Test	Moderate deficit	Mild deficit	Mild deficit
Verbal Fluency	Mild to moderate deficit; may be increased rate of intrusions	Moderate deficit in number of items named increased rate of perseverations, possible loss of set	Mild deficit
Token Test	Deficit absent or mild on simpler items, moderate for multi-stage items	Deficit absent or mild	Deficit absent or mild
BDAE Complex Ideational Material	Deficit absent or mild on simpler items, moderate to severe for items dependent on memory	Deficit absent or mild	Deficit absent or mild
Learning and Memory			
WMS-R Logical Memory	Moderate to severe deficit in immediate recall; <50% retention on delay; may be intrusions, confabulation; may confuse elements of two stories	Mild to moderate deficit; retention ≥50%	Mild to moderate deficit; retention ≥50%
WMS-R Visual Reproduction	Moderate to severe deficit in immediate recall; <50% retention on delay; whole figures may be omitted; others with marked distortion; occasional perseveration of designs or elements	Mild to moderate deficit in immediate recall; ≥50% retention on delay; details may be distorted or omitted, but gestalt of the figure typically preserved	Mild to moderate deficit in immediate recall; ≥50% retention on delay; details may be distorted or omitted, but gestalt of the figure typically preserved
Auditory Verbal Learning Test; California Verbal Learning Test; or Fuld Object Memory Evaluation	Moderate to severe deficit in recall on first trial and in rate of acquisition; <50% recall on short or long delay; may be increased rate of intrusions; little benefit from cues; moderate deficit on recognition testing	Mild to moderate deficit on first trial and in rate of acquisition; >50% recall on short or long delay; mild to moderate benefit from cues; may be increased rate of perseverations	Mild to moderate deficit on first trial and in rate of acquisition; >50% recall on short or long delay; mild to moderate benefit from cues; may be increased rate of perseverations
Benton Visual Retention Test	Moderate to severe deficit; may omit whole figures; marked distortion or errors of perserveration	Mild to moderate deficit; may omit minor figures; may be some distortion of major figures	Mild to moderate deficit; may omit minor figures; may be some distortion of major figures

Visuospatial skills			
Clock drawing	Mild to severe deficit; may perseverate numbers or distort number placement; concrete in hand placement (e.g., for 3:40, large hand pointing to 4).	Deficit absent or mild; minor errors in number or hand placement	Deficit absent or mild; minor errors in number or hand placement
WAIS-R Block Design	Mild to severe deficit; may string out blocks or fail to reproduce square pattern	Mild to moderate deficit; slowed rate of performance; errors more likely to involve details of pattern than gestalt; may be mild apraxia	Mild to moderate deficit; slowed rate of performance; errors more likely to involve details of pattern than gestalt; may give up or show poor effort on difficult items
Rey-Osterreith Complex Figure	Mild to severe deficit; may fail to reproduce underlying rectangular structure of figure; may omit or distort major components of design	Mild to moderate deficit; errors more likely to involve details of pattern than the gestalt	Mild to moderate deficit; errors more likely to involve details of pattern than the gestalt
Executive functions and reasoning			
Wisconsin Card Sort	Mild to severe deficit; slowed rate of learning of categories; problems shifting categories; increased perseverative errors	Mild to severe deficit; slowed rate of learning of categories; problems shifting categories; increased perseverative errors	Mild to moderate deficit; slowed rate of learning of categories and problems shifting; may show poor effort
Stroop Color Word Test	Mild to moderate deficit on interference trial	Mild to moderate deficit in speed of color or word naming and on interference trial	May be mild deficit in speed of color or word naming; mild to moderate deficit on interference trial
WAIS-R Digit Symbol	Mild to moderate deficit; may copy items out of prescribed sequence or lose set as task progresses	Mild to moderate deficit due to slowing of response	Mild to moderate deficit due to slowing of response
Trail-making Test	Mild to severe deficit; may be unable to maintain alternating sequence	Mild to moderate deficit; may be unable to maintain alternating sequence; slowing of visual search or motor response	Mild to moderate deficit; may be unable to maintain alternating sequence; may be slowing of visual search or motor response
WAIS-R Similarities	Mild to moderate deficit; may lose set as task progresses	Deficit absent or mild	Deficit absent or mild
Proverbs	Mild to moderate deficit	Deficit limited to most abstract or unfamiliar items	Deficit limited to most abstract or unfamiliar items
Motor functions			
Finger tapping	Deficit absent or mild	Mild to severe deficit	Deficit absent or mild
Spontaneous speech	Normal rate and volume	May be slowed rate, reduced volume, dysarthria, stuttering	May be slowed rate and volume
Fine motor behavior	Deficit absent or mild	Movements may be slow and awkward; possible agraphia	Possible slowing
Gross motor behavior	Normal	Gait may be slowed, balance impaired	Gait may be slowed

a WAIS-R, Wechsler Adult Intelligence Scale-Revised; WMS-R, Wechsler Memory Scale-Revised; BDAE, Boston Diagnostic Aphasia Examination.

Butters, Granholm, Salmon, Grant, & Wolfe, 1987; Hodges, Salmon, & Butters, 1991).

Deficits on tests of executive function and on complex psychomotor speeded tasks are also common in mild AD. Storandt et al. (1984) and Storandt and Hill (1989) found Digit Symbol and Trail-making Part A, in combination with tests of memory and language, to be highly effective in discriminating mild AD from normal aging. A more recent study (Lafleche & Albert, 1995) with very mildly impaired AD patients (mean MMSE = 25, mean MDRS = 126) failed to find significant differences from controls on Trails A, but did for Trails B. This same study failed to find significant group differences for WAIS-R Similarities or a proverbs test, but noted deficits among AD patients on additional measures of set shifting, self-monitoring, and sequencing. Concurrent manipulation of information was proposed as the unifying requirement among executive function tasks sensitive to AD. These findings concur with an earlier longitudinal report (Grady et al., 1988) that found executive function deficits antedating language or spatial impairments in the progressive decline of AD.

In Table 2, several functions are listed as mildly to severely impaired in early AD. The wide range of expected performances reflects differences between individuals in non-memory functions impaired in early stages of disease. Table 3 provides a more detailed summary of expected performance profiles in mild AD.

Patients with possible AD (see McKhann et al.,

Table 3. Summary of Neuropsychological Test Findings in Alzheimer's Disease[a]

Typical presentation
Disproportionate loss of secondary, explicit memory, accompanied by:
    deficits in cognitive flexibility and speeded perceptual-motor integration
    deficits in language production and comprehension
    visuospatial impairments
Contraindications
Any of the following in early stages of illness:
    focal neurological signs and symptoms
    motor impairments (e.g., gait disturbance, tremor)
    speech problems
    severe attention deficits
Variations in presentation (present in some cases)
    Moderate deficits in attention and short-term memory
    Depression, psychosis, anxiety, or agitation
    Differential severity of language vs. visuospatial impairments
Most informative tests
Secondary memory measures
    Quantitative deficit relative to age/education norms on all such tests
    Qualitative features present in many cases
        Logical Memory—intrusions, confabulation; >50% decline on delayed recall
        Associate Learning—intrusions; additional decline on delayed recall
        California Verbal Learning Test—shallow learning curve; delayed recall impaired, free or cued; false positive errors on
            recognition testing
        Object Memory Evaluation—impairment in storage as well as retrieval; impaired recognition relative to norms.
        Visual Reproduction—omission of complete figure; gross distortions; perseveration of one design to the next
Semantic memory/language processes
    Quantitative deficit relative to age/education norms.
    Qualitative features present in many cases
        Boston Naming Test—marked circumlocation; remote semantic associations; perseverations
        Controlled Oral Word Association—perseveration; loss of set
        Picture description—fluent, but many vague terms; word-finding problems
Cautions
Very early Alzheimer's disease cannot be reliably identified by cognitive tests.
Autopsy is required to confirm Alzheimer's pathology.

[a]Adapted by permission from La Rue (1992, p. 196). Copyright 1992 by Plenum Press.

1984) or questionable AD (see Berg, 1988) exhibit the same types of impairments, but to milder degrees, and for these individuals, history of decline may be variable or uncertain. Average neuropsychological scores for groups of patients of this type fall between those of normal elderly persons and patients with mild AD (Storandt & Hill, 1989), and no single test or set of tests reliably distinguishes these individuals from controls. On longitudinal follow-up, however, a substantial proportion (just under 70% in a 7-year follow-up; Rubin, Morris, Grant, & Vendegna, 1989) of such persons develop more severe deficits and eventually meet diagnostic criteria for AD.

The possibility that AD might be identified in preclinical stages by neuropsychological tests is attracting considerable attention. La Rue and Jarvik (1980, 1987) were among the first to address this question with long-term longitudinal follow-up. In a sample of aging twins, performance on tests of vocabulary, verbal reasoning, and psychomotor speed in early old age (mean = 70 years) was related to development of dementia in late old age (mean = 85 years), with those in the lowest performance quartiles at age 70 later diagnosed with dementia more often than their better performing peers.

More recent studies have focused on subtle memory changes which may serve as precursors of a more general dementia. A prospective study of very old, cognitively normal elderly (Masur, Silwinski, Lipton, Blau, & Crystal, 1994) found that recall scores from either the Object Memory Evaluation or the Selective Reminding Test, as well as some language and visuospatial measures, were predictive of dementia 1 or more years before clinical onset of the disorder. Another recent longitudinal study (Bondi et al., 1994) suggested that poor learning, proclivity for intrusion errors, and diminished delayed recall on the CVLT may serve as markers for the subsequent development of dementia, particularly in individuals with familial risk for AD.

Although this research is intriguing, it is important to note that the predictive utility of the test findings noted above is modest (e.g., positive predictive value = 68% in the study by Masur et al., 1994), and the range of time over which prediction has been demonstrated is typically quite short (e.g., 1 to 3 years). Two recent studies in addition to the earlier work of La Rue and Jarvik (1980, 1987) have

shown predictive associations over longer intervals of time (Linn et al., 1995; Zonderman et al., 1995). However, in light of the modest retest stability of memory performance among normal elderly adults, as discussed below, caution is advised in drawing conclusions about the predictive validity of cognitive tests vis-à-vis new-onset dementia. Additional long-term studies are needed, and the age ranges across which prediction can be expected need to be better established.

Subcortical Dementia

Although there is overlap in neuropsychological performance in mild Alzheimer's disease and subcortical dementing disorders, the relative prominence of specific impairments is likely to differ. The characteristics noted in Table 2 are applicable for the two subcortical disorders most commonly observed in old age, that is, Parkinson's disease and vascular dementia of the lacunar infarct or Binswanger's disease.

Parkinson's Disease (PD). Among PD patients in very early stages of disease who have not yet begun to take medications, the most prominent deficits are in psychomotor speeded performance and selected executive functions. Reaction times are about 30% slower in early PD patients compared to age-matched controls, and similar slowing is noted on more complex speeded tasks such as trail-making (Hietanen & Teravainen, 1986). On the Wisconsin Card Sorting Test, early PD patients make more perseverative errors and identify fewer categories than controls (Lees & Smith, 1983). On verbal fluency testing, overall output may be normal, but problems are observed in shifting from one letter category to the next, and an increase in perseverative errors may be observed (Lees & Smith, 1983). Memory problems may also be noted, but the severity of impairment is generally less than that seen in early AD; on list learning tests, deficits are most apparent in learning trials, with final performance levels similar to those of controls (Weingartner, Burns, Diebel, & Le Witt, 1984).

In moderate stages of illness, when patients have typically been on medication for several years, a broader pattern of impairments is likely to be observed. Tests that combine motor speed requirements with cognitive flexibility and/or visuospatial processing demands are most severely impaired, but nonspeeded tasks are also likely to show at least mild impairment (Huber, Freidenberg, Shuttleworth, Paulson, & Christy, 1989; Pirozzolo, Hansch, Mortimer, Webster, & Kuskowski, 1982). Nonetheless, most moderately ill PD patients score in the normal or low normal range on mental status examinations, verbal intelligence tests, and untimed memory tests such as Logical Memory.

Recent studies suggest that treatment with L-dopa may selectively improve performance on tests that are sensitive to frontal lobe function. The most recent of these investigations (Owen et al., 1995) showed mild facilitation of planning accuracy (but not planning latency or working memory) on the Tower of London task in nondemented, medicated PD patients compared to those who were not on medication. This provides some support for the hypothesis that certain executive function deficits in PD may be a direct result of damage to striatal dopaminergic projections or of dopamine loss in the prefrontal cortex.

A minority of PD patients (10% to 20%) exhibit more severe, broadly based deficits, including impairment of learning and memory. Whether these cases reflect a more severe form of PD pathology or result from other coexisting brain impairment (e.g., Alzheimer's disease, Lewy body disease) is unclear. Even in these more severe cases, however, motor disability (e.g., alteration in speech and writing ability; Cummings, Darkins, Mendez, Hill, & Benson, 1988) and certain executive function deficits (e.g., imitation of motor sequences, Wisconsin Card Sorting Test performance; Freedman & Oscar-Berman, 1986; Huber, Shuttleworth, Paulson, Bellchambers, & Clapp, 1986) are relatively more prominent in PD patients than in Alzheimer's patients.

Table 4 summarizes in greater detail expected patterns of neuropsychological performance in PD. The diagnosis of PD is normally made on the basis of neurological assessment. However, neuropsychological testing may be requested to determine whether problems with cognitive impairment as reported by medical staff or family members are characteristic of PD or some other disorder. Also, such testing may be helpful to the patient and family in clarifying the limits of impairment for a given individual and in suggesting changes in daily routines to minimize the impact of these changes.

Table 4. Summary of Neuropsychological Test Findings in Parkinson's Disease[a]

Typical presentation
Disproportionate slowing and change in cognitive flexibility, accompanied by:
  mild memory deficit
  speech problems
  visuospatial impairment
Contraindications
Any of the following in early stages of illness:
  severe memory impairment
  severe attentional deficit
  deficits in language comprehension
  loss of verbal intellectual ability
Most informative tests
Cognitive flexibility/attentional switching
  Reduced speed of performance relative to age/education norms
  Qualitative features present in many cases
    Wisconsin Card Sort—perseveration; difficulty in inferring or switching categories
    Trails B—difficulty comprehending task; loss of set
List-learning tests
  Storage, recognition, and rate of forgetting within normal limits
  Impaired consistency of retrieval
  Impaired recall of serial position
  Low rate of intrusion errors
Cautions
Only a rough parallel should be expected between the severity of motor symptoms and the extent of cognitive loss.
Depression is commonly observed and may exacerbate cognitive problems.
10%–20% of patients have diffuse cognitive problems that are hard to distinguish from Alzheimer's disease.

[a]Adapted by permission from La Rue (1992, p. 218). Copyright 1992 by Plenum Press.

Vascular Dementia (VaD).

The multiple causes of vascular dementia (e.g., large cortical infarcts, multiple small subcortical infarcts, or deep white matter disease) and variable course of the disease have rendered it difficult to specify neuropsychological test outcomes characteristic of vascular dementia.

Early studies suggested that intellectual impairment and memory impairment are less severe on the average in multi-infarct dementia (MID) than in AD (e.g., Perez et al., 1975), but that the presentation is heterogeneous. Loewenstein and colleagues (1991) reported similar mean performance for MMSE-matched MID and DAT groups on all tests but the Object Memory Evaluation, on which the DAT patients showed poorer learning and made more intrusion errors. On tests of language function, MID patients may exhibit more dysarthria and reiterative speech disturbance (e.g., stuttering and echolalia) and produce fewer words and shorter clauses during picture description (Hier, Hagenlocker, & Shindler, 1985; Powell, Cummings, Hill, & Benson, 1988). Verbal fluency tests and confrontation naming may be less likely to distinguish vascular from Alzheimer's-type dementia than analysis of narrative discourse.

Russell and Polakoff (1993) reported statistically significant differentiation of small groups of men with AD versus those with a history of transient ischemic attack (TIA) based on WAIS-R profiles and on motor measures from the Halstead-Reitan battery, with TIA patients performing worse on motor tasks than those with AD. However, in a replication study comparing AD and MID patients, only the Halstead-Reitan motor measures successfully distinguished the groups. This study equated the overall level of performance for AD and TIA or MID patients by statistical correction; with this general correction, no difference was noted for the two types of dementia on verbal and figural memory tests.

Diagnostic criteria for VaD recommended by an international work group (Román et al., 1993) state that memory impairment must be present, accompanied by deficits in at least two other domains. This report emphasized subcortical dysfunction as underlying many of the clinical features in VaD and stated that deficits on tasks assessing psychomotor speed, executive function deficits, and mood or personality changes support a diagnosis of VaD (p. 253). No specific battery of neuropsychological tests was recommended to confirm a diagnosis of VaD, but examiners were encouraged to test each major cognitive domain, with special attention to measures that have sensitivity in detecting subcortical lesions and in evaluating language and motor functions.

The possibility that subtle frontal/subcortical deficits may precede clinically significant dementia in patients with mild cerebrovascular disease has been illustrated in two recent studies. In a sample of healthy elderly adults, those with deep white matter lesions exceeding a certain threshold (affected area > 10 mc^2) scored lower than those with minimal or moderate white matter changes on several measures sensitive to frontal lobe function (Digit Span, Wisconsin Card Sorting Test and Auditory Consonant Trigrams), but not on tests assessing global mental status, intelligence, memory, visuospatial ability, or language (Boone et all., 1992). A prospective study (Wolfe, Linn, Babikian, Knoefel, & Albert, 1990) demonstrated deficits among nondemented older adults with multiple small lacunar infarcts relative to controls in shifting mental set (the Visual Verbal Test), response inhibition (Stroop Color-Word Interference Test), executive function (semantic clustering on the CVLT), and verbal fluency, and more of these subjects showed apathetic behavior. However, several other measures that might be expected to tap frontal functioning (reciprocal motor programming and vigilance tests) did not distinguish participants with and without lacunar infarcts.

Cummings (1993) described five parallel but segregated circuits linking the frontal lobes with subcortical structures, each with somewhat unique clinical manifestations (e.g., executive function deficits with lesions of the dorsolateral prefrontal circuits, disinhibition with lesions of the orbitofrontal circuit). In VaD, several of these circuits may be affected, producing a broad, but variable, set of behavioral dysfunctions.

While it is not possible to specify a typical pattern of neuropsychological findings in VaD, some general guidelines can be stated. For vascular dementia patients who have suffered multiple large infarcts, deficits commensurate with the location and extent of infarction should be expected. For those whose cerebrovascular pathology is limited to lacunar infarcts or who have extensive deep white matter disease, deficits would be expected to parallel those of PD more closely than those of DAT. A high rate of inter-test scatter is not specific to vascular dementia and cannot be used to identify this condition or to differentiate it from normal aging or Alzheimer's disease.

Depression

Cognitive deficits are commonly reported among patients with major depression, but the severity and specificity of impairments varies from study to study (for reviews, see Caine, 1986; Lamberty & Bielianuskas, 1993; La Rue, 1992). Some investigations, especially with depressed outpatients, report little or no impairment relative to nondepressed controls (e.g., Niederehe, 1986; Reisberg, Ferris, Gerogotas, de Leon, & Schneck, 1982), whereas others report mild to moderate deficits in several areas (e.g., King, Cox, Lyness, & Caine, 1995; Lyness, Eaton, & Schneider, 1994). A recent epidemiologic study of several hundred elderly community residents observed significant associations, adjusted for health and demographic variables, between self-rated depression and neuropsychological measures of memory, verbal fluency, psychomotor speed, and cognitive flexibility, and even the MMSE (La Rue, Swan, & Carmelli, 1995).

Table 5 summarizes findings to be expected in major depression of moderate or greater severity. While most recent studies corroborate this listing of relatively impaired and unimpaired functions, one investigation has reported a sparing of memory, constructional ability, and basic attention in depressed elderly outpatients, while noting mild weaknesses in information-processing speed and executive functions (Boone et al., 1995). In contrast, Lachner, Statzger, and Engel (1994) found that older depressed patients scored lower than controls on each of seven memory measures, including the AVLT and Selective Reminding Test. Only a few memory measures (recognition after short and long delay, and delayed recall) reliably distinguished depressed and demented individuals. Kaszniak and Christenson (1994) emphasize that neuropsychological distinction of dementia and depression can be difficult at times; they list historical and behavioral features and qualitative aspects of cognitive performance that may help in differentiation.

Assessing Mood, Personality, and Everyday Function

Although differentiation among brain syndromes relies heavily on assessment of cognitive performance, many cases also require assessment of mood and personality and an estimate of ability to perform activities of daily living (ADL). A formal, standardized evaluation of these domains can provide a valuable baseline for follow-up comparisons and for planning and monitoring the results of interventions.

Table 5. Summary of Neuropsychological Test Findings in Geriatric Depression[a]

Typical presentation
Depressed mood or pervasive loss of interest, accompanied by:
  mild memory deficit
  mild to moderate visuospatial impairment
  reduced abstraction and cognitive flexibility
Contraindications
Depressive symptoms mild or questionable
Problems in language comprehension
Severe memory deficit
Behavior during testing
Self-critical of performance; may underestimate ability or reject
  positive comments from the examiner
Complaints of fatigue or physical distress, often accompanied by
  an objective loss of stamina
Complaints of poor concentration, but usually can attend to tasks
  if encouraged.
Most informative tests
List-learning tests
  Storage, recognition, and rate of forgetting close to normal
  Mild to moderate impairments in recall
  Low rate of intrusion errors
  Benefit from cueing and encoding enhancement
Intelligence testing
  Verbal IQ close to normal levels
  Digit span ≤ other verbal subtests
  Mild to moderate impairment on Performance subtests, due
    primarily to slowing, carelessness, or refusal to complete
    the task
Cautions
Cognitive loss may be linked more closely to global dysfunction
  than to severity of depression per se.
Depression often coexists with organic brain disorder.
10%–20% of patients with diffuse cognitive problems that are
  hard to distinguish from Alzheimer's disease or other organic
  dementias.

[a]Adapted by permission from La Rue (1992, p. 280). Copyright 1992 by Plenum Press.

Mood and Personality

Core features of personality remain stable with normal aging, and as a result, age differences on scales such as the second version of the Minnesota Multiphasic Personality Inventory (MMPI-2) are minimal (Butcher et al., 1991). This scale can be used effectively with older persons, provided that the educational level is high enough to permit appropriate comprehension and that cognitive impairment is absent or very mild. Often, geropsychologists prefer more focused rating instruments to evaluate the severity of particular types of symptoms such as depression. Several well known depression rating scales have been validated for use with older adults (for reviews, see Gallagher, 1986; Yesavage, 1986), including the Beck Depression Inventory (Beck, Ward, Mendelson, Mock, & Erbaugh, 1961), the Geriatric Depression Scale (Yesavage et al., 1983), and the Hamilton Depression Rating Scale (Hamilton, 1967), and application of these or related instruments typically improves detection of depression in older patients in general medical settings.

Assessing mood and personality in memory-impaired patients presents special difficulties as patients may be unable to reliably describe or recall their feelings or behaviors. Several tools have been developed to assist in this situation, most being completed entirely by, or with the assistance of, relatives or other caregivers. The Neuropsychology Behavior and Affect Profile is one of the most comprehensive of these instruments; it asks relatives to rate different mood and behavioral symptoms of the patient before and after brain injury and has been normed for older and younger adults (Nelson et al., 1989). For individuals with dementia, tools such as the Cornell Scale of Depression in Dementia (Alexopoulos, Abrams, Young, & Shamoian, 1988) may be useful, as may the noncognitive subscale from the Alzheimer's Disease Assessment Scale (Rosen, Mohs, & Davis, 1984). For all instruments that rely on ratings by relatives, it is important to keep in mind that lay caregivers often perceive patients as having more problems with mood or affect than professional raters do, and family members who are themselves depressed or anxious also tend to rate the patients they are caring for higher on these dimensions (e.g., La Rue, Watson, & Plotkin, 1992).

Rating ADL

Structured rating scales have also been developed to measure the ability of older persons to perform basic self-care activities or higher-level activities essential to independent living (for a review, see Kemp & Mitchell, 1992). These, too, are generally completed by relatives or other caregivers. Two of the better known scales of this type are the Instrumental Activities of Daily Living scale (Lawton & Brody, 1969), which covers independent living skills such as meal preparation, use of medications, and financial management, and the Blessed Dementia Rating Scale (Blessed, Tomlinson, & Roth, 1968), which assesses practical everyday functions (e.g., finding one's way in the neighborhood) as well as mood and personality changes. Another scale that ranks both functional problems and changes in behavior and mood and assesses caregivers' level of distress in response to difficulties in these areas is the Memory and Behavior Problems Checklist, now available in revised form (Teri et al., 1992).

Instruments such as the Direct Assessment of Functional Status scale (see Loewenstein, Rubert, Argüelles, & Duara, 1995) circumvent possible rater bias by asking patients to directly perform basic activities such as telling time, using a telephone, making change, or balancing a checkbook. Designed for use with elderly persons with mild to moderate dementia, outcomes on this scale correlate significantly but modestly with observer-rated ADL measures.

Variability, Stability, and Change

Intertest Scatter

It is a common clinical practice to interpret discrepancies in performance across different measures as an indicator of impairment; however, recent data convincingly illustrate that caution is needed in drawing inferences based on inter-test scatter.

Nearly one half (48.7%) of the WAIS-R standardization sample exhibited differences of seven or more points between scale scores for their highest and lowest subtests (Matarazzo & Prifitera, 1989). The reliability of WAIS-R difference scores (e.g., discrepancies between verbal and performance quotients) is lower than that of individual scores (Matarazzo & Herman, 1984), and well-educated persons and those over 65 exhibit greater scatter across subtests than do younger adults with average education.

Data from MOANS (Ivnik, Smith, Malec, Petersen, & Tangalos, 1995) document the extent of scatter among cognitively normal older adults (ages 55 to 85+ years). The initial sample consisted of 502 persons without mental disorder; retest data obtained 1 to 5 years later (mean = 3.7 years) were available for 248 persons still judged to be cognitively intact. Among five factors of intellectual and memory performance derived from the WAIS-R, WMS-R, and AVLT, differences between factor scores of 20 or more points (approximately 2 standard deviations) were noted for 10% to 20% of the sample, and 10 or more points for 37% to 53% percent of the sample. Particularly striking was the relative independence of Verbal Comprehension and Retention scores ($r = .28$), raising doubts about interpreting discrepancies between intelligence and retention as an indication of memory impairment.

Performance profiles for detecting particular brain syndromes, based on discrepancies between test scores, have occasionally been proposed for geriatric application. For example, Fuld (1984) identified a profile based on the relative ranking of seven WAIS subtests that appeared useful in distinguishing between Alzheimer's-type and multi-infarct dementia. However, subsequent studies have generally reported low sensitivities of the Fuld profile to Alzheimer's disease and instability of the profile over time (Goldman, Axelrod, Giordani, Foster, & Berent, 1992).

Stability and Change over Time

Geropsychological assessments often call for reexamination after a few months or a year if borderline deficits are observed on first testing, if everyday complaints or dysfunctions persist despite initially adequate performance, or if specific treatments or interventions have been prescribed. To interpret retest results, it is important to be able to estimate the extent of negative change (due to aging or age-related factors) and positive change (due to practice) that is typical of older samples. Until recently, this has been difficult to do because of a paucity of data on older groups on clinically relevant measures and extended periods of time.

Data from descriptive longitudinal studies of older samples often show small declines in mean scores on cognitive tests over a period of a few years (e.g., Schaie, 1990, 1994; Taylor, Miller, & Tinklenberg, 1992; Zelinski, Gilewski, & Schaie, 1993). However, these changes are not large by clinical standards, and few subjects show declines on most or all measures. A long-term longitudinal study

headed by Werner Schaie examined the proportion of individuals in different age groups from 25 to 88 years who showed stability or decline (defined as a loss in performance equal to greater than one standard error of measurement) in different cognitive abilities across successive 7-year intervals (Schaie, 1990, 1994). The percentage who remained stable in performance on at least three of five cognitive tests measuring verbal and arithmetic abilities, visuospatial skill, abstract reasoning, and motor speed ranged from over 90% for ages 53 to 60 to over 75% for ages 75 to 81. Stability was clearly the typical outcome, even for the oldest group.

Ivnik and colleagues (1995) examined stability of performance on clinical tests of intelligence and memory in normal older adults. Test–retest correlations were very high for WAIS-R Full-Scale, Verbal, and Performance IQs ($r = .86$, .86, and .79, respectively) and moderately high for summary indices derived from the WMS-R ($r = .74$, .61, .78, .72, for Verbal, Visual, and Memory indices, and for the Attention/Concentration index, respectively). These results, based on a mean retest interval of 3.7 years, compare favorably with the reliability coefficients reported by Wechsler (1981, 1987) for intervals of a few weeks. Indices of delayed recall derived from the WMS-R and AVLT had stability coefficients of .66 and .71, respectively, but percent retention estimates derived from these instruments were quite unstable ($r = .42$ and .39 for the WMS-R and AVLT, respectively). Shared variance between first and second testings for pairs of specific abilities ranged from .50 for Verbal Comprehension and Learning factors to a low of only .11 for Learning and Retention factors. The authors concluded that there is considerable shifting in specific performances for normally aging individuals across intervals of a few years, and that for certain measures (e.g., percent retention), change may be more of the norm than stability.

Youngjohn and Crook (1993) examined practice effects in healthy older adults (50 to 77 years) participating in a year-long medication trial. A battery of memory tests was administered an average of seven times using different but equivalent forms of the test instruments. Significant improvements occurred on all seven tests of everyday memory, despite the use of parallel forms, with effect sizes ranging from 2% to 44%. At a long-term follow-up conducted 3 years after the end of the drug study, performance declined to levels closer to the initial baseline, and as a result, the investigators proposed a retest interval of 3 years to minimize practice effects on secondary memory tasks.

In a companion group retested only once after an interval of 4.6 years, slight declines were noted on some tests, but on others, mean scores were slightly higher at the second testing. The relative lack of decline over time in everyday memory performance was the outcome that Youngjohn and Crook found most noteworthy. In another recent study with a 4-year test–retest interval, slight decline was noted on a majority of memory tests for all subjects over the age of 70 but for only 59% of subjects in their 60s (Taylor et al., 1992), and at a 1-year retest on the WAIS-R (Snow, Tierney, Zorzitto, Fisher, & Reid, 1989), normal persons in their 60s and early 70s were more likely to show gains in summary scores than declines (60% vs. 33%).

Predicting Everyday Function

Neuropsychologists are often asked to offer an opinion as to a patient's ability to perform specific functional tasks such as driving or functioning safely in a global manner in an independent living setting.

Comparatively little research has been directed at establishing the validity of neuropsychological tests for predicting performance of real-life tasks by older adults. Pertinent studies have shown modest relationships between scores on brief mental status examinations and informant ratings of patient abilities to perform everyday activities (e.g., Reed et al., 1989; Warren et al., 1989), with weaker associations noted for mildly demented individuals. When outcomes of more extensive mental status assessment or neuropsychological testing are compared to directly assessed functional abilities (e.g., Loewenstein, Rubert, et al., 1995; McCue et al., 1990; Nadler et al., 1993), significant associations are observed, but neuropsychological scores generally account for less than 50% of the variance in functional activity ratings.

Researchers familiar with this area (e.g., Grisso, 1994; Loewenstein, Rubert, et al., 1995)

have urged caution in using neuropsychological tests as a basis for major decisions regarding functional capacity. Functional performance measures and reports of family and other caregivers should be used in conjunction with cognitive and medical tests to provide a thorough understanding of an individual's functional strengths and limitations. This recommendation applies to assessment of general competence for independent care and to more specific functional areas such as financial management and driving.

Culturally Diverse Assessment

Examiners are often in a quandary about interpreting test outcomes for persons whose language or cultural background differs from that of the populations on which the tests were standardized and normed. Although more attention is being paid to cultural diversity in test development and validation, comparatively few studies focus on older persons, and those that do often involve small and select samples that may not be representative of more general populations. In general, this research suggests that education has a greater impact on cognitive test performance than ethnicity. Nonetheless, small performance differences associated with language or cultural background are observed on certain measures.

Some MMSE items may be biased against populations whose primary language is not English or whose cultural identification differs from that of normative samples, which are largely white and middle-class. Ethnicity and language effects were noted in a comparison of white and Hispanic adults on orientation to county and state, attention and calculation items, and repetition of a specified phrase (Escobar et al., 1986). Another recent study found that the MMSE misclassified more cognitively normal Hispanic elderly as impaired than a memory test based on learning and recall of 10 common objects (Loewenstein, Duara, Argüelles, & Argüelles, 1995). In a multicultural epidemiologic survey (Wilder et al., 1995), the MMSE and most other mental status exams misclassified as impaired a majority of nondemented elderly with less than 4 years of education. Anthony et al. (1982) reported comparatively few differences in performance on the MMSE for medically ill white and African-American elderly when differences in education were taken into account. By contrast, a study of community residing adults (Fillenbaum, Heyman, Williams, Prosnitz, & Burchett, 1990) found the specificity of the MMSE for detecting dementia to be much lower for African Americans than for white adults (59% vs. 94%, respectively). Fortunately, some of the MMSE items most sensitive to Alzheimer's disease (delayed recall and design copying) appear to be less affected by ethnicity and education differences than other items.

A newer mental status examination, the Cognitive Abilities Screening Instrument (CASI), has been developed with the potential to modify test items to suit the language, dialect, and cultural, educational, and geographic background of different study populations (Teng et al., 1994). The CASI is composed of 20 questions drawn from established dementia screening measures, including the Hasegawa Dementia Screening Scale (Hasegawa, 1983), the MMSE, and the Modified Mini-Mental State Exam (Teng & Chui, 1987), and an additional question assessing judgment. Some of the original items were altered or replaced when item difficulty varied across different countries, when there were problems in translating the item into other languages, or when standardized administration or scoring was lacking. The CASI currently has several versions adapted to specific locales in the United States and Japan, and more are being developed. Most recently, the CASI has been adapted for use in a study of dementia among Chinese elderly with little or no education (Liu et al., 1994).

Within the United States, there is an expanding database on performance of Spanish-speaking older adults, both normal and cognitively impaired, on neuropsychological tests that have gone through a back-translation process. On many measures, equivalent performance has been observed for Spanish- and English-speaking groups (Loewenstein, Argüelles, Argüelles, & Linn-Fuentes, 1994; Taussig, Henderson, & Mack, 1992) when differences in average educational attainment are statistically controlled. However, on a few widely used tests, mean performance differences favoring non-Hispanic whites have been observed.

Community residing Spanish-speaking older adults scored lower on the Vocabulary and Sim-

ilarities subscales of the Escala de Inteligencia Wechsler Para Adultos (EIWA) (Wechsler, 1968) than non-Hispanic elders tested on WAIS-R versions of these subscales (Lopez & Taussig, 1991); the same study documented differences in favor of English-speaking participants on WAIS-R Digit Span and Block Design. Normal elderly Spanish speakers of Cuban descent performed less well on delayed recall of a list of grocery items than English-speaking individuals and generated fewer relevant items on a test of verbal fluency that entailed naming of words beginning with the letters F, A, and S (Loewenstein et al., 1994). Taussig et al. (1992) also found differences favoring normal English-speaking as opposed to Spanish-speaking individuals on the FAS test and on the Boston Naming Test. In their attempts to interpret these outcomes, investigators have pointed to possible differences between cultural or linguistic groups in the salience of specific test items (e.g., grocery lists to be remembered or the Boston Naming Test stimuli), the orthographic complexity of certain language tasks (e.g., FAS naming), and the strategies used for chunking numbers in Spanish- versus English-speaking environments (possibly affecting Digit Span).

Loewenstein, Duara, et al. (1995) reported an absence of differences in performance on the Object Memory Evaluation (Fuld, 1981) for Cuban-American elders compared to non-Hispanic white Americans. Moreover, a single cutting score proved highly effective in both cultural/linguistic groups for distinguishing mildly demented from nondemented participants. Although no data are provided, the authors mention that preliminary findings support the appropriateness of the Object Memory Evaluation for normal African-American elderly, and a previous study supports the utility of this procedure for Japanese elderly (Fuld, Muramoto, Blau, Westbrook, & Katzman, 1988). Considering the importance of learning and memory assessment in clinical geropsychology, these outcomes are encouraging. However, Taussig et al. (1992) observed small but statistically significant differences in Object Memory Evaluation performance for English- and Spanish-speaking patients with AD, despite equivalent performance of normal Spanish- and English-speaking controls. In a cognitively normal community sample, La Rue, Ortiz, Romero, Liang, and Lindeman (1995) noted significant differences between Hispanic elderly adults and non-Hispanic whites on the Object Memory Evaluation, but the magnitude of separation was less on this test than on measures assessing attention, verbal fluency, visuospatial performance, speed, and cognitive flexibility.

Ardila, Rosselli, and Puente (1994) have validated cognitive tests in a Spanish-speaking population outside of the United States (Colombia). This team has methodically developed normative data for a battery of commonly used tasks that are relevant for older ages and lower educational levels. Their work provides a model for similar, large-scale validation attempts in other countries and cultures.

Summary and Conclusions

In the next few years, we are likely to witness increasing pressure for cost-efficient screening of cognitive impairment in geriatric patient populations. A diverse set of instruments is available for this purpose, and selection among alternatives will vary with the characteristics of the individual being assessed or the population being served. In our experience, a standardized cognitive mental status exam is the most versatile and informative approach, and the MMSE, the best known and most widely used of such measures, is still a good choice for many situations. To be applied and interpreted correctly, brief instruments often require a greater knowledge base on the part of the practitioner than lengthier test batteries (cf. Lezak, 1995), and it will be important for training programs to fully acquaint students with the use of screening tools. Screening of normal older persons is a valuable adjunct to training with clinical groups.

Neuropsychological test results often provide an important component of the information needed to diagnose neuropsychiatric disorders. Although precise neuropsychological profiles cannot be specified for conditions such as Alzheimer's disease, vascular dementia, or geriatric depression, the relative prominence of deficits varies across these conditions, making it possible to state whether results are consistent with a particular disorder or atypical of that condition. Coexisting illness can confuse the picture, as can premorbid idiosyncrasies in cognitive strengths and impairments. A thorough understanding of premorbid ability is crucial to interpreting outcomes of any single assessment, and caution is needed in interpreting results when historical information is conflicting or ambiguous. Integration of testing outcomes with historical, psychosocial, and medical diagnostic information is the key to beneficial application of neuropsychological testing. This is best taught through mentoring and supervised experience and is difficult to communicate in brief workshops or general courses.

Repeat assessment is very useful in diagnosing progressive conditions in early stages. Among cognitively normal persons, discrepancies of one standard deviation or more across specific performances are not unusual, and mild deficits in performance on a particular test may not prove stable on repeat assessment. In retesting older persons 6 months to a year after first assessment, most scores should be stable or slightly improved. Deficits that persist across testings are important, as are declines on multiple indicators of one or more abilities.

High priority areas for future work include (1) continuing to extend age norms (e.g., to age 80 and older) for commonly used tests in diverse populations; (2) taking a closer look at neuropsychological performance of poorly educated older persons, or the development of new measures better suited for such populations; (3) more research on the gray area between normal aging changes and very early dementia to clarify the conditions under which mild deficits are likely to progress; and (4) more research on the relationship between neuropsychological test outcomes and competence in everyday activities, especially complex activities such as driving, financial management, or medical decision-making.

References

Alexopoulos, G. S., Abrams, R. C., Young, R. C., & Shamoian, C. A. (1988). Cornell Scale for Depression in Dementia. *Biological Psychiatry, 23,* 271–284.

American Psychiatric Association. (1994). *Diagnostic and statistical manual of the American Psychiatric Association* (4th ed.). Washington, DC: Author.

Anthony, J. C., La Resche, L., Niaz, U., Von Korff, M., & Folstein, M. (1982). Limits of the ''Mini-Mental State'' as a screening test for dementia and delirium among hospital patients. *Psychological Medicine, 12,* 317–326.

Ardila, A., Rosselli, M., & Puente, A. E. (1994). *Neuropsychological evaluation of the Spanish speaker.* New York: Plenum Press.

Bak, J. S., & Greene, R. L. (1980). Changes in neuropsychological functioning in an aging population. *Journal of Consulting and Clinical Psychology, 48,* 395–399.

Ballard, E. L., Nash, F., Raiford, K., & Harrell, L. E. (1993). Recruitment of black elderly for clinical research studies of dementia: The CERAD experience. *The Gerontologist, 33,* 561–565.

Beck, A. T., Ward, C. H., Mendelson, M., Mock, J., & Erbaugh, J. (1961). An inventory for measuring depression. *Archives of General Psychiatry, 4,* 561–571.

Berg, L. (1988). Mild senile dementia of the Alzheimer type: Diagnostic criteria and natural history. *Mount Sinai Journal of Medicine, 55,* 87–96.

Blessed, G., Tomlinson, B. E., & Roth, M. (1968). The association between quantitative measures of dementia and of senile change in the cerebral grey matter of elderly subjects. *British Journal of Psychiatry, 114,* 797–811.

Bondi, M. W., Monsch, A. U., Galasko, D., Butters, N., Salmon, D. P., & Delis, D. C. (1994). Preclinical cognitive markers of dementia of the Alzheimer type. *Neuropsychology, 8,* 374–384.

Boone, K. B., Miller, B. L., Lesser, I. M., Mehringer, C. M., Hill-Gutierrez, E., Goldberg, M. A., & Berman, N. G. (1992). Neuropsychological correlates of white-matter lesions in healthy elderly subjects. *Archives of Neurology, 49,* 549–554.

Boone, K. B., Lesser, I. M., Miller, B. L., Wohl, M., Berman, N., Lee, A., Palmer, B., & Back, C. (1995). Cognitive function in older depressed outpatients: Relationship of presence and severity of depression to neuropsychological test scores. *Neuropsychology, 9,* 390–398.

Brantjes, M., & Bouma, A. (1991). Qualitative analysis of the drawings of Alzheimer patients. *Clinical Neuropsychologist, 5,* 41–52.

Brown, F. M., III, & Wiggins, J. B., Jr. (1994). A survey of clinicians' practices with older adults. In M. Storandt & G. R. VandenBos (Eds.), *Neuropsychological assessment of dementia and depression in older adults* (pp. 177–182). Washington, DC: American Psychological Association.

Butcher, J. N., Aldwin, C. M., Levenson, M. R., Ben-Porath, Y. S., Spiro, A., III, & Bosse, R. (1991). Personality and aging: A study of MMPI-2 among older men. *Psychology and Aging, 6,* 361–370.

Butters, N., Granholm, E., Salmon, D., Grant, I., & Wolfe, J. (1987). Episodic and semantic memory: A comparison of amnesic and demented patients. *Journal of Clinical and Experimental Neuropsychology, 9,* 447–497.

Butters, N., Salmon, D. P., Cullum, C. M., Cairns, P., Troster, A. I., Jacobs, D., Moss, M., & Cermak, L. S. (1988). Differentiation of amnesic and demented patients with the Wechsler Memory Scale-Revised. *Clinical Neuropsychologist, 2,* 121–132.

Caine, E. D. (1986). The neuropsychology of depression: The pseudodementia syndrome. In I. Grant & K. M. Adams (Eds.), *Neuropsychological assessment of neuropsychiatric disorders* (pp. 221–243). New York: Oxford University Press.

Christensen, J., Hadzi-Pavlovic, D., & Jacomb, P. (1991). The psychometric differentiation of dementia from normal aging: A meta-analysis. *Psychological Assessment, 3,* 147–155.

Crum, R. M., Anthony, J. C., Bassett, S. S., & Folstein, M. F. (1993). Population-based norms for the Mini-Mental State Examination by age and educational level. *Journal of the American Medical Association, 269,* 2386–2391.

Cullum, C. M., Thompson, L. L., & Smernoff, E. N. (1993). Three-word recall as a measure of memory. *Journal of Clinical and Experimental Neuropsychology, 15,* 321–329.

Cummings, J. L. (1993). Frontal-subcortical circuits and human behavior. *Archives of Neurology, 50,* 873–880.

Cummings, J. L., & Benson, D. R. (1984). Subcortical dementia: Review of an emerging concept. *Archives of Neurology, 41,* 874–879.

Cummings, J. L., Darkins, A., Mendez, M., Hill, M. A., & Benson, D. F. (1988). Alzheimer's disease and Parkinson's disease: Comparison of speech and language alterations. *Neurology, 38,* 680–684.

Delis, D. C., Kramer, J. H., Kaplan, E., & Ober, B. A. (1987). *The California Verbal Learning Test* (Research ed.) New York: Psychological Corporation.

Erickson, R. C., Ermon, P., & Hebber, N. (1992). A bibliography of normative articles on cognition tests for older adults. *The Clinical Neuropsychologist, 6,* 98–102.

Escobar, J. I., Burnam, A., Karno, M., Forsythe, A., Landsverk, J., & Golding, J. M. (1986). Use of the Mini-Mental State Examination (MMSE) in a community population of mixed ethnicity. *Journal of Nervous and Mental Disease, 174,* 607–614.

Eslinger, P. J., Damasio, A. R., Benton, A. L., & Van Allen, M. (1985). Neuropsychologic detection of abnormal mental decline in older persons. *Journal of the American Medical Association, 253,* 670–674.

Fillenbaum, A., Heyman, A., Williams, K., Prosnitz, B., & Burchett, B. (1990). Sensitivity and specificity of standardized screen of cognitive impairment and dementia among elderly black and white community residents. *Journal of Clinical Epidemiology, 43,* 651–660.

Folstein, M. F., Folstein, S. E., & McHugh, P. R. (1975). "Mini-Mental State": A practical guide of grading the cognitive state of patients for the clinician. *Journal of Psychiatric Research, 12,* 189–198.

Freedman, M., & Oscar-Berman, M. (1986). Comparative neuropsychology of cortical and subcortical dementia. *Canadian Journal of Neurological Sciences, 13,* 410–414.

Freedman, M., Leach, L., Kaplan, E., Winocur, G., Shulman, K. I., & Delis, D. C. (1994). *Clock drawing: A neuropsychological analysis.* New York: Oxford University Press.

Fuld, P. A. (1981). *The Fuld Object Memory Evaluation.* Chicago: Stoelting Instrument Company.

Fuld, P. A. (1984). Test profile of cholinergic dysfunction and of Alzheimer type dementia. *Journal of Clinical Neuropsychology, 6,* 380–392.

Fuld, P. A., Muramoto, O., Blau, A. D., Westbrook, L. E., & Katzman, R. (1988). Cross-cultural and multi-ethnic dementia evaluation by mental status and memory testing. *Cortex, 24,* 511–519.

Galasko, D., Klauber, M. R., Hofstetter, C. R., Salmon, D. P., Lasker, B., & Thal, L. J. (1990). The Mini-Mental State Examination in the early diagnosis of Alzheimer's disease. *Archives of Neurology, 47*, 49–52.

Gallagher, D. (1986). Assessment of depression by interview methods and psychiatric rating scales. In L. W. Poon (Ed.), *Handbook for clinical memory assessment of older adults* (pp. 202–212). Washington, DC: American Psychological Association.

Golden, C. J., Hammeke, T. A., & Purisch, A. D. (1980). *The Luria-Nebraska Neuropsychological Battery manual.* Los Angeles: Western Psychological Services.

Goldman, R. S., Axelrod, B. N., Giordani, B. J., Foster, N., & Berent, S. (1992). Longitudinal sensitivity of the Fuld cholinergic profile to Alzheimer's disease. *Journal of Clinical and Experimental Neuropsychology, 14*, 566–574.

Grady, C. L., Haxby, J. V., Horwitz, B., Sundaram, M., Berg, G., Schapiro, M., Friedland, R. P., & Rapoport, S. I. (1988). Longitudinal study of the early neuropsychological and cerebral metabolic changes in dementia of the Alzheimer type. *Journal of Clinical and Experimental Neuropsychology, 10*, 576–596.

Grisso, T. (1994). Clinical assessments for legal competence of older adults. In M. Storandt & G. R. VandenBos (Eds.), *Neuropsychological assessment of dementia and depression* (pp. 119–140). Washington, DC: American Psychological Association.

Hamilton, M. (1967). Development of a rating scale for primary depressive illness. *British Journal of Social and Clinical Psychology, 6*, 278–296.

Harper, R. B., Chacko, R. C., Kotik-Harper, D., & Kirby, H. B. (1992). Comparison of two cognitive screening measures for efficacy in differentiating dementia from depression in a geriaetric inpatient population. *Journal of Neuropsychiatry, 4*, 178–184.

Hasegawa, K. (1983). The clinical assessment of dementia in the aged: A dementia screening scale for psychogeriatric patients. In M. Bergener, U. Lehr, E. Lang, & R. Schmitz-Scherzer (Eds.), *Aging in the eighties and beyond* (pp. 207–218). New York: Springer.

Haxby, J. V., Raffaele, K., Gillette, J., Schapiro, M. B., & Rapoport, S. I. (1992). Individual trajectories of cognitive decline in patients with dementia of the Alzheimer type. *Journal of Clinical and Experimental Neuropsychology, 14*, 575–592.

Heaton, R. K., Grant, I., & Matthews, C. G. (1991). *Comprehensive norms for an expanded Halstead-Reitan Battery.* Odessa, FL: Psychological Assessment Resources.

Hier, D. B., Hagenlocker, K., & Shindler, A. G. (1985). Language disintegration in dementia: Effects of etiology and severity. *Brain and Language, 25*, 117–133.

Hietanen, M., & Teravainen, H. (1986). Cognitive performance in early Parkinson's disease. *Acta Neurologica Scandinavica, 73*, 151–159.

Hodges, J. R., Salmon, D. P., & Butters, N. (1991). The nature of the naming deficit in Alzheimer's and Huntington's disease. *Brain, 114*, 1547–1558.

Huber, S. J., Shuttleworth, E. C., Paulson, G. W., Bellchambers, M. J. G., & Clapp, L. E. (1986). Cortical vs. subcortical dementia. *Archives of Neurology, 43*, 392–394.

Huber, S. J., Freidenberg, D. O., Shuttleworth, E. C., Paulson, G. W., & Christy, J. A. (1989). Neuropsychological impairments associated with severity of Parkinson's disease. *Journal of Neuropsychiatry, 1*, 155–158.

Huff, F. J., Becker, J. T., Belle, S. H., Nebes, R. D., Holland, A. L., & Boller, F. (1987). Cognitive deficits and clinical diagnosis of Alzheimer's disease. *Neurology, 37*, 1119–1124.

Ivnik, R. J., Malec, J. F., Smith, G. E., Tangalos, E. G., Petersen, R. C., Kokmen, E., & Kurland, L. T. (1992). Mayo's Older Americans Normative Studies: Updated AVLT norms for ages 56 to 97. *The Clinical Neuropsychologist, 6*(Suppl.), 83–104.

Ivnik, R. J., Smith, G. E., Malec, J. F., Peterson, R. C., & Tangalos, E. G. (1995). Long-term stability and intercorrelations of cognitive abilities in older persons. *Psychological Assessment, 7*, 155–161.

Jacobs, D., Troster, A. I., Butters, N., Salmon, D. P., & Cermak, L. S. (1990). Intrusion errors on the Visual Reproduction Test of the Wechsler Memory Scale and the Wechsler Memory Scale-Revised: An analysis of demented and amnestic patients. *Clinical Neuropsychologist, 4*, 177–191.

Kaszniak, A. W. (1986). The neuropsychology of dementia. In I. Grant & K. M. Adams (Eds.), *Neuropsychological assessment of neuropsychiatric disorders* (pp. 172–220). New York: Oxford University Press.

Kaszniak, A. W., & Christenson, G. D. (1994). Differential diagnosis of dementia and depression. In M. Storandt & G. R. VandenBos (Eds.), *Neuropsychological assessment of dementia and depression* (pp. 81–118). Washington, DC: American Psychological Association.

Katzman, R., Brown, T., Fuld, P., Peck, A., Schechter, R., & Schimmel, H. (1983). Validation of a short orientation-memory-concentration test of cognitive impairment. *American Journal of Psychiatry, 140*, 734–739.

Kemp, B. J., & Mitchell, J. (1992). Functional assessment in geriatric mental health. In J. E. Birren, R. B. Sloane, & G. D. Cohen (Eds.), *Handbook of mental health and aging* (2nd ed., pp. 672–697). San Diego, CA: Academic Press.

Kiernan, R. J., Mueller, J., Langston, J. W., & Van Dyke, C. (1987). The Neurobehavioral Cognitive Status Examination: A brief but quantitative approach to cognitive assessment. *Annals of Internal Medicine, 107*, 481–485.

King, D. A., Cox, C., Lyness, J. M., & Caine, E. D. (1995). Neuropsychological effects of depression and age in an elderly sample: A confirmatory study. *Neuropsychology, 9*, 399–408.

Kupke, T., Revis, E. S., & Gantner, A. B. (1993). Hemispheric bias of the Mini-Mental State Examination in elderly males. *The Clinical Neuropsychologist, 7*, 210–214.

Lachner, G., Statzger, W., Engel, R. R. (1994). Verbal memory tests in the differential diagnosis of depression and dementia: Discriminative power of seven test variations. *Archives of Clinical Neuropsychology, 9*, 1–14.

Lafleche, G., & Albert, M. S. (1995). Executive function deficits in mild Alzheimer's disease. *Neuropsychology, 9*, 313–320.

Lamberty, G. J., & Bielianuskas, L. A. (1993). Distinguishing between depression and dementia in the elderly: A review of neuropsychological findings. *Archives of Clinical Neuropsychology, 8*, 149–170.

La Rue, A. (1992). *Aging and neuropsychological assessment*. New York: Plenum Press.

La Rue, A., & Jarvik, L. F. (1980). Reflections of biological changes in the psychological performance of the aged. *Age, 3*, 29–32.

La Rue, A., & Jarvik, L. F. (1987). Cognitive function and prediction of dementia in old age. *International Journal of Aging and Human Development, 25*, 79–89.

La Rue, A., Watson, J., & Plotkin, D. P. (1992). Retrospective accounts of dementia symptoms: Are they reliable? *The Gerontologist, 32*, 240–245.

La Rue, A., Ortiz, I., Romero, L., Liang, H., & Lindeman, R. (1995, November). *Neuropsychological performance of Hispanic and non-Hispanic elderly in New Mexico*. Paper presented at the annual meeting of the Gerontological Society of America, Los Angeles, CA.

La Rue, A., Swan, G. E., & Carmelli, D. (1995). Cognition and depression in a cohort of aging men: Results from the Western Collaborative Group Study. *Psychology and Aging, 10*, 30–33.

Lawton, M. P., & Brody, E. M. (1969). Assessment of older people: Self-maintaining and instrumental activities of daily living. *The Gerontologist, 9*, 179–186.

Lees, A. J., & Smith, E. (1983). Cognitive deficits in the early stages of Parkinson's disease. *Brain, 106*, 257–270.

Lezak, M. D. (1995). *Neuropsychological assessment* (3rd ed.). New York: Oxford University Press.

Libon, D. J., Swenson, R. A., Barnoski, E. J., & Sands, L. P. (1993). Clock drawing as an assessment tool for dementia. *Archives of Clinical Neuropsychology, 8*, 405–415.

Linn, R. T., Wolf, P. A., Bachman, D. L., Knoefel, M. D., Cobb, J. L., Belanger, A. J., Kaplan, E. F., & D'Agostino, R. B. (1995). The "preclinical phase" of probable Alzheimer's disease. *Archives of Neurology, 52*, 485–490.

Liu, H. C., Chou, P., Lin, K. N., Wang, S. J., Fuh, J. L., Lin, H. C., Liu, C. Y., Wu, G. S., Larson, E. B., White, L. R., Graves, A. B., & Teng, E. L. (1994). Assessing cognitive abilities and dementia in a predominantly illiterate population of older individuals in Kinmen. *Psychological Medicine, 24*, 763–770.

Loewenstein, D. A., D'Elia, L., Guterman, A., Eisdorfer, C., Wilkie, F., La Rue, A., Mintzer, J., & Duara, R. (1991). The occurrence of different intrusive errors in patients with Alzheimer disease, multiple cerebral infarctions, and major depression. *Brain and Cognition, 16*, 104–117.

Loewenstein, D. A., Argüelles, T., Argüelles, S., & Linn-Fuentes, P. (1994). Potential cultural bias in the neuropsychological assessment of the older adult. *Journal of Clinical and Experimental Neuropsychology, 16*, 623–629.

Loewenstein, D. A., Duara, R., Argüelles, T., & Argüelles, S. (1995). The utility of the Fuld Object Memory Evaluation in the detection of mild dementia among Spanish-speaking and English-speaking groups. *American Journal of Geriatric Psychiatry, 3*, 300–307.

Loewenstein, D. A., Rubert, M. P., Argüelles, T., & Duara, R. (1995). Neuropsychological test performance and prediction of functional capacities among Spanish-speaking and English-speaking patients with dementia. *Archives of Clinical Neuropsychology, 10*, 75–88.

Logue, P. E., Tupler, L. A., D'Amico, C., & Schmitt, F. A. (1993).

The Neurobehavioral Cognitive Status Examination: Psychometric properties in use with psychiatric inpatients. *Journal of Clinical Psychology, 49*, 80–89.

Lopez, S. R., & Taussig, I. M. (1991). Cognitive-intellectual functioning of Spanish-speaking impaired and nonimpaired elderly: Implications for culturally sensitive assessment. *Psychological Assessment, 3*, 448–454.

Luria, A. R., & Majovski, L. V. (1977). Basic approaches used in American and Soviet clinical neuropsychology. *American Psychologist, 32*, 959–968.

Lyness, S. A., Eaton, E. M., & Schneider, L. S. (1994). Cognitive performance in older and middle-aged depressed outpatients and controls. *Journal of Gerontology: Psychological Sciences, 49*, P129–P136.

Masur, D. M., Silwinski, M., Lipton, R. B., Blau, A. D., & Crystal, H. A. (1994). Neuropsychological prediction of dementia and the absence of dementia in healthy elderly persons. *Neurology, 44*, 1427–1432.

Matarazzo, J. D., & Herman, D. O. (1984). Base rate data for the WAIS-R: Test-retest stability and VIQ-PIQ differences. *Journal of Clinical Neuropsychology, 6*, 351–366.

Matarazzo, J. D., & Prifitera, A. (1989). Subtest scatter and premorbid intelligence: Lessons from the WAIS-R standardization sample. *Psychological Assessment, 1*, 186–191.

Mattis, S. (1988). *Dementia Rating Scale: Professional manual*. Odessa, FL: Psychological Assessment Resources, Inc.

McCue, M., Goldstein, G., & Shelly, C. (1989). The application of a short form of the Luria-Nebraska Neuropsychological Battery to discrimination between dementia and depression in the elderly. *International Journal of Clinical Neuropsychology, 11*, 21–29.

McCue, M., Rogers, J. C., & Goldstein, G. (1990). Relationships between neuropsychological and functional assessment in elderly psychiatric patients. *Rehabilitation Psychology, 35*, 91–99.

McInnes, W. D., Gillen, R. W., Golden, C. J., Graber, B., Cole, J. K., Uhl, H. S. M., & Greenhouse, A. H. (1983). Aging and performance on the Luria-Nebraska Neuropsychological Battery. *International Journal of Neuroscience, 19*, 179–190.

McKhann, G., Drachman, D., Folstein, M., Katzman, R., Price, D., & Stadlin, E. M. (1984). Clinical diagnosis of Alzheimer's disease: Report of the NINCDS-ADRDA work group under the auspices of the Department of Health and Human Services Task Force on Alzheimer's Disease. *Neurology, 34*, 939–944.

Milberg, W. P., Hebben, H., & Kaplan, E. (1986). The Boston process approach to neuropsychological assessment. In I. Grant & K. M. Adams (Eds.), *Neuropsychological assessment of neuropsychiatric disorders* (pp. 65–86). New York: Oxford University Press.

Mitrushina, M., & Satz, P. (1991). Effect of repeated administration of a neuropsychological battery in the elderly. *Journal of Clinical Psychology 47*, 790–801.

Morris, J. C., Heyman, A., Mohs, R. C., Hughes, J. P., van Belle, G., Fillenbaum, G., Mellitis, E. D., & Clark, C. (1989). The Consortium to Establish a Registry for Alzheimer's Disease (CERAD). *Neurology, 39*, 1159–1165.

Nadler, H. D., Richardson, E. D., Malloy, P. R., Marran, M. E., & Brinson, E. H. (1993). The ability of the dementia rating scale to predict everyday functioning. *Archives of Clinical Neuropsychology, 8*, 449–460.

Nelson, L. D., Satz, P., Mitrushina, M., van Gorp, W., Cicchetti, D., Lewis, R., & Van Lancker, D. (1989). Development and validation of the Neuropsychology Behavior and Affect Profile. *Psychological Assessment, 1*, 266–272.

Niederehe, G. (1986). Depression and memory impairment in the aged. In L. W. Poon (Ed.), *Handbook for clinical memory assessment of older adults* (pp. 226–237). Washington, DC: American Psychological Association.

Osato, S., Yang, J., & La Rue, A. (1993). The Neurobehavioral Cognitive Status Examination: An exploratory study with older psychiatric inpatients. *Neuropsychiatry, Neuropsychology, and Behavioral Neurology, 1*, 221–230.

Owen, A. M., Sahakian, B. J., Hodges, J. R., Summers, B. A., Polkey, C. E., & Robbins, T. W. (1995). Dopamine-dependent frontostriatal planning deficits in early Parkinson's disease. *Neuropsychology, 9*, 126–140.

Perez, F. I., Rivera, V. M., Meyers, J. S., Gay, J. R. A., Taylor, R. L., & Mathew, N. T. (1975). Analysis of intellectual and cognitive performance in patients with multi-infarct dementia, vertebrobasilar insufficiency with dementia, and Alzheimer's disease. *Journal of Neurological and Neurosurgical Psychiatry, 38*, 533–540.

Pirozzolo, F. J., Hansch, E. C., Mortimer, J. A., Webster, D. D., & Kuskowski, A. (1982). Dementia in Parkinson disease: A neuropsychological analysis. *Brain and Cognition, 1*, 71–83.

Powell, A. L., Cummings, J. L., Hill, M. A., & Benson, F. (1988). Speech and language alterations in multi-infarct dementia. *Neurology, 38*, 717–719.

Román, G. C., Tatemichi, T. K., Erkinjuntti, T., Cummings, J. L., Masdeu, J. C., Garcia, J. H., Amaducci, L., Orgogozo, J.-M., Brun, A., Hofman, A., Moody, D. M., O'Brien, M. D., Yamaguchi, T., Grafman, J., Drayer, B. P., Bennett, D. A., Fisher, M., Ogata, J., Kokmen, E., Bermejo, F., Wolf, P. A., Gorelick, P. B., Bick, K. L., Pajeau, A. K., Bell, M. A., DeCarli, C., Culebras, A., Korczyn, A. D., Bogousslavsky, J., Hartmann, A., & Scheinberg, P. (1993). Vascular dementia: Diagnostic criteria for research studies. Report of the NINDS-AIREN International Workshop. *Neurology, 43*, 250–260.

Reed, B. R., Jagust, W. J., & Seab, J. P. (1989). Mental status as a predictor of daily living in Alzheimer's disease. *The Gerontologist, 29*, 804–807.

Reisberg, B., Ferris, S. H., Gerogotas, A., de Leon, M. J., & Schneck, M. K.. (1982). Relationship between cognition and mood in geriatric depression. *Psychopharmacology Bulletin, 18*, 191–193.

Reitan, R. M., & Wolfson, D. (1993). *The Halstead-Reitan Neuropsychological Test Battery: Theory and clinical interpretation*. Tempe, AZ: Neuropsychology Press.

Rey, A. (1964). *L'examen clinique en psychologie*. Paris: Presses Universitaires de France.

Rosen, W. G., Mohs, R. C., & Davis, K. L. (1984). A new rating scale for Alzheimer's disease. *American Journal of Psychiatry, 141*, 1356–1364.

Rubin, E. H., Morris, J. C., Grant, E. A., & Vendegna, T. (1989). Very mild senile dementia of the Alzheimer type. *Archives of Neurology, 46*, 379–382.

Russell, E. W., & Polakoff, D. (1993). Neuropsychological test patterns in mean for Alzheimer's and multi-infarct dementia. *Archives of Clinical Neuropsychology, 8*, 327–344.

Ryan, J. J., Paolo, A. M., & Oehlert, M. E. (1989, June). Dementia screening: A tale of two tests. *VA Practitioner, 51*–54.

Salmon, D. P., Riekkinen, P. J., Katzman, R., Zhang, M., Jin, H., & Yu, E. (1989). Cross-cultural studies of dementia: A comparison of Mini-Mental State Examination performance in Finland and China. *Archives of Neurology, 46*, 769–772.

Schaie, K. W. (1990). Intellectual development in adulthood. In J. E. Birren & K. W. Schaie (Eds.), *Handbook of the psychology of aging* (3rd ed., pp. 291–309). San Diego, CA: Academic Press.

Schaie, K. W. (1994). The course of adult intellectual development. *American Psychologist, 49*, 304–313.

Scherr, P. A., Albert, M. A., Funkenstein, H. H., Cook, N. R., Hennekens, C. H., Branch, L. G., White, L. R., Taylor, J. O., & Evans, D. A. (1988). Correlates of cognitive function in an elderly community population. *American Journal of Epidemiology, 128*, 1084–1101.

Schwamm, L. H., Van Dyke, C., Kiernan, R. J., Merrin, E. L., & Mueller, J. (1987). The Neurobehavioral Cognitive Status Examination: Comparison with the Cognitive Capacity Screening Examination and the Mini-Mental State Examination in a neurosurgical population. *Annals of Internal Medicine, 107*, 486–491.

Smith, G. E., Petersen, R. C., & Ivnik, R. J. (1991, February). *Internal consistency and construct validity of the Dementia Rating Scale*. Poster presented at the annual meeting of the International Neuropsychology Society, San Antonio, TX.

Snow, W. G., Tierney, M. C., Zorzitto, M. L., Fisher, R. H., & Reid, D. W. (1989). WAIS-R test-retest reliability in a normal elderly sample. *Journal of Clinical and Experimental Neuropsychology, 11*, 423–428.

Spreen, O., & Strauss, E. (1991). *A compendium of neuropsychological tests: Administration, norms, and commentary*. New York: Oxford University Press.

Storandt, M. (1994). General principles of assessment of older adults. In M. Storandt & G. R. VandenBos (Eds.), *Neuropsychological assessment of dementia and depression in older adults* (pp. 7–32). Washington, DC: American Psychological Association.

Storandt, M., & Hill, R. D. (1989). Very mild senile dementia of the Alzheimer type: 2. Psychometric test performance. *Archives of Neurology, 46*, 383–386.

Storandt, M., & VandenBos, G. R. (Eds.). (1994). *Neuropsychological assessment of dementia and depression in older adults*. Washington, DC: American Psychological Association.

Storandt, M., Botwinick, J., Danziger, W. L., Berg, L., & Hughes, C. P. (1984). Psychometric differentiation of mild senile dementia of the Alzheimer type. *Archives of Neurology, 41*, 497–499.

Sunderland, T., Hill, J. L., Mellew, A. N., Lawlor, B. A., Gundersheimer, J., Newhouse, P. A., & Grafman, J. H. (1989). Clock drawing in Alzheimer's disease: A novel measure of dementia severity. *Journal of the American Geriatrics Society, 37*, 725–729.

Taussig, I. M., Henderson, V. W., & Mack, W. (1992). Spanish translation and validation of a neuropsychological battery: Performance of Spanish- and English-speaking Alzheimer's disease patients and normal comparison subjects. *Clinical Gerontologist, 2,* 95–108.

Taylor, J. L., Miller, T. P., & Tinklenberg, J. R. (1992). Correlates of memory decline: A 4-year longitudinal study of older adults with memory complaints. *Psychology and Aging, 7,* 185–193.

Teng, E. L., & Chui, H. C. (1987). The Modified Mini-Mental State (3MS) examination. *Journal of Clinical Psychiatry, 48,* 314–318.

Teng, E. L., Hasegawa, K., Homma, A., Imai, Y., Larson, E., Graves, A., Sugimoto, K., Yamaguchi, T., Sasaki, H., Chiu, D., & White, L. R. (1994). The Cognitive Abilities Screening Instrument (CASI): A practical test for cross cultural epidemiological studies of dementia. *International Psychogeriatrics, 6,* 45–60.

Teri, L., Truax, P., Logsdon, R., Uomoto, J., Zarit, S., & Vitaliano, P. P. (1992). Assessment of behavioral problems in dementia: The revised Memory and Behavior Problems Checklist. *Psychology and Aging, 7,* 622–631.

Tierney, M. C., Snow, G., Reid, D. W., Zorzitto, M. L., & Fisher, R. H. (1987). Replication and extension of the findings of Storandt and co-workers. *Archives of Neurology, 44,* 720–722.

Tuokko, H., Hadjistavropoulos, T., Miller, J. A., & Beattie, B. L. (1992). The Clock Test: A sensitive measure to differentiate normal elderly from those with Alzheimer disease. *Journal of the American Geriatrics Society, 40,* 579–584.

Uhlmann, R. F., Larson, E. B., Rees, T. S., Koepsell, T. D., & Duckert, L. G. (1989). Relationship of hearing impairment to dementia and cognitive dysfunction in older adults. *Journal of the American Medical Association, 261,* 1916–1919.

Warren, E. J., Grek, A., Conn, D., Herrmann, H., Icyk, E., Kohl, J., & Silberfeld, M. (1989). A correlation between cognitive performance and daily functioning in elderly people. *Journal of Geriatric Psychiatry and Neurology, 2,* 96–100.

Wechsler, D. (1968). *Escala de Inteligencia Wechsler para Adultos.* New York: Psychological Corporation.

Wechsler, D. (1981). *Wechsler Adult Intelligence Scale-Revised.* New York: Psychological Corporation.

Wechsler, D. (1987). *Wechsler Memory Scale-Revised.* New York: Psychological Corporation.

Weingartner, H., Burns, S., Diebel, R., & Le Witt, P. A. (1984). Cognitive impairments in Parkinson's disease: Distinguishing between effort-demanding and automatic cognitive processes. *Psychiatry Research, 11,* 223–235.

Welsh, K. A., Butters, N., Hughes, J., Mohs, R., & Heyman, A. (1991). Detection of abnormal memory decline in mild cases of Alzheimer's disease using CERAD neuropsychological measures. *Archives of Neurology, 48,* 278–281.

Welsh, K. A., Butters, N., Mohs, R. C., Beekly, D., Edland, S., Fillenbaum, G., & Heyman, A. (1994). The Consortium to Establish a Registry for Alzheimer's Disease (CERAD). Part V. A normative study of the neuropsychological battery. *Neurology, 44,* 609–614.

Whitehouse, P. J. (1986). The concept of subcortical and cortical dementia: Another look. *Annals of Neurology, 19,* 1–6.

Wilder, D., Cross, P., Chen, J., Gurland, B., Lantigua, R. A., Teresi, J., Bolivar, M., & Encarnacion, P. (1995). Operating characteristics of brief screens for dementia in a multicultural population. *American Journal of Geriatric Psychiatry, 3,* 96–107.

Wolfe, N., Linn, R., Babikian, V. L., Knoefel, J. E., & Albert, M. L. (1990). Frontal systems impairment following multiple lacunar infarcts. *Archives of Neurology, 47,* 129–132.

Yesavage, J. A. (1986). The use of self-rating depression scales in the elderly. In L. W. Poon (Ed.), *Handbook for clinical memory assessment of older adults* (pp. 213–217). Washington, DC: American Psychological Association.

Yesavage, J., Brink, T., Rose, T., Lum, O., Huang, O., Adey, V., & Leirer, V. (1983). Development and validation of a geriatric depression screening scale: A preliminary report. *Journal of Psychiatric Research, 17,* 37–49.

Youngjohn, J. R., & Crook, T. H., III. (1993). Stability of everyday memory in age-associated memory impairment: A longitudinal study. *Neuropsychology, 7,* 406–416.

Zelinski, E. M., Gilewski, M. J., & Schaie, K. W. (1993). Individual differences in cross-sectional and 3-year longitudinal memory performance across the adult life span. *Psychology and Aging, 8,* 176–186.

Zonderman, A. B., Giambra, L. M., Arenberg, D., Resnick, S. M., Costa, P. T., Jr., & Kawas, C. H. (1995). Changes in immediate visual memory predict cognitive impairment. *Archives of Clinical Neuropsychology, 10,* 111–124.

25

Memory Assessment of the Older Adult

LINDA S. ROCKEY

Introduction

Neuropsychological assessment of the older adult often presents unique challenges to the clinician, who must frequently find ways to modify evaluation techniques. This is especially true when the neuropsychologist must assess an older individual's memory functioning. Because results of memory testing play a pivotal role in predicting the future level of independence of the patient, the neuropsychologist should be well-versed in the areas of memory research and psychometric theory (test reliability and validity) and their interplay in determining viable measures which will comprehensively assess an individual's memory functioning.

To this end, this chapter explores the nature and types of memory currently assessed by the neuropsychologist (verbal memory, nonverbal memory, immediate recall, delayed recall, etc.); reviews the aging research literature with regard to the essential differences in decline typically associated with normal aging and those that result from pathology and disease (a review of the research on age-associated memory impairment); and illuminates some of the differences observed in memory functioning in older adults with temporal lobe pathology, frontal lobe pathology, diencephalic lesions, and diffuse disease. Additionally, this chapter will familiarize the reader with the available tools currently used to assess memory functioning.

Above all, this chapter seeks to evoke continued interest among practicing clinical neuropsy-

chologists who are searching for answers to the question of how best to assess memory functioning in the older adult, especially in light of the rapid increase in the older adult population as we advance toward the 21st century. By continuously exploring the ecological and predictive validity of our current memory assessment techniques, we will be in a better position to identify those unique and special "extra-test" needs of the older individual, especially issues that challenge the reliability of our results, such as fatigue, inattention, depression, and demotivation.

Comprehensive Memory Assessment

The importance of a thorough memory assessment within the overall evaluation of an older adult's cognitive functioning cannot be overemphasized. In searching for cognitive strengths and weaknesses within this important domain, the neuropsychologist should distinguish between various types of memory functioning, namely, verbal memory, nonverbal memory, and immediate recall and delayed recall. These distinctions are important not only to provide diagnostic clarity (right hemisphere vs. left hemisphere dysfunction, cortical vs. subcortical atrophy, etc.), but also to ensure that the assessor does not miss some early sign of disease by failing to comprehensively review memory functioning in all of these areas. Equally, assessment of memory functioning in all of these domains is important in order to arrive at ecologically useful treatment and planning suggestions that are tailored spe-

LINDA S. ROCKEY • Geriatric Care Services, Lutheran Affiliated Services, Mars, Pennsylvania 16046-0928.

cifically to the individual and caregiver and that can be readily implemented within his or her contextual circumstances. Moreover, as La Rue (1992) suggests, a sound memory assessment assists the clinician in distinguishing those aspects of memory loss that may be associated with "normal forgetfulness" for the older person, and those that comprise a disorder (p. 95).

Before distinguishing between various types of memory, it is important to note that memory may not exist solely within certain regions or stores within the brain, but may be conceived as an active process of reconstruction in which certain triggers of an event are woven together within the contextual circumstances in which they arise (Kolb & Whishaw, 1990). A clinician assessing a patient who is experiencing difficulty in recalling brief stories in the context of a cognitive evaluation, for example, should not readily assume that he or she will never be able to recall events mediated within the verbal realm. Similarly, a clinician may find that an individual may be unable to copy the Rey-Osterrieth Complex Figure, however, he or she may well be able to identify photographs of famous faces. For a more thorough discussion of this issue, the reader is encouraged to review Kolb and Whishaw (1990).

Assessment of various facets of memory (verbal and visual memory, immediate recall and delayed recall) is important because everyday events are mediated both verbally and visually. It is incumbent upon the clinician, therefore, to select measures that will appropriately assess the domains of verbal and visual memory and that will answer questions relevant to the nature of the presenting problem and the purpose of the evaluation.

Types of Memory

Verbal Memory

Verbal memory is typically associated with dominant left hemisphere functioning and is naturally mediated by language. The neuropsychologist assesses verbal memory by presenting one or two brief stories in which the individual must first encode and then later retrieve the details and content (and indirectly the tone) of the stories presented. Assessment of this aspect of free recall enables the clinician to directly assess the individual's ability to recount events as they are told to him or her, without the initial use of recognition or contextual cues.

Another important contribution made by neuropsychologists in assessing an individual's verbal retention is his or her ability to recognize recent information presented via list-learning tasks. An individual may first be asked to freely recall a list of approximately 10 to 12 words presented across multiple trials in order to assess free recall, and then be requested to distinguish between those words presented and those not presented during testing. This latter aspect of verbal memory designed to assess the individual's recognition skills is important in distinguishing between dementias of varying etiology.

An individual who is unable to freely recall any of the words presented to him or her, for example, but who can later identify such words when provided with recognition cues is likely to be experiencing deficits in the area of retrieval, but not in the area of encoding verbal data (Lovell & Nussbaum, 1994). This pattern of performance is typical of persons with frontal and subcortical damage, for example, resulting from frontal lobe disorders or disorders of the basal ganglia (Lovell & Nussbaum, 1994). Conversely, impairment of performance in both free recall and recognition is thought to be characteristic of medial temporal lobe damage. Individuals with Alzheimer's disease, for example, often exhibit this pattern of performance (Lovell & Nussbaum, 1994).

Important neuropsychological measures useful in determining the extent of an individual's verbal memory using short stories include the Logical Memory subtests of the Wechsler Memory Scale-Revised (WMS-R; Wechsler, 1987), while tests designed to assess an individual's list-learning skills and recognition memory might include the California Verbal Learning Test (Delis, Kramer, Kaplan, & Ober, 1987), the Rey Auditory Verbal Learning Test (Rey, 1964), and the Hopkins Verbal Learning Test (Brandt, 1991).

Although the utility and applicability of these tests for the older adult will be discussed later in this chapter, it is important to note here that in terms of ecological validity, the Logical Memory subtests of the WMS-R have been noted to be one of the best predictors of real-life memory functioning among traditional memory tests according to some studies (e.g., Sunderland & Watts, 1986); the Rivermead Behavioral Memory Test (Wilson, Cockburn, & Baddeley, 1985) also has good ecological validity.

Nonverbal Memory

In addition to the assessment of an individual's ability to remember verbally mediated material, assessment of his or her memory capacity in the area of visuospatial processing is also essential. Because difficulties in the ability to recall visuospatial material are often the result of nondominant right hemisphere damage, exploration of this domain is important.

To proceed, the clinician first assesses the individual's constructional skills, determining whether the individual can freely copy an abstract visual design. Next, the assessor must determine the individual's ability to recall those designs presented following removal of the stimuli and a brief delay.

Neuropsychological measures useful in assessing visual memory include the Rey-Osterrieth Complex Figure (Rey, 1964), the Benton Visual Retention Test (Benton, 1974), and the Visual Reproduction sections of the WMS-R (Wechsler, 1987). An explanation of the efficacy of these tests in assessing visual memory functioning will also be provided later in this chapter.

Assessment of an individual's ability to retain figural material and/or to freely recall or recall with cueing such material is often useful in determining the most appropriate manner (verbally or visually mediated material) of presenting important information to the patient (medical regimens, etc.), and it can serve as a useful adjunct in planning treatment strategies.

Primary and Secondary Memory

Another distinction often made in assessing memory functioning is that between primary memory or immediate recall of material and secondary or long-term memory functioning. To assess long-term memory, the clinician asks the individual to recall both verbal and visual material (usually presented approximately 20 to 30 min earlier) in order to assess his or her capacity to store and recall data provided.

A distinction between long-term memory within the testing situation and remote memory within the contextual sphere must also be made. While the clinician can assess the individual's retention capacity within the testing situation, for example, it is also helpful to assess the person's ability to recall important earlier periods in his or her life. Here, the skills of the assessing clinician become readily apparent. The skilled clinician, for example, will often include an assessment of at least some aspects of long-term memory via the process of an in-depth clinical interview. The clinician may ask the older person, for example, about events surrounding his or her early life (e.g., "Where did you attend school?"; "What was your first grade teacher's name?"; "What type of work did you do?"; "When did you get married?"). While a few measures exist to facilitate assessment of an individual's remote memory (e.g., the Famous Faces Test and the Famous Events Test; Albert, Butters, & Levin, 1979), they are often confounded by the multiple, varying levels of exposure of older adults to the stimuli, as well as by cultural, economic, and educational variables.

Thus, understanding the distinction in types of memory is essential for the clinician who must comprehensively measure an individual's functioning in all of these respective areas.

Memory in Normal Aging

Memory changes that normally occur in the fifth and sixth decades of life (Albert, 1988) as well as those changes that may occur in later decades of life must be differentiated from those aspects of memory functioning frequently associated with disease processes. Perhaps these differences represent only a matter of degree, or they may involve varying comprehensive *differences of style* in information processing, as well as differences in the depth, level, and sophistication of information processing.

Recent research has begun to highlight essential differences between normal memory functioning and those related to various disease processes. La Rue's (1992) work on cognition and aging suggests age-related deficits in sensory memory such that older adults are likely to require a longer exposure time to sensory stimuli in order to adequately encode and register them. Similarly, older persons are thought to perform more slowly on tasks that require the processing and accessing of information from primary (immediate) or secondary (delayed) memory than are their younger associates. Albert (1988), however, aptly notes that the relationship between primary and secondary memory "is presently viewed as interactive" (p. 39), while Craik (1984) points out that encoding strategies influence retrieval; hence, the relationship between the two is co-constitutive. Further, older adults compared to younger adults exhibit less elaborate strategies for encoding information that typically aid in efficient retrieval (La Rue, 1992).

Possible causes for differences in memory performance between younger and older adults include distraction or inattention at the time of initial processing of the material, lack of specification regarding the parameters of the information to be encoded, lack of enhanced sophistication in cognitive skills in general (that is, less well delineated awareness of meta-analytic strategies secondary to cultural and educational variables), and lack of available time to store information at later ages.

Moreover, extensive research dating back to the mid-1960s seems to support the notion that older individuals encode and categorize material in ways that are perhaps more concrete and less essential, thus, possibly missing significant nuances and tones of the situation that may aid in their retrieval (Craik & Lockhart, 1972). Hence, the older individual may approach familiar stimuli as if they are novel or unique.

While such changes in the processing of information for recall are often associated with normal aging, it would be remiss not to mention Albert's (1988) review of the literature in this area wherein she aptly suggests that "while older individuals do not spontaneously use elaborate encoding strategies to improve retrieval, they are capable of doing so, and when they do, age differences in secondary memory are reduced" (p. 43). Additionally, other investigators (Craik & Lockhart, 1972; Weingartner et al., 1981) have pointed out that improved organization of the material at the time of storage often aids in retrieval irrespective of age.

Further, work by Craik and McDowd (1987) has demonstrated that differing intra-individual variables may well contribute to the presence or absence of age-associated memory decline. Examples of such factors include cultural variables, socioeconomic factors, the individual's history of academic achievement and intelligence, personality variables, history of disease and tendencies to comply with medical regimes, and career and occupational opportunities.

These intra-individual differences signify that not all persons will experience memory decline at the same rate, or even at all. A comprehensive review by Ratcliff and Saxton (1994), however, clearly supports the notion that there is a decline in memory functioning "of substantial proportion" with increasing age (p. 146).

These same authors describe the nature of such memory decline, pointing out that age tends to negatively influence delayed recall to a greater extent than immediate recall and that visuospatial data is less well remembered than material of a verbal nature (p. 156).

Based on the above review, it becomes important to ask whether memory is likely to be improved by training. Reviews in this area, however, have not met with much promise (La Rue, 1992). It appears, for example, that while training may have some initial positive effects, it is particularly labor-intensive, and the benefits that are accrued often are not maintained over any prolonged period of time (La Rue, 1992).

Future research might address the question of whether training might have at least some implicit and "vicarious" effects. Perhaps the individual might benefit from "learning about learning," or from training aimed at increasing self-efficacy, thus, enhancing his or her motivation to maximize whatever cognitive strengths and strategies he or she presently maintains and uses. Moreover, it may be worthwhile to consider whether opportunities for training might encourage more active interaction and stimulation with the environment, thereby altering an individual's locus of control (from that of a passive or dependent approach frequently associated with the elderly, whether accurate or not, to the more active, independent view of self which incorporates a belief in the ability to alter one's immediate environment). Training that enables the older person to gain at least a "perceived" sense of mastery and efficacy in life might lead to some early positive results.

Age-Associated Memory Impairment (AAMI)

In reviewing the associations between normal decline in memory functioning and decline associated with pathological aging, Ratcliff and Saxton (1994) have made useful observations. Distinguishing between "age-appropriate forgetting" (a decline in memory based on comparison with younger cohorts) and age-inappropriate forgetfulness (a notable decline based on comparison with same-age peers), these authors support the notion of a decline in certain aspects of memory functioning with aging, although they readily suggest the necessity of viewing age-associated memory impairment in light of the individual's premorbid intellectual and educational functioning, his or her history of physical problems and diseases, and available memory standards with similar age cohorts.

Most importantly, while previous research has generally, though appropriately, been based on comparison with younger age norms (up to the age of 74), it is now recognized by gerontological and neuropsychological professionals that standardized norms for those over the age of 74 are needed. Moreover, that varied concepts of aging are necessary, as suggested by Ratcliff and Saxton (1994), cannot be overstressed. As they point out, aging research must begin to focus on the processes involved in remembering as a key to distinguishing between memory changes associated with normal aging and those associated with disease. (See Ratcliff & Saxton, 1994, for a more thorough review in this area.)

The Influence of Pathophysiology on Memory Functioning

Having distinguished between some of the general changes in memory functioning typically associated with normal aging, it is now important to highlight some of the more specific difficulties that may arise secondary to impairment in essential regions of the brain. With the advent of brain-scanning techniques such as computerized tomography (CT), magnetic resonance imaging (MRI), positron emission tomography (PET), and single photon emission computerized tomography (SPECT), ready and easy identification of which brain areas are involved in disease states is possible. Regions often associated with memory dysfunction include the temporal cortex, the medial thalamus, mammillary bodies, and the basal forebrain (Kolb & Whishaw, 1990).

Within the temporal lobe, areas thought to contribute to memory dysfunction when damaged include the hippocampus, the amygdala, and the entorhinal cortex. Influencing the afferent connections to the hippocampus, damage to the entorhinal cortex is frequently implicated in memory loss associate with Alzheimer's disease (Kolb & Whishaw, 1990). Similarly, substructures within the hippocampus (CA1, CA2, CA3) serve as connecting links that are especially vulnerable to damage caused by epilepsy and vascular atrophy, often associated with amnestic disorders (Kolb & Whishaw, 1990). Lastly, the amygdala is thought to play a major role in the interconnections between emotion and memory and may also be affected by cerebrovascular disease and head trauma (Kolb & Whishaw, 1990).

In addition to the temporal neocortex, the frontal lobes may also contribute to memory dysfunction. It has been suggested that the frontal lobes are significant in the planning, organizing, and sequencing of events, as well as in separating events of memory in time (Squire, 1987). Memory dysfunction associated with frontal lobe impairment is often clinically manifested in poor free recall but normal recognition memory, suggestive of a retrieval deficit. This is in contrast to medial-temporal lobe-related memory deficits in which both free recall and recognition memory are impaired. This suggests that the medial-temporal lobe is important for encoding mechanisms (Cummings, 1989). Errors of omission or commission (false-positive and false-negative errors on list-learning tasks), errors of intrusion, and susceptibility to interference when intervening tasks are incorporated within the testing situation are also likely following damage to this area (Craik & McDowd, 1987). Similarly, focal cortical lesions may produce long-term memory deficits, while diencephalic lesions are common with Korsakoff's syndrome.

Finally, other causes of memory loss include head injuries, alcoholism, depression, electroconvulsive therapy (ECT), concussion, vitamin B_{12} deficiencies, thyroid dysfunction, infantile amnesias, and posttraumatic stress disorder (Kolb & Whishaw, 1990).

In a testing situation, individuals with medial-temporal lobe dysfunction usually associated with Alzheimer's disease often demonstrate impairments in free verbal recall and verbal recognition, visual recall and recognition, and ability to learn new material. They may equally confabulate details when they have difficulty recalling the material presented to them, demonstrate perseveration, exhibit decreased verbal fluency at either the letter or category levels (typically this occurs at the category level in more advanced stages), and show a general impoverishment in their ability to integrate verbal and visual material (Terry, Katzman, & Bick, 1994).

In contrast, individuals presenting with frontal lobe impairment demonstrate difficulties in planning and sequencing, perseveration, reduced verbal fluency (usually in the case of left hemisphere frontal damage), impaired mental flexibility, fatigue, a tendency to be stimulus-bound, and limited insight into their cognitive deficits. Apathy or depression may result depending on the level and extent of frontal lobe involvement. Individuals fitting this pattern also exhibit a limited attention span. Table 1 depicts types of memory dysfunction associated with damage to various brain regions. (For a more thorough review of memory deficits associated with temporal or frontal lobe involvement, see Lovell and Nussbaum, 1994.)

Assessing Memory Functioning of the Older Adult

While there are many available neuropsychological measures designed to assess an individual's memory functioning, such measures are not always readily applicable to the older individual who may exhibit difficulties with vision, hearing, and endurance (La Rue, 1992). (For a helpful review of available neuropsychological tests to assess memory functioning, see Lezak, 1983.)

The WMS-R (Wechsler, 1987) uses brief verbal stories that assess an individual's thematic free verbal recall. Since recent norms for individuals over the age of 74 were established (Ivnik et al., 1992), the WMS-R verbal memory subtests have

Table 1. Memory Dysfunction Associated with Various Brain Regions[a]

Brain region	Disease (Examples)	Memory dysfunction
Medial-temporal	Alzheimer's disease	Impaired recall and recognition memory
Thalamus Dorsal-medial, nuclei	Stroke Alcohol	Impaired recall and recognition memory; temporal gradient
Frontal lobe	Parkinsonism Depression	Impaired recall but intact recognition memory

[a]For more information, see Lovell & Nussbaum (1994).

become more efficacious in assessing an older individual's memory functioning.

Issues that may confound the use of the WMS-R, and other measures as well, include the individual's attention span, energy level, motivation, audiological processing, and extent and awareness of memory decline or denial. An elderly person, for example, who has some awareness of his or her memory deficits might refuse to repeat whatever he or she can recall of the presented stories; hence, it is incumbent upon the assessor to make the testing situation as nonthreatening and as informative as possible.

Among the available list-learning tests mentioned previously, the Hopkins Verbal Learning Test (HVLT; Brandt, 1991) is the most "user-friendly" and applicable (but probably less predictive of real life) measure for the elderly individual. The HVLT uses 12-word list, compared to 15 or 16, for the AVLT and CVLT, respectively, and three memory trials instead of five. Similarly, the recognition portion of the HVLT is easily administered and allows for a quicker assessment of memory functioning even for those elderly with limited endurance. The HVLT provides a discrimination index to aid in assessing the individual's recognition memory and his or her ability to positively identify only those aspects verbally presented. There are also multiple versions of the HVLT which allow for repetition of the test without as great a concern for practice effects. A disadvantage of the HVLT is its lack of normative data, a clear strength of the CVLT and AVLT.

Several tests can be used to assess nonverbal memory, including the Visual Reproduction portions of the WMS-R (Wechsler, 1987), the Rey-Osterrieth Complex Figure Test (Rey, 1964), portions of the Benton Visual Retention Test (Benton, 1974), the Rivermead Behavioral Memory Test (Wilson et al., 1985) and Recognition Memory Test (Warrington, 1984). These procedures require the individual to retain abstract visual material immediately and following a 20- to 30-min delay. Problems that may confound results on these measures for the older individual include limited vision or other visual difficulties, constructional problems, attentional problems, or problems with organizing visual stimuli that are characteristic of frontal lobe impairment. The complexity of the Rey figure drawing, for example, may increase the frustration of the elderly individual who may not be readily amenable to testing due to any of the above reasons.

Additionally, it is important to point out that a correlation has been found between the Visual Reproduction portions of the WMS-R and the Logical Memory sections of the WMS-R, suggesting a "loading" of verbal memory when using this visual memory test. Hence, assessment of visual memory might include tests of visual memory that are less influenced by verbal mediation.

Lastly, the Fuld Object Memory Evaluation (Fuld, 1977) may show promise because it requires "guaranteed stimulus processing" and has a selective reminding format. It also provides comparisons between older individuals living in the community and those living in nursing homes, although nursing home residents do not necessarily represent a homogeneous group. Table 2 provides a list of available tests, along with their respective validities and norms. (For further discussion of this issue, see Lovell and Nussbaum, 1994 and Chapter 24, this volume.)

The issues of face validity and ecological validity that may confound the assessment of memory functioning in the elderly must also be considered. The possible dissimilarity between testing completed by the neuropsychologist and the individual's everyday functioning has led neuropsychologists to explore the applicability of favoring functional assessments of patients with geropsychiatric disorders (Rogers, Holm, Goldstein, McCue, & Nussbaum, 1994). These findings support the use of multidisciplinary approaches in assessing an older individual's ability to live independently, manage his or her finances, or plan for his or her future.

In light of the above possible limitations of assessing memory functioning for the older individual, the assessor must often adjust the testing battery (from a fixed battery approach to a process-oriented approach; see La Rue, Chapter 24 of this volume), use only key aspects of certain tests as opposed to the whole test, combine a variety of assessment measures, and complete the neuropsychological assessment across several days and at various times when necessary. By conducting the assessment with an eye toward limitations the individual might present (e.g., inefficient attention/concentration, fatigue, decreased endurance), the neuropsychologist will arrive at a more adequate, reliable, and informative picture of the older individual's cognitive strengths and weaknesses.

Future Directions

This chapter has explored various types of memory functioning, summarized the essential differences between typical declines associated with normal aging and those associated with memory dysfunction, illustrated the differences observed in memory dysfunction typical of damage to various brain regions, and discussed an array of tests and measures available to the clinical neuropsychologist in assessing memory functioning in the older adult.

Still needed for advancing and promoting interest and work in the areas of neuropsychology and aging are additional age-appropriate norms, ecologically valid and "user-friendly" tests that will match the endurance and motivation of the older adult, refined diagnostic nomenclature and classification schemes to aid in improved specification of normal and abnormal aging processes, and broadened theoretical and scientific paradigms in the areas of gerontology and neuropsychology such that a focus on memory in normal aging will be standard.

Table 2. Neuropsychological Tests Used in Assessing
Memory Functioning for the Older Adult

Test[a]	Reference	Available norms	Strengths/weaknesses
AVLT	(Rey, 1964; Ivnik et al., 1992)	13–97 years	Good measure of verbal learning and memory Gives recognition memory information Brief administration Adequate norms for "old-old"
CERAD	(Morris et al., 1989)	65+ years	List-learning test Based on large sample Good diagnostic criteria Not applicable for those with significant visual impairment "User-friendly" for the elderly
CVLT	(Delis, Kramer, Kaplan, & Ober, 1987)	17–80 years	Good measure of verbal learning and memory Gives recognition memory information Long and complex Inadequate norms for "old-old"
Fuld	(Fuld, 1977)	79–79 years 80-89 years	Useful for community and nursing home residents Provides chance to observe word-finding, verbal fluency, stereognosis, and left–right orientation Assesses storage, retrieval, consistency of retrieval, and failure to recall even after reminders Guaranteed stimulus processing Separate scores for assessing long-term recall Inadequate norms for "old-old"
HVLT	(Brandt, 1991)	19–77 years	"User-friendly" for the elderly Alternate forms of the test No norms for delayed recall Inadequate norms for "old-old"
RBMT	(Wilson, Cockburn, & Baddeley, 1985)	5–95 years	Assesses memory impairment using analogues of everyday memory situations Good ecological validity Short, easy to administer Four parallel versions available
RMT	(Warrington, 1984)	18–70 years	Compares verbal and nonverbal performance independent of constructional ability Long and complex Test stimuli are "dated"
ROCF	(Rey, 1964)	6–85 years	Assesses visual memory while "factoring out" constructional abilities Good norms for older adults May be too complex
WMS-R	(Wechsler, 1987; Ivnik et al., 1992)	16–94 years	Good test of general, verbal, and visual memory Good ecological validity for memory stories Provides scoring for delayed recall Norms available for "old-old" Visual subtests prone to verbal mediation Forms are not interchangeable Longer administration time No parallel forms available

[a]AVLT, Auditory Verbal Learning Test; CERAD, Consortium to Establish a Registry for Alzheimer's Disease; CVLT, California Verbal Learning Test; Fuld, Fuld Object Memory Evaluation; HVLT, Hopkins Verbal Learning Test; RBMT, Rivermead Behavioral Memory Test; RMT, Recognition Memory Test; ROCF, Rey-Osterrieth Complex Figure (Rey, 1964); WMS-R, Wechsler Memory Scale-Revised.

ACKNOWLEDGMENTS

The author gratefully acknowledges the contributions of Dr. Graham Ratcliff and Dr. Paul Nussbaum for their provision of clinical and editorial expertise in the preparation of this chapter.

References

Albert, M. S. (1988). *Geriatric neuropsychology* (pp. 39–44). New York: Guilford Press.

Albert, M. S., Butters, N., & Levin, J. (1979). The retrograde amnesia of patients with alcoholic Korsakoff's disease. *Archives of Neurology, 36,* 211–216.

Benton, A. L. (1974). *Revised Visual Retention Test* (4th ed.). New York: The Psychological Corporation.

Brandt, J. (1991). The Hopkins Verbal Learning Test: Development of a new verbal memory test with six equivalent forms. *The Clinical Neuropsychologist, 5,* 125–142.

Craik, F. I. M. (1984). Age differences in remembering. In L. R. Squire & N. Butters (Eds.) *Neuropsychology of memory* (pp. 3–12). New York: Guilford Press.

Craik, F. I. M., & Lockhart, R. S. (1972). Levels of processing: A framework for memory research. *Journal of Verbal Learning and Verbal Behavior, 11,* 671–684.

Craik, F. I. M., & McDowd, J. M. (1987). Age differences in recall and recognition. *Journal of Experimental Psychology, Learning, Memory, and Cognition, 13,* 474–479.

Cummings, J. (1989). Dementia and depression: An evolving enigma. *The Journal of Neuropsychiatry and Clinical Neurosciences, 1,* 236–242.

Delis, D., Kramer, J. H., Kaplan, E., & Ober, B. A. (1987). *The California Verbal Learning Test-Adult Version.* San Antonio, TX: The Psychological Corporation.

Fuld, P. A. (1977). *Fuld Object Memory Evaluation.* Chicago: Stoelting.

Ivnik, R., Malec, J., Smith, G., Tangalos, E., Petersen, R., Kokmen, E., & Kurland, L. (1992). Mayo's older Americans normative studies: WMS-R norms for ages 56 to 94. *The Clinical Neuropsychologist, 6,* 49–82.

Kolb, B., & Whishaw, I. (1990). *Fundamentals of human neuropsychology.* New York: W. H. Freeman and Co.

La Rue, A. (1992). *Aging and neuropsychological assessment.* New York: Plenum Publishing.

Lezak, M. D. (1983). *Neuropsychological assessment* (2nd ed.). New York: Oxford University Press.

Lovell, M. R., & Nussbaum, P. D. (1994). Neuropsychological assessment. In *Textbook of geriatric neuropsychiatry.* Washington, DC: American Psychiatric Press, Inc.

Morris, J. C., Heyman, A., Mohs, R. C., Hughes, J. P., van Belle, G., Fillenbaum, G., Mellits, E. D., Clark, C., and the CERAD Investigators (1989). The consortium to establish a registry for Alzheimer's disease (CERAD). *Neurology, 39,* 1159–1165.

Ratcliff, G., & Saxton, J. (1994). Age-associated memory impairment. In *Textbook of geriatric neuropsychiatry.* Washington, DC: American Psychiatric Press, Inc.

Rey, A. (1964). *L'Examen clinique en psychologie.* Paris: Press Universitaires de France.

Rogers, J., Holm, M., Goldstein, G., McCue, M., & Nussbaum, P. (1994). Stability and change in functional assessment of patients with geropsychiatric disorders. *The American Journal of Occupational Therapy, 48,* 914–918.

Squire, L. R. (1987). *Memory and the brain.* New York: Oxford University Press.

Sunderland, A., & Watts, K. (1986). Subjective memory assessment in test performance in elderly adults. *Journal of Gerontology, 41,* 376–384.

Terry, R. D., Katzman, R., & Bick, K. (1994). *Alzheimer's disease.* New York: Raven Press.

Warrington, E. K. (1984). *Recognition Memory Test.* NFER: Nelson Publishing Company.

Wechsler, D. (1987). *Wechsler Memory Scale-Revised.* New York: The Psychological Corporation.

Weingartner, H., Kaye, W., Smallberg, S. A., Ebert, M., Gillin, J. C., & Sitaram, N. (1981). Memory failures in progressive idiopathic dementia. *Journal of Abnormal Psychology, 90,* 187–196.

Wilson, B. A., Cockburn, J., & Baddeley, A. (1985). *The Rivermead Behavioral Memory Test.* Reading, England: Thames Valley Test Co.; Gaylord, MI: National Rehabilitation Services.

26

The Relationship between Neuropsychology and Functional Assessment in the Elderly

MICHAEL McCUE

Introduction

Typically, neuropsychological assessment has been used to predict various diagnostic parameters. In the elderly, referrals are often made to psychologists for the purpose of facilitating diagnosis of psychiatric or organic conditions, such as depression or Alzheimer's disease. However, psychologists are routinely requested to make recommendations about patients' functional capacity for the purpose of aftercare planning. This request becomes particularly relevant in the case of the impaired elderly patient, where a decision is needed about whether an individual is capable of living independently and can return home following hospitalization, whether a person will need assistance, or whether he or she should be admitted to an institutional care facility. Major issues typically involve modifications needed in the home for the patient who returns there, or the particular level of institutional care needed. The problem is usually the self-care capability of the patient. In the case of the psychiatric or neurological patient, self-care capacity is often not a function of physical limitations such as loss of sensory or motor function, but cognitive limitations, such as impairment of memory, judgment, or communicative abilities. It is often quite difficult to determine whether a patient's functional, self-care capacities while in the hospital are sufficiently in-

tact to plan for a return to relatively independent living. It is likewise difficult to predict the least restrictive level of care needed, if continued institutionalization is indicated. These difficulties sometimes make for inappropriate types of placement, particularly in those instances in which patients are sent to nursing homes on the basis of limitations of self-care capacity and need not be there.

Neuropsychological assessment typically provides information regarding pattern and level of performance among cognitive, perceptual, and motor domains including orientation and attention, language, memory, spatial ability, problem-solving ability, and perceptual-motor skills. Traditionally, it has been used to assist in the diagnosis of diseases or insults to the central nervous system. In a sense, neuropsychological assessment may be viewed as an extension of the neurological evaluation that emphasizes the status of higher cortical functions. It thereby stands in contrast to functional assessment which typically has to do with specific content areas, such as the ability to dress, ambulate safely, manage money and use a checkbook, cook, or use some device, such as a telephone or home appliance. Functional assessment deals with direct relationships between functional skills and specific environments and performance demands.

The relationship between these two orientations is complex, since a particular functional content area usually involves a number of the specific skills typically evaluated by neuropsychological tests. There is no direct correspondence between

MICHAEL McCUE • Center for Applied Neuropsychology, Pittsburgh, Pennsylvania 15222.

performance in a single cognitive or sensorimotor domain and performance of a functional task. For example, using a telephone would require, at a minimum, short-term memory, motor, and language skills. From a clinical standpoint, neuropsychologists are often asked to offer opinions concerning specific functional capacities of patients based upon results of neuropsychological tests. These requests usually concern functions that are relatively complex cognitively, but they may also concern rather basic self-care skills involving matters of hygiene and mobility. However, the process of making judgments about function based upon neuropsychological test results is generally a matter of forming subjective opinions or inferences, rather than using results of research in which relationships have been empirically demonstrated. It therefore is important to understand relationships between neuropsychological test performance and functional skills. The process is further complicated in that the demands of the task at hand and the environment are highly individualized and situationally specific. Unless accounted for clinically, predictions about function may be confounded by environmental and situational constraints that cannot be replicated in the test setting.

Making clinical inferences based upon relationships between abilities and skills, as measured by formal neuropsychological tests, and *level* of function in a natural environment is also a consequential matter. One might surmise that neuropsychological tests, in stressing assessment of cognitive function, would be most strongly associated with functional skills that have major information-processing components. However, most neuropsychological batteries contain measures of elementary perceptual and motor skills which may be predictive of functional activities that do not have major cognitive demands. Thus, while the strongest relationships between neuropsychological test performance and everyday function may be anticipated to involve cognitively complex activities, it is nonetheless possible that tests of elementary perceptual and motor skills in particular may be predictive of levels of independence in performing more basic activities of daily living (ADL).

This chapter addresses the relationship between neuropsychological and functional assessment in the elderly. The discussion will survey existing research on the relationship between test performance and functional abilities, provide a definition of functional assessment as it relates to the elderly, and present recommendations for maximizing functional utility of neuropsychological assessment in working with this population.

Review of Research on the Relationship between Neuropsychological Test Data and Functional Abilities

A number of studies have been conducted in an attempt to examine the relationship between clinical rating scales commonly used with elderly patients for assessing the range and severity of cognitive limitations. Weintraub, Baratz, and Mesulam (1982) attempted to form associations between cognitive tasks (subtests of the Wechsler Adult Intelligence Scale, the Mattis Dementia Rating Scale, and Clock Drawing) and the Record of Independent Living, devised by the authors. They categorized ADL problems into initiation, memory, and visuopractic skill components, finding that while extent of cognitive deficit was not necessarily associated with ADL dysfunction in early Alzheimer's disease patients, patterns of cognitive impairment were found to parallel patterns of ADL difficulties.

Nadler, Richardson, Malloy, Marran, and Brinson (1993) examined the ability of the Dementia Rating Scale (DRS) (Mattis, 1988) to predict everyday functioning of 50 geriatric patients who were referred for neuropsychological assessment of possible dementia. Results of correlational and regression analyses revealed significant predictive relationships between the DRS and functional domains of self-care, safety, money management, cooking, medication administration, and community utilization assessed by simulation during inpatient hospitalization. The most salient predictor from the DRS was performance on the Initiation/Perseveration subscale. Vitaliano, Breen, Albers, Russo, and Prinz (1984) attempted to assess degree to which cognitive test scores could predict functional competence in patients with senile dementia of the Alzheimer's type (SDAT). They used measures of attention, calculation, and memory from the Mini-Mental State Examination (MMSE; Folstein,

Folstein, & McHugh, 1975) and the Dementia Rating Scale to predict behavioral maintenance (e.g., feeding, dressing), communication (talking, listening), and recreation (reading, writing, hobbies) as measured by the Record of Independent Living (Weintraub et al., 1982). The authors reported that it was possible to predict behavioral competence in areas such as recreation and maintenance behavior using measures of attention and memory, but only with certain constraints. The researchers pointed out that, due to the degree of redundancy found across various functional dimensions, detailed analyses of functioning may not be required. However, the study appears limited by the lack of specificity and comprehensiveness in instrumentation used to measure cognitive skills as well a lack of clearly developed hypotheses linking specific areas of cognitive functioning with performance of functional tasks.

Reed, Jagust, and Seab (1989) evaluated the relationship between scores on MMSE and physical and instrumental ADL as reported by caregivers. Patients in this study were 59 geriatric patients divided into two severity groups based on MMSE scores. Results for the entire sample revealed that the MMSE was predictive of both physical and instrumental ADL. However, when the low- and high-functioning patients were addressed independently, the MMSE was only marginally associated with ADL in the low-functioning group, and no significant association was observed in the high-functioning group.

Studies which evaluate the relationship of neuropsychological testing (as opposed to clinical rating scales) are of greater interest because they can evaluate complex cognitive and sensorimotor functions in depth. In a study of elderly hospitalized patients with dementia, depression, or mixed neurological conditions, McCue, Rogers, and Goldstein (1990) used an abbreviated form of the Luria-Nebraska Neuropsychological Battery (McCue, Shelly, & Goldstein, 1985) to predict functional abilities assessed in the home 2 weeks following discharge by an occupational therapist. This study indicated that neuropsychological assessment was a valid predictor of those ADL that have a strong cognitive component. Results revealed a significant predictive relationship between specific neuropsychological skill measures and the ability to perform higher-level, cognitive-based daily living functions (e.g., using the telephone, balancing a checkbook) and a limited relationship to personal care tasks (such as bathing and hygiene).

Baum, Edwards, Yonan, and Storandt (1995) selected patients from an Alzheimer's disease registry and evaluated the predictive relationship between a standard neuropsychological battery and several measures of ADL including performance testing and simulations. Results indicated that while functional behavior was significantly correlated with neuropsychological test performance, specific tasks were not associated with specific neuropsychological tests. The study also found that performance on routinized overlearned functional tasks was not likely to be related to neuropsychological test performance.

Searight, Dunn, Grisso, Margolis, and Gibbons (1989) used the Halstead-Reitan (Reitan & Wolfson, 1985) battery to predict daily living skills of 40 geriatric patients with suspected dementia. This study used canonical correlations and multiple regression analyses to test the relationship between neuropsychological measures and ratings by informants in 16 independent living dimensions. While general relationships were observed, predictions about specific skills from neuropsychological tests was not supported. In what appears to be a related study using the same patient population, Dunn, Searight, Grisso, Margolis, and Gibbons (1990) attempted to predict a different measure of functional outcome. The study used a performance test of ADL abilities, the Community Competence Scale (CCS) (Anderten, 1981). Results suggested a moderately strong relationship between neuropsychological and ADL functioning. The Speech Sounds Perception test, Seashore Rhythm test, and the Memory score from the Tactual Performance test were found to be consistently and significantly related to measures of ADL functioning.

There are additional studies in which neuropsychological test batteries are used to predict outcome in terms of functional capacities. Psychological tests such as the WAIS, the Wechsler Memory Scale, the Bender Gestalt Visual Motor test, and the Hand Test have been used with some success in the prediction of general level of self-care in the elderly (Ben-Yishay, Gerstman, Diller, & Haas, 1970;

Breen, Larson, Reigler, Vitaliano, & Lawrence, 1984; Hayslip & Panek, 1983; Wolber & Lira, 1981). Features of studies which relate psychological or neuropsychological procedures to functional outcome are described in Table 1.

To summarize, studies which focus on the relationship of neuropsychological test performance and performance in response to daily living demands reveal a great deal of diversity in elements of design, approaches to neuropsychological assessment or predictor variables, outcome criteria, outcome environments, and approaches to identifying and quantifying outcome. Unfortunately, very few of the studies address key issues of ecological validity and utility, that is, what one can say about an individual's particular test performance that will predict what an individual can or cannot do with respect to purposeful activity and in response to specific task and environmental demands in real-world situations. The reason for this is that most studies reviewed use either nonspecific or summary predictor variables (such as IQ scores or impairment indices) and global, nonspecific measures of outcome from clinical rating scales. So results generally report strong relationships between general indices of verbal problem-solving and memory and summary scores on a clinician-coded rating scale. While reporting the presence of a relationship between predictor and outcome variables, these studies provide little information other than that general cognitive status seems to be related to the ability to perform daily living tasks, and they say nothing about how measures of specific neuropsychological functions relate to the ability to meet specific environmental demands.

There are studies that use fairly specific sets of predictors to predict global outcomes. For example, in studies by Searight et al. (1989) and Dunn et al. (1990), the Halstead-Reitan tests were used to predict either clinician rating of functional skills or analog ADL functional performance. While these studies strengthen our knowledge of the relationship between specific neuropsychological parameters and outcome, they still fall short of providing support for neuropsychological tests as predictors of specific capacities in the real world.

Studies in which measures of specific brain functions are contrasted, by design, with specific real-world demands are desired. The McCue et al. (1990) study is unique in its use of specific sets of neuropsychological predictors and direct observations of specific functional behaviors performed by the patient in his or her own home. This study may establish a relationship between measures of neuropsychological ability and the actual performance demands of the real world.

Overall, there is evidence for a relationship between neuropsychological tests and general types of outcome such as dependence/independence in ADL. However, the findings are not strong enough to support definitive predictions about any given individual's capacity to care for self or to perform instrumental tasks. Nor is the data available to validate the ability of neuropsychological tests to predict how an individual might function in response to specific demands such as balancing a checkbook, paying rent, or operating a piece of equipment. Too many of the studies employ rather nonspecific predictors, global outcome measures, or both. In order to respond to the need to establish validity of neuropsychological tests to predict specific outcome, improvements must be made in both predictor and outcome measures, as well as basic design aspects. Examples of promising work can be seen in the emerging literature on the prediction of driving ability, which typically uses very specific sets of neuropsychological predictors and specific outcomes like driving performance, either in a simulator or on the road.

While acknowledging that most psychological and neuropsychological tests were not developed to predict behavior in the natural environment and that extensive validation does not exist for this purpose, there is increasing evidence to suggest that standardized measurement of cognitive and behavioral skills on psychological and neuropsychological tests is well correlated with performance in the daily living environment. Furthermore, the ability to make such predictions about real-world behavior is enhanced when test data are combined with specific knowledge about the environment (and the demands which exist within that environment). Finally, when inferences are made about functional abilities from psychological tests, further testing of such inferences or working hypotheses is required through functional assessment.

Table 1. Summary Characteristics of Studies of the Relationship between Neuropsychological Assessment and ADL Functions

Investigator (year)	Design	Subject population (n)	Predictor instrument	Criterion instrument	Results
Baum, Edwards, Yonan, & Storandt (1995)	Canonical correlations tested the relationship between neuropsychological measures and three simulated measures of functional performance administered several weeks later in an OT clinic.	Patients with no dementia (n = 69), very mild dementia (n = 25), moderate dementia (n = 24), severe dementia (n = 3) selected from Alzheimer patient registry (n = 126)	Neuropsychological battery: WMS-R subscales, WAIS-R subscales, Benton Visual Retention Test, Trail-making Test, Crossing-off Test, Boston Naming Test	Manual Apraxia Battery (Edwards, Deuel, Baum, & Morris, 1992) Simulated ADL Battery (Potvin et al., 1972) Kitchen Task Assessment (Baum, Edwards, & Morrow-Howell, 1993)	Functional behavior was substantially correlated with neuropsychological performance. Specific tasks were not associated with specific neuropsychological tests. Well-routinized motor tasks (procedural memory) were unrelated to neuro-psychological test performance.
Ben-Yishay, Gerstman, Diller, & Haas (1970)	Subjects were administered a psychometric evaluation 2 weeks post admission to a rehabilitation facility. Three outcome criteria were obtained at the time of discharge. A multiple regression equation was completed yielding 27 variables.	Left hemiparetic stroke patients (n = 69)	WAIS, Bender-Gestalt, sensory and motor tasks, Purdue pegboard	Assessment of ambulation, self-care, and length of rehabilitation treatment	The psychometric variables contributed significantly to the prediction of outcomes of ambulatory and self-care, and to a lesser degree, length of rehabilitation.
Breen, Larson, Reigler, Vitaliano, & Lawrence (1984)	Standard psychological tests of IQ and memory were correlated with ADL items on a dementia rating scale	Elderly community residents (57–88 years) with senile dementia of the Alzheimer's type (SDAT) (n = 21)	WAIS, WMS, Mini-Mental State Exam (MMSE)	DRS self-care items (Blessed, Tomlinson, & Roth, 1968)	In demented patients, significant correlations were noted between self-care capacity and WAIS WIQ ($r = .74$; $p = .0005$), WAIS FSIQ ($r = -.75$; $p = .005$), and the WMS MQ ($r = -.63$; $p = .005$).
Dunn, Searight, Grisso, Margolis, & Gibbons (1990)	Canonical correlations and regression equations were used to assess the relationship between neuropsychological test performance and a test of ADL comprising knowledge of fact, comprehension, and demonstration of simulated activities (CCS)	Geriatric patients suspected of dementia (n = 40)	Halstead-Reitan Battery (Reitan & Wolfson, 1985)	Community Competence Scale (CCS) (Anderten, 1981)	Results suggested a moderately strong relationship between neuropsycho-logical and ADL functioning. Speech Sounds Perception, Seashore Rhythm, and Tactual Performance Memory were most consistently and significantly related to measure of ADL functions.

Study	Description	Sample	Measures	Results
Eastwood, Lautenschlaeger, & Corbin (1983)	Psychological measures of mental status were correlated with changes in self-care, personality, and habits over a 6-month period and at 1-year follow-up.	Octogenarians from home, retirement, and nursing home settings (mean age = 82) (n = 60)	Mental Status Questionnaire (MSQ) (Kahn, Goldfarb, Pollock, & Gerber, 1960), Present State Examination (PSE) (Fink, Green, & Bender, 1952) / Dementia Rating Scale (DRS) (Blessed, Tomlinson, & Roth, 1968)	Significant correlations were found between the MSQ and the DRS ($r = .60$; $p = .001$). The predictive ability of the tests were felt to be compromised by mental status changes at one year's follow-up.
Ferm (1974)	Investigated the behavioral manifestations of degrees of dementia through correlations analyses	Psychogeriatric patients (mean age = 76.4) (n = 124)	Dementia Test (Isaacs & Walkey, 1964) / Behavioral variables including communication, orientation in space, and recognition of persons; rated by nursing staff	Dementia test scores correlated well with the ability to communicate ($r = 82$), orientation in space ($r = .76$), and recognition of persons ($r = .74$).
Hayslip & Panek (1983)	A projective personality test was administered to establish its validity in measuring differences in relationships between mental status and physical self-maintenance.	Institutionalized elderly adults (mean age = 83.87) (n = 52)	MSQ (Kahn et al., 1960), Hand Test (Wagner, 1962) / Physical Self-Maintenance Scale (PSMS) (Lawton & Brody, 1969)	Thirteen of 25 Hand Test variables were found to correlated significantly with a total dependency score on the PSMS.
Hersch (1979)	Inpatient elderly subjects were rated on a dementia scale which was correlated with results of a geriatric rating scale of daily functioning ability.	Elderly with progressive dementia (n = 55)	Extended Scale for dementia (ESDS) (More defined version of the Mattis Dementia Rating Scale) / London Psychogeriatric Rating Scale (PRS) (Hersch, Kral, & Palmer, 1978)	A correlation of .62 was reported between ESDS and behavioral ratios of daily functioning on the LPRS.
Lawton & Brody (1969)	Mental status evaluation was correlated with social workers' ratings of personal self-care, instrumental self-care, and behavior and adjustment.	Elderly applicants to a long-term care institution, age 60 and over (n = 180)	MSQ (Kahn et al., 1960) / Physical Self-Maintenance Scale (PSMS) (Lowenthal, 1964), Instrumental Activities of Daily Living (IADL), ratings of behavior and adjustment	The following correlations were noted: MSQ with PSMS ($r = .38$), MSQ with IADL ($r = .48$), and MSQ with behavior and adjustment ($r = .58$).
McCue, Rogers, & Goldstein (1990)	Pearson correlations and multiple regression were used to examine the relationship between neuropsychological performance and ADL functioning in the home 2 weeks following discharge.	Geropsychiatric inpatients with suspected dementia (n = 58)	Luria-Nebraska Neuropsychological Battery-Short Form (McCue et al., 1985). / Performance Assessment of Self-Care Skills (PASS) (Rogers, Holm, Goldstein, McCue, & Nussbaum, 1994).	Significant predictive relationships were demonstrated between neuropsychological measures and higher-level, cognitively oriented ADL tasks while low relationships were noted with personal care tasks.

(continued)

Table 1. (*Continued*)

Investigator (year)	Design	Subject population (n)	Predictor instrument	Criterion instrument	Results
Nadler, Richardson, Malloy, Marran, & Brinson (1993)	Regression analyses were used to assess the relationship between DRS and a standardized measure of ADL (OTEPS) administered during an inpatient hospital stay.	Geriatric patients referred for neuropsychological assessment to rule out dementia (n = 50)	DRS (Mattis, 1988)	Occupational Therapy Evaluation of Performance and Support (OTEPS)	Results revealed significant predictive relationships between the DRS and functional domains. Initial perseveration subscale was most strongly associated with functional abilities.
Reed, Jaqust, & Seab (1989)	Univariate analysis and multiple regression were used to evaluate the relationship between Mini-Mental State Examination (MMSE) and physical and instrumental ADL in two severity groups.	Patients with progressive dementia with no other history of psychiatric/medical problems with MMSE scores >14 (n = 59)	Mini-Mental State Examination (MMSE) (Folstein, Folstein, & McHugh, 1975)	Lawton's (1971) Physical and Instrumental ADL scales	In the whole sample, significant regression coefficients were obtained for both physical ADL (−.60) and instrumental ADL (.63). For low-functioning patients, significant association with physical (r = .68) and instrument (r = .51) ADL. Neither regression was significant for the high-functioning groups.
Searight, Dunn, Grisso, Margolis, & Gibbons (1989)	Canonical correlations and multiple regression tested the relationships between neuropsychological measures and rating by informants of 16 independent living dimensions (SCILS)	Geriatric patients suspected of dementia (n = 40)	Halstead-Reitan Battery (Reitan & Wolfson, 1985)	Scale of Competence in Independent Living Skills (SCILS)	Neuropsychological tests were globally related to daily living skills; predictors about specific skills from NP tests may be unwarranted.
Skurla (1984)	Examined the ability of a global mental status measure to predict self-care in Alzheimer's disease patients	Patients with SDAT (mean age = 65.4) (n = 9)	Hughes Evaluation Clinical Scale for Staging Dementia (CDR) (Hughes, Berg, Danziger, Coben, & Martin, 1982)	Four situational tests (dressing, purchasing, making coffee, telephoning)	A significant relationship was found between the CDR and self-care (Kendall's tau = 0.59; p = .027)
Smyer, Hofland, & Jonas (1979)	Validation study of the SPMSQ for predicting self-care capacity using discriminate analysis procedures	Elderly residents of intermediate care facilities and home care programs (mean age = 75.3) (n = 181)	Short Portable Mental Status Questionnaire (SPMSQ) (Pfeiffer, 1978)	OARS-ADL Scale Activities of Daily Living Scale (Katz, Ford, Moskowitz, Jackson, & Jaffee, 1963)	The SPMSQ was found to correctly classify 70.01% of the subjects into three levels of functioning, minimal or no impairment, moderate impairment, and severe impairment.

Study	Description	Sample	Measures	Functional measure	Results
Vitaliano, Breen, Albers, Russo, & Prinz (1984)	Examined the predictive validity of attention and memory items of mental status tests for activities of daily living	Elderly subjects with SDAT and living in the community (n = 34)	Mini-Mental State Exam (MMSE), (Folstein, Folstein, & McHugh, 1975), DRS (Mattis, 1988)	Record of Independent Living (Weintraub, Baratz, & Mesulam, 1982)	Cognitive behaviors including attention and recognition were found to predict self-maintenance.
Weintraub, Baratz, & Mesulam (1982)	Selected cognitive tests and the Record of Independent Living were administered to determine associations between the two sets of measures.	Early Alzheimer's disease patients, ages 54–72 (n = 7)	Parts of WAIS, DRS, clock drawing	Record of Independent Living (unpublished)	Extent of impairment noted on predictor was not associated with extent of ADL deficit. Patterns of impairment were related.
Wilson, Grant, Witney, & Kerridge (1973)	Subjects were administered a mental status questionnaire and were rated on several psychiatric dimensions by a physician. Correlation analyses between mental status and ADL measures were performed.	Female hospitalized elderly (mean age = 79.4) with multiple medical diagnosis (n = 100)	Mental Status Questionnaire (MSQ) (Kahn et al., 1960), physician's ratings of psychiatric variables	Performance test of seven personal and instrumental self-care tasks	MSQ and physician's ratings of "dementia" were highly related to self-care capacity (no correlation coefficients reported)
Winograd (1984)	Mental status measures were correlated with investigator ratings of self-care ability.	Nursing home residents (mean age = 87) with multiple medical diagnosis (n = 56)	Short Portable Mental Status Questionnaire (SPMSQ), Mental Competence Scale (MCS) (Fisher & Pierce, 1967)	Ability to dress, eat, and walk rated by the investigator	Correlations were found between self-ability and the SPMSQ ($r = .37$; $p = .005$) and the MCS ($r = .47$; $p = .001$).
Wolber & Lira (1981)	Performance on a single test of visual-motor integration was correlated with performance measures of basic living skills	Inpatient residents of a geriatric unit of a state psychiatric hospital (n = 35)	Bender-Gestalt Test	Basic Living Skills Assessment (Wolber & Lira, 1981)	An increase in visual-motor impairment was significantly related with a decrease in basic living skills ($r = -.623$; $p = .001$).

Functional Assessment Defined

Functional assessment may be defined as "the analysis and measurement of specific behaviors that occur in real environments and are relevant to life or vocational goals" (Halpern & Fuhrer, 1984). Functional assessment always involves an interaction between purposeful or "goal-directed" behavior and environmental conditions such as people, rules, physical barriers, or schedules. Because demands placed upon a person differ from one environment to another, and from one task to another, functional assessment is always a highly individualized process.

Functional assessment is undertaken to determine the *impact* of disease or disability on behavior. Neurological evaluations, psychiatric evaluations, and neuropsychological testing are measures of disability. In contrast, functional assessment, which relates to purposeful behavior such as cooking a meal, is a measure of the degree of impediment. The *environmental specificity* and *goal directedness* of functional assessment separate it from other types of assessment. Put simply, functional assessment is the measurement of what persons can or cannot do (their strengths and weaknesses) in particular situations, under certain conditions, and in light of unique demands.

The goal of functional assessment in the elderly is to identify unique obstacles to effective functioning. Obstacles occur when deficits associated with disease or disability (e.g., prospective memory) interfere with the elderly individual's ability to meet demands and conditions imposed by the environment in which he or she must function (e.g., live with limited supports in the home), the goal the person aspires to attain (e.g., community independence), or the specific task requirements of a particular situation the individual must master (e.g., maintain a complex medication regime). The challenge of functional assessment is not only to identify the individual's strengths and weaknesses, but to fully understand the demands and conditions of the environment in which the individual expects to function. The purpose is to delineate functional obstacles that are likely to occur so that rehabilitation intervention might be systematically applied.

Functional assessment should reveal information about assets and limitations or potential problem areas. Functional limitations should be conceptualized in behavioral, rather than diagnostic terms. For example, "an inability to dress independently" is preferable to "apraxia." When possible, active involvement of the elderly individual in the assessment process should be encouraged to improve validity and reliability of information gathered; to enhance the individual's understanding of and investment in rehabilitation; and to assist the person in gaining more accurate self-appraisal and insight into strengths and limitations and subsequent need for intervention or accommodation.

Approaches to Functional Assessment in the Elderly

Functional assessment is accomplished with elderly individuals through a variety of approaches. Each of these assessment procedures can be used to evaluate how an individual might respond in the face of real-life problems and demands. These activities may require the individual to deal with multiple priorities, unforeseen circumstances, and interpersonal interactions. The following discussion addresses direct observation in the natural environment, situational and simulated assessments, as well as use of rating scales and other mechanisms for eliciting observations on functional performance of elderly individuals. Functional observation procedures are typically the purview of the occupational therapist. However, the psychologist's expertise is uniquely valuable in interpreting and understanding complex performance in the face of cognitive demands.

Undoubtedly, the most effective way of understanding functional capacity in performing a particular task, or in responding to a specific environmental demand, is to directly observe individuals actually performing the task in their natural environment over a period of time. The individual's ability to perform in his or her own environment may be markedly different from performance in other settings and should be assessed through direct observation. Furthermore, observations may provide more valid results than self-report measures in persons with impaired cognition, which may interfere with their ability to accurately assess their own functioning.

Observations can be completed in the individual's home or community setting, depending on the questions to be addressed. In order to fully understand complex cognitive behaviors, observations should be made in the context of cognitive domains (e.g., memory, language) and should consider areas of strength as well as those that pose difficulty. To make the best use of data from observations in the natural environment (and to allow for inferences about or to generalize to other functional abilities not directly observed), the *process* an individual engages in to meet environmental and task demands should be observed. Observation of process variables such as organizational abilities, communication style, and endurance may provide more relevant data than traditional measurement of productivity or task outcome. Observation in the natural environment also provides an opportunity to observe the individual's spontaneous use of compensatory strategies or accommodations, as well as possible problem situations that might easily lend themselves to such.

The process of observing an elderly person in his or her natural environment poses a risk of confounding the individual's typical response or performance style. Effort must be made to minimize this effect by making the individual comfortable and through nonobtrusive observation. There may be opportunities for an evaluator to participate in activities around the individual, such as conversing with a spouse, rather than merely observing.

Situational assessment of functional abilities in simulated environments is also frequently used to assess ADL skills of the elderly patient. This approach has the flexibility of being conducted in a hospital setting, in the patient's room, or in specially designed simulated home environments. Difficulties associated with direct assessment in the home such as cost and staffing requirements are minimized through the use of simulations. However, the elderly individual is likely to be less flexible, cognitively and emotionally. As a result, the individual's performance in a simulated setting may not reflect his or her actual capacity (or incapacity) to perform the task. For example, in the person's kitchen, location of utensils and ingredients is very

familiar. Finding necessary materials is an overlearned, automatic process at home, whereas, if the individual is required to perform in a simulated kitchen, the cognitive demands of learning and remembering the location of materials is introduced into the task. Failure to meet these cognitive demands (memory and learning), rather than the requirements of the task itself (cooking), may interfere with adequacy of performance, and subsequently validity of the functional assessment. In this case, it may be falsely determined that the individual cannot prepare a meal and is therefore not independent in this aspect. Care must be taken to understand possible threats to validity of simulations in functional assessment. Despite potential confounds, simulations offer the opportunity to directly observe functional skills.

Interviewing informants is another way of obtaining information about functional abilities and competencies in the natural environment without the expense of direct observation. Spouses, housemates, caregivers, and adult children can provide rich information on how an elderly individual goes about performing a task, how the individual's environment is structured, what obstacles he or she encounters, as well as the supports the individual needs and has access to.

The manner of questioning is important in that it may influence the response. For example, asking an informant whether an individual "can" perform a task may produce a different (and perhaps less accurate) response than asking if the person regularly "does" a task. Asking about *how* an individual goes about a task (the approach, strategies, and accommodations used) can provide the neuropsychologist with information to make generalization about other functional skills and future behaviors.

Rating scales and questionnaires represent a very common approach to quantifying functional behaviors and obtaining information from informants in a structured fashion. Rating scales may be completed by clinical staff or informants who have firsthand knowledge of the individual's functional skill level. Instruments such as the OARS-IADL scale (Duke University Center for the Study on Aging, 1978) have been commonly used in an attempt to quantify elderly individuals' functional capacities through clinician ratings. A wide variety of format and item content is seen in rating scales used with the elderly. Many of the scales focus primarily on basic ADL items, including mobility, self-care, feeding, and hygiene; these scales may be less useful to the psychologist. Scales that focus on higher level skills, such as instrumental activities of daily living (e.g., balancing a checkbook, planning a meal, responding to mail) are more relevant to the neuropsychologist, and the use of such instruments may facilitate the functional assessment process. Table 2 presents a list of rating scales that address functional capacities in the elderly.

Use of Neuropsychological Assessment to Generate Inferences about Functional Capacities in the Elderly

The nature of functional activities of daily living is such that any content area generally involves several cognitive, perceptual, and motor requirements. For example, as Weintraub et al. (1982) have pointed out, such activities as dressing have initiation, memory, and visuopractic skill components. Thus, the individual may have difficulty initiating dressing behavior, forget where clothes are kept, or

Table 2. Functional Assessment Rating Scales

ADL scale	Type of rating	Content area
Barthel index (Mahoney & Barthel, 1965)	Clinician rated scale based upon judgment (interview) and observation	Basic ADL items useful in rehabilitation settings
Instrumental ADL scale (Lawton, 1982)	Clinician rating by judgment (interview) or observation	More complex instrumental ADL items including cooking, shopping, housekeeping
Framingham Disability scale (Jette & Branch, 1981)	Clinical rating by interview	Broad range of activities of self-care to more involved physical functioning (e.g., lifting)
Katz ADL scale (Katz, Ford, Moskowitz, Jackson, & Jaffee, 1963)	Clinician rating by judgment (interview) or observation	Basic ADL skill functions
Kenny Self-Care Scale (Schoening et al., 1965)	Clinical rating by judgment or patient self-rating	Self-care and ambulation items
Older Americans Resources Multidimensional Functional Assessment Activities of Daily Living Scale (OARS-ADL) (Duke University Center for the Study on Aging, 1978)	Clinician rating based upon judgment (interview) and observation	Broad range of physical (e.g., eating, personal hygiene) and instrumental ADL activities (e.g., ability to shop, manage medication)
Patient Assessment of Own Functioning Inventory (PAOFI) (Heaton & Pendleton, 1981)	Patient self-rating and informant forms	Wide range of cognitive and sensorimotor tasks related to neurological/neuropsychological functioning (not designed specifically for the elderly)
Patient Competency Rating scale (PCRS) (Fordyce, 1983)	Patient self-rating and informant forms	Wide range of cognitive and sensorimotor tasks related to neurological/neuropsychological functioning (not designed specifically for the elderly)
Performance test of ADL (Kruiansky & Gurland, 1976)	Clinician rating by judgment (interview)	Self-care, mobility and transfers
Performance Assessment of Self-Care Skills (Rogers, 1987)	Clinician observation of specific ADL behaviors in the natural setting	Wide range of basic ADL including mobility and personal self-care (bathing), and higher level instrumental abilities (use telephone, balance checkbook)

don clothes in a way that is not spatially correct (e.g., putting on trousers backward). This multi-ability nature of most everyday activities makes it necessary to develop some model for relating those activities to level and pattern of cognitive skills. Ideally, the neuropsychological tests should predict the content deficit as well as the specific pattern of underlying neuropsychological deficits. For example, for a particular patient, tests should be able to predict that a patient has difficulty with dressing because of visuopractic difficulties and not because of a memory problem regarding location of his or her clothing or initiation of dressing behavior. Different patterns may be predicted for other patients.

When it is stated that neuropsychological test performance should be predictive of ADL status, this does not mean that prediction should be restricted to specific content areas. Obviously, the best predictor of how an individual should do at a particular content area, such as dressing, would be the level of specific task performance at some previous time. Thus, the best predictor of how well a patient dresses at occasion B would ordinarily be how well dressing was accomplished at occasion A. Rather, test performance should predict specific cognitive deficits that may have implications for performance in certain content areas (e.g., communication skills). Therefore, during treatment or disposition planning, it becomes possible to identify appropriate placements and develop particular accommodation and management strategies based on identification of particular problem areas and the cognitive deficits associated with them. Inferences that particular patterns of neuropsychological tests performance are in fact associated with performance of functional activities are commonly made on theoretical grounds rather than on the basis of empirical demonstrations. A systematic understanding of the individual's cognitive strengths and weaknesses is likely to contribute greatly to clinical predictions made about functional skills. It is understood that the underlying cognitive structures needed to perform any practical task may be extremely variable, depending on the specificity of the task demands.

One could argue that prediction of skill level of some specific activity of daily living can be best assessed by observing the patient perform the activity itself. While there obviously is merit to that view, neuropsychological tests may have the capacity to predict a variety of behaviors involving, for example, short-term memory and perceptual-motor coordination rather than predicting behavior in single specific content areas. Therefore, neuropsychological testing may provide a more efficient prognostic tool relative to assessing each specific skill. Furthermore, within the context of a specific skill, even slight variations in task requirements might make the difference between success and failure. Thus, while functional assessment can determine how an individual will perform a specific task in a specific situation, it is uncertain whether assessment of this skill will generalize to other situations or other slightly different tasks. Neuropsychological tests, in consideration of their generic nature, may help one to understand the patients's abilities over a variety of functional tasks and situations.

Neuropsychological assessment for functional purposes then becomes a process of generating clinical inferences about what an individual is likely to be able to do and not do and about the specific support and accommodations the individual may require for task completion. These inferences or clinical hypotheses about real-world competencies posed on the basis of psychological and neuropsychological tests require knowledge and expertise in three areas. First, clear clinical knowledge of the skills and abilities that are being measured is required. In the case of the elderly patient, behaviors might be those associated with neurocognitive disease and disability. For example, in order to make predictions about how difficulties in memory would interfere with fiscal management of personal affairs, one would need a thorough appreciation for the types, degree, and intensity of disorders of memory. Secondly, predictions are contingent upon a clear understanding of what the tests measure, including the limitations of the instruments used. Such expertise includes an appreciation for the range of behaviors required for adaptive or intact performance and strong interpretive skills for addressing difficulties or performance failures. Finally, an understanding of and appreciation for the demands of the situation or environment one is attempting to make predictions about is absolutely critical. Performance on standardized tests must be related to the demands of environment for the test to be functionally relevant. For example, the clinician must know that adherence to a medically advised diet requires a patient to be adept in organizational skills, planning, judgment, and initiation, along with basic cooking and shopping skills.

Psychologists and neuropsychologists are typically well trained and experienced in the tests used and in understanding cognition. However, in order to generate sound hypotheses about functional abilities from psychological and neuropsychological tests, the psychologist or neuropsychologist must either develop knowledge and expertise in evaluating the demands of the environment or obtain this information in the referral and dialogue process. This may be done by conferring with other professionals (e.g., occupational therapy) or by talking with informants familiar with the environmental and task demands faced by the patient. Without a clear sense of the outcome environment, test scores are of limited use in understanding how an individual will function in everyday living environments.

might be associated with diseases of the elderly, but determining how the disease or disability impairs or impedes independent living functioning. It is often the case that cognitive manifestations of disability are not easily quantified, and the impact of specific cognitive deficits is difficult to ascertain. Assessment must provide not just diagnostic formulations, but rather detail as to how deficits might interact with task and environmental demands to affect the individual's functioning in real-life situations.

While acknowledging that most psychological and neuropsychological tests were not developed to predict behavior in the natural environment and that extensive validation does not exist for this purpose, there is increasing evidence to suggest that standardized measurement of cognitive and behavioral skills on psychological and neuropsychological tests are well correlated with performance in the daily living and work environments. Furthermore, the ability to make such predictions about real-world behavior is enhanced when test data are combined with specific knowledge about the environment and its demands.

Summary

The problems encountered by elderly individuals with medical, neurological, and psychiatric disorders frequently relate to functional capacity. Functional assessment is required to make predictions about functional skills and limitations and to identify rehabilitation and independent living needs. Direct and simulated observation procedures can be used to address functional questions, but these approaches may be costly and require the expertise of occupational therapists. Furthermore, findings may fail to generalize to situations and demands not directly observed, particularly when observations are not made by individuals who have an appreciation for how brain–behavior relationships may influence the conduct of complex cognitive behaviors in the environment. Rating scales and informant interviews may also provide an economical and valid source of functional information. The neuropsychologist also can make significant contributions to the determination of functional capacity.

A critical component of the assessment process is establishing not only the appropriate diagnosis, or elucidation of the cognitive deficits that

References

Anderten, P. S. (1981). *Psychological testing* (5th ed.). New York: MacMillan.

Baum, C., Edwards, D. F., & Morrow-Howell, N. (1993). Identification and measurement of productive behaviors in senile dementia of the Alzheimer type. *The Gerontologist, 33*, 403–408.

Baum, C., Edwards, D., Yonan, C., & Storandt, M. (1995). The relation of neuropsychological test performance to performance of functional tasks in dementia of the Alzheimer type. *Archives of Clinical Neuropsychology, 11*(I), 69–75.

Ben-Yishay, Y., Gerstman, L., Diller, L., & Haas, A. (1970). Prediction of rehabilitation outcomes from psychometric parameters in left hemiplegics. *Journal of Consulting and Clinical Psychology, 34*, 436–441.

Blessed, G., Tomlinson, B. E., & Roth, M. (1968). The association between quantitative measures of dementia and of senile change in the cerebral gray matter of elderly subjects. *British Journal of Psychiatry, 114*, 797.

Breen, A. R., Larson, E. B., Reigler, B. V., Vitaliano, P. P., & Lawrence, G. L. (1984). Cognitive performance and functional competence in coexisting dementia and depression. *Journal of the American Geriatrics Society, 32*, 132–137.

Duke University Center for the Study on Aging. (1978). *Multidimensional functional assessment: the OARS methodology* (2nd ed.). Durham, NC: Duke University Press.

Dunn, E. J., Searight, H. R., Grisso, T., Margolis, R. B., &

Gibbons, J. L. (1990). The relation of the Halstead-Reitan Neuropsychological Battery to functional daily living skills in geriatric patients. *Archives of Clinical Neuropsychology, 5,* 103–117.

Eastwood, M. S., Lautenschlaeger, E., & Corbin, S. (1983). A comparison of clinical methods for assessing dementia. *Journal of the American Geriatrics Society, 31,* 342–347.

Edwards, D. F., Deuel, R. K., Baum, C. M., & Morris, J. C. (1992). A quantitative analysis of apraxia in senile dementia of the Alzheimer's type: State related difference in prevalence and type. *Dementia, 2,* 142–149.

Ferm, L. (1974). Behavioral activities in demented geriatric patients. *Gerontologica Clinica, 16,* 185–194.

Fink, M., Green, M., & Bender, M. (1952). The face-hand test as a diagnostic sign of organic mental syndrome. *Neurology 2,* 46.

Fisher, J., & Pierce, R. C. (1967). Dimensions of intellectual functioning in the aged. *Journal of Gerontology, 22,* 166–173.

Folstein, M. F., Folstein, S. E., & McHugh, P. R. (1975). "Mini-mental state." A practical method for grading the cognitive state of patients for the clinician. *Journal of Psychiatric Research, 12,* 189–198.

Fordyce, D. J. (1983). Psychometric assessment of denial of illness in brain injured patients. Paper presented at the 91st Annual Convention of the American Psychological Association, Anaheim, CA.

Halpern, A. S., & Fuhrer, M. J. (1984). *Functional assessment in rehabilitation.* Baltimore, MD: Paul H. Brooks Publishing Co.

Hayslip, B., & Panek, P. E. (1983). Physical self-maintenance, mental status, and personality in institutionalized elderly adults. *Journal of Clinical Psychology, 39,* 479–485.

Heaton, R. K., & Pendleton, M. G. (1981). Use of neuropsychological tests to predict adult patients' everyday functioning. *Journal of Consulting and Clinical Psychology, 49*(6), 807–821.

Hersch, E. L. (1979). Development and application of the extended scale for dementia. *Journal of the American Geriatrics Society, 27,* 348–354.

Hersch, E. L., Kral, V. A., & Palmer, R. B. (1978). Clinical value of the London Psychogeriatric Rating Scale. *Journal of the American Geriatrics Society, 26,* 348.

Hughes, C. P., Berg, L., Danziger, W., Coben, L. A., & Martin, R. L. (1982). A new clinical scale for the staging of dementia. *British Journal of Psychiatry, 140,* 556–572.

Isaacs, B., & Walkey, F. A. (1964). The measurement of mental impairment in geriatric practice. *Gerontologica Clinica, 6,* 114–123.

Jette, A. M., & Branch, L. G. (1981). The Farmingham Disability Study. II. Physical disability among the aging. *American Journal of Public Health, 71,* 1211–1216.

Kahn, R. L., Goldfarb, A. I., Pollock, M., & Gerber, I. E. (1960). The relationship of mental and physical status in institutionalized aged persons. *American Journal of Psychiatry, 117,* 120–124.

Katz, S., Ford, A. B., Moskowitz, R. W., Jackson, B. A., & Jaffee, M. W. (1963). Studies of illness in the aged: The index of ADL: A standardized measure of biological and psychosocial function. *Journal of the American Medical Association, 185,* 914–919.

Kruiansky, J., & Gurland, B. (1976). The performance test of activities of daily living. *International Journal of Aging and Human Development, 7,* 343–352.

Lawton, M. P. (1971). The functional assessment of elderly people. *Journal of the American Geriatric Society, 19,* 465–481.

Lawton, M. P. (1982). A research and service oriented multilevel assessment instrument. *Journal of Gerontology, 37,* 91–99.

Lawton, M. P., & Brody, E. (1969). Assessment of older people: Self-maintaining and instrumental activities of daily living. *The Gerontologist, 9,* 179–186.

Lowenthal, M. F. (1964). *Lives in distress.* New York: Basic Books.

Mahoney, F. I., & Barthel, D. W. (1965). Functional evaluation: The Barthel Index. *Maryland State Medical Journal, 14*(2), 61–65.

Mattis, S. (1988). *Dementia Rating Scale.* Odessa, FL: Psychological Assessment Resources, Inc.

McCue, M., Shelly, C., & Goldstein, G. (1985). A proposed short form of the Luria-Nebraska Neuropsychological Battery oriented toward assessment of the elderly. *International Journal of Clinical Neuropsychology, 7*(2), 96–101.

McCue, M., Rogers, J. C., & Goldstein, G. (1990). Relationships between neuropsychological and functional assessment in elderly psychiatric patients. *Rehabilitation Psychology, 35,* 91–99.

Nadler, J. D., Richardson, E. D., Malloy, P. F., Marran, M. E., & Brinson, M. E. H. (1993). The ability of the dementia rating scale to predict everyday functioning. *Archives of Clinical Neuropsychology, 8,* 449–460.

Pfeiffer, E. (1978). A short portable mental status questionnaire for the assessment of organic brain deficit in elderly patients. *Journal of the American Geriatrics Society, 21,* 433–441.

Potvin, A. R., Tourellotte, W. W., Dailey, J. S., Albers, J. W., Walker, J. E., Pew, R. W., Henderson, W. G., & Snyder, D. N. (1972). Simulated activities of daily living examination. *Archives of Physical Medicine and Rehabilitation, 50,* 476–486.

Reed, B. R., Jaqust, W. J., Seab, J. P. (1989). Mental status as a predictor of daily function in progressive dementia. *The Gerontologist, 29*(6), 804–807.

Reitan, R. M., & Wolfson, D. (1985). *The Halstead-Reitan Neuropsychological Test Battery: Theory and clinical interpretation.* Tucson, AZ: Neuropsychology Press.

Rogers, J. C. (1987). *Performance Assessment of Self-Care Skills (PASS).* Unpublished performance test.

Rogers, J. C., Holm, M. B., Goldstein, G., McCue, M., & Nussbaum, P. (1994). Stability and change in functional assessment of patients with geropsychiatric disorders. *The American Journal of Occupational Therapy, 48,* 914–918.

Schoening, H. A., Anderegg, L., Bergstrom, D., Fonda, M., Steinke, N., & Ulrich, P. (1965). Numerical scoring of a self-care status of patients. *Archives of Physical Medicine Rehabilitation, 46,* 689–697.

Searight, H. R., Dunn, E. J., Grisso, T., Margolis, R. B., & Gibbons, J. L. (1989). The relation of the Halstead-Reitan Neuropsychological Battery to ratings of everyday functioning in a geriatric sample. *Neuropsychology, 3,* 135–145.

Skurla, E. (1984). *A qualitative study of the functioning of patients with Alzheimer's disease in activities of daily living.*

Unpublished master's thesis, University of North Carolina, Chapel Hill.

Smyer, M. A., Hofland, B. F., & Jonas, E. A. (1979). Validity study of the short portable mental status questionnaire for the elderly. *Journal of the American Geriatrics Society, 27,* 263–269.

Vitaliano, P. P., Breen, A. R., Albers, M. S., Russo, J., & Prinz, P. N. (1984). Memory, attention, and functional status in community-residing Alzheimer type dementia patients and optimally healthy aged individuals. *Journal of Gerontology, 39,* 58–64.

Wagner, E. E. (1962). The Hand Test: Manual for administration, scoring, and interpretation. Los Angeles: *Western Psychological Services.*

Weintraub, S., Baratz, R., & Mesulam, M. (1982). Daily living activities in the assessment of dementia. In S. Corkin et al. (Eds.), *Aging: Vol. 19. Alzheimer's disease: A report of progress.* New York: Raven Press.

Wilson, L. A., Grant, K., Witney, G. P., & Kerridge, D. F. (1973). Mental status of elderly hospital patients related to occupational therapist's assessment of activities of daily living. *Gerontologica Clinica, 15,* 197–202.

Winograd, C. H. (1984). Mental status tests and the capacity for self care. *Journal of the American Geriatrics Society, 32,* 49–61.

Wolber, G., & Lira, F. T. (1981). Relationship between bender designs and basic living skills of geriatric psychiatric patients. *Perceptual and Motor Skills, 52,* 16–18.

Neuroimaging in Normal Aging and Dementia

ERIN D. BIGLER

In the work-up of the dementia patient, contemporary neuroimaging in the form of routine computerized tomography (CT) and/or magnetic resonance (MR) imaging has become an essential procedure (Caselli, 1995; Corey-Bloom et al., 1995; Kucharczyk, Moseley, & Barkovich, 1994; Osborn, 1994). While neuroimaging studies do not provide definitive tests for the diagnosis of a dementing disorder, they do permit the determination of presence/absence of cerebral atrophy (a hallmark sign in many dementing illnesses) and the detection of potentially treatable factors producing dementia-like problems (i.e., tumors, vascular abnormalities, chronic subdural hematomas, infection, etc.). Although not definitive of a particular dementing illness, there are characteristics observed in neuroimaging studies that aid in the differential diagnosis of a dementing illness (i.e., Alzheimer's disease [AD] vs. multi-infarct dementia [MID]). Additionally, the degree of degenerative change observed on brain imaging typically has some relationship to symptom severity and also may aid in monitoring progression. These various topics form the basis of this chapter. However, because dementing illnesses are superimposed on an aging brain, neuroimaging findings in normal aging will be discussed first.

Neuroimaging and Normal Aging

Conception inaugurates a rapid development of central nervous system (CNS) tissue that ulti-

mately forms the infant brain. Throughout childhood a dynamic growth pattern dominates brain development which includes synaptic interconnectedness and myelination (Jernigan & Tallal, 1990; Jernigan, Trauner, Hesselink, & Tallal, 1991). Head circumference growth curves (see DeMyer, 1994) indirectly demonstrate dynamic brain growth throughout infancy, with rapid tapering off by adolescence. During this dynamic growth phase, brain growth fills the cranium, and cranial vault capacity responds in direct proportion to brain growth. Thus, when brain growth stabilizes in adolescence, so does cranial vault capacity and head size. This is an important point to note because head size is related to intracranial volume which is related to brain volume. In degenerative dementias, as the brain shrinks in volume, cerebrospinal fluid (CSF) spaces between the inner table of the skull and brain surface become more prominent. Since the original size of the brain essentially fills the cranial fault, except for the space occupied by CSF, an increase in CSF is an indication of brain wasting. Thus, an indirect measure of original brain size may be obtained by determining intracranial volume, and the amount of brain atrophy can be calculated by subtracting brain volume from intracranial volume or by subtracting CSF volume from intracranial volume.

Since the laws of aging and entropy apply to all, "normal" aging effects on the brain are inescapable. Thus, neuroimaging assessment of the dementia patient has to be performed in the context of what effects normal aging has on brain structure. Recently, we used quantitative MR methods to address the issue of normal aging (see Blatter et al.,

ERIN D. BIGLER • Department of Psychology, Brigham Young University, Provo, Utah 84602; and LDS Hospital, Salt Lake City, Utah 84103.

1995) and the relationship of normal aging to intellectual decline (Bigler, Johnson, Jackson, & Blatter, 1995). In the Blatter et al. study, we examined various cerebral structures by decade in normal volunteers from 16 to 65 years of age. As can be seen in Figure 1, there is steady decline in total brain volume with a corresponding increase in CSF with increase in age. In contrast (not shown, see Blatter et al., 1995), as would be expected, total intracranial volume (the volume within the skull) remains stable with the aging process. Thus, declining brain volume with aging represents an actual shrinkage of brain mass and corresponding increase in CSF space. Somewhat surprising, this decline in brain mass begins early, apparently in the fourth decade of life. This decrease initially follows a fairly linear pattern and then speeds up during senescence (see Blatter et al., 1995; Jernigan, Archibald, et al., 1991; Jernigan, Press, & Hesselink, 1990). Interestingly, this decline in brain volume with aging matches the

decline of more fluid aspects of intelligence (i.e., Performance IQ) that steadily decline with age (Bigler et al., 1995). This relationship is depicted in Figure 2. Thus, the decline in brain mass, in other words, the development of cerebral atrophy, is a normal process of aging and relates to certain declines in cognitive function that are age-dependent. Accordingly, any clinical imaging study of the brain must take into account the normal aging process and any deviation from the normal.

In Figure 3, a representative prototype scan has been selected from the Blatter et al. (1995) study for each decade to visually demonstrate these changes over time. Ventricular system and cortical CSF spaces remain relatively stable with aging, but there is also more variability. These "normal" aging changes represent a diagnostic problem for the radiologist who must provide a clinical interpretation of scan data. For example, just in Figure 3, the degree of "atrophy" in the 56–65 age range, which is "normal" for that age, would not necessarily be considered so normal in a 16-year-old individual. Also, when neuroimaging studies are being evaluated in the work-up of a dementia patient, careful attention is typically directed to the sylvian fissure, because sylvian fissure prominence is a sign of frontal and/or temporal lobe degeneration. However, Jernigan, Archibald, et al. (1991); Jernigan, Salmon, Butters, and Hesselink (1991); and Shear et al. (1995) have demonstrated that in normal aging, the sylvian fissure becomes distinctly more prominent. Shear et al. (1995) also have demonstrated the prominence of ventricular increase with age. Thus, when clinically reviewing scans in cases of suspected or confirmed dementia, the clinician always has to keep in mind the issue of "normal" aging and the age of the patient.

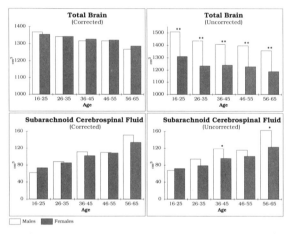

FIGURE 1. Bar graph depiction of age-related morphometric changes in total brain volume and whole brain subarachnoid cerebrospinal fluid (CSF) in normal, nondemented individuals over five decades. The right upper and lower graphs represent values uncorrected for head size, and the left upper and lower graphs represent values corrected for head size. Note that without correcting for head size, males have larger brain volume at each decade. However, by correcting for head size this difference vanishes. The most important factor demonstrated by these graphs is that brain volume changes with age, with a steady decline in volume for each decade investigated. Since CSF space increases as brain volume declines, volume of subarachnoid CSF will be the inverse of brain volume. Graphs have been adapted from Blatter et al. (1995). Asterisks represent significant gender differences at the $p \leqslant .01$ level.

Alzheimer's Disease

From a neuroimaging standpoint, of all the neurodegenerative dementias, AD is the most prevalent and probably the most researched disorder (Braffman, 1994; Corey-Bloom et al., 1995). Typically, either MR or CT imaging studies of the AD patient depict cerebral atrophy and ventricular dilation (see Figure 4). Brain atrophy is present because as cellular degeneration occurs, brain volume is

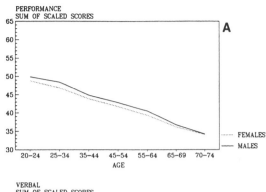

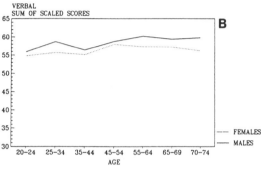

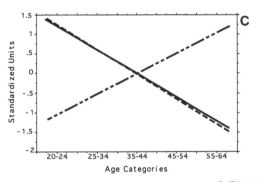

	Regression Equation	Coefficient of Determination
Ave. Brain Volume	y = - 0.61x + 1.83	.93
Ave. PIQ-ss	y = - 0.63x + 1.89	.99
Ave. VIQ-ss	y = 0.52x - 1.57	.69

FIGURE 2. (A) Lifespan graph depicting the decline of Performance IQ (PIQ) as measured by the Wechsler Adult Intelligence Scale-Revised (WAIS-R) based on the study of Kaufman, Kaufman-Packer, McLean, and Reynolds (1991). Note the steady decline of PIQ over each decade. (B) Lifespan graph depicting no decline in WAIS-R Verbal IQ scores. Bigler et al. (1995) noted that the rate of decline in PIQ scores matched the rate of decline in total brain volume with age and this relationship is depicted in (C). Note that the slope of decline is almost identical between loss of brain mass and drop in nonverbal, perceptual motor function (PIQ). Since perceptual-motor changes appear to be more specific to age-related changes, these results suggest that the basis may be related to the inexorable decline in brain structure with age.

lost. Jernigan, Salmon, et al. (1991) have demonstrated through quantitative MR techniques that the degenerative changes that produce volume loss in AD are rather uniform, but particularly apparent in the mesial cortices.

In a recent study involving identical twins discordant for AD, we were able to demonstrate these classic changes in the AD-affected twin when compared to the asymptomatic twin (Plassman et al., 1995). Figure 5 demonstrates these findings. It is possible to coregister the images, and those areas common to aging *per se* would show considerable overlap between the twins. In contrast, areas more susceptible to the effects of AD would show disproportionate atrophy. Thus, the places where the gray scale images fuse represent the areas common to aging. In contrast, the areas that do not share a common color in the merged images in Figure 4 represent regions of greater atrophy presumably related to the disease process in the affected twin. This study demonstrates considerable communality in the aging brains of identical twins, again emphasizing the need to interpret scans in the elderly against the backdrop of the aging process.

Another recent development in imaging of AD is the examination of white matter changes; the changes are thought to be due in large part to vascular abnormalities. In one of the most comprehensive studies to date, Skoog and colleagues (see Skoog, 1994; Skoog, Nilsson, Palmertz, Andreasson, & Svanborg, 1993; Skoog, Palmertz, & Andreasson, 1995) have demonstrated a significant vascular component in terms of white matter lesions in the aging population and AD. An illustration of such white matter lesions can be seen in Figure 6. White matter lesions in the healthy elderly correlate with a decrease in attention and speed of mental processing (Ylikoski et al., 1993) which likely aggravate these cognitive problems in the AD subject. Vascular factors probably play a much more significant role in AD than heretofore considered because of the possible role of the apolipoprotein E ε4 allele (ApoE) in vascular abnormalities and AD (Breitner et al., 1995; Small, Mazziotta, & Collins, 1995). The relationship between presence of the ApoE genotype and neuroimaging findings is unknown at the time of this writing.

The relationship of neuroimaging findings in AD to cognitive symptoms and/or neuropsycho-

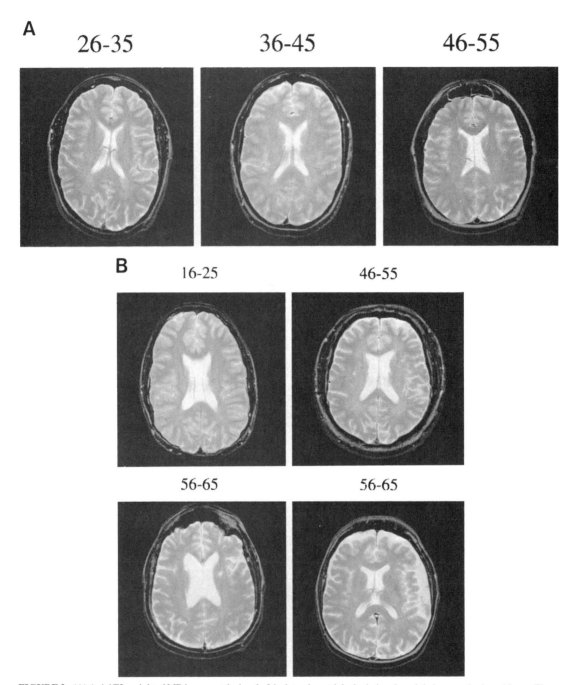

FIGURE 3. (A) Axial T2-weighted MR images at the level of the lateral ventricle depicting the subtle increase in size with age. These images were selected from Blatter et al. (1995) as ventricle size measures most closely matched the mean for that decade. Each axial view is based on a subject from his or her respective decade. Contrast the subject in the 46–55 decade with the subject in the 26–35 decade, and it is obvious that there are some increases in overall ventricular size. (B) From the same data set described above, the most prominent outlier in terms of total CSF space for three of the decades is present. Note that all these individuals were "normal" with no history of neurologic disease or disorder, yet they have enlarged ventricular space and/or cortical CSF. Also note there are white matter hyperintensities in the 46–55 and 56–65 group. The figure in the lower righthand corner demonstrates prominent CSF space in an otherwise normal individual. These studies demonstrate the variability that may accompany "normal" aging.

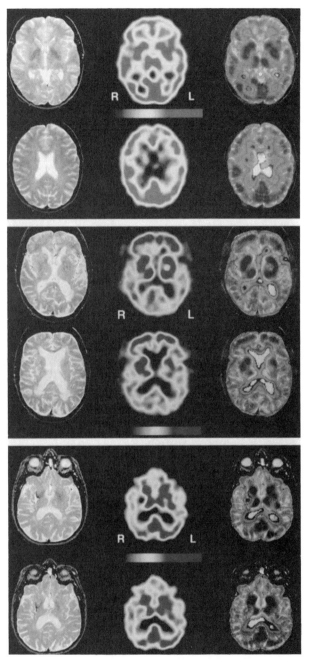

FIGURE 4. (Top) SPECT perfusion images and corresponding level MR scans of a normal control, a 71-year-old woman with normal neuropsychological testing and no significant medical or psychiatric history. The patient's MR scan (left) and SPECT scan (middle) are shown, along with superimposed MR and SPECT data (right). (Middle) SPECT perfusion images and MR scans of a 78-year-old patient with dementia whose neuropsychological and neurological exams suggested Alzheimer's disease and in whom there had been a 2.5-year decline in level of function. (Bottom) SPECT and MR scans of a 76-year-old woman with a 2.5-year history of dementia with stepwise progression and a past history of vascular disease whose clinical history, presentation, and neuropsychological results were consistent with a diagnosis of multi-infarct dementia. Reproduced with permission from Jagust, Johnson, and Holman (1995) and Little, Brown, and Company.

"Unaffected" Twin   Normal
Age-Matched   AD Twin

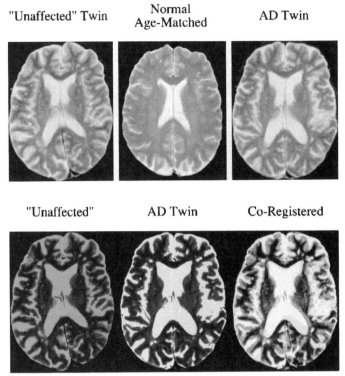

"Unaffected"   AD Twin   Co-Registered

FIGURE 5. Comparison of MR image analysis in a twin set discordant for Alzheimer's disease. The twins were in their mid-60s when imaged. Note the similarity in brain morphology, but that the AD twin has slightly larger ventricles and prominent cortical sulci. The original images are presented on top and the enhanced images highlighting the contrast between white versus gray matter and CSF are presented below, so that the two images could be coregistered and a combined image presented. The combined image clearly demonstrates the similarities of the two images, particularly at the level of the ventricular system, sylvian fissure, and interhemispheric fissure. This illustration underscores the importance of examining brain imaging studies in the patient with AD symptoms against the patient with normal age-related changes. In this example, since these were identical twins raised together in the same environment, the "unaffected" twin demonstrates the changes more attributable to age whereas the "affected" twin demonstrates more of what could be attributable to neuropathological changes associated with the disease process. Because they are identical twins and because of the genetic loading that occurs with AD, it is not known if the unaffected twin will become an incident case or not. At the time of this writing the unaffected twin was starting to exhibit some neurobehavioral changes that may be the harbinger of an ensuing AD.

logical deficits has been elusive. Numerous studies have attempted to examine the relationship between cerebral atrophy and cognitive change in AD (see Bigler, 1988; Corey-Bloom et al., 1995). Although a wide variety of outcomes have been reported, it is obvious that a linear relationship does not exist. In other words, while there is some relationship between the degree of cerebral atrophy and cognitive impairment, severe atrophy does not necessarily predict severe deficit. This point is well illustrated in Figure 7. Magnetic resonance imaging demonstrates severe atrophy in this patient with probable AD. However, when first evaluated, her Full Scale IQ score (FSIQ) was 122 on the Wechsler Adult

Intelligence Scale-Revised (WAIS-R), with a memory quotient (MQ) of 103 on the Wechsler Memory Scale. Over a 6-year period her level of functioning deteriorated significantly, and her last assessment indicated an FSIQ of 80 with an MQ of 66 (Naugle, Cullum, & Bigler, 1990).

Why is there not a more linear relationship between the degree of degenerative change and cognitive performance? Several factors are at play that help explain this lack of relationship. First, educational attainment and vocational history appear to be mitigating factors, not only in terms of the onset of AD symptoms, but also in terms of progression of AD. In several important studies in this

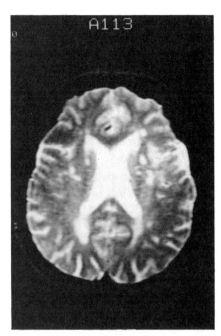

FIGURE 6. Multiple white matter hyperintensities on a T2-weighted axial image. Note the indistinct boundaries separating the anterior and posterior parts of the lateral ventricular system and surrounding white matter. The greatest changes in white matter may be observed in the periventricular regions. Also note the variable size and the scattered, random appearance of the hyperintensities. These types of changes are often seen in multi-infarct dementia.

domain, Stern and colleagues (1995) have demonstrated that educational attainment and vocational experience may provide a reserve that delays the clinical manifestation of AD. For example, the patient discussed in Figure 7 had advanced degrees in English and was a schoolteacher for 35 years, prior to retirement. There is speculation that more complex cognitive functions may have requirements for greater redundancy in the brain, thereby providing a substrate for multiple pathways for performing similar cognitive functions (see Bigler, 1996). If this is the case, then a relationship may exist between complexity of neural organization and the age at which AD symptoms are expressed. Schofield, Mosesson, Stern, and Mayeux (1995) have examined this hypothesis by evaluating intracranial size in AD subjects and the subjects' ages at the time of onset. As discussed in the opening statements, there is a robust (approaching unity) linear relationship be-

tween intracranial size and brain volume. Katzman et al. (1988) observed that elderly women studied at autopsy who manifested histologic changes of AD, but who were cognitively intact at the time of their death, had larger brains than cognitively impaired women with similar pathologic changes. The concept here is that complexity may relate to size, and relative size may have some "protective" influence because of redundancy. Schofield et al. (1995) demonstrated such a relationship. Age at onset of AD symptoms correlated positively ($r = .48$) with intracranial area. Obviously, while a significant finding, slightly less that one quarter of the variance is explained by this factor, suggesting a multiplicity of other factors at play as well. It is conceivable that as imaging technology methods improve, an algorithm will be developed that may provide greater diagnostic precision than what is currently available. As of this writing, we will have to accept the global clinical indicators of cerebral atrophy in AD as being *supportive* of the diagnosis of AD, but not *diagnostic*. Likewise, studies have shown that progression of AD is better detected by neuropsychological tests than by neuroimaging (Naugle et al., 1990). The reason for this is that degenerative and metabolic changes have to progress to the point of detection by the rather gross measures of imaging (i.e., changes in tissue less than 1 mm are not going to be detected by MR imaging, but such small lesions may literally involve millions of neural cells or pathways). In contrast, disruption of certain cognitive functions (i.e., memory) may be more notable and more easily detected by neuropsychological procedures because of the dependence of cognitive functions on functional units in the brain. Thus as neurons fail, their failure is first expressed in disruption and/or loss of function whereas neuronal degeneration and tissue loss take place over a more extended period of time.

Pick's Disease

In Pick's disease, typically there is marked regional atrophy of the brain, particularly observed in frontal or temporal regions. In the case presented in Figure 8, marked temporal lobe atrophy is evident. Although far from diagnostic, the typical neuroimaging distinction between Pick's disease and AD lies with the more focal presentation of atrophy

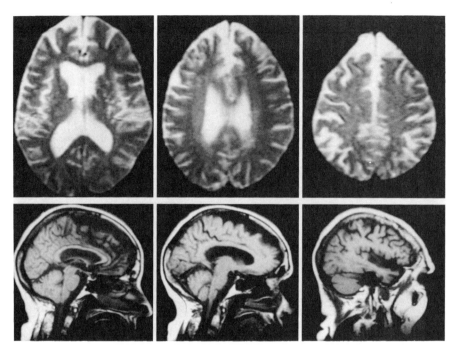

FIGURE 7. (Top) Axial views of an AD patient who initially presented with symptoms more consistent with depression than cognitive decline, but who then went on to exhibit a more classic deterioration consistent with AD. Note the prominence of the ventricular system and interhemispheric fissure. Also, there is asymmetric cortical atrophy in that the frontal regions of the brain are disproportionately affected. (Bottom) Sagittal views again depicting the greater prominence of frontal atrophy along with distinct atrophic changes in the temporal lobe (lower righthand corner). Even though prominent atrophy was present on original imaging, here initial neuropsychological studies indicated relatively preserved function (see Naugle et al., 1990). The point to make with this figure is that at any given point in time there may be only weak relationships between the degree of cortical atrophy and related neuropsychological impairment.

associated with Pick's disease. Although AD may result in marked frontal and/or temporal lobe atrophy, atrophy associated with AD tends to be more bilateral and symmetric. By contrasting Figure 8 with Figure 7, it is apparent that the Pick's patient displays more focal (right side) temporal atrophy than the more uniform, symmetric atrophy seen in the AD patients.

Multi-Infarct Dementia or Vascular Dementia (VaD)

In the traditional sense, multi-infarct or vascular dementia (MID/VaD) is supposed to present with more abrupt symptom onset than observed with AD or Pick's. Likewise, cognitive decline associated with MID is supposed to be more "stair-stepped" or "stepwise," meaning that the deterioration in cog-

nitive function follows an intermittent pattern of abrupt impairment (thought to be associated with acute vascular change, i.e., infarct) followed by stability, until the next pathologic vascular effect occurs. This also results in a more "patchy" presentation of clinical signs, symptoms, and neuropsychological deficits. The typical CT/MR neuroimaging pattern is one of small infarcts and/or white matter changes (so-called leukoaraiosis) and atrophic changes. These changes are usually distinguishable from large infarcts following a specific cerebrovascular accident (CVA), which often are not sufficient to produce a dementia (although they may be a precursor to more progressive vascular changes, such as that seen in the poststroke elderly hypertensive patient who goes on to develop a progressive VaD). Likewise, with an isolated CVA, typically there is improvement and stability over time. In contrast, with MID/VaD the cerebrovascu-

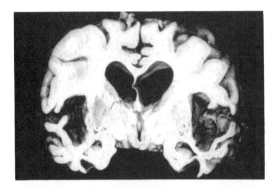

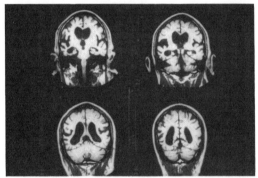

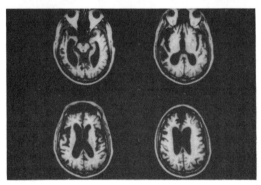

FIGURE 8. (Top) Postmortem coronal section of a patient who had Pick's disease. Note the very prominent sylvian fissure and the marked temporal lobe atrophy. (Middle and bottom) MR images from a patient with Pick's disease. Note the prominence of the ventricular system, particularly the temporal horns (a sign of temporal lobe wasting). While patients with Pick's disease clearly show some generalized neuropathological changes, more focal atrophy is typically present in one lobe or region, most often either the frontal or temporal lobes. The MR studies were supplied by Helena Chang Chui, M.D., Rancho Los Amigos Medical Center-University of Southern California.

lar changes are progressive, manifested in predictable deterioration. Figure 4 presents an MR scan from a typical MID patient contrasted with a normal control and an AD scan. As previously presented, Figure 4 depicts the relationship of MR findings in MID with metabolic changes as demonstrated by single photon emission computerized tomography (SPECT) imaging. It is important to note that SPECT imaging studies indicate more extensive perfusion changes than would be predicted by just the presence of any given lesion. This suggests that the pathophysiologic disruption that occurs in the brain of the MID patient is greater than the sum of identifiable lesions on anatomic imaging such as CT and MR. Also, note from Figure 4 that it is difficult to differentiate MID from AD on SPECT imaging alone.

As discussed previously, part of the underlying pathology in AD may be mediated by the vascular network. Accordingly, it may be that the distinction between AD and MID is not be as clear as was once thought, and neuroimaging studies appear to support this contention. This may relate to the difficulty in distinguishing the significance of degenerative brain changes from vascular changes in aging and dementia (Skoog, 1994). In fact, some of the degenerative changes thought to be strictly related to AD may be mediated via vascular changes. Vascular changes also may mediate age-related mild cognitive decline (Ylikoski et al., 1993) and dysphoric mood seen in depressed elderly who are not demented (Nussbaum, Kaszniak, Allender, & Rapcsak, 1995). However, vascular findings observed on neuroimaging studies may just be the harbinger of a later developing dementia (see Nussbaum et al., 1995).

Huntington's Disease

The genetic disorder Huntington's disease (HD) is another progressive degenerative disorder but has its expression much earlier in life than typically observed with all other syndromes discussed in this chapter. Accordingly, even though a marked dementia eventually ensues, HD typically is not considered in the same light as other degenerative disorders, such as Alzheimer's. Huntington's disease is characterized by specific degenerative changes at the level of the basal ganglia, which produce choreoathetoid movements and focal changes (basal ganglia) along with global degenerative changes (cerebral atrophy). As would be expected, based on morphometric MR studies, Jernigan, Salmon, et al. (1991) demonstrated that the greatest reductions in HD brain structure were in the basal ganglia. However, generalized atrophy was also noted. Figure 9 presents a postmortem coronal section from an HD patient depicting wasting of the caudate nucleus with associated ventricular expansion. An axial MR is also presented, again depicting the expansion of the ventricular system and caudate atrophy. As will be discussed below with Parkinson's disease, HD is considered to produce a so-

called subcortical dementia because of the proclivity of the neuropathologic changes at the basal ganglia level.

Asymmetric Cortical Degeneration (ACD) Syndromes

The syndromes discussed above all have core clinical characteristics associated with their neuropathologic presentations. Prior to the contemporary aging/degenerative disease perspective, the prevailing thought was that the major dementing illnesses were Alzheimer's, Pick's, and MID. The three-part distinction was clinically based on whether symptom presentation was slow and insidious (e.g., Alzheimer's), abrupt with stair-stepped decline (e.g., MID), or focal (e.g., Pick's). However, as initially discussed by Mesulam (1987), there are degenerative syndromes that present with focal onset and symptomatology but do not necessarily fit the traditional pattern of the three characterizations mentioned above. For example, Mesulam (1987) described several cases of progressive aphasia, without the typical memory and visual-spatial problems observed with AD. Some of these cases have now progressed to autopsy, and interestingly, histopathological studies have indicated degenerative changes similar to AD in some of the cases (see Benson & Zaias, 1991). That these focal degenerative syndromes are an Alzheimer's variant remains a possibility (see Caselli, 1995). Caselli and Jack (1992) propose that the term "asymmetric cortical degeneration" (ACD) be used (see also Caselli, Jack, Petersen, Wahner, & Yanaghihara, 1992). For ACD classification, Caselli and Jack (1992) suggest that slowly progressive focal symptoms must be present but without the frank dementia seen with classic Alzheimer's disease. Caselli (1995) reviews the various syndromes. From a neuroimaging perspective, one expects to observe more focal atrophic changes associated with the clinical presentation of the patient. The focal changes may be superimposed on a background of more generalized atrophy. For example, in the case already shown in Figure 7, this retired schoolteacher presented with problems of initiation, which were initially mistaken for depression. Her original imaging studies (see Naugle et al., 1990) exhibited distinct frontal atrophy super-

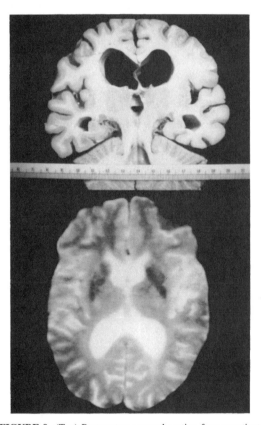

FIGURE 9. (Top) Postmortem coronal section from a patient who had Huntington's disease. Note the prominence of the ventricular system, which in part is related to a combination of changes including subcortical (basal ganglia) and cortical atrophy. (Bottom) Axial MR view of a patient with Huntington's disease exhibiting ventricular increase and atrophic basal ganglia changes.

imposed on nonspecific cortical atrophy, but her initial neuropsychological testing was considered to be within normal limits and not indicative of AD. However, as the syndrome progressed it became more Alzheimer's-like, and the degenerative changes became widespread. Accordingly, based on the clinical exam and neuropsychological testing, wherein focal pathology is suggested, neuroimaging studies should be examined for findings of focal atrophy that may correspond to the patient's clinical presentation.

Parkinson's Disease (PD)

The old, traditional view of PD was that its effect on cognition was minimal in comparison to motor deficits. Accordingly, from this historical perspective, PD per se was not considered a primary dementing illness. However, contemporary views of PD and dementia are that PD is often associated with changes in cognition and that a form of a "subcortical" dementia may be associated with PD (Mayeaux, Stern, Rosen, & Leventhal, 1981; Whitehouse, Lerner, & Hedera, 1994). As with the other dementing illnesses, neuroimaging studies are not diagnostic of the disorder, but rather used to rule out treatable causes for the dementia symptoms (e.g., presence of tumor) and to look for age-related

changes (Osborn, 1994). In the classic nondemented PD patient MR imaging may be negative, or changes/signal irregularities may be seen in basal ganglia structures, particularly the substantia nigra. Even though the locus of neuropathological changes occurs subcortically, significant cortical atrophy may be observed as well. As more prominent sulcal enlargement is observed in combination with nonspecific ventricular expansion, the likelihood that cognitive and neurobehavioral features of dementia associated with PD are present is greater.

Dementia Associated with Head Injury

Significant trauma to the brain results in atrophic changes, typically manifested by ventricular enlargement and sulcal widening (see Figure 10; Bigler, 1996). It is of interest to note that one of the by-products of neuronal degeneration induced by trauma is β-amyloid (Roberts et al., 1994). Beta-amyloid is also one of the degenerative by-products associated with AD (see Oda, Lehrer-Graiwer, Finch, & Pasinetti, 1995). Furthermore, various epidemiologic studies have demonstrated an association between history of significant head injury and AD. In the elderly individual with a history of head injury, it may be difficult to distinguish between some of the nonspecific degenerative changes asso-

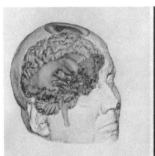 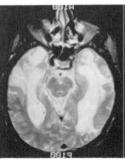 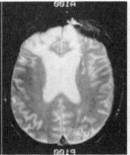 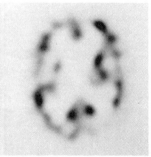

FIGURE 10. Dementia associated with posttraumatic brain injury. (Left) Three-dimensional reconstruction depicting the brain inside the cranium with distinctly dilated ventricles as a sign of generalized cortical atrophy and residual bifrontal wasting, as depicted by the darker shade of gray in the frontal region. (Middle) Axial MR views of T2-weighted images depicting ventricular enlargement and frontal-temporal lobe wasting. (Right) SPECT scan depicting multiple areas of cortical hypoperfusion, particularly in frontal-temporal and occipital regions. Prior to this patient's head injury, which was sustained in a 30-foot fall from a scaffold, the patient was an independent building contractor with a high school education (estimated premorbid IQ=100). After the injury, his IQ scores on various tests were in the 60–70 range. While the enlargement of the ventricular system in traumatically related injury may appear similar to what is observed with aging and the various dementing illnesses, the presence of cortical atrophy and encephalomalacic changes associated with old cortical contusions is distinct for trauma and not degenerative disease.

ciated with the aging process (increased cortical CSF and ventriculomegaly) and what is residual from trauma (compare Figure 10 with the other figures in this chapter). Where clearly demarcated cortical contusions or hemorrhagic lesions have occurred, those type of lesions are readily delineated from age-related degenerative changes (see again Figure 10).

Summary

Contemporary neuroimaging studies of the aging brain are capable of demonstrating structural as well as metabolic brain changes. Although not diagnostic of a specific dementia, there are characteristic changes observed on brain imaging studies with various dementing illnesses. Imaging findings always have to be viewed against the backdrop of normal aging, which produces its own set of changes that can be observed in neuroimaging studies. Atrophic changes in the brain identified on neuroimaging do relate to cognitive status, but the relationship is nonlinear and multifactorial. Accordingly, clinical caution is recommended when interpreting the relationship of neuroimaging-defined brain atrophy and neuropsychological outcome.

References

Benson, D. F., & Zaias, B. W. (1991). Progressive aphasia: A case with postmortem correlation. *Neuropsychiatry, Neuropsychology and Behavioral Neurology, 4*, 215–223.

Bigler, E. D. (1988). Neuropsychological and computed tomographic identification in dementia. In H. A. Whitaker (Ed.), *Neuropsychological studies of nonfocal brain damage* (pp. 61–85). New York: Springer-Verlag.

Bigler, E. D. (1996). Brain morphology and intelligence. *Developmental Neuropsychology, 11*, 377–403.

Bigler, E. D., Johnson, S. C., Jackson, C., & Blatter, D. D. (1995). Aging, brain size and I.Q. *Intelligence, 21*, 109–119.

Blatter, D. D., Bigler, E. D., Gale, S. D., Johnson, S. C., Anderson, C. V., Burnett, B. M., Parker, N., Kurth, S., & Horn, S. (1995). Quantitative volumetric analysis of brain MR: Normative data base spanning 5 decades of life. *American Journal of Neuroradiology, 16*, 241–251.

Braffman, B. (1994). Neurodegenerative disorders. In J. Kucharczyk, M. Moseley, & A. J. Barkovich (Eds.), *Magnetic resonance neuroimaging* (pp. 217–243). Boca Raton, FL: CRC Press.

Breitner, J. C. S., Welsh, K. A., Gau, B. A., McDonald, W. M., Steffens, D. C., Saunders, A. M., Magruder, K. M., Helms, M. J., Plassman, B. L., Folstein, M. F., Brandt, J., Robinette, C. D., & Page, W. F. (1995). Alzheimer's disease in the National Academy of Sciences-National Research Council Registry of aging twin veterans: III. Detection of cases, longitudinal results, and observations on twin concordance. *Archives of Neurology, 52*, 763–771.

Caselli, R. J. (1995). Focal and asymmetric cortical degeneration syndromes. *The Neurologist, 1*, 1–19.

Caselli, R. J., & Jack, C. R., Jr. (1992). Asymmetric cortical degeneration syndromes. A proposed clinical classification. *Archives of Neurology, 49*, 770–780.

Caselli, R. J., Jack, C. R., Jr., Petersen, R. C., Wahner, H. W., & Yanaghihara, T. (1992). Asymmetric cortical degenerative syndromes: Clinical and radiologic correlations. *Neurology, 42*, 1462–1468.

Corey-Bloom, J., Thal, L. J., Galasko, D., Folstein, M., Drachman, D., Raskind, M., & Lanska, D. J. (1995). Diagnosis and evaluation of dementia. *Neurology, 45*, 211–218.

DeMyer, W. (1994). Microcephaly, micrencephaly, megalocephaly, and megalencephaly. In K. F. Swaiman (Ed.), *Pediatric neurology* (pp. 205–218). St. Louis, MO: Mosby.

Jagust, W. J., Johnson, K. A., & Holman, B. L. (1995). SPECT perfusion imaging in the diagnosis of dementia. *Journal of Neuroimaging, 5*, S45–S52.

Jernigan, T. L., & Tallal, P. (1990). Late childhood changes in brain morphology observable with MRI. *Developmental Medicine and Child Neurology, 32*, 379–385.

Jernigan, T. L., Press, G. A., & Hesselink, J. R. (1990). Methods for measuring brain morphologic features on magnetic resonance images: Validation and normal aging. *Archives of Neurology, 47*, 27–32.

Jernigan, T. L., Archibald, S. L., Berhow, M. T., Sowell, E. R., Foster, D. S., & Hesselink, J. R. (1991). Cerebral structure on MRI, Part I: Localization of age-related changes. *Biological Psychiatry, 29*, 55–67.

Jernigan, T. L., Salmon, D. P., Butters, N., & Hesselink, J. R. (1991). Cerebral structure on MRI, Part II: Specific changes in Alzheimer's and Huntington's diseases. *Biological Psychiatry, 29*, 68–81.

Jernigan, T. L., Trauner, D. A., Hesselink, J. R., & Tallal, P. A. (1991). Maturation of human cerebrum observed in vivo during adolescence. *Brain, 114*, 2037–2049.

Katzman, R., Terry, R., DeTeresa, R., Brown, T., Davies, P., Fuld, P., Renbing, X., & Peck, A. (1988). Clinical, pathological, and neurochemical changes in dementia: A subgroup with preserved mental status and numerous neocortical plaques. *Annals of Neurology, 23*, 138–144.

Kaufman, A. S., Kaufman-Packer, J. L., McLean, J. E., & Reynolds, C. R. (1991). Is the pattern of intellectual growth and decline across the adult life span different for men and women? *Journal of Clinical Psychology, 47*, 802–812.

Kucharczyk, J., Moseley, M., & Barkovich, A. J. (1994). Magnetic resonance neuroimaging. Boca Raton, FL: CRC Press.

Mayeaux, R., Stern, Y., Rosen, J., & Leventhal, J. (1981). Depression, intellectual impairment and Parkinson's disease. *Neurology, 31*, 645–650.

Mesulam, M.-M. (1987). Primary progressive aphasia: Differentiation from Alzheimer's disease. *Annals of Neurology, 22,* 533–534.

Naugle, R. I., Cullum, C. M., & Bigler, E. D. (1990). Evaluation of intellectual and memory function among dementia patients who were intellectually superior. *The Clinical Neuropsychologist, 4,* 355–374.

Nussbaum, P. D., Kaszniak, A. W., Allender, J., & Rapcsak, S. (1995). Depression and cognitive decline in the elderly: A follow-up study. *The Clinical Neuropsychologist, 9,* 101–111.

Oda, T., Lehrer-Graiwer, J., Finch, C. L., & Pasinetti, G. M. (1995). Complement and β-amyloid (AB) neurotoxicity in vitro: A model for Alzheimer's disease. *Alzheimer's Research, 1,* 29–34.

Osborn, A. G. (1994). *Diagnostic neuroradiology.* St. Louis, MO: Mosby.

Plassman, B. L., Welsh, K. A., Abildskov, T., Johnson, S. C., Anderson, C. V., Bigler, E. D., & Breitner, J. C. (1995). Merging methods: MRI volumetric studies in monozygotic twin pairs discordant for Alzheimer's disease. *Archives of Clinical Neuropsychology, 19,* 377.

Roberts, G. W., Gentleman, S. M., Lynch, A., Murray, L., Landon, M., & Graham, D. I. (1994). B-amyloid protein deposition in the brain after severe head injury: Implications for the pathogenesis of Alzheimer's disease. *Journal of Neurology, Neurosurgery and Psychiatry, 57,* 419–425.

Schofield, P. W., Mosesson, R. E., Stern, Y., & Mayeaux, R. (1995). The age at onset of Alzheimer's disease and an intracranial area measurement. *Archives of Neurology, 52,* 95–98.

Shear, P. K., Sullivan, E. V., Mathalon, D. H., Lim, K. O., Davis, L. F., Yesavage, J. A., Tinklenberg, J. R., & Pfefferbaum, A. (1995). Longitudinal volumetric computed tomographic analysis of regional brain changes in normal aging and Alzheimer's disease. *Archives of Neurology, 52,* 392–402.

Skoog, I. (1994). Risk factors for vascular dementia: A review. *Dementia, 5,* 137–144.

Skoog, I., Nilsson, L., Palmertz, B., Andreasson, L.-A., & Svanborg, A. (1993). A population-based study of dementia in 85-year-olds. *New England Journal of Medicine, 328,* 153–158.

Skoog, I., Palmertz, B., & Andreasson, L.-A. (1995). The prevalence of white-matter lesions on computed tomography of the brain in demented and nondemented 85-year-olds. *Journal of Geriatric Psychiatry and Neurology, 7,* 169–175.

Small, G. W., Mazziotta, J. C., & Collins, M. T. (1995). Apolipoprotein E type 4 allele and cerebral glucose metabolism in relatives at risk for familial Alzheimer's disease. *Journal of the American Medical Association, 273,* 942–947.

Stern, Y., Alexander, G. E., Prohovnik, I., Stricks, L., Link, B., Lennon, M. C., & Mayeux, R. (1995). Relationship between lifetime occupation and parietal flow: Implications for a reserve against Alzheimer's disease pathology. *Neurology, 45,* 55–60.

Whitehouse, P. J., Lerner, A., & Hedera, P. (1994). Dementia. In K. M. Heilman & E. Valenstein (Eds.), *Clinical neuropsychology* (pp. 603–645). New York: Oxford University Press.

Ylikoski, R., Ylikoski, A., Erkinjuntti, T., Sulkava, R., Raininko, R., & Tilvis, R. (1993). White matter changes in healthy elderly persons correlate with attention and speed of mental processing. *Archives of Neurology, 50,* 818–824.

28

Electroencephalography in the Elderly

HARRY W. McCONNELL, PETER J. SNYDER, AND JAMES VALERIANO

Introduction

The electroencephalogram (EEG) reflects the electrical activity of the underlying cerebral cortex. The invention of EEG largely resulted from the work of the German psychiatrist Hans Berger (1873–1941). Berger first showed that rhythmic ("spike-and-wave") electrical activity, now considered to be the hallmark of an epileptic seizure, can be recorded from the surface of the brain. Four principal EEG rhythms have been described in routine EEG recording: delta (< 4 Hz), theta (4–7 Hz), alpha (8–13 Hz), and beta (14–30 Hz).

The major EEG rhythms seen in the awake adult at rest are the alpha and beta rhythms. The alpha rhythm consists of sinusoidal 8–13 Hz waves, it disappears with drowsiness and sleep, and it is also blocked by opening the eyes and by being alerted. The alpha rhythm is seen mostly over the posterior head areas. The beta rhythm may be widely distributed or limited to the frontal or posterior areas. The beta rhythm is any waveform over 13 Hz and, like the alpha rhythm, disappears in drowsiness and in sleep. Other EEG rhythms seen in the normal awake adult include (1) the mu rhythm

(arch-shaped waves of 7–11 Hz seen in less than 10% of EEGs and usually in young adults); (2) lambda waves (sharp transients in the occipital regions of some subjects when they look at objects with substantial visual detail); (3) vertex sharp transients (this type of waveform occurs rarely in awake adults, but more commonly in normal sleep); (4) kappa rhythm (bursts of low amplitude waves which originate from the temporal areas of some subjects who are engaged in mental activity, and thus rarely seen in routine recordings); and (5) posterior theta rhythms, slow alpha variants, and rhythmical slow waves rarely seen in routine recordings with awake adults (for review, see Fisch, 1991, pp. 213–228). Spikes and sharp waves (except for vertex sharp transients and lambda waves), slow waves of less than 8 Hz, abnormally low or high amplitude waveforms, and marked changes in the frequency or reactivity of the alpha rhythm are the major abnormalities seen in the EEG of an awake subject.

In normal sleep, the slower waves on EEG are generally associated with the "deeper" stages of sleep. Listed in Table 1 are the five distinct EEG stages associated with normal sleep. These sleep stages cycle throughout the night, usually about four times per night (see reviews by Hughes, 1981, and Fisch, 1991, for further description of EEG characteristics). In the elderly, sleep onset may be associated with slow waves beginning when alpha activity has ceased, sleep delta is diminished overall (decreased amount of time in stages III and IV), and

HARRY W. McCONNELL • Institute of Epileptology, Maudsley Hospital, London SE5 8AZ, England. PETER J. SNYDER AND JAMES VALERIANO • Department of Neurology, Medical College of Pennsylvania and Hahnemann University–Allegheny Campus, Pittsburgh, Pennsylvania 15212.

Table 1. Five EEG Stages of Normal Sleep

Sleep stage	Associated EEG changes
Stage 1: Drowsiness	Decrease in alpha rhythm
Stage 2: Light sleep	Theta rhythm, especially posteriorly; vertex sharp transients and sleep spindles (14 Hz) seen, the combination of which are called "k complexes"
Stage 3: Moderately deep sleep	Symmetrical delta waves (<50%)
Stage 4: Deepest sleep	More than 50% delta rhythms
REM stage: Rapid eye movements	Movements of eyes; sleep stage during which most (but not all) dreaming takes place; low-voltage EEG patterns

rapid eye movement (REM) sleep may also decrease to less than 20% of total sleep time by age 70–80 years (Fisch, 1991).

In interpreting the EEG it is very important to pay attention to potential sources of artifact which frequently occur and may erroneously look like true EEG abnormalities. The most common sources of such artifact are muscle movement, interference from power sources ("60–cycle artifact"), electrode movement, electrode problems ("electrode popping"), eye movement, sweating, pulse wave artifact, tongue movements, electrocardiogram (EKG) artifacts, and artifacts arising from voltage surges, faulty equipment, swallowing, tremors, or respiration. The lack of recognition of such sources of artifact may lead to misinterpretation of EEG abnormalities, and hence the electroencephalographer is continually on the lookout for the technical quality of the EEG record he or she is reviewing.

The EEG is a useful adjunct to the clinical examination for suspected epilepsy, delirium, dementia, stupor, and coma. It must, however, always be used along with the clinical history and examination findings when considering any of these diagnoses. A normal EEG, for example, does not rule out the possibility of a seizure disorder, as 40% of patients with definite epilepsy will not show a paroxysmal disturbance on EEG recording. Nonetheless, the advent of EEG has led to radical improvements in patient care in that it provides a painless, noninvasive method for diagnosing a variety of conditions, as will be described below.

Age-Related EEG Changes

Many investigators have noted an increased incidence of EEG abnormalities in normal aging subjects. Hughes and Cayaffa (1977) reviewed the EEGs of 420 neurologically normal patients who underwent EEG over a 12-year period and whose symptoms were believed to have a psychogenic or other non-neurological basis. They noted that the distribution of the major frequency of the background rhythm showed a shift of the peak from 9 Hz to 10 Hz from the first to the second decade of life, followed by a flattening of this peak over the next two decades and an increase in slower alpha activity by the seventh decade of life, with a gradual shift back to 9 Hz. They also noted an increase in sharp waves and slow waves in the elderly, as well as a decrease in photic driving. The incidence of sharp wave or spike paroxysms rose from 2% to 10–11% after the fifth decade. Several other studies have also noted higher rates of focal abnormalities in the elderly which generally have not been associated with neuropsychological abnormalities (Busse, Barnes, Friedman, & Kelty, 1956; Silverman, Busse, & Barnes, 1955), although other investigators have demonstrated subclinical abnormalities (Visser, 1987). Torres, Faoro, Loewenson, and Johnson (1983) found 52% of their normal asymptomatic elderly subjects to have an identifiable EEG abnormality. This finding is consistent with several earlier reports, although some more recent studies have found a lower incidence (e.g., 29% incidence reported by Soininen, Partanen, Helkala, & Riekkinen, 1982), depending on how the EEG abnormalities are defined and the characteristics of the normal subjects studied.

Whether these EEG abnormalities relate to neural aging per se or, more likely, to pathological changes associated with aging is not certain. Hubbard, Sunde, and Goldensohn (1976) found EEG changes in their group of centenarians similar to those seen in studies of somewhat younger elderly (slowing of posterior alpha-mean 8.62 Hz, some diffuse slowing, and focal slow wave activity, usually left temporal in origin) and suggest that the EEG changes seen in the elderly are not relentlessly progressive and are related more to pathological processes associated with aging. The more recent 5-year follow-up study by Shigeta et al. (1995)

would also be consistent with this view. Hughes (1987), Niedermeyer (1987a), Fenton (1994), and Klass and Brenner (1995) have reviewed the changes that are commonly found for specific EEG waveforms in the elderly, and these are summarized in Table 2.

Clinical Use of EEG in the Elderly

In the geriatric population, EEG is primarily useful for the evaluation of suspected seizures and changes in mental state. The latter includes episodic losses of consciousness, stupor, coma, delirium, and dementia.

The main indication for obtaining an EEG in the elderly is in the investigation of a possible seizure disorder. As the EEG may not necessarily show any abnormalities between episodes, prolonged EEG monitoring for 24 or 48 hr, or longer, using ambulatory or continuous video-EEG monitoring is frequently useful for maximizing the chances of obtaining an episode of seizure activity. In surgical candidates, this may at times be done with grid placement or depth electrodes since the surface EEG may miss deep epileptic foci. Ambulatory

Table 2. EEG Changes in the Elderly[a]

Focal abnormalities	Description	Significance
Temporal slowing; temporal sharp activity	Brief trains of 3–8 Hz often mixed with faster frequencies Mild to moderate sharp transients More common on the left than on the right	Usually of no clinical significance May support diagnosis of cerebrovascular disease or be related to ischemic involvement of hippocampus
Slowing of alpha rhythm	Decline from 9.7 to 9.0 Hz between ages of 60 and 90 Decreased alpha voltage Decreased reactivity of alpha Mu rhythm also less prevalent	May be of no clinical significance or may related to mental decline and early dementia
Bilateral anterior slow activity "anterior bradyarrhythmia"	Delta (1.5–2.5 Hz) seen anteriorly Usually seen in drowsiness or light sleep Must be distinguished from frontal intermittent rhythmic delta activity (FIRDA)	May reflect vascular disease or transient deterioration of health
Diffuse slowing	Mixed delta and theta (3–5 Hz)	May relate to cerebrovascular insufficiency or to development of delirium or dementia
Increased fast activity	Increased beta (14–30 Hz) activity Accentuated over central regions Females have more beta than males Voltage may also be attenuated	Not associated with mental decline May be related to preservation of mental functioning
Decline in hyperventilation changes	Decrease in (normal) symmetrical delta and theta patterns Elderly with temporal slow transients may have these accentuated with hyperventilation	May relate to decreased physical ability to hyperventilate or to autonomic instability
Decline in photic-driving responses	Decreased incidence and quality of photic driving	Significance unknown
Changes in nocturnal sleep patterns	Decreased sleep efficiency Increased awakenings Decreased stages 3 and 4 sleep	No clinical significance
Changes in evoked response patterns	Increased P300 latency (1.36 ms/yr) and decreased amplitude in healthy aging May have increased auditory and visual response latencies; must control for peripheral receptor changes	Ongoing research into relationship to intellectual decline

[a]Adapted from Klass & Brenner, 1995; Niedermeyer, 1987a; Fisch, 1991; and Hughes, 1987.

recordings may, in particular, be marred by movement artifacts which may make the tracing difficult to interpret. Recordings from the newer digital 16-channel units represent a significant advance over the older 8-channel analogue systems and produce data that are less fraught by artifact. These systems generally have automated seizure and slow wave detection devices which tend to greatly overestimate the occurrence of spikes and slowing, and the "final call" must be made by an experienced neurophysiologist, who should also take into consideration the clinical state of the patient at the time of recording.

Prolonged EEG monitoring has traditionally been done on an inpatient basis, but the recent advent of ambulatory EEG time-linked to video has only recently made this procedure feasible on an outpatient basis. Limited outpatient monitoring for 6 to 8 hr is also becoming more common. The use of photic stimulation, hyperventilation, sleep deprivation, or sedative-induced sleep may also help to bring out EEG abnormalities during routine EEG testing. In cases of suspected nonepileptic seizure-like events (NESLEs) of psychogenic origin, some centers will also make use of suggestion to provoke an episode during EEG monitoring. The term NESLE is preferred by these authors over the more common term "pseudoseizures" for many of the same reasons that Nussbaum has discussed in Chapter 17 of this volume regarding the use of the term "pseudodementia." The term pseudoseizure often has pejorative connotations for both patients and staff and thus has a significant impact on psychological transference and countertransference in the treatment of these patients. A normal EEG during a NESLE is thus very useful clinically in that it helps to redirect treatment to the underlying cause of the events. As mentioned above, deeper epileptic foci are not always detected on surface EEG, and this possibility underscores the importance of considering EEG findings in the context of the clinical event being monitored at the time. Depth recording is not indicated in evaluating NESLEs and should be reserved for surgical candidates only. The recent advent of longer lasting isotopes used as contrast material has made ictal single photon emission computerized tomography (SPECT) a useful adjunct to surface EEG in such cases.

When a seizure disorder is confirmed with ictal or interictal recording, the EEG can be very useful in ascertaining whether there is a single seizure focus that may be amenable to surgery (although it is rare for geriatric epilepsy patients to be considered for elective surgical treatment of medically refractory epilepsy [see Chapter 18, this volume]), whether the seizure disorder is multifocal, and whether there exists a primary generalized epilepsy. Information about specific types of epilepsy can also sometimes be inferred from close examination of the EEG (e.g., 3-Hz spike-and-wave activity seen in absence seizures).

In the evaluation of stupor and coma, the EEG may show generalized slowing indicative of an encephalopathy or may show asymmetrical or focal abnormalities suggestive of encephalitis. In hepatic encephalopathy, as well as in other metabolic encephalopathies, the posterior rhythm may be preserved, generalized triphasic waves may be seen, and the degree of slowing parallels the rise in blood ammonia (Burns, 1991). The EEG abnormalities are generally restricted to the temporal lobes in herpes encephalitis, and they tend to be seen unilaterally in about 80% of cases. In addition to giving clues to the etiology of stupor or coma, the degree of coma usually correlates with the degree of slowing.

The EEG is one of the most sensitive indicators of delirium and may give clues to the underlying etiology. Low-voltage activity with posterior slowing and bursts of theta may be seen in acute renal failure; hyperthyroidism may show an acceleration of alpha rhythm, and hypocalcemia may show slowing with bursts of spikes. Medication may be the primary cause of delirium and may be suspected by the evaluation of the EEG. Phenothiazines, for example, may decrease beta activity while increasing the slow activity, alpha, and voltage; benzodiazepines will increase beta activity and, in toxic amounts, increase slow activity (Burns, 1991). Jacobson, Leuchter, and Walter (1993), among others, have found quantitative EEG (QEEG) to be helpful in distinguishing delirium from dementia. They noted that among patients suffering from senile dementia of the Alzheimer's type (SDAT), in comparison to patients with delirium secondary to various conditions, there is a shift in the spectrum toward the slower frequencies, with an increase in theta and delta activity and a decrease in beta activity. Koponen, Partanen, Paakkonen, Mattila, and Riekkinen (1989) showed the percentage of alpha activity to correlate linearly with their patients' Mini-Mental State Examination (MMSE) scores, and that relative spectral power is an important variable distinguishing normal from encephalopathic cases.

In evaluating specific causes of dementia, the EEG can be a useful tool; it can also be used to differentiate cognitive changes related to depression versus other causes of dementia. In the early stages of senile dementia of the Alzheimer's type (SDAT), the EEG is often normal. As the condition progresses, there is often a decrease in amplitude and amount of beta activity over the frontal region, with an increased amount of temporal theta. Additionally, over time the posteriorly dominant alpha rhythm will decrease in frequency, and the temporal theta rhythm will become more pronounced. These changes can sometimes help distinguish SDAT from another common form of dementia, multi-infarct dementia (MID). In the latter, the alpha rhythm may remain intact further into the disease (Fenton, 1994), and focal abnormalities will be more prominent. Eventually, in MID, the alpha frequency will decrease. However, if focal findings are prominent, especially if they are asymmetric, MID would be the more likely of the two diagnoses.

One other type of dementia with very specific findings is Jakob-Creutzfeldt disease (JCD). With JCD, an early slowing of the background rhythm is often seen, but the most characteristic abnormality is the occurrence of a high-voltage, repetitive, sharp wave discharge. This discharge may be seen unilaterally at first, but with an eventual progression to bilateral involvement. Initially, these sharp waves may be time-locked with the patient's myoclonic jerks, but eventually they occur independent of them. The absence of this type of discharge in a patient with a mild dementia mitigates strongly against the diagnosis of Jakob-Creutzfeldt disease.

Recently, many investigators have used various measures derived from QEEG in evaluating

Table 3. EEG Findings in Dementia[a]

Etiology	EEG findings
Senile dementia of the Alzheimer's type (SDAT)	Diffuse slowing with frontal and temporal accentuation
	Slowing of posterior rhythm
	May be normal in very early stages
Pick's type dementia	Usually normal in early stages
	Alpha rhythm better preserved than in SDAT
	Later slowing of posterior basic rhythm and eventually diffuse slowing
Huntington's chorea	Progressive decrease in amplitude (correlates with caudate nucleus involvement)
	Diffuse slowing as disease progresses
	Juvenile form may show either normal EEG for years or spike-and-wave-like discharges
	May be associated with generalized asynchronous slow waves
Progressive supranuclear palsy	Bilateral rhythmic delta with frontal accentuation
	Slowing of posterior basic rhythm (6–7 Hz)
	Usually normal in early stages
	Markedly decreased REM and poor development of spindles and k complexes
Multi-infarct dementia (MID)	Diffuse slowing with focal features, often asymmetries
	Alpha rhythm better preserved than in SDAT
Jakob-Creutzfeldt disease (JCD)	Biphasic and triphasic periodic generalized complexes occurring at 0.5–1.0s intervals
Normal pressure hydrocephalus	EEG often normal
	May be associated with generalized or focal slow waves
	Generalized slow waves are often synchronous (in contrast to bisynchronous slow waves which may be seen in obstructive hydrocephalus)

[a]Adapted from reviews by Klass & Brenner, 1995; Niedermeyer, 1987a; Fisch, 1991; and Hughes, 1987.

dementia, and the QEEG may prove a valuable clinical tool in the future (Giaquinto & Nolfe, 1986; Leuchter et al., 1993; Leuchter & Holschneider, 1994). Niedermeyer (1987b), and Fenton (1994) have reviewed the principal EEG abnormalities seen in various types of dementia, and these are listed in Table 3.

Conclusion

The EEG undergoes various changes throughout the aging process. Focal changes are common and usually include temporal slow and sharp wave activity. These are usually of no clear clinical significance, although there is some debate as to their relation to cognitive deficits and to possible underlying cerebrovascular disease. Why these focal abnormalities are so frequently localized to the left temporal lobe is not known. Other changes seen with aging include the slowing of the posterior alpha dominant frequency, which may relate to intellectual decline. Bilateral anterior slow activity and diffuse slowing may occur and may be related to vascular disease or to mental deterioration. The increased beta activity seen in some elderly may relate to a relative preservation of mental functioning. Elderly women tend to have a higher parasagittal mean frequency in comparison to elderly men (Brenner, Ulrich, & Reynolds, 1995). These changes, which can all be seen in asymptomatic elderly patients, need to be taken into account when evaluating the EEG in this age group. The EEG is most useful for the evaluation of elderly patients with suspected seizure disorders, stupor, coma, delirium, and dementia. Finally, the clinical history and examination must always be taken into account in evaluating the EEG and its meaning for an individual patient.

ACKNOWLEDGMENTS

The authors thank Ms. Nicole Ceravolo for her assistance in preparing this manuscript.

References

Brenner, R., Ulrich, R., & Reynolds, C. (1995). EEG spectral findings in healthy, elderly men and women—sex differences. *Electroencephalography and Clinical Neurophysiology, 94*, 1–5.

Burns, A. (1991). Electroencephalography and imaging. In R. Jacoby & C. Oppenheimer (Eds.), *Psychiatry in the elderly* (pp. 255–257). Oxford, England: Oxford University Press.

Busse, E., Barnes, R., Friedman, E., & Kelty, E. (1956). Psychological functioning of aged individuals with normal and abnormal EEGs. I. A study of nonhospitalized community volunteers. *Journal of Nervous and Mental Diseases, 124*, 135–141.

Fenton, G. W. (1994). Electroencephalography. In J. Copland, M. Abou-Saleh, & D. Blazer (Eds.), *Geriatric psychiatry*. Chichester: John Wiley & Sons.

Fisch, B. J. (1991). *Spelman's EEG primer*. Amsterdam: Elsevier Press.

Giaquinto, S., & Nolfe, G. (1986). The EEG in the normal elderly. *Electroencephalography and Clinical Neurophysiology, 63*, 540–546.

Hubbard, O., Sunde, D., & Goldensohn, E. (1976). The EEG in centenarians. *Electroencephalography and Clinical Neurophysiology, 40*, 407–417.

Hughes, J. (1981). *EEG in clinical practice*. Boston: Butterworth Press.

Hughes, J. (1987). Normal limits in the EEG. In A. Halliday, S. Butler, & R. Paul (Eds.), *A textbook of clinical neurophysiology* (pp. 145–150). Chichester: John Wiley & Sons.

Hughes, J., & Cayaffa, J. (1977). The EEG in patients at different ages without organic cerebral disease. *Electroencephalography and Clinical Neurophysiology, 42*, 776–788.

Jacobson, S., Leuchter, A., & Walter, D. (1993). Conventional and quantitative EEG in the diagnosis of delirium among the elderly. *Journal of Neurology, Neurosurgery, and Psychiatry, 56*, 153–158.

Klass, D. W., & Brenner, R. P. (1995). Electroencephalography of the elderly. *Journal of Clinical Neurophysiology, 12*, 116–131.

Koponen, H., Partanen, J., Paakkonen, A., Mattila, E., & Riekkinen, P. (1989). EEG spectral analysis in delirium. *Journal of Neurology, Neurosurgery, and Psychiatry, 52* 980–985.

Leuchter, A., & Holschneider, D. (1994). Quantitative electroencephalography: Neurophysiological alterations in normal aging and geriatric neuropsychiatric disorders. In E. Coffey & J. Cummings (Eds.). *The American psychiatric press textbook of geriatric Neuropsychiatry* (pp. 215–240). Washington, DC: American Psychiatric Press, Inc

Leuchter, A., Cook, I., Newton, T., Dunkin, J., Walter, D. O., Rosenberg-Thompson, S., Lachenbruch, P. A., & Weiner, H. (1993). Regional differences in brain electrical activity in dementia. *Electroencephalography and Clinical Neurophysiology, 8*, 385–395.

Niedermeyer, E. (1987a). EEG and old age. In Niedermeyer & F. L. da Silva (Eds.). *Electroencephalography*. Baltimore: Urban & Schwarzenberg.

Niedermeyer, E. (1987b). EEG and dementia. In E. Niedermeyer & F. L. da Silva (Eds.), *Electroencephalography*. Baltimore: Urban & Schwarzenberg.

Shigeta, M., Julin, P., Almkvist, O., Basun, H., Rudberg, V., & Wahlund, L. (1995). EEG in successful aging: A 5-year follow-up study from the eight to ninth decade of life. *Electroencephalography and Clinical Neurophysiology, 95*, 77–83.

Silverman, A., Busse, E., & Barnes, R. (1955). Studies in the process of aging: EEG findings in 400 elderly subjects. *Electroencephalography and Clinical Neurophysiology, 7*, 67–74.

Soininen, H., Partanen, V., Helkala, E., & Riekkinen, P. (1982). EEG findings in senile dementia and normal aging. *Acta Neurologica Scandinavica, 65*, 59–70.

Torres, F., Faoro, A., Loewenson, R., & Johnson, E. (1983). The EEG of elderly subjects revisited. *Electroencephalography and Clinical Neurophysiology, 56*, 391–398.

Visser, S. (1987). EEG and senescence. *The London Symposium, 39*, (EEG Suppl.), 403–406.

V

Treatment Interventions and the Older Patient

29

Psychotherapy with Older Adults

Theoretical Issues, Empirical Findings, and Clinical Applications

JENNIFER J. BORTZ AND KEVIN P. O'BRIEN

Introduction

Compared to the general population, older adults often experience greater excess disability due to a variety of emotional disturbances and formal psychiatric disorders. There is increasing evidence that much of this unnecessary suffering can be ameliorated by a variety of psychotherapeutic interventions (Teri & McCurry, 1994). However, there are factors unique to older adults that affect the recognition of emotional disorders in late life as well as the availability, delivery, and effectiveness of mental health services. This chapter begins with an overview of key issues relevant to psychotherapy with older adults, beginning with accessibility and utilization of mental health services in this population. This is followed by a selective review of relevant clinical, empirical, and theoretical issues in the diagnostic categories of late-life depression, anxiety, and substance abuse. The chapter concludes with a discussion of suggested guidelines for therapeutic interventions with older adults, with particular attention to psychiatric disability in individuals with neurological disorders.

Current Trends and Issues

There are three trends that may dramatically alter our ability to provide mental health services in

the near future: the aging of the demographic profile; a decline in the number of professionals who are adequately trained to serve this growing population; and the encroachment of reimbursement restrictions and financial disincentives for treating mental disorders in older adults.

Approximately 12% of the U.S. population is currently over the age of 65, and a dramatic increase in the size of this age cohort is predicted in the next few decades (Lazenby & Letsch, 1990). By the year 2030, a growth rate three times that of the general population will result in a 21% prevalence of older adults (Gerety, 1994; Waldo, Sonnefeld, McHusick, & Arnett, 1988). This translates to approximately 69.8 million individuals over the age of 65 and 8.4 million over the age of 85 (see Malmgren, 1994, p. 18). Currently, over one third of all health care spending is accounted for by individuals over the age of 65 (Lazenby & Letsch, 1990). This figure will undoubtedly increase as medical advances and other factors extend the life expectancy (see review by Gerety, 1994).

Results of several recent epidemiologic studies suggest that members of the "baby boom" generation may have higher rates of emotional disturbance, including depression, anxiety, and chemical dependency, compared to the current elderly cohort at similar ages. For example, information derived from the application of life-table methodology and analysis of the Epidemiologic Catchment Area (ECA) data indicate that cohorts born after World War II may experience higher rates of major depression with a lower age of onset relative to older age

JENNIFER J. BORTZ AND KEVIN P. O'BRIEN • Barrow Neurological Institute, St. Joseph's Hospital and Medical Center, Phoenix, Arizona 85013-4496.

cohorts. Although methodological artifacts must be considered in the interpretation of these data (see discussion and review by Klerman & Weissman, 1989), such findings point to an impending crisis— that significant rates of psychopathology in the younger cohort may persist into the senior years within a system that is aggressively working to reduce expenditures and to restrict mental health services for older adults.

Current policies and trends suggest that there may not be sufficient numbers of adequately trained professionals to meet the needs of a burgeoning elderly population. This problem is reflected in the scope of academic curricula offered to medical students among whom "fewer than 5% have had either a focused experience in geriatric medicine or preclinical didactic instruction in geriatrics" (Gerety, 1994, p. 594). Bias against this specialization appears throughout the continuum of professional training as significantly fewer physicians choose postresidency fellowships in geriatrics than in other specialties such as cardiology. Due to reduced demand, in 1994 the Bureau of Health Professions eliminated the funding of almost two thirds of the fellowship training programs in geriatric medicine. If this trend continues, a significant shortfall of qualified geriatricians is anticipated by the year 2040 (Gerety, 1994). This has important implications for the appropriate identification of psychiatric symptoms in older adults and subsequent referral for psychotherapeutic assessment and treatment, since referrals for therapeutic intervention are often initiated by physicians who provide primary care for geriatric patients. Adequate training and supervised experience in psychotherapy for late-life disorders are similarly lacking in psychology graduate school programs and clinical internship curricula (Teri & Logsdon, 1992).

One possible reason for the predicted shortfall in qualified geriatric specialists is that financial disincentives exist under Medicare's current funding system. There is an increasing trend toward decreasing costs by reducing lengths of stay for inpatient psychiatric hospitalizations. This has a particular impact on the elderly, since Medicare's reimbursement rates for outpatient services are typically much lower than those of commercial insurance companies. Furthermore, under the existing Medicare fee schedule, longer office visits are reimbursed at a lower dollar amount per unit of encounter time than are shorter ones. Thus, health care professionals who see patients with more complex disorders earn less than those who treat healthier patients who require shorter visits (Gerety, 1994). Medicare's most recent Current Procedural Terminology (CPT) code allows billing for 5- to 15-min visits for medication management, enabling physicians who provide pharmacological interventions to see more patients per hour and thus mitigate the lowered reimbursement rates (Koenig, George, & Schneider, 1994). However, this strategy is not available to providers of the more time-intensive psychoeducational, cognitive, and behavioral therapies.

Depression

The number of published studies on psychotherapy with the healthy elderly is limited. Empirical and clinical papers on this topic have focused almost exclusively on mood disorders, and more recently on anxiety and substance abuse. There are even fewer studies that focus on patients with medical or neurological disease. In the following discussion, prevalence and prognosis, clinical significance, treatment barriers, and empirical outcome studies for these disorders are briefly summarized. Theoretical issues and types of treatment strategies are then reviewed, followed by a discussion of intervention guidelines and proposed modifications for older adults.

Prevalence and Prognosis

As in younger adults, depression is the most common emotional disorder presenting in late life (Butler, Lewis, & Sutherland, 1991). Estimates of clinically diagnosable depression range from 2–10% for major depression (Blazer, Hughes, & George, 1987) to 20–30% for less severe depressive illness and adjustment disorders (Butler et al., 1991). Multiple factors account for this variability in prevalence estimates, including (1) inconsistent application and choice of diagnostic criteria, (2) limitations of diagnostic instruments to adequately assess depression in medically ill and elderly populations, (3) overlap of depressive symptoms with a variety of chronic illnesses, (4) differences in sampling procedures, and (5) time intervals selected for prevalence and incidence estimates. Despite these methodological confounds, the fact that depression is a major health problem of older adults is indisputable.

Longitudinal studies investigating the course of late-life depression are few in number. The majority of existing reports document a relatively poor prognosis for untreated depression in the elderly, characterized by frequent and prolonged relapses (see review by Burvill, Stampfer, & Hall, 1986). For example, in one study of 64 elderly patients meeting *Diagnostic and Statistical Manual of Mental Disorders* third edition (*DSM-III*) criteria for major affective disorder, only 31% remained in good health, while 69% of these patients were determined to be "chronically impaired" or underwent frequent relapses at 6–24 months follow-up (Magni, Palazzolo, & Bianchin, 1988). According to the National Institute of Mental Health (NIMH) ECA study, advanced age, changes in health status and disability, sleep disturbance, and availability of formal support services have been shown to significantly affect onset and chronicity of depressive symptoms in older adults (see Kennedy, Kelman, & Thomas, 1991).

Clinical Significance

Differential diagnosis of depression in late life is complicated by an extensive overlap between signs and symptoms of normal aging, primary affective disorders, adverse reactions to medications, and neurological disease (Brown, Scott, Bench, & Dolan, 1994; Jenike, 1988). Perhaps the most compelling evidence of the clinical significance of depression in older adults is the incidence of completed suicide. In 1988, the completed suicide rate was 26.5 per 100,000 individuals between the ages of 80 and 84. This is more than twice the rate of 12.4 per 100,000 documented in the general population. Perhaps most alarming is the fact that over 75% of these individuals saw their primary care physician within 1 month prior to their death, and that most were experiencing their first episode of major depression which was neither treated nor apparently recognized by their physician (Conwell, Rotenberg, & Caine, 1990; National Institutes of Health [NIH], 1992).

Barriers to Treatment

Multiple treatment barriers have been blamed for the grim prognosis of depression in this age cohort. While progress has been made in understanding late-life depression, many obstacles to obtaining effective treatment persist. These barriers include undertreatment by primary care physicians, noncompliance with prescribed medication regimens, patients' reluctance to seek treatment for psychiatric illness, ageism in society and in the mental health community, and a paucity of research on the efficacy of psychotherapeutic interventions with older adults, particularly those with neurological or medical comorbidity.

General medicine physicians provide up to half of all outpatient mental health care (Regier et al., 1993). However, findings from studies examining physician care practices with regard to rate of detection and treatment of depression in older adults are sobering. In a recent investigation, Rogers, Wells, Meredith, Sturm, and Burnam (1993) found that less than half of the elderly patients in their sample received any form of counseling for acute episodes of depression. Significant problems in the prescribing practices for antidepressants have also been reported. These include discrepancies between self-reported treatment preferences and actual practice (Meredith, Wells, & Camp, 1994), frequent prescriptions for subtherapeutic dosage levels (Wells, Katon, Roberts, & Camp, 1994), and a reluctance to prescribe antidepressants for individuals with medical comorbidities (Lustman, Griffith, & Clouse, 1988). Undertreatment of depression by primary care physicians has also been attributed to limited training and clinical skill in the diagnosis and treatment of mental illness, attitudinal biases, and overreliance on biomedical models of psychological disorders (Alexopoulous, 1992; Callahan, Nienaber, Hendrie, & Tierney, 1992).

The treatment of choice for late-life depression is pharmacotherapy (NIH, 1992). The most recent class of antidepressants, selective serotonin reuptake inhibitors (SSRIs), holds several advantages in this age group. They have relatively few side effects because of their specificity for serotonin receptors. Also SSRIs have limited, if any, anticholinergic, antihistaminic, or alpha1-adrenergic reactions and do not appear to interfere with cognitive function (Dunner, 1994). Such advances hold considerable promise for regulating biochemical abnormalities associated with depression in the elderly. Still, even the best of antidepressant therapies are not considered to be a panacea given the potential adverse side effects (e.g., nausea, agitation, potential drug interactions) and numerous chronic diseases for which antidepressant drugs are contraindicated (Drevets, 1994; Dunner, 1994; Khan, Mirolo, Mirolo, & Dobie, 1993).

Medication noncompliance has been identified as another key obstacle in treating late-life depression. According to the NIH consensus statement, up to 70% of elderly patients take only 50–75% of the prescribed medication dose. Saltzman (1995) reported a similar rate of 40–75% medication noncompliance in this age group that he attributed to three primary causes: overuse and abuse, forgetting, and alteration of schedules and doses. Consequently, pharmacological treatment may not be indicated in some patients, and in others, treatment with drugs may first require interventions to enhance medication compliance. This provides a strong argument for the need to address the broader issues of life changes—such as the loss of loved ones, decline in physical health, and changes in psychosocial status—associated with depressive symptoms, rather than considering potential risks inherent to medication therapy alone.

Patients' attitudes toward treatment for affective disturbances contribute to the discouraging statistics regarding undertreatment and poor prognosis of late-life depression. For example, Waxman (1986) surveyed 88 senior center participants about their attitudes and practices regarding mental health services. Although 29% of the respondents endorsed symptoms of mild to moderate levels of depression, only 3% actually received treatment from a psychologist or psychiatrist for their symptoms. Sixty-three percent of subjects participating in the study reported that they would not inform a health professional about severe symptoms in the future, although 71.8% indicated that they would

tell a health professional about the onset of cardiac symptoms. Ninety percent reported that they would contact a family physician rather than a mental health professional if they chose to pursue treatment for depression. Finally, a similar majority identified general physicians, rather than psychologists or psychiatrists, as the "most effective" professional for treating depression or dementia (p. 296). The fact that older adults either do not seek treatment or choose to seek treatment from professionals who may not be adequately trained to manage emotional disorders deserves further attention and systematic investigation.

Doubts concerning psychotherapy as an effective treatment for emotional disorders in late life are not limited to older adults. Tacit beliefs that treatment efforts directed at the psychological problems of the elderly are "not worth the candle" (Freud, 1924) appear to persist among mental health professionals and extend equally to the general public (Zivian, Larsen, Gekowski, Knox, & Hatchette, 1994; Zivian, Larsen, Knox, Gekowski, & Hatchette, 1992). Thus, despite empirical evidence to the contrary, beliefs discounting the value and benefit of psychotherapy in older adults exist in many facets of today's society.

Unfortunately, the fields of psychological treatment and research have similarly failed to address the mental health problems of the elderly. Recently, Scogin and McElreath (1994) conducted a meta-analysis of published research on controlled psychosocial treatments for depression in older adults. Three methods were used in their literature search: (1) a computer search on key words and synonyms pertaining to treatment of depression in older adults from 1975 to 1990; (2) a literature search from 1970 to 1988 on journals considered likely to publish studies related to the treatment of late-age depression; and (3) a search of references listed in the articles located by the first two methods. A total of 17 articles—an average of only one per year—were retrieved. Importantly, results of this study found psychosocial treatments for depressive symptoms to be quite effective, with effect sizes comparable to depression treatments for other age groups. However, this small number of controlled studies not only underscores the lack of empirical and clinical interest in this patient population, but also emphasizes the limited scope of our scientific knowledge about nonpharmacologically based treatment in this arena.

Empirical Studies of Treatment Efficacy

In an era when mental health services are progressively shrinking in a rapidly aging society, establishing effective treatments for late-life depression presents a major challenge to health care providers. Recent outcome studies have supported the efficacy of group therapy in treating late-life depression. Gallagher-Thompson, Hanley-Peterson, and Thompson (1990) examined the frequency of depression relapse associated with brief cognitive, behavioral, and psychodynamic psychotherapy at posttreatment, 12- and 24-month followup. The percentage of patients who failed to meet research diagnostic criteria (RDC; Spitzer, Endicott, & Robins, 1978) for depressive disorder in each modality was 52%, 58%, and 70%, respectively. No differences emerged in the effectiveness of the three treatment protocols. The authors note that these figures are comparable to those documented in treatment studies with younger depressed patients and support the long-term benefit of psychotherapy in late life. Arean et al. (1993) examined the relative efficacy of social problem-solving therapy (PST) and reminiscence therapy (RT) in 74 subjects over the age of 55 who met RDC criteria for unipolar major depressive disorder. Subjects were randomly assigned to one of the two treatment conditions or to a wait-list control group. Therapy patients participated in 12 weekly sessions, with measures of self-report and observer-based depression administered at baseline, posttreatment, and 3-month follow-up. Results indicated significant reductions in depressive symptoms in both PST and RT conditions relative to controls. In addition, a greater number of PST patients demonstrated sufficient change to classify depression as improved or in remission relative to RT participants following completion of the study.

Beutler and colleagues (1987) investigated both relative and combined effectiveness of alprazolam and group cognitive therapy in 56 patients presenting with a first episode of unipolar depression. Subjects were assigned to one of four treatment conditions: medication only, placebo, cognitive therapy plus medication, and cognitive therapy plus placebo. Psychotherapy subjects completed a total of 20 group sessions. Results demonstrated a decrease in self-report of depressive symptoms and in electrophysiological indices of sleep impairment associated with cognitive group therapy. Medication assignment did not significantly affect these measures. Of note, differential changes were not documented on psychiatrists' ratings of depression severity (i.e., Hamilton Rating Scale for Depression [HAM-D]; Hamilton, 1967). The authors submit three findings other than patients' subjective ratings of improvement that support the effectiveness of psychotherapy in this patient sample: (1) continued benefit at 12-week follow-up, (2) concordance between subjective report and objective measures of sleep disturbance, and (3) greater motivation for continuing treatment, manifested by lower drop-out and dissatisfaction ratings in group versus medication-only conditions. This last point may be particularly important, given the estimates of low medication compliance in this age group, as discussed previously.

For many older adults, optimal treatment of depression may involve a combination of behavioral and pharmacological therapies. The efficacy of combining interpersonal psychotherapy (IPT) and medication therapy has been documented in a series of studies by Reynolds and colleagues (1994). For example, Reynolds et al. (1992) examined response and relapse rates of 61 elderly patients with moderate to severe recurrent depression. Subjects received approximately 9 weeks of acute therapy, consisting of combined medication and interpersonal psychotherapy, followed by 16 weeks of continuation therapy tapered to biweekly and finally triweekly sessions. Upon completion of continuation therapy, 65.7% of patients initially enrolled in the study and 78.7% of patients who fully completed the study were classified as treatment responders (i.e., HAM-D scores ≤ 10). Three patients (5%) achieved partial remission, with HAM-D scores between 11 and 14, and 16.4% were considered to be treatment failures, with HAM-D ratings of 15 or higher. Discontinuation of nortriptyline during the double-blind transition to maintenance therapy resulted in a relapse rate of 25%.

Systematic assessment of the differential and combined effectiveness of these therapies is beginning to emerge in the literature. Reynolds and colleagues are conducting an ongoing series of controlled investigations on the differential and combined prophylactic value of antidepressant therapy and IPT in reducing the risk of recurrent depression in older adults (Reynolds et al., 1992, 1994). Preliminary results thus far indicate benefit in all treatment conditions over placebo in preventing recurrence following 1 year of maintenance therapy. In summary, these findings support psychotherapy as an effective and lasting treatment for advanced age depression.

Anxiety

Prevalence and Prognosis

Anxiety disorders are common in late life, yet remain among the least studied (Sheikh, 1994). Blazer and colleagues' analysis of the Epidemiologic Catchment Area Program (ECAP) survey data revealed a 6-month prevalence of 19.7% for all anxiety disorders and a lifetime prevalence of 34.1% in individuals age 65 and older (Blazer, George, & Hughes, 1991). Lifetime prevalence rates of specific anxiety disorders range from a low of 0.29% for panic disorder to 16.1% for simple phobias. Because epidemiologic studies only include individuals who meet formal diagnostic criteria (e.g., *DSM-III-R*), current prevalence figures most likely underestimate the magnitude of the clinical problem due to exclusion of individuals with subsyndromal or subclinical states (Flint, 1994; Smith, Sherrill, & Colenda, 1995; Weiss, 1994). Information on the long-term course and prognosis of late-life anxiety disorders is virtually absent in the published literature (Sheikh, 1994).

Clinical Significance

Anxiety syndromes which occur in late life may be obscured by coexisting medical symptoms or viewed as a normal or expected aspect of aging. Weiss (1994) and others strongly challenge the validity of the latter view and emphasize the need for careful diagnosis and appropriate intervention of psychiatric symptoms in the elderly.

Proper diagnosis and treatment of anxiety disorders in the elderly are important for a variety of reasons. First, anxiety is often the presenting symptom in a wide range of otherwise asymptomatic medical disorders (e.g., cardiovascular, endocrinological, pulmonary, neurological). Second, anxiety disorders may produce medical complications in older adults, including cardiac arrhythmias and insomnia (see review by Sheikh, 1994). Early recognition and treatment of these disorders also may reduce the financial burden to society given the association between generalized anxiety disorders and excess medical and health care costs (Souetre et al., 1994).

Barriers to Treatment

Factors similar to those in late-life depression hinder efforts to adequately treat anxiety in older adults, including underrecognition and undertreatment by primary care physicians, medication noncompliance and inconsistent dosing, biases among the elderly against psychiatric or psychological treatment, and current treatment emphasis on pharmacological interventions. While several studies indicate that pharmacological treatment of late-life anxiety is effective (Sheikh, 1992, 1994; Smith et al., 1995; Tueth, 1993), issues of polypharmacy, drug interaction, medication side effects, and compliance discussed earlier with regard to depression are equally relevant here. Consequently, psychotherapeutic interventions may be the primary treatment choice for patients unable or unwilling to comply with a pharmacological regimen. Psychotherapy may also be a key adjunctive therapy to medication in effecting important behavioral changes.

Symptoms of anxiety may actually facilitate, rather than hinder, treatment-seeking behavior since they are often viewed by older adults as signs of medical illness. In our clinical experience, initial treatment that targets somatic features of emotional disorders are often better tolerated than those that primarily focus on patients' affective experience. Empirical support has been documented for treatment of select somatic symptoms which may be nonspecific signs of emotional distress. For example, preliminary results of a study investigating cognitive behavioral interventions for insomnia in older adults revealed not only that these procedures were effective, but that patients perceived these procedures to be enjoyable and nonthreatening (Friedman, Bliwise, Yesavage, & Salom, 1991). Other studies have similarly supported the effectiveness of behavioral treatments for late-life insomnia (see review by Engle-Friedman, Bootzin, Hazelwood, & Tsau, 1992).

Empirical Studies of Treatment Efficacy

Clinical research on the treatment of anxiety and related disorders is limited to case reports and a few studies investigating the application of specific therapeutic techniques for alleviating somatic symptoms of anxiety and depression. For example, relaxation training procedures have been successful in ameliorating a range of anxiety symptoms in older adults (Deberry, 1982; Sallis, Lichstein, Clarkson, Stalgaitis, & Campbell, 1983). Two common procedures, progressive relaxation (PR) and imaginal relaxation (IR), are known to be effective in younger patients with medical comorbidities (e.g., Decker, Cline-Elsen, & Gallagher, 1992; Gustafson, 1992). Progressive relaxation involves a series of systematic tensing and releasing of various muscle groups with concomitant attention to associated physiological changes. Imaginal relaxation techniques are varied and usually involve procedures in which one imagines pleasant scenes, events, or sensations. To our knowledge, only one controlled group study examining the efficacy of these procedures in older adults has been published. Scogin, Rickard, Keith, Wilson, and McElreath (1992) compared the efficacy of progressive versus imaginal relaxation procedures in a group of community dwelling older adults. Subjects were randomly assigned to one of three treatment conditions: PR, IR, or delayed treatment control (DC). Therapy subjects completed a series of four training sessions and 1-month follow-up. Relative to subjects in the delayed control condition, participants in the two training conditions reported a significant decrease in psychiatric symptoms. Both treatment groups produced lower scores on the state anxiety component of the State-Trait Anxiety Inventory (STAI; Spielberger, Gorsuch, & Lushene, 1970) and on the Symptom Checklist-90-Revised (SCL-90-R; Derogatis, 1977). No differences emerged in subjects' self-report of more long-standing anxiety, as indicated by comparable scores on the Trait scale of the STAI. Mixed results were found at follow-up, with continued improvement indicated by lower SCL-90-R scores, but higher scores on the State scale. The clinical utility of this study was to document the effectiveness of IR for patients in whom progressive muscle relaxation techniques are contraindicated, specifically in individuals with arthritis. The utility of these procedures in ameliorating symptoms of anxiety appears promising, but requires further empirical verification.

Obsessive–Compulsive Disorder

While it is unusual for obsessive–compulsive disorder (OCD) to first declare itself in late life, a significant number of older patients with preexisting OCD present for treatment in clinical settings (Jenike, 1991). The lifetime prevalence rate of OCD is approximately 3.3% in the general population and 2% for older adults (Blazer et al., 1991). Psychotherapy treatment studies of OCD in older adults consist of anecdotal case reports (e.g., Wise & Griffies, 1995; Woods & Britton, 1985). Several studies in which pharmacological intervention has been combined with exposure and response prevention have shown positive results (Riggs & Foa, 1993; Rowan, Holborn, Walker, & Siddiqui, 1984). In a recent review paper on OCD in the elderly, a case study was presented to illustrate successful amelioration of OCD symptoms through patient education, exposure and response prevention, and SSRI therapy (Calamari, Faber, Hitsman, & Poppe, 1994). Unfortunately, the methodology employed in these investigations does not allow for the separation of therapeutic effects attributed to psychotherapeutic interventions versus pharmacological treatment.

Alcoholism and Drug Abuse

A strong correlation between alcoholism and anxiety exists in the general population (Finlayson, Hurt, Davis, & Morse, 1988; Kushner, Sher, & Beitman, 1990). While this relationship does not hold in the current elderly cohort, impending demographic shifts over the next few decades may alter this trend. For these reasons, we have included the following discussion on alcohol and drug abuse in the elderly. A comprehensive review of substance abuse disorders in the elderly is presented in Chapter 9 of this volume.

Prevalence and Prognosis

Until recently, the extent of alcohol and drug dependence in older adults was not fully appreciated due to multiple factors, including (1) inaccurate beliefs that lifetime substance abusers died prematurely or spontaneously recovered before entering late adulthood, (2) the fact that symptoms of alcoholism can imitate symptoms of other medical disorders, (3) the failure of clinicians to recognize substance abuse disorders and make appropriate referrals for evaluation and treatment, and (4) the underreporting of drinking problems by older adults due to memory impairment, discouragement about recovery, and shame associated with the belief that substance abuse is immoral (Atkinson & Ganzini, 1994).

Prevalence data on alcoholism in the elderly are limited and inconsistent. Community-based prevalence rates range from 6% to 14% for heavy use and 1% to 17% for problematic use (Atkinson, 1990). One-month prevalence rates also vary according to gender, with ECA estimates of 1.8% and 0.3% for males and females, respectively, over age 65 (Regier et al., 1988). Methodological problems contributing to discordant prevalence estimates include (1) the lack of clear operational definitions for alcoholism, (2) difficulty in measuring alcohol use, (3) problems inherent to self-report indices, (4) impact of individual difference variables, and (5) differences in sample characteristics due to clinical setting (Czarnecki, Russell, Cooper, & Salter, 1990; Fleming, Bruno, Barry, & Fost, 1989; Liberto, Oslin, & Ruskin, 1992; Miller, Belkin, & Gold, 1991).

Surprisingly, the ECA data revealed a virtual absence of drug abuse/dependence in adults over the age of 65 (0.0, Regier et al., 1988). The clinical course and prognosis of substance abuse in the elderly is unknown.

Clinical Significance

The signs and symptoms of substance use/abuse may be difficult to detect due to their ability to imitate symptoms of other geriatric illnesses. For example, poor grooming, erratic changes in mood or behavior, frank depression, or bladder and bowel incontinence may be a result of unsuspected alcohol or drug use/abuse, but may also be associated with systemic disease, focal neurological disorder, or dementing illness (Atkinson & Ganzini, 1994). Chronic alcohol use/abuse also may cause or exacerbate existing medical problems which in turn may lead to increased disability, reduced adaptive functioning, and emotional distress. Potential medical complications include a decline in nutritional status, liver disease, peptic ulcer disease, gastritis, pancreatitis, cardiomyopathy, insomnia, and injury due to falls (see Liberto et al., 1992). Of particular concern, alcohol-related disorders may precipitate the development of neurological syndromes such as alcoholic dementia, Wernicke's encephalopathy, and Korsakoff's syndrome, which may each produce profound cognitive deficits (Kolb & Whishaw, 1990). Alcohol use/abuse also has been associated with the presence of depressive symptoms and with increased suicide risk in the aged (Conwell et al., 1990). Increased stress, retirement, death of a spouse, and health problems have been identified as factors that contribute to increased alcohol consumption or relapse after periods of sobriety in the elderly (Finlayson et al., 1988).

Precipitants of prescription drug dependence include insomnia, persistent family discord, and chronic pain syndromes (Atkinson & Ganzini, 1994). The latter finding is significant given that chronic pain is present in a substantial number of aged adults (see Closs, 1994). Finally, while illicit drug use is quite rare in the elderly, use of over-the-counter (OTC) medication is common. It has been estimated that over two thirds of older adults use at least one type of OTC medication on a regular basis (Miller et al., 1991). Consequently, multiple factors apparently predispose older adults to overreliance on or frank abuse of prescription and/or OTC medications.

Empirical Studies of Treatment Efficacy

Controlled trials examining treatment efficacy for substance abuse disorders in the elderly are scant. In a recent review of the literature, Liberto and colleagues (1992) cited only three treatment outcome studies which included older adults. Recently, the treatment efficacy of an inpatient program specifically designed for older alcoholics was compared to a traditional inpatient alcohol treatment program (Kashner, Rodell, Ogden, Guggenheim, & Karson, 1992). The older alcoholic rehabilitation program (OAR) focused on establishing peer relationships, building self-esteem, and setting time-limited goals. Both treatment groups showed improvement in the number of patients maintaining abstinence at follow-up, with higher abstinence rates documented for older OAR participants. This study illustrates the benefit of interventions that are tailored to the needs of the older adult population.

No systematic studies examining the treatment outcome for drug abuse in older adults have been reported.

Psychotherapeutic Approaches: Theoretical Issues and Clinical Applications

Assessment and evaluation are key steps preceding the implementation of psychotherapeutic interventions (Maloney & Ward, 1976; Weiner, 1976). Clinical assessment reflects the theoretical orientation and sophistication of the evaluator. Consequently, both assessment and psychotherapeutic work with the elderly require an understanding of developmental issues; medical, neuropsychological, and pharmacological aspects; and basic psychotherapeutic techniques.

Behavior Therapy

Behavior therapies, founded on classic learning theories, view behavior as the product of specific antecedent stimuli and consequential events (see Leahey & Harris, 1989). In this conceptualization, target behaviors are altered through interventions derived from systematic assessment and analysis of social–environmental interactions. Traditional behavioral interventions embrace a wide range of techniques to effect behavioral change, including participant modeling, self-monitoring, systematic desensitization, behavioral rehearsal, token reinforcement, behavior modification, and

stimulus control strategies (e.g., Franks & Barbrack, 1991; Haynes, 1991). The effectiveness of behavior therapies in altering maladaptive or dysfunctional behavior in older adults has been documented in a variety of settings. Successful treatment interventions have included stimulus control procedures to decrease incidents of wandering behavior and increase social interaction, as well as contingency management techniques to increase exercise participation and independent eating and to reduce urinary incontinence (Fisher & Carstensen, 1990; Keating, Schulte, & Miller, 1988; Yu, Kaltreider, Hu, & Craighead, 1991).

In addition to altering such target behaviors, traditional learning theories have been used to effect broader clinical issues with older adults. Empirical data supporting the effectiveness of behavioral interventions in the elderly are primarily derived from studies of late-life depression. Classic behavior theory predicts a cycle of stimulus–response contingencies in which increased depression is a consequence of a decrease in positive person–environment interactions and/or increased aversive interactions (Lewinsohn, Antonuccio, Steinmetz, & Teri, 1984). The focus of therapeutic intervention is to alter maladaptive behavior by increasing exposure and participation in pleasant events and minimizing aversive interactions.

Cognitive Behavior Therapy

Cognitive therapies are founded upon the assumption that many disorders result from idiosyncratic patterns of thinking, attitudes, and beliefs. Techniques derived from these therapies have been particularly effective in treating late-life depression. Two of the major cognitive theories applicable to older adults are the learned helplessness model formulated by Seligman and colleagues (Overmier & Seligman, 1967; Maier & Seligman, 1976) and Beck's (1967) cognitive theory of depression.

Based on a series of animal learning studies, Seligman posited that individuals exposed to uncontrollable situations may develop deficits in motivation, learning, and emotional responsivity. Eventually these individuals come to believe that their responses are independent of environmental outcomes. This perception of uncontrollability then generalizes to new situations, producing maladaptive behavior and low self-efficacy expectations manifested as clinical depression (see Abramson, Seligman, & Teasdale, 1978). Empirical support for this model (and subsequent reformulations) has been documented in experimental studies and in investigations of clinically depressed college students (e.g., Hiroto & Seligman, 1975; Metalsky, Abramson, Seligman, Semmel, & Peterson, 1982; Peterson & Seligman, 1984). According to the learned helplessness model, depression in older adults is associated with a perceived loss of control that has generalized from past experiences of unpredictable and uncontrollable losses (e.g., loss of a spouse or loved one, physical decline, retirement). In support of this theory, a recent study documented a significant relationship between intensity of hopelessness and suicidal behavior in older adults with recurrent depression (Rifai, George, Stack, Mann, & Reynolds, 1994).

Beck's cognitive theory of depression (Beck, 1967, 1976; Beck, Rush, Shaw, & Emery, 1979) posits that negative cognitions and biases represent a psychological predisposition derived from traumatic early childhood experiences of loss. In turn, these negative experiences condition future responses to stress (Brown & Harris, 1978; Lloyd, 1980) and foster the development of depressogenic cognitive schemas. Consistent with a diathesis-stress model, this schema remains dormant until the individual is exposed to idiosyncratic stressors which render the person vulnerable to the emergence of a depressive syndrome. Eventually unrealistic and negative distortions about the self, world, and future (Beck's negative triad) come to dominate the depressive's thoughts and actions. By far, the majority of outcome studies involving psychotherapeutic interventions with older adults have involved therapies based on Beck's cognitive distortion model. The therapeutic focus of these approaches is on systematically challenging and modifying dysfunctional thoughts, attitudes, and beliefs. In addition to decreasing depressive symptoms, adaptations of this approach have been quite successful in the treatment of late-life insomnia (e.g., Morin, Kowatch, Barry, & Walton, 1993).

A related theory of late-life depression is the social problem-solving model developed by Nezu and colleagues (Nezu, 1987; Nezu & Perri, 1989). According to this model, depression results from breakdowns in problem-solving skills which arise from ineffective coping under stress. Nezu's social problem-solving therapy (PST) consists of five components. First, there exists a set of orienting responses that includes "beliefs, assumptions, appraisals, and expectations concerning life's problems and one's own general problem-solving ability" (Nezu & Perri, 1989, p. 408). The remaining components involve a set of skills or goal-directed tasks which allow for successful solutions to stressful problems: problem definition and formulation, generation of alternative solutions, decision-making, and solution implementation and verification. Therapeutic efforts are directed toward increasing the depressive's motivation in the problem orientation process by modifying beliefs or attitudes that hinder the ability to produce effective problem-solving responses. Nezu and colleagues have recently documented the utility of this model in treating late-life depression (Arean et al., 1993).

In summary, the efficacy of cognitive behavior therapies in treating older adults has received considerable empirical support. The continued popularity of these approaches in working with older patients has been attributed to their focus on patient education, emphasis on active interchange between the therapist and patient, and their time-limited course (Blazer, 1989).

Psychodynamic Therapies

Traditional dynamic psychotherapies emerged from the work of early object relations theorists, including Freud, Abraham, Klein, and Winnecott. The central tenet of such theories is that our interpersonal relationships, rooted in early caretaking experiences, create a complex internal world shaped by both conscious and unconscious mental processes. Pathological states and behavior are considered to be overt manifestations of unresolved internal or psychodynamic conflicts. More recent theorists have emphasized the importance of the concept of the self (e.g., Grossman, 1982; Kernberg, 1982; Kohut, 1971, 1977). Revised constructs have led to the development of a new phenomenological approach, in which cognitive and affective processes are incorporated into the more traditional analytic framework. Discussion and exploration of these beliefs within the therapeutic relationship is therefore intended to disconfirm patients' pathological expectations (see review by Blatt & Lerner, 1991). Grief, guilt, reactions to loss, and central issues that reflect the patient's "chronically endured pain" (Mann, 1973) are typical themes explored within a dynamic framework.

The complexity of traditional dynamic therapies requires careful patient selection in order to promote therapeutic change. Myers (1991) identified several criteria used to determine which patients would benefit from psychoanalytic psychotherapy and psychoanalysis in late life. These criteria include the individual's degree of object relatedness, attunement to unconscious processes, depth of motivation for change, and additional factors such as sufficient intellectual level, success experiences in at least one area of life, and capacity to tolerate strong affect. Diagnostic contraindications for dynamic therapy include individuals who present with severe emotional disturbances, such as psychoses, borderline or narcissistic personality disorders, drug or alcohol abuse, chronic depression, and acute suicidal ideation and intent (Rosenberg, 1985). Support for the efficacy of traditional dynamic therapies in late life has been documented in multiple case reports (e.g., Nemiroff & Colarusso, 1985; Sadavoy & Leszcz, 1987), but has not been systematically assessed. Nonetheless, these findings are in keeping with Abraham's strong contention that "the age of the neuroses is more important than the age of the patient" (Abraham, 1919/1953)

Two other psychoanalytically based approaches to treating depression in late life are life review and reminiscence therapies. Although both therapies are considered useful in alleviating psychological distress in older adult patients, neither has been reliably tested under well-controlled conditions. They are included in this text because of their unique application and potential benefit to elderly patients.

Life review therapy (Butler, 1963) is a systematic approach that draws heavily from Erikson's stage theory of development. The purpose of this approach is to reexperience, rework, and resolve old conflicts in order to integrate life experiences and thereby restore ego integrity (Lewis & Butler, 1974). Therapeutic techniques associated with life review include requests that the patient tape or write an autobiography which allows the therapist to identify key points of emphasis and exclusion. Other tools used to facilitate this process include review of photographs or other personal memorabilia. Evaluation and analysis of important life experiences is thus believed to provide a sense of closure, meaning, fulfillment, and resolution to one's life. The efficacy of this approach in treating late-life depression has been empirically documented (e.g., Goldwasser, Aurbach, & Harkins, 1987; Rattenbury & Stones, 1989).

Reminiscence therapy is a closely related therapeutic process that is often confused with life review. Unlike life review, the focus of reminiscence therapy is on the recollection and sharing of life memories as a means to enhance self-esteem and social intimacy, rather than to directly resolve dynamic conflicts (Teri & McCurry, 1994). Authors advocating this approach maintain that late-life depression is preceded by multiple experiences of loss, rejection, and exposure to negative life events (e.g., Mueller, Edwards, & Yarvis, 1977). The psychosocial consequences to the elderly are purportedly exacerbated by a lack of skill and/or opportunity to engage in adaptation following serious life events. Thus, the purpose of intervention is twofold: (1) eliciting a retrospective account of meaningful dimensions of life, and (2) using this account to overcome intrusion and avoidance previously inhibiting clear recollection of past events (Horowitz, Wilner, Marmar, & Krupnick, 1980). This procedure reportedly has been successfully used by a range of mental health professionals, including social workers and nursing staff, in both institutionalized and outpatient settings (Hewett, Asamen, Hedgepeth, & Dietch, 1991; Soltys & Coats, 1994).

At least one study demonstrated the efficacy of structured versus unstructured reminiscence training in depressed elderly subjects compared to a group of control subjects who engaged in conversation only (Fry, 1983). Participants in the structured program evidenced greater improvement of depressive symptoms, increased self-confidence, and greater perceived personal adequacy relative to subjects in the unstructured reminiscence condition. Both treatment groups demonstrated significant improvement relative to controls.

Therapeutic Considerations and Modifications for Healthy and Cognitively Intact Elderly

Assessment Issues

The importance of the initial diagnostic assessment in treatment selection and planning cannot be overstated. Information gathered in this phase of treatment is critical to providing appropriate and effective treatment of emotional disorders in late life. We begin our discussion of three topics under this final section with a framework for clinical decision-making developed by Sadavoy (1994). This section is followed by a selected review of general considerations and recommendations for psychotherapy with neurologically intact older adults. We conclude this chapter with a discussion that highlights treatment issues and modifications

for neurologically impaired patients based upon assessment of the patients' neuropsychological restrictions and competencies.

Sadavoy's Model

In light of the varied and complex issues associated with emotional disorders in late life, Sadavoy (1994) emphasizes the "therapeutic necessity" of employing treatment strategies with older adults that are both interactive and integrative. To this end, Sadavoy formalized a decision-making schema that details important features of clinical assessment and provides pathways to facilitate sound therapeutic recommendations for elderly patients (see Figure 1). The five major decision-making stages of this model are summarized below.

In the first stage of Sadavoy's model, issues relevant to various treatment modalities are investi-

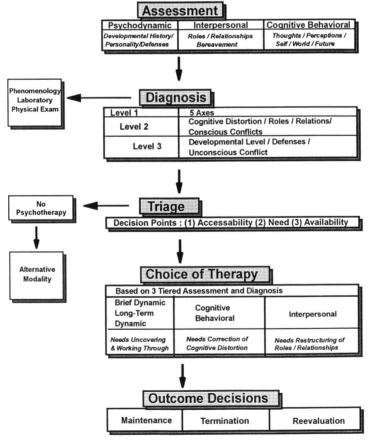

FIGURE 1. Sadavoy's psychotherapy decision pathway.

gated. Within the psychodynamic realm, patients' developmental history, personality structure, and defense mechanisms are explored. The author appropriately emphasizes that developmental history is often omitted in the assessment of older adults, despite the importance of this information in understanding patients' strengths and weaknesses, ability to cope with past stressors, and typical or habitual patterns of behavior. These issues may significantly affect the clinician's ability to identify key therapeutic issues and to make well-founded decisions regarding the appropriateness of the patient for psychodynamic treatment. In our experience, the *process* of gathering a detailed developmental history serves important clinical purposes. Perhaps most importantly, it provides structure for the therapist to enter into an increasingly personal and intimate discussion with the patient. This enhances rapport and helps establish a productive working alliance. Social roles, relationships with others, and losses are similarly evaluated in the context of assessing changes in interpersonal relationships associated with the stress of life transitions and aging, as well as assessing more static or long-standing patterns of social interaction. Finally, patients' attitudes, beliefs, and perceptions of the self, world, and future are elicited. Attention to themes associated with aging, such as physical and mental competencies, abandonment, and bereavement, is likely to provide insight into the nature and extent of cognitive distortion amenable to cognitive behavioral interventions.

The second stage of assessment encompasses three levels of diagnostic formulation. The first level entails formal diagnosis of emotional status according to a traditional multi-axial system. The second and third levels indicate diagnostic conclusions regarding the patient's behaviors and thought processes and the level of emotional maturity reflected by the patient's defense mechanisms and internal conflicts.

The third stage of evaluation involves triage decisions regarding the appropriateness of both the patient and the clinical problem for psychotherapeutic intervention. At this point, decisions are made as to treatment accessibility, need, and availability. Accessibility is determined by physical status, "mental frailty," and the ability to overcome both attitudinal and environmental treatment barriers. Decisions of need depend on whether the clinical problem requires active intervention, or whether sufficient improvement is likely to occur in the absence of formal treatment due to the natural course of resolution and/or availability of preexisting resources. Availability is determined by surveying treatments which are at hand to treat the patient's emotional disorder.

The next decision-making stage involves selecting an optimal therapeutic approach. This decision is based upon information gathered and analyzed in the earlier stages of assessment and diagnosis. Given the paucity of empirically based guidelines, selection of the therapeutic modality is typically based upon the therapist's knowledge about the nature of the patient's problem and the efficacy of a given approach in treating a specific patient. An important point highlighted by Sadavoy (1994) is that the choice of a given therapy should not preclude inclusion of, or a change to, another therapeutic approach. The fluidity of this system provides sufficient flexibility for establishing fundamental elements of therapy and adapting to potential changes or reevaluations of health and cognitive/emotional status.

The last stage represents the final pathway leading to outcome decisions regarding therapeutic maintenance, termination, and reevaluation. Endpoint decisions may vary according to the therapeutic modality(ies).

Treatment Issues

In the absence of significant health or physical disabilities, traditional psychotherapeutic approaches require minimal, if any, modification in their application to healthy older adults. However, therapists working with elderly patients should be aware of issues that may affect treatment efficacy, including the potential need to modify fundamental approaches, the need to attend to problems or complications associated with sensory deficits, and the need to minimize the impact of attitudinal barriers on the working alliance and therapeutic process.

Gallagher and Thompson (1983) offer the following guidelines in the application of cognitive behavioral interventions to problems of late-life depression: (1) the assumption of an active role by the therapist in socializing the older adult into treatment, (2) the implementation of strategies that enhance the learning ability of the patient (e.g., multi-modal presentation of information, use of age and personally relevant examples in therapy, and minimizing risk aversion, which may impede a patient's willingness and ability to seek novel rewarding experiences), and (3) the careful preparation for termination by the gradual tapering of sessions. Other authors have stressed the importance of setting specific therapeutic goals, the need for greater therapist involvement in the therapeutic process, and the need for therapists to directly confront problems associated with patient passivity (e.g., Pfeiffer, 1976; Weiner, 1975). While similar issues may arise in treating younger patients, they often demand a greater amount of therapeutic attention in older adults.

Another important consideration in working with older adults is age-related declines in auditory and visual processing abilities. Primary sensory deficits can significantly interfere with the patient's ability to participate in psychotherapeutic assessment and treatment efforts. For example, high-frequency hearing loss increases with age and occurs in approximately 60% of individuals ages 71 to 80 (Davis, Ostri, & Parving, 1990). If unrecognized, such deficits may adversely affect the patient's ability to understand therapeutic discussions and respond to the therapist's rapport-building efforts and otherwise disrupt the therapeutic process. Even subtle auditory deficits may lead to overestimation of psychopathology and to unnecessary or inappropriate treatment (Kreeger, Raulin, Grace, & Priest, 1995; Stein, 1990). Declines in vision occur in the course of normal aging (Hazzard, Andres, Bierman, & Blass, 1990) and may similarly complicate cognitive and therapeutic assessment. In one study, 13% of patients with age-related macular degeneration experienced visual hallucinations unrelated to primary psychiatric disorder (Holroyd et al., 1992). History of stroke, lowered cognitive status, living alone, and bilaterally impaired visual acuity were associated with the presence of hallucinations. Such patients are likely to be at greater risk for error in diagnostic classification and for inappropriate treatment referral. These age-related changes can result in spuriously low scores on formal tests of neuropsychological functioning and lead to erroneous inferences about the cognitive status of older adults (Lezak, 1995, p. 135). Assessment procedures may require modifications that take into account slower speed of information processing, such as stimulus pacing and providing ample time for the patients to respond (Botwinick, 1981). Practical yet often overlooked suggestions in therapeutic work with sensory-impaired older adults include making explicit inquiries regarding the need and use of functional hearing aids and glasses, speaking in a lowered pitch, and using large and high-contrast print for educational or other therapeutic purposes.

Establishment of a strong working alliance is one of the most important therapeutic tasks regardless of age. However, more time and effort is typically devoted to rapport-building with older adults, due to a variety of attitudinal factors and other treatment barriers. In our clinical experience, initial efforts to "normalize" the patient's experience of psychological distress are often critical to the development of a good working relationship. Discussing depression or anxiety as a more intense, though treatable, version of distress experienced by all adults may be particularly helpful in dispelling patients' beliefs that they are "crazy" or "weak" for seeking psychological services. This is not to be confused with endorsing the fallacy that emotional distress is an expected or normal part of the aging process. Depression, anxiety, and other emotional disorders of late life result in *excess* burden and are not considered endemic to proceeding through later developmental stages.

Therapeutic Considerations and Modifications for Cognitively Impaired Elderly

Assessment Issues

As previously discussed, the first step of the treatment selection and planning process is diagnostic assessment. Emotional and behavioral sequelae are common in a variety of neurological disorders. For example, mood disorders, personality changes, and explosive behavior are frequent concomitants of Huntington's disease (Mendez, 1994); apathy, depression, and behavior dyscontrol may be concomitants of stroke and of frontal lobe insults (Stuss, Gow, & Hetherington, 1992); nondominant hemisphere damage may produce impaired comprehension of emotional prosody and expression (Blonder, Bowers, & Heilman, 1991; Starkstein, Federoff, Price, Leiguarda, & Robinson, 1993); and depression is evidenced in approximately 40% of patients with Parkinson's disease (Cummings, 1992) and in approximately 17–29% of patients with Alzheimer's disease (AD) (Teri & Wagner, 1992). Thus, formal assessment of both emotional and cognitive functions is an important step in treatment planning for older adults with known or suspected neurological disorders.

There are at least two major reasons that underscore the need for a detailed cognitive evaluation of elderly patients who present with psychiatric complaints. First, depression and anxiety may herald an undeclared dementing illness (Seigel & Gershon, 1986). There is a high degree of overlap among signs of normal aging, affective disorders, and neurological illness in this cohort. For example, the most common emotional reaction associated with AD is depression. The signs and symptoms of depression in AD are usually similar to those of younger depressives, including depressed mood, alterations in appetite and sleep behaviors (particularly increased nighttime awakenings), anhedonia, and social isolation and withdrawal. Moreover, depression in the elderly is commonly manifested as subjective complaints and/or documented impairment of cognitive decline that resolves with treatment (Cummings, 1989). Thus, one of the most challenging diagnostic problems is differentiating a treatable depression from an irreversible dementia. As emphasized by Kaszniak and Christenson (1994), "the risks of misdiagnosis, and the potential benefits of accurate diagnosis, make strong arguments for the importance of careful diagnostic evaluation."

Three primary goals for the formal assessment of geriatric patients are (1) to establish the individual's cognitive and behavioral strengths and weaknesses, (2) to interpret findings from a diagnostic perspective, and (3) to develop treatment and rehabilitation recommendations based on the neuropsychological examination findings (La Rue, 1992). As with younger patients, a broad range of cognitive domains should be evaluated. These include, but are not limited to, attention and concentration, language, general intelligence, judgment, abstract reasoning and executive functioning, learning and memory, visuospatial skills, fine motor speed, co-

ordination and strength, as well as functional strengths and deficits (Kaszniak, 1990; Lezak, 1995; Lovell & Nussbaum, 1994). It is also important to assess potential restrictions in insight and deficit awareness due to neurological compromise and to appreciate the relative contribution and/or potential confound of psychological defense mechanisms such as denial (see Prigatano & Schacter, 1991).

In addition to providing diagnostic information, neuropsychological findings play an important role in therapeutic decision-making. Returning to Sadavoy's multi-stage model, cognitive decline, concurrent illness, and general frailty are identified as factors that can significantly influence the patient's ability to successfully engage in psychotherapy. Neuropsychological evaluation provides a systematic means of obtaining this important information. It also provides a baseline from which important changes in cognition can be detected over time. For example, remission of memory impairment over the course of treatment for depression would suggest a nondementing illness, whereas a progressive deterioration in mnestic and other cognitive functions would suggest a degenerative dementia. Neuropsychological examination also enhances the therapeutic relationship, for it shows that the patient's cognitive complaints are taken seriously. In patients with a primary affective disorder or the dementia syndrome of depression (formerly termed "pseudodementia"), neuropsychological findings may allay the patient's fears regarding the severity of perceived impairment. In all, formal assessment of cognitive status not only facilitates sound treatment decisions, but may also help develop a meaningful and clinically effective therapeutic alliance.

Treatment Issues

Psychotherapy is often a useful means of ameliorating excess disability in older adults, although the range of psychotherapeutic approaches for individuals with neurological disorders may be more restricted than for those without cognitive impairment. To date, the utility of psychotherapeutic interventions in cognitively impaired elderly has received little empirical attention. Current understanding of treatment issues is largely an extension of a sparse literature on the effectiveness of behavioral interventions in treating the emotional and behavioral sequelae of AD.

A review of psychotherapeutic interventions with AD patients was recently detailed by Bonder (1994). Multiple treatment options, similar to those employed with neurologically intact adults, are available to individuals in the early stages of a dementing illness. Treatment goals may be varied, but often include providing emotional support, developing and augmenting existing coping mechanisms, enhancing existing intellectual abilities, and restoring a sense of ego integrity, self-efficacy, and mastery.

Several treatment modifications may be necessary to compensate for restrictions in higher cerebral functions associated with AD. Memory dysfunction, impaired abstract reasoning, and restrictions in language processing are typical features of AD, although the severity and constellation of deficits vary over the course of the illness (Cummings & Benson, 1992). Solomon and Szwabo (1992) note that verbal therapies may need to be modified for these patients. They advise therapists to use concrete rather than abstract interpretations and to avoid paradoxical interventions. Confrontation should be highly selective and carefully worded to avoid confusion and paranoid reactions. To compensate for memory impairment in AD, Bonder (1994) highlights the need for frequent repetition of themes and specific information, review and restatement, and shorter but more frequent therapy sessions. Note-taking, audiotaping of selected information, and providing patients with written summary statements of key points addressed during the therapy session are tools which similarly may lessen the effects of memory impairment. In late stages of the disease, verbal interventions become increasingly more difficult. Several authors have suggested that encouraging patients to engage in expressive arts (e.g., art, music, and movement therapies) allows for improved communication and pleasurable experiences which may otherwise be missed (Lipe, 1991; Smith, 1992).

The Seattle Protocol for Behavioral Treatment of Depressed Demented Patients is an example of how traditional therapies have been successfully modified for this clinical population (see Teri, 1986, 1991; Teri & Uomoto, 1991). The protocol is based upon classic learning theory, with the intent of identifying experiences which are potentially enjoyable and increasing patients' involvement in these positive activities. Patients and caregivers initially receive instruction to facilitate basic understanding of the treatment rationale, to broaden existing knowledge about the nature of AD, and to develop a working knowledge about the fundamental tenets of behavior change. Ongoing educational instruction is used to promote patient and caregiver skill in the development and implementation of strategies to increase the patient's participation in pleasant activities. Additional instruction is provided to address behavioral and practical problems, to maximize patients' cognitive and functional abilities, and to reduce caregiver burden. Toward the end of treatment, plans are made for the maintenance and generalization of treatment gains following termination. A major component of the Seattle protocol is caregiver involvement. For patients in moderate to severe stages of AD, the caregiver role is expanded such that the caregiver actively participates in the structuring of daily activities, monitors the patient's mood and activity level, and reinforces the patient's participation in pleasurable events. This important modification allows for continued treatment beyond the scope of traditional therapies. Additionally, this approach reduces caregiver burden, a major precipitant of institutionalization (e.g., Steele, Rovner, Chase, & Folstein, 1990). Preliminary results of this research documented improvement in both patient and caregiver depression (Teri, 1994).

Summary and Conclusions

The psychological, social, health, and economic needs of older adults are multifaceted and often underrecognized. Psychological assessment and treatment planning for this population require considerable gathering, sorting, integration, and interpretation of clinically relevant information. To this end, Sadavoy's (1994) decision-making schema emphasizes integration of data from varied sources, details important features of clinical assessment, and provides pathways to facilitate sound psychotherapeutic recommendations for elderly patients.

There is a small but growing body of literature supporting the efficacy of a variety of psychotherapeutic interventions for late-life emotional disorders. An even more limited but increasing amount of empirical data have similarly demonstrated the effectiveness of psychological techniques for elderly patients with neurologically based cognitive impairment. Although most psychotherapeutic techniques can be used with otherwise healthy elderly patients with little or no modifications, substantial alterations may be required when interventions are applied to individuals with neurological disorders. In this regard, the neuropsychological evaluation plays an important role in the formulation of sound psychotherapeutic treatment plans. The need to alter established techniques to account for changes in physical and/or neuropsychological functioning in older adult patients should also be considered.

Further empirical work documenting treatment efficacy of late-life emotional disorders is needed. Controlled studies are required to determine which techniques are best suited to both cognitively intact and neurologically impaired elderly. In these times of cost containment, professionals working with geriatric patients must further scientific advances and advocate for appropriate services for this population.

References

Abraham, K. (1953). The applicability of psycho-analytic treatment to patients at an advanced age. In *Selected papers*. New York: Basic Books. (Original work published 1919).

Abramson, L. Y., Seligman, M. E. P., & Teasdale, J. D. (1978). Learned helplessness in humans: Critique and reformulation. *Journal of Abnormal Psychology, 87*, 49–74.

Alexopoulous, G. S. (1992). Geriatric depression reaches maturity. *International Journal of Geriatric Psychiatry, 7*, 305–362.

Arean, P. A., Perri, M. G., Nezu, A. M., Schein, R. L., Christopher, F., & Joseph, T. X. (1993). Comparative effectiveness of social problem-solving therapy and reminiscence therapy for depression in older adults. *Journal of Consulting and Clinical Psychology, 61*(6), 1003–1010.

Atkinson, R. M. (1990). Aging and alcohol use disorders: Diagnostic issues in the elderly. *International Psychogeriatrics, 2*, 55–72.

Atkinson, R. M., & Ganzini, L. (1994). Substance abuse. In E. C. Coffey & J. L. Cummings (Eds.), *Textbook of geriatric neuropsychiatry*. Washington, DC: American Psychiatric Press.

Beck, A. (1967). *Depression: Clinical, experimental, and theoretical aspects*. New York: Harper & Row.

Beck, A. T. (1976). *Cognitive therapy and the emotional disorders*. New York: International Universities Press.

Beck, A. T., Rush, A. J., Shaw, B. F., & Emery, G. (1979). *Cognitive therapy of depression: A treatment manual*. New York: Guilford Press.

Beutler, L. E., Scogin, F., Kirkish, P., Schretlen, D., Corbishley, A., Hamblin, D., Meredith, K., Potter, R., Bamford, C. R., & Levenson, A. I. (1987). Group cognitive therapy and alprazolam in the treatment of depression in older adults. *Journal of Consulting and Clinical Psychology, 55*, 550–556.

Blatt, S. J., & Lerner, H. (1991). Psychodynamic perspectives on personality theory. In M. Hersen, A. E. Kazdin, & A. S. Bellack (Eds.), *The clinical psychology handbook* (2nd ed.). New York: Pergamon Press.

Blazer, D. (1989). Medical intelligence, current concepts: Depression in the elderly. *The New England Journal of Medicine, 320*(3), 164–166.

Blazer, D., Hughes, D. C., & George, L. K. (1987). The epidemiology of depression in an elderly community population. *The Gerontologist, 27*, 281–287.

Blazer, D., George, L. K., & Hughes, D. (1991). The epidemiology of anxiety disorders: An age comparison. In C. Saltzman & B. D. Lebowitz (Eds.), *Anxiety in the elderly*. New York: Springer.

Blonder, L. S., Bowers, D., & Heilman, K. M. (1991). The role of the right hemisphere in emotional communication. *Brain, 114*, 1115–1127.

Bonder, B. R. (1994). Psychotherapy for individuals with Alzheimer's disease. *Alzheimer's Disease and Related Disorders, 8*(Suppl. 3), 75–81.

Botwinick, J. (1981). Neuropsychology of aging. In S. B. Filskov & T. J. Boll (Eds.), *Handbook of clinical neuropsychology*. New York: John Wiley and Sons.

Brown, G. W., & Harris, T. (1978). *Social origins of depression: A study of psychiatric disorders in women*. New York: Free Press.

Brown, R. G., Scott, L. D., Bench, C. J., & Dolan, R. J. (1994). Cognitive function in depression: Its relationship to the presence and severity of intellectual decline. *Psychological Medicine, 2*(4), 829–847.

Burvill, P. W., Stampfer, H., & Hall, W. (1986). Does depressive illness in the elderly have a poor prognosis? *Australian and New Zealand Journal of Psychiatry, 20*, 422–427.

Butler, R. N. (1963). The life review: An interpretation of reminiscence in the aged. *Psychiatry, 26*, 65–76.

Butler, R. N., Lewis, M. I., & Sutherland, T. (1991). *Aging and mental health: Positive psychosocial and biomedical approaches* (4th ed.). Columbus, OH: Charles E. Merrill.

Calamari, J. E., Faber, S. D., Hitsman, B. L., & Poppe, C. J. (1994). Treatment of obsessive compulsive disorders in the elderly: A review and case example. *Journal of Behavior Therapy and Experimental Psychiatry, 25*(2), 95–104.

Callahan, M., Nienaber, N. A., Hendrie, H. C., & Tierney, W. M. (1992). Depression of elderly outpatients: Primary care physicians' attitudes and practice patterns. *Journal of General Internal Medicine, 7*, 26–31.

Closs, S. J. (1994). Pain in elderly patients: A neglected phenomenon? *Journal of Advanced Nursing, 19*, 1072–1081.

Conwell, Y., Rotenberg, M., & Caine, E. D. (1990). Completed suicide at age 50 and over. *Journal of the American Geriatrics Society, 38*, 640–644.

Cummings, J. L. (1989). Dementia and depression: An evolving enigma. *Journal of Neuropsychiatry Clinical Neurosciences, 1*(3), 236–242.

Cummings, J. L. (1992), Depression in Parkinson's disease: A review. *American Journal of Psychiatry, 149*, 443–454.

Cummings, J. L., & Benson, D. F. (1992). *Dementia: A clinical approach* (2nd ed.). Boston: Butterworth-Heinemann.

Czarnecki, D. M., Russell, M., Cooper, M. L., & Salter, D. (1990). Five year reliability of self-reported alcohol consumption. *Journal of Studies on Alcohol, 51*, 68–76.

Davis, A. C., Ostri, B., & Parving, A. (1990). Longitudinal study of hearing. *Acta Otolaryngologica (Stockholm), 476*(Suppl.), 12–22.

Deberry, S. (1982). The effects of meditation-relaxation on anxiety and depression in a geriatric population. *Psychotherapy: Theory, Research, and Practice, 4*, 512–521.

Decker, T. W., Cline-Elsen, J., & Gallagher, M. (1992). Relaxation therapy as an adjunct in radiation oncology. *Journal of Clinical Psychology, 48*(3), 388–393.

Derogatis, L. R. (1977). *The SCL-90-R: Administration, scoring and procedures manual.* Baltimore, MD: Clinical Psychometric Research.

Drevets, W. C. (1994). Geriatric depression: Brain imaging correlates and pharmacologic considerations. *Journal of Clinical Psychiatry, 55*(9, Suppl. A), 71–81.

Dunner, D. L. (1994). Therapeutic considerations in treating depression in the elderly. *Journal of Clinical Psychiatry, 55*(12, Suppl.), 48–58.

Engle-Friedman, M., Bootzin, R. R., Hazelwood, L., & Tsau, C. (1992). An evaluation of behavioral treatments for insomnia in the older adult. *Journal of Clinical Psychology, 48*(1), 77–90.

Finlayson, R. E., Hurt, R. D., Davis, L. J., & Morse, R. M. (1988). Alcoholism in elderly persons: A study of the psychiatric and psychosocial features of 216 patients. *Mayo Clinic Proceedings, 63*, 761–768.

Fisher, J. E., & Carstensen, L. L. (1990). Behavior management of the dementias. *Clinical Psychology Review, 10*, 611–629.

Fleming, M. R., Bruno, M., Barry, K., & Fost, N. (1989). Informed consent, deception, and the use of disguised alcohol questionnaires. *American Journal of Drug and Alcohol Abuse, 15*, 309–319.

Flint, A. J. (1994). Epidemiology and comorbidity of anxiety disorders in the elderly. *American Journal of Psychiatry, 151*(5), 640–649.

Franks, C. M., & Barbrack, C. R. (1991). Behavior therapy with adults: An integrative perspective for the nineties. In M. Hersen, A. E. Kazdin, & A. S. Bellack (Eds.), *The clinical psychology handbook* (2nd ed., pp. 551–556). Elmsford, NY: Pergamon Press.

Freud, S. (1924). On psychotherapy. In *Collected Papers* (Vol. 1). London: Hogarth Press.

Friedman, L., Bliwise, D. L., Yesavage, J. A., & Salom, S. R. (1991). A preliminary study comparing sleep restriction and relaxation treatments for insomnia in older adults. *Journal of Gerontology: Psychological Sciences, 46*, 1–8.

Fry, P. S. (1983). Structured and unstructured reminiscence training and depression among the elderly. *Clinical Gerontologist, 3*, 15–37.

Gallagher, D. E., & Thompson, L. W. (1983). Cognitive therapy for depression in the elderly: A promising model for treatment and research. In L. D. Breslau & M. R. Haug (Eds.), *Depression and aging: Causes, care, and consequences.* New York: Springer Publishing Company.

Gallagher-Thompson, D., Hanley-Peterson, P., & Thompson, L. W. (1990). Maintenance of gains versus relapse following brief psychotherapy for depression. *Journal of Consulting and Clinical Psychology, 58*(3), 371–374.

Gerety, M. B. (1994). Health care reform from the view of a geriatrician. *The Gerontologist, 34*(5), 590–597.

Goldwasser, A. N., Aurbach, S. M., & Harkins, S. W. (1987). Cognitive, affective, and behavioral effects of reminiscence group therapy on demented elderly. *International Journal of Aging and Human Development, 25*(3), 209–222.

Grossman, W. I. (1982). The self as fantasy: Fantasy as theory. *Journal of the American Psychoanalytic Association, 30*, 919–938.

Gustafson, R. (1992). Treating insomnia with a self-administered muscle relaxation training program: A follow-up. *Psychological Reports, 70*(1), 124–126.

Hamilton, M. (1967). Development of a rating scale for primary depressive illness. *British Journal of Social and Clinical Psychiatry, 6*, 278–296.

Haynes, S. N. (1991). Behavioral assessment. In M. Hersen, A. E. Kazdin, & A. S. Bellack (Eds.), *The clinical psychology handbook* (2nd ed., pp. 430–464). Elmsford, NY: Pergamon Press.

Hazzard, W. R., Andres, R., Bierman, E. L., & Blass, J. P. (1990). (Eds). *Principles of geriatric medicine and gerontology* (2nd ed.). New York: McGraw-Hill.

Hewett, L. J., Asamen, J. K., Hedgepeth, J. & Dietch, J. T. (1991). Group reminiscence with nursing home residents. *Clinical Gerontologist, 10*(4), 69–72.

Hiroto, D. S., & Seligman, M. E. P. (1975). Generality of learned helplessness in man. *Journal of Personality and Social Psychology, 31*, 311–327.

Holroyd, S., Rabins, P. V., Finkelstein, D., Nicholson, M. C., Chase, G. A., & Wisniewski, S. C. (1992). Visual hallucinations in patients with macular degeneration. *American Journal of Psychiatry, 149*(12), 1701–1706.

Horowitz, M. J., Wilner, M., Marmar, C., & Krupnick, J. (1980). Pathological grief and the activation of latent self-images. *American Journal of Psychiatry, 137*(10), 1152–1157.

Jenike, M. A. (1988). Depression and other psychiatric disorders. In M. S. Albert & M. B. Moss (Eds.), *Geriatric neuropsychology.* New York: Guilford Press.

Jenike, M. A. (1991). Geriatric obsessive-compulsive disorder. *Journal of Geriatric Psychiatry and Neurology, 4*, 34–39.

Kashner, T. M., Rodell, D. E., Ogden, S. R., Guggenheim, F. G., & Karson, C. N. (1992). Outcomes and costs of two VA inpatient treatment programs for older alcoholic patients. *Hospital and Community Psychiatry, 43*(10), 985–989.

Kaszniak, A. W. (1990). Psychological assessment of the aging individual. In J. E. Birren & K. W. Schaie (Eds.), *Handbook of the psychology of aging* (3rd ed.). New York: Academic Press.

Kaszniak, A. W., & Christenson, G. D. (1994). Differential diagnosis of dementia and depression. In M. Storandt & G. R.

VandenBos (Eds.), *Neuropsychological assessment of dementia and depression in older adults: A clinician's guide.* Washington, DC: American Psychological Association.

Keating, J. C., Schulte, E. A., & Miller, E. (1988). Conservative care of urinary incontinence in the elderly. *Journal of Manipulative and Physiological Therapeutics, 11*(4), 300–308.

Kennedy, G. J., Kelman, H. R., & Thomas, C. (1991). Persistence and remission of depressive symptoms in late life. *American Journal of Psychiatry, 148*(2), 174–178.

Kernberg, O. (1982). The theory of psychoanalytic psychotherapy. In S. Slipp (Ed.), *Curative factors in dynamic psychotherapy* (pp. 1–21). New York: McGraw-Hill.

Khan, A., Mirolo, J., Mirolo, M. H., & Dobie, D. J. (1993). Depression in the elderly: A treatable disorder. *Geriatrics, 48*(Suppl. 1), 14–17.

Klerman, G. L., & Weissman, M. M. (1989). Increasing rates of depression. *Journal of the American Medical Association, 261*(15), 2229–2235.

Koenig, H. G., George, L. K., & Schneider, R. (1994). Mental health care for older adults in the year 2020: A dangerous and avoided topic. *The Gerontologist, 34*(5), 674–679.

Kohut, H. (1971). *The analysis of the self.* New York: International Universities Press.

Kohut, H. (1977). *The restoration of the self.* New York: International Universities Press.

Kolb, B., & Whishaw, I. Q. (1990). *Fundamentals of human neuropsychology* (3rd ed.). New York: W. H. Freeman and Company.

Kreeger, J. L., Raulin, M. L., Grace, J., & Priest, B. L. (1995). Effect of hearing enhancement on mental status ratings in geriatric psychiatric patients. *American Journal of Psychiatry, 152*(4), 629–631.

Kushner, M. G., Sher, K. J., & Beitman, B. D. (1990). The relation between alcohol problems and anxiety disorders. *American Journal of Psychiatry, 147*, 685–695.

La Rue, A. (1992). *Aging and neuropsychological assessment.* New York: Plenum.

Lazenby, H. C., & Letsch, S. W. (1990). National health expenditures, 1989. *Health Care Finance Review, 12*, 1–26.

Leahey, T., & Harris, R. J. (1989). *Human learning* (2nd ed.). Englewood Cliffs, NJ: Prentice Hall.

Lewinsohn, P. J., Antonuccio, D. O., Steinmetz, J., & Teri, L. (1984). *The coping with depression course.* Eugene, OR: Castalia Publishing.

Lewis, M. I., & Butler, R. N. (1974). Life-review therapy: Putting memories to work in individual and group therapies. *Geriatrics, 29*, 165–173.

Lezak, M. D. (1995). *Neuropsychological assessment* (3rd ed.). New York: Oxford University Press.

Liberto, J. G., Oslin, D. W., & Ruskin, P. E. (1992). Alcoholism in older persons: A review of the literature. *Hospital and Community Psychiatry, 43*(10), 975–984.

Lipe, A. W. (1991). Using music therapy to enhance the quality of life in a client with Alzheimer's dementia: A case study. *Music Therapy Perspective, 9*, 102–105.

Lloyd, C. (1980). Life events and depressive disorder reviewed: I. Events as predisposing factors. II. Events as precipitating factors. *Archives of General Psychiatry, 37*, 529–548.

Lovell, M. R., & Nussbaum, P. D. (1994). Neuropsychological assessment. In E. C. Coffey & J. L. Cummings (Eds.), *Textbook of geriatric neuropsychiatry.* Washington, DC: American Psychiatric Press.

Lustman, P. J., Griffith, L. S., & Clouse, R. E. (1988). Depression in adults with diabetes: Results of a 5-year follow-up study. *Diabetes Care, 11*(8), 605–612.

Magni, G., Palazzolo, O., & Bianchin, G. (1988). The course of depression in elderly outpatients. *Canadian Journal of Psychiatry, 33*(1), 21–24.

Maier, S. F., & Seligman, M. E. (1976). Learned helplessness: Theory and evidence. *Journal of Experimental Psychology: General, 105*, 3–46.

Malmgren, R. (1994). Epidemiology of aging. In E. C. Coffey & J. L. Cummings (Eds.), *Textbook of geriatric neuropsychiatry* (pp. 17–33). Washington, DC: American Psychiatric Press.

Maloney, M. P., & Ward, M. P (1976). *Psychological assessment.* New York: Oxford University Press.

Mann, J. (1973). *Time-limited psychotherapy.* Cambridge, MA: Harvard University Press.

Mendez, M. F. (1994). Huntington's disease: Update and review of neuropsychiatric aspects. *International Journal of Psychiatry in Medicine, 24*(3), 189–208.

Meredith, L. S., Wells, K. B., & Camp, P. (1994). Clinician specialty and treatment style for depressed outpatients with and without medical comorbidities. *Archives of Family Medicine, 3*, 1065–1072.

Metalsky, G. I., Abramson, L. Y., Seligman, M. E. P., Semmel, A., & Peterson, C. (1982). Attributional styles and life events in the classroom: Vulnerability and invulnerability to depressive mood reactions. *Journal of Personality and Social Psychology, 43*, 612–617.

Miller, N. S., Belkin, B. M., & Gold, M. S. (1991). Alcohol and drug dependence among the elderly: Epidemiology, diagnosis, and treatment. *Comprehensive Psychiatry, 32*(2), 153–165.

Morin, C. M., Kowatch, R. A., Barry, T., & Walton, E. (1993). Cognitive-behavior therapy for late-life insomnia. *Journal of Consulting and Clinical Psychology, 61*(1), 137–146.

Mueller, D. P., Edwards, D. W., & Yarvis, R. M. (1977). Stressful life events and psychiatric symptomatology: Change or undesirability? *Journal of Health and Social Behavior, 18*, 307–317.

Myers, W. A. (1991). Psychoanalytic psychotherapy and psychoanalysis with older patients. In W. A. Myers (Ed.), *New techniques in the psychotherapy of older patients.* Washington, DC: American Psychiatric Press.

National Institutes of Health. (1992). Diagnosis and treatment of depression in late life. *Journal of the American Medical Association, 268*(8), 1018–1024.

Nemiroff, R. A., & Colarusso, C. A. (1985). *The race against time: Psychotherapy and psychoanalysis in the second half of life.* New York: Plenum Press.

Nezu, A. M. (1987). A problem solving formulation of depression: A literature review and proposal of a pluralistic model. *Clinical Psychology Review, 7*, 121–144.

Nezu, A. M., & Perri, M. G. (1989). Social problem-solving therapy for unipolar depression: An initial dismantling investigation. *Journal of Consulting and Clinical Psychology, 57*(3), 408–413.

Overmier, J. B., & Seligman, M. E. P. (1967). Effects of inescapable shock upon subsequent escape and avoidance learning. *Journal of Comparative and Physiological Psychology, 63*, 23–33.

Peterson, C., & Seligman, M. E. P. (1984). Causal explanations as a risk factor for depression: Theory and evidence. *Psychological Review, 91*, 347–374.

Pfeiffer, E. (1976). Psychotherapy with elderly patients. In L. Bellak & T. Karasu (Eds.), *Geriatric psychiatry: A handbook for psychiatrists and primary care physicians* (pp. 191–205). New York: Grune & Stratton.

Prigatano, G. P., & Schacter, D. L. (Eds.). (1991). *Awareness of deficit after brain injury: Clinical and theoretical issues.* New York: Oxford University Press.

Rattenbury, D., & Stones, M. J. (1989). A controlled evaluation of reminiscence and current topics discussion groups in a nursing home context. *The Gerontologist, 29*, 768–771.

Regier, D. A., Boyd, J. H., Burke, J. D., Rae, D. S., Myers, J. K., Kramer, M., Robins, L. N., George, L. K., Karno, M., & Locke, B. Z. (1988). One-month prevalence of mental disorders in the United States. *Archives of General Psychiatry, 45*, 977–986.

Regier, D. A., Narrow, W. E., Rae, D. S., Manderscheid, R. W., Lock, B. A., & Goodwin, F. K. (1993). The de facto US mental and addictive disorders service system: Epidemiologic catchment area prospective 1-year prevalence rates of disorders and services. *Archives of General Psychiatry, 50*(2), 85–94.

Reynolds, C. F., Frank, E., Perel, J. M., Imber, S. D., Cornes, D., Morycz, R. K., Mazumdar, S., Miller, M. D., Pollock, B. G., Rifai, A. H., Stack, J. A., George, C. J., Houck, R. P., & Kupfer, D. J. (1992). Combined pharmacotherapy and psychotherapy in the acute and continuation treatment of elderly patients with recurrent major depression: A preliminary report. *American Journal of Psychiatry, 149*(12), 1687–1692.

Reynolds, C. F., Frank, E., Perel, J. M., Miller, M., Cornes, C., Rifai, A. H., Pollock, B. G., Mazumdar, S., George, C. J., Jouck, P. R., & Kupfer, D. J. (1994). Treatment of consecutive episodes of major depression in the elderly. *American Journal of Psychiatry, 151*(12), 1740–1743.

Rifai, A. H., George, C. J., Stack, J. A., Mann, J. J., & Reynolds, C. F. (1994). Hopelessness in suicide attempters after acute treatment of major depression in late life. *American Journal of Psychiatry, 1515*(11), 1687–1690.

Riggs, D. S., & Foa, E. B. (1993). Obsessive compulsive disorder. In D. H. Barlow (Ed.), *Handbook of clinical disorders* (2nd ed., pp. 189–239). New York: Guilford Press.

Rogers, W. H., Wells, K. B., Meredith, L. S., Sturm, R., & Burnam, A. (1993). Outcomes for adult depressed outpatients under prepaid and fee-for-service financing. *Archives of General Psychiatry, 50*, 517–525.

Rosenberg, S. E. (1985). Brief dynamic psychotherapy for depression. In E. E. Beckham & W. R. Leder (Eds.), *Handbook of depression: Treatment, assessment, and research.* Dorsey Press: Homewood, IL.

Rowan, V. C., Holborn, S. W., Walker, J. R., & Siddiqui, A. R. (1984). A rapid multi-component treatment for an obsessive-

compulsive disorder. *Journal of Behavior Therapy and Experimental Psychiatry, 15*(4), 347–352.

Sadavoy, J. (1994). Integrated psychotherapy for the elderly. *Canadian Journal of Psychiatry, 39*(8, Suppl. 1), 19–26.

Sadavoy, J., & Leszcz, M. (1987). *Treating the elderly with psychotherapy: The scope for change in later life.* Madison, CT: International Universities Press.

Sallis, J. F., Lichstein, K. L., Clarkson, A. D., Stalgaitis, S., & Campbell, M. (1983). Anxiety and depression management for the elderly. *International Journal of Behavior Geriatrics, 1*, 3–12.

Saltzman, C. (1995). Medication compliance in the elderly. *Journal of Clinical Psychiatry, 56*(Suppl. 1), 18–30.

Scogin, F. R., & McElreath, L. (1994). Efficacy of psychosocial treatments for geriatric depression: A quantitative review. *Journal of Consulting and Clinical Psychology, 62*(1), 69–74.

Scogin, F. R., Rickard, H. C., Keith, S., Wilson, J., & McElreath, L. (1992). Progressive and imaginal relaxation training for elderly persons with subjective anxiety. *Psychology and Aging, 7*(3), 419–424.

Seigel, B., & Gershon, S. (1986). Dementia, depression, and pseudodementia. In H. J. Altman (Ed.), *Alzheimer's disease: Problems, prospects, and perspectives* (pp. 29–44). New York: Plenum.

Sheikh, J. I. (1992). Anxiety disorders and their treatment. *Clinics in Geriatric Medicine, 8*(2), 411–426.

Sheikh, J. I. (1994). Anxiety disorders. In E. C. Coffey & J. L. Cummings (Eds.), *Textbook of geriatric neuropsychiatry.* Washington, DC: American Psychiatric Press.

Smith, B. B. (1992). Treatment of dementia: Healing through cultural arts. *Pride Institute Journal of Long Term Home Health Care, 11*, 37–45.

Smith, S. L., Sherrill, K. A., & Colenda, C. C. (1995). Assessing and treating anxiety in elderly persons. *Psychiatric Services, 46*(1), 36–59.

Solomon, K., & Szwabo, P. (1992). Psychotherapy for patients with dementia. In J. E. Morley, R. M. Coe, R. Strong, & G. T. Grossberg (Eds.), *Memory function and aging-related disorders.* New York: Springer.

Soltys, F. G., & Coats, L. (1994). The SolCos Model: Facilitating reminiscence therapy. *Journal of Gerontological Nursing, 20*(11), 11–16.

Souetre, E., Lozet, J., Cimarosti, I., Martin, P., Chignon, J. M., Ades, J., Tignol, J., & Darcourt, G. (1994). Cost of anxiety disorders: Impact of comorbidity. *Journal of Psychosomatic Research, 38*(1), 151–160.

Spielberger, C. D., Gorsuch, R. L., & Lushene, R. E. (1970). *State-Trait Anxiety Inventory.* Palo Alto, CA: Consulting Psychologists Press.

Spitzer, R. L., Endicott, J., & Robins, E. (1978). Research Diagnostic Criteria (RDC): Rationale and reliability. *Archives of General Psychiatry, 35*, 773–782.

Starkstein, S. E., Federoff, J. P., Price, T. R., Leiguarda, R. C., & Robinson, R. G. (1993). Apathy following cerebrovascular lesions. *Stroke, 24*(11), 1625–1630.

Starkstein, S. E., Federoff, J. P., Price, T. R., Leiguarda, R. C., & Robinson, R. G. (1994). Neuropsychological and neuroradiologic correlates of emotional prosody comprehension. *Neurology, 44*(3, Pt. 1), 515–522.

Steele, C., Rovner, B., Chase, G. A., & Folstein, M. (1990). Psychiatric symptoms and nursing home placement of patients with Alzheimer's disease. *American Journal of Psychiatry, 147*(8), 1049–1051.

Stein, L. M. (1990). Acquired hearing impairment among older females with psychopathology. *Journal of the American Academy of Audiology, 1*, 1–44.

Stuss, D. T., Gow, C. A., & Hetherington, C. R. (1992). "No longer Gage": Frontal lobe dysfunction and emotional changes. *Journal of Consulting and Clinical Psychology, 60*(3), 349–359.

Teri, L. (1986, August). *Treating depression in Alzheimer's disease: Teaching the caregiver behavioral strategies.* Paper presented to the American Psychological Association, Washington, DC.

Teri, L. (1991). Behavioral assessment and treatment of depression in older adults. In P. Wiscocki (Ed.), *Handbook of clinical behavior therapy with the elderly client* (pp. 225–243). New York: Plenum.

Teri, L. (1994). Behavioral treatment of depression in patients with dementia. *Alzheimer's Disease and Associated Disorders, 8*(3), 66–74.

Teri, L., & Logsdon, R. G. (1992). The future of psychotherapy with older adults. *Psychotherapy, 29*, 81–87.

Teri, L., & McCurry, S. M. (1994). Psychosocial therapies. In E. C. Coffey & J. L. Cummings (Eds.), *Textbook of geriatric neuropsychiatry.* Washington, DC: American Psychiatric Press.

Teri, L., & Uomoto, J. (1991). Reducing excess disability in dementia patients: Training caregivers to manage patient depression. *Clinical Gerontologist, 10*, 49–63.

Teri, L., & Wagner, A. (1992). Alzheimer's disease and depression. *Journal of Consulting and Clinical Psychology, 60*, 379–391.

Tueth, M. J. (1993). Anxiety in the older patient: Differential diagnosis and treatment. *Geriatrics, 48*, 51–54.

Waldo, D. R., Sonnefeld, S. T., McHusick, D. R., & Arnett, R. H. (1988). Health expenditures by age group, 1977 and 1987. *Health Care Finance Review, 10*, 111–120.

Waxman, H. M. (1986). Community mental health care for the elderly—a look at the obstacles. *Public Health Reports, 10*(3), 294–300.

Weiner, I. B. (1975). *Principles of psychotherapy.* New York: John Wiley and Sons.

Weiner, I. B. (1976). *Clinical methods in psychology.* New York: John Wiley and Sons.

Weiss, K. J. (1994). Management of anxiety and depression syndromes in the elderly. *Journal of Clinical Psychiatry, 55*(2, Suppl.), 5–12.

Wells, K. B., Katon, W., Roberts, S., & Camp, P. (1994). Use of minor tranquilizers and antidepressant medications by depressed outpatients: Results from the Medical Outcomes Study. *American Journal of Psychiatry, 15*, 694–700.

Wise, M. G., & Griffies, W. S. (1995). A combined treatment approach to anxiety in the medically ill. *Journal of Clinical Psychiatry, 56*(2, Suppl.), 14–19.

Woods, R. T., & Britton, P. G. (1985). *Clinical psychology with the elderly.* Rockville, MD: Aspen.

Yu, L. C., Kaltreider, D. L., Hu, T., & Craighead, W. E. (1991). Impact of a behavior therapy on the psychological status of incontinent elderly nursing home residents: Quantitative and qualitative assessment. In W. A. Myers (Ed.), *New techniques in the psychotherapy of older patients* (pp. 181–202). Washington, DC: American Psychiatric Press, Inc.

Zivian, M. T., Larsen, W., Knox, V. J., Gekowski, W., & Hatchette, V. (1992). Psychotherapy for the elderly: Psychotherapists' preferences. *Psychotherapy, 29*(4), 668–674.

Zivian, M. T., Larsen, W., Gekowski, W., Knox, V. J., & Hatchette, V. (1994). Psychotherapy for the elderly: Public opinion. *Psychotherapy, 31*(3), 492–502.

30

Behavior Modification of Older Adults

ANTHONY J. GORECZNY

Introduction

Behavior modification principles have enjoyed a relatively short but storied history of success in ameliorating behavior management difficulties. Although human beings have made attempts since ancient times to explain human behavior, it was not until recently that a formalized discipline and set of principles to guide human behavior became established (Krasner, 1990). Most historians credit John B. Watson and his 1913 treatise, "Psychology as the Behaviorist Views it," as the catalyst of the behavioral movement, a movement that focuses on objective observation of behavior and deemphasizes conscious processes. Although Watson has often received recognition as the founder of behaviorism, some authors have noted that the movement toward behaviorism was already in progress when Watson championed this approach, but that Watson's works served to catapult it forward (Kazdin, 1978; Samelson, 1981).

The behavior modification approach to therapy focuses on objective, observable behaviors; implementation of scientifically validated treatment techniques; and continual monitoring of the target behavior to verify efficacy of treatment. The purpose of the present chapter is to elucidate principles used in behavior modification, briefly review techniques to assess the efficacy of behavior change principles used, provide an overview of why these principles

ANTHONY J. GORECZNY • Department of Behavioral Sciences, University of Indianapolis, Indianapolis, Indiana 46227.

are applicable to older adults, and review some studies that have used these principles.

Basic Principles

Although most psychologists have a keen understanding of the basic principles of behavior modification, mental health professionals who operate primarily from psychodynamic or medical models of psychiatric care may have only a limited understanding of these concepts (Corrigan, MacKain, & Liberman, 1994). Therefore, a brief review of these principles appears warranted. Interested readers who want a more detailed description than provided here can refer to one of the many excellent books on behavior modification (e.g., Bellack, Hersen, & Kazdin, 1990).

Four of the most basic principles of behavior modification appear in the 2×2 grid displayed in Figure 1. *Reinforcement* is any contingency that increases the likelihood that an organism will repeat a certain behavior. There are two forms of reinforcement: positive reinforcement and negative reinforcement. Positive reinforcement refers to the administration of a pleasant or positive consequence contingent upon display of a certain behavior. Negative reinforcement, on the other hand, is removal of a negative or noxious stimulus contingent upon display of a certain behavior. Negative reinforcement is *not* punishment. *Punishment* is presentation of a noxious stimulus contingent upon display of a certain behavior.

	Administer	Remove
Positive Consequence	Positive reinforcement	Time Out/ Response Cost
Negative Consequence	Punishment	Negative reinforcement

FIGURE 1. Basic principles of behavior modification.

Examples of these three concepts help to illustrate their action. An example of positive reinforcement is a word of encouragement or praise for having accomplished a certain feat. An example of negative reinforcement is a patient who continually pleads with a physician until the physician decides to appease the patient by prescribing Valium. In this instance, the patient negatively reinforced the physician's behavior by removing the pleading behavior. The unfortunate consequence of this action is that it increases the likelihood that the physician will prescribe Valium again in the future and that the physician's behavior will be the result more of negative reinforcement and less of clinical indication. An example of punishment is a health care provider verbally insulting a patient for "asking too many questions." The unfortunate consequence of this is that patients then often stop asking appropriate questions and subsequently fail to comply with providers' "orders" without informing the providers.

The fourth principle from Figure 1 is *time out* or *response cost*. Time out is removal of an individual, contingent upon display of a specific target behavior, from an environment in which he or she is able to obtain rewards and moving that individual to an environment in which no rewards are available. The time out period is a limited time period, after which the individual is able to return to the prior environment. Response cost is removing something of value from the individual contingent upon display of a certain behavior. An example of this includes a fine for speeding.

The four basic principles above represent the basis for the remaining tenets of behavior modification. Additional principles include extinction, shaping, discrimination training, generalization, maintenance, modeling, and differential reinforcement. Extinction is removal of reinforcement from a previously reinforced behavior (Poling, 1985). The effect is that the organism will slowly stop displaying the previously reinforced behavior. However, prior to reduction in that behavior, there is an "extinction

burst," a relatively short period of time during which the frequency and/or strength of the behavior increases. Also, there is a period of spontaneous recovery; that is, after the frequency of the targeted behavior has decreased, a short burst in increased frequency of the behavior occurs. Clinicians working to extinguish behaviors must be very careful not to reinforce the behavior during either of these times because such reinforcement will only increase the strength of the bond between reinforcement and the behavior, thereby increasing the difficulty of later extinguishing that behavior.

Shaping is the gradual learning of a desired response in successive approximations to the response (Wolf, Risley, & Mees, 1964). For example, a health care provider who wants to teach a reclusive older adult who is new to a facility to interact with others would first reinforce smaller behaviors, such as looking up at other residents or taking a step toward him or her. Once the patient was consistently engaging in those behaviors for the reward, the health care team would then set a new goal that uses a behavior, such as any non-negative verbal comment made to others, that moves the patient forward toward the ultimate goal of interacting with other residents. This pattern would continue until the patient had successfully performed the final goal.

Discrimination training is teaching an organism to respond with a certain behavior in one setting but not in settings where it would be inappropriate. For example, when teaching social interaction skills, one might want to retrain a head-injured individual the importance of laughing only at appropriate times. Therefore, discrimination training involves administering reinforcement when the patient is laughing at a joke or funny story but not when someone is relating a sad or hurtful story or when someone gets injured.

Generalization training is almost the opposite of discrimination training. Often, patients who learn a behavior limit it to the setting in which they had learned that behavior; the behavior becomes bound only to the stimuli of the training sessions. Generalization training involves having patients take what they learned in one setting and applying it to another equally appropriate setting.

Maintenance is the process of ensuring that patients continue to display appropriate behaviors they learned during treatment sessions after treatment has ended. Probably the best way to increase the likelihood of maintenance is through behavioral trapping (Baer & Wolf, 1970). This involves teaching patients behaviors that will likely earn them rewards and reinforcement (e.g., the approval of others) in their natural environments. Thus, when training is complete, the behavior will persist because of rewards the patients are receiving while naturally interacting in their regular environment.

Modeling is the process of teaching a behavior by having the patient observe someone else performing the desired behavior (Bandura, 1969). Although patients actually learn the behavior just by watching, actual performance of the behavior by the patient may require some reinforcement as well (Bandura, 1965). Use of multiple models (Meichenbaum, 1971) and similarity of the models to the patient (Kornhaber & Schroeder, 1975) increase the likelihood that modeling will prove successful.

Differential reinforcement involves providing reinforcement for one behavior while at the same time extinguishing another behavior or set of behaviors (Dietz, Repp, & Dietz, 1976; Singh, Dawson, & Manning, 1981). There are multiple types of differential reinforcement schedules. Two of these schedules (differential reinforcement of incompatible behavior and differential reinforcement of other behavior) have as the goal replacing one behavior with another, and two schedules (differential reinforcement of low-rate behavior and differential reinforcement of high-rate behavior) have as the goal changing the rate or frequency of a behavior.

Differential reinforcement of incompatible behavior (DRI) operates by reinforcing a behavior that is inconsistent with the behavior one is trying to eliminate. For example, for a patient who spends most of the day lying down in bed, DRI might involve reinforcing the patient only when the patient is standing or walking. A differential reinforcement of other behavior (DRO) operates by reinforcing the patient for not displaying the target behavior. Therefore, a patient with dementia who displays significant wandering behavior might receive reinforcement for staying in a certain area without walking away from the area for a specified period of time.

Differential reinforcement of low-rate behavior is best for a behavior that the health care team

would like a patient to display at a specified low frequency. Under this paradigm, patients receive reinforcement for behavior up to a certain rate, but all responses of that behavior over the predetermined rate get extinguished. An example might be brushing one's teeth. The team might decide to reinforce a patient for brushing in the morning, after meals, and at nighttime but at no other time. Differential reinforcement of high-rate behavior can be a useful technique to get a patient to display desired behavior at a higher rate than currently exhibited. For example, patients who underwent shaping to get them to engage in social activity might subsequently have to spend a certain number of hours in social activities (greater than the number currently spent) in order to receive the reinforcement.

Assessment of Other Factors

The basic principles briefly discussed above form the basis of intervention via behavior modification. However, prior to intervention and as part of an ongoing assessment throughout intervention, it is important for the treatment team to assess other factors as well. These include assets and limitations of patients, environmental supports and restrictions, and motivators.

Throughout the above section, the term reinforcement (or reinforcer) appears. However, it is very important to remember that what is reinforcing for one patient will not be for another and may even be a punishment. Treatment teams and individual health care providers must be careful not to attempt to apply the same contingency to each patient and expect to get similar results. Although special time with a ward staff member may be a reinforcer for one patient, another patient, who prefers solitude, may find this "special time" unpleasant.

In addition to an individual's set of reinforcers, treatment team members must be careful to also conduct an evaluation of the social context in which the patient will be living. Although many places give "lip service" to this aspect of care, very few actually conduct the comprehensive evaluations necessary to ensure that a patient's environment is optimally suitable to his or her needs. Much of the reason for this is likely the changing health care climate, which has decreased the availability of resources to conduct such evaluations (Goreczny & O'Halloran, 1995).

Evaluation of patients' social and physical environments may get overlooked. Nonetheless, an examination of these aspects will help determine whether behavior modification (or other intervention) will be effective. For example, although retraining an elderly individual on performance of activities of daily living (ADL) might prove to be very effective while an inpatient, the physical layout of the home may not permit the patient to engage in the full spectrum of behaviors; a patient who is unable to traverse steps will have a very difficult time completing ADL if the only bathroom is on the second floor of the home while the patient's bedroom is on the first floor. Also, a caregiver who may not want a patient to get better for reasons of financial disability loss or fear of losing control over the patient will certainly sabotage any efforts to help the patient improve. On the other hand, overly solicitous caregivers may inadvertently reinforce disability in an effort to be helpful (see Lousberg, Schmidt, & Groenman, 1992).

General Standards for Using Behavioral Principles

Although all of the above behavior modification principles will work effectively when properly implemented, there is a general tendency to favor the use of punishment and time out and to minimize the use of reinforcement principles because of the quick results that punishment produces. Reliance on punishment as the primary means of treatment is directly opposite the optimal use of behavior modification principles.

One of the primary problems with the use of punishment is that there are many subsequent negative consequences. One of these is some form of undesired emotional reaction, such as anger. Another problem is that the punishment becomes paired with the punisher. Thus, the punisher becomes someone to avoid. In a therapeutic setting, such consequences will undoubtedly have a negative impact on the patient–therapist relationship and limit the amount of information that patients are willing to share with their therapists. Health care

providers inadvertently punish patient behaviors in many ways, often rendering patient–therapist communication ineffectual. Another problem with punishment is that there is often a displayed aggression that occurs, and a punished patient (or staff member) may take out frustration on someone who is unlikely to retaliate. Finally, punishment often results in power struggles, and patients may display passive–aggressive behaviors that affect their health or the milieu of the ward.

For these reasons, the following guidelines may help to produce the desired behavioral response: First, use positive reinforcement as the primary tool to shape and change behaviors. Second, rather than using punishment to suppress behavior, rely on extinction when possible. Third, use punishment procedures (including time out and response cost) mostly when behaviors are dangerous or disruptive to the learning process. Finally, whenever using either punishment or extinction, reinforcement procedures should also be used. While punishment and/or extinction teaches what not to do, reinforcement procedures teach what to do and will help replace the behavior that has been eliminated.

Measurement of Behavior

Another important, though often unappreciated, concept is that of identifying and measuring target behavior(s). There are generally three classes of behaviors to measure: motoric, physiological, and cognitive. Motoric behaviors are those that involve some body movement (e.g., walking, verbal insults, positive social interaction). Physiological measures are those that assess some aspect of body physical state (e.g., heart rate, muscle tension, and catecholamine level). Finally, cognitions are those reports of one's thoughts. Cognitive measures are the least objective.

There are various ways to measure the three classes of behaviors, including observation (either in vivo or during role-playing), self-report, video- or audiotaping, self-monitoring, test scores, polygraph readings, or measures from blood/urine samples. The specific behavior one wants to measure will largely determine the method used. For example, measuring heart rate in response to an anxiety-provoking stimulus will require physiological methods, but measurement of an individual's actual behavior toward that stimulus could involve the patient's self-report, a videotape, or actual observation.

When choosing a method of measurement, it is generally best to avoid self-report because of the many questions surrounding its reliability and validity, though there are also many sources of error in direct observation (Hartmann & Wood, 1990). In order to assess effects of a behavior modification program, the clinician must use measures that are observable, repeatable, reliable, and valid and that have standardized administration and scoring procedures. Measures that have significant practice effects are not acceptable because of the multiple measures required when instituting a behavior modification.

Implementing the Behavior Modification Program

Prior to implementing any behavior modification program, it is important for the health care team to conduct a functional analysis of the environment and the behavior. To do this, one must first identify the target behavior of the modification program (e.g., verbally insulting behavior or positive socialization). The goal may be to decrease verbally insulting behavior or to increase positive socialization. The next step is to analyze the topography of this behavior. This includes frequency and severity measures.

It is also important to analyze the environment in which the behavior is occurring and to specifically identify how that environment may be affecting the target behavior. Most important is to identify any discriminative stimuli of the behavior, the effects the behavior has on the environment, and any reinforcement that might be naturally sustaining the behavior. Such a functional analysis might help a treatment team recognize that they had originally intended to target the wrong behavior. For example, consider the scenario in Figure 2. As in this example, it is possible that one patient's aggressive behavior always follows the verbal insults of another patient. Targeting the physically aggressive behavior is likely to be less effective than targeting the verbal insults. The reason for this is that the discrim-

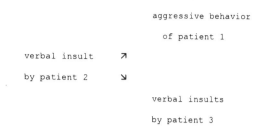

FIGURE 2. Simplified example of functional analysis of aggressive behavior.

inative stimuli (or prompts) for the aggressive behavior will remain, and termination of the treatment program will only permit the prompts to regain their control over the aggressive behavior. Thus, the most appropriate target behavior in this example would be verbal insults of patient 2 instead of the more salient and original target—the aggression of patient 1. In this example, targeting the verbal insults of patient 2 will also likely reduce those of patient 3, a beneficial side effect of spending a little additional time to appropriately perform a functional analysis and identify the best target behavior. The utility of such a functional analysis has received some critical review (Haynes, 1986). However, proper behavioral assessment allows teams to take an idiographic approach to treatment and objectively display therapeutic results (Barrett, Johnston, & Pennypacker, 1986).

Assessment of Intervention Effects

To assess intervention effects, it is helpful to use some type of experimental design. In this way, the treatment team can have increasing confidence that their treatment plan was the responsible agent of change. However, designs using large control groups are often impractical or cost-inefficient. With the current health care changes and increasing emphasis on cost containment, control group outcome studies have become even more difficult to conduct than they were years ago.

Nonetheless, the need for proving efficacy of treatments has increased. One set of procedures ideally suited to assess clinical effects with low cost to the treatment team is the group of designs called *single case* or *small N subject* designs. These designs permit objective verification of treatment effects on a small scale and offer many advantages over the larger control group designs (Barrett et al., 1986). One advantage is that only one subject (or just a few subjects) is necessary for implementation. In these designs, subjects serve as their own controls. Another advantage of these designs is that the team can change the treatment as necessary. These designs do not confine treatment team members to implementing only a certain package at predetermined intervals. The team is able to change the treatment, add a component, or dismantle a treatment package according to the best interest of the patient.

Another advantage of single case designs over group designs is that there is no intersubject variability. There is also more ability to assess intrasubject variability with single subject designs than there is with group designs (Hersen & Barlow, 1976). For example, if a subject has a large change (either in the desired direction or in the opposite direction), the treatment team can try to identify the discriminative stimuli responsible for that change. In a group design, however, the large change of one person might appear only as a small change (or no change) in the group statistics and get overlooked by treatment team members.

Once the treatment team has identified a target behavior or behaviors, it is imperative to obtain baseline data on the identified behavior or behaviors. This baseline data will serve as the initial criterion by which the treatment team can ascertain the effectiveness of any intervention. Ideally, the baseline period consists of at least three data points and is relatively stable (Barlow & Hersen, 1973; Sidman, 1960). It would not be possible to identify any trends in the targeted behavior with less than three data points. Also, an unstable baseline makes determination of the effects of intervention difficult, if not impossible.

Two particularly problematic baseline patterns are increasing or decreasing baseline and variable baseline. Decreasing baseline is most problematic for assessing the effects of an intervention designed to decrease the targeted behavior. For example, consider the case of a treatment team that has targeted a patient's yelling behavior in an attempt to decrease it. If the baseline amount of yelling is already decreasing at the time of implementation of the inter-

vention, it would take a large effect to indicate that the intervention had any impact on the behavior. On the other hand, with a stable baseline we have more confidence in stating that changes that occur in the targeted behavior following intervention were the result of intervention. Even this is not certain, however, because there may have been some other change that occurred at the same time as the implementation of the intervention, and this may have been the responsible agent of change. (This problem receives further attention below.) The best way to deal with a decreasing or increasing baseline is to wait until the behavior produces a stable period of three data points. This may be difficult in some circumstances, especially if the behavior is dangerous or when staff are pressuring the treatment team to make an intervention quickly.

Variable baseline also presents the problem of determining whether or not an intervention was effective. One way to deal with variable baseline is to average several data points together to find a stable baseline and to then use that method of measurement (i.e., averaging three data points to produce one measurement point) throughout the measurement period. However, this may obscure identifying the sources of variability.

Single Case Designs

For a more detailed review of single case designs, the reader may consult one of the many excellent sources on the topic (Hersen, 1990; Hersen & Barlow, 1976). The most basic type of single case design is the A–B design. This design consists of two phases: baseline followed by treatment. The problem with this most basic design is that even though the behavior may have changed following initiation of treatment, it is possible that some factor other than the treatment itself had the main effect on behavior. For example, it is possible that removal of a patient from the ward or introduction of a new staff member at the same time as initiation of treatment produced the therapeutic change. (Although reason for the improvement may be of minimal concern for clinical and administrative staff who just wanted to see the change, behavioral scientists must consider reasons for change from both a theoretical perspective and for use in future consultations.)

One way to ascertain whether treatment had any therapeutic benefit is to withdraw treatment and determine the effects of this on the target behavior. This is an A–B–A design. The primary problem with this design is the ethical concern of ending intervention on a no-treatment phase. Thus, one way to counter this is to reinstate treatment (an A–B–A–B design) and once again show the therapeutic effect. Such a design presents a powerful argument for effects of treatment. There are numerous variations of these designs (e.g., A–B–A–C–A–B, A–B–A–C–A–BC, where C is a second treatment intervention and BC represents combining treatments B and C). One particularly noteworthy example is the B–A–B design. This design is particularly useful when the patient is displaying a behavior that needs to come under immediate control or when staff are too restless to allow for measurement of an adequate baseline.

The above designs present problems for clinicians or administrators who feel uncomfortable with the idea of removing (or withholding) a potentially effective therapy (this is the second A phase) and for treatments that might maintain themselves without specific therapeutic intervention (e.g., teaching an anxious older adult relaxation skills or other anxiety reduction skills that do not involve medication). Therefore, an alternative design is the multiple baseline design. In this design, the treatment team chooses several patients or several behaviors in the same patient to target with the same intervention. After collecting baseline data on all patients (or behaviors), the treatment team targets one of the patients for the intervention and institutes treatment only with this patient while continuing to collect data on all other patients in the study. After a period of several data points, the treatment team initiates intervention with the second patient while still continuing intervention for the first patient. The treatment team repeats this process until all patients are receiving intervention. Demonstration of the effectiveness of intervention is present when the identified patients change their behaviors only after having been the target of intervention (see Figure 3).

Multiple baseline designs can focus on multiple behaviors, patients, or settings. This presents clinicians with the advantages of being able to treat several patients with the same intervention without

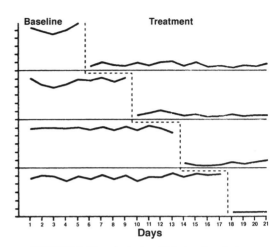

FIGURE 3. Hypothetical multiple baseline design.

having to withdraw treatment in order to provide strong evidence of therapeutic efficacy.

Another design is the changing criterion design. Treatment teams using this design set a specified criterion that the patient must meet in order to receive reinforcement. Once the patient has consistently displayed the behavior with the predetermined criterion, team members change the criterion for reinforcement, and the pattern continues until the treatment has achieved the final goal. This type of design is especially good for behaviors that require gradual acquisition or elimination. Such a behavior might be increasing the level of physical activity in an older adult. A physician and psychologist could collaborate on such an endeavor, making sure that the patient's physical condition can tolerate an additional increase prior to implementation.

Token Economies

Token economies have been useful therapeutic techniques (Kazdin, 1977). Unfortunately, their use in recent years has declined. With the increasing number of older adults in need of residential services, this type of treatment may, once again, prove to be a useful adjunct to therapy. In this treatment program, patients receive tokens for previously determined behaviors. The patients can then "cash in" their tokens for services, privileges, goods, or other rewards.

The first step in developing a token economy is to develop a contingency contract that details the specific behaviors for which patients will receive tokens, sanctions or penalties, bonus clauses, and potential rewards and their costs. When possible, it is best to negotiate the contract with patients. This generally will improve performance, teach them how to negotiate with staff, teach patients that they have some control, and teach flexibility to both staff and patients. In addition to the regular therapeutic effects of token economies, some side effects of these systems may include positive changes in non-target behaviors and in staff attitudes.

The Need for Behavior Modification with Older Adults

As many authors have emphasized and as indicated by health demography statistics, the number of individuals in the United States over age 65 and the percentage of the United States population over age 65 is growing at a very fast pace (Rowe & Katzman, 1992). Unquestionably, one of the clear reasons is improved medical technology and health care, permitting individuals who would have normally died from conditions such as strokes, myocardial infarctions, or head injuries to live longer than they would have prior to the recent medical advances (Goreczny, 1995).

One of the consequences of improved care, however, is that a different set of problems has developed—the need to rehabilitate and care for disabled individuals or those individuals who have lost some of their physical or mental abilities or, in many cases, evidence both physical and mental health problems. Unquestionably, physical health problems affect our mental health and cognitive abilities. Also, older adults have a greater likelihood of developing physical health problems than younger adults or children. Therefore, the likelihood of developing mental health difficulties is also greater.

Although behavior modification principles discussed above may seem obvious to some readers, many, if not most, health care providers take these principles for granted and either do not use them

in their work or administer them improperly. Unfortunately, patients are often better at using basic behavior modification principles than are health care professionals, and health care professionals often inadvertently shape undesired behavior in their patients, as illustrated earlier in the chapter. Nonetheless, problems from which older adults suffer may make them uniquely appropriate for behavior modification strategies.

Cardiovascular Changes

One of the most recognized changes in the human body as we age involves the cardiovascular system. The risk of myocardial infarction increases with advancing age, and there are recognized physiological changes in the cardiovascular system that affect cardiovascular functioning (Gribbin, Pickering, Sleight, & Peto, 1971). Finally, medical procedures themselves designed to ameliorate cardiovascular deficiencies may produce iatrogenic cognitive impairment. For example, there is a risk of cerebral damage resulting from open heart surgery (Savageau, Stanton, Jenkins, & Frater, 1982; Savageau, Stanton, Jenkins, & Klein, 1982; Sontaniemi, Monomen, & Hokkanen, 1986) and from cardiac transplantation (Nussbaum & Goldstein, 1992). Most importantly and most relevant to the current chapter, a recent study (Nussbaum, Allender, & Copeland, 1995) revealed that cardiac transplant candidates evidence verbal learning deficits and that these deficits correlated with patients' ejection fractions, a measure of cardiac output. The implications of this study are that patients with low cardiac output may have difficulty learning new verbally mediated tasks or instructions (i.e., medical regimen). Whether the same relationship holds for nonverbally mediated instructions remains unanswered. Nonetheless, this does highlight the fact that cardiovascular changes will likely affect future behavior and subsequent attempts to modify such behavior.

Neuropsychological Impairment

Although most older adults remain essentially intact cognitively for most, if not all, of their lives (Birren & Renner, 1980), age-related cognitive decrements do occur (Katzman & Terry, 1992). Of significance is that changes generally represent decrements in effortful processing (Nussbaum, 1995), and the hippocampus, which is important for learning new information, also suffers age-related changes (Hoyer, 1990; Lim, Zipursky, Murphy, & Pfefferbaum, 1990). In addition, older adults are susceptible to head injuries as a result of falls, and they are more likely than younger adults to have negative outcomes associated with such falls (Holden, 1984).

Noteworthy is a recent study (Goldstein & McCue, 1995) that confirmed previously reported differences in functional outcome ratings by head-injured individuals and their informants. Data from this study and others (cf. Chelune, Heaton, & Lehman, 1986; Ranseen, Bohaska, & Schmitt, 1990) indicate that head-injured individuals are inaccurate reporters of their behavior. Although these studies did not specifically address head injuries in older adults, there is no reason to believe that the results would be less prominent among older adults than among younger adults. In fact, one could argue that it is more likely older adults, relative to their younger cohorts, would inaccurately judge their behavior after a head injury due to the increased risk of negative outcomes following head injury in older adults, as noted earlier.

Thus, not only do older adults suffer from "normal" age-related changes in cognitive functioning, but they also are at risk for head injuries that may leave their abilities to accurately judge their behaviors impaired. Therefore, behavior modification techniques appear to have an especially important place among nonpharmaceutical therapies because the emphasis of behavior modification techniques is on changing behavior, not on developing insight into problems so that subsequent behavior change might ensue. Older adults with cognitive deficits, especially those with head injuries, might find it difficult to process complex material, but may respond to specific behavioral instructions and use of behavior modification principles, which do not require effortful processing or insight.

Some Examples

Although behavior modification principles are very appropriate for use with older adults, there have been relatively few published examples of such interventions. The majority of published studies focus on training urinary retention and on minimizing disruptive behavior. Thus, this section first reviews these studies and then highlights studies that have used behavior modification for other purposes.

Urinary Retention

Between 30% and 50% of older adults suffer from urinary incontinence (Diokno, Brock, & Brown, 1986; Ouslander, 1990), and incontinence is the second leading risk factor for institutionalization (Brazda, 1983). Therefore, it is not surprising that there is a fair amount of research on this problem, especially because nursing staff report it as a very difficult and frustrating problem to manage (Hu, 1990; Yu & Kaltreider, 1987). Primary behavioral interventions include scheduled voiding, prompted voiding, and biofeedback-assisted pelvic floor muscle training. Each of these has shown success, especially when combined with response-contingent reinforcement. However, success generally means a reduction in the frequency of voiding or the amount of urine voided during incontinence episodes, not complete cessation of incontinence, and maintenance of the gains may require implementation of a staff management program (see, for example, Engel et al., 1990).

For example, in a variant of the multiple baseline design, Schnelle (1990) assessed the implementation of a program of prompted voiding and reinforcement for continence using two groups. After obtaining baseline readings, one group received intervention and the second group continued to undergo evaluation of their bedwetting. During a subsequent phase, both groups received intervention. The results indicated that the percent of hourly checks that indicated wetness decreased for each group, but only when the group received intervention. Although many of the studies conducted, similar to the Schnelle study above, have used research staff to conduct the intervention, a few recent studies have also shown that regular nursing staff (Colling, Ouslander, Hadley, Eisch, & Campbell, 1992) or regular multidisciplinary treatment teams (McDowell, Burgio, Dombrowski, Locher, & Rodriquez, 1992) can effect positive changes in level of continence. Thus, it is possible to implement behavior modification procedures for treatment of urinary incontinence in applied settings and to achieve therapeutic results in these settings.

Although behavior modification procedures are able to significantly reduce frequency of incontinence episodes and amount of urine voided during such episodes, they have not as yet been able to eliminate the problem. Also, there remain some questions about maintenance of these interventions and comparative efficacy between different types of behavior modification techniques. Finally, current computer technology offers some opportunities for improvement over current behavior modification treatments of incontinence (Werner, 1995).

Aggressive/Disruptive Behavior

Aggressive or disruptive behavior is one of the most frequent symptoms in older adults with dementia (Eisdorfer et al., 1992) and those in nursing homes (Zimmer, Watson, & Treat, 1984), who often have some dementia. Unfortunately, the treatment most often prescribed for these patients is pharmacotherapy (Maletta, Mattow, & Dysken, 1991), which is beneficial for only a limited number of patients (Risse & Barnes, 1986), and older adults who display disruptive behaviors need more nursing care than those who do not exhibit such behaviors (National Center for Health Statistics, 1981). Additionally, dementia and agitated/aggressive behaviors are risks factors for placement in nursing homes and for caregiver distress (Blume, Persely, & Mintzer, 1992).

Unfortunately, nursing staff often are the victims of aggressive behavior in nursing homes. In an effort to identify nursing staff members' perceptions of the primary disruptive behaviors among nursing home residents and the strategies used to treat these behaviors, Whall, Gillis, Yankou, Booth, and Beel-Bates (1992) conducted a survey of nursing staff members. The results indicate that the three procedures most frequently used by staff members to deal with disruptive behaviors are verbal discussion (66% of staff), chemical restraints (50%), and physical restraints (43%). Staff also used behavior modification techniques, but only on a limited basis: time out (40%), extinction (17%), differential reinforcement of other behavior (3%). Given that the majority of disruptive behaviors are ones not generally dangerous to patients or staff (the main exception was hitting/slapping), these figures are especially disturbing.

Fortunately, there is evidence that proper training can reduce the number of aggressive behaviors and increase the appropriate use of behavior modification strategies. One study (Colenda & Hamer, 1991) showed that prior to an in-service training, the primary staff intervention for aggression consisted of one-to-one supervision. Staff then received training in behavior modification and use of psychotropic drugs for older adults, with an encouragement to use p.r.n. ("as-needed") medications with violent patients who "began to telegraph aggressive behavior" (p. 289). Review of records indicated a 23.6% decrease in aggressive behaviors, with the primary decrease coming from dementia patients. Also of interest, the primary self-reported means of dealing with aggressive behavior changed. For dementia patients, p.r.n. medications became the primary staff intervention, and for nondementia patients, removal of patient (a form of time out) became the primary staff intervention. Thus, staff in-service trainings can alter behavior of staff and patients in dealing with aggressive behavior. Another report describing a behavioral intensive care unit (BICU) revealed that with appropriate behavior modification interventions, BICU staff were able to eliminate the need for medication to control aggressive and wandering behaviors among some case study examples (Mintzer et al., 1993).

There are many other examples of studies that have used behavior modification or multicomponent treatments that include behavior modification to treat aggressive behavior among older adults (e.g., Bakke et al., 1994; Davis & Boster, 1988; Hinchliffe, Hyman, Blizard, & Livingston, 1992; Mishara & Kastenbaum, 1973; Rapp, Flint, Herrmann, & Proulx, 1992). Thus, there is no question that behavior modification techniques can help ameliorate aggressive behavior difficulties among older adults, even if the patients have significant cognitive impairment. There remain, however, numerous areas for future research. For example, additional studies to compare how behavior modification strategies compare against pharmacotherapy, the use of behavioral assessment strategies for evaluating the effects of pharmacotherapy, and the ability to train caregivers in the implementation of behavior modification strategies are just a few areas in need of research.

Health Behaviors

The majority of behavior modification techniques used with older adults involve elimination of "negative" behaviors, such as aggressiveness or incontinence. There has been relatively little research on the acquisition of health promoting behaviors among older adults. Although many studies that emphasize acquisition of health behaviors include older adults in the sample, very few studies have actually attempted to determine if age affects acquisition of these behaviors.

One of the areas of significant importance is that of exercise. A recent study revealed that 80% of older adults have at least one chronic illness that may have an impact on level of physical activity (King, 1991). The decline in exercise among older adults may reduce strength, flexibility, balance, and cardiovascular capacity, thereby affecting ability to conduct regular daily tasks (Dubbert & Stetson, 1995) and contributing to the increase in falls. Thus, maintenance of regular physical activity among older adults is important if they are to remain independent (Buschner & de Lateur, 1991). Fortunately, one recent study (Neff, Bill-Harvey, Shade, Iezzi, & DeLorenzo, 1995) indicated that through the use of videotaped modeling procedures, staff could increase exercise participation for as much as 6 months. Using a modified multiple baseline design, Neff and colleagues (1995) also demonstrated that exercise participation improved gait and balance of the participants.

Another area ripe for research is improving dietary practices of older adults. Because dietary habits relate to both cancer and coronary artery disease, two of the leading causes of death among older adults (Ho, Lee, & Meyskens, 1991; Kannel, 1986), this is an important consideration. In one of the few studies assessing effects of behavior modification on food choices of older adults, Stock and Milan (1993) introduced prompts, feedback about number of healthy food choices made, and social reinforcement contingent upon report of having chosen healthy foods in an effort to increase the percentage of healthy foods chosen among targeted

patients. Investigators used a single case experimental design to determine the efficacy of intervention and found that the treatment package did indeed result in a substantial increase in the percentage of healthy choices made by targeted individuals. Another study assessing behavioral training, didactics, and provision of emotional support on older adults with diabetes used a two-group multiple baseline design to determine effects on blood glucose levels and dietary adherence (Robison, 1993). This study also revealed that behavior modification procedures used were effective in meeting dietary objectives. In addition, as a positive consequence, subjects evidenced lower blood glucose levels compared to pretreatment levels. Follow-up results revealed sustained glucose results at 12 and 24 weeks but an increasing number of diet deviations by 48 weeks. Thus, the few studies conducted on behavior modification of older adults' eating behavior have shown that they are amenable to change with these techniques. It remains unknown, however, whether these changes have any appreciable effect on subsequent health status.

Summary

The literature on behavior modification with older adults is still very much in its infancy. Although behavior modification techniques have enjoyed good success over the roughly 80 years of their existence within the behavior therapy discipline, there remain few studies that have specifically targeted older adults.

Future areas of research for behavior modification with older adults abound. For example, although research has clearly shown the efficacy of behavior modification techniques in reducing aggressive/disruptive behavior, the extent of their applicability remain ambiguous. Also, there is the possibility of using behavioral assessment methodology in evaluating pharmacotherapy (e.g., Burgio & Hawkins, 1991), especially because psychoactive drugs can differentially affect individuals based on age (Andersson, Antonsson, Corin, Swahn, & Fridlund, 1995). Implementation of behavior modification programs, such as token economies, may become increasingly important, especially since federal mandates have encouraged the use of behavior modification and other nonpharmacological treatments for control of behavior problems among nursing home residents (Burgio & Bourgeois, 1992).

Beyond behavior modification itself, there is a significant need for evaluation of psychopathology and coping among older adults. Such issues will undoubtedly affect the efficacy of behavior modification attempts and may play a role in many of the problems older adults exhibit. For example, there is very little information on anxiety in older adults (Hersen & Van Hasselt, 1992; Hersen, Van Hasselt, & Goreczny, 1993). Much of the motoric and disruptive movements often associated with nondemented older adults may be symptomatology of an anxiety disorder. In addition, although one study noted that older adults report feeling less "stressed" than do younger adults (Nussbaum & Goreczny, 1994), a recent study revealed that older adults, relative to their younger cohorts, have greater psychophysiological reactivity to a mental arithmetic stressor (Goreczny, Keen, & Walter, 1996). Thus, changing physiologies of older adults and their beliefs in their coping abilities may affect the outcome of behavior modification programs.

Another area for future research is modification of health behaviors of older adults. Although there has been some initial speculation that older adults do not respond to behavior therapies aimed at improving health status as well as younger adults do, there are studies that indicate a different picture; older adults are able to use behavior modification strategies to improve exercise participation and healthy dietary choices. In addition, recent research has revealed that older adults are able to benefit from smoking cessation attempts (Fincham, 1992) and strategies aimed at reducing blood pressure (Pearce, Engel, & Burton, 1989) as well as treatments to reduce headaches (Holroyd & French, 1995). The evaluation of cardiac rehabilitation programs and behavior modification of patients in such programs represents another exciting area for investigation (Stetson, Frommelt, Boutelle, & Cole, 1995).

Evaluating behavior modification treatment differences between patients with dementia versus those without dementia is another area for future consideration. Recent research has revealed that patients with dementia may actually evidence increased symptomatology when participating in a structured group activity designed to increase their socialization (Walter, DeYoung, Masciantonio, & Goreczny, 1994). The importance of finding ways to increase socialization among both community dwelling and nursing home residents is an area that must receive future attention if we want to continue to service the needs of our older adults (Hersen, Van Hasselt, & Segal, 1995; Ungvari & Hantz, 1991).

Finally, there are many basic studies about the patient–provider relationship that warrant investigation. For example, how do patients affect providers' behaviors and vice versa? Investigation into this interaction may provide information that will not only be applicable to older adults, but also to the health care industry in general. Also of interest to all practitioners (and administrators and health policy experts) is how staff training and implementation of basic behavior modification principles at the organizational level affect health behaviors of patients. Although behavior modification principles are undoubtedly effective, much work remains to convince policy makers and administrators of their effectiveness in changing staff and patient behaviors and outcomes.

References

Andersson, E., Antonsson, M., Corin, B., Swahn, B., & Fridlund, B. (1995). The preventive effect of lithium therapy on bipolar patients, with special reference to gender and age. *International Journal of Rehabilitation and Health, 1,* 203–209.

Baer, D. M., & Wolf, M. M. (1970). The entry into natural contingencies of reinforcement. In R. Ulrich, T. Stachnik, & J. Mabry (Eds.), *Control of human behavior* (Vol. 2, pp. 319–324). Glenview, IL: Scott-Foresman.

Bakke, B. L., Kvale, S., Burns, T., McCarten, J. R., Wilson, L., Maddox, M., & Cleary, J. (1994). Multicomponent intervention for agitated behavior in a person with Alzheimer's disease. *Journal of Applied Behavior Analysis, 27,* 175–176.

Bandura, A. (1965). Influence of model's reinforcement contingencies on the acquisition of imitative responses. *Journal of Personality and Social Psychology, 1,* 589–595.

Bandura, A. (1969). *Principles of behavior modification.* New York: Holt, Rinehart, & Winston.

Barlow, D. H., & Hersen, M. (1973). Single-case experimental designs: Uses in applied clinical research. *Archives of General Psychiatry, 29,* 319–325.

Barrett, B. H., Johnston, J. M., & Pennypacker, H. S. (1986). Behavior: Its units, dimensions, and measurement. In R. O. Nelson & S. C. Hayes (Eds.), *Conceptual foundations of behavioral assessment* (pp. 156–200). New York: Guilford Press.

Bellack, A. S., Hersen, M., & Kazdin, A. E. (1990). *International handbook of behavior modification and therapy* (2nd ed.). New York: Plenum.

Birren, J. E., & Renner, J. (1980). Concepts and issues of mental health and aging. In J. E. Birren & R. B. Sloane (Eds.), *Handbook of mental health and aging* (pp. 3–33). Englewood Cliffs, NJ: Prentice-Hall.

Blume, L., Persely, N., & Mintzer, J. (1992). The prevalence of dementia: The confusion of numbers. *American Journal of Alzheimer's Care and Related Disorders Research, May/June,* 3–18.

Brazda, J. F. (1983). Washington report. The nation's health.

Burgio, L. D., & Bourgeois, M. (1992). Treating severe behavioral disorders in geriatric residential settings. *Behavioral Residential Treatment, 7,* 145–168.

Burgio, L. D., & Hawkins, A. M. (1991). Behavioral assessment of the effects of psychotropic medications on demented nursing home residents. *Behavior Modification, 15,* 194–212.

Buschner, D. M., & de Lateur, B. J. (1991). The importance of skeletal muscle strength to physical function in older adults. *Annals of Behavioral Medicine, 13,* 133–140.

Chelune, G. J., Heaton, R. K., & Lehman, R. A. W. (1986). Neuropsychological and personality correlates of patients' complaints of disability. In G. Goldstein & R. E. Tarter (Eds.), *Advances in clinical neuropsychology* (Vol. 3, pp. 95–126). New York: Plenum Press.

Colenda, C. C., & Hamer, R. M. (1991). Antecedents and interventions for aggressive behavior of patients at a geropsychiatric state hospital. *Hospital and Community Psychiatry, 42,* 287–292.

Colling, J., Ouslander, J., Hadley, B. J., Eisch, J., & Campbell, E. (1992). The effects of patterned urge-response toileting (PURT) on urinary incontinence among nursing home residents. *Journal of the American Geriatrics Society, 40,* 135–141.

Corrigan, P. W., MacKain, S. J., & Liberman, R. P. (1994). Skills training modules: A strategy for dissemination and utilization of a rehabilitation innovation. In J. Rothman & E. Thomas (Eds.), *Intervention research* (pp. 317–352). Chicago: Haworth Press.

Davis, D. L., & Boster, L. (1988). Multifaceted therapeutic interventions with violent inpatients. *Hospital and Community Psychiatry, 39,* 867–869.

Dietz, S. M., Repp, A. C., & Dietz, D. E. D. (1976). Reducing inappropriate classroom behavior of retarded students through three procedures of differential reinforcement. *Journal of Mental Deficiency Research, 20,* 155–170.

Diokno, A. C., Brock, B. M., & Brown, M. B. (1986). Prevalence of urinary incontinence and other urological symptoms in the noninstitutionalized elderly. *Journal of Urology, 136,* 1022.

Dubbert, P. M., & Stetson, B. A. (1995). Exercise and physical activity. In A. J. Goreczny (Ed.), *Handbook of health and rehabilitation psychology* (pp. 255–274). New York: Plenum.

Eisdorfer, C., Cohen, D., Paveza, G. J., Ashford, J. W., Luchins, D. J., Gorelick, P. B., Hirschman, R. S., Freels, S. A., Levy, P. S., Semla, T. P., & Shaw, H. A. (1992). An empirical evaluation

of the Global Deterioration Scale for staging Alzheimer's disease. *American Journal of Psychiatry, 140,* 190–194.

Engel, B. T., Burgio, L. D., McCormick, K. A., Hawkins, A. M., Scheve, A. A. S., & Leahy, E. (1990). Behavioral treatment of incontinence in the long-term care setting. *Journal of the American Geriatrics Society, 38,* 361–363.

Fincham, J. E. (1992). The etiology and pathogenesis of detrimental health effects in elderly smokers. *Journal of Geriatric Drug Therapy, 7,* 5–21.

Goldstein, G., & McCue, M. (1995). Differences between patient and informant functional outcome ratings in head-injured individuals. *International Journal of Rehabilitation and Health, 1,* 25–35.

Goreczny, A. J. (1995). Introductory statement—Forging ahead into the 21st century: Issues in rehabilitation. *International Journal of Rehabilitation and Health, 1,* 1–3.

Goreczny, A. J., & O'Halloran, C. M. (1995). The future of psychology in health care. In A. J. Goreczny (Ed.), *Handbook of health and rehabilitation psychology* (pp. 663–676). New York: Plenum.

Goreczny, A. J., Keen, A., & Walter, K. (in preparation). Psychophysiological reactivity among younger versus older adults.

Gribbin, B., Pickering, T. G., Sleight, P., & Peto, R. (1971). Effect of age and blood pressure on baroflex sensitivity in man. *Circulation Research, 29,* 424–431.

Hartmann, D. P., & Wood, D. D. (1990). Observational methods. In A. S. Bellack, M. Hersen, & A. E. Kazdin (Eds.), *International handbook of behavior modification and therapy* (2nd ed., pp. 107–138). New York: Plenum Press.

Haynes, S. N. (1986). The design of intervention programs. In R. O. Nelson & S. C. Hayes (Eds.), *Conceptual foundations of behavioral assessment* (pp. 386–429). New York: Guilford Press.

Hersen, M. (1990). Single-case experimental designs. In A. S. Bellack, M. Hersen, & A. E. Kazdin (Eds.), *International handbook of behavior modification and therapy* (2nd ed., pp. 175–210). New York: Plenum Press.

Hersen, M., & Barlow, D. H. (1976). *Single case experimental designs: Strategies for studying behavior change.* New York: Pergamon Press.

Hersen, M., & Van Hasselt, V. B. (1992). Behavioral assessment and treatment of anxiety in the elderly. *Clinical Psychology Review, 12,* 619–640.

Hersen, M., Van Hasselt, V. B., & Goreczny, A. J. (1993). Behavioral assessment of anxiety in older adults: Some comments. *Behavior Modification, 17,* 99–112.

Hersen, M., Van Hasselt, V. B., & Segal, D. L. (1995). Social adaptation in older visually impaired adults: Some comments. *International Journal of Rehabilitation and Health, 1,* 49–60.

Hinchliffe, A. C., Hyman, I., Blizard, B., & Livingston, G. (1992). The impact on carers of behavioural difficulties in dementia: A pilot study on management. *International Journal of Geriatric Psychiatry, 7,* 579–583.

Ho, E. E., Lee, F. C. Y., & Meyskens, F. L., Jr. (1991). An exploratory study of attitudes, beliefs and practices related to the interim dietary guidelines for reducing cancer in the elderly. *Journal of Nutrition for the Elderly, 10,* 31–49.

Holden, U. (1984). Head injury and older people. In U. Holden (Ed.), *Neuropsychology and aging* (pp. 154–176). New York: New York University Press.

Holroyd, K. A., & French, D. J. (1995). Recent developments in the psychological assessment and management of recurrent headache disorders. In A. J. Goreczny (Ed.), *Handbook of health and rehabilitation psychology* (pp. 3–30). New York: Plenum.

Hoyer, C. C. (1990). Brain glucose and energy metabolism during normal aging. *Aging, 2,* 245–258.

Hu, T. (1990). Impact of urinary incontinence on health-care costs. *Journal of American Geriatrics Society, 38,* 292–295.

Kannel, W. B. (1986). Nutritional contributors to cardiovascular disease in the elderly. *Journal of the American Geriatrics Society, 34,* 27–36.

Katzman, RE., & Terry, R. (1992). Normal aging of the central nervous system. In R. Katzman & J. W. Rowe (Eds.), *Principles of geriatric neurology* (pp. 18–58). Philadelphia: Davis.

Kazdin, A. E. (1977). *The token economy: A review and evaluation.* New York: Plenum Press.

Kazdin, A. E. (1978). *History of behavior modification: Experimental foundations of contemporary research.* Baltimore: University Park Press.

King, A. C. (1991). Physical activity and health enhancement in older adults: Current status and future prospects. *Annals of Behavioral Medicine, 13,* 87–90.

Kornhaber, R. C., & Schroeder, H. E. (1975). Importance of modeling similarity on extinction of avoidance behavior in children. *Journal of Consulting and Clinical Psychology, 5,* 601–607.

Krasner, L. (1990). History of behavior modification. In A. S. Bellack, M. Hersen, & A. E. Kazdin (Eds.), *International handbook of behavior modification and therapy* (2nd ed., pp. 3–25). New York: Plenum.

Lim, K. O., Zipursky, R. B., Murphy, G. M., & Pfefferbaum, A. (1990). In vivo quantification of the limbic system using MRI: Effects of normal aging. *Psychiatry Research, 35,* 15–26.

Lousberg, R., Schmidt, A. J., & Groenman, N. H. (1992). The relationship between spouse solicitousness and pain behavior: Searching for more experimental evidence. *Pain, 51,* 75–79.

Maletta, G., Mattow, K. M., & Dysken, M. (1991). Guidelines for prescribing psychoactive drugs in the elderly: Part I. *Geriatrics, 46,* 40–47.

McDowell, B. J., Burgio, K. L., Dombrowski, M., Locher, J. L., & Rodriquez, E. (1992). An interdisciplinary approach to the assessment and behavioral treatment of urinary incontinence in geriatric outpatients. *Journal of the American Geriatrics Society, 40,* 370–374.

Meichenbaum, D. (1971). Examination of model characteristics in reducing avoidance behavior. *Journal of Personality and Social Psychology, 17,* 298–307.

Milan, M. A. (1990). Applied behavior analysis. In A. S. Bellack, M. Hersen, & A. E. Kazdin (Eds.), *International handbook of behavior modification and therapy* (2nd ed., pp. 67–84). New York: Plenum.

Mintzer, J. E., Lewis, L., Pennypaker, L., Simpson, W., Bachman, D., Wohlreich, G., Meeks, A., Hunt, S., & Sampson, R. (1993). Behavioral intensive care unit (BICU): A new concept in the management of acute agitated behavior in elderly demented patients. *The Gerontologist, 33,* 801–806.

Mishara, B. L., & Kastenbaum, R. (1973). Self-injurious behavior and environmental change in the institutionalized elderly. *International Journal of Aging and Human Development, 4,* 133–145.

National Center for Health Statistics. (1981). Characteristics of nursing home residents' health status and care received. *National Nursing Home Survey* (Department of Health and Human Services Publication No. PHS 81-1712). Washington, DC: U.S. Government Printing Office.

Neff, N. A., Bill-Harvey, D., Shade, D., Iezzi, M., & DeLorenzo, T. (1995). Exercise participation with videotaped modeling: Effects on balance and gait in elderly residents of care facilities. *Behavior Therapy, 26,* 135–151.

Nussbaum, P. D. (1995). Aging: Issues in health and neuropsychological functioning. In A. J. Goreczny (Ed.), *Handbook of health and rehabilitation psychology* (pp. 583–603). New York: Plenum.

Nussbaum, P. D., & Goldstein, G. (1992). Neuropsychological sequelae of cardiac transplantation: A preliminary review. *Clinical Psychology Review, 12,* 475–484.

Nussbaum, P. D., & Goreczny, A. J. (1994). Self-appraisal of stress level and related psychopathology. *Journal of Anxiety Disorders, 9,* 463–472.

Nussbaum, P. D., Allender, J., & Copeland, J. (1995). Verbal learning in cardiac transplant candidates: A preliminary report. *International Journal of Rehabilitation and Health, 1,* 5–12.

Ouslander, J. G. (1990). Urinary incontinence in nursing homes. *Journal of the American Geriatrics Society, 38,* 289–291.

Pearce, K. L., Engel, B. T., & Burton, J. R. (1989). Behavioral treatment of isolated systolic hypertension in the elderly. *Biofeedback and Self-Regulation, 14,* 207–217.

Poling, A. (1985). Extinction. In A. S. Bellack & M. Hersen (Eds.), *Dictionary of behavior therapy techniques* (p. 124). Elsford, NY: Pergamon Press.

Ranseen, J., Bohaska, L., & Schmitt, F. (1990). An investigation of anosognosia following traumatic head injury. *International Journal of Clinical Neuropsychology, 12,* 29–36.

Rapp, M. S., Flint, A. J., Herrmann, N., & Proulx, G. B. (1992). Behavioural disturbances in the demented elderly: Phenomenology, pharmacotherapy and behavioural management. *Canadian Journal of Psychiatry, 37,* 651–657.

Risse, S. C., & Barnes, R. (1986). Pharmacologic treatment of agitation associated with dementia. *Journal of the American Geriatrics Society, 34,* 368–376.

Robison, F. F. (1993). A training and support group for elderly diabetics: Description and evaluation. *Journal of Specialists in Group Work, 18,* 127–136.

Rowe, J. W., & Katzman, R. (1992). Principles of geriatrics as applied to neurology. In R. Katzman & J. W. Rowe (Eds.), *Principles of geriatric neurology* (pp. 3–17). Philadelphia: Davis.

Samelson, F. (1981). Struggle for scientific authority: The reception of Watson's behaviorism, 1913–1920. *Journal of the History of the Behavioral Sciences, 17,* 399–425.

Savageau, J. A., Stanton, B., Jenkins, C. D., & Frater, R. W. M. (1982). Neuropsychological dysfunction following open heart surgery. II. A six-month reassessment. *Journal of Thoracic and Cardiovascular Surgery, 84,* 595–600.

Savageau, J. A., Stanton, B., Jenkins, C. D., & Klein, M. D. (1982). Neuropsychological dysfunction following elective cardiac operation. I. Early assessment. *Journal of Thoracic and Cardiovascular Surgery, 84,* 585–594.

Schnelle, J. F. (1990). Treatment of urinary incontinence in nursing home patients by prompted voiding. *Journal of the American Geriatrics Society, 38,* 356–360.

Sidman, M. (1960). *Tactics of scientific research: Evaluating experimental data in psychology.* New York: Basic Books.

Singh, N. N., Dawson, M. J., & Manning, P. (1981). Effects of spaced responding DRL on the stereotyped behavior of profoundly retarded persons. *Journal of Applied Behavior Analysis, 14,* 521–526.

Sontaniemi, K. A., Monomen, H., & Hokkanen, T. E. (1986). Long term cerebral outcome after open heart surgery: A five year neuropsychological follow-up study. *Stroke, 17,* 410–416.

Stetson, B. A., Frommelt, S. J., Boutelle, K. N., & Cole, J. (1995). Exercise-related thoughts in cardiac exercise programs: A study of exercise adherent cardiac rehabilitation patients. *International Journal of Rehabilitation and Health, 1,* 125–136.

Stock, L. Z., & Milan, M. A. (1993). Improving dietary practices of elderly individuals: The power of prompting, feedback, and social reinforcement. *Journal of Applied Behavior Analysis, 26,* 379–387.

Ungvari, G. S., & Hantz, P. M. (1991). Social breakdown in the elderly: I. Case studies and management. *Comprehensive Psychiatry, 32,* 440–444.

Walter, K., DeYoung, R., Masciantonio, M. P., & Goreczny, A. J. (1994). Efficacy of a structured group activity program for demented and non-demented psychiatric inpatients. Paper presented at the Greater Pittsburgh Sixth Annual Clinical Nursing Research Conference, Pittsburgh, PA.

Watson, J. B. (1913). Psychology as the behaviorist views it. *Psychological Review, 20,* 158–177.

Werner, G. (1995). Computer applications in behavioral medicine. In A. J. Goreczny (Ed.), Handbook of health and rehabilitation psychology (pp. 605–635). New York: Plenum.

Whall, A. L., Gillis, G. L., Yankou, D., Booth, D. E., & Beel-Bates, C. A. (1992). Disruptive behavior in elderly nursing home residents: A survey of nursing staff. *Journal of Gerontological Nursing, 18,* 13–17.

Wolf, M. M., Risley, T. R., & Mees, H. L. (1964). Application of operant conditioning procedures to the behavior problems of an autistic child. *Behaviour Research and Therapy, 1,* 305–312.

Yu, L. C., & Kaltreider, D. L. (1987). Stressed nurses dealing with incontinent patients. *Journal of Gerontological Nursing, 13,* 27–30.

Zimmer, J. G., Watson, N., & Treat, A. (1984). Behavioral problems among patients in skilled nursing facilities. *American Journal of Public Health, 74,* 1118–1121.

31

Elderly Caregivers and Care Receivers

Facts and Gaps in the Literature

Introduction

Meeting the needs of families caring for elders at home continues to be a major challenge as we move into the 21st century. The tremendous expansion of the older population will mean that ever more families will be involved in providing some amount of care for aged parents, grandparents, spouses, siblings, and adult children. By 2010 the baby boomers will contribute their mass to the 65 and older group and by 2030 will have a dramatic effect on the numbers of individuals over 85 (Hooyman & Kiyak, 1993). Since fewer members of that generation got married and stayed married, and since many tended to have one or no children, the impact of that generation on society will be great (Dychtwald & Flower, 1988). Initially, "boomers" will be primary caregivers to parents and grandparents. Later, their small families will be their caregivers.

Although the continued expansion of the older population is a phenomenon of minorities as well as of whites, the caregiving literature has paid too little attention to the needs of poor elderly and minority caregiving families. The proportion of the population age 65 and older is increasing. It was 9.2% in 1960, 12.6% in 1990, and is projected to grow to 17.7% in 2020 and to 22.9% in 2050 (Angel & Hogan, 1994). The ethnic minority population is

SHARON M. WALLSTEN • Duke University School of Nursing, Duke University Medical Center, Durham, North Carolina 27710.

expected to grow more rapidly than the population of whites, so that the population proportion of African Americans and other minorities would increase from 10.2% in 1990 to 15.3% in 2020 and to 21.3% in 2050 (Angel & Hogan, 1994). Minority older Americans continue to be overrepresented in the group with incomes below the poverty line. Among elder whites, 10% have a below-poverty income. Corresponding percentages for minorities are as follows: Asian Americans, 14%; Hispanics, 23%; Native Americans, 35%; and African Americans, 36% (Hooyman & Kiyak, 1993). Very little is known about the circumstances in which caregiving occurs in these minority and/or poor households. Jackson (1994) urged gerontological researchers to place more emphasis on race, culture, ethnicity, gender, and social and economic status, so that the needs of all peoples can be better understood and appropriate services can be provided.

This chapter begins by describing demographic trends and their potential impact on caregivers and their care recipients. Next, it considers facts and gaps in the caregiving literature as they pertain to broadening the knowledge base to include minorities, in particular African Americans, and to include other understudied populations. This section contains an overview of deficiencies in research, trends regarding minority caregiving, a discussion of the importance of comparing caregivers to non-caregivers, and the need for an in-depth look at elder spouse caregivers. The chapter concludes with a look at caregiver and care receiver interactions and with a summary and implications of findings for researchers and practitioners.

Demographic Changes and Their Implications for Caregiving

Life Expectancy, Morbidity, and Living Arrangements

Knowledge and pharmacological control of infectious disease, sophisticated technology, and attention to healthy lifestyles have contributed to an ever increasing number of people living into the oldest years. In 1980, Fries suggested that average life expectancy was increasing toward the maximum possible because preventive approaches to chronic illness were postponing or preventing certain disease processes. He described a "rectangularization" of the life span; at some point the life span will stay approximately constant at a biological limit; morbidity years will occupy a smaller proportion of the life span, and people will be older when first experiencing manifestations of chronic disease. Refuting Fries's predictions, Schneider and Brody (1983) provided evidence that the life span was increasing, that the number of the very old was increasing rapidly, but that chronic diseases occupy a larger percentage of the life span, necessitating increased health care needs in later life. Using the National Health Interview Survey from 1958 to 1985, Verbrugge (1989) found that cohorts of middle-aged (45–64) and older adults (65 and over) reported increased short-term disability and increased days of restricted activity in each successive survey. Thus, over a 27-year period, morbidity rates increased for life-threatening and non-life-threatening diseases; however mortality rates did not change. Fries's predictions may be realized in future cohorts (including the baby boomers) who are more likely to have participated in disease prevention behaviors such as eating low-fat diets and engaging in exercise.

Older Adults as Caregivers and Care Receivers

Although an individual's ability to function independently is based on many factors including psychological, cognitive, sensory, social, eco- nomic, and physical disease, the two factors thought to have the greatest direct impact on independent functioning are physical and cognitive functioning (Guralnik & Simonsick, 1993). In 1987, approximately 13% of older adults living in the community needed help with basic self-care, or activities of daily living (ADL) such as toileting and bathing, and 17.5% were limited in interactive functions which facilitate community independence or in instrumental activities of daily living (IADL) such as using a telephone, paying bills, and food preparation (Rakowski & Pearlman, 1995). The majority of people in need of some help with IADL or ADL receive it from informal sources in the community. Although 59% of elders with five to seven losses in ADL receive care in nursing homes, 41% with equally high levels of disability receive care in the home (Guralnik & Simonsick, 1993; Hing & Bloom, 1990). Chances for disability increase dramatically with advancing age: whereas 9% of males and 10% of females in the 65–74 age group require some help from another person while living at home, 14% of males and 21% of females in the 75–84 age group require help, and 31% of males and 37% of females in the 85+ age group need help. Although the proportion of disabled men and women are similar for the 65–74 age group, women have greater disability at higher age groups (Guralnik & Simonsick, 1993; Schneider & Guralnik, 1990). Males are more likely to die at younger ages from life-threatening disease, and women have more years to accrue more disabling conditions (Markides & Mindel, 1987). Therefore it can be inferred that married men are more likely to be living with a spouse and more likely to be cared for by their spouse (Kasper, 1988). On the other hand, married male caregivers are more likely to be among the oldest of caregivers.

Overall, approximately 5 million elderly persons living in the community require some amount of long-term care, and the majority of the care is provided by families. This figure is projected to increase to 7.2 million by 2000, 10.1 million by 2020, and 14.4 million by 2050 (Hooyman & Kiyak, 1993). The majority of people turn to a spouse or children for help (Kasper, 1988). In descending order of frequency, primary caregivers include spouses, children, other relatives, and friends/neighbors (Cantor, 1983; Johnson, 1983; Stone, Cafferata, & Sangl, 1987). It is also becoming increasingly apparent that many spouses, other relatives, and friends who are primary caregivers are themselves in their aged years (Gatz, Bengston, & Blum, 1990; S. M. Wallsten, 1995).

Longer life expectancy has increased the probability that middle-aged persons have living parents and grandparents. Over 25% of the women born in the 1930s who reach their 60th birthday will have mothers still living, and 10% of women over the age of 65 will have a child who is over age 65. Many such women will have a living parent and be a grandparent simultaneously (Hooyman & Kiyak, 1993). Moreover, because most middle-aged adults have grown up with fewer siblings than did their own parents, they have a smaller prospective network of support from kin (Gatz et al., 1990). With over half of married middle-aged women working and an even greater proportion of unmarried middle-aged women working, families with elder parents and/or grandparents experience competing demands on their time.

As reported by Kasper (1988), women continue to have longer life expectancies from birth than men; once they reach age 65, women average 19 more years of life and men average 15. However, these added years present new problems to some women living alone, especially those with disabling conditions. Continued independence relies upon factors such as having caregivers from informal and/or formal sources as well as having someone willing to coordinate these efforts. It is not surprising then that elderly people living alone are at greater risk for entering a nursing home as their ADL needs increase (Kasper, 1988).

Using 1987 U.S. Bureau of the Census data, Kasper (1988) reported that 15.1 million people 65 years of age or older (54%) live with spouses; 4.4 million (16%) live with children, other relatives, or friends; and 8.5 million (30%) live alone. Angel and Hogan (1994) provide data showing living arrangements of elderly persons in 1989 by ethnicity and race. Within ethnic groups, similar percentages of African-American and white elderly live alone (31.2% vs. 32.0%, respectively). However, more than half (55.3%) of whites and only a little over a third (36.7%) of African Americans live with a spouse. This is in part attributed to the lower life expectancy of African-American males and the higher percentage of older African-American females who are widowed. In addition, rates of di-

vorce and separation in the younger years for African Americans are higher than in other groups (Hooyman & Kiyak, 1993). Angel and Hogan also show that while 32.1% of African-American elderly persons live with others, only 12.7% of whites do.

Looking at the percentages of African-American and white elderly living alone, 37% of African Americans and 26% of whites have no living children, 18% of African Americans and 19% of whites have one child upon whom they can rely, and 45% of African Americans and 55% of whites have two or more children. Contrary to widely held beliefs about having extensive support networks, African Americans living alone appear to have fewer family members upon whom they can rely (Hooyman & Kiyak, 1993; Kasper, 1988).

It has been estimated that 19% of elderly living alone are poor compared to 10% of those living with others and 4% of couples (Kasper, 1988). However, of those elderly living alone and in poverty, 57.4% are African Americans and 18.2% are whites. Of those elderly living in poverty with a spouse, 14.9% are African Americans and 4.6% are whites. Noteworthy is that a greater percentage of impoverished African Americans (14.9%) live with others than do whites (4.6%) (Angel & Hogan, 1994), possibly placing increased financial strain on their families. Despite the greater likelihood of poverty when living alone or with others, and the decreased likelihood of having someone to rely on when living alone, African-American elders 65 years of age and older comprised only 7% of nursing home residents in 1985 whereas 92.2% were white and less than 1% were of another race (National Center for Health Statistics, 1989).

With four out of five persons 65 and older having at least one chronic condition, many elderly caregivers themselves suffer from chronic illness (Besdine, 1990). Guralnik, LaCroix, Everett, and Kovar (1989) examined nine commonly reported chronic illnesses from the Supplement on Aging of the National Health Interview Survey and found substantial comorbidity in persons 65 and older, which increased with age. Problems that could affect caregiving, such as cardiovascular disease, arthritis, dementia, hearing, visual impairment, and osteoporosis, are more prevalent in older people than in younger people (Rowe, 1985). It follows then that elderly caregivers and care recipients are both highly likely to have physical and/or cognitive problems; yet circumstances are such that one member of the pair thinks of himself/herself as the caregiver rather than the care recipient.

Geller, Delfs, Rabins, and Reichel (1995) estimated that 1% of the population has dementia at age 65, 10% at age 75, and 25% to 30% at age 85. Heyman et al. (1991) reported significantly higher prevalence of dementia in African Americans than in whites in their study of community residents of a five-county area in North Carolina. Subjects were drawn from the sample of the Duke Established Populations for Epidemiological Studies of the Elderly (EPESE), a longitudinal study of a stratified sample of community residents 65 years of age and older. The authors speculated that the fivefold higher rates observed in African Americans and verified through neurological exam may be related to their history of significantly higher reported rates of stroke and hypertension. The authors reviewed two other studies that examined dementia in African-American and white populations. One study (Schoenberg, Anderson, & Haerer, 1985) showed that severe dementia was more prevalent among women than among men and more prevalent among African Americans than among whites. The other, smaller study (Folstein, Anthony, Parhad, Duffy, & Gruenberg, 1985) found dementia prevalence the same in both groups, but dementia caused by cerebrovascular disease was more frequent among African Americans. Considering that the racial composition of nursing home residents 65 and older is overwhelmingly white, and keeping in mind the higher disability rates among African Americans, it is possible that African-American care recipients and caregivers in the community have greater physical and cognitive problems than their white counterparts. Hence, African-American and other ethnic minority caregivers potentially face great challenges in fulfilling their basic needs. It seems particularly important to examine the circumstances in which African Americans and other minorities receive care in the community.

Caregiving Is a Dynamic Process

The caregiving process is not static. Each member of the caregiver and care recipient dyad can have acute and/or chronic problems that improve or worsen, and, of course, this happens within the context of other ongoing life experiences and changes over time. Unfortunately, cross-sectional designs are not likely to provide important insights into this transitional process. It is often the case that functional deficiencies in ADL and/or IADL stem from cognitive dysfunction as well as other problems such as stroke, hip fracture, and arthritis. The mental and physical health of both members of the caregiving relationship must be considered. A subtle change in conditions may produce insurmountable strain leading to dangerous or compromised caregiving conditions. Families often consider nursing home placement as a last resort, thereby waiting until conditions have worsened considerably (Quinn & Tomita, 1986).

Abusive and neglectful situations arise from many sources, including the closeness of the relationship, nature of the past relationship, kinds of adjustments needed, kinds of responsibilities added, sense of control over the situation, social network, and experience with the caregiving role (Quinn & Tomita, 1986). For example, on May 7, 1995, the *St. Petersburg Times* in Florida reported the story of a 71-year-old woman who was cared for by her son and who was reported to police by an anonymous friend. The woman was found on her couch "covered in her own feces and crawling with worms, ants, roaches and maggots … her flesh in places was rotting away." Her 40-year-old son had provided care for 2 years and left her in one position for 6 months (Landry, 1995). A follow-up report on May 9 based on an interview with the woman's daughter who lived in a nearby county indicated that she had not seen her mother for 6 months because of childcare issues and her own job caring for a diabetic, blind, double-amputee elderly woman (P. F. Wallsten, 1995). This family had limited involvement with a formal health care system. We know little about what is happening with this segment of the population that is falling through the cracks of the current health care system.

Trends in early hospital discharges often necessitate elderly caregivers' accommodation to highly taxing and complex care requirements (McCann, 1988). In some situations, conditions work out well or to some level of acceptability, but in others, conditions worsen, promoting isolation and despair resulting in neglectful and abusive situations. Millions of older adults are being discharged "sicker and quicker" (p. 314), and home care services are unable to respond to meet the need. With almost no Medicare coverage for rehabilitative and social support services, extended care in the home, however complex the needs, may fall increasingly to unskilled, untrained family members, friends, and neighbors (Estes & Rundall, 1992). Clearly, societal conditions propel us to fill the gaps in caregiving research.

The need for care in the community has had great impact on the formal caregiving industry as well as on informal care providers. Watkins and Kirby (1987) reported 5,953 home health agencies certified to provide Medicare and Medicaid services in 1988—double the number that were certified in 1981. However, in 1988 there were approximately 11,000 home care agencies in the United States, suggesting that almost half the agencies were unlicensed and uncertified. Moreover, the National Institute of Nursing Research Priority Expert Panel on Long-term Care (1994) found few studies that evaluated quality and outcomes of care. In addition to lacking quality control on certified and uncertified health agencies, we have little information about the quality and outcomes of care provided by family and friends.

Facts and Gaps in the Literature

Several authors have reviewed the caregiving literature and identified major trends (despite differences in methodologies among studies) and deficiencies. Baumgarten (1989) reviewed 28 studies in which the study sample was composed of caregivers of patients with Alzheimer's disease or another dementing disorder. Problems which were uncovered pervaded much of the caregiving literature. These problems included unrepresentative samples, preponderance of cross-sectional studies, paucity of work with comparison groups, use of global multidimensional scoring, and use of instruments related only to caregiving so that comparisons to noncaregiving controls could not be made. Baumgarten alerted researchers that an inherent danger in cross-sectional work is that it provides a snapshot of "survivors," or the "healthy caregiver effect" (p. 1141)—those who become caregivers at similar

time periods but did not make it into the sample may represent a less hearty group or may represent a group affected by other life circumstances and who dropped out of the role at an earlier time point. This same phenomenon may also apply to the care receivers; those who have multiple or more complex problems may die sooner or may be transferred to other settings earlier, leaving heartier survivors able to adapt to the care recipient role.

Wright, Clipp, and George (1993) argue that little is known about long-term health effects on caregivers because cross-sectional studies cannot untangle physical and emotional problems prior to the caregiving situation. Malonebeach and Zarit (1991) suggested that future research should include defining caregiving, using sociodemographic variables in analyses, paying attention to the broader family context of caregiving, and including information on the care recipient. Schulz, Visintainer, and Williamson (1990) reviewed 34 studies of psychiatric and physical effects of caregiving. They noted definite trends of increases in psychiatric measures over population norms or control groups, but no trend was clearly evident in physical health effects. The authors concluded that morbidity effects attributable to caregiving are inconclusive and that a major problem stems from sample biases. Not only are samples small, but they are often drawn from groups of people seeking help (i.e., those who are distressed); yet the most distressed may be too incapacitated to even seek help.

Although considerable research has described the composition of caregivers, the impact of caregiving on daily life, and the stressful and demanding nature of the role, a good deal of our understanding about caregiving stems from research on caregivers of patients with Alzheimer's disease or related cognitive impairments (Baumgarten et al., 1992; Deimling & Bass, 1986; Fitting, Rabins, Lucas, & Eastham, 1986; George & Gwyther, 1986; Lawton, Moss, Kleban, Glicksman, & Rovine, 1991; Wallsten & Snyder, 1990; Zarit, Reever, & Bach-Peterson, 1980). Not only are samples drawn from nonrandom groups (such as support groups) which tend not to include representative numbers of lower income caregivers or minorities, but few include non-caregiving comparison groups. This also pertains to many studies with samples of physically and cognitively impaired patients (Cattanach & Tebes,

1991; Chenoweth & Spencer, 1986; Clipp & George, 1990; Deimling, Bass, Townsend, & Noelker, 1989; Fitting et al., 1986; Gallagher, Rose, Rivera, Lovett, & Thompson, 1989; Lawton et al., 1991; Poulshock & Deimling, 1984; Strawbridge & Wallhagen, 1991). Moritz, Kasl, and Ostfeld (1992) and Moritz, Kasl, and Berkman (1989) used samples recruited for the Yale Health and Aging Study (one of the five EPESE sites) to determine whether there were health, social, and psychological consequences of living with a cognitively impaired elderly spouse. Though the sample was representative of the geographic area, the study was not intended as a caregiving study, and the authors, then, did not know whether one of the spouses even considered herself or himself a caregiver. The possibility remains that the cognitively impaired spouse may have been the caregiver in some circumstances. Deimling and Bass (1986) sampled households in Cleveland and 10 surrounding counties which included a racial mix of 25% African Americans and 75% whites. Unfortunately, the authors did not report having examined race or socioeconomic factors in the analyses. With little focus in caregiving research on race and socioeconomic factors, we have learned relatively little about lower income caregivers or caregivers who have never entered or have not remained in any formal health care organization. There is good reason to expect differences in the impact of home caregiving on lower income people and on African Americans, who are disproportionately in the lower income group.

Physical Health and Income

Several facts suggest that the physical health of low income caregivers age 65 and older is poorer than that of corresponding people in the middle-income class. In general, the percentage of older persons reporting major activity limitations is greatest among those persons living in poverty (Longino, Warheit, & Green, 1989). Approximately 24% of older people with yearly incomes less than $20,000 report "excellent" health whereas 41% with incomes of $20,000 and above report "excellent" health (National Center for Health Statistics, 1994).

In 1990, the proportion of elderly African Americans living in poverty was 33.8% compared to 10.1% of white elderly (Chen, 1994). Markides

and Mindel (1987) suggest that because of greater disadvantages throughout the life course, fewer African Americans have the opportunity to live to advanced age; therefore, fewer of the less hearty individuals survive. However, when elderly respondents rate their own health, only 9% of African Americans report "excellent" health whereas 16% of whites report "excellent" health. Similarly, while 18% of African Americans report "poor" health, only 8% of whites report this (National Center for Health Statistics, 1994). Moreover, elderly African Americans report having major activity limitations at a rate of one and one third times that of whites (National Center for Health Statistics, 1994).

The 1982 National Long Term Care Survey (NLTCS) and Informal Caregivers Survey (ICS) reported by Stone, Cafferata, and Sangl (1987) was one of the first widely based random sample of potential caregivers. Reports of this research have finally given us more accurate glimpses of conditions existing in the general population. The NLTCS was conducted by telephone by the Bureau of the Census for the Department of Health and Human Resources to estimate personal characteristics and use of health services by community dwelling disabled persons in the United States. Surveyors telephoned a random sample of 36,000 persons from files listing all Medicare enrollees. The ICS participants were those who indicated upon the first contact that they received help from an individual at least 14 years of age in at least one activity of daily living. In addition to confirming prior findings with respect to relationships of the informal caregivers to the recipients, the ICS provided valuable insights into the nature of caregiving among the population in general, including minorities and people in lower income groups. The majority of informal caregivers were female, with adult daughters comprising 29%, wives 23%, and husbands 13% of the overall sample. Wives accounted for 60% of the female primary caregivers and husbands accounted for 55% of the male primary caregivers. The average age of caregivers was 57.3 years, 25% were between 65 and 74 years, and 10% were over 74 years. The oldest caregivers were husbands, with an average age of 74, and they reported spending the greatest number of hours fulfilling caregiving responsibilities. Only about 50% had any informal or paid help. Many of the caregivers themselves suffered from one or more chronic diseases, and one third rated their health as "fair" or "poor." In addition, although the majority rated their incomes in the low to middle range, about one in three had incomes in the poor or near poor categories (Macken, 1986; Stone et al., 1987). Results of this study point to the need to study caregivers who are not readily identifiable: those from lower socioeconomic groups, subgroups such as males and minorities, those not represented in volunteer study samples, and people not identified in formal care practices or support groups.

Attention to Ethnicity

In recent years, the caregiving literature has given more attention to issues related to ethnicity. Although some of these studies include nonrepresentative samples or exclude white control groups, they provided greater understanding for the caregiving circumstances of minorities and poorer populations (Chatters, Taylor, & Jackson, 1986; Gibson & Jackson, 1987; Picot, 1995; Taylor & Chatters, 1986). Several studies used samples and methodology that enabled comparisons between African-American and white caregivers on income, education, and other factors (Hinrichsen & Ramirez, 1992; Miller, McFall, & Campbell, 1994; Mui, 1992; Wallsten, 1995). The studies suggest that there are some interesting differences and similarities between African-American and white caregivers.

Miller et al. (1994) reported findings from the cross-sectional and longitudinal components of the 1982–1984 NLTCS. Findings showed that regardless of the sources of care in 1982, race differences emerged in 1984: Whites were less likely to be deceased, more likely to be institutionalized, and less likely to rely only on informal helpers. Among African Americans and whites who had no help in 1982, whites were less likely to have help in 1984. However, among those who had help in 1984, whites were more likely to have a combination of formal and informal help than African Americans. Several points of interest emerged in the 1984 description of the sample. Whites were better educated and had better incomes. African Americans were more likely to receive Medicaid, reported greater problems with IADL, and had almost double the percentage of signs of dementia. Analyses were performed to assess the extent to which racial differences could be explained by other sources, but few differences in change patterns from 1982 to 1984 emerged between African Americans and whites. The authors suggest that the interdependence of race, income, and other dimensions are important to examine as predictors of long-term care use.

Mui (1992) used data from the National Long-term Care Channeling Demonstration (1982–1984) to examine strain among African American and white daughter caregivers. She found African-American care recipients to be more functionally impaired than whites. African-American caregivers had lower incomes than whites and were less likely to be married. They also reported less strain than whites although the caregiving role demand was higher. For white women, poor quality of the parent relationship and conflicts at work and in other relationships were predictors of strain, and for African Americans, poor perceived health, lower caregiving role demands, unavailability of respite support, and conflicts in relationships were predictors of strain.

In the first of a two-wave longitudinal study, Young and Kahana (1995) examined the role of race in the well-being of caregivers after an older family member suffered a heart attack. Patients 45 and over were recruited from seven hospitals in a major metropolitan area during hospitalization for a myocardial infarction. African-American caregivers were younger, were less likely to be caring for a spouse, had less education, and were in worse health. Their patients had greater numbers of ADL and IADL limitations, and caregivers provided greater numbers of caregiving hours. Interestingly, although caregivers reported similar support and formal services, African Americans had better attitudes despite greater burden scores. Levels of depression between the groups were similar. Depression was correlated with age (younger caregivers were more depressed), caregiver health (better health, the more depressed), and attitude toward the elder (more depressed, the less favorable attitude). Unfortunately, it appears that a direct measure of income was not included in the study. The authors suggest that an interaction between socioeconomic status (SES) and race may occur, and that race may have an indirect effect on outcomes. They discuss potentially important relationships that may exist between race, attitudes, and caregiving behavior.

Hinrichsen and Ramirez (1992) compared 119

African-American and 33 white primary caregivers of dementia patients recruited from diverse settings in the New York City area. White patients were more likely than African Americans to be married, and African Americans were more likely to be widowed or single. African-American patients were of a lower social class with lower incomes and were more likely to receive Medicaid. Whereas white caregivers were equally divided among adult children and spouses, the majority of African-American caregivers were adult children. African-American and white caregivers did not significantly differ on social class. High social class was associated with more needs met by the formal care system. Similar to other studies, African-American caregivers report lower levels of burden (although they also report needing more services), more unmet needs due to lack of supportive services, and fewer services provided exclusively by family members. Though not a significant finding, they tended to report more formal care and more mixed services (formal and family). (The authors comment that in New York state, being poor gives one entrance into the Medicaid system which provides many kinds of in-home services.) Race had no relationship with coping strategies or with seeking professional help, however African Americans made less use of active dementia management strategies, perceived less burden, and had less desire to institutionalize. The authors argue that comparison made on race is only the first step in trying to untangle multiple influences due to culture, economics, and social class. They suggest that culture is multifaceted in itself, encompassing values, beliefs, practices, and other aspects. In summary, African-American caregivers reported less strain than their white counterparts, although they reported greater economic difficulties and greater numbers of health problems of their patients. Contrary to prior research, these studies suggest that despite greater difficulties faced by African-American caregivers, extensive support from African-American families may not be significantly different from that provided by white families.

Comparing Caregivers and Non-Caregivers

Two limiting factors in much of the research on strain or burden are the exclusion of non-caregiving comparison groups and the use of assessment instruments designed only for caregivers (Baumgarten et al., 1992; George & Gwyther, 1986; Moritz, Kasl, & Berkman, 1989). Thus, it cannot be determined whether the strain of caregiving is any greater than the strains and difficulties thrust upon non-caregivers of similar ages and backgrounds. These problems were addressed by George and Gwyther (1986), Wallsten and Snyder (1990), and Baumgarten et al. (1992) by including non-caregiving comparison groups and by studying outcome variables that can be compared between the groups. Baumgarten et al. (1992) compared psychological and physical health problems of caregivers and non-caregivers. They looked at a sample of spouses or child caregivers of patients with dementia recruited from a geriatric assessment clinic. The non-caregivers were recruited from families of patients who were undergoing cataract surgery but who were without dementia or severe impairments; the non-caregivers were identified as the potential spouse or adult child to provide care if the patient became disabled. Major findings showed significantly higher depression and physical illness scores for caregivers than for non-caregivers. Although the measurement tools were not specific for caregivers, and there was a non-caregiving control group, there were important limitations of the study that may have biased the results. Namely, all patients were receiving care at the same hospital, and they were obviously all among people who actively seek help (Schulz et al., 1990).

George and Gwyther (1986), who measured physical health by self-ratings and number of physician visits, found no differences between primarily middle-class caregivers and non-caregivers on these two indicators. But they found striking differences in psychological indicators, with caregivers averaging almost three times as many stress symptoms as non-caregivers. A major problem in using self-rated health as an absolute health status indicator (as George and Gwyther did) is that elderly respondents tend to rate their health relative to "how bad things could be" rather than provide an objective evaluation. Also, because the elderly expect disabilities and diseases as a normal part of aging, they frequently underreport important symptoms (Rowe, 1985). Moreover, because caregivers are so overwhelmed by their caregiving responsibilities, they may ignore their own health needs and not make medical appointments for themselves.

In an attempt to gather objective and self-report measures, Kiecolt-Glaser, Dura, Speicher, Trask, and Glaser (1991) assessed depression, self-reported infectious illness episodes (verified by physicians), and immune function determined by blood assays. Measures were obtained for 69 caregivers of dementia patients and a matched group of 69 controls. Participants were recruited from sources including support groups, respite care programs, newspaper ads, and church groups. Caregivers and controls did not differ on total number of illnesses, however, caregivers reported greater incidence of depressive disorders, greater numbers of days of illness episodes, and more physician visits for these episodes and showed more negative immunological changes. Of great interest is that caregivers who reported lower levels of social support at the first interview and who were most distressed by behaviors of their care recipients showed the greatest immunological declines.

Wallsten's (1995) study is a three-wave longitudinal study of spousal caregivers of elders 65 and older and non-caregiver controls. Subjects for the study were drawn from the EPESE, a longitudinal study based on a stratified sample of 4,162 community residents age 65 and older and living in a five-county area of the central Piedmont area of North Carolina (Cornoni-Huntley, Blazer, Service, & Farmer, 1990). Participant caregivers had to be married to the EPESE sample member, consider herself/himself a caregiver, and have a spouse (EPESE sample member) who could not do at least one ADL or two IADL or who was cognitively impaired. The non-caregivers met the same criteria except they considered themselves non-caregivers, and the EPESE sample member could have no ADL impairment, only one IADL impairment, and no known cognitive impairment. Years of caregiving ranged from less than 1 year to 40 years, with a mean of 5.3 years and a mode of 2 years. Both caregivers and non-caregivers were married for approximately 47 years. Regardless of caregiver/non-caregiver status, the majority of people did not discuss with their partner what they would do if one could not provide care in the home for the other. Caregivers' and non-caregivers' ages were similar, but spousal care recipients were significantly older than their caregivers (M = 78.8 vs. 74.8). Caregivers and their controls reported similar numbers of visits for medical care, and there was no difference in their re-

ported need for care beyond what they were currently receiving. Although caregivers and non-caregivers reported similar numbers of diseases (M = 3.7 vs. 3.6, respectively), caregivers reported significantly greater numbers of health symptoms than controls (M = 4.9 vs. 3.8, respectively). Also, although caregivers and non-caregivers were responsible for taking their own medications (M = 3.64, M = 2.83, respectively), the majority of caregivers were also responsible for giving medications to their spouses, whereas non-caregivers did not engage in this activity. Caregivers rated their overall health as being worse than did their peers, and they performed worse than their peers on a physical performance task that used many movements needed in caregiving. The incomes of the caregivers were significantly lower, as were their ratings about their satisfaction with income. Incomes of African-American caregivers were lower than the incomes of white caregivers and non-caregivers. Caregivers reported worse control over their environment than did their non-caregiving peers (M = 16.90 vs. 17.80, respectively). Although in some regards caregivers were similar to non-caregiving controls, they differed in ways that can have direct impact on the quality of caregiving tasks.

Pruchno and Potashnik (1989) interviewed caregivers of spouses diagnosed with Alzheimer's disease or related disorders who were identified from community outreach institutions such as churches, synagogues, and community service organizations. They compared their results to a large population-based study, the National Health Interview Study conducted by the National Center for Health Statistics. Mental health measures were significantly worse for caregivers than for non-caregivers, and certain physical health measures were worse as well. Interestingly, they found that caregivers reported similar or fewer visits for medical care; the authors suggested that caregivers may have too little time to seek out care.

Using Wallsten's (1987) Routines, Uplifts, Challenges, and Hassles List (RUCHL), (Wallsten, 1992–1993; Wallsten & Snyder, 1990) it was found that negative ratings were significantly higher for caregivers than for non-caregivers. In addition, negative ratings of daily non-caregiving experiences correlated with psychological symptoms for both caregivers and non-caregivers. Positive ratings did not differ between groups, correlate with symptoms, or provide a buffering effect against psychosomatic symptoms. At a qualitative level, caregivers and non-caregivers differentially labeled items on the RUCHL as routines, uplifts, challenges, and hassles. For example, events that were challenges for caregivers were rated as uplifts for non-caregivers. In a study by Wallsten (1992–1993), few non-caregivers, but at least 50% of caregivers, endorsed "non-events" as hassles items, that is, experiences that caregivers were unable but longed to do, such as working on hobbies or relaxing. Likewise, Chenoweth and Spencer (1986) found that for caregivers, inability to engage in customary leisure or social activities was strongly associated with feelings of burden.

Spouse Caregivers

Very elderly male caregivers are providing care for their spouses, and we know little about them. According to Shanas (1979a,b), the main source of help for bedfast elders living in the community is spouses, with children as the next largest source. Elders turn first to their families for help and last to community institutions. Chatters et al. (1986) cautions that although spouses are ideally suited to care for each other, they may do so to the exclusion of finding additional help. Moreover, Cantor (1983) maintains that spouses are the highest risk caregivers. They usually are older than other caregivers, have lower incomes, and are in poorer health. According to Colerick and George (1986), spouses are the last to give up their role as caregiver despite, in many circumstances, being frail and old themselves. Though there have been few studies of husband caregivers, certain patterns have been reported. In a study of caregivers taking part in a homemaker service provided by the New York City Department for the Aging, Cantor (1983) found that slightly more than half of spouse caregivers were males, who in most instances lived alone with the ill spouse. As noted earlier (Stone et al., 1987), husband caregivers are the oldest caregivers and spend the greatest number of extra hours fulfilling caregiving tasks. Also, they provide about 50% of the care with no informal or paid assistance. A study of service utilization (Caserta, Lund, Wright, & Redburn, 1987) found that 70.5% of respondents not using services were spouse caregivers. They found that spouses were older, had higher burden scores, and devoted greater amounts of time to caregiving than did non-spouse caregivers. In addition, most non-users reported household yearly incomes of under $30,000. The most common reason for non-use was a perceived lack of need; financial reasons for non-use were least often cited. It may be that these lower income spouse caregivers were receiving adequate informal support from neighbors, friends, and family, but we have no data on this.

In Wallsten's (1987) study, spouse caregivers reported becoming increasingly lonely as their spouses became less communicative. They described this as losing their "best friend"; they could no longer confide in their spouses or receive their love and understanding. Also, spouses described loneliness stemming from changes in health status of kin and close friends; some had recently died, and others were ill or caring for an ill family member themselves.

According to Wallsten and Snyder (1990), Wallsten (1992–1993), and Poulshock and Deimling (1984), the caregiver's perception of the impact of caregiving is of prime importance in understanding caregiver burden. The degree to which social networks change as the patients impose ever greater demands on the primary caregiver may greatly affect the caregiver's perception of stress. In some cases, friends and neighbors may begin to withdraw from such awesome demands, leaving the spouse more and more isolated. According to Lee (1979), confidants play a significant role as a source of morale for elderly people, even if the interaction is by means of telephone contacts. Clearly, the kinds of changes brought about in the network over time are important to understand; they can be assessed best in a longitudinal rather than a cross-sectional study.

In a 2-year study of husband and wife caregivers' subjective burdens, Zarit, Todd, and Zarit (1986) reported that wife caregivers initially reported significantly greater burden than husbands, but this difference disappeared at the second interview. The authors suggest that the wives may have learned to cope better than or more like the husbands. Caregiving wives report anecdotally that upon first becoming caregivers, they felt great strain from having to take on financial functions they had never before done; however, they later felt relief and pride that they were capable of learning about them and carrying them out. Perhaps this change accounted for some of the differences between the first and second interview. Although Zarit et al. (1980) reported no differences in feelings of burden between husband and wife caregivers, other studies suggest some differences. According to Pruchno and Resch (1989), there are many reasons why current male elderly caregivers are faced with more problems than female caregivers; namely, current elderly women were socialized to be nurturing and family-oriented whereas males were socialized more toward jobs and other external responsibilities. Thus, women would view caregiving roles as more familiar whereas caregiving would be much more foreign to males.

Not all researchers agree with these assumptions. Guttman (1987) suggests that in the postparental years, men become more nurturing and family-oriented and women become more assertive and instrumental. Thus, the caregiving role in the elder years may lend itself more to the male's developmental pattern than the female's. In Wallsten's (1987) study, middle-income wife caregivers expressed longing for the kind of life they had anticipated for their retirement years—to travel and engage in other pleasurable experiences. Similarly, Zarit et al. (1986) suggest that older women resent becoming caregivers to their husbands because they look forward to their elder years for their own personal opportunities and growth. Pruchno and Resch (1989) also found caregiving wives to be more depressed and more burdened than husbands. They found caregiving husbands to be more invested in the marital relationship than wives. The husbands reported that the care they were giving their sick wives was an expected role after years of being tended to by their wives. More research is needed to understand husband/wife differences in the dynamics of the caregiving role, in the use of social support networks, and in the use of paid and unpaid formal supports.

Caregiver and Care Receiver Interactions

The severity of the care receiver's symptoms is not entirely predictive of the caregiver's report of burden or the caregiver's decision to institutionalize his or her relative. There is increasing evidence that the caregiver's unique perceptions of the conditions at hand play a primary role in his or her interpretation of a symptom or event as a stressor (Colerick & George, 1986; Deimling & Bass, 1986; George & Gwyther, 1986; Lazarus & Folkman, 1984; Poulshock & Deimling, 1984; Zarit et al., 1980). Factors such as the physical and mental status of caregiver and care receiver, the amount of control the caregiver has over his/her environment, coping strategies of the caregiving dyad, social networks, and financial status may play important intermediary roles in the perception of an event. Zarit et al. (1986) reported that the patient's behaviors were not related to burden, but rather to the lack of caregiver's personal time, fears about the patient's further deterioration, and the patient's great dependence on the caregiver. Similar conclusions were reached by Colerick and George. Also Zarit et al. (1980) found that for dementia patients' caregivers, the patient's duration of illness and behaviors were unrelated to stress but were associated with social supports or continuity in meaningful relationships.

Poulshock and Deimling (1984) made a strong case for addressing caregivers' subjective interpretation of burden stemming from problems due to elders' impairments. They found that subjective reports of burden were linked to the elders' impairments, family relationships, and caregivers' activities. Similarly, in a study by Deimling and Bass (1986), the results suggested that cognitive incapacity of the care receiver does not directly affect caregiver stress; rather, cognitive impairment had a significant indirect effect through the patient's disruptive social and behavioral functions. The authors speculated that caregivers may perceive these behaviors as a need to increase supervision of the patient. Therefore, the stressor may have been the nature of supervision and not the behavioral symptoms directly.

Several studies have pointed to patient behaviors as being significantly related to caregiver burden and institutionalization (Knopman, Kitto, Deinard, & Heiring, 1988; Sanford, 1975). In a study of 50 geriatric admissions to a London hospital which were due to the relatives' inability to cope with the patients, Sanford found that caregivers reported least tolerance for sleep disturbance, immobility, wandering, aggressive behaviors, and fecal incontinence. Interestingly, Wallsten (1987) found that the most frequent kind of caregiving experiences that caregivers described as hassles were specific behaviors of their patients, such as pacing, aimless wan-

dering, combativeness, irritability, and constant demands for the caregiver to repeat everything he or
she said. Clearly, it is important to understand what
combination of factors increases caregivers' perception of stress in caregiving activities and in everyday experiences and ultimately what brings the
caregivers to the point of institutionalizing the patient. Perhaps income and lack of institutional
placement options explain the "indefatigable"
caregivers (Knopman et al., 1988), that is, those
caregivers whose patients have reached advanced
stages of disease and have similar risk factors as
institutionalized patients, yet who make the decision to keep the patients at home.

Rhythmicity and Meshing of Caregiver and Care Receiver Interactions

Although the concept of interactional-devel-
opmental learning is usually applied to child development (Cairns, Green, & MacCombie, 1980), it
can as easily be applied to adult caregiving situations in which the caregiver's and care receiver's
responses to one another, to a large extent, are
driven by their past relationship and current ex-
changes and responses. Researchers have explored
the kinds of behaviors and problems care receivers
present that pose the most difficulties for caregivers,
but we know little about the nature of the caregiver/
care receiver interactions that affect the well-being
of both (i.e., the rhythmicity of interactions). With
elder caregivers having to meet their own health
care needs in addition to their care recipient's, previous balances may be challenged. Wallsten (1995)
found that the mean number of health problems
reported by caregivers and their care recipients was
similar ($M = 3.7$ vs. 3.6, respectively). It is not
surprising, then, that in the second wave of the
longitudinal study, some previously designated
caregivers had become care recipients, and in a few
situations, both had become simultaneous caregivers and care recipients for the other. Indeed, the
caregiving process is dynamic, and the caregiving
relationship needs further investigation.

Niederehe and Fruge (1984) noted the lack of
attention given to qualitative interactions between
patients and caregiving family members as a major
shortcoming in the literature. Niederehe and Scott
(1987) showed that caregivers' difficulties were not
associated with patient dysfunctions, but rather with
contextual variables such as less contact with confidants and other social supports and a less satisfactory relationship with the patient. Preliminary findings by Niederehe (1990), who analyzed videotaped
sessions of caregivers and patients performing specific tasks, suggested that caregivers who are more
distressed show more negative than positive emotion in interactions.

Several researchers report that the past relationship between caregivers and care receivers influences the degree of depression or burden caregivers feel. Pallett (1990) points out that family
caregiving is not an isolated event but takes place
within a historical context, which can facilitate or
complicate the caregiving process. A relationship
built upon dislike or ambivalence will be displayed
differently in caregiving interactions than a relationship built upon love, respect, and reciprocity.
Motenko (1989) reported that perceived change for
the worse in marital closeness was associated with
lower gratification from caregiving, and perceived
continuity of the marital relationship was associated
with greater gratification. Also, wives who gave
care out of reciprocity and love were highly grati-
fied, whereas those who gave care out of feelings
of responsibility had low gratification scores. Yet, in
the study by Pruchno and Resch (1989), caregiving
wives who reported low levels of depression and
burden were less emotionally invested in their relationships with their husbands than those who reported higher levels of depression and burden.

Hirschfield (1983) defined "mutuality in caregivers of persons with dementia" as the ability to
derive gratification in the relationship with the patient by virtue of the care receiver's existence without expecting any other kind of reciprocal response.
Hirschfield predicted that high levels of mutuality
would allow caregivers to continue their roles despite difficult situations. So few studies have been
done in this area that Hirschfield's predictions are
far from definitive. Rather, current findings tend to
support the hypothesis that positive caregiving interactions stem from historical or current perception
of reciprocity in the relationship. Archbold, Stewart, Greenlick, and Harvath (1990) found that mutuality ameliorated certain kinds of role strain, such as
that associated with direct care, but not economic
strain.

In a series of questions asked of each spouse in the dyad about their feelings of mutuality and regard for the other, Wallsten (1995) found that non-caregivers and their spouses reported similar feelings of regard for each other, whereas caregivers reported their feelings of regard for their spouses as significantly worse.

Niederehe and Fruge (1984) urge researchers to go beyond the accepted notion that caregivers are burdened and to explore the associations driving the caregiver/care receiver dyad. We have little understanding of the factors that contribute to positive interactions between caregivers and their care receivers. Moreover, we do not have insights into the kinds of interactions that correlate with burden level and whether such interactions are influenced by race, income, or gender.

Conclusions

Health care providers can use the caregiving literature, despite its gaps, to help older adults care for their family members. Demographics related to the aging population are such that every health care provider of an adult 50 years of age and over should assume that their client is in a potential caregiving or care-receiving situation. This outcome is even more likely with minority families who show stronger tendencies to maintain their elders in the community rather than in a nursing home. The individual seeking professional health care may have symptoms related to or compounded by the strain of caregiving. The older the individual, the more likely that he or she is to have personal health problems while trying to provide care to a relative. Although caregivers may not volunteer the information, when asked, they may feel relieved to talk about their situation and be grateful for any referrals for help in the community.

Reserachers have provided rich information about the complexities of caregiving, and now a leap forward must be taken. The use of representative samples will move the field forward and make the data more usable for program development. With relatively few minority elders in nursing homes, many families in poorer socioeconomic groups must be adapting to highly stressful home caregiving circumstances, and to date little is known about this process.

Whenever appropriate, control groups should be used so that comparisons can be made between caregivers and non-caregivers. This procedure will allow the researcher to separate usual strains in daily experiences from those imposed on caregivers. For example, in Wallsten's (1995) study, caregivers and non-caregivers were of similar age, but caregivers reported greater numbers of health problems and performed worse on physical function tests. Both longitudinal design and inclusion of a control group allow for important comparisons. Because spouses tend to be the eldest of caregivers, attention should be given to understanding the dynamics behind the dyadic relationship. Most older adults have disabilities in more than one domain, and the combination of limitations prescribes a good deal of the caregiving tasks (Silliman & Sternberg, 1988). For example, an individual with a stroke or hip fracture requires different kinds of care than does someone with diabetes or dementia. Furthermore, a physically impaired care receiver may have different kinds of demands placed upon him or her when the caregiver is cognitively impaired. Spousal caregiving may also be influenced by the kinds of tasks each member of the dyad did prior to disability. There is much to be learned within the domain of spousal caregivers, as well as in any dyadic caregiving situation.

With growing numbers of elderly people receiving care in the community from relatives and others, it is urgent that conditions in the greater population be examined. We must uncover the conditions of caregiving that heretofore have been neglected: in older caregiving couples, minorities, and people in poor economic groups. It is essential that we use representative samples and longitudinal designs to facilitate the examination of the process of caregiving—the interactions of those involved as caregiver and care receiver. In this way, we can go to the next step and apply our understanding and knowledge about caregiving conditions to program development for all elders.

ACKNOWLEDGMENTS

Preparation of this chapter was supported by the National Institute of Health, National Institute Of Aging Grant #5 R29 AGO9777-03.

References

Angel, J. L., & Hogan, D. P. (1994). The demography of minority aging populations. In J. S. Jackson (Chair), *Minority elders: Five goals toward building a public policy base*. Washington, DC: The Gerontological Society of America.

Archbold, P. G., Stewart, B. J., Greenlick, M. R., & Harvath, T. (1990). Mutuality and preparedness as predictors of caregiver role strain. *Research in Nursing and Health, 13*, 375–384.

Baumgarten, M. (1989). The health of persons giving care to the demented elderly: A critical review of the literature. *Journal of Clinical Epidemiology, 42*(12), 1137–1148.

Baumgarten, M., Battista, R. N., Infante-Rivard, C., Hanley, J. A., Becker, R., & Gauthier, S. (1992). *Journal of Clinical Epidemiology, 45*(1), 61–70.

Besdine, R. W. (1990). Clinical evaluation of the elderly. In W. R. Hazzard, E. L. Bierman, & J. P. Blass (Eds.), *Principles of geriatric medicine and gerontology* (pp. 175–183). New York: McGraw-Hill.

Cairns, R. B., Green, J. A., & MacCombie, D. J. (1980). The dynamics of social development. In E. C. Simmel (Ed.), *Early experiences and early behavior: Implications for social development*. New York: Academic Press, Inc.

Cantor, M. H. (1983). Strain among caregivers: A study of experience in the United States. *The Gerontologist, 23*, 597–604.

Caserta, M. S., Lund, D. A., Wright, S. D., & Redburn, D. E. (1987). Caregivers to dementia patients: The utilization of community services. *The Gerontologist, 27*, 209–214.

Cattanach, L., & Tebes, J. K. (1991). The nature of elder impairment and its impact on family caregivers' health and psychosocial functioning. *The Gerontologist, 31*, 246–255.

Chatters, L. M., Taylor, R. J., & Jackson, J. S. (1986). Aged blacks' choices for an informal helper network. *Journal of Gerontology, 41*, 94–100.

Chen, Y. P. (1994). Improving the economic security of minority persons as they enter old age. In J. S. Jackson (Chair), *Minority elders: Five goals toward building a public policy base*. Washington, DC: The Gerontological Society of America.

Chenoweth, B., & Spencer, B. (1986). Dementia: The experience of family caregivers. *Gerontological Society of America, 26*, 267–272.

Clipp, E. C., & George, L. K. (1990). Caregiver needs and patterns of social support. *Journal of Gerontology: Social Sciences, 45*, S102–111.

Colerick, E. J., & George, L. K. (1986). Predictors of institutionalization among caregivers of patients with Alzheimer's disease. *Journal of the American Geriatrics Society, 34*, 483–489.

Cornoni-Huntley, J., Blazer, D. G., Service, C., & Farmer, M. E. (Eds.). (1990). *Established populations for epidemiologic studies of the elderly*. NIH Publication No. 90-495. Bethesda, MD: National Institute on Aging.

Deimling, G. T., & Bass, D. M. (1986). Symptoms of mental impairment among elderly adults and their effects on family caregivers. *Journal of Gerontology, 41*(6), 778–784.

Deimling, G. T., Bass, D. M., Townsend, A. L., & Noelker, L. S. (1989). Care-related stress: A comparison of spouse and adult-child caregivers in shared and separate households. *Journal of Aging and Health, 1*, 67–82.

Dychtwald, K., & Flower, J. (1988). *Age-wave: The challenges and opportunities of an aging America*. New York: Bantam Books.

Estes, C. L., & Rundall, T. G. (1992). Social characteristics, social structure, and health in the aging population. In M. G. Ory, R. P. Abeles, & P. D. Lipman (Eds.), *Aging, health, and behavior*. Newbury Park, CA: Sage.

Fitting, M., Rabins, P., Lucas, M. J., & Eastham, R. (1986). Caregivers for dementia patients: A comparison of husbands and wives. *The Gerontologist, 26*, 248–252.

Folstein, M., Anthony, J. C., Parhad, I., Duffy, B., & Gruenberg, E. M. (1985). The meaning of cognitive impairment in the elderly. *Journal of the American Geriatrics Society, 33*, 228–235.

Fries, J. F. (1980). Aging, natural death, and the compression of morbidity. *New England Journal of Medicine, 303*, 130–135.

Gallagher, D., Rose, J., Rivera, P., Lovett, S., & Thompson, L. W. (1989). Prevalence of depression in family caregivers. *The Gerontologist, 29*, 449–456.

Gatz, M., Bengston, V. L., & Blum, M. J. (1990). Caregiving families. In J. E. Birren & K. W. Schaie (Eds.), *Handbook of the psychology of aging*. San Diego, CA: Academic Press, Inc.

Geller, L. N., Delfs, J., Rabins, P. B., & Reichel, W. (1995). Alzheimer's disease: Biological aspects. In W. Reichel (Ed.), *Care of the elderly: Clinical aspects of aging*. Baltimore: Williams & Wilkins.

George, L. K., & Gwyther, L. P. (1986). Caregiver well-being: A multidimensional examination of family caregivers of demented adults. *The Gerontologist, 26*, 253–259.

Gibson, R. C., & Jackson, J. S. (1987). The health, physical functioning, and informal supports of the black elderly. *The Milbank Quarterly, 65*, 421–454.

Guralnik, J. M., & Simonsick, E. M. (1993). Physical frailty in older Americans. *The Journal of Gerontology, 48*, (Special issue), 3–10.

Guralnik, J. M., LaCroix, A. Z., Everett, D. F., & Kovar, M. G. (1989). Aging in the eighties: The prevalence of comorbidity and its association with disability. *Advance Data from Vital and Health Statistics of the National Center for Health Statistics, 170*, 1–8.

Guttman, D. (1987). *Reclaimed powers: Towards a psychology of men and women in later life*. New York: Basic Books.

Heyman, A., Fillenbaum, G., Prosnitz, B., Raiford, K., Burchett, B., & Clark, C. (1991). Estimated prevalence of dementia among elderly black and white community residents. *Archives of Neurology, 48*, 594–598.

Hing, E., & Bloom, B. (1990). *Long-term care for the functionally dependent elderly*. Vital Health Statistics, Series 13, No. 104. Washington, DC: National Center for Health Statistics.

Hinrichsen, G. A., & Ramirez, M. (1992). Black and white dementia caregivers: A comparison of their adaptation, adjustment, and service utilization. *The Gerontologist, 32*, 375–381.

Hirschfield, M. (1983). Homecare versus institutionalization:

Family caregiving and senile brain disease. *International Journal of Nursing Studies, 20,* 23–32.

Hooyman, N. R., & Kiyak, H. A. (1993). *Social gerontology.* Boston: Allyn and Bacon.

Jackson, J. S. (1994). Preface. *Minority elders: Five goals toward building a public policy base.* Washington, DC: The Gerontological Society of America.

Johnson, C. L. (1983). Dyadic family relations and social support. *The Gerontologist, 4,* 377–383.

Kasper, J. D. (1988). *Aging alone—profiles and projections.* The Commonwealth Fund Commission on Elderly People Living Alone. New York: The Commonwealth Fund.

Kiecolt-Glaser, J., Dura, J. R., Speicher, C. E., Trask, O. J., & Glaser, R. (1991). Spousal caregivers of dementia victims: Longitudinal changes in immunity and health. *Psychosomatic Medicine, 53,* 345–362.

Knopman, D. S., Kitto, J., Deinard, S., & Heiring, J. (1988). Longitudinal study of death and institutionalization in patients with primary degenerative dementia. *Journal of American Geriatrics Society, 26,* 108–112.

Landry, S. (1995, May 7), Mother found deteriorating in son's home. *St. Petersburg Times,* p. B1.

Lawton, M. P., Moss, M., Kleban, M. H., Glicksman, A., & Rovine, M. (1991). A two-factor model of caregiving appraisal and psychological well-being. *Journal of Gerontology, 46,* P181–189.

Lazarus, R. S., & Folkman, S. (1984). *Stress, appraisal, and coping.* New York: Springer.

Lee, G. (1979). Children and the elderly. *Research on Aging, 1,* 335–370.

Longino, C. F., Warheit, G. J., & Green, J. A. (1989). Class, aging, and health. In K. S. Markides (Ed.), *Aging and health: Perspectives on gender, race, ethnicity, and class.* London: Sage.

Macken, C. L. (1986). A profile of functionally impaired elderly persons living in the community. *Health Care Financing Review, 4*(4), 33–49.

Malonebeach, E. E., & Zarit, S. H. (1991). Current research issues in caregiving to the elderly. *International Journal of Aging and Human Development, 32*(2), 103–114.

Markides, K. S., & Mindel, C. H. (1987). *Aging and ethnicity.* Newbury Park, CA: Sage.

McCann, J. J. (1988). Long term home care for the elderly: Perceptions of nurses, physicians, and primary caregivers. *Quality Review Bulletin, March,* 66–74.

Miller, B., McFall, S., & Campbell, R. T. (1994). Changes in sources of community long-term care among African-American and white frail older persons. *Journal of Gerontology, 49,* S14–24.

Moritz, D. J., Kasl, S. V., & Berkman, L. F. (1989). The health and impact of living with a cognitively impaired elderly spouse: Depressive symptoms and social functioning. *Journal of Gerontology: Social Sciences, 44,* S17–27.

Moritz, D. J., Kasl, S. V., & Ostfeld, A. M. (1992). The health impact of living with a cognitively impaired elderly spouse: Blood pressure, self-rated health, and health behaviors. *Journal of Aging and Health, 4*(2), 244–267.

Motenko, A. K. (1989). The frustrations, gratifications, and well-being of dementia caregivers. *The Gerontologist, 29*(2), 166–172.

Mui, A. C. (1992). Caregiver strain among black and white daughter caregivers: A role theory perspective. *The Gerontologist, 32,* 201–212.

National Center for Health Statistics. (1989). *Nursing home utilization by current residents: United States, 1985.* Vital and Health Statistics, Series 13, No. 102 (DHHS Publication No. PHS 89-1763) Hyattsville, MD: USDHHS, PHS, Centers for Disease Control, National Center for Health Statistics.

National Center for Health Statistics. (1994). *Current estimates from the National Health Interview Survey, 1992.* Vital and Health Statistics, Series 10, No. 189 (DHHS Publication No. PHS 94-1517). Hyattsville, MD: USDHHS, PHS, Centers for Disease Control, National Center for Health Statistics.

National Institute of Nursing Research Priority Expert Panel on Long-term Care. (1994). *Long-term care for older adults: Developing knowledge for practice.* Washington, DC: U.S. Department of Health and Human Services.

Niederehe, G. (1990). *Communication patterns and caregiver distress in senile dementia.* Paper presented at 43rd Annual Scientific Meeting of the Gerontological Society of America, November 17, Boston.

Niederehe, G., & Fruge, E. (1984). Dementia and family dynamics: Clinical research issues. *Journal of Geriatric Psychiatry, 17,* 21–56.

Niederehe, G., & Scott, J. (1987). Psychological and family factors influencing caregiver stress in senile dementia. *The Southwestern: The Journal of Aging for the Southwest, 4,* 48–58.

Pallett, P. J. (1990). A conceptual framework for studying family caregiver burden in Alzheimer's-type dementia. *Image, 22,* 52–58.

Picot, S. J. (1995). Rewards, costs, and coping of African American caregivers. *Nursing Research, 44,* 147–152.

Poulshock, S. W., & Deimling, G. T. (1984). Family caring for elders in residence: Issues in the measurement of burden. *Journal of Gerontology, 39,* 230–239.

Pruchno, R. A., & Potashnik, S. L. (1989). Caregiving spouses: Physical and mental health in perspective. *Journal of the American Geriatrics Society, 37,* 697–705.

Pruchno, R. A., & Resch, N. L. (1989). Husbands and wives as caregivers: Antecedents of depression and burden. *The Gerontologist, 29,* 159–165.

Quinn, M. J., & Tomita, S. K. (1986). *Elder abuse and neglect.* New York: Springer.

Rakowski, W., & Pearlman, D. (1995). Demographic aspects of aging. In R. Reichel (Ed.), *Care of the elderly: Clinical aspects of aging.* Baltimore: Williams & Wilkins.

Rowe, J. W. (1985). Medical progress: Health care of the elderly. *New England Journal of Medicine, 312,* 827–835.

Sanford, J. R. A. (1975). Tolerance of debility in elderly dependents by supporters at home: Its significance for hospital practice. *British Medical Journal, 3,* 471–473.

Schneider, E. L., & Brody, J. (1983). Aging, natural death and the compression of morbidity: Another view [Editorial]. *New England Journal of Medicine, 309*(14), 854–855.

Schneider, E. L., & Guralnik, J. M. (1990). The aging of America: Impact on health care costs. *Journal of the American Medical Association, 263*, 2335–2340.

Schoenberg, B. S., Anderson, D. W., & Haerer, A. V. (1985). Severe dementia: Prevalence and clinical features in a biracial U.S. population. *Archives of Neurology, 42*, 740–743.

Schulz, R., Visintainer, P., & Williamson, G. M. (1990). Psychiatric and physical morbidity effects of caregiving. *Journal of Gerontology, 45*, 181–191.

Shanas, E. (1979a). Social myth as hypothesis: The case of the family relations of old people. *Gerontologist, 19*, 3–9.

Shanas, E. (1979b). The family as the support system in old age. *The Gerontologist, 19*, 169–174.

Silliman, R. A., & Sternberg, J. (1988). Family caregiving: Impact of patient functioning and underlying causes of dependency. *The Gerontologist, 28*, 377–382.

Stone, R., Cafferata, G. L., & Sangl, J. (1987). Caregivers of the frail elderly: A national profile. *The Gerontologist, 27*, 616–626.

Strawbridge, W. J., & Wallhagen, M. I. (1991). Impact of family conflict on adult child caregivers. *The Gerontologist, 31*, 770–777.

Taylor, R. J., & Chatters, L. M. (1986). Church-based informal support among elderly blacks. *The Gerontologist, 26*, 637–642.

U.S. Department of Commerce. (1987). *Estimates based on data from the March 1987 current population survey.* Washington, DC: U.S. Bureau of the Census.

Verbrugge, L. (1989). Recent, present, and future health of American adults. *Annual Review of Public Health, 10*, 333–361.

Wallsten, P. F. (1995, May). I had no idea it had approached this. *St. Petersburg Times*, p. B3.

Wallsten, S. M. (1987). *Interactive factors in stress: Difference between caregivers' and noncaregivers' perception of stress in daily experiences.* Unpublished doctoral dissertation, North Carolina State University, Raleigh.

Wallsten, S. M. (1992–1993). Comparing patterns of stress in daily experiences of elderly caregivers and noncaregivers. *The International Journal of Aging and Human Development, 37*(1), 55–68.

Wallsten, S. M., & Pantez, A. T. (1995). *Caregiving couples and their noncaregiving peers: Some first year findings.* Paper presented at 48th Annual Scientific Meeting of the Gerontological Association of America, Los Angeles, CA.

Wallsten, S. M., & Snyder, S. (1990). A comparison of elderly family caregivers' and noncaregivers' perception of stress in daily experiences. *Journal of Community Psychology, 18*, 228–238.

Watkins, V., & Kirby, W. (1987). Health care facilities participating in Medicare and Medicaid programs. *Health Care Financing Review, 9*(2), 101–105.

Wright, L. K., Clipp, E. C., & George, L. K. (1993). Health consequences of caregiver stress, *Medicine, Exercise, Nutrition, and Health, 2*, 181–195.

Young, F. R., & Kahana, E. (1995). The context of caregiving and well-being outcomes among African and Caucasian Americans. *The Gerontologist, 35*, 225–232.

Zarit, S. H., Reever, K. E., & Bach-Peterson, J. (1980). Relatives of the impaired elderly: Correlates of feelings of burden. *The Gerontologist, 20*, 649–655.

Zarit, S., Todd, P., & Zarit, J. (1986). Subjective burden of husbands and wives as caregivers: A longitudinal study. *The Gerontologist, 26*, 260–266.

32

Geriatric Psychopharmacology

An Update and Review

BEN ZIMMER AND GEORGE GROSSBERG

Introduction

Whether one is a strict "structure–function" neuropsychiatrist or whether one interprets neuropsychiatry in a more liberal fashion, skilled clinicians in both camps know that despite the clear and logical principles of medicating affective, behavioral, and cognitive disturbances in late life, the ideal pharmacotherapist often must be creative and sometimes violate these principles even as he or she observes the most basic tenet of medicine of *princeps non sincere*.

The aging of developed societies has indeed led to increasingly significant numbers of elderly people with mental disorders. Currently, epidemiologic studies document the prevalence of mental disorders in those over age 65 to be in the range of 12–15% (Regier, Boyd, & Burke, 1988). Nuances in the presentation of affective, anxiety, cognitive, and psychotic disorders of the *Diagnostic and Statistical Manual of Mental Disorders* fourth edition (*DSM-IV*; American Psychiatric Association, 1994), however, led to their underdiagnosis and undertreatment.

This chapter will look at the choice of pharmacologic interventions available to treat late-life anxiety, affective, cognitive, and psychotic disturbances of the older adult. Among the disorders,

BEN ZIMMER • Geriatric Psychiatry Program, Department of Psychiatry, and Allegheny Neuropsychiatric Institute, Medical College of Pennsylvania and Hahnemann University–Allegheny Campus, Pittsburgh, Pennsylvania 15212. GEORGE GROSSBERG • Division of Geriatric Psychiatry, Department of Psychiatry and Human Behavior, St. Louis University, St. Louis, Missouri 63104.

current treatment choices will be pointed out including suggestions for augmented strategies.

Geriatric Pharmacology Principles

In prescribing any psychotropic medication, Larson and Zorc (1989) have suggested three common principles:

1. *Make an accurate diagnosis prior to treatment.* Diagnosing a patient prior to initiating drug care enables the physician to focus on presenting symptoms and provides the precision needed to determine the correct drug for that patient. This is especially true for elderly patients, who may present with complex symptoms related to physical illness or other nonpsychotropic drugs. The primary care clinician may take some time to assess a differential diagnosis and should consult with a psychiatrist if doubt remains.

2. *Make full use of the available variety of agents and regimens.* The physician should consider the symptoms and history of the patient in order to choose the most appropriate psychotropic drug with the least amount of potential side effects.

3. *Prescribe the lowest possible dose at the beginning, during maintenance, and at the end of treatment.* The physician should start with a low dose and increase the amount gradually until treated symptoms improve. Once target symptoms subside, the physician should at-

483

tempt to reduce the frequency of administration and the dosage. If the drug must be maintained for more than 6 months, the dosage should be kept as low as possible, and regular drug "holidays" (1 to 3 days per week without medication) can be attempted. These respites from drug treatment may reduce side effects without compromising efficacy. Physicians should be aware, however, that sometimes medication may need to be maintained over a prolonged period.

Pharmacokinetics and Pharmacodynamics

Any discussion about pharmacotherapy in the elderly must be preceded by definitions and a brief review of late-life pharmacodynamics and pharmacokinetics.

Pharmacodynamics refers to the effect of the drug or psychoactive substance on the body via its target receptors. Unfortunately, the influence of aging on the biochemical and physiologic effects of drugs and their mechanisms of action is largely unknown. Indeed, for such good clinical studies, it is difficult to accurately quantitate drug effects in persons without the use of invasive techniques.

Pharmacokinetics refers to the process of drug absorption, distribution, and elimination from the body. It refers to what the body does to the drug.

Greene (1988) has described many physiologic as well as pathologic changes that occur with aging which seem to significantly influence drug pharmacokinetics properties.

> Absorption of drugs from the gastrointestinal (GI) tract is not generally affected by aging, but in a few instances, because of elevation in gastric acidity seen in many of the elderly, it can be increased or decreased. Aging results in a relative increase in body lipid content, thereby increasing the distribution volume of lipid-soluble agents and decreasing distribution of water-soluble ones. Serum albumin, "the drug carrier," is often reduced in elderly patients and, therefore, the "free" (and active) fraction of certain drugs in serum increases and alters the therapeutic range. Both cardiac output and renal function decrease predictably in the elderly, resulting in diminished clearance of many drugs. Alterations in renal function are not always recognized. In addition, because of changes in muscle mass and the ratio of body

fat to weight, serum creatinine is less reliable as a predictor of renal function. Hepatic metabolic capacity may also decline with age and, therefore, result in decreased clearance of certain metabolized agents. (p. 15)

Koche-Weser, Greenblatt, and Sellers (1982) have also described additional changes that occur with aging that may affect drug pharmacokinetics.

> The mechanisms controlling hepatic biotransformation of drugs and their alterations with old age are considerably more complex than those involved in renal excretion. Hepatocytes carry out many biotransformation (Phase 1—preparation; Phase II—synthetic) reactions that contribute to the removal of drugs and other foreign chemicals. With the exception of the plasma albumin concentration the usual clinical tests of hepatic function reported in laboratory screening profiles are not importantly altered in healthy elderly persons and do not necessarily reflect drug-metabolizing capacity. The function of the hepatic microsomal enzymes responsible for Phase I oxidative drug metabolism (principally hydroxylation and N-dealkylation) may be importantly impaired in old age, leading to reduced total drug clearance and higher steady-state plasma concentrations, especially during multiple dosing. On the other hand, studies of biotransformations of the Phase II glucuronide-conjugation capacity have not shown them to be affected significantly by advancing age. Moreover, elderly patients may exhibit increased sensitivity to effects of drugs that are even within the therapeutic range. (p. 1083)

The above does not even address the 40–45% reduction in hepatic flow (as well as absolute and relative decrease in liver size) in old age and its major effect—a decreased clearance of a number of commonly used drugs. Ironically, changes in drug clearance in old age are not necessarily predictable consequences of well-understood alterations of hepatic function (Koche-Weser et al., 1982).

Moreover, with the enormous growth of thymoleptic, neuroleptic, and sedative hypnotic classes of agents in the last 5 to 10 years, the cytochrome P450 enzyme system that metabolizes these agents has received increased attention (see Table 1). Pharmacokinetic and pharmacodynamic drug interactions have become more important with the availability of the new selective serotonin reuptake inhibitors (SSRIs) and serotonin norepinephrine reuptake inhibitors (SNRIs). As we have discussed, drug metabolism is normally a multistep process involving both drug oxidation and conjugation of

Table 1. P450 Isoenzymes: Potential Drug Interaction[a]

Isoenzyme	Metabolizes		Inhibited by	Other features
2D6	Antiarrhythmics	SSRIs	Fluoxetine	5–10% of Caucasians are
	Encainide	Fluoxetine	Paroxetine	slow or fast metabolizers
	Flecainide	N-desmethylcitalopram	Sertraline	
	Mexiletine	Norfluoxetine	(weakest)	
	Propafenone	Paroxetine		
	Antipsychotics	Tricyclic antidepressants		
	Clozapine	Amitriptyline		
	Haloperidol	Clomipramine		
	Perphenazine	Desipramine		
	Reduced haloperidol	Imipramine		
	Risperidone	N-desmethyl-clomipramine		
	Thioridazine	Nortriptyline		
	Zuclopenthixol	Trimipramine		
	β-Blockers	Miscellaneous		
	Alprenolol	Amiflamine		
	Bufuralol	Guanoxan		
	Metoprolol	4-Hydro-amphetamine		
	Propranolol	Indoramin		
	Timolol	Methoxyphenamine		
	Opiates	Perhexiline		
	Codeine	Phenformin		
	Dextromethorphan	N-Propyl-ajmaline		
	Ethylmorphine	Tomoxetine		
		Terfenadine		
		Venlafaxine		
1A2	Amitriptyline	Paracetamol	Fluvoxamine	—
	Caffeine	Phenacetin	Grapefruit juice	
	Clomipramine	Propranolol		
	Clozapine	Theophylline		
	Imipramine			
3A4	Antiarrhythmics	Calcium channel blockers	Astemizole	Potentially dangerous
	Lidocaine	Diltiazem	Fluoxetine	arrhythmias for those
	Propafenone	Felodipine	Fluvoxamine	taking antihistamines;
	Quinidine	Nifedipine	Grapefruit juice	tricyclics, venlafaxine
	Anticonvulsants	Verapamil	Ketoconazole	less likely to inhibit;
	Carbamazepine	Nonsedating antihistamines	Nefazodone	carbamazepine induces
	Antidepressants	Astemizole	Sertraline	
	Nefazodone	Terfenadine		
	Sertraline	Miscellaneous		
	Venlafaxine	Cyclosporine		
	Some tricyclics	Cortisol		
	Benzodiazepines	Dexamethasone		
	Alprazolam	Erythromycin		
	Midazolam	Ethinylestradiol		
	Triazolam	Tamoxifen		
2C19	Citalopram	Mephobarbital	Fluoxetine	
	Clomipramine	Omeprazole	Sertraline	
	Diazepam	Proguanil		
	Hexobarbital	Propranolol		
	Imipramine			

[a]Reproduced with permission from Gelenberg (1995).

the oxidative products (Brosen, 1990). The cytochrome P450 system oxidizes a variety of chemicals, including endogenous substrates such as prostaglandins, fatty acids, and steroids and exogenous substrates such as lipophilic drugs. Cytochrome P450 is composed of a group of related enzymes or isoenzymes located in the endoplasmic reticulum (Gonzalez & Gelboin, 1992), predominantly in the liver and gut wall. While the metabolism of many therapeutically useful drugs has been associated with a specific P450 isoenzyme, the enzymes involved in the metabolism of most drugs still remain to be defined. More than one enzyme may be involved in the metabolism of a specific drug, and the enzyme's metabolic activity may show different degrees of specificity for a particular substrate.

There are many important known drug interactions. Antacids decrease the absorption of phenothiazine and benzodiazepine. Cimetidine, on the other hand, decreases the metabolism of benzodiazepines. Neuroleptics can increase serum glucose, necessitating alteration in diabetic medication. Carbamazepine and antibiotics, particularly erythromycin, can cause neurotoxicity, dizziness, vomiting, ataxia, and blurry vision. Lithium carbonate plus nonsteroidal anti-inflammatory agents can cause lithium toxicity as can lithium with diuretics. As can be seen in Table 1, a wide variety of drugs will inhibit P450 enzymes, including some that are also substrates. The difference between status as a substrate for a specific isoenzyme and status as an inhibitor should be recognized. While all substrates can be potential inhibitors, the reverse is not necessarily true. For example, quinidine is a potent inhibitor of CYP2D6, but is apparently not metabolized by this enzyme (DeVane, 1994; Guengerich, Muller-Enoch, & Blair, 1986; Mikus, Ha, & Vozeh, 1986). With these pharmacologic principles as a background, we can now focus on the various general disorders.

Anxiety

Background

Unlike the primary affective disorders (major depressive disorders or bipolar affective disorders), primary anxiety disorders rarely present initially in late life. On the other hand, anxiety symptoms occur frequently in a variety of primary psychiatric disorders and as part of many primary medical conditions. It is also our experience that the first episode of anxiety in the elderly is often the manifestation of an organic condition.

Ironically though, anxiety disorders are the mostcommonofallpsychiatricdisordersamong elderly people, although there does tend to be a trend downward for both men and women. There is a high correlation between anxiety and medical illness for both men and women in late life, and this relationship is not entirely dependent on the correlation between age and physical health. Further, anxiety as a symptom is much more common than anxiety disorder as defined by *DSM-IV*. Sexual dysfunction, somatization, and hypochondriasis are frequently associated with symptoms of anxiety among elders.

New onset of late-life anxiety spans the gamut of all the organic brain syndromes and is a principal feature of late-life depression. Indeed, the most common psychiatric disorder causing anxiety in late life is depression. As many as 70% of patients of any age with major depression have significant anxiety (Sussman, 1988). Even carefully performed evaluations may be unable to consistently differentiate anxiety from depression, and the overlap between these disorders is becoming more apparent.

Panic disorder which occurs for the first time in later life is relatively uncommon. The Epidemiologic Catchment Area (ECA) found no cases in elderly men and a prevalence rate of approximately 0.2% in elderly women. This raises the question of what happens to people with panic disorders as they get older. Do they become depressed? Do they "outgrow" their pathology? Are there higher mortality rates? Certainly, insight into answering this question will provide an important piece of information regarding the life span for the clinical course of panic disorders.

Phobic disorders are considerably more common, with prevalence rates of approximately 6% for older women and 3% for older men. However, ECA data show wide variability at various geographic sites, with some phobias showing rates six times greater at one site than at another.

It has been well established that benzodiazepines are effective in the treatment of nonpsychotic anxiety, and some of the benzodiazepines display great anxiolytic potency (Braestrup & Neilsen, 1982; Rickels, 1982). Although most widely prescribed as anxiolytics, anticonvulsants, muscle relaxants, and hypnotics, benzodiazepines have also been used in the treatment of alcohol withdrawal syndrome and as premedication in anesthesia (Baldessarini, 1985; Tallman et al., 1980). The benzodiazepines are different pharmacologically and clinically. Schatzberg and Cole (1986) divide the anxiolytic benzodiazepines into three subclasses on the basis of structure: *2-keto* (chlordiazepoxide, diazepam, prazepam, chlorazepate, halazepam and the hypnotic flurazepam); *3-hydroxy* (oxazepam, lorazepam, and the hypnotic temazepam); and *triazolo* (alprazolam and the hypnotic triazolam) (see Figure 1). The pharmacokinetic properties (i.e., half-lives) vary among these classes as well as the tricyclic antidepressants and major tranquilizers (discussed below), in part reflecting differences in their modes of metabolism. The 2-keto drugs and their active metabolites are oxidized in the liver, a slow process as previously discussed, especially in the elderly. Differences among these compounds revolve around the rates of absorption and specific active metabolites which also feed into another phase of metabolism, that is, conjugation.

In addition, competition by other drugs relative to the oxidative process will result in further delay in metabolism. The three hydroxy compounds are metabolized via direct conjugation with a glucuronide radical, a more rapid process than oxidation and one also not involving the formation of active metabolites. The two major examples of this subclass are oxazepam and lorazepam, which have shorter half-lives and, therefore, are important in the geriatric population.

Finally, while the triazolo compounds are also oxidized, their active metabolites are limited and are less affected by slow metabolism. On the other hand, they too are affected by slower competitive oxidation reactions.

The above discussion has not taken into account the hydrophilic and lipophilic properties of the drugs and their effects on the rates of absorption and distribution—important factors in the selection of an anxiolytic drug in the elderly. Drugs that are more lipophilic (such as the 2-keto agent diazepam)

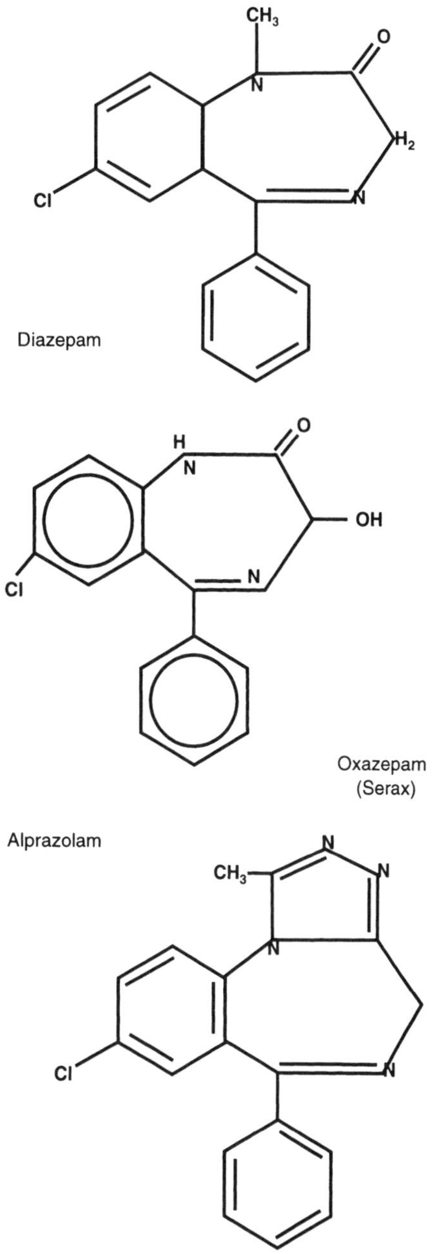

FIGURE 1. The anxiolytic benzodiazepines.

will enter the brain more quickly, but also disappear in the body fat. Less lipophilic compounds (such as the 3-hydroxy compounds, e.g., lorazepam) are more hydrophilic and will produce clinical effects more slowly, but in a sustained fashion (Schatzberg & Cole, 1986).

Efficacy and Safety

Until recently, benzodiazepines were felt to be equivalent in terms of overall clinical efficacy (Gershon & Eison, 1987). One of the newest benzodiazepine derivatives, alprazolam, a triazolobenzodiazepine, has been shown to be effective for generalized anxiety and, in preliminary trials, to be more effective in reducing panic disorder and agoraphobia with panic attacks and phobic avoidance (Greenblatt, Selkis, & Koche-Weser, 1982) than other benzodiazepines. In addition, it reduces anticipatory anxiety much like the other benzodiazepines.

Benzodiazepines are relatively safe, the most common side effect being sedation, which can be managed in part by dose reduction. Therapeutic and toxic doses are widely separated, but their interaction with other central nervous system (CNS) depressants, especially alcohol, poses a major problem. Their absorption and tendency to produce CNS depression are enhanced by the presence of alcohol (Ascione, 1978; Bellantuono, Reggi, & Tognoni, 1980).

Of concern, especially when one considers the cognitively compromised elderly, is that benzodiazepines can cause significant but reversible cognitive impairment. The most pronounced of these is anterograde amnesia, which can be a source of anxiety. All benzodiazepines can potentially produce amnesic effects, but these effects are reported to be more frequent with short half-life agents such as triazolam. In a controversial report, Morris and Read (1987) described transient global amnesia (TGA) in three individuals using triazolam. Their report led to other reports of amnesia secondary to even single doses of triazolam, and most without an association with alcohol (Cohen, 1988; DiMaio, 1988; Ewing, 1988; Radack, 1988).

Adverse effects on balance and reaction time may increase the risk of accidents. Control of balance diminishes with age, but benzodiazepines directly affect motor coordination, inducing ataxia. Indeed, the risk of falls and hip fractures is significantly increased in elderly patients taking long half-life benzodiazepines such as flurazepam (Ray, Griffin, & Downey, 1989).

Physical and psychological addiction can be a problem with benzodiazepines as withdrawal symptoms have been observed especially upon abrupt discontinuation of high doses. Predicting tolerance and withdrawal, however, is not straightforward. Although tolerance is a real phenomenon, it is of interest that some patients, including many elderly, actually do not develop tolerance and still respond to a given daily dose over many years. Withdrawal symptoms would seem to be more problematic with benzodiazepines of high potency and high receptor affinity, such as lorazepam and alprazolam. Ironically, oxazepam, which is similar in lipid solubility and half-life to lorazepam, appears to produce less in the way of withdrawal symptoms (Lader, 1982a,b; Schatzberg & Cole, 1986). Cumulative effects have been associated with chronic administration (Greenblatt & Shader, 1974; Harvey, 1980; Marks, 1978). Golombok (1988), looking at a battery of cognitive and psychomotor performance tests on several groups of benzodiazepine users and non-users, has speculated that long-term use of benzodiazepines may lead to posterior cortical dysfunction. Moreover, Lader and colleagues (1984) have reported on long-term benzodiazepine exposure leading to increased cerebral ventricular size.

In order to minimize the risk of severe withdrawal symptoms, benzodiazepine therapy should never be stopped abruptly, but rather slowly tapered. Patients taking rapidly eliminated drugs, such as lorazepam, and more specifically alprazolam (Zipursky, Baker, & Zimmer, 1985), should be cautioned against running out of medication or deliberately abstaining from taking their medication. The resulting symptoms can be severe, adversely affecting medical and psychiatric conditions.

Severity of withdrawal increases when drugs with short half-lives are involved and is related to duration of treatment. Patients using a benzodiazepine for more than 8 months are five times more likely to experience withdrawal symptoms than those using the drug for less than a month. Physical dependence, however, can develop in as little as 2 weeks, at therapeutic doses. Compounds with shorter half-lives, such as lorazepam or alprazolam, are especially difficult to discontinue in some patients (Sussman, 1988).

Buspirone, an azaspirodecanedione and non-benzodiazepine (see Figure 2), has been available since the early to mid-1980s (Lader, 1980) and is

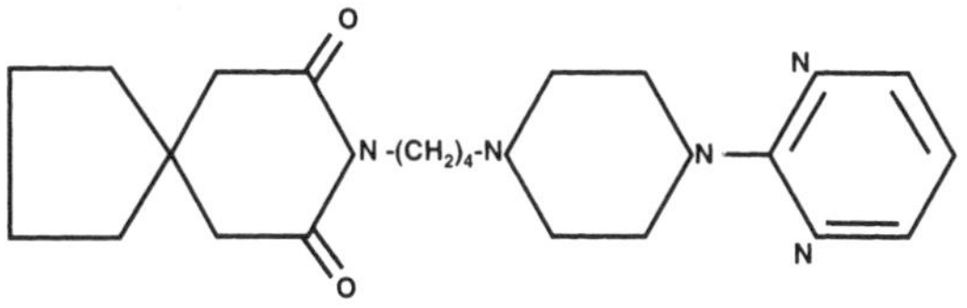

Graphic formula of buspirone

FIGURE 2. Nonbenzodiazepines.

efficacious in mild to moderate generalized anxiety. It is not effective for panic. Unlike the benzodiazepines, it cannot be taken on an "as needed" basis, nor does it have an immediate effect when taken. It may in fact require 2–4 weeks for optional anxiolytic effect. In the elderly, it is dosed at 5–10 mg three times daily. Buspirone indirectly affects the gamma-aminobutyric acid (GABA)–benzodiazepine receptor complex. Buspirone, a 5-HT 2A partial agonist, influences serotonergic, noradrenergic, cholinergic, and dopaminergic activity in the brain. Its main side effects are gastrointestinal.

Buspirone (up to 30 mg/day) can be used in first-onset generalized anxiety. Short-term use of benzodiazepines such as lorazepam, oxazepam, or alprazolam may be useful for immediate intervention and relief of both general anxiety disorder (GAD) and panic disorder. The high-potency benzodiazepines (alprazolam and clonazepam) have demonstrated efficacy for panic disorder in placebo-controlled trials (Ballenger, Burros, & DuPont, 1988). Oxazepam may be started at 10 to 20 mg per day, with a gradual increase in dosage up to (but rarely) 45 mg per day. Lorazepam and alprazolam may be started at 0.25 mg two or three times per day up to 4 mg/day. Secondary amine tricyclic antidepressants (such as nortriptyline) or SSRIs can be used for panic disorder. Indeed, SSRIs have become the drug of choice for panic disorder despite a paucity of controlled trials (Gorman, Liebowitz, & Fyer, 1987; Schneider, Liebowitz, & Davies, 1990). Again, we remind the reader of the lack of good controlled studies of the treatment of anxiety disorders in the elderly.

Other medications that are useful for panic disorder include the tricyclic antidepressants (imipramine, desipramine, nortriptyline), SSRIs (e.g., fluoxetine, sertraline, paroxetine, fluvoxamine), and

monoamine oxidase inhibitors (MAOIs) (e.g., phenelzine). Lithium carbonate, buspirone, beta blockers, neuroleptics, and the atypical antidepressants trazodone and bupropion have not been shown to be useful with panic disorder.

Depression

Background

Much of this section has been adapted from Franson, Renner, and Grossberg (1994). Estimates relative to the prevalence of major depression, or clinically significant depression, in individuals older than 65 have varied. The current thinking is that 2% to 3% of older adults meet the criteria for major depression, which is actually lower than the rate seen in younger adults (Gurland, 1976). Women tend to have higher rates of depression in all age groups, but there may not be a statistically significant difference in rates of depression between the sexes after the age of 65. In addition to those older individuals meeting criteria for major depression, nearly one in five nursing home residents meet the criteria for major depression, and 20% to 35% of older adults with significant medical illness are depressed (Grossberg et al., 1990; Moffie & Paykel, 1975). Twenty-seven percent of elderly persons experience dysphoria and/or a subsyndromal affective disorder (Blazer, 1989). It is crucial for practitioners to recognize and vigorously treat depression in older adults, because individuals older than 65 account for 25% of all suicides in the United Sates (Grossberg & Nakra, 1986). Older patients with mood disorders are less likely to seek medical attention (Shapiro et al., 1984), be referred to a mental health specialist (Borson et al., 1986; Coyne, 1995), or receive an optimal therapeutic intervention (Shamoian, 1985). With prompt, effective treatment, however, between 80% and 90% of late-life depressions respond to therapy (Grossberg & Nakra, 1986; Jenike, 1988). Because of the recent development of the newer antidepressants, we review the pros and cons of the use of various antidepressants in the elderly, with a particular emphasis on side effects to consider and appropriate dosing for this age group.

Treatment

Cyclic Antidepressants

The mainstays of antidepressant therapy have been the tricyclic antidepressants, which date back more than 30 years. The cyclic antidepressants can be separated into designated classes by chemical structure: piperazine (amoxapine), triazolopyridine (trazodone), tetracyclic (maprotiline), and tricyclics. The tricyclics can be further designated as tertiary or secondary amines. Tricyclic tertiary amines include amitriptyline, imipramine, and doxepin, and secondary amines include desipramine, protriptyline, and nortriptyline. By dividing these agents by chemical structure, it becomes easier to distinguish and remember the traits of the various agents (see Figure 3).

Tricyclic Tertiary Amines. Most clinicians have found these agents to have high anticholinergic properties which are potentiated in the elderly. This increased sensitivity can lead to increased sedation and confusion and possibly manifest as delirium (Watanabe & Davis, 1990). The use of the tricyclic tertiary amines may also lead to disturbances in cardiac conduction secondary to prolongation of the QT interval of the electrocardiogram (EKG). The elderly may be at a higher risk of manifesting clinically significant conduction abnormalities. This is believed to be caused by two principal physiological changes: the alterations in conduction secondary to the patient's concomitant underlying cardiac disease and the alterations in pharmacokinetics that lead to increased serum concentrations and cardiac toxicity (Jenike, 1989). These potentially serious adverse effects combined with the growing availability of other antidepressants does not warrant the routine use of the tertiary amines in the elderly.

Tricyclic Secondary Amines. The secondary amines desipramine and nortriptyline are monomethylated derivatives of the parent compounds imipramine and amitriptyline, respectively. These antidepressants have less than half the anticholinergic effects of their parent compounds, and they have been extensively studied in the elderly (Jenike, 1989). Although serum concentrations are inconsistent with the clinical effect for most anti-

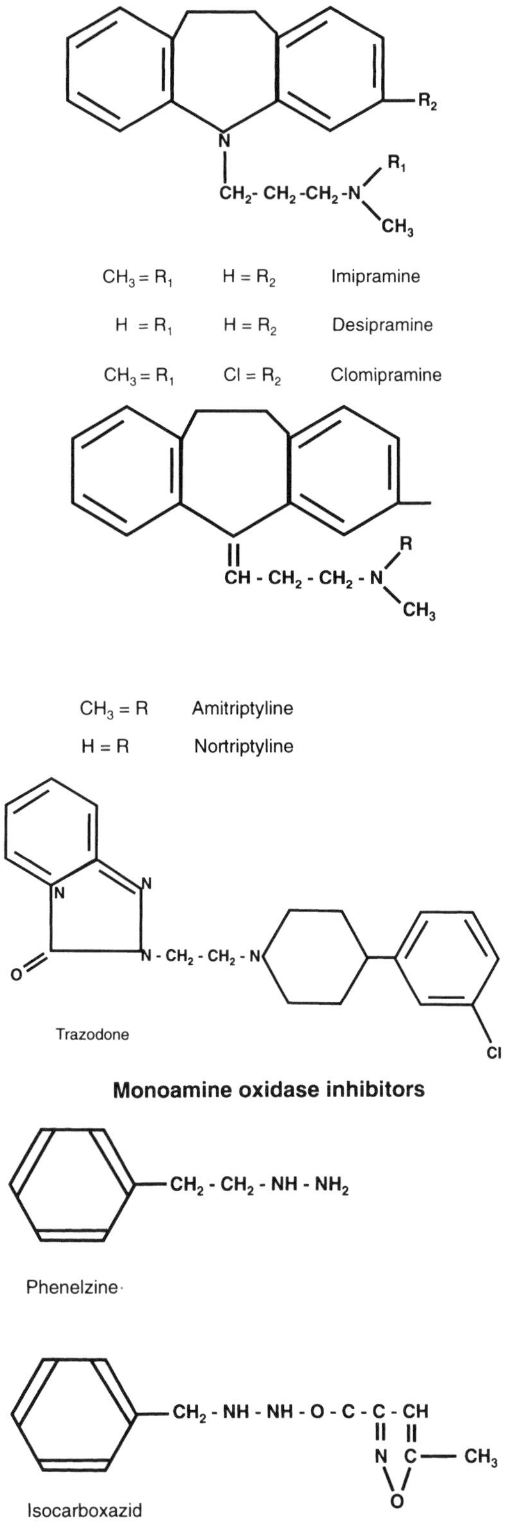

$CH_3 = R_1$	$H = R_2$	Imipramine
$H = R_1$	$H = R_2$	Desipramine
$CH_3 = R_1$	$Cl = R_2$	Clomipramine

$CH_3 = R$	Amitriptyline
$H = R$	Nortriptyline

Trazodone

Monoamine oxidase inhibitors

Phenelzine

Isocarboxazid

FIGURE 3. Older antidepressants.

depressants, reliable therapeutic levels have been-described for the secondary amines (nortriptyline, 50 to 150 ng/ml; desipramine, > 125 ng/ml).

Therapeutic drug level monitoring has been advocated to reduce the risk of toxicity associated with the cyclic antidepressants. Nevertheless, in a study by Preskorn (1989) it was found that toxicity occurred at the same rate between groups that had therapeutic drug monitoring and those whose doses were titrated to effect. Given the high cost of therapeutic drug monitoring, therefore, its routine use is not warranted with the exception of the secondary amines. Because higher serum drug concentrations are likely to lead to more adverse drug reactions, however, it is a general rule of thumb to "start low and go slow" when initiating antidepressant therapy in the elderly. Nortriptyline is approximately twice as strong as desipramine, and initial doses should start at 10 mg for the elderly. These doses should be given at bedtime to avoid complications from the possible sedative, anticholinergic, and orthostatic effects.

Trazodone, Amoxapine, Maprotiline. Trazodone, amoxapine, and maprotiline are sometimes described as second-generation antidepressants. Amoxapine is the demethylated derivative of the antipsychotic loxapine. Amoxapine has not been shown to be an effective antipsychotic, even in psychotic depression. The elderly, however, are at an increased risk of developing extrapyramidal side effects from a metabolite that blocks dopamine, which can lead to akinesia and pseudoparkinsonism (Jenike, 1989). Amoxapine has also been linked to tardive dyskinesia—it should be avoided. Less adverse cardiovascular drug reactions have been associated with amoxapine use.

Trazodone is a triazolopyridine with a short elimination half-life of 5 hr. Due to its sedative and antiagitation effects, it may be dosed at night and in divided doses during the day generally at 50 to 150 mg daily and occasionally up to 400 mg daily. Trazodone is associated with orthostatic hypotension more than other antidepressants. Priapism is an unfortunate but rare side effect of trazodone and may require surgical intervention for relief of penile tumescence.

Maprotiline is a tetracyclic antidepressant. Like the tricyclic secondary amines, maprotiline is believed to act by blocking norepinephrine reuptake. The accumulation of maprotiline's metabolite is associated with an increased risk for seizures (Bressler & Katz, 1993). Initial dosages of 25 to 50 mg daily should be maintained for 2 weeks prior to increases in dosages.

Monoamine Oxidase Inhibitors

The monoamine oxidase inhibitors (MAOIs) include the hydrazine (phenelzine), nonhydrazine (tranylcypromine), and reversible MAOIs (meclobemide). The reversible MAOIs are not yet available in the United States. These agents inhibit metabolism of the biogenic amines of the central nervous system—norepinephrine, serotonin, and dopamine. The MAOIs are often used only for treatment-resistant depression due to the limitations on lifestyle secondary to the drug–drug and drug–food interactions. The hypertensive crisis that results from these interactions leads to avoidance of these antidepressants by clinicians. The adverse effect profile of MAOIs, however, is less threatening to the geriatric population than that of the tricyclic antidepressants. Late orthostatic hypotension can be the most troubling adverse effect, because this may lead to an increased risk of falls in the elderly (Salzman, 1993). The MAOIs may be either activating or sedating, with tranylcypromine tending to be more activating, but also shorter in duration of action.

Newer Antidepressant Agents

Antidepressant medications other than cyclic antidepressants and MAOIs are also referred to as second- or third-generation antidepressants. These medications include the SSRIs, bupropion, venlafaxine, and nefazodone (see Figure 4). Although they often are grouped together to differentiate them from the first-generation antidepressants, they have diverse chemical structures.

The increasing interest in these antidepressants has been primarily the result of their more benign side effect profile. Because they have a very low potency for blocking muscarinic, α_1, noradrenergic, and H_1 histaminergic receptors, they do not seem to produce anticholinergic effects or postural hypotension and have minimal cardiac effects. These anti-

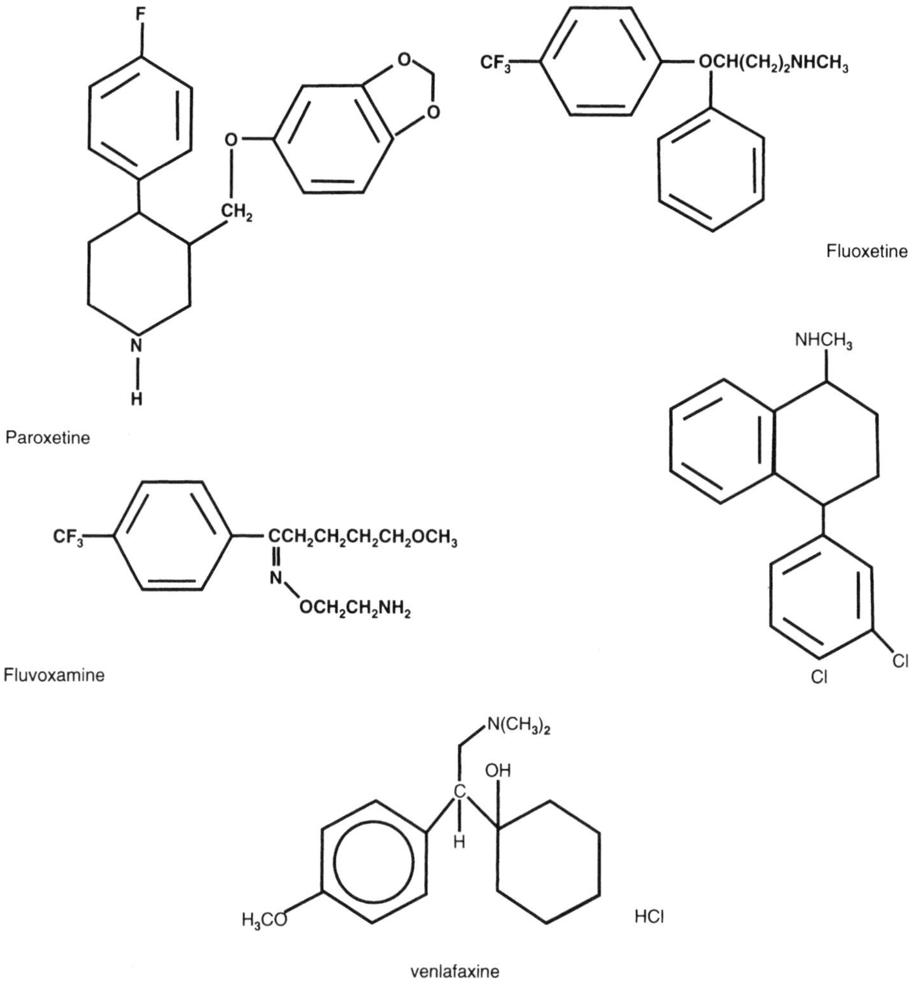

FIGURE 4. Newer antidepressants.

depressants do have some specific adverse effects including nausea, diarrhea, nervousness, and insomnia. In cases of overdose, however, they generally are safer than first-generation antidepressants.

Selective Serotonin Reuptake Inhibitors

The SSRIs are so termed because they inhibit the reuptake of serotonin to a much greater degree than norepinephrine. The currently marketed drugs in this class include fluoxetine, sertraline, paroxetine, and fluvoxamine. They vary in length of elimination half-life and intensity of side effects (DeVane, 1992). Usually the SSRIs are administered in the morning due to stimulating effects, but they may be administered in the evening if the patient experiences hypersomnia or sedation, which occurs more often with some of the agents. There are similarities in the side effect profile of the SSRIs. They all cause nausea (15% to 35% incidence) and vomiting to a greater extent than the tricyclics (Grimsley & Jann, 1992; Rickels & Schweizer, 1990; Wagner, Plekkenpol, Gray, Vraskamp, & Essers, 1992). Nausea is the most common side effect of these drugs, and for most of them, insomnia is relatively frequent also. Both the nausea and insomnia tend to dissipate over time as the drugs continue to be taken. Headache is also a common side effect of this class of drugs and may increase in frequency over time. Fluoxetine appears to be distinct among the SSRIs in producing a relatively high incidence of insomnia, nervousness, restlessness, and anxiety (Rickels & Schweizer, 1990). Fluvoxamine seems to produce agitation and anxiety at a particularly low rate (Wagner et al., 1992). Another important difference between most SSRIs and older antidepressants is the induction of weight gain with the older agents. This side effect can lead to problems with patient compliance. Most SSRIs have an anorectic effect and do not cause any clinically significant weight gain (Harto-Traux, Stern, Miller, Sato, & Cato, 1983). Paroxetine may be unique among SSRIs in having no clinically significant anorectic effect (Dechant & Clissold, 1991), and weight gain has been reported in patients being treated with paroxetine over time (Frazer, 1994; Grimsley & Jann, 1992). Sertraline seems to produce the least disruption in sleep architecture and is the least inhibitory of P450 2D6 cytochromes.

In general, the "tolerability" of the SSRIs is superior to that of the tricyclics. The different side effect profile of the SSRIs which leads to their increased tolerability might make this class of drug particularly useful for the geriatric depressive. However, the efficacy of the SSRIs remains to be established (Frazer, 1994).

Fluoxetine generally is dosed at 10 to 20 mg daily or every other day in the elderly, but because it is available in a liquid form it may be dosed as low as 5 mg daily. Given that fluoxetine has an elimination half-life of up to 85 hr, however, clearance may take up to 2 weeks in the elderly. The SSRIs currently marketed include sertraline and paroxetine. Sertraline is dosed at 50 to 150 mg daily, but it has a shorter elimination half-life of only 26 hr. Paroxetine, dosed at 10 to 40 mg daily in the elderly, has the shortest elimination half-life of 21 hr and has been reported as minimally anxiogenic (Dunner & Dunbar, 1992; Sheehan, Dunbar, & Fuell, 1992).

Bupropion

Bupropion, a monocyclic phenylaminoketone, is a unique antidepressant that inhibits the reuptake of dopamine more potently than norepinephrine or serotonin (Montgomery, 1993). Bupropion is a stimulating antidepressant dosed at 75 to 100 mg three times daily as therapeutically necessary. The elimination half-life of bupropion is only 10 hr. There has been concern regarding the reportedly increased tendency of bupropion to produce seizures as compared with cyclic antidepressants, although this attribution has been debated (Rosenstein, Nelson, & Jacobs, 1993). Bupropion can cause nervousness and insomnia, but does not cause the weight gain associated with the older antidepressants (Harto-Traux et al., 1983).

Psychostimulants, methylphenidate, and dextroamphetamine are related structurally to bupropion. Methylphenidate is the preferred stimulant for the elderly due to its shorter elimination half-life of 2 to 4 hr, as compared with 11 to 12 hr for dextroamphetamine. Methylphenidate is generally dosed in the morning at 5 mg daily, with an additional 5 mg at noon as therapeutically necessary, although doses as high as 30 to 40 mg daily have been used in the elderly. Both methylphenidate and bupropion may be particularly useful for the apathetic medically ill elderly, especially when a more rapid response is preferred.

Venlafaxine

Venlafaxine is a novel phenethylamine antidepressant notable for its strong inhibition of both norepinephrine and serotonin reuptake. It has a rapid onset of action in animal models (Montgomery, 1993), as well as a dose-related time course of improvement (Schweizer, Weise, Clary, Fox, & Rickels, 1991). Doses of 37.5 to 150 mg twice daily may be optimal. Patients treated with venlafaxine had more headaches, nausea, and hypertension than patients treated with tricyclic antidepressants, but they had a significantly lower incidence of dry mouth, dizziness, and tremor. Studies indicate that venlafaxine has potential for use in refractory depression and that it protects against relapse for as long as 12 months, but double-blind trials are needed to establish efficacy (Montgomery, 1993). No clinical trials of venlafaxine have yet been conducted in the elderly.

Nefazodone hydrochloride (a phenylpiperazine derivative) has a chemical structure that is distinctly different from the tricyclic antidepressants, MAOIs, SSRIs, venlafaxine, and bupropion. Within the serotonergic synapse, nefazodone blocks serotonin type 2 (5-HT$_2$) receptors postsynaptically and inhibits 5-HT reuptake presynaptically. These two mechanisms allow for increased availability of serotonin to interact with other 5-HT receptors. Within the norepinephrine synapse, nefazodone blocks norepinephrine reuptake presynaptically. With chronic administration, nefazodone also downregulates 5-HT$_2$ receptors. Nefazodone has also been shown to antagonize α_1-adrenergic receptors. However, nefazodone has not demonstrated affinity for α_2- and β-adrenergic, 5-HT$_{1a}$ cholinergic, dopaminergic, or benzodiazepine receptors. Controlled clinical trials have shown nefazodone to be as effective as conventional therapy in relieving depression. The recommended initial dose of nefazodone for patients 65 years or older or those who are medically debilitated is 25–50 mg twice daily. Patient response should be carefully assessed after a week of nefazodone therapy. In most elderly patients, nefazodone should be titrated to a dose of at least 100 mg twice daily. Analysis of data of patients 65 years or older who were enrolled in premarketing clinical trials indicate that the optimal therapeutic response to nefazodone is obtained at doses of 200 mg to 400 mg daily (Bristol-Myers Squibb, data on file, 1992). Results of these trials also indicate that there were no significant qualitative or quantitative differences in safety and tolerability profiles in young versus elderly patients treated with nefazodone. Nefazodone appears to be weight neutral and is not associated with sexual dysfunction (Anton et al., 1994; Eison, Eison, Torrente, Wright, & Yocca, 1990).

One of the major differences among the SSRIs and SNRIs is their ability to inhibit P450 enzymes. Fluoxetine and paroxetine at their usually effective minimum dose produce substantial inhibition of P450 2D6. The possible effects of fluoxetine and the other SSRIs on 3A3/4 and 2C19 has not been sufficiently studied to comment with confidence. Nonetheless, sertraline at its usually effective minimum dose (50 mg/day) has substantially less effects on diazepam clearance than does fluoxetine and would be expected to have less effects on alprazolam clearance. Fluvoxamine, indicated primarily for obsessive–compulsive disorder (up to 200 mg/day) is the only SSRI that produces substantial inhibition of the P450 enzyme 1A2 in vitro (Brosen et al., 1993). Like other antidepressants, SSRIs are likely to have

their clearance accelerated to a clinically significant extent by enzyme inducers such as carbamazepine and phenytoin (Pollock, 1994).

Venlafaxine has no known clinically relevant effect on any P450 enzyme. Its in vitro potency for inhibiting the P450 enzyme 2D6 is two orders of magnitude weaker than that of paroxetine and fluoxetine. Given its plasma concentrations at its clinically effective antidepressant doses, venlafaxine would not be expected to produce any effect on the functional integrity of 2D6 in patients taking clinically relevant antidepressant doses. Nonetheless, formal studies are needed to confirm this.

Venlafaxine is dependent on several P450 enzymes for its biotransformation and clearance, including 2D6 and 3A3/4. Therefore, fluoxetine may increase the plasma levels of venlafaxine and/or its metabolites when patients are abruptly switched from fluoxetine to venlafaxine. Whether such an effect occurs, to what extent, or with what frequency is unknown. Even if it does occur, the issue should be a tolerability matter rather than a toxicity issue since venlafaxine has a wide therapeutic index. If it occurs, then tolerability problems may occur, since high doses and hence high levels of venlafaxine can be associated with dose-limiting problems such as gastrointestinal distress. If such an interaction does occur, any clinical consequence should be avoidable by appropriate dose adjustment. As with other antidepressants, the metabolism of venlafaxine is likely to be induced by the same drugs (e.g., carbamazepine, phenytoin) that induce the metabolism of other antidepressants. Hence, dose adjustment would be necessary to compensate for the increased clearance rate.

Nefazodone is an inhibitor of P450 111A4, and, therefore, the manufacturer lists its coadministration with terfenadine or astemizole (Hismanal), another nonsedating antihistamine, as contraindicated. Under normal conditions, terfenadine and astemizole are totally metabolized, with little parent compound detectable in plasma. When the IIIA4 isoenzyme is inhibited, however, the parent antihistamine can accumulate, potentially leading to prolonged cardiac QTC of the EKG intervals and possibly lethal cardiac arrhythmias. The triazolobenzodiazepines triazolam (Halcion) and alprazolam (Xanax) also are metabolized by the liver's IIIA4 system. When these agents are coadministered with nefazodone, their plasma concentrations increase, with potential for adverse clinical effects. Other benzodiazepines (e.g., lorazepam) not metabolized by the IIIA4 isoenzyme are not affected by coadministration with nefazodone (Pollock, 1994).

Depression Prescription Recommendations

While Richelson (1994) has commented that thymoleptics are now as readily available as antibiotics, it is clear that their method of prescription should not be similar.

It is ironic that after 30 years of antidepressant availability, we are only now becoming aware of how antidepressants should be prescribed. Greden (1993) recently reviewed the recurrent depression data of David Kupfer, M.D., in adults and concluded that major depression is much more recurrent than we previously have thought. From Kupfer's data, Greden recommended lifetime antidepressant medication for patients over the age of 50, patients over 40 with two previous distinct depressive episodes, and for anyone with three previous depressive episodes. Patients also need to be maintained on the same dosage of antidepressant medication that helped bring about resolution. Episodes need to be not just partially resolved, but completely concluded.

Even using the most liberal criteria, Gershon, Plotkin, and Jarvik (1988) could only find 25 placebo-controlled antidepressant studies for late-life depression and fewer for "so-called neuropsychiatric depression." Most of clinical practice among board-certified geriatric psychiatrists is based on these studies as well as extrapolations from a younger population.

In dealing with the depressed geriatric patient, we recommend starting with an SSRI, SNRI, or nefazodone depending on the initial target symptoms. If the patient is anergic, we have found venlafaxine to be a useful agent starting at 75 mg a day (37.5 mg morning and afternoon) and advancing up to 200 mg a day in the elderly. Sertraline at similar dosage per 24 hr, but dosed once a day, can also be tried, but it seems to create the greatest amount of gastrointestinal distress and may need to be toler-

ated briefly or given with yogurt in the beginning. Prozac at a dose of 10 to 30 mg can also be tried. Paroxetine, an agent for the more agitated depressives, can be dosed in the morning or at suppertime (we prefer supper) starting at 10 mg and advancing after 1 week up to 20 mg or even 30 mg by the second week. We have little experience with nefazodone in the geriatric population but it may have efficacy in anxious depression. If one SSRI or SNRI cannot be tolerated or is not successful, an alternative one can be tried. If the patient is very depressed and even melancholic, the tricyclics nortriptyline and desipramine have been shown to be effective (Roose, 1994). The SSRI can be augmented with tricyclics or trazodone. Bupropion can be used even as a first-line treatment successfully and safely in anergic depressives. In our hands, we have used bupropion safely, even in brain injury, and have not seen any seizure activity even in this vulnerable population. We have also used bupropion as an intermediate between SSRIs and MAOIs so that we would not need to wait the 4 weeks between the administration of SSRIs and MAOIs. The MAOIs still have their utility in elderly depressives. Augmenting strategies seem more simple than changing medication, but experiences with lithium in the elderly have not been remarkable (Flint & Rifat, 1994; Zimmer, Rosen, Thornton, Perel, & Reynolds, 1991) nor documented thoroughly.

There is no data regarding the treatment of elderly dysthymics and subsyndromal depressives or the potential efficacy of treating even minor "medical" illness depression (Burvill, 1995). Indeed, within the past 2 years, two major studies of poststroke depression and post-myocardial infarction depression (Frasure-Smith, 1995) have reported depression (even minor depression) to be a predictor of mortality. Markowitz, Kocasis, and Moran (1992) and Hellerstein et al. (1993) have already reported on the efficacy of thymoleptics in the treatment of dysthymia. We recommend the use of thymoleptics in comorbid medical conditions and depression (even minor depressives).

Antidepressants can be a safe and effective treatment for late-life depression. Care should be taken to select the appropriate agent from the vast armament available to suit the needs of the patient. It is important to recognize that some antidepressants have not been extensively studied in the elderly. Starting with lower dosages and titrating to effect slowly will avoid many of the hazards of using this class of agents.

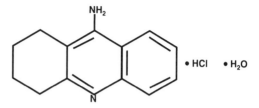

FIGURE 5. Cognex (tacrine).

Dementia

Background

Dementia in the United States affects from 6% to more than 12% of the elderly population. Prevalence rates for probable Alzheimer's disease range from 2% in Baltimore to 12.3% in east Boston. Whether these discrepancies are due to real geographic differences or differences in interviewees or interview instruments is still unclear.

Epidemiological Catchment Area studies estimate that people over 65 residing in the noninstitutionalized community have prevalence rates of approximately 5% for severe cognitive impairment. However, prevalence was approximately 3% for those between the ages of 65 and 69 and 48% for those over the age of 85. Alzheimer's disease is thought to affect over 4 million people at a cost of more than $100 billion a year. Recent estimates of the annual care of Alzheimer's patients based on nursing home care or other care, including medications, is about $47,000 per patient (Rice, 1993).

Dementia of the Alzheimer's type is a disorder of progressive brain deterioration resulting in cognitive decline and increasing impairment. Rarely striking before age 65, Alzheimer's disease may afflict as many as half of those who survive through their mid-80s and accounts for half of the dementias. There is no cure, but in 1993 the U.S. Food and Drug Administration approved tacrine (Cognex; see Figure 5) as a palliative.

Alzheimer's disease selectively attacks cholinergic neurons. Tacrine reversibly inhibits brain acetylcholinesterase, preventing the breakdown of acetylcholine from presynaptic neurons. In Alzheimer's patients, tacrine should increase cholinergic transmission in neurons that are not yet destroyed. The most beneficial dose of tacrine is 30–40 mg four times a day, given to patients with mild to moderate disease.

In an editorial, Winker (1994) noted that the benefit of tacrine is roughly equivalent to rolling back the deterioration of Alzheimer's disease by about 6 months. Once the clock is reset however, the cognitive decline continues. Moreover, if the drug is stopped, the patient loses the 6-month margin. Winker points out a number of qualifications about tacrine therapy. In addition to the fact that many patients cannot tolerate the dosage required for benefit, the drug must be given four times daily and blood must be drawn every 2 weeks for at least 3 months to monitor serum alanine aminotransferase (ALT). The cost of the drug is estimated to be $112 per month, while each ALT assay costs between $16 and $37.

Tacrine is metabolized by the liver enzyme P450 IA2, which is also involved in the metabolism of cimetidine and theophylline. Cimetidine appears to elevate blood levels of tacrine, and tacrine elevates blood levels of theophylline. Probably by acting on the same liver isoenzyme, smoking lowers blood levels of tacrine (Winker, 1994).

Other medication interventions specifically aimed at cognitive deficits include serotonin receptor agonists, anti-Parkinson's oxidase inhibitors, and different thymoleptic agents. Thymoleptic agents have not only been used to treat the cognitive deficits, but also to treat concurrent or underlying depression.

Even if the disease that causes a person's dementia cannot be cured, psychiatric symptoms and behavioral problems associated with it usually can and should be addressed. These problems can be alleviated with changes in the person's daily activities, modifications to his or her environment, training for caregivers in how to respond, in some cases counseling and relaxation therapies for the patient, and medication.

In addition, we cannot forget that many people with Alzheimer's disease also have other medical conditions unrelated or only peripherally related to their disease. Any coexisting medical condition can exacerbate a patient's cognitive, behavioral, and self-care deficits and complicate his or her care. Conversely, treatment of the condition can maintain or restore the person's physical health and maximize his or her functioning.

Although costly and encumbered with complications, tacrine is all that is currently available to reverse, even temporarily, the cognitive decline in patients with Alzheimer's disease. Patients and caregivers must be told what is involved in a trial of this cholinergic agent, which seems worth considering in selected cases.

Psychosis

Background

As mentioned above, many of the behavioral complications of Alzheimer's disease and the vascular dementias can be managed with medications. Before discussing the management of these disorders, we first discuss the psychotic disorders. This background serves well to a discussion of the behavioral disturbances in the dementias.

About 1% of the people in the world develop schizophrenia, the most disabling of mental illnesses. Like most mental illnesses, schizophrenia has the status of a syndrome (a group of symptoms) rather than a well-defined disease. These symptoms are often classified as positive (psychotic hallucinations and delusions) and negative (apparent loss of emotional expressiveness and responsiveness, lack of spontaneity and curiosity, and difficulty in initiating purposeful actions). Cognitive disorganization (confused thought and speech) may be regarded as either positive or negative, but there is increasing evidence that it may belong in a separate category. These three groups of symptoms might be based on different brain pathways, or the same disorder of information processing might underlie all three (*DSM-IV*).

Psychosis found in elderly chronic schizophrenics, combined with acute paraphrenic pathology (Almeida, 1995), are observed in less than 0.5% of the elderly population, although many of these individuals are so disruptive that it appears that these illnesses are more common than they really are. Until recently, American psychiatrists were reluctant to diagnose schizophrenia with onset after age 45. The *DSM-IV-R* indeed reintroduced the idea of "late-onset schizophrenia." Unrecognized until a few years ago and controversial today, late-onset schizophrenia is gaining acceptance as a valid diagnostic entity that warrants serious clinical and research attention.

Although females present with late-onset schizophrenia more than males by a 2:1 ratio (Jeste et al., 1995), early and late-onset schizophrenias present with a similar range of symptoms. As is characteristic of paranoid schizophrenia, many patients have bizarre delusions, that is, delusions that are completely incongruent with reality. However, some patients have only nonbizarre delusions. Investigations with symptom rating scales have not confirmed an earlier clinical impression that patients with late-onset schizophrenia have fewer negative symptoms than younger patients.

Several conditions should be considered in the differential diagnosis of delusions in an older patient. First, the psychiatrist should rule out early-onset psychosis that may have been missed until middle age. Jeste et al. (1995) make the diagnosis only in patients who have had no evidence of early schizophrenia or a prodromal illness, no decline in function related to psychiatric symptoms, and no psychiatric symptoms, and no psychiatric hospitalization or chronic treatment with a psychotropic drug before the age of 45.

New-onset mood disorders are more common than schizophrenia in the middle-aged and elderly. Affective symptoms are also common in patients with late-onset schizophrenia, and primary affective disorders are diagnosed or ruled out using the same criteria as in younger patients.

Late-onset schizophrenia differs from delusional disorder in several respects. Bizarre delusions, prominent auditory hallucinations, and significant decline in overall function associated with bizarre behavior are not features of a delusional disorder. These phenomena are often present in late-onset schizophrenia.

Organic syndromes must be ruled out using a standard medical history, physical and neurologic examinations, and appropriate laboratory and diagnostic imaging studies looking for endocrinopathy and brain tumors. A progressive decline in cognitive function and the presence of a memory deficit are indicative of dementia (Jeste et al., 1995).

Similar to the first-generation antidepressants, which are dominated by the tricyclic thymoleptics, the first-generation antipsychotics or major tranquilizers have four major classes, two of which are tricyclic (Figures 6 and 7). The four major groups of the antipsychotics are the tricyclic phenothiazines, thioxanthene derivatives, nontricyclic butyrophenones and dibenzodiazepines. Other less important groups include the indolic compounds and the amine depleting agents. The phenothiazines themselves are divided into three subclasses on the basis of their side chains and include the low-potency aliphatic piperidine compounds such as thioridazine and the more potent piperazine compounds includ-

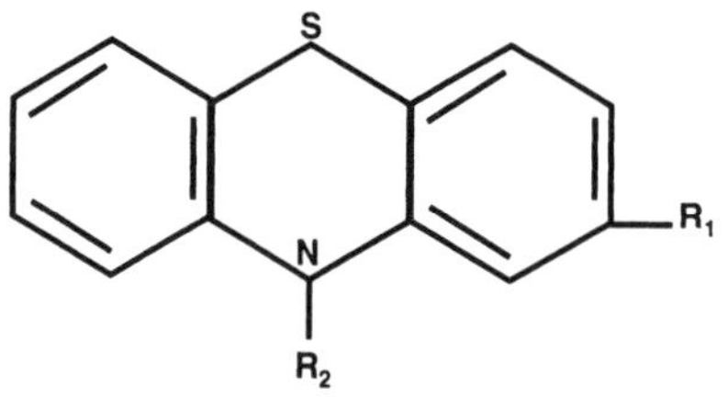

Phenothiazine nucleus

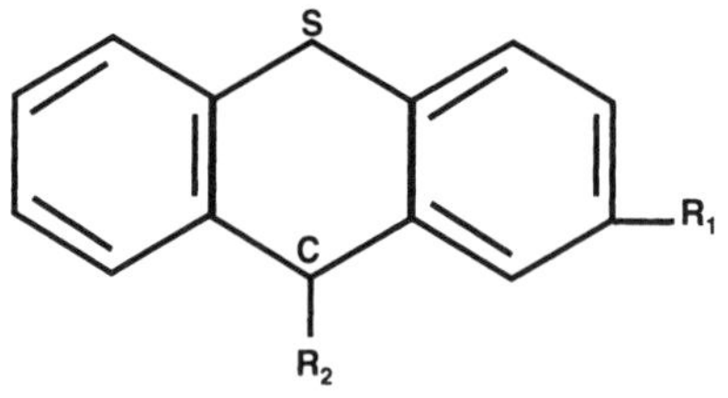

(Alternative) Phenothiazine nucleus

R_2 can be many different side chains
ie; $R_2 = CH_2 - CH_2 - CH_2 - CH_2 - N(CH_3)_2$

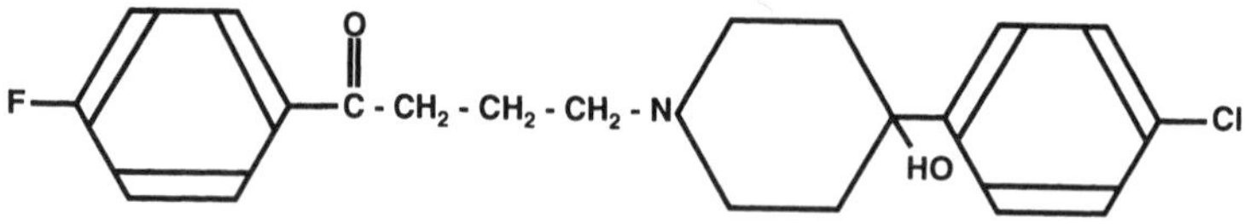

Butyrophenones: Haloperidol (Haldol)

IDOLIC COMPOUNDS

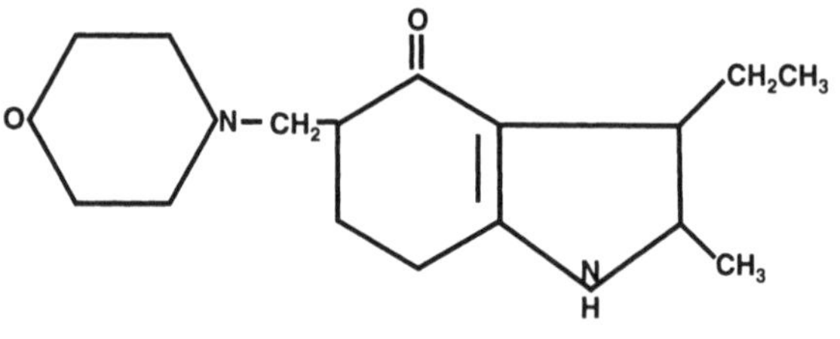

Molindone (Moban)

FIGURE 6. Traditional antipsychotics.

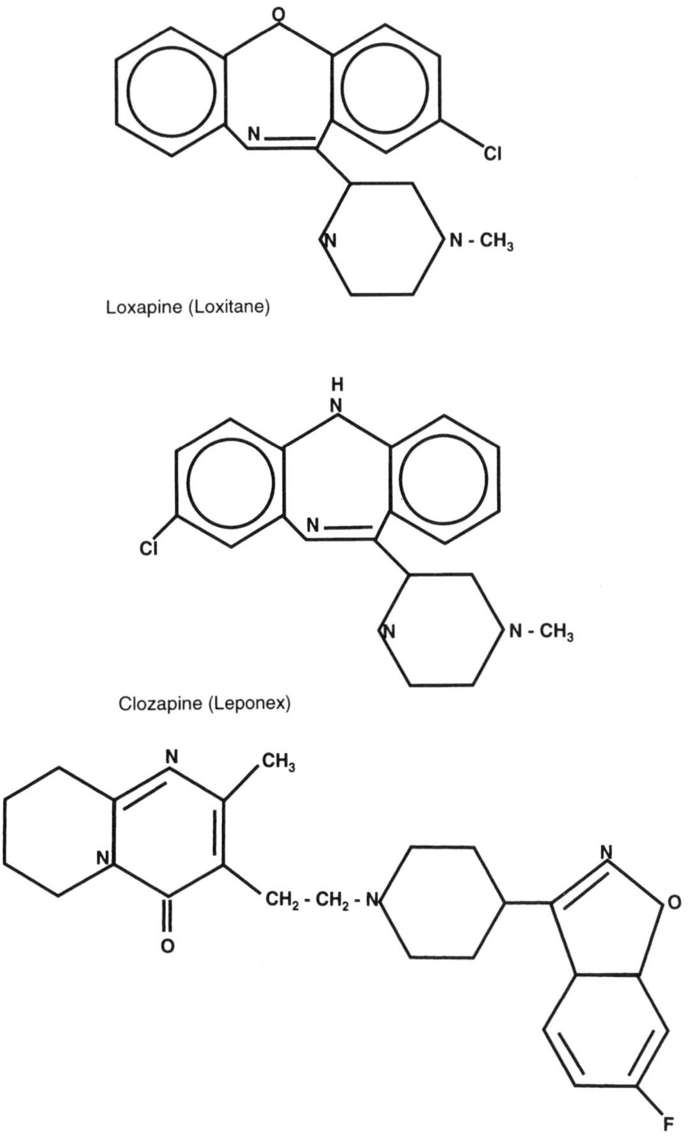
O
N
Cl
N
N - CH3
Loxapine (Loxitane)
H
N
N
Cl
N
N - CH3
Clozapine (Leponex)
N
CH3
N
O
CH2 - CH2 - N
N
O
F

FIGURE 7. Atypical (newer) antipsychotics.

ing fluphenazine, trifluoperazine, and perphenazine (Meltzer, 1992).

Late-onset schizophrenia is responsive to the same antipsychotic agents used in younger patients. However, lower doses should be used, both because they are highly effective in this population and because older patients are at greater risk of side effects and adverse drug interactions. Typically the effective dose of antipsychotic medication for late-onset schizophrenia is less than 200 mg chlorpromazine or its equivalent, which is significantly lower than the dose used in younger patients (Jeste, Locro, Gilbert, Kline, & Kline, 1993). Even with low-dose therapy, tardive dyskinesia (TD) develops in 30% of patients over age 45 after a year of treatment. Indeed, in a group of patients with a mean age of 66 years treated with relatively low doses of neuroleptics, Jeste et al. (1995) found a high incidence of TD: 26% developed TD after 12 months of treatment, 52% developed it after 24 months, and 60% after 36 months of treatment. Cumulative amounts of neuroleptics, especially the very potent ones; a history of alcohol abuse or dependency; and baseline subtle subcortical dysfunction appear to be the most significant risk factors for TD (Jeste et al., 1995).

Psychiatrists should prescribe antipsychotics cautiously in older patients who are taking other medications that may have anticholinergic or sedative effects. Since conventional antipsychotic medications are equally effective in controlling positive symptoms, the choice among them should be based on their side effect profile. For example, for a man with prostatic hypertrophy, the clinician may prefer to administer a high-potency antipsychotic such as haloperidol or perphenazine because of the reduced potential for anticholinergic side effects. A patient with parkinsonism might do better with a low-potency antipsychotic such as thioridazine or chlorpromazine to reduce the likelihood of extrapyramidal (parkinsonian) symptoms (EPS) (Jeste et al., 1993; Meltzer, 1992).

Older patients tend to respond well to antipsychotic medications, particularly with respect to positive symptoms; the established antipsychotic drugs are less effective in controlling negative symptoms in late-onset illness. There has been little experience with newer antipsychotic drugs in late-onset schizophrenia, as newer agents are typically tested and prescribed initially in the young.

Patients with late-onset schizophrenia often need to continue drug therapy for prolonged periods and are likely to suffer a relapse if they stop taking medication. The clinician should treat the acute symptoms and then maintain the patient on the lowest possible dose. Once the patient is stabilized, the dose should be lowered. If the patient tolerates the lower dose, it should be reduced even further. Finally, discontinuation of medication can be attempted cautiously.

The newer atypical antipsychotics were developed to deal with the problems of "treatment-resistant schizophrenia" (Brenner et al., 1990), neuroleptic intolerance, and TD. Treatment-resistant schizophrenia may be characterized by (1) persistent delusions, hallucinations, or thought disorder; or (2) pervasive negative symptoms such as withdrawal, anhedonia, poverty of thought content, defect in volition, and lack of energy. When at least one of the positive symptoms is present to a marked extent, or several of the negative symptoms are present to at least a moderate extent in combination with slight to moderate positive symptoms, there is little dispute that such patients are resistant to treatment and are candidates for alternative forms of therapy, especially novel drug treatments. When only negative symptoms are present or when positive symptoms are mild, or when there is a partial improvement from a more severely ill state, elements of both treatment responsiveness and resistance are present. Subjective considerations and level of social function play a major role in determining the modification of the treatment regimen in such cases.

Treatment-resistant schizophrenia makes us consider the phenomenology of schizophrenia, other psychosis, and late-life schizophrenia, as well as the specificity of the site of action of the traditional neuroleptics and the newer atypical antipsychotics. In addition to treatment-resistant patients, neuroleptic-intolerant patients usually derive limited benefit from neuroleptic drugs. This is usually due to parkinsonian side effects or moderate to severe TD or tardive dystonia.

Tardive dyskinesia may be considered a type of neuroleptic intolerance. In mild forms, patients may tolerate the symptoms of TD surprisingly well. There is evidence that its severity may not be progressive (Gardos, Pereny, Cole, Samu, & Kallos, 1983; Kane et al., 1984). In such cases, the presence of TD does not necessarily mean that neuroleptic treatment should be discontinued, but only that dosage should be lowered to the least amount needed to achieve remission of psychotic symptoms. It is conceivable, however, that less than optimal relief of psychosis results from such a strategy. In a small group of patients, TD may be severe, progress rapidly, or be intolerable. After clinical testing confirmed its effectiveness as an antipsychotic with few or no EPS (Hippius, 1980), clozapine (a dibenzodiazepine), like loxapine, was introduced in the early 1960s in a number of Western European countries. Unfortunately, problems with agranulocytosis and subsequent death (Amsler, Teerenhoui, Bartha, Harjula, & Vuppio, 1993) delayed its release in the United States and worldwide when its dramatic efficacy in neuroleptic-resistant schizophrenia was repeatedly demonstrated (Janicah, David, Preskorn, & Ayd, 1993; Lindstrom, 1988; Meltzer, 1989).

Clozapine is available in 25 mg and 100 mg tablets in the United States. The usual starting dose is 25 mg once or twice a day. In some European countries, a parenteral preparation for intramuscular use is available; however, it is known to cause local pain at the injection site.

It is possible to start clozapine on outpatients with close monitoring of blood pressure, pulse, and sedation to determine when the dose can be raised, but this requires good cooperation from patients and their families or caregivers. Many clinicians will find it safest and most convenient to begin clozapine treatment on an inpatient basis. The dose of clozapine is gradually increased by 25 mg every other day until it reaches 100 mg. It can then be increased by 50 mg every other day until a dose of 300 to 450 mg/day is reached, usually by the end of 2 weeks. The dose usually should not exceed 450 to 600 mg/day because the risk of seizures is dose-related (see below). If response at 600 mg/day is unsatisfactory, dosage can be further increased up to a maximum of 900 mg/day. There are no fixed-dose studies to determine optimal dosage. It may be possible to lower the dosage during the maintenance phase. The dosage of clozapine required in the elderly is less than that in younger patients.

Unfortunately, despite the dramatic, truly life-saving aspects of clozapine, there is controversy regarding its usage. Debate continues on whether the improvement in negative symptoms is independent of its effect on positive symptoms and whether it is worth subjecting patients to clozapine's risk of agranulocytosis (Carpenter, Conley, Buchanon, Breier, & Tomminga, 1995). Debate also continues regarding clozapine's ability to independently treat the negative symptoms of schizophrenia, how long one should wait before abandoning the clozapine intervention, and how to exactly taper and discontinue other neuroleptics with the addition of clozapine.

Risperidone was introduced into the United States in late 1994 to address symptom resistance, the negative symptoms of schizophrenia, and the acute and latent movement disorders which negated clozapine's positive effects. Risperidone is a benzisoxazole compound that, like clozapine, is about 100 times as potent in antagonizing 5-HT$_2$ as D$_2$ receptors (Borison, Diamond, & Pathiraja, 1992). It has been estimated that 5 mg of risperidone has an antipsychotic effect equivalent to about 400 mg of clozapine (Borison, Diamond, & Pathiraja, 1992). In chronically and acutely ill schizophrenic patients, risperidone in doses of 2 to 6 mg/day has been found to be at least as effective as haloperidol in treating positive symptoms and superior in relieving negative symptoms (Anderson, True, & Ereshefsky, 1993; Chouinard, Jones, & Remington, 1993; Muller-Spahn, 1992).

Risperidone, which has an elimination half-life of about 20 hr and a bioavailability of about 66% (Huang, Van Peer, & Woestenborghs, 1993), is metabolized by the P450 2D6 system to 9-hydroxy-risperidone, a clinically active metabolite (Huang et al., 1993). Studies in schizophrenic patients suggest a therapeutic window, at least for negative symptoms, with doses lower than 2 mg/day being largely ineffective and a declining response rate, possibly due to the emergence of EPS, as daily doses approach 16 mg (Anderson et al., 1993; Borison, Pathiraja, & Diamond, 1992). The optimal daily dose for negative symptoms of schizophrenia appears to be about 6 mg (Chouinard et al., 1993; Marder, 1992). Doses for other disorders have not been studied. Because improvement at a given dose of risperidone may continue gradually over 7 months or so (Borison, Pathiraja, & Diamond, 1992), caution is warranted before changing the treatment in slow responders.

Blockade of D$_2$ receptors by risperidone has been said to be low enough at doses below 10 mg/day to minimize the risk for EPS and TD. Chouinard et al. (1993) and Borison et al. (1992) found that the incidence of EPS with doses of risperidone up to 16 mg/day was equivalent to that with placebo and significantly less than with haloperidol and that preexisting TD was improved. Most other studies agree that the risk for EPS is low with risperidone and that risperidone might be a treatment for TD (Claus, Bollen, & De Cuyper, 1992; Janssen, Niemegeers, & Awouters, 1988). However, although receptor binding studies are performed in animal in vitro or ex vivo preparations, and extrapolation to intact humans is inexact at best, Hollister (1994) notes that 50% of D$_2$ receptors are occupied at a dose of 1 mg risperidone, suggesting that higher doses might block enough of these receptors in the basal ganglia to produce EPS. Some clinicians are encountering more EPS than would be predicted from much of the published literature and more than is seen with clozapine. On the other hand, clinical experience with any form of EPS in patients who were previously taking classical neuroleptics, especially neuroleptics with long half-lives and active metabolites, may reflect inadequate washout of the neuroleptic (Safferman, Lieberman, & Pollack, 1993).

More predictable adverse effects of risperidone (Borrison, Diamond, & Pathiraja, 1992; Borison, Pathiraja, & Diamond, 1992; Chouinard et al., 1993) include sedation, weakness, insomnia, and problems with concentration and memory. Insomnia, ataxia, salivation, prolactinemia, and elevated liver function may also occur. Risperidone has had placebo-controlled comparative treatment trials to clozapine and haloperidol. At 4 mg and 8 mg doses, it has been shown as effective as clozaril and haloperidol (Marder, 1992). Unfortunately, there still exists a group of treatment-resistant patients who respond better to clozapine.

Positive treatment trials (but uncontrolled) of risperidone in psychotic elderly are beginning to appear (Aranson, Lingam, & Hasanat, 1995; Goldberg, 1995), showing its effectiveness in treating agitation and delusions in dementia and schizophrenia, but reminding us that risperidone does not eliminate movement disorders in those in whom it is already present and can cause movement disorders at higher than 2 mg doses in the elderly. In the elderly and in patients who are medically compromised or exquisitely sensitive to EPS, risperidone should be started as low as 0.25 mg twice daily and pushed to 2 mg/day. Since the half-life is 20 to 23 hr, it can be dosed to once per day. Weight gain is less than with clozapine, and sedation is about as low as that with haloperidol. Men have erectile and ejaculatory problems that are dose-related.

If a patient has not had a clozapine trial, has severe treatment-resistant schizophrenia, and is doing poorly, then it is reasonable to try risperidone before clozapine. Unfortunately, once clozapine has been tried, risperidone seems to have less efficacy, and some patients become dysphoric. The latter could be related to cholinergic overload once clozapine is withdrawn.

Other Psychoses

Psychosis is not just confined to late-life schizophrenia and includes bipolar affective disorder, major depression with psychotic features, the so-called delusional disorders, paraphrenia, and the dementias. When trying to understand the phenomenology of psychosis in dementia, the so-called positive and negative symptoms of schizophrenia can also be found in dementia.

Suspiciousness and paranoia have been identified in 20% to 25% of people with Alzheimer's disease. Similarly, visual and auditory hallucinations have been found in 25% of people with Alzheimer's disease and other dementing diseases. On the other hand, 50% to 75% of people with Alzheimer's disease are withdrawn and have reduced emotional responsiveness.

Other behavioral complications such as aggression, angry outbursts, assaultiveness, wandering, repetitive manipulation of objects, and vegetative symptoms such as disturbed sleep and incontinence are frequent correlates of dementia (Deutsch & Rovner, 1991). Agitation, sundowning, and the catastrophic reaction too are often discussed in connection with dementia. Agitation, found in 25–89% of people with Alzheimer's disease as defined by the American Psychiatric Association's (1987) psychiatric glossary is characterized by excessive motor activity, usually nonpurposeful, and is associated with internal tension, dread, and an inability to find the right words. Agitation is common in mood disorders and toxic states so it is often misdiagnosed as an anxiety disorder. In the elderly, agitation may be an early sign of an organic mental disorder. Furthermore, elderly patients in nursing homes and hospitals typically exhibit increased restlessness, confusion, and verbal deterioration in the late afternoon, a phenomenon termed "sundowning."

Moreover, in 1952, Goldstein described the "catastrophic reaction" as part of the characteristic emotional reactions which emerge when a brain-injured or impaired patient is faced with problems which tax his or her ability.

> [They] may overreact in an anxious aggressive manner or alternatively become quiet, sullen, and withdrawn. The catastrophic reaction may occur without warning, but usually is heralded by increasing anxiety and tension. The patient looks dazed and starts to

fumble, whereas a moment before he was calm and amiable, he now shows an intense affective response, varying from irritability and temper to outbursts of crying and despair. Autonomic disturbance is seen in the form of flushing, sweating, or trembling. He may become evasive, where further questions are concerned or show a sudden aimless restlessness. The catastrophic reaction develops simultaneously with the attempt to perform the task in which he fails, and not following the performance. It, therefore, does not represent the patient's response to the awareness that he has failed, but an awareness of the brain's limitation. To avoid this unpleasant reaction, the brain injured patients develop a variety of avoidant type behaviors. (Kolb & Brodie, 1982, p. 304)

Although nonintrusive behavioral interventions are gaining acceptance among geriatric health care professionals for the treatment of behavioral excess and deficits, the most common intervention is pharmacotherapy with psychotropics (Cohen-Mansfield & Billing, 1986), most commonly with the neuroleptic class of compounds. In the 1980s, it was suggested that physicians should consider a trial of benzodiazepines prior to the use of neuroleptics (Raskin, 1985), particularly in the treatment of nonpsychotic behavioral disturbances (Peabody, Warner, Whiteford, & Hollister, 1987).

Risse and Barnes (1986) conclude in their review that benzodiazepines have not been studied well in older demented patients with behavioral disturbances, although uncontrolled studies have reported generally favorable results. Covington (1975), on the other hand, comparing the effectiveness of thioridazine and diazepam in geriatric patients with various symptoms of "senility," reported some deterioration of patients receiving diazepam. Other researchers have looked at the comparative efficacy of benzodiazepines with mixed results (Coccaro, 1990). Judging from the previous research, it is clear that the efficacy of the benzodiazepine anxiolytics for controlling geriatric behavior problems has not been firmly established by placebo-controlled studies.

Neuroleptic medications are often effective in managing agitated behaviors, although studies have demonstrated that the efficacy is modest. In a meta-analysis of controlled trials (Schneider, Pollock, & Lyness, 1990) found that 18% of dementia patients with agitation benefited from neuroleptic treatment beyond that of placebo. As in the treatment of psy-chosis of schizophrenia, there is no clear difference in efficacy among neuroleptic agents. Research studies and clinical experience have shown that some patients do not respond to neuroleptic treatment, and a small proportion worsen behaviorally when treated.

Sultzer (1995) recently reported on a double-blind comparison of trazodone versus haloperidol for the treatment of agitated behavior in elderly individuals with dementia. The 10-week trial showed both drugs to have equal efficacy. An interesting finding was the item analysis showing that nonaggressive motor symptoms (pacing, general restlessness) responded preferentially to haloperidol, whereas repetitive behaviors, verbal aggression, negativism, and opposition to assistance preferentially responded to trazodone. It is obvious that further studies are warranted.

Tariot et al. (1994) have recently reported on the efficacy of carbamazepine for agitation in nursing home patients in a nonsystematized, placebo-controlled cross-over trial conducted in 25 patients in two nursing homes. In another recent report by Lott, McElroy, and Keys (1995) valproic acid too was found to be efficacious when compared to placebo for agitation in dementia.

Other medications have been reported to be effective for the treatment of agitated behaviors. Unfortunately nearly all those published are open trials with small numbers of patients and without a comparison group of active drug placebo. Other medications commonly used to manage agitated behaviors include the beta blockers with their potential cardiac problems, antimanic and anticonvulsant agents, and the new serotonin uptake inhibitors. Alteration of serotonergic activity has been implicated in reduction of aggression, irritability, and impulsivity; this suggests that this group of agents might be the most promising for the treatment of so-called agitation.

The most frequently prescribed first-line antipsychotics are the high-potency compounds haloperidol, thiothixene, and perphenazine. Clozapine is reserved for resistant late-life schizophrenia or psychosis secondary to Parkinson's disease. Though relatively new, risperidone has been tried in late-life schizophrenia (Aranson et al., 1995; Goldberg, 1995) and its promise of efficacy for positive and negative symptoms and the safety and low incidence of parkinsonian and dyskinetic side effects would seem to make it a good first-line agent for any late-life psychoses.

Conclusion

This chapter has focused on psychopharmacology strategies to deal with geriatric behavioral disturbances. Suggesting general principles and ideas, we have really only dealt more fully with one neuropsychiatric area, namely dementia, and have not dealt with specific neuropsychiatric illnesses such as Parkinson's disease, stroke, or head injury. Because of the paucity of good studies despite good practical clinical interventions, we have also not dealt with the developing area of sleep disorders and the vast armament of agents available. Generally, sleep abnormalities occur in the context of the major categories of psychiatric problems discussed in this chapter. The newer hypnotic agent zolpidem, or Ambien, seems to have a rapid onset and short duration of action. The geriatric dose is normally 5 mg at bedtime. This drug seems safe and particularly helpful if taken on an occasional basis. Changes in electroconvulsive therapy (ECT) and the new specific insight and problem-solving psychotherapies cannot and should not be ignored when thinking about pharmacologic interventions.

We have described the most up-to-date pharmacologic interventions for late-life behavioral disturbances. In the future more focused placebo-controlled and comparative studies are needed, so that effective interventions can be found.

References

Alexopoulos G. S., Meyers, B. S., Young, R. C., Chester, J., Feder, M., & Einborn, A. (1995). Anxiety in geriatric depression, effects of age and cognitive impairment. *American Association for Geriatric Psychiatry, 3*(2), 108–117.

Almeida, O. P. (1995a). Psychotic states arising in late life (late paraphrenia): Psychopathology and nosology. *British Journal of Psychiatry, 66,* 205–214.

Almeida, O. P. (1995b). Psychotic states arising in late life (late paraphrenia): The role of risk factors. *British Journal of Psychiatry, 166,* 215–228.

American Psychiatric Association. (1987). *Diagnostic and statistical manual of mental disorders* (3rd ed., rev.). Washington, DC: Author.

American Psychiatric Association. (1994). *Diagnostic and statistical manual of mental disorders* (4th ed.). Washington, DC: Author.

Amsler, H. A., Teerenhoui, L., Bartha, E., Harjula, K., & Vuppio, P. (1993). Agranulocytosis in patients treated with clozapine: A study of the Finnish epidemic. *Acta Psychiatrica Scandinavica, 56,* 241–248.

Anderson, C. B., True, J. E., & Ereshefsky, L. (1993, May 25). Risperidone dose, plasma level and response [Abstract NR217:113]. In *New research program and abstracts of the 146th annual meeting of the American Psychiatric Association.* San Francisco: APA.

Anton, S., Robinson, D. S., Roberts, D. L., Kensler, T. T., English, P. A., & Archibald, D. G. (1994). Long-term treatment of depression with nefazodone. *Psychopharmacology Bulletin, 30*(2), 165–169.

Aranson, S. M., Lingam, V., & Hasanat, A. (1995). *Risperidone in geropsychiatry: Review of early experience in two public hospitals.* Poster presented at the American Psychiatric Association 148th annual meeting, Miami, Florida.

Ascione, F. J. (1978). Benzodiazepines and alcohol. *Drug Therapy, 9,* 58–71.

Baldessarini, R. J. (1985). *Chemotherapy in psychiatry, principles and practice,* Cambridge, MA: Harvard University Press.

Ballenger, J. C., Burros, G. D., & DuPont, R. (1988). Alprazolam in panic disorder and agoraphobia: Results from a multicenter trial. I. Efficacy in short-term treatment. *Archives of General Psychiatry, 455,* 413–422.

Bellantuono, C., Reggi, V., & Tognoni, G. (1980). Benzodiazepines: Clinical pharmacology and therapeutic use. *Drugs, 19,* 195–219.

Blazer, D. (1989). Epidemiology of "depression" in later life. *Journal of Geriatric Psychiatry and Neurology, 22,* 35–52.

Borison, R. L., Diamond, B. I., & Pathiraja, A. (1992). Clinical overview of risperidone. In H. Y. Meltzer (Ed.), *Novel antipsychotic drugs* (pp. 233–239). New York: Raven Press.

Borison, R. L., Pathiraja, A. P., & Diamond, B. I. (1992). Risperidone: Clinical safety and efficacy in schizophrenia. *Psychopharmacology Bulletin, 28,* 213–218.

Borson, S., Barnes, R. A., Kukull, W. A., Okimoto, J. T., Veith, R. C., Inui, T. S., Carter, W., & Raskind, M. A. (1986). Symptomatic depression in elderly medical outpatients. 1. Prevalence, demography, and health-service utilization. *Journal of the American Geriatrics Society, 34,* 341–347.

Braestrup, C., & Neilsen, M. (1982). Anxiety. *Lancet, 2,* 1030–1034.

Brenner, H. D., Deneker, S. J., Goldstein, M. J., Hubbard, J. W., Keegan, D. L., Druger, G., Kulhanek, F., Liberman, R. P., Malm, U., & Midha, K. K. (1990). Defining treatment refractoriness in schizophrenia. *Schizophrenia Bulletin, 16,* 551–562.

Bressler, R., & Katz, M. D. (1993). Drug therapy for geriatric depression. *Drugs and Aging, 3*(3), 195–219.

Brosen, K. (1990). Recent developments in hepatic drug oxidation, implications for clinical pharmacokinetics. *Clinical Pharmacokinetics, 18,* 220–239.

Brosen, K., Skjelbo, E., & Rasmussen, B. B. (1993). Fluvoxamine is a potent inhibitor of cytochrome P4501A2. *Biochemical Pharmacology, 45*(6), 1211–1214.

Burvill, P. W. (1995). Prevalence of depression after stroke: The Perth community stroke study. *British Journal of Psychiatry, 166*, 320–327.

Carpenter, W. T., Jr., Conley, R. R., Buchanon, R. W., Breier, A., Tomminga, C. A (1995, June). Patient response and resource: Clozapine treatment of schizophrenia. *American Journal of Psychiatry, 152*, 827–832.

Chouinard, G., Jones, B., & Remington, G. (1993). A Canadian multicenter placebo controlled study of fixed doses of risperidone and haloperidol in the treatment of chronic schizophrenic patients. *Journal of Clinical Psychopharmacology, 13*, 25–40.

Claus, A., Bollen, J., & De Cuyper, H. (1992). Risperidone versus haloperidol in the treatment of chronic schizophrenic inpatients: A multicentre double-blind comparative study. *Acta Psychiatric Scandinavica, 85*, 295–305.

Coccaro, E. F. (1990). Pharmacologic treatment of noncognitive behavioral disturbances in elderly demented patients. *American Journal of Psychiatry, 147*, 1640–1645.

Cohen, M. (1988). You don't have to be a neuroscientist to forget everything with triazolam—but it helps [Letter to the editor]. *Journal of the American Medical Association, 259*(3), 352.

Cohen-Mansfield, J., & Billing, N. (1986). Agitated behaviors in the elderly. *Journal of the American Geriatrics Society., 34*, 711–721.

Covington, J. S. (1975). Alleviating agitation, apprehension, and related symptoms in geriatric patients: A double blind comparison of phenothiozine and benzodiazepine. *Southern Medical Journal, 68*, 719–724.

Coyne, J. C. (1995, January). Nondetection of depression by primary care physicians reconsidered. *General Hospital Psychiatry, 17*, 3–12.

Dechant, K. L., & Clissold, P. (1991). Paroxetine: A review of its pharmacodynamic and pharmacokinetic properties, and therapeutic potential in depressive illness. *Drugs, 41/42*, 225–253.

Deutsch, L. H., & Rovner, B. W. (1991). Agitation and other noncognitive abnormalities in Alzheimer's disease. *Psychiatric Clinics of North America, 14*, 341–351.

DeVane, C. L. (1992). Pharmacokinetics of the selective serotonin reuptake inhibitors. *Journal of Clinical Psychiatry, 53* (Suppl. 2), 13.

DeVane, C. L. (1994). Pharmacogenetics and drug metabolism of newer antidepressant agents. *Journal of Clinical Psychiatry, 55*(12, Suppl.), 38–45.

DiMaio, L. (1988). You don't have to be a neuroscientist to forget everything with triazolam—but it helps [Letter to the editor]. *Journal of the American Medical Association, 259*(3), 351.

Dunner, D. L., & Dunbar, G. C. (1992). Optimal dose regimen for paroxetine. *Journal of Clinical Psychiatry, 53* (Suppl.), 21–26.

Eison, A. S., Eison, M. S., Torrente, J. R., Wright, R. N., & Yocca, E. D. (1990). Nefazadone: Preclinical pharmacology of a new antidepressant. *Psychopharmacology Bulletin, 26*, 311–315.

Ewing, J. A. (1988). You don't have to be a neuroscientist to forget everything with triazolam—but it helps [Letter to the editor]. *Journal of the American Medical Association, 259*(3), 350.

Flint, A. J., & Rifat, S. L. (1994). A prospective study of lithium augmentation in antidepressant-resistant geriatric depression. *Journal of Clinical Psychopharmacology, 14*, 353–356.

Franson, K. L., Renner, J. A., & Grossberg, G. T. (1994). A practical guide to the use of antidepressants in the elderly. *Clinical Geriatrics, 2*, 39–49.

Frasure-Smith, N. (1995). Depression and 18-month prognosis after myocardial infarction. *Circulation, 91*, 999–1005.

Frazer, A. (1994). Antidepressant drugs [review article]. *Depression, 2*, 1–19.

Gardner, M. J., Ronfeld, R. A., & Wilner, K. D. (in Press). Sertraline has minimal effects on the pharmacokinetics and protein binding of diazepam in healthy volunteers. *Clinical Pharmacokinetics.*

Gardos, G., Pereny, A., Cole, J. O., Samu, I., & Kallos, M. (1983). Tardive dyskinesia: Changes after three years. *Journal of Clinical Psychopharmacology, 3*, 315–318.

Gershon, S., & Eison, A. S. (1987). The ideal anxiolytic. *Psychiatric Annals, 17*(3), 156–170.

Gershon, S. C., Plotkin, D. A., & Jarvik, L. F. (1988). Antidepressant drug studies, 1964–1986: Empirical evidence for ongoing patients. *Journal of Clinical Psychopharmacology, 8*, 311–322.

Goldberg, R. J. (1995). *Risperidone for dementia-related disturbed behavior in nursing home residents: A clinical experience.* Poster presented at the American Psychiatric Association 148th annual meeting.

Goldstein, K. (1952). The effect of brain damage on the personality. *Psychiatry, 15*, 245–260.

Golombok, S., Moodley, P., & Lader, M. (1988). Cognitive impairment in long-term benzodiazepine users. *Psychological Medicine, 18*, 365–374.

Gonzalez, F. J., & Gelboin, H. V. (1992). Human cytochromes P450: evolution and cDNA-directed expression. *Environmental Health Perspectives, 98*, 81–85.

Gorman, J., Liebowitz, M. R., & Fyer, A. J. (1987). An open trial of fluoxetine in the treatment of panic disorder. *Journal of Clinical Psychiatry, 7*, 329–332.

Greden, J. F. (1993). Antidepressant maintenance medications: When to discontinue and how to stop. *Journal of Clinical Psychiatry, 54* (Suppl. 8), 39–45.

Greenblatt, A. J., Selkis, E. M., & Koche-Weser, J. (1982). Medical intelligence: Drug disposition in old age. *New England Journal of Medicine, 306*(18), 1081–1088.

Greenblatt, D. J., & Shader, R. I. (1974). Benzodiazepines in medical practice. New York: Raven Press.

Greene, W. L. (1988). Therapeutic drug monitoring: Practical and clinical consideration in the elderly patient. *Clinical Report on Aging, 2*(2), 14–16.

Grimsley, S. R., & Jann, M. W. (1992). Paroxetine, sertraline and fluoxetine: New selective serotonin reuptake inhibitors. *Clinical Pharmacy, 11*, 930–957.

Grossberg, G. T., & Nakra, R. (1986). Treatment of depression in the elderly. *Comprehensive Therapy, 12*(10), 16–22.

Grossberg, G. T., Hassan, R., Szwabo, P. A., Morley, J. E., Nakra, B. R., Bretscher, C. W., Zimny, G. H., & Solomon, K. (1990). Psychiatric problems in the nursing home. St. Louis University Geriatric Grand Rounds clinical conference. *Journal of American Geriatrics Society, 38*(8), 907–917.

Guengerich, F. P., Muller-Enoch, D., & Blair, I. A. (1986). Oxidation of quinidine by human livery cytochrome P-450. *Molecular Pharmacology, 30,* 287–295.

Gurland, B. J. (1976). The comparative frequency of depression in various adult age groups. *Journal of Gerontology, 3*(3), 283–292.

Harto-Traux, N., Stern, W. C., Miller, L. L., Sato, T. L., & Cato, A. E. (1983). Effects of bupropion on body weight. *Journal of Clinical Psychiatry, 44,* 183–186.

Harvey, S. C. (1980). Hypnotics and sedatives. In A. G. Gilman, L. S. Goodman, & A. Gilman (Eds.), *Pharmacological basis of therapeutics* (6th ed., pp. 391–447). New York: Macmillan Publishing Co.

Hellerstein, D. J., Yanowitch, P., Rosenthal, J., Samstag, L. W., Mauer, M., & Kasch, K. (1993). A randomized double-blind study of fluoxetine versus placebo in the treatment of dysthymia. *American Journal of Psychiatry, 150,* 1169–1175.

Hippius, H. (1980). The history of clozapine. *Psychopharmacology, 99*(Suppl.), S3–S5.

Hollister, L. E. (1994). New psychotherapeutic drugs. *Journal of Clinical Psychopharmacology, 14,* 50–63.

Huang, M. L., Van Peer, A., & Woestenborghs, R. (1993). Pharmacokinetics of the novel antipsychotic agent risperidone and the prolactin response in healthy subjects. *Clinical Pharmacology Therapy, 54,* 257–268.

Janicah, P. G., David, J. M., Preskorn, S. H., & Ayd, F. J., Jr. (1993). *Principles and practice of psychopharmacotherapy* (p. 107). Baltimore: Williams & Wilkins.

Janssen, P. A., Niemegeers, C. J., & Awouters, F. (1988). Pharmacology of risperidone (R 64 766), a new antipsychotic with serotonin-S2 and dopamine-D2 antagonistic properties. *Journal of Pharmacology Experimental Therapy, 244,* 685–693.

Jenike, M. A. (1988). Assessment and treatment of affective illness in the elderly. *Journal of Geriatric Psychiatry and Neurology, 1*(2), 89–107.

Jenike, M. A. (1989). Treatment of affective illness in the elderly with drugs and electroconvulsive therapy. *Journal of Geriatric Psychiatry, 22*(1), 77–112.

Jeste, D. V., Locro, J. P., Gilbert, P. L., Kline, J., & Kline, N. (1993). Treatment of late life schizophrenia with neuroleptics. *Schizophrenia Bulletin, 19*(4), 817–838.

Jeste, D. V., Harris, M. J., Krull, A., Kuck, J., McAdams, L. A., & Heaton, R. (1995). Clinical and neuropsychological characteristics of patients with late-onset schizophrenia. *American Journal of Psychiatry, 152,* 772–730.

Kane, J. M., Woerner, M., Weinhold, P., Wegner, J., Kinon, B., & Borenstein, M. (1984). Incidence of tardive dyskinesia. Five-year data from a prospective study. *Psychopharmacology Bulletin, 20,* 387–389.

Koche-Weser, J., Greenblatt, D. J., & Sellers, E. M. (1982). Medical intelligence; Drug therapy-drug disposition in old age. *New England Journal of Medicine, 306*(18), 1081–1088.

Kolb, L. C., & Brodie, K. (1982). *Modern clinical psychiatry* (10th ed., pp. 299–311). Philadelphia: Saunders.

Lader, M. (1982a). Psychological effects of buspirone. *Journal of Clinical Psychiatry, 43* (12, Sec. 2), 62–67.

Lader, M. (1982b). Summary and commentary. In E. Usdin, F.

Kolnick, J. F. Tallman, et al. (Eds.), *Pharmacology of benzodiazepine* (pp. 53–60). New York: Macmillan Press.

Lader, M. H., Ron, M., & Petursson, H. (1984). Computed axial brain tomography in long-term benzodiazepine users. *Psychological Medicine, 14,* 203–206.

Larson, D. B., & Zorc, J. J. (1989, August). Prescribing psychotropics in the nursing home. *Geriatric Medicine Today, 8,* 42–51.

Lindstrom, L. H. (1988). The effect of long-term treatment with clozapine in schizophrenia: A retrospective study in 96 patients treated with clozapine for up to 13 years. *Acta Psychiatric Scandinavica, 77,* 524–529.

Lott, A. D., McElroy, S. L., & Keys, M. A. (1995). Valproate in the treatment of behavioral agitation in elderly patients with dementia. *Journal of Neuropsychiatry and Clinical Neuroscience, 7*(3), 314–319.

Marder, S. R. (1992). Risperidone; clinical development: North American results. *Clinical Neuropharmacology, 15*(Suppl. 1, pt. A), 92A–93A.

Markowitz, J. C., Kocasis, J. H., & Moran, M. E. (1992). Interpersonal deficits and TCA response in dysthymia. In *New research abstracts,* 145th Annual Meeting of the American Psychiatric Association. Washington, DC: American Psychiatric Association.

Marks, J. (1978). *The benzodiazepines: Use, overuse, misuse, abuse.* London: MTP Press.

Meltzer, H. Y. (1989). Duration of a clozapine trial in neuroleptic-resistant schizophrenia [Letter to editor]. *Archives of General Psychiatry, 46,* 672.

Meltzer, H. Y. (1992). Treatment of the neuroleptic-nonresponsive schizophrenic patient. *Schizophrenia Bulletin, 18*(3), 515–541.

Mikus, G., Ha, H. R., & Vozeh, S. (1986). Pharmacokinetics and metabolism of quinidine in extensive and poor metabolisers of sparteine. *European Journal of Clinical Pharmacology, 31,* 69–72.

Moffie, H. S., & Paykel, E. S. (1975). Depression in medical inpatients. *Britain Journal of Psychiatry, 126.* 346–353.

Montgomery, S. A. (1993). Venlafaxine: A new dimension in antidepressant pharmacotherapy. *Journal of Clinical Psychiatry, 54*(3), 119–126.

Morris, H. H., & Read, A. E. (1987). Traveler's amnesia: Transient global amnesia secondary to triazolam. *Journal of the American Medical Association, 258,* 945–946.

Muller-Spahn, R. (1992). Risperidone in the treatment of chronic schizophrenic patients: An international double-blind parallel-group study versus haloperidol. *Clinical Neuropharmacology, 15*(Suppl. 1, Pt. A), 90–91.

Peabody, C. A., Warner, D., Whiteford, H. A., & Hollister, L. E. (1987). Neuroleptics and the elderly. *Journal of the American Geriatrics Society, 35,* 232–238.

Pollock, B. G. (1994). Recent developments in drug metabolism of relevance to psychiatrist. *Harvard Review of Psychiatry, 2,* 204–213.

Preskorn, S. H. (1989). Tricyclic antidepressants: The whys and hows of therapeutic drug monitoring. *Journal of Clinical Psychiatry, 50*(Suppl. 7), 34–42.

Radack, H. B. (1988). You don't have to be a neuroscientist to forget everything with triazolam—but it helps. *Journal of the American Medical Association, 259*(3), 351.

Raskin, D. E. (1985). Antipsychotic medication and the elderly. *Journal of Clinical Psychiatry, 46,* 36–40.

Ray, W. A., Griffin, M. R., & Downey, W. (1989). Benzodiazepines of long and short elimination half-life and the risk of fractures. *Journal of the American Medical Association, 262,* 3303–3307.

Regier, D. A., Boyd, J. H., & Burke, J. D., Jr. (1988). One month's prevalence of mental disorders in the United States. *Archives of General Psychiatry, 45,* 977–986.

Rice, D. P. (1993). Economic burden of Alzheimer's disease care. *Health Affairs, 12*(2), 164–176.

Richelson, E. (1994). Pharmacology of antidepressants—Characteristics of the ideal drug. *Mayo Clinic Proceedings, 69,* 1069–1081.

Rickels, K. (1982). Benzodiazepines in the treatment of anxiety. *American Journal of Psychotherapy, 36,* 350–370.

Rickels, K., & Schweizer, E. (1990). Clinical overview of serotonin reuptake inhibitors. *Journal of Clinical Psychiatry, 51,* 1–12.

Risse, S. C., & Barnes, R. (1986). Pharmacological treatment of agitation associated with dementia. *Journal of the American Geriatrics Society, 34,* 368–376.

Roose, S. P., Glassman, A. H., Attia, E., & Woodring, S. (1994). Comparative efficacy of selective serotonin reuptake inhibitors and tricyclics in the treatment of melancholia. *American Journal of Psychiatry, 151,* 1735–1739.

Rosenstein, D. L., Nelson, J. C., & Jacobs, S. C. (1993). Seizures associated with antidepressants: A review. *Journal of Clinical Psychiatry, 54*(8), 289–299.

Safferman, A. Z., Lieberman, J. A., & Pollack, S. (1993). Akathisia and clozapine treatment [Letter]. *Journal of Clinical Psychopharmacology, 13,* 286–287.

Salzman, C. (1993). Pharmacologic treatment of depression in the elderly. *Journal of Clinical Psychiatry, 54*(Suppl. 2), 23–28.

Schatzberg, A. F., & Cole, J. O. (1986). *Manual of clinical psychopharmacology.* Washington, DC: American Psychiatric Press.

Schneider, F. R., Liebowitz, M. R., & Davies, S. O. (1990). Fluoxetine in panic disorder. *Journal of Clinical Psychopharmacology, 10,* 119–121.

Schneider, L. S., Pollock, V. E., & Lyness, S. A. (1990). A metaanalysis of controlled trials of neuroleptic treatment in dementia. *Journal of the American Geriatrics Society, 38,* 553–563.

Schweizer, E., Weise, C., Clary, C., Fox, I., & Rickels, K. (1991). Placebo-controlled trial of venlafaxine for the treatment of major depression. *Journal of Clinical Psychopharmacology, 11*(4), 233–236.

Shamoian, C. A. (1985). Assessing depression in elderly patients. *Hospital and Community Psychiatry, 36,* 338–339.

Sheehan, D., Dunbar, G. C., & Fuell, D. L. (1992). The effect of paroxetine on anxiety and agitation associated with depression. *Psychopharmacology Bulletin, 28*(2), 139–143.

Sultzer, D. L. (1995). Treatment of delusions and agitation: Neuroleptics and trazodone. In *New Research Abstracts* (148th Annual Meeting of the American Psychiatric Association, Miami, Florida, p. 186). American Psychiatric Association Press.

Sussman, N. (1988). Diagnosis and drug treatment of anxiety in the elderly. *Geriatric Medicine Today, 7*(10), 37–51.

Tallman, J. F., Paul, S. M., Skolnick, P., & Gallagher, D. W. (1980). Receptors for the age of anxiety: Pharmacology of the benzodiazepines. *Science, 207,* 274–281.

Tariot, P. N., Erb, R., Leibovici, A., Podgorski, C. A., Cox, C., Asnis, J., Kolassa, J., & Irvine, C. (1994). Carbamazepine treatment of agitation in nursing home patients with dementia: A preliminary study. *American Geriatrics Society, 42,* 1160–1166.

Wagner, W., Plekkenpol, B., Gray, T. E., Vraskamp, H., & Essers, H. (1992). Review of fluvoxamine safety database. *Drugs, 43,* 48–54.

Watanabe, M., & Davis, J. M. (1990). Pharmacotherapeutic considerations in the elderly psychiatric patient. *Psychiatric Annals, 20*(8), 423–432.

Winker, A. (1994). Tacrine for Alzheimer's disease; Which patient, what dose? *Journal of the American Medical Association, 271,* 1023–1024.

Zimmer, B., Rosen, J., Thornton, J. E., Perel, J. M., & Reynolds, C. F. (1991). Adjunctive lithium carbonate in nortriptyline-resistant elderly depressed patients. *Journal of Clinical Psychopharmacology, 11,* 254–256.

Zipursky, R. B, Baker, R. W., & Zimmer, B. (1985). Alprazolam withdrawal delirium unresponsive to diazepam: Case report. *Journal of Clinical Psychiatry, 46*(8), 344–345.

33

Electroconvulsive Therapy

BENOIT H. MULSANT AND JOHN A. SWEENEY

Introduction

Older patients with severe depression often present with psychosis, suicidality, or food refusal requiring rapid treatment. They are also less likely to respond to selective serotonin reuptake inhibitors (Roose, Glassman, Attia, & Woodring, 1994) or to tolerate the anticholinergic and cardiac side effects of tricyclic antidepressants. Thus, while age per se does not constitute an indication for, or a predictor of, favorable response to electroconvulsive therapy (ECT), older patients are particularly likely to meet the current indications for ECT (American Psychiatric Association, 1990; Sackeim, 1994). As a result, 16% of inpatients 65 years of age and older with a mood disorder are treated with ECT, and the elderly constitute more than one third of ECT recipients even though they represent less than 10% of hospitalized psychiatric patients (Thompson, Weiner, & Myers, 1994). This chapter reviews the indications and contraindications for ECT in late life, discusses management of the older patient receiving ECT, and reviews the literature on cognitive effects of ECT.

Indications for ECT

In 1938, electroconvulsive therapy (ECT) became one of the first effective somatic psychiatric treatments available. To this day, it remains one of the most controversial. For this reason, ECT is usually used when pharmacotherapy has been ineffective. However, ECT may be used as a first line-

treatment (1) when a rapid response is needed, for instance, to treat an actively suicidal patient or a depressed patient refusing fluids, food, or medications; (2) when a patient presents with a recurrence of a disorder that has responded to ECT but not to medications in the past; and (3) when a patient requests to be treated with ECT rather than medications (American Psychiatric Association, 1990).

Electroconvulsive therapy is mostly used to treat major depressive episodes due to any mood disorder (including mood disorders due to general medical conditions). It can also be used to treat other conditions when they have not responded to pharmacotherapy, including mixed or manic episodes, schizophrenia and other psychoses in the presence of catatonia, or prominent depressive symptoms associated with dementia. In a few cases, ECT has been used to treat other psychiatric disorders or some physical disorders (e.g., treatment-resistant Parkinson's disease).

Contraindications for ECT

While there are no absolute contraindications to ECT, it should not be used when its associated risks outweigh its potential benefits. Electroconvulsive therapy requires repeated induction of general anesthesia, and during the procedure, intracranial pressure, heart rate, and blood pressure (and thus, myocardial demand of oxygen) are increased (Knos & Sung, 1993). Therefore, the following physical conditions are associated with a very high risk for serious morbidity or mortality and are considered as contraindications to ECT in almost all cases:

1. Contraindications to general anesthesia

BENOIT H. MULSANT AND JOHN A. SWEENEY • Western Psychiatric Institute and Clinic and Department of Psychiatry, University of Pittsburgh School of Medicine, Pittsburgh, Pennsylvania 15213.

2. Space-occupying cerebral lesion (or other conditions) associated with increased intracranial pressure
3. Retinal detachment
4. Recent intracerebral hemorrhage or ischemic stroke
5. Bleeding or unstable aneurysm or vascular malformations
6. Pheochromocytoma
7. Recent (i.e., within 12 weeks) myocardial infarction

In the absence of these contraindications, modern ECT techniques, including careful medical assessment of risks and intensive monitoring and management of physiologic side effects, have made ECT a safe treatment in older patients, even in the presence of comorbid physical illness or dementia (Burke, Rubin, Zorumski, & Wetzel, 1987; Gaspar & Samarasinghe, 1982; Godber, Rosenvinge, Wilkinson, & Smithies, 1987; Mulsant, Rosen, Thornton, & Zubenko, 1991; Nelson & Rosenberg, 1991; Price & McAllister, 1989; Rice, Sombrotto, Markowitz, & Leon, 1994; Stoudemire, Hill, Morris, Martino-Saltzman, & Lewison, 1993; Weiner, 1983; Zielinski, Roose, Devanand, Woodring, & Sackeim, 1993; Zubenko et al., 1994). Poor health status rather than advancing age increases risks for medical complications associated with ECT. Elderly patients are at greater risks for prolonged postictal confusion and interictal delirium, in particular when they suffer from a degenerative or vascular dementia (Mulsant et al., 1991). However, elderly patients presenting with dementia syndrome of depression may experience a dramatic improvement in cognition when treated with ECT (Mulsant et al., 1991; Stoudemire et al., 1991). Thus cognitive impairment should not constitute by itself a contraindication to ECT.

Baseline Evaluation Prior to Initiation of ECT

A thorough psychiatric evaluation (including a detailed history of previous treatment) establishes and documents the indications for ECT. An assessment of cognitive functions prior to treatment helps monitor potential cognitive changes induced by ECT. Minimally, it should include a general screening test such as Folstein's Mini-Mental State Examination (Folstein, Folstein, & McHugh, 1975), a test of attention such as the Trail-making test (Reitan, 1958), and measures of remote and recent memory. In order to assess adequately the risk/benefit ratio of ECT and/or to optimize the patient's condition to decrease medical risks of ECT, a fairly thorough medical work-up is needed prior to initiating ECT. In all patients, it should include a complete history and physical examination, a battery of blood tests (serum electrolytes, BUN, creatinine, CBC with differential, liver function tests, metabolic profile, thyroid function tests, and thyroid stimulating hormone), an electrocardiogram (EKG), chest and spinal x-rays, and brain imaging (computerized axial tomography [CT] scan or magnetic resonance imaging [MRI]) if it has not been obtained since the onset of the psychiatric disorders being treated. Besides ruling out some of the contraindications listed above, this work-up can identify various abnormalities that put a patient at higher risk for adverse effects. For instance, low sodium (in particular below 120 meq/L) increases risk for prolonged seizure (Finlayson, Vieweg, Wilkey, & Cooper, 1989; Greer & Stewart, 1993). Low potassium or preexisting cardiac conduction defects increase risk for arrhythmia. Spinal x-rays will detect and document preexisting vertebral compression fractures or osteoporosis that put a patient at higher risk for a new compression fracture. Further assessment may be needed in some patients. For instance, a cardiologist familiar with ECT and its specific cardiac risks should be consulted to assist in assessment and management of patients with significant cardiac disease.

Procedures for ECT Treatment

Electroconvulsive therapy devices and procedures have been discussed in detail elsewhere (American Psychiatric Association, 1990). To prepare a patient prior to his or her first treatment, the evaluation described above should be completed, and the patient's medical status should be optimized. Benzodiazepines, other sedatives or hypnotics, and anticonvulsants (when clinically possible) should be tapered since they increase the seizure threshold and may decrease efficacy of ECT (Pettinati, Stephens, Willis, & Robin, 1990). Lithium should be discontinued since it increases risks for interictal delirium. Other psychotropics may be continued during ECT; with the exception of neuroleptics in schizophrenic patients, there is no convincing empirical evidence that the combination of psychotropic medications with ECT increases its efficacy. Furthermore, in some patients, psychotropic medications may increase risk for adverse effects (e.g., arrhythmia, delirium).

Standards for consent depend on legislation of the state. If a patient is considered incompetent to consent to ECT, legal proceedings may be required. The written consent document should include both the frequent minor adverse effects of ECT (i.e., headaches, muscle pain, postictal transient confusion) and the rarer but more significant ones (i.e., death, arrhythmia and other cardiac events, spinal compression fractures, interictal delirium, and persistent memory complaint).

On the day of ECT, a patient should receive nothing orally for at least 6 hr prior to a treatment, except for medications that can be given with a sip of water. To manage significant anxiety or agitation prior to ECT, intramuscular (IM) medications can be used 30 min prior to transfer to the ECT room. After the patient is discharged from the recovery room, he or she should remain under constant observation until the postictal confusion has cleared.

To minimize risks of interictal confusion, treatment is usually initiated in older patients with unilateral ECT (i.e., with placement of electrodes over the nondominant hemisphere), except in patients who have previously responded to bilateral but not unilateral ECT or who are so sick that the most definitive treatment is needed (e.g., a catatonic patient refusing fluids and food). If a patient shows no or minimal improvement after five or six unilateral treatments, electrode placement should be switched to bilateral (i.e., bitemporal). Regardless of electrode placement, brief pulse (square wave) stimuli are routinely used since their efficacy is similar to sine wave stimuli but they are less likely to induce significant cognitive adverse effects (Abrams, 1992; American Psychiatric Association, 1990). Similarly, optimization of stimulus intensity, based on a systematic determination of each patient's seizure threshold, has been shown to improve efficacy and to decrease cognitive impairment (Sackeim et al., 1993).

Typically, treatments are administered three times a week. Mood and cognition should be carefully assessed on the days post-ECT. If significant confusion persists on the days post-ECT, any psychotropic medications the patient is still receiving should be discontinued, further ECT treatment should be held until confusion resolves, and upon resuming ECT, frequency of treatments should be decreased to twice a week (Lerer et al., 1995).

Typically ECT is discontinued once a patient's mood is back to baseline or when it reaches a plateau after two consecutive treatments. Generally an ECT course consists of six to twelve treatments, although some patients (particularly schizophrenic patients) may require more treatments.

Continuation and Maintenance Therapy after ECT

About three fourths of older depressed patients treated with ECT respond well (Mulsant et al., 1991). There is minimal data related to efficacy of continuation and maintenance therapy in patients who have responded to ECT (Mulsant, Singhal, & Kunik, 1996; Sackeim et al., 1990). However, controlled studies strongly indicate that depressed patients who respond to pharmacotherapy do better when they continue to take full dose antidepressant medication for at least 4 months and when they are subsequently maintained on the same treatment. Thus, as a general rule, patients with major depression who respond to ECT receive full dose antidepressant pharmacotherapy after completing ECT. In patients who were treated with ECT after failing an adequate antidepressant medication trial, an antidepressant from a different class should be selected and combination pharmacotherapy should be considered. For example, for a patient who has failed to respond to a tricyclic antidepressant with therapeutic blood levels for 6 or more weeks, a selective serotonin reuptake inhibitor combined with lithium, venlafaxine, or a monoamine oxidase inhibitor (MAOI) could be selected as continuation/maintenance pharmacotherapy. In patients who have not received an adequate antidepressant medication trial prior to being treated with ECT, a "first-line" antidepressant such as a selective serotonin reuptake inhibitor or a secondary tricyclic antidepressant could be selected as continuation/maintenance therapy.

In patients who suffer from bipolar disorder, antidepressants are usually combined with lithium or an anticonvulsant. Patients who presented initially with a psychotic depression may need an antidepressant combined with a neuroleptic at a moderate to high dose for 6 to 12 months following ECT (Aronson, Shukla, & Hoff, 1987). However, in the absence of data demonstrating the superiority of such a combination over an antidepressant alone (or over an antidepressant combined with lithium), patients need to be informed about the risk of tardive dyskinesia (Sweet et al., 1995).

In a small number of selected patients who exhibit a good response to ECT but relapse rapidly despite adequate continuation pharmacotherapy, continuation ECT can be used. Typically, this consists of ECT given on an outpatient basis every 2 to 4 weeks for 2 to 6 months. Although the safety of this strategy has been supported by some published case series (Dubin, Jaffe, Roemer, Lipschutz, & Spencer, 1989; Grunhaus, Pande, & Haskett, 1990; Jaffe et al., 1990; Thienhaus, Margletta, & Bennett, 1990; Thornton, Mulsant, Dealy, & Reynolds, 1990), its efficacy has not yet been validated by a controlled study.

Cognitive Effects of ECT

Electroconvulsive therapy can cause significant transient cognitive impairment (Calev & Phil, 1994; Rosen, Mulsant, & Nebes, 1992; Russ, Ackerman, Burton, & Shindledecker, 1990; Squire, 1986). The most prominent deficit occurs in the area of memory function, but verbal fluency, language skills, and psychomotor speed can also be adversely affected (Khan, Mirolo, Hughes, & Bierut, 1993). A large number of animal studies have confirmed the association between ECT and memory loss (Fochtmann, 1994). In fact, studying behavioral effects of electrically induced seizures is a common method for studying neurobiology of memory and amnestic states (Ray & Barrett, 1969; Squire & Spanis, 1964).

Animal studies have documented differences in degree of memory impairment resulting from variation in intensity and waveform of the electrical current used to generate seizures (Spanis & Squire, 1981). Clinical studies have also investigated effects of different types of electrical current waveforms used in ECT on severity of memory impairment (Sackeim, Devanand, & Prudic, 1991). Use of brief pulse instead of sine wave current appears to cause less cognitive impairment (Daniel, Weiner, & Crovitz, 1983; Weiner, Rogers, Davidson, & Squire, 1986). Memory impairments are more severe with higher electrical current intensity (Ottosson, 1960; Sackeim et al., 1993), particularly when electrical current intensity significantly exceeds that needed to produce a seizure (Sackeim et al., 1991). Improved procedures for titrating intensity and controlling waveform and duration of electrical current have reduced adverse cognitive effects of ECT. However, the greatest reduction in adverse cognitive effects from ECT has been realized by the widely used method of unilateral rather than bilateral stimulation. While some spatial memory deficits commonly result from administering ECT to the nondominant hemisphere, verbal memory losses that are particularly distressing and disruptive for patients' day-to-day functioning are much less pronounced than those associated with bilateral ECT (Cannicott & Waggoner, 1967; Dornbush, Abrams, & Fink, 1971; Fraser & Glass, 1980).

Importantly, available research indicates that adverse memory effects following ECT are short-lasting, even following bilateral treatment. While memory for events preceding ECT treatment by a few days can be lost permanently, psychometric studies of memory function after a course of ECT have failed to identify any persisting impairment in the ability to learn and remember new information, or in any other neuropsychological function (Pettinati & Bonner, 1984). Memory impairments evident within the first few weeks of treatment are no longer evident 6 months after the last ECT treatment (Squire & Chace, 1975; Squire, Slater, & Miller, 1981). Even patients who have received large numbers of ECT treatments (over 100) do not appear to demonstrate persistent neuropsychological deficits (Devanand, Verma, Tirumalasetti, & Sackeim, 1991). These observations parallel findings from prospective CT and MRI studies which have failed to identify any structural anatomic abnormalities associated with ECT (Devanand, Dwork, Hutchenson, Bolwig, & Sackeim, 1994).

One important caveat remains before accepting the conclusion that ECT does not cause any enduring neuropsychological deficits. There appears to be some disparity between subjective reports of memory functioning and objective measures of memory loss after ECT. Patients treated with ECT sometimes describe themselves as having cognitive impairments after ECT that are inconsistent with results of objective cognitive tests (Freeman & Kendell, 1980). It has been difficult to determine whether patient reports of cognitive problems greater than those observed in psychometric studies reflect deficits that are missed by the tests, residual depression that causes low self-esteem and feelings of general inadequacy that influence self-reports of cognitive function, subtle side effects from antidepressant medications, or other factors (Pettinati & Rosenberg, 1984). Weeks, Freeman, and Kendell (1980) reported similar objectively assessed residual cognitive deficits in patients who had been treated with antidepressant medications or ECT during their most recent acute episode of illness. Based on this observation, Freeman, Weeks, and Kendell (1980) argued that complaints of memory loss are most likely the result of residual depression or adverse effects from antidepressant medications, rather than any adverse result of ECT. It is difficult to prove that there are no enduring cognitive deficits associated with ECT, but to date investigators have not identified any cognitive function that is significantly impaired by ECT in any enduring fashion. The consistent failure of psychometric research to identify any such deficits, including several studies using large batteries of neuropsychological tests sensitive to subtle deficits, suggests that any such residual impairments are not likely of sufficient severity to have significant effects on posttreatment socio-occupational functioning.

Conclusion

In conclusion, when administered properly, ECT is an effective and safe treatment for older patients with severe depression, even in the pres-ence of comorbid physical illness or dementia. While elderly patients are more prone than younger patients to develop transient confusion (in particular, with bilateral ECT), cognitive impairment occurring in the context of a severe depression may resolve with successful treatment of the depression with ECT. How to prevent relapse of depression following ECT (i.e., what constitutes optimal continuation therapy) is probably the most pressing research issue related to ECT at the present time.

References

Abrams, R. (1992). *Electroconvulsive therapy* (2nd ed.). New York: Oxford Univesity Press.

American Psychiatric Association. (1990). Task Force on Electroconvulsive Therapy. *The practice of electroconvulsive therapy: Recommendations for treatment, training, and privileging*. Washington, DC: American Psychiatric Association Press.

Aronson, T. A., Shukla, S., & Hoff, A. (1987). Continuation therapy after ECT for delusional depression: A naturalistic study of prophylactic treatments and relapse. *Convulsive Therapy, 3*, 251–259.

Burke, W. J., Rubin, E. H., Zorumski, C. F., & Wetzel, R. D. (1987). The safety of ECT in geriatric psychiatry. *Journal of the American Geriatrics Society, 35*, 516–521.

Calev, A., & Phil, D. (1994). Neuropsychology and ECT: Past and future research trends. *Psychopharmacology Bulletin, 30*, 461–469.

Cannicott, S. M., & Waggoner, R. W. (1967). Unilateral and bilateral electroconvulsive therapy. *Archives of General Psychiatry, 16*, 229–232.

Daniel, W. F., Weiner, R. D., & Crovitz, H. F. (1983). Autobiographical amnesia with ECT: An analysis of the roles of stimulus wave form, electrode placement, stimulus energy, and seizure length. *Biological Psychiatry, 18*, 121–126.

Devanand, D. P., Verma, A. K., Tirumalasetti, F., & Sackeim, H. A. (1991). Absence of cognitive impairment after more than 100 lifetime ECT treatments. *American Journal of Psychiatry, 148*, 929–932.

Devanand, D. P., Dwork, A. J., Hutchenson, E. R., Bolwig, T. G., & Sackeim, H. A. (1994). Does ECT alter brain structure? *American Journal of Psychiatry, 151*, 957–970.

Dornbush, R., Abrams, R., & Fink, M. (1971). Memory changes after unilateral and bilateral convulsive therapy (ECT). *British Journal of Psychiatry, 119*, 75–78.

Dubin, W. R., Jaffe, R. L., Roemer, R. A., Lipschutz, L., & Spencer, M. (1989). Maintenance ECT in coexisting affective and neurologic disorders. *Convulsive Therapy, 5*, 162–167.

Finlayson, A. J. R., Vieweg, W. V. R., Wilkey, W. D., & Cooper, A. J. (1989). Hyponatremic seizure following ECT. *Canadian Journal of Psychiatry, 34*, 463–464.

Fochtmann, L. J. (1994). Animal studies of electroconvulsive therapy: Foundations for future research. *Psychopharmacology Bulletin, 30,* 321–444.

Folstein, M. F., Folstein, S. E., & McHugh, P. R. (1975). Mini mental state: A practical method for grading the cognitive state of patients for the clinician. *Journal of Psychiatric Research, 12,* 189–198.

Fraser, R. M., & Glass, I. B. (1980). Unilateral and bilateral ECT in elderly patients. *Acta Psychiatrica Scandinavica, 62,* 13–31.

Freeman, C. P. L., & Kendell, R. E. (1980). ECT: I. Patients' experiences and attitudes. *British Journal of Psychiatry, 137,* 8–16.

Freeman, C. P. L., Weeks, D., & Kendell, R. E. (1980). ECT: II: Patients who complain. *British Journal of Psychiatry, 137,* 17–25.

Gaspar, D., & Samarasinghe, L. A. (1982). ECT in psychogeriatric practice—a study of risk factors, indications and outcome. *Comprehensive Psychiatry, 23,* 170–175.

Godber, C. Rosenvinge, H., Wilkinson, D., & Smithies, J. (1987). Depression in old age: prognosis after ECT. *International Journal of Geriatric Psychiatry, 2,* 19–24.

Greer, R. A., & Stewart, R. B. (1993). Hyponatremia and ECT. *American Journal of Psychiatry, 150,* 1272.

Grunhaus, L., Pande, A. C., & Haskett, R. F. (1990). Full and abbreviated courses of maintenance electroconvulsive therapy. *Convulsive Therapy, 6,* 130–138.

Jaffe, R., Dubin, W., Shoyer, B., Roemer, R., Sharon, D., & Lipschutz, L. (1990). Outpatient electroconvulsive therapy: Efficacy and safety. *Convulsive Therapy, 6,* 231–238.

Khan, A., Mirolo, M. H., Hughes, D., & Bierut, L. (1993). Electroconvulsive therapy. *The Psychiatric Clinics of North America, 16,* 497–513.

Knos, G. B., & Sung, Y. F. (1993). ECT anesthesia strategies in the high risk medical patient. In A. Stoudemire & B. S. Fogel (Eds.), *Psychiatric care of the medical patient* (pp. 225–240). New York: Oxford University Press.

Lerer, B., Shapira, B., Calev, A., Tubi, N., Drexler, H., Kindler, S., Lidsky, D., & Schwartz, J. E. (1995). Antidepressant and cognitive effects of twice-versus three-times-weekly ECT. *American Journal of Psychiatry, 152,* 564–570.

Mulsant, B. H., Rosen, J., Thornton, J. E., & Zubenko, G. S. (1991). A prospective naturalistic study of electroconvulsive therapy in late-life depression. *Journal of Geriatric Psychiatry and Neurology, 4,* 3–13.

Mulsant, B. H., Singhal, S., & Kunik, M. (1996). New developments in the treatment of late-life depression. In R. E. Hales & S. C. Yudovsky (Eds.), *Practical clinical strategies in treating depression and anxiety disorders in a managed care environment* (pp. 55–61). Washington, DC: American Psychiatric Association.

Nelson, J. C., & Rosenberg, D. R. (1991). ECT treatment of demented elderly patients with major depression: A retrospective study of efficacy and safety. *Convulsive Therapy, 7,* 157–165.

Ottosson, J. O. (1960). Experimental studies of the mode of action of electroconvulsive therapy. *Acta Psychiatrica Scandinavica Supplement, 145,* 103–141.

Pettinati, H. M., & Bonner, K. M. (1984). Cognitive functioning in depressed geriatric patients with a history of ECT. *American Journal of Psychiatry, 141,* 49–52.

Pettinati, H. M., & Rosenberg, J. (1984). Memory self-ratings before and after electroconvulsive therapy: Depression versus ECT induced. *Biological Psychiatry, 19,* 539–549.

Pettinati, H. M., Stephens, S. M., Willis, K. M., & Robin, S. E. (1990). Evidence for less improvement in depression in patients taking benzodiazepines during unilateral ECT. *American Journal of Psychiatry, 147,* 1029–1035.

Price, T. R., & McAllister, T. W. (1989). Safety and efficacy of ECT in depressed patients with dementia: A review of clinical experience. *Convulsive Therapy, 5,* 61–74.

Ray, O. S., & Barrett, R. J. (1969). Step-through latencies in mice as a function of ECT-test interval. *Biology and Behavior, 4,* 583–586.

Reitan, R. M. (1958). Validity of the trailmaking test as an indicator of organic brain damage. *Perceptual and Motor Skills, 8,* 271–276.

Rice, E. H., Sombrotto, L. B., Markowitz, J. C., & Leon, A. C. (1994). Cardiovascular morbidity in high-risk patients during ECT. *American Journal of Psychiatry, 151,* 1637–1641.

Roose, S. P., Glassman, A. H., Attia, E., & Woodring, S. (1994). Comparative efficacy of selective serotonin reuptake inhibitors and tricyclics in the treatment of melancholia. *American Journal of Psychiatry, 151,* 1735–1739.

Rosen, J., Mulsant, B. H., & Nebes, R. D. (1992). A pilot study of interictal cognitive changes in elderly patients during ECT. *International Journal of Geriatric Psychiatry, 7,* 407–410.

Russ, M. J., Ackerman, S. H., Burton, L., & Shindledecker, R. D. (1990). Cognitive effects of ECT in the elderly: Preliminary findings. *International Journal of Geriatric Psychiatry, 5,* 115–118.

Sackeim, H. A. (1994). Use of electroconvulsive therapy in late-life depression. In L. S. Schneider, C. F. Reynolds, III, B. D. Lebowitz, & A. J. Friedhoff (Eds.), *Diagnosis and treatment of depression in late life: Results of the NIH Consensus Development Conference* (pp. 259–277). Washington, DC: American Psychiatric Press, Inc.

Sackeim, H. A., Prudic, J., Devanand, D. P., Decina, P., Kerr, B., & Malitz, S. (1990). The impact of medication resistance and continuation pharmacotherapy on relapse following response to electroconvulsive therapy in major depression. *Journal of Clinical Psychopharmacology, 10,* 96–104.

Sackeim, H. A., Devanand, D. P., & Prudic, J. (1991). Stimulus intensity, seizure threshold, and seizure duration: Impact on the efficacy and safety of electroconvulsive therapy. *The Psychiatric Clinics of North America, 14,* 803–843.

Sackeim, H. A., Prudic, J., Devanand, D. P., Kiersky, J. E., Fitzsimons, L., Moody, B. J., McElhiney, M. C., Coleman, E. A., & Settembrino, J. M. (1993). Effects of stimulus intensity and electrode placement on the efficacy and cognitive effects of electroconvulsive therapy. *New England Journal of Medicine, 328,* 839–846.

Spanis, C. W., & Squire, L. R. (1981). Memory and convulsive stimulation: Effects of stimulus waveform. *American Journal of Psychiatry, 138,* 1177–1181.

Squire, L. R. (1986). Memory functions as affected by electroconvulsive therapy. *Annals of the New York Academy of Sciences, 462,* 307–314.

Squire, L. R., & Chace, P. M. (1975). Memory functions six to nine months after electroconvulsive therapy. *Archives of General Psychiatry, 32,* 1557–1564.

Squire, L. R., & Spanis, C. (1964). Long gradient of retrograde amnesia in mice: Continuity with the findings in humans. *Behavioral Neuroscience*, *98*, 345–348.

Squire, L. R., Slater, P. C., & Miller, P. L. (1981). Retrograde amnesia and bilateral electroconvulsive therapy. *Archives of General Psychiatry*, *38*, 89–95.

Stoudemire, A., Hill, C. D., Morris, R., Martino-Saltzman, D., Markwalter, H., & Lewison, B. (1991),. Cognitive outcome following tricyclic and electroconvulsive treatment of major depression in the elderly. *American Journal of Psychiatry*, *148*, 1336–1340.

Stoudemire, A., Hill, C. D., Morris, R., Martino-Saltzman, D., & Lewison, B. (1993). Long-term affective and cognitive outcome in depressed older adults. *American Journal of Psychiatry*, *150*, 896–890.

Sweet, R. A., Mulsant, B. H., Gupta, B., Rifai, A. H., Pasternak, R. E., McEachran, A., & Zubenko, G. S. (1995). Duration of neuroleptic treatment and prevalence of tardive dyskinesia in late life. *Archives of General Psychiatry*, *52*, 478–486.

Thienhaus, O. J., Margletta, S., & Bennett, J. A. (1990). A study of the clinical efficacy of maintenance ECT. *Journal of Clinical Psychiatry*, *51*, 141–144.

Thompson, J. W., Weiner, R. D., & Myers, C. P. (1994). Use of ECT in the United States in 1975, 1980, and 1986. *American Journal of Psychiatry*, *151*, 1657–1661.

Thornton, J. E., Mulsant, B. H., Dealy, R., & Reynolds, C. F. (1990). A retrospective study of maintenance electroconvulsive therapy in a university-based psychiatric practice. *Convulsive Therapy*, *6*, 121–129.

Weeks, D., Freeman, C. P. L., & Kendell, R. E. (1980). ECT:III: Enduring cognitive deficits? *British Journal of Psychiatry*, *137*, 26–37.

Weiner, R. D. (1983). ECT in the physically ill. *Journal of Psychiatric Treatment and Evaluation*, *5*, 457–462.

Weiner, R. D., Rogers, H. J., Davidson, J. R. T., & Squire, L. R. (1986). Effects of stimulus parameters on cognitive side effects. *Annals of the New York Academy of Sciences*, *462*, 315–325.

Zielinski, R. J., Roose, S. P., Devanand, D. P., Woodring, S., & Sackeim, H. A. (1993). Cardiovascular complications of ECT in depressed patients with cardiac disease. *American Journal of Psychiatry*, *150*, 904–909.

Zubenko, G. S., Mulsant, B. H., Rifai, A. H., Sweet, R. A., Pasternak, R. E., Marino, L., & Tu, X. M. (1994). Impact of acute psychiatric inpatient treatment on major depression in late life and prediction of response. *American Journal of Psychiatry*, *151*, 987–994.

34

Memory Rehabilitation

MERYL A. BUTTERS, ELIZABETH SOETY, AND JAMES T. BECKER

Introduction

The multifactorial nature of memory processing may be responsible for its particular vulnerability to disruption as individuals age (Craik, 1986; Moscovitch & Winocur, 1992). Memory "loss" is the most common cognitive complaint among healthy elderly (Chaffin & Herrmann, 1983; Sunderland, Watts, Baddeley, & Harris, 1986), and it is also the hallmark of many forms of progressive dementia such as Alzheimer's disease (AD) (Albert & Moss, 1988; Nebes, 1992). As a result, attempts have been made over recent years to develop and apply methods to improve the memory functioning of normal elderly individuals and to remediate the memory deficits (and the effects on daily living) of demented patients.

The purpose of this chapter is to describe the nature and extent of memory rehabilitation in elderly individuals. First, basic memory concepts and their relations to one another are reviewed. Using these concepts as a framework, the second section highlights the nature of memory problems and the findings on memory rehabilitation in normal elderly. The third section reviews the nature of memory impairment in AD and some attempts that have been made at remediation. Finally, future directions for research in memory rehabilitation with the elderly will be discussed.

MERYL A. BUTTERS, ELIZABETH SOETY, AND JAMES T. BECKER • Department of Psychiatry, University of Pittsburgh School of Medicine, Pittsburgh, Pennsylvania 15213.

Basic Memory Concepts

Memory processing and memory loss have been studied from numerous perspectives, and many conceptual frameworks have been developed to explain the various findings. A few of the more well-developed concepts in the cognitive neuropsychological literature are particularly relevant when considering practical methods to improve memory.

Perhaps the most important conceptual issue involves distinctions between various memory systems and their respective processing systems. There is substantial evidence from studies with amnesic and demented patients, as well as normal individuals, for the existence of multiple, distinct forms of mnemonic processing, and this work has been reviewed extensively (see Schacter, 1985, 1987). At a basic level, there appear to be at least two types of mnemonic processing, termed "explicit" and "implicit" by Graf and Schacter (1985) or "declarative" and "procedural" by Squire (1987) (See Figure 1). The major feature that distinguishes these forms of memory from one another can be defined as conscious awareness. Information processed by the explicit system (left side of Figure 1) is accessible to conscious recall while the implicit system (right side of Figure 1) does not require the conscious recollection of previous experience. Implicit or procedural memory is exhibited when performance on a task is facilitated by a previous experience, regardless of whether there is any conscious recollection of the previous experience. An example of a form of implicit memory is perceptual-motor skill learning. Another type of implicit memory can be detected using priming tasks (Diamond & Rozin, 1984; Jacoby & Dallas, 1981; Warrington & Weiskrantz, 1974). Under these conditions, sub-

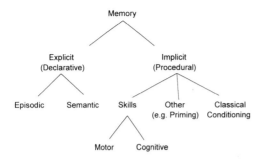

FIGURE 1. Memory systems. Adapted from Squire (1987).

jects may demonstrate memory for information (e.g., with reduced reaction time in lexical decision tasks) without being able to explicitly recall the information.

By contrast, "explicit" memory processes and systems are capable of the intentional and active production of specific target information using either recall or recognition procedures. The explicit system has been divided into "episodic" and "semantic" components (Tulving, 1972), because initially the episodic system was the one most extensively studied, but the dichotomy has received further support from studies of brain-damaged patients (Kinsbourne & Wood, 1975; Schacter & Tulving, 1982).

These dichotomies have direct relevance to rehabilitation potential. Patients with organic amnesia appear to have relatively selective loss of episodic memory—semantic memory and implicit systems often function normally (Milner, Corkin, & Teuber, 1968; Starr & Philipps, 1970). Patients with progressive fluent aphasia (i.e., semantic dementia) appear to have selective impairment in the semantic system; Alzheimer's disease patients, by contrast, are generally impaired in all realms of explicit memory with some forms of implicit memory spared (Bondi & Kaszniak, 1991; Eslinger & Damasio, 1986; Heindel, Salmon, Shults, Walicke, & Butters, 1989).

In contrast to the impairments seen in these patients with "cortical" dementia syndromes (Cummings & Benson, 1992), patients with "subcortical" dementia such as those arising from Lewy body dementia, progressive supranuclear palsy, and Huntington's disease have a substantially greater impairment on some implicit learning tasks, particularly perceptual-motor learning (Bondi & Kaszniak, 1991; Heindel et al., 1989).

Given the distinctive patterns of impairment that can occur in syndromes affecting memory and learning, it is critical to have information on the qualitative aspects of performance available at the time of rehabilitation planning. Data from prospective studies comparing the rehabilitation potential of different memory-impaired subjects are not extensive, so the nature of the differences in such potential is unclear. Nevertheless, there are strong conceptual reasons for tailoring the rehabilitation strategy to the patient's cognitive capacity with specific reference to the pattern of impaired and spared cognitive processes (Wilson, 1989).

Normal Aging

Memory Characteristics

The decline in memory functioning in older adults largely affects explicit, episodic memory and appears to be related to failure to spontaneously organize material during encoding. That is, while the basic ability to learn and remember information appears relatively unaffected by aging, certain metacognitive processes clearly decline with advancing age (Backman, 1989). For example, elderly individuals may fail to organize material, resulting in shallow encoding. Older adults do not use organizational strategies as often or as efficiently as their younger counterparts (Hultsch, 1971, 1974; Rankin, Karol, & Tuten, 1984; Sanders, Murphy, Schmitt, & Walsh, 1980; Worden & Meggison, 1984). Moreover, it has been suggested that there is a decline in the recoding (Tulving, 1983) or reprocessing of material after initial encoding with age. Younger adults engage in numerous spontaneous recoding operations, which result in richer, more elaborate memory traces and therefore maximize memory performance (Backman, 1989). Older adults are also more affected by divided attention tasks (Kinsbourne, 1980; for a review, see Hartley, 1992), perhaps reflecting impairment in "executive" processes. These executive functions are critical for integration and coordination of cognitive operations, and their loss can have a direct impact on memory functions (Baddeley, 1986; Della Sala & Logie,

1993). However, by relearning to use such methods (and putting them more under conscious control), older adults can improve their recall of information. A few studies have focused on training elders in the use of memory strategies.

Memory Retraining

There have been many laboratory studies on the effect of aging on memory, as well as on the use of mnemonic strategies to improve memory in younger individuals (Cermak, 1975; Higbee, 1993; Lorayne & Lucas, 1974). However, the literature on the use of memory remediation or compensation methods with the elderly is very scant (for reviews, see Backman, 1989; Greenberg & Powers, 1987: West, 1989; West & Tomer, 1989; Wilson, 1989; Yesavage, Lapp, & Sheikh, 1989). The results have been mixed, but in general, the evidence suggests that older adults can be trained in self-initiated compensation methods, and these methods have improved explicit memory. In most of the successful studies, normal elderly individuals have used remediation methods that have largely focused on internal, effortful, explicit encoding methods that help organize or associate information, which results in a deeper level of encoding. It is generally accepted that the deeper information is processed, or the more it is semantically analyzed at the time of encoding, the better it is recalled (Craik & Lockhart, 1972; Craik & Tulving, 1975). Thus far, the focus of much of the retraining work has been on two methods, each of which involves the use of visual imagery. These techniques are the *method of loci* and *face–name association*. Other mnemonic techniques, such as the visually based peg system (Mason & Smith, 1977) and the verbally based PQRST (Preview-Question-Read-State-Test) (Wilson & Moffat, 1984), have not been validated sufficiently with older adults.

Visual Imagery

Visual imagery is by far the most studied approach to memory remediation in the elderly. Although the data are limited (Poon, Walsh-Sweeney, & Fozard, 1980), it appears that elderly individuals are able to produce images of the same quality as younger individuals (Hartley, 1982). However, in some studies older adults exhibit deficits in the use of imagery (Hulicka & Grossman, 1967; Mason & Smith, 1977; Pavio, 1971; Poon et al., 1980; Winograd & Simon, 1980). In addition, while the use of bizarre imagery is effective in aiding recall for younger individuals, elderly individuals are generally not receptive to forming images that are bizarre (Poon & Walsh-Sweeney, 1981; Yesavage, 1985). Nevertheless, many studies have demonstrated that training in the use of visual imagery methods can be an effective tool for enhancing memory in the elderly (see Poon et al., 1980, and Yesavage et al., 1989, for reviews).

There are several mnemonic methods that make use of imagery. One well-studied strategy is the method of loci, in which one associates mental images of items to be remembered with mental images of locations for items (Higbee, 1979; Hrees, 1986; Yates, 1966). As told by Cicero, the method was developed based on an experience of a Greek poet, Simonides, circa 500 B.C. Simonides was speaking at a banquet when he was given a message that there was someone outside waiting for him. While he was outside, the roof over the banquet collapsed, killing everyone beyond recognition. Simonides was asked to identify the bodies and was able to do so by remembering the places at which people had been sitting. So, when using the method of loci, an individual identifies a series of images which he or she has memorized or overlearned (usually one's home or a familiar route). To use the method, an individual forms a visual association between the first item on the list or first fact in a series and the first image on the route. Subsequent items to be remembered are associated with subsequent images along the route. When it is time to recall the information, one takes an imaginary walk around the house or travels along the route and each of the familiar spots serves as a retrieval cue for the item to be remembered. Several studies have found that the method of loci enhances recall in older adults (Anschutz, Camp, Markley, & Kramer, 1985; Robertson-Tchabo, Hausman, & Arenberg, 1976; Rose & Yesavage, 1983; Yesavage & Rose, 1984b).

The face–name mnemonic is another example of a visual imagery technique that can be successfully taught (Yesavage & Jacob, 1984; Yesavage et al., 1989; Yesavage & Rose, 1984a; Yesavage, Rose, & Bower, 1983; Zarit, Cole, & Guider, 1981; Zarit,

Gallagher, & Kramer, 1981) to address a common memory complaint of older individuals—remembering people's names (Zelinski, Gilewski, & Thompson, 1980; Yesavage et al., 1983). Briefly, the technique consists of three steps: (1) identifying a prominent feature, (2) transforming the name into a concrete image, and (3) forming a visual image associating the feature with the name–image. For example, if "Butters" was the name to be recalled and the person had light, wavy hair, the image might be butter dripping from the individual's hair. The recall phase then consists of (1) recognizing the prominent physical feature (light, wavy hair), (2) using this feature as a retrieval cue to recall the image–name association (the liquid dripping), (3) reconstructing the transformed name from the image (the liquid was butter), and finally (4) decoding the name from the transformation (Butters).

Verbal Organization

There are relatively few studies of the effectiveness of verbal strategies in improving the memory of older adults. Some researchers have found that the verbal elaborations of the elderly are not as accurate as those of younger adults (Pearlmutter, 1979; Puglisi, Park, & Smith, 1987; Rabinowitz & Ackerman, 1982; Rankin & Collins, 1985), so training should focus on the creation of specific associations with personal meaning. Moreover, there is evidence that training in verbal mediation can improve memory in younger individuals (Catino, Taub, & Borkowski, 1977; DeLeon, 1974; Hellebusch, 1976; Hulicka & Grossman, 1967), and in one study, training in verbal elaboration methods was especially effective for long-term retention (as long as retrieval cues were present, as they often are in the environment) (West & Tomer, 1989). In addition, the elderly are likely to already use verbal methods (Hulicka, Sterns, & Grossman, 1967; Rowe & Schnore, 1971; Treat, Poon, & Fozard, 1981; Weinstein, Duffy, Underwood, MacDonald, & Gott, 1981). Because verbal skills and semantic memory networks remain intact in older individuals, methods that rely on elaboration by associating new information with known information could be helpful.

For example, difficulty remembering the names of familiar people is a very common com-

plaint among elderly individuals (Yesavage et al., 1983; Zelinski et al., 1980). To help elderly individuals improve face–name learning, Yesavage and colleagues (1983) had subjects engage in a semantic orienting task (judging the pleasantness of faces) in addition to interactive imagery (imagining a prominent feature interacting with a concrete word related to the last name). They found that adding the semantic orienting task enhanced the retention of the names.

First-letter associations, or acronyms, have yielded mixed results when used by the elderly. To form first-letter associations, one simply takes the first letter of items to be remembered and forms a word or a meaningful sentence out of them (e.g., "HOMES" for the Great Lakes). Harris (1980) and Lovelace (1984) successfully employed the technique as an organizational strategy, however, the technique was not helpful in improving recall in other training studies (Hellebusch, 1976; Hultsch, 1969). The figure alphabet method (a phonetic system for number recall) has also been used successfully (Smith, Heckhausen, Kliegl, & Baltes, 1984).

Multimodal Approach

As noted earlier, the goal of many of the compensatory techniques is to increase depth of processing of information to be remembered. Interestingly, Backman (1985) and Backman and Nilsson (1984, 1985) found that age differences in recall were eliminated when subjects were required to recall a series of subject-performed tasks (Cohen 1981). One explanation for these findings is that the performed tasks are multimodal, with subjects' visual and tactile systems involved, in addition to the auditory/verbal processing of task instructions that occurs. After reviewing a variety of subject-performed task experiments, Backman (1986) concluded that age differences were most pronounced when the presentation was unimodal, were reduced in bimodal presentation, and were eliminated in multimodal presentation. Greenberg and Powers (1987) also addressed the issue of multimodality in their review of the literature on memory rehabilitation with the elderly and concluded that the multimodal approach facilitates performance in older adults.

Yesavage et al.'s (1983) study on teaching the face–name association accompanied by other methods is a good example of the usefulness of multimodal encoding methods. Although the initial presentation of the face–name stimuli is only bimodal, the subjects were asked to generate elaborations in the visual modality (images) and verbal modalities (personality, like or dislike) to increase depth of processing. In fact, the effect of relaxation training, imagery training, and semantic elaboration used in combination with face–name association was found to be stable at a 6-month follow-up (Sheikh, Hill, & Yesavage, 1986).

Indirect Memory Training Methods

Preliminary training in the skills needed to acquire compensation methods seems to enhance their ultimate effect (Yesavage & Rose, 1983). For example, to address the relatively superficial processing of visual images in older adults, subjects were trained in imagery skills before learning imagery mnemonics. The authors found that this strategy enhanced the older adults' subsequent use of imagery mnemonics (Yesavage et al., 1983).

Training individuals to attend to stimuli (e.g., noticing details of information to be remembered) may also be helpful. When taught several techniques designed to improve attention, such as selective attention exercises (list learning with verbal interference) and sensory awareness exercises (examination of various colored pictures with instructions to identify details), recall of the information to be remembered was improved relative to the control condition (Yesavage & Rose, 1983).

Relaxation training has been used as an additional pretraining measure to address the performance anxiety experienced by many elderly individuals during the process of learning another memory enhancing technique. Relaxation training can reduce anxious ruminations, thereby improving attention and increasing available memory processing capabilities. The effectiveness of the face–name learning technique was improved with relaxation training prior to learning the technique (Yesavage & Jacob, 1984). Studies by Zarit and co-workers (Zarit, Cole, & Guider, 1981; Zarit, Gallagher, & Kramer, 1981) applied relaxation training in addition to other motivation and attention methods to address memory complaints in older adults and found improvement similar to that achieved with organization techniques. Individual anxiety levels may prove to be an important consideration when implementing relaxation training. One study reported that only individuals with initially high levels of anxiety showed improvement in memory performance with relaxation training (Yesavage, Rose, & Spiegel, 1982). Thus, as with any remediation program, individual differences must be taken into consideration when planning a memory rehabilitation program (Wilson, 1989).

Retrieval

All of the methods discussed thus far affect the encoding of information to be remembered, increasing the amount of material stored and, hence, the amount of information available for retrieval. None of the methods is of benefit once encoding has taken place. An important point to be made is that most of the internal strategies typically used by the elderly are *retrieval* strategies. For example, most individuals, young and old, spontaneously use mental retracing and alphabetic searching to aid retrieval (Cavanaugh, Grady, & Perlmutter, 1983). However, to some extent, retrieval declines with age (Burke & Light, 1981; Kausler, 1982). Lovelace (1984) found that the only internal retrieval strategy used by older adults with any frequency was mental retracing. Nevertheless, training in retrieval methods is beneficial. Training in verbal elaboration methods (first-letter association for remembering text, simple association for remembering object locations, and name sentences for remembering names and faces) is especially effective for long-term retention, as long as retrieval cues are present (which they often are in the environment) (West & Tomer, 1989).

External Aids

In contrast to the internal compensatory methods highlighted thus far, external aids are those devices that actually store information or that act as cues to retrieve internally stored information (Harris, 1984). Examples of external aids that store information include shopping lists, notebooks, and computers. External aids substitute for memorization and are used as an extension of one's internal memory. Unfortunately, very few studies have attempted to train older adults in the use of these aids. One reason for this dearth of research may be that many elderly individuals, to some extent, already employ such strategies (Cavanaugh et al., 1983).

Most of the studies that have addressed the use of external aids that store information have involved training brain-injured, memory-impaired individuals. For example, a few investigators have successfully demonstrated the use of a personal computer as an external aid in younger memory-impaired individuals (Kirsch, Lajiness, Levine, & Schneider, 1990; Kirsch, Levine, Fallon-Krueger, & Jaros, 1987; Kirsch et al., 1988). Sohlberg and Mateer (1989) describe a theoretically based, systematic program that they have developed to train memory-impaired patients in the use of a notebook. The program attempts to systematically train individuals using standard learning principles, and it is based on the assumption that many amnesic patients retain some ability to learn new information. The authors believe that in this case, their program relies on patients' generally intact ability to learn new *procedures*—specifically learning to use the notebook and not to recall what is in the notebook (i.e., the episodic memories). They emphasize that while the particular sections in a notebook must be chosen to fit the needs of an individual patient, the training program includes standard steps which are applied regardless of the specific contents. The steps include acquisition, application, and adaptation. The program not only encompasses how, when, and where to use the notebook, but perhaps most importantly, carries over the training outside the clinic and into natural settings. The authors describe in detail a successful case study using their approach. While both the attempt to develop a training program based on theoretical principles and the preliminary results are encouraging, larger group studies are needed.

Another category of external devices consists of those that act as cues to retrieve *internally* stored information (Harris, 1984). Examples include instruments such as cooking timers and calendars with holidays identified. These types of devices serve best as prospective memory aids, as they cue an individual when some task must be performed. These types of aids interact with an individuals' internal memory system in a way that external aids, which simply store information (such as lists), do

not. While these sorts of systems may be useful for "forgetful," but not amnesic, subjects, they are probably less useful in individuals who would have difficulty remembering the task to be performed even after having been cued to perform it.

There are several potential problems that apply to all external memory aids that should be considered. First, some aids such as computers require a high level of cognitive functioning to operate and thus can be challenging for some elderly individuals. Second, memory-impaired individuals may forget to use the aid. Lastly, many individuals reject the use of aids due to lack of motivation, lack of awareness of their memory deficit, or sensitivity to the stigma of having memory problems, which gets confirmed each time they rely upon a device.

Limitations

There are numerous limitations of the current knowledge base. First, most studies have been performed with experimental materials (e.g., word lists, paired associates) in the laboratory and have little demonstrated ecological validity. In a related vein, many of the methods studied may be too complicated and impractical for elderly individuals to use in daily life. Moreover, while most of these strategies enhance short-term recall of information, in some studies their use has not affected delayed recall. Finally, follow-up data, in terms of generalization, long-term use, or efficacy of training, is frequently lacking.

Recommendations

First, to overcome many of the limitations inherent in internal strategies, the clinician should encourage the use of external aids (notebooks, calendars, lists). When internal strategies are trained, one should target specific problems and focus on increasing elaboration of encoding (visual or verbal) or on training in retrieval. Preliminary training in skills needed to perform encoding strategies, relaxation training to reduce anxiety and increase ability to learn the methods, and attention training to increase awareness of features and thus depth of encoding may enhance performance. Finally, these methods should be implemented thoroughly, one at a time.

Alzheimer's Disease

Memory Characteristics

Alzheimer's disease (AD) is characterized by a progressive loss of episodic and semantic memory and other cognitive abilities, accompanied by relative preservation of procedural learning ability. Individuals with AD exhibit a progressive decline in independent functioning (Form, 1994; Skurla, Rogers, & Sunderland, 1988; Teunisse, Derix, & van Crevel, 1991). Caregiver burden is a major factor in the decision to institutionalize demented patients (Colerick & George, 1986). If patients' level of functioning can be maximized, it may delay institutionalization. Few researchers have studied the effect of training patients in functional skills, and even fewer have employed established methods based on learning theory and emergent knowledge from cognitive neuropsychology.

Memory Retraining

Attempts at memory remediation with AD patients, best described as prolonging maximal functioning, have been very rare but are increasing. Most of the research has used the same methods that have been used in the normal elderly (Beck et al., 1985; Diesfeldt, 1984; Zarit, Zarit, & Reever, 1982). That is, most attempts to improve memory in AD have focused on improving episodic memory by enhancing encoding (e.g., repetition, visual imagery, verbal mediation). Given that the primary deficit is in storage of information (Delis et al., 1991; Knopman & Ryberg, 1989; Wilson, Bacon, Fox, & Kaszniak, 1983), it is not surprising that many of these attempts to increase the quality of encoding have met with limited success. Nevertheless, there has been some preliminary work on other potential approaches.

External Aids

Attempts at training AD patients in the use of external memory aids have been extremely scarce. However, diaries, reality orientation boards, and signposts have helped to maintain personal information and orientation facts in senile dementia patients (Hanley, 1981). Bourgeois (1990) conducted a study in which she trained caregivers to train patients in the use of a memory aid. The aid consisted of a notebook which contained facts about themselves and their lives, organized by conversation topic. The subjects learned to use the memory aid with conversational partners and improved the quality of their conversations. In another study, an alarm watch with an hourly chime was used in one study to remind an AD patient to look at his daily program (Kurlychek, 1983).

Environmental Modifications

Environmental modifications are relatively easy to achieve, but the extent of their benefit has not been sufficiently addressed. One study of 80 elderly demented women in a long-stay hospital ward combined verbal orientation training and signposts at different locations in the ward. The orientation training consisted of verbal description of the particular areas and individual coaching with the patient regarding the use of the particular area. This combination training proved to be effective, and the improvements were maintained at a 3-month follow-up (Hanley, 1981). These findings were replicated in homes for the aged by Gilleard, Mitchell, and Riordan (1981).

Exploiting Procedural Memory Ability

In contrast to their impairments in explicit memory, AD patients are able to acquire some kinds of new information through implicit memory, which does not require conscious recollection. There are a number of forms of implicit memory that appear to remain intact throughout much of the course of AD. For example, AD patients' ability to learn motor skills appears to be spared (Eslinger & Damasio, 1990; Heindel et al., 1989). Karlsson, Backman, Nilsson, Winblad, and Osterlind (1989) and, in a follow-up study, Herlitz, Adolfsson, Backman, and Nilsson (1991) investigated the ability of AD patients and controls to recall tasks under a variety of learning conditions, including hearing the tasks described verbally and performing the tasks themselves (subject-performed tasks; SPT). All subjects recalled the most material under the SPT condition. More importantly, motor action during learning enhanced recall even in severely demented AD patients. Moreover, in AD, the ability to use cues to improve performance on motor tasks is preserved longer than are other forms of memory. Another study (Josephsson et al., 1993) actually exploited AD patients' ability to acquire motor skills by demonstrating improved functional skills in three out of four AD patients. The authors developed individualized programs to train specific dining skills that deemphasized episodic and semantic memory and were more dependent on procedural motor skills. Each training program also provided environmental guidance (a form of cueing to aid recall) and was developed based on individuals' habits and motivations.

Another method that helps AD patients acquire new information, spaced retrieval, appears to be related to implicit memory, but does not involve the motor system (Landauer & Bjork, 1978; Schacter, Rich, & Stampp, 1985). In the spaced retrieval method, information to be remembered is retrieved repeatedly at increasingly longer intervals of time. Camp and McKitrick (1992) used the spaced retrieval method to improve AD patients' memory for location of objects and face naming. The level of success with AD patients using spaced retrieval has led to the explanation that the method requires little cognitive effort and primarily relies on the implicit memory system.

Some investigators have successfully used methods that rely on implicit memory to teach new information to patients with nonprogressive amnesia. One approach in particular, called the method of vanishing cues, is worth noting because it may be useful in AD patients. Glisky, Schacter, and Tulving (1986a,b) developed the method of vanishing cues, which takes advantage of patients' implicit memory ability to respond to word fragments. This method initially provides subjects with correct answers and then systematically diminishes the letters (cues) across trials. However, subjects are always provided with as many cues as necessary to produce the correct response. Amnesic patients successfully mastered a computer vocabulary and various computer operations with this method (Glisky et al., 1986a,b), despite impaired ability to explicitly recall the training sessions. Butters, Glisky, and Schacter (1993) successfully employed a variation of the vanishing cues procedure to teach a group of amnesic patients information about a fictitious corporation. Thus, amnesic patients can acquire complex knowledge and retain it over several months. This method may be equally useful with AD patients.

Nevertheless, it is important to note that even with this successful training method, amnesic patients performed far more poorly than control subjects on several transfer tasks. These results suggest that memory training with amnesic individuals (and likely with AD patients as well) must be "domain-specific." That is, training programs must be carefully designed to neither require nor anticipate generalization.

A final promising approach to teaching memory-impaired patients which may be useful in AD, is termed "errorless learning." Errorless learning is accomplished by any training method that limits the opportunity for subjects to commit errors. Errorless learning has its origins in animal learning experiments by Terrace (1963, 1966), who found that pigeons could learn to discriminate colored keys if they were prevented from committing errors. Using a similar errorless learning procedure, Sidman and Stoddard (1967) taught mentally handicapped children to discriminate between circles and ellipses. More recently, other researchers (Baddeley & Wilson, 1994; Wilson, 1992; Wilson, Baddeley, Evans, & Shiel, 1994) have found that subjects with severe memory disorders exhibited greater learning and better retention with an errorless learning procedure as compared to conventional learning methods. Anecdotal evidence of the functional significance of errorless learning is available from Moakes (1988), who reported that his severely amnesic wife successfully learned to cook and run the house independently, drive a limited number of routes, and resume her job as a secretary, following training that involved extensive repetition, limited recourse to episodic memory, and limited errors. Baddeley and Wilson (1994) point out that procedural learning is based on emitting the strongest response from a range of possible responses with varying salience. If errors occur when learning a procedural task, the repeated erroneous responses become strengthened across trials, and learning is impeded. Thus, all learning, including procedural learning should be enhanced by error elimination.

Recommendations

The foregoing literature leads to a number of recommendations regarding memory retraining in AD. Specific problems should be trained directly, without requiring generalization for success. Goals should be practical and should take patient and caregiver motivation into account. The caregiver should be involved in the training, if appropriate. If possible, the focus should be on environmental manipulation, such as eliminating confusing items and adding cues to help direct patients. Conscious memorization of a technique or of the task itself should not be required for success. Instead, reliance on preserved abilities such as motor learning and use of spaced retrieval should be emphasized. Training should be extensive and thorough and should minimize the opportunity to make errors.

Future Directions

Memory Remediation for Normal Elderly

Future research should first focus on overcoming the limitations of past studies. In particular, tasks should be more practical or ecologically valid. Also, individuals who have been trained should be followed for a period of time to assess maintenance of the acquired skills. It may be that "booster sessions" are necessary to help maintain criterion levels of performance. Generalization, both across materials and settings, is extremely important to study. The solution may be to provide training on more ecologically relevant tasks in an individual's everyday environment and therefore incorporate generalization into the training.

Memory Remediation in AD

There has been theoretical and empirical progress in the development of memory rehabilitation methods with amnesic individuals (e.g., studies employing errorless learning, spaced retrieval, and the method of vanishing cues), and some of these techniques are beginning to be used with AD patients in a limited fashion. Further studies that focus on exploiting preserved abilities to compensate for deficits that impair AD patients' everyday functioning are critical.

ACKNOWLEDGMENTS

This work was supported in part by a Research Scientist Development Award, Level II (MH-0177) to James T. Becker. Support was also provided to Meryl Butters by the MHCRC for the study of Late Life Mood Disorders (Charles F. Reynolds, III, PI; MH-52247) and to Meryl Butters and Elizabeth Soety by a V.A. Rehabilitation Research Development Service Award (Steven Graham, PI; VA-B785-RC).

References

Albert, M. S., & Moss, M. B. (1988). *Geriatric neuropsychology.* New York: Guilford Press.

Anschutz, L., Camp, C. J., Markley, R. P., & Kramer, J. J. (1985). Maintenance and generalization of mnemonics for grocery shopping by older adults. *Experimental Aging Research, 11,* 157–160.

Backman, L. (1985). Further evidence for the lack of adult age differences on free recall of subject-performed tasks: The importance of motor action. *Human Learning, 4,* 79–87.

Backman, L. (1986). Adult age differences in cross-modal recoding and mental tempo, and older adults' utilization of compensatory task conditions. *Experimental Aging Research, 12,* 135–140.

Backman, L. (1989). Varieties of memory compensation by older adults in episodic remembering. In L. W. Poon, B. Wilson, & D. Rubin (Eds.), *Everyday cognition in adulthood and latelife* (pp. 509–544). Cambridge, England: Cambridge University Press.

Backman, L., & Nilsson, L. G. (1984). Aging effects in free recall: An exception to the rule. *Human Learning, 3,* 53–69.

Backman, L., & Nilsson, L. G. (1985). Prerequisites for lack of age differences in memory performance. *Experimental Aging Research, 11,* 67–73.

Baddeley, A. (1986). *Working memory.* Oxford, England: Oxford University Press.

Baddeley, A., & Wilson, B. A. (1994). When implicit learning fails: Amnesia and the problem of error elimination. *Neuropsychologia, 32,* 53–68.

Beck, C. K., Heacock, P., Thatcher, R., Mercer, S. O., Sparkman, C., & Roberts, M. A. (1985, July). *Cognitive skills remediation with Alzheimer's patients.* Paper presented at the 13th International Congress of Gerontology, New York, NY.

Bondi, M. W., & Kaszniak, A. W. (1991). Implicit and explicit memory in Alzheimer's disease and Parkinson's disease. *Journal of Clinical and Experimental Neuropsychology, 13,* 339–358.

Bourgeois, M. S. (1990). Enhancing conversation skills in patients with Alzheimer's disease using a prosthetic memory aid. *Journal of Applied Behavior Analysis, 23,* 29–42.

Burke, D. M. & Light, L. L. (1981). Memory and aging: The role of retrieval processes. *Psychological Bulletin, 90,* 513–546.

Butters, M. A., Glisky, E. L. & Schacter, D. L. (1993). Transfer of new learning in memory-impaired patients. *Journal of Clinical and Experimental Neuropsychology, 15,* 219–230.

Camp, C. J. & McKitrick, L. A. (1992). Memory interventions in Alzheimer's-type dementia populations: Methodological and theoretical issues. In R. L. West & J. D. Sinnot (Eds.), *Everyday memory and aging: Current research and methodology* (pp. 155–172). New York: Springer-Verlag.

Catino, C., Taub, S. I., & Borkowski, J. G. (1977). Mediation in children and the elderly as a function of memory capabilities. *The Journal of Genetic Psychology, 130,* 35–47.

Cavanaugh, J. C., Grady, J. G., & Perlmutter, M. P. (1983). Forgetting and use of memory aids in 20- and 70-year-olds' everyday life. *International Journal of Aging and Human Development, 17,* 113–122.

Cermak, L. S. (1975). *Improving your memory.* New York: McGraw-Hill.

Chaffin, R., & Herrmann, D. J. (1983). Self reports of memory abilities by old and young adults. *Human Learning, 2,* 17–28.

Cohen, R. L. (1981). On the generality of some memory laws. *Scandinavian Journal of Psychology, 22,* 267–282.

Colerick, E., & George, L. (1986). Predictors of institutionalization among caregivers of patients with Alzheimer's disease. *Journal of the American Geriatrics Society, 34,* 493–498.

Craik, F. I. M. (1986). A functional account of age differences in memory. In F. Klix & H. Hagendord (Eds.), *Human memory and cognitive capabilities: Mechanisms and performances* (pp. 409–422). Amsterdam: Elsevier.

Craik, F. I. M., & Lockhart, R. S. (1972). Levels of processing: A framework for memory research. *Journal of Verbal Learning and Verbal Behavior, 11,* 671–684.

Craik, F. I. M., & Tulving, E. (1975). Depth of processing and the retention of words in episodic memory. *Journal of Experimental Psychology: General, 104,* 268–294.

Cummings, J. L., & Benson, F. D. (1992). *Dementia: A clinical approach (2nd ed.).* Boston: Butterworth-Heinemann.

DeLeon, J. M. (1974). *Effects of training in repetition and mediation on paired-associate learning and practical memory in the aged.* Unpublished Ph.D. dissertation, University of Hawaii.

Delis, D. C., Massman, P. J., Butters, N., Salmon, D. P., Kramer, J. H., & Cermak, L. (1991). Profiles of demented and amnesic patients on the California Verbal Learning Test: Implications for the assessment of memory disorders. *Psychological Assessment: A Journal of Clinical and Consulting Psychology, 3,* 19–26.

Della Sala, S. D., & Logie, R. H. (1993). When working memory does not work: The role of working memory in neuropsychology. In F. Boller & J. Grafman (Eds.), *Handbook of neuropsychology* (pp. 1–62). Amsterdam: Elsevier.

Diamond, R., & Rozin, P. (1984). Activation of existing memories in the amnesic syndrome. *Journal of Abnormal Psychology, 12,* 105–111.

Diesfeldt, H. F. A. (1984). The importance of encoding instructions and retrieval cues in the assessment of memory in senile dementia. *Archives of Gerontology and Geriatrics, 3,* 51–57.

Eslinger, P. J., & Damasio, A. R. (1986). Preserved and motor learning in Alzheimer's disease: Implications for anatomy and behavior. *Journal of Neuroscience, 6,* 3006–3009.

Form, A. F. (1994). Disability in dementia: Assessment, prevention, and rehabilitation. *Disability and Rehabilitation, 16,* 98–109.

Gilleard, C., Mitchell, R. G., & Riordan, J. (1981). Ward orientation training with psychogeriatric patients. *Journal of Advanced Nursing, 6,* 96–98.

Glisky, E. L., Schacter, D. L., & Tulving, E. (1986a). Computer learning by memory-impaired patients: Acquisition and retention of complex knowledge. *Neuropsychologia, 24,* 313–328.

Glisky, E. L., Schacter, D. L., & Tulving, E., (1986b). Learning and retention of computer-related vocabulary in memory-impaired patients: Method of vanishing cues. *Journal of Clinical and Experimental Neuropsychology, 8,* 292–312.

Graf, P., & Schacter, D. L. (1985). Implicit and explicit memory for new associations in normal and amnestic patients. *Journal of Experimental Psychology: Learning, Memory, and Cognition, 11,* 501–518.

Greenberg, C., & Powers, S. A. (1987). Memory improvement among adult learners. *Educational Gerontology, 13,* 263–280.

Hanley, I. G. (1981). The use of signposts and active training to modify ward disorientation in elderly patients. *Journal of Behavioral Therapy and Experimental Psychiatry, 12,* 241–247.

Harris, J. E. (1980). Memory aids people use: Two interview studies. *Memory and Cognition, 8,* 31–38.

Harris, J. E. (1984). Methods of improving memory. In B. A. Wilson & N. Moffat (Eds.), *Clinical management of memory problems* (pp. 46–62). Rockville, MD: Aspen.

Hartley, A. A. (1992). Attention. In F. I. M. Craik & T. A. Salthouse (Eds.), *The handbook of aging and cognition* (pp. 3–50). Hillsdale, NJ: Erlbaum.

Hartley, J. T. (1982). *Semantic characteristics of older and younger persons' visual images.* Paper presented at the meeting of the Gerontological Society of America, Boston, MA.

Heindel, W. C., Salmon, D. P., Shults, C. W., Walicke, P. A., & Butters, N. (1989). Neuropsychological evidence for multiple implicit memory systems: A comparison of Alzheimer's, Huntington's and Parkinson's disease patients. *Journal of Neuroscience, 9,* 582–587.

Herlitz, A., Adolfsson, R., Backman, L., & Nilsson, L. G. (1991). Cue utilization following different forms of encoding in mildly, moderately, and severely demented patients with Alzheimer's disease. *Brain and Cognition, 15,* 119–130.

Hellebusch, S. J. (1976). *On improving learning and memory in the aged: The effects of mnemonics on strategy, transfer, and generalization.* Dissertation Abstract (1459-B Order No. 76-19, 465), University of Notre Dame.

Higbee, K. L. (1993). *Your memory: How it works and how to improve it.* New York: Paragon.

Higbee, K. L. (1979). Recent research on visual mnemonics: Historical roots and educational fruits. *Review of Educational Research, 49,* 611–629.

Hrees, R. A. (1986). *An edited version of mnemonics from antiquity to 1985: Establishing a foundation for mnemonic-based pedagogy with particular emphasis on mathematics.* Unpublished. Ph.D. dissertation, Indiana University.

Hulicka, I. M., & Grossman, J. L. (1967). Age group comparisons for the use of mediators in paired-associate learning. *Journal of Gerontology, 22,* 46–51.

Hulicka, I. M., Sterns, H., & Grossman, J. (1967). Age-group comparisons of paired-associate learning as a function of paced and self-paced association and response times. *Journal of Gerontology, 22,* 274–280.

Hultsch, D. F. (1969). Adult age differences in the organization of free recall. *Developmental Psychology, 1,* 673–678.

Hultsch, D. F. (1971). Organization and memory in adulthood. *Human Development, 14,* 16–29.

Hultsch, D. F. (1974). Learning to learn in adulthood. *Journal of Gerontology, 29*(3), 302–308.

Jacoby, L. L., & Dallas, M. (1981). On the relationship between autobiological memory and perceptual learning. *Journal of Experimental Psychology: General, 110,* 306–340.

Josephsson, S., Backman, L., Borell, L., Bernspang, B., Nygard, L., & Ronnberg, L. (1993). Supporting everyday activities in dementia: An intervention study. *International Journal of Geriatric Psychiatry, 8,* 395–400.

Karlsson, T., Backman, L., Nilsson, L. G., Winblad, B., & Osterlind, P.O. (1989). Memory improvement at different stages of Alzheimer's disease. *Neuropsychologia, 27,* 737–742.

Kausler, D. H. (1982). *Experimental psychology and human aging.* New York: John Wiley.

Kinsbourne, M. (1980). Attentional dysfunction and the elderly: Theoretical models and research perspectives. In L. W. Poon, J. L. Fozard, L. S. Cermak, D. Arenberg, & L. W. Thompson (Eds.), *New directions in memory and aging: Proceedings of the George Talland Memorial Conference.* Hillsdale, NJ: Lawrence Erlbaum.

Kinsbourne, M., & Wood, F. (1975). Short-term memory process and the amnestic syndrome. In D. Deutsch & J. A. Deutsch (Eds), *Short-term memory* (pp. 259–291). New York: Academic Press.

Kirsch, N. L., Lajiness, R., Levine, S. P., & Schneider, M. (1990). Performance of functional activities with the aid of task guidance systems [Abstract]. *Journal of Clinical and Experimental Neuropsychology, 12,* 65.

Kirsch, N. L., Levine, S. P., Fallon-Krueger, M., & Jaros, L. A. (1987). The microcomputer as an "orthotic" device for patients with cognitive deficits. *Journal of Head Trauma Rehabilitation, 2,* 77–86.

Kirsch, N. L., Levine, S. P., Lajiness, R., Mossaro, M., Schneider, M., & Donders, J. (1988). Improving functional performance with computerized task guidance systems. *Proceedings of the 11th Annual Conference on Rehabilitation Technology,* Montreal, Canada.

Knopman, D. S., & Ryberg, S. (1989). A verbal memory test with high predictive accuracy for dementia of the Alzheimer type. *Archives of Neurology, 46,* 141–146.

Kurlychek, R. T. (1983). Use of a digital alarm chronograph as a memory aid in early dementia. *Clinical Gerontologist, 1,* 93–94.

Landauer, T. K., & Bjork, R. A. (1978). Optimum rehearsal patterns and name learning. In M. M. Grunberg, P. E. Morris, & R. N. Sykes (Eds.), *Practical aspects of memory* (pp. 625–632). London: Academic Press.

Lorayne, H., & Lucas, J. (1974). *The memory book.* New York: Ballantine Books.

Lovelace, E. A. (1984, August). *Reported mnemonics and perceived memory changes with aging.* Paper presented at a meeting of the American Psychological Association, Toronto.

Mason, S. E., & Smith, A. D. (1977). Imagery in the aged. *Experimental Aging Research, 3,* 17–32.

Milner, B., Corkin, S., & Teuber, J. L. (1968). Further analysis of the hippocampal amnesic syndrome: A 14 year follow-up study of H.M. *Neuropsychologia, 61,* 215–234.

Moakes, D. (1988). *The viewpoint of the career.* Paper presented at the Amnesia Association Course on Memory and Amnesia, Isle of Thorns Conference Center, East Sussex, England.

Moscovitch, M. C., & Winocur, G. (1992). The neuropsychology of memory and aging. In F. I. M. Craik & T. A. Salthouse (Eds.), *The handbook of aging and cognition* (pp. 315–372). Hillsdale, NJ: Erlbaum.

Nebes, R. D. (1992). Cognitive dysfunction in Alzheimer's disease. In F. I. M. Craik & T. A. Salthouse (Eds.), *The handbook of aging and cognition* (pp. 373–446). Hillsdale, NJ: Erlbaum.

Pavio, A. (1971). *Imagery and verbal processes.* New York: Holt, Rinehart & Winston.

Pearlmutter, M. (1979). Age differences in adults' free recall, cued recall, and recognition. *Journal of Gerontology, 34,* 533–539.

Poon, L. W., & Walsh-Sweeney, L. (1981). Effects of bizarre and interacting imagery on learning and retrieval of the aged. *Experimental Aging Research, 7,* 65–70.

Poon, L. W., & Walsh-Sweeney, L., & Fozard, J. L. (1980). Memory skill training for the elderly: Salient issues on the use of imagery mnemonies. In L. W. Poon, J. L. Fozard, L. S. Cermak, D. Arenberg, & L. W. Thompson (Eds.), *New directions in memory and aging: Proceedings of the George Talland Memorial Conference.* Hillsdale, NJ: Lawrence Erlbaum.

Puglisi, J. T., Park, D. C., & Smith, A. D. (1987). Picture associations among older and young adults. *Experimental Aging Research, 13,* 115–116.

Rabinowitz, J. C., & Ackerman, B. P. (1982). General encoding of episodic events by elderly adults. In F. I. M. Craik & S. Trehub (Eds.), *Aging and cognitive processes* (pp. 145–154). New York: Plenum.

Rankin, J. L., & Collins, M. (1985). Adult age differences in memory elaboration. *Journal of Gerontology, 40,* 451–458.

Rankin, J. L., Karol, R., & Tuten, C. (1984). Strategy use, recall, and recall organization in young, middle-aged, and elderly adults. *Experimental Aging Research, 10*(4), 193–196.

Robertson-Tchabo, E. A., Hausman, C. P., & Arenberg, D. (1976). A classic mnemonic for older learners: A trip that works! *Educational Gerontology, 1,* 215–226.

Rose, T. L., & Yesavage, J. A. (1983). Differential effects of a list-learning mnemonic in three age groups. *Gerontology, 29,* 293–298.

Rowe, E. J., & Schnore, M. M. (1971). Item concreteness and reported strategies in paired-associate learning as a function of age. *Journal of Gerontology, 26,* 470–475.

Sanders, R. E., Murphy, M. D., Schmitt, F. A., & Walsh, K. K. (1980). Age differences in free recall rehearsal strategies. *Journal of Gerontology, 35,* 550–558.

Schacter, D. L. (1985). Multiple forms of memory in humans and animals. In N. M. Weinberger, J. L. McGaugh, & G. Lynch (Eds.), *Memory systems of the brain* (pp. 351–379). New York: Guilford Press.

Schacter, D. L. (1987). Implicit memory: History and current status. *Journal of Experimental Psychology: Learning, Memory, & Cognition, 13,* 501–518.

Schacter, D. L., Rich, S. A., & Stampp, M. S. (1985). Remediation of memory disorders: Experimental evaluation of the spaced retrieval technique. *Journal of Clinical and Experimental Neuropsychology, 7,* 79–96.

Schacter, D. L., & Tulving, E. (1982). Memory, amnesia, and the episodic-semantic distinction. In R. L. Isaacson & N. E. Spear (Eds.), *The expression of knowledge* (pp. 35–65). New York: Plenum Press.

Sheikh, J. I., Hill, R. D., & Yesavage, J. A. (1986). Long-term efficacy of cognitive training for minimal memory impairment: A six-month follow-up study. *Journal of Developmental Neuropsychology, 2*, 413–421.

Sidman, M., & Stoddard, L. T. (1967). The effectiveness of fading in programming simultaneous form discrimination for retarded children. *Journal of the Experimental Analysis of Behavior, 10*, 3–15.

Skurla, E., Rogers, J. C., & Sunderland, T. (1988). Direct assessment of activities of daily living in Alzheimer's disease: A controlled study. *Journal of the American Geriatrics Society, 36(2)*, 97–103.

Squire, L. (1987). *Memory and brain.* New York: Oxford.

Smith, J., Heckhausen, J., Kliegl, R., & Baltes, P. B. (1984, November). *Cognitive reserve capacity, expertise, and aging: Plasticity of digit span performance.* Paper presented at the meeting of the Gerontological Society of America, San Antonio, TX.

Sohlberg, M. M., & Mateer, C. A. (1989). *Introduction to cognitive rehabilitation: Theory and practice.* New York: Guilford.

Starr, A., & Phillips, L. (1970). Verbal and motor memory in the amnestic syndrome. *Neuropsychologia, 8*, 75–88.

Sunderland, A., Watts, K., Baddeley, A. D., & Harris, J. E. (1986). Subjective memory assessment and test performance in elderly adults. *Journal of Gerontology, 28*, 376–384.

Teunisse, S., Derix, M. M. A., & van Crevel, H. (1991). Assessing the severity of dementia. *Archives of Neurology, 48*, 274–277.

Terrace, H. S. (1963). Discrimination learning with and without "errors." *Journal of the Experimental Analysis of Behavior, 6*, 1–27.

Terrace, H. S. (1966). Stimulus control. In W. K. Honig (Ed.), *Operant behavior: Areas of research and application* (pp. 271–344). New York: Appleton-Century-Crofs.

Treat, N. J., Poon, L. W., & Fozard, J. L. (1981). Age, imagery, and practice in paired-associate learning. *Experimental Aging Research, 7*, 337–342.

Tulving, E. (1972). Episodic and semantic memory. In E. Tulving & W. Donaldson (Eds.), *Organization of memory* (pp. 381–403). New York: Acacemic Press.

Tulving, E. (1983). *Elements of episodic memory.* New York: Oxford University Press.

Warrington, E. K., & Weiskrantz, L. (1974). The effect of prior learning on subsequent retention in amnesic patients. *Neuropsychologia, 12*, 419–428.

Weinstein, C. E., Duffy, M., Underwood, V. L., MacDonald, J., & Gott, S. P. (1981). Memory strategies reported by older adults for experimental and eveyday learning tasks. *Educational Gerontology, 7*, 205–213.

West, R. L. (1989). Planning practical memory training for the aged. In L. W. Poon, B. Wilson, & D. Rubin (Eds.), *Everyday cognition in adulthood and latelife* (pp. 573–579). Cambridge, England: Cambridge University Press.

West, R. L., & Tomer, A. (1989). Everyday memory problems of healthy older adults: Characteristics of a successful interven-tion. In G. C. Gilmore, P. J. Whitehouse, & M. L. Wykle (Eds.), *Memory, aging and dementia: Theory, assessment, and treatment* (pp. 74–98). New York: Springer Publishing Company.

Wilson, B. (1989). Designing memory-therapy programs. In L. W. Poon, B. Wilson, & D. Rubin (Eds.), *Everyday cognition in adulthood and latelife* (pp. 615–638). Cambridge, England: Cambridge University Press.

Wilson, B., & Moffat, N. (1984). Rehabilitation of memory for everyday life. In J. E. Harris & P. E. Morris (Eds.), *Everyday memory, actions and absent-mindedness* (pp. 207–233). London: Academic Press.

Wilson, B. A. (1992). Rehabilitation and memory disorders. In L. Squire & N. Butters (Eds.), *Neuropsychology of memory* (2nd ed., pp. 315–321). New York: Guilford.

Wilson, B. A., Baddeley, A., Evans, J., & Shiel, A. (1994). Errorless learning in the rehabilitation of memory impaired people. *Neuropsychological Rehabilitation, 4*, 307–326.

Wilson, R. S., Bacon, L. D., Fox, J. H., & Kaszniak, A. W. (1983). Primary and secondary memory in dementia of the Alzheimer type. *Journal of Clinical Neuropsychology, 5*, 337–344.

Winograd, E., & Simon, E. W. (1980). Visual memory and imagery in the aged. In L. W. Poon, J. L. Fozard, & L. S. Cermak (Eds.), *New directions in memory and aging: Proceedings of the George Talland Memorial Conference.* Hillsdale, NJ: Lawrence Erlbaum.

Worden, P. E., & Meggison, D. L. (1984). Aging and the category-recall relationship. *Journal of Gerontology, 39*, 322–324.

Yates, F. (1966). *The art of memory.* London: Routledge & Kegan Paul, Ltd.

Yesavage, J. A. (1985). Nonpharmacological treatments for memory losses with normal aging. *American Journal of Psychiatry, 142*, 600–605.

Yesavage, J. A., & Jacob, R. (1984). Effects of relaxation and mnemonics on memory, attention and anxiety in the elderly. *Experimental Aging Research, 10*, 211–214.

Yesavage, J. A., Lapp, D., & Sheikh, J. I. (1989). Mnemonics as modified for use by the elderly. In L. W. Poon, B. Wilson, & D. Rubin (Eds.), *Everyday cognition in adulthood and latelife* (pp. 598–611). Cambridge, England: Cambridge University Press.

Yesavage, J. A., & Rose, T. L. (1983). Concentration and mnemonic training in elderly subjects with memory complaints: A study of combined therapy and order effects. *Psychiatry Research, 9*, 157–167.

Yesavage, J. A., & Rose, T. L. (1984a). The effects of a face-name mnemonic in young, middle-aged, and elderly adults. *Experimental Aging Research, 10*, 55–57.

Yesavage, J. A., & Rose, T. L. (1984b). Semantic elaboration and the method of loci: A new trip for older learners. *Experimental Aging Research, 10*, 155–159.

Yesavage, J. A., Rose, T. L., & Bower, G. H. (1983). Interactive imagery and affective judgments improve face–name learning in the elderly. *Journal of Gerontolgoy, 38*, 197–203.

Yesavage, J. A., Rose, T. L, & Spiegel, D. (1982). Relaxation training and memory improvement in elderly normals: Correlation of anxiety ratings and recall improvement. *Experimental Aging Research, 8*, 195–198.

Zarit, S. H., Cole, K. D., & Guider, R. L. (1981). Memory training strategies and subjective complaints of memory in the aged. *The Gerontologist, 21,* 158–164.

Zarit, S. J., Gallagher, D., & Kramer, N. (1981). Memory training in the community aged: Effects on depression, memory complaint, and memory performance. *Educational Gerontology, 6,* 11–27.

Zarit, S. H., Zarit, J. M., & Reever, K. E. (1982). Memory training for severe memory loss: Effects on senile dementia patients and their families. *Gerontologist, 4,* 373–377.

Zelinski, E. M., Gilewski, M. J., & Thompson, L. W. (1980). Do laboratory tests relate to self-assessment of memory ability in young and old? In L. W. Poon, J. L. Fozard, L. S. Cermak, D. Arenberg, & L. W. Thompson (Eds.), *New directions in memory and aging: Proceedings of the George Talland Memorial Conference* (pp. 519–550). Hillsdale, NJ: Lawrence Erlbaum.

35

Guardianship and the Elderly

DANIEL A. KRAUSS AND BRUCE D. SALES

The increasing size and proportion of the elderly, individuals 65 and older, in the U.S. population is a well-documented trend (Fell, 1994; Friedman & Savage, 1988; Polivka, 1991; Rein, 1992; Tor, 1993). While in 1980 the elderly constituted roughly 11% of the U.S. population or 25.5 million people, in 1990 they made up 13% of the population or 31 million people, and it is projected that by the year 2030 they will represent nearly 22% of the population or 65 million people (Scogin & Perry, 1986). The 85 and older age group represents the fastest growing segment not only of the elderly population, but also of all age groups (Fell, 1994; Iris, 1988; Polivka, 1991; Smyer, 1993).

The aging of our population or "graying of America" has serious legal, psychological, and policy implications. While some aging individuals will be able to maintain physical and mental health, a disproportionate number of those 65 and older will develop physical disabilities, cognitive impairments, or both. The likelihood of experiencing these conditions also continues to increase as one reaches older ages (Smyer, 1993). For example, dementia commonly associated with Alzheimer's disease, the most common form of dementia among the elderly, is estimated to affect 1% of those ages 65 to 74, 7% of those ages 74 to 85, and over 25% of those over 85 years of age (Polivka, 1991). Many of these impairments may leave elderly individuals temporarily or chronically unable to effectively care for themselves. The chronic degenerative course of Alzheimer's disease will inevitably compromise

one's ability to exercise important decision-making skills as well as care for oneself (Marson, Schmitt, Ingram, & Harrell, 1994).

The comorbidity of mental illness and physical disability may also reduce an older individual's ability to perform activities of daily living, since the severity, duration, and recovery from a physical disability or mental illness is negatively affected by the existence of another condition. Additionally, the loss of social support and the economic changes often associated with aging predispose the elderly to both mental and physical illness and may inhibit their recovery from the illnesses or their adjustment to them (Iris, 1988; Smyer, 1993). For all these reasons, older individuals with physical and mental illnesses, more so than individuals in younger age groups, will likely experience difficulty caring for themselves, managing their money, and exercising appropriate judgment in making important life decisions.

Perhaps the most important mechanism the law has created for responding to these problems is *guardianship*—the appointment of a legal guardian by the state to care for and make decisions for an incapacitated person. Not surprisingly, the vast majority of guardian determinations involve the elderly, and as the size of the elderly population continues to grow, guardianship is likely to become an increasingly important and commonplace legal proceeding. Yet, while some elderly will benefit from the legal appointment of a guardian, the current process is fraught with errors and may do more harm than good. In this chapter we (1) describe the origins and purpose of guardianship, (2) examine recent legal reforms in guardianship, (3) highlight important psychological and neuropsychological

DANIEL A. KRAUSS AND BRUCE D. SALES • Department of Psychology, University of Arizona, Tucson, Arizona 85721.

assessment issues in guardianship proceedings, and (4) suggest a reconceptualization of guardianship assessment and of the institution of guardianship.

Guardianship

Origin and Purpose

Guardianship involves the appointment by the court of an individual, the *guardian*, to control the finances of, make important decisions for, and monitor the self-care skills of a person, the *ward*, who is deemed not to possess the legal competency to perform these tasks for himself or herself. A legal guardian, then, is an individual "lawfully invested with the power, and charged with the duty of, taking care of the person and managing the property and rights of another who ... is considered incapable of managing his/her own affairs." (Black's Law Dictionary, 1990, p. 488). In the majority of guardianship hearings, the petitioner for guardianship, the person who brings the potential ward's inabilities to the attention of the court and seeks guardianship responsibilities, is a family member. In guardianship hearings involving the elderly, a family member (a spouse, child, or grandchild of the ward) is most commonly appointed by the court as guardian (Fell, 1994; Friedman & Savage, 1988; Melton, Petrila, Poythress, & Slobogin, 1987; Tor, 1993; Tor & Sales, 1996).

This delegation by the state of a ward's rights to the guardian is justified under the *parens patriae* doctrine. Parens patriae literally means parent of the country, and this doctrine was traditionally used to allow the state to act as a legal parent to protect the interests of those who were unable to protect themselves. Children and the insane were among those presumed to lack the competency to perform a number of different and necessary functions, and consequently, the state allowed a parent or an appointed guardian to act on their behalf. Today, the law presumes that adults are legally competent until proven otherwise. In the guardianship context, this means that the individual petitioning the court for guardianship bears the burden of proving that an individual is incapable of performing self-care and/or financial duties (Sacks, 1994).

Importance of Autonomy and Its Health Implications

At its heart, a guardianship determination involves balancing an individual's right to autonomy and self-determination with state-sponsored paternalism (Fell, 1994). The right to make important life decisions, even if it seems foolish to others, is one of our culture's most sacred and protected rights (Rein, 1992). This control over one's life is removed, however, once the court ascertains that a legal guardian is appropriate. Once appointed, the legal guardian gains the power to determine what are reasonable choices for his or her ward. It is important to note that this loss of control and autonomy may be quite substantial and might produce outcomes which are not comparable to that which individuals might choose for themselves. Studies have shown that guardians do not tend to make the same decisions as their wards in many instances, even when they are explicitly told to attempt to mirror their judgment (Melton et al., 1987).

Furthermore, the ward's loss of control and autonomy may have significant health implications (Fell, 1994; Rodin, 1986). Research has shown that actual control or a sense of control is an important determinant of the physical and mental health of the elderly, and that a loss of control adversely affects many individuals' health (Rodin, 1986). Therefore, the actual or perceptual loss of rights associated with guardianship could have a substantial negative impact on the physical and mental health of an elderly ward.

Guardianships in Practice

While every state recognizes a legal mechanism for the appointment of a legal guardian for individuals who are unable to care for themselves or manage their property (Grisso, 1986; Sacks, 1994), each state has it own requirements for the appointment of a guardian. All 50 states and the District of Columbia have promulgated their own statutory definitions of guardianship (Parry & Hurme, 1991; Thomas, 1994; Tor, 1993; Weiler, Helms, & Buckwalter, 1993). In addition, some jurisdictions further differentiate between *guardianship*, in which an individual is legally given power over only a ward's self-care needs, and *conservatorship*, in which an individual is legally designated to act only in financial matters. In contrast, other jurisdictions use one term, guardianship or conservatorship, to refer to both conditions (Fell, 1994; Iris, 1988; Parry & Hurme, 1991; Tor, 1993; Tor & Sales, 1996; Weiler et al., 1993). In this chapter, guardianship will refer to proceedings in which guardians are appointed to perform financial and/or self-care needs for incompetent persons. Conversely, *competency* refers to the legal capacity of an individual to perform certain actions (Grisso, 1986; Marson et al., 1994; Melton et al., 1987).

There are two types of guardianship: (1) full or plenary guardianship and (2) limited guardianship. By far the most common, full guardianship permits the guardian to exercise control over all the ward's personal and financial interests. A limited guardianship, on the other hand, recognizes specific areas in which the ward is incapable of performing tasks adequately and allows the guardian control over these areas (Parry & Hurme, 1991; Sacks, 1994; Tor, 1993; Tor & Sales, 1996). For example, a mildly demented individual might be fully capable of handling his personal care, but unable to manage his complex financial matters. In this case, a judge might appoint a limited guardian to maintain control only over financial concerns while the ward would still control decisions relevant to his or her care. This is an unusual case, however; judges consistently fail to approve anything other than plenary guardianships even when it is clearly appropriate to do so (Friedman & Savage, 1988; Keith & Wacker, 1993).

The appointment of a plenary guardian necessarily removes a ward's right to manage his or her property and care for himself or herself. In addition, a successful full guardianship adjudication can also produce the concomitant loss of other significant rights, including the right to marry, drive an automobile, contract, choose a residence, and make medical treatment decisions (Fell, 1994; Hommel, Wang, & Bergman, 1990; Melton et al., 1987). These restrictions go well beyond financial management and self-care and are serious infringements on a ward's autonomy and right to make important life decisions. One commentator has noted that the appointment of a plenary guardian leaves a ward with less rights than a convicted felon (Rein, 1992), while another remarked that full guardianships could be

viewed as "institutionalization without walls" (Tor & Sales, 1996).

Legal Reforms in Guardianship

For some time, guardianship and guardianship proceedings have come under increased scrutiny and have been soundly criticized by scholars (Anderer, 1990; Hurme, 1991; Massad & Sales, 1981; Melton et al., 1987; Rein, 1992; Sales et al., 1982; Scogin & Perry, 1986; Smyer, 1993; Tor, 1993; Tor & Sales, 1996). As a legal proceeding that involves the potential loss of significant autonomy and civil rights, guardianship determinations have been characterized as having too few procedural protections for the participants, vague statutory standards, and an overreliance on medical testimony (Anderer, 1990). Scogin and Perry (1986) succinctly noted that guardianship hearings have been rubber stamp procedures in which guardianship was too easily obtained, too restrictive, and too difficult to revoke.

As a result of the criticism leveled against guardianship practices, many states have made substantial changes in both the procedural due process protections afforded to the proposed ward and the substantive statutory definitions contained in guardianship laws. Although it is beyond the scope of this chapter to discuss them all, a number of the more important changes will be highlighted (for an excellent review, see Hommel et al., 1990).

Criticism and Reform of Legal Procedures

Traditional guardianship adjudications were characterized by: (1) limited or no notice to the proposed ward concerning the hearing. Notice is supposed to alert the ward of the hearing, explain the purpose of the hearing, describe the rights that might be lost as a result of the hearing, and describe the ward's rights to contest allegations in petition; (2) absence of the proposed ward at the hearing; (3) failure of the proposed ward to have appointed counsel; (4) appointment of counsel that acts as a *guardian ad litem*, an individual that represents the best interest of the client rather than the actual interest of the client (it is believed by many lawyers that guardianship is in the best interest of the client);

(5) relaxed evidentiary standards. Evidence was allowed that would be prohibited from use in most other legal cases; (6) conclusory guardianship petitions simply reciting the guardianship statute rather than presenting specific reasons why guardianship should be granted; and (7) limited cross-examination of witnesses (Melton et al., 1987).

Consequently, most guardianship hearings were uncontested, nonadversarial determinations in which the proposed ward was not even present, no evidence was presented against guardianship, no one represented the proposed ward's interests, and full (plenary) guardianship was granted. These proceedings allowed a significant deprivation of an individual's liberties with limited procedural protection.

To make matters worse, review and revocation of guardianship was nonexistent (Nolan, 1984). Once guardianship was granted by the court it was unlikely that the ward would ever regain important rights. In subsequent hearings, the burden of proving that he or she no longer needed a guardian fell to the ward. Meeting this burden of proof was nearly impossible. Because the original guardianship hearing contained so little evidence, any judge reviewing the case later would have little knowledge as to why the original guardianship had been granted and, therefore, no means by which to determine if it was still necessary (Keith & Wacker, 1993).

Today, as the result of reforms, many state guardianship statutes now mandate (1) express notice of an upcoming hearing to the proposed ward, (2) the presence of the proposed ward at the hearing, (3) the appointment of counsel for the ward, and (4) a specific statement of evidence that supports guardianship for the proposed ward (Hommel et al., 1990; Keith & Wacker, 1993). Yet, even with these procedural changes, guardianship continues to be granted in over 90% of cases, and many of these procedural protections continue not to be followed (Keith & Wacker, 1993; Rein, 1992). Further, a recent study has found that the only factor that reliably leads to limited guardianship or to successfully challenging guardianship is the ward's hiring of his or her own lawyer (Keith & Wacker, 1993). Conversely, the appointment of counsel was determined to increase the likelihood of guardianship being granted because appointed counsel continues to act as a guardian ad litem, rather than

advocating against the imposition of guardianship (Keith & Wacker, 1993).

Criticism and Reforms of the Substantive Basis of Guardianship

As previously mentioned, all states have promulgated their own guardianship statutes and requirements for guardianship. The substantive basis for the imposition of guardianship can be categorized as causal, decisional, or functional (Tor, 1993; Tor & Sales, 1996).

Causal Statutes

Causal or traditional guardianship statutes equate financial, personal, and decisional incompetency with mental or physical labels attached to the proposed ward. In these statutes, the mere presence of the label of a mental or physical disability is enough to justify the finding of legal incompetency and the need for a guardian (Tor & Sales, 1996). In essence, traditional guardianship statutes are classification-oriented—all individuals with a particular mental or physical condition are appropriate for full guardianship (Tor & Sales, 1996). These traditional standards suffer from a multitude of faults. Probably the most glaring error of traditional statutes is that no evidence is necessary that an alleged condition adversely affects the proposed ward's abilities to perform activities of daily living that underlie his or her need for a guardian. These conditions were assumed to, rather than proven to, affect a ward's ability to care for himself or herself, manage his or her finances and property, and make important decisions (Tor & Sales, 1996). In fact, many statutes contain "old age" as a legitimate category for the appointment of a guardian.

Further, traditional statutes fail to recognize both variability within a specific disease or disability and variability in individual reactions to mental illness and disability. For example, an individual in the early stages of dementia commonly associated with Alzheimer's disease might need little if any help in managing the tasks of daily living while an individual with advanced dementia might be incapable of performing any of these tasks. Further, an individual with ample social and economic support is often able to cope with many physical and mental disabilities better than one who lacks such advantages (Fell, 1994; Nolan, 1984; Smyer, 1993).

Decisional Statutes

Following harsh criticism by scholars of causal guardianship statutes, many states adopted decisional statutes that use a formulation proposed by the Uniform Probate Code (UPC). In these statutory schemes, the term "incompetency" was replaced by "incapacitation" in order to remove the stigmatization that was thought to be associated with incompetence and connote the limited, potentially transitory nature of the impairment (Tor & Sales, 1996). Yet, incapacitation can be associated with many of the same mental and physical conditions that were included in traditional statutes, such as mental illness, mental deficiency, physical illness or disability, *advanced age*, chronic use of drugs, chronic intoxication, or other cause (Hommel et al., 1990).

These new statutes also adopted a decisional definition of incapacity: An incapacitated person is one who lacks "sufficient understanding or capacity to make or communicate responsible decisions concerning his person" (Tor & Sales, 1996, Uniform Probate Code 5-103(7)(Suppl. 1993). The use of the terms "understanding," "communicate," and "responsible decisions" highlights the UPC-based guardianship statute's emphasis on the link between mental and physical conditions and decision-making ability. Unfortunately, although appropriate decision-making is one important aspect of evaluating the need for a guardian, it does not encompass the ward's other behaviors that justify the granting of a guardianship. Specifically, these statutes do not mention the ability to care for oneself and manage one's finances which can also justify the imposition of a guardian by the court. In addition, under these statutes, plenary guardians could be appointed for mildly demented persons who are decisionally impaired, but who are fully capable of performing self-care tasks. In other words, under the UPC standard, wards could lose important rights (i.e., right to marry, right to live outside an institution, etc.) through a legal proceeding that does not expressly address their ability to perform these functions.

Finally, UPC-based guardianship standards also fail to clarify what constitutes "reasonable decisions" or "understanding." Without concrete guidelines for these terms, judges are likely to make these determinations in accord with their own beliefs or defer to expert testimony. Psychologists, psychiatrists, and neuropsychologists are identically challenged in evaluating an individual's ability to make decisions. No score on a mental status exam or on any other psychological device, in and of itself, should be used to determine if an individual makes reasonable decisions (Marson et al., 1994). As a consequence of their lack of clarity, UPC-based guardianships decisions will necessarily be inconsistent from one jurisdiction to another, one judge to another, and one mental health expert to another.

Functional Statutes

In attempting to alleviate many of the problems associated with both causal and decisional guardianship statutes, a growing number of states have adopted statutes that emphasize a ward's actual behavioral or functional inabilities or incapacities. Functional guardianship statutes, therefore, focus on what actions and behaviors a ward may not be able to perform, rather than solely upon what conditions a potential ward suffers from or the potential ward's capacity to make "reasonable" decisions. Functional statutes list crucial, specific activities of daily living and financial management in their statutory definitions (Nolan, 1984). For example, the District of Columbia's guardianship statute specifies that individuals not able to "meet essential requirements for physical health and safety" are those individuals who are incapable of undertaking actions necessary "to provide health care, food, shelter, clothing, personal hygiene, and other care without which serious physical injury is more likely than not to occur" (DC Code 21-2011 (16)).

Functional guardianship statutes also have the potential to be more ecologically valid than either causal or UPC guardianship statutes. That is, they can ask how effectively a proposed ward performs concrete, everyday skills in his or her actual environment (Tor, 1993). Functional skills are the manifest abilities or inabilities that underlie the need for a legal guardian. Mental illness and physical disability might increase the probability that individuals cannot perform important life activities, but these conditions, by themselves, do not necessitate that these tasks and activities cannot be adequately accomplished.

Functional statutes also have been praised for recognizing the possibility of partial incapacitation, using more objective criteria, and emphasizing ecological validity in assessments and guardianship judgments (Anderer, 1990; Tor, 1993). Under a functional statute, it is possible and likely that a proposed ward could be found to be incapable of performing some specific tasks, but not others. For example, a proposed ward could be unable to obtain adequate health care, but could be able to provide for his or her own shelter, clothing, and hygiene. These specific criteria and findings afford the judge guidelines to tailor and limit the guardianship to the needs of each individual (Nolan, 1984).

The use of objective criteria also improves the guardianship process in a number of ways. Objective and specified criteria promote consistency in judicial decision-making by constraining judges to make decisions based on requirements expressly contained in statutes, rather than based on their own beliefs about reasonable decision-making, financial management, and personal care (Tor, 1993). Explicit requirements also help mental health practitioners offer more focused, pragmatic, and empirically valid opinions about a potential ward's abilities. At least in theory, functional assessments are more consistent with the expertise and training of a subset of mental health practitioners. Gerontologists, geriatric nurses, social workers, occupational therapists, psychologists, and physicians all have experience with and are specifically trained to assess the functional deficits of patients (Nolan, 1984). Consequently, they are prepared to offer more directly relevant and more "expert" opinions in functional guardianship proceedings.

Functionalization of guardianship criteria could and should also lead to the development of specific assessment instruments that are designed to incorporate the skills contained within functional guardianship statutes and that reliably and validly measure them. This in turn should lead to more accurate expert opinions, because they will at least be partially based on an objective instrument rather than a practitioner's subjective beliefs about incapacitation. The development of standardized instruments could also aid in promoting even greater consistency in judicial decision-making (Tor, 1993). Cutoff scores, scores that signify a statistically significant deviation from the norm for an age group, could be calculated for the different skills pertinent to guardianship. This information could be used to help determine the severity of a deficit and determine at what levels a deficit might warrant guardianship.

Parenthetically, it should be noted that the development of standardized guardianship assessment instruments has already begun. The Community Competency Scale developed by Loeb (1983) is a 16-scale assessment instrument designed specifically to target the skills and abilities contained in guardianship statutes (Grisso, 1986; Melton et al., 1987; Schwartz & Barone, 1992). It is not designed with one specific functional guardianship statute in mind, however, but is based on expert opinions on what skills should be assessed in any guardianship proceeding (Grisso, 1986; Melton et al., 1987; Schwartz & Barone, 1992).

Although functional statutes are a considerable improvement over causal and decisional standards, they could potentially increase the number of individuals for whom guardianship might be sought. Using this approach, many older individuals who suffer from no discernible disease or definable disorder could be found to lack the explicitly defined personal self-care skills, financial management skills, or appropriate decision-making skills, and thereby, deemed to require a guardian. If these individuals, however, are truly incapable of performing important tasks, a guardianship, if adequately tailored and limited, could be beneficial to them.

Yet, functional statutes still pose significant problems for both legal and psychological professions. Statutory reforms and objective requirements are well and good in theory, but if in practice the legal system continues to treat guardianship as a nonadversarial, rubber stamp process, they will have little impact. In the same vein, explicitly specifying the skills and abilities that compose guardianship serves little point if courts continue to be unwilling to take the time and effort to grant limited guardianships and adapt them to the strengths and weaknesses of the proposed ward. Unfortunately, this is a recurring problem (Tor & Sales, 1996).

Perhaps the gravest problem with functional

statutes is that they fail to link functional incapacities to their cause and remediations. Without specifying why or knowing why proposed wards cannot adequately perform certain activities, it is impossible to limit the guardianship to the appropriate degree. For example, there are a multitude of reasons why a given individual might be unable to manage his or her finances effectively (e.g., impaired short-term memory, lack of mathematical training, or dementia). Each of these possibilities should have different implications for the appointment of a guardian. Thus, before guardianship is granted, questions such as the following need to answered: What is the cause(s) of the deficit?; Is training likely to improve the skill?; What type of training is appropriate?; Is the deficit likely to be transitory, stable, or progressive?; Is greater social support likely to affect the deficit?; Has the individual developed any adaptations to cope with the problem?; Can any adaptations be developed that can effectively remedy the problem without guardianship? In sum, functional guardianship statutes alone cannot solve the problems associated with guardianship.

Psychological and Neuropsychological Guardianship Assessment Issues

Perhaps the largest nonlegal problem for the successful implementation of functional guardianship statutes and causal and decisional statutes as well are the assessments of prospective and adjudicated wards. Psychological and neuropsychological assessments conducted for the courts present a number of fundamental difficulties for both psychological and legal practitioners. Not the least of these problems is that legal definitions are not intended to and do not directly correspond to psychological constructs, assessment instruments, and nomenclature (Anderer, 1990; Grisso, 1986; Marson et al., 1994; Melton et al., 1987). For example, in the criminal context, the legal definition of "insanity" does not accurately reflect any particular mental illness. Consequently, labeling a defendant as "psychotic," "paranoid schizophrenic," or as "borderline" does not effectively answer the question of whether the defendant is legally insane. Analogously, the determination of mental illness does not

directly substitute for a decision about legal competency or incompetency (Appelbaum & Grisso, 1995a; Grisso, 1986; Marson et al., 1994; Melton et al., 1987). In Appelbaum and Grisso's (1995a,b,c) study of competency of the mentally ill to make treatment decisions, they found that over 50% of schizophrenics and 76% of those considered to be clinically depressed were judged legally competent to make hypothetical treatment decisions.

Conversely, the majority of psychological and neuropsychological assessment instruments were not designed to address legal questions (Grisso, 1986; Marson et al., 1994). As a result, a specific verbal IQ score on the Wechsler Adult Intelligence Scale-Revised (WAIS-R) does not resolve the question of whether an individual is legally competent to stand trial. That is not to say that the results obtained by psychological diagnosis and assessment techniques cannot contribute to the determination of legal questions, but rather that these findings alone should not be portrayed as providing scientific answers to legal questions.

In fact, Grisso (1986) argues that a complete translation and operationalization of legal concepts into psychological constructs may not be possible, because legal decisions necessarily involve a value and normative judgment by the court, which no mechanical, psychological formulation can ever approximate. Following this logic, a standardized guardianship assessment instrument can never replace the traditional hearing process because the judge, not the scientist, must decide at what level an incapacitation becomes great enough to warrant guardianship. Again, this does not mean that the attempted operationalization and objective measurement of legal standards is useless. Rather, it means that this measurement process should be viewed as a way to enhance and inform judicial decision-making.

Beyond the general assessment problems, psychological assessment for guardianship also presents a number of specific assessment concerns. First, guardianship involves the assessment of a legal competency or incapacitation. Competency and capacity assessments require the examiner to predict future abilities or inabilities based on an interview and other behavioral samples conducted at a particular time and place. The assessor is called upon to predict how a proposed ward will in the future take care of himself or herself, manage his or her financial affairs, and make decisions. This determination must be based on the potential ward's self-report, the impressions of his or her friends and relatives, and the evaluator's own assessment. Unfortunately, behavioral incapacities are not static (Anderer, 1990), but vary over time depending on a multitude of factors, including the potential ward's environment, social support, mood, health, and self-efficacy beliefs. These factors make the accurate prediction of future behavioral incapacities extremely difficult, although this problem could be attenuated somewhat by frequent reassessment and more active reviews of guardianship arrangements.

Second, as previously mentioned, functional guardianship assessment involves the evaluation of a number of divergent skills. Assessing whether a proposed ward has self-care skills, financial management skills, and decisional skills may be extremely time-consuming and beyond the expertise of one individual. A geriatric nurse or an occupational therapist may be the most qualified assessor of self-care skills, while a neuropsychologist might be a more appropriate assessor of decisional capabilities. One potential solution to this problem is the development of integrated interdisciplinary assessment teams (Hafemeister & Sales, 1984).

Third, the psychological or neuropsychological assessment of decision-making is a difficult task. It is not clear what level of mental or logical dysfunction is necessary to legally constitute a decisional impairment. At the two extremes this assessment seems relatively easy. A "normal" individual should be able to make decisions for himself or herself, while someone in the last stages of dementia commonly associated with Alzheimer's disease clearly does not have this capability. Yet, individuals who have moderate degrees of cognitive impairment represent a more difficult problem for the legal system and assessors.

In the informed consent context, Roth, Meisel, and Lidz (1977) have suggested a decisional hierarchy of competency. This same order was used by Appelbaum and Grisso (1995a,b,c) in their study of competency of the mentally disordered to make treatment decisions. It seems appropriate to also use their structure in the assessment of decision-making for guardianship (Anderer, 1990). At the lowest level of the hierarchy is the ability of an individual

to communicate a choice. At this level, if individuals can simply express a choice, then they are competent. The second level of competency requires that the individual make a choice consistent with a reasonable person in similar circumstances, that is, the individual's choice seems reasonable to others. To reach the third level, an individual must show that he or she appreciates the consequences of his or her decision. At the fourth level, an individual must exhibit the capacity to make decisions based on rational reasons—that is, the ability to use logical processes to compare alternatives and weigh them effectively to reach a decision. Finally, at the fifth or highest level, individuals must show that they can choose based on an "understanding" of the situation and possible alternatives. In assessing treatment competency, this was operationalized by testing whether an individual was able to remember important words and phrases, comprehend the essential nature of important information, and state the sequence of events that would occur with treatment (Appelbaum & Grisso, 1988).

This framework has already been used by Marson et al. (1994) to assess competency to make treatment decisions in cognitively normal elderly patients, mildly demented Alzheimer's patients, and moderately demented Alzheimer's patients. Marson et al. (1994) found that normal elderly adults performed better than both Alzheimer's groups on the highest two decisional levels, and that the mildly demented Alzheimer's patients also achieved significantly higher scores than the moderately demented Alzheimer's patients on the two highest decision levels. The normal elderly group also obtained higher scores than the moderately demented Alzheimer's group, but did not score higher than the mildly impaired Alzheimer's group on the third level of the decisional hierarchy.

This study and its results have a number of important implications for guardianship. The decisional levels proposed by Roth, Meisel, and Lidz (1977) seem to offer a quantifiable means of assessing individuals' decision-making abilities. This framework could then allow the court to choose what level of decision-making ability is appropriate for different legal decisions.

Another implication is that in addition to the different hierarchical levels reflecting different levels of cognitive functioning (i.e., the cognitively normal elderly participants were able to outperform the mildly and moderately demented Alzheimer's patients, and the mildly demented Alzheimer's patients were able to outperform the moderately demented Alzheimer's patients), they also reflect different types and levels of physiological dysfunction (Marson et al., 1994). The linking of decisional impairment with physiological deficits would lead to more appropriate guardianships by forcing the guardianship order to be limited to specified deficits. This limitation would, in turn, focus the guardian's training and remediation of the ward on these deficits, and consequently, lead to a better chance of the ward's recovery of these functional abilities. To accomplish this goal, the decisional levels could be compared to scores on a standardized neuropsychology battery to determine which neuropsychological inabilities relate to difficulties with different decisional levels. Once the relationship between neuropsychological deficits and decisional levels is established, existing literature on neuropsychological incapacities could be used to reach treatment, remediation, coping, and guardianship decisions.

Rein (1992) has suggested that the level of decisional ability an individual must evidence may differ as a function of the importance of the decision. Using this schema, instead of stating that individuals are decisionally impaired, a psychological or neuropsychological assessor would describe the levels at which individuals perform adequately and at which they exhibit deficits. Using this information, the onus of determining if the decisional impairment is sufficient enough to warrant a guardian would fall on the court and not the assessor.

A fourth specific problem with guardianship evaluations is that they are confounded by both the proposed ward's affective state and characteristics of the disease process. Many elderly persons suffer from depression—the second most common mental illness among the elderly (the first is dementia)—and from the concomitant decline in accomplishing self-care tasks, managing their finances, and engaging in adequate decision-making (Smyer, 1993). While partial paralysis caused by a stroke might impair an individual's personal self-care, the depression commonly associated with this illness may further reduce these skills and induce significant decisional deficits. Depression has also been found to lower individuals' scores on a wide variety of psychological assessment instruments (La Rue, 1992). Consequently, it is incumbent on a guardianship evaluator to determine if depression is present, what effects if any it has on the evaluation, the amenability of the depression to treatment, and the likely change in the individual's abilities with proper treatment.

Chronic progressive illnesses also present difficulties for guardianship evaluators. The most chronic form of dementia in the elderly, Alzheimer's disease, has an extremely variable course but inevitably leads to incompetency (Marson et al., 1994). Because guardianship decisions are generally not reviewed regularly (or at all) (Keith & Wacker, 1993; Tor & Sales, 1996), an evaluator may be tempted to suggest, or a court might grant, full guardianship when it is not necessary at the time of the hearing but will likely be necessary sometime in the future. A more appropriate course of action would be for the evaluator to explain to the court the problems associated with degenerative illness, to make an assessment of the individual's current functioning, and to ask the court to require periodic review of the guardianship arrangements, making changes when appropriate.

Fifth, the lack of the use of standardized assessment instruments by guardianship evaluators has important implications. As already noted, only one instrument has been designed specifically to assess the need for guardianship. As a result, the skills assessed by commonly used evaluation techniques (e.g., intelligence tests) may not be appropriate for guardianship determinations (Grisso, 1986). These instruments frequently lack appropriate standardization and age-appropriate norms (La Rue, 1992). This makes it impossible to determine if a potential elderly ward is actually performing skills less adequately than other individuals of the same age.

Sixth, and finally, the one standardized instrument* developed for guardianship proceedings, the Community Competency Scale (Loeb, 1983), which does provide a convenient summarization of skills associated with guardianship, cannot explain why

---

*There are other instruments that are available for use in guardianship assessments. These are not considered in this chapter because they were not specifically designed to evaluate the skills associated with guardianship (e.g., Kane & Kane, 1981).

the deficits that it records exist. Without knowing what is causing an individual's incapacitation, the court is not capable of limiting and tailoring the guardianship adequately. Further, this instrument reviews a multitude of skills in short period of time—within 60–90 min (Grisso, 1986; Melton et al., 1987; Schwartz & Barone, 1992). As a consequence, scores obtained on these instruments might not accurately reflect how individuals perform these skills in their home environment (when they are not being watched) and over extended periods of time.

A New Conceptualization for the Guardianship Standard

A new emphasis on functional incapacities and the need for more objective assessment criteria are, and will be, important developments for the appropriate administration of guardianships. Yet, they are only part of the solution to the current problems. For example, Smyer (1993) and Anderer (1990) have argued that guardianship requires a three-level analysis: (1) A mental illness or physical disability must be linked to (2) a decisional impairment, and this decisional impairment or the original disorder must be causally related to (3) observable functional impairments. They contend that without this causal analysis, guardianship cannot be limited effectively. Following the logic of Smyer and Anderer, guardianship orders should be disorder- and behavior-specific. Mental illnesses and physical disabilities tend to affect decisional and other abilities differently. A stroke might have a significant impact on an individual's ability to perform self-care tasks while having lesser or minimal effects on an individual's capacity to make decisions. Limited guardianships that mandate remediation, coping, and training for wards may be appropriate answers to incapacities caused by some disorders and inappropriate answers for others. Similarly, some illnesses are likely to cause transitory incapacitation for which a time- and skill-limited guardianship would be beneficial. On the other hand, chronic degenerative illness may require guardianship orders that are subject to frequent review, reanalysis, modification, and extension.

Grisso (1986) has advocated an even more complex framework for the analysis of guardian-ship and other legal assessments. Grisso's formulations focus on (1) functional impairment (observable and measurable behaviors that the individual can and cannot accomplish); (2) context (the specific situations in which these behaviors must be performed); (3) causal link (the origins, stability, and probability of remediation of the deficits); (4) interaction (the discrepancy between the functional abilities and the environmental demands); and (5) judgment (the legal decision when the discrepancy between demands and environment is sufficiently great to warrant action). As opposed to the Smyer and Anderer framework, Grisso's structure highlights the importance of additional, individual-specific factors to be considered in guardianship evaluation. An evaluation of "context" and "interaction" can and should incorporate knowledge of a given individual's social support, economic stability, coping skills, and self-efficacy beliefs. Without weighing these factors, guardianships are likely to be poorly tailored to an individual's needs.

While Smyer, Anderer, and Grisso present more effective analysis strategies for determining the need for guardianship and its appropriate scope, the most prominent deficiency may lie in its conceptualization. The notion that one hearing should determine an individual's incapacities in three distinct and largely unrelated areas is ill conceived. Although decision-making is an overlapping component of both financial management and self-care, there are a number of decision-making skills that exist apart from the financial and self-care components of guardianship. Decisions such as the right to marry, choose a residence, consent to medical treatment, participate in research, compose a will, or create a living will can be taken from a ward when guardianship is granted.

In addition, decision-making can itself represent a functional impairment. An individual may be able to perform specified functions appropriately for an assessment, but a decisional deficit could indicate that the individual will not be able to perform these functions adequately in a different environment or in the future. Therefore, without a separate decisional assessment, a subset of individuals who are in need of a guardian would remain undetected. Finally, evaluating decision-making entails different assessors and assessment techniques than other aspects of guardianship.

In the interest of preserving the autonomy of potential wards (and possibly their psychological and physical health), one solution might be to dissolve guardianship into its components and mandate that distinct findings be delineated. These findings should be defined using disorder-specific behavioral information relevant to each category of behaviors that the court wishes to restrict. As previously mentioned, the Roth, Meisel, and Lidz (1977) decisional hierarchy might be one appropriate method to determine if an individual exhibits a sufficient level of cognitive impairment to require decisional guardianship for each disorder-specific behavior. Furthermore, multidisciplinary assessments (Hafemeister & Sales, 1984) should be required. Although a neuropsychologist is probably the most qualified to assess decisional skills, a geriatric nurse, a gerontologist, or an occupational therapist is likely better qualified to evaluate functional impairments that characterize the other aspects of guardianship.

Another alternative might be to expressly remove from a guardian's powers the decision-making aspects that do not relate to the ward's personal self-care and financial management. Thus, the ward's rights to consent to medical treatment or to marry, for example, would no longer be under the auspices of an appointed guardian. The ability of a ward to make each of these decisions would have to be decided as the need arose in separate hearings. This solution may be expensive and inefficient, but it would also protect a ward from losing rights that were not specifically addressed in a guardianship hearing and/or which relate to unimpaired abilities. Although not relating directly to decisional rights, one state, North Dakota, explicitly prohibits the guardian from making substituted judgments on behalf of the ward in regard to certain rights (to vote, to marry, to drive a car, or to testify) unless a specific finding is made by a court. Similarly, certain decisional rights could also require a specific finding by the court.

Beyond recognizing the importance of decisional abilities, mandating separate hearings or distinct findings would also serve to focus the proceedings more accurately on appropriate skills or deficits. The skills underlying each area would likely receive more direct attention, and the determinations of the court would likely be more individualized. Although these hearings would be more time-consuming, they would substantially increase the probability that "limited" guardianship was the rule rather than the exception. These distinct hearings would force the courts to start with a "limited" guardianship in one area and adjudicate other areas only if necessary.

Conclusions and Future Directions

It must be recognized that even if sufficient information is obtained to address the proposed ward's competency in limited domains, the legal system might still be unwilling to make limited guardianships the norm. Determining whether insufficient analysis and information causes the predominance of full guardianship or whether some aspect of the legal system causes this problem are empirical questions that still need to be addressed. For example, even with detailed information about prospective wards, courts often have too little time and resources to consider this information when fashioning, monitoring, and reviewing guardianship orders.

On the other hand, even if courts maintain their present notions of guardianship, the proceedings and decisions can be made more beneficial to the participants in a variety of ways. Legally, the courts could more effectively enforce due process requirements such as notice, presence of the proposed ward at the hearing, representation by counsel, increased evidentiary standards, and elimination of boilerplate statements in petitions for guardianship. Researchers also could determine which of these factors or other factors or approaches (e.g., pre-hearing negotiation conferences) might lead to more limited guardianships.

Additionally, all states should consider a new type of guardianship—one that explicitly incorporates disorder evaluations in the context of specific behavioral domains. Researchers could then design instruments to objectively assess the decision-making and behavioral skills expressed in these statutes which would improve psychological and neuropsychological assessments of guardianship. At a minimum, however, appropriate evaluations for guardianship hearings should be at least based on the Grisso framework. In addition to specifying what functional impairments exist, the assessors should highlight (1) the causal relationship between the impairment and any disorders (including the likely stability, progression, and amenability to treatment and remediation of both the disorder and the decisional and behavioral deficits); (2) the context in which the functional deficits exist; and (3) the interaction between an individual's coping skills, economic support, and social support as well as the demands of the individual's environment. This differentiation may require separate assessment techniques and the recognition that one evaluator may not be able to effectively address all three issues.

Finally, and perhaps most importantly, the legal system must realize, and psychologists must try to communicate, that guardianship involves very significant autonomy and self-determination issues. Full guardianships based on rubber stamp procedures and granted out of well-meaning benevolence are unlikely to be in the actual interest of the participants. Unnecessary revocation of important rights may well do more harm than good. Physical and psychological health are likely to be damaged by overextensive guardianship orders. Guardianship should be a beneficial alternative to institutionalization for the elderly rather than simply institutionalization without walls.

References

Anderer, S. J. (1990). A model for determining competency in guardianship proceedings. *Mental and Physical Disability Law Reporter, 14,* 107–114.

Appelbaum, P., & Grisso, T. (1988). Assessing patient's capacity to consent to treatment. *New England Journal of Medicine, 319,* 1635–1638.

Appelbaum, P., & Grisso, T. (1995a). The MacArthur treatment study I. *Law and Human Behavior, 19,* 105–126.

Appelbaum, P., & Grisso, T. (1995b). The MacArthur treatment study II. *Law and Human Behavior, 19,* 127–148.

Appelbaum, P., & Grisso, T. (1995c). The MacArthur treatment study III. *Law and Human Behavior, 19,* 149–174.

Black's Law Dictionary. (6th ed.). (1990). St. Paul, MN: West Publishing Company.

Fell, N. (1994). Guardianship and the elderly: Oversight notoverlooked. *University of Toledo Law Review, 25,* 189–204.

Friedman, L., & Savage, M. (1988). Taking care of the law of conservatorship in California. *University of Southern California Law Review, 61,* 273–290.

Grisso, T. (1986). *Evaluating competencies, forensic assessments and instruments.* New York: Plenum Press.

Hafemeister, T., & Sales, B. (1984). Interdisciplinary evaluations for guardianship. *Law and Human Behavior, 8,* 335.

Hommel, P., Wang, L., & Bergman, J. (1990). Trends in guardianship reform: Implications for the medical and legal professions. *Law, Medicine, and Health Care, 18,* 213–220.

Hurme, S. B. (1991). *Steps to enhance guardianship monitoring.* Washington, DC: American Bar Association Commission on the Legal Problems of the Elderly.

Iris, M. (1988). Guardianship and the elderly: A multiperspective view of the decision-making process. *The Gerontologist, 28*(Suppl.), 39–45.

Kane, R., & Kane, R. (1981). *Assessing the elderly: A practical guide to measurement.* Lexington, MA: Lexington Books.

Keith, P. M., & Wacker, R. R. (1993). Guardianship practices and outcomes of hearings for older persons. *The Gerontologist, 33,* 81–87.

La Rue, A. (1992). *Aging and neuropsychological assessment.* New York: Plenum Press.

Loeb, P. A. (1983). *Validity of the Community Competency Scale with the elderly.* Unpublished doctoral dissertation, St. Louis University.

Marson, D. C., Schmitt, F., Ingram, K., & Harrell, L. (1994). Determining the competency of Alzheimer's patient to consent to treatment and research. *Alzheimer's Diseases and Associated Disorders Supplement, 8,* 5–18.

Massad, P. M., & Sales, B. D. (1981). Guardianship and deinstitutionalization. *American Behavioral Scientist, 24,* 755–770.

Melton, G., Petrila, J., Poythress, N., & Slobogin, C. (1987). *Psychological evaluations for the courts.* New York: Guilford Press.

Nolan, B. S. (1984). Functional evaluations of the elderly in guardianship evaluations. *Law, Medicine, and Health Care, 12,* 210–217.

Parry, J. W., & Hurme, S. B. (1991). Guardianship monitoring and enforcement nationwide. *Mental and Physical Disability Law Reporter, 15,* 304–309.

Polivka, L. (1991). In Florida the future is now: Aging issues and policies in the 1990's. *Florida State University Law Review, 18,* 401–436.

Rein, J. E. (1992). Preserving dignity and self-determination of the elderly in the face of competing interests and grim alternatives: A proposal for statutory refocus and reform. *George Washington Law Review, 60,* 1810–1887.

Rodin, J. (1986). Aging and health: Effects of the sense of control. *Science, 233,* 1271–1276.

Roth, L., Meisel, A., & Lidz, C. (1977). Tests of competency to consent to treatment. *American Journal of Psychiatry, 134,* 279–284.

Sacks, D. (1994). Guardianship: Issues and legislative trends. *Practicing Law Institute, 231,* 37–87.

Sales, B. D., Powell, D. M., & Van Duizend, R. (1982). *Disabled persons and the law.* New York: Plenum Press.

Schwartz, J. J., & Barone, D. F. (1992). Assessing civil competency in the elderly. *Forensic Science, 37,* 938–941.

Scogin, F., & Perry, J. (1986). Guardianship proceedings with older adults: The role of functional assessment and gerontologists. *Law and Psychology Review, 10,* 123–128.

Smyer, M. (1993). Aging and decision-making capacity. *Generations, 17,* 51–56.

Thomas, B. L. (1994). Guardianship and the vulnerable elderly. *Journal of Gerontology Nursing, 20,* 10–16.

Tor, P. (1993). Finding incompetency in guardianship: Standardizing the process. *Arizona Law Review, 35,* 739–764.

Tor, P., & Sales, B. D. (1996). Guardianship for incapacitated individuals. In B. Sales & D. Shuman (Eds.), *Law, mental health, and mental disorder.* Pacific Grove, CA: Brooks/Cole.

Weiler, K., Helms, L., & Buckwalter, K. (1993). Guardianship petitions for adults and elder adults. *Journal of Gerontology Nursing, 19,* 15–25.

36

Conclusion

PAUL DAVID NUSSBAUM

The intent of this handbook is to first underscore the importance of the field of aging for health care and second to address specific domains of expertise within the field in order to provide a reference point for continued study. As such, the handbook illustrates a generally traditional methodology for communication within the medical and academic professions. The reader is encouraged to note, however, that normal aging is positioned as the lead section. This small gesture is meant to be symbolic of the greater need to refocus attention on understanding the variability of "normality" across the life span which should enhance appreciation of disease and pathology in late life. Further, the content of the handbook is interdisciplinary, spanning geriatric medicine, psychology, neuropsychology, psychiatry, neuropsychiatry, neurology, gerontology, law, and nursing. This reflects the belief that integrated, interdisciplinary study and clinical practice is the appropriate approach with the older adult population. Finally, the handbook is meant to convey the importance of bridging theory and conceptualization of aging to applied practice with older persons and society, something that remains a challenge for health care and academia.

In underscoring the broad import of the field of aging for the 21st century, this editor reasserts the need for the paradigm shift articulated in the introduction. From such critical thought and debate, a more integrated and comprehensive field of aging may emerge, one that better operationalizes theory and bridges the major factors discussed in the introduction.

Aging is now recognized as a major social and political topic for the United States. Indeed, the demographic revolution now under way will affect nearly all aspects of life with a clear need for increased understanding and appreciation of the strengths and limitations of the older adult. In preparing for the increased number of seniors, a fundamentally different paradigm of aging was proposed in the introduction of this handbook. At present, aging is typically framed from the perspective of disease, dependency, and fear. These perceptions are likely the consequence of society's overreliance on the health care field (itself a disease-driven system) to define aging. The proposed paradigm of aging considers health care to be one aspect of a more comprehensive approach to understanding the process of growing older. Indeed, consideration of social, educational, religious, political, and familial factors will likely result in a more accurate understanding of aging. It is proposed that a more optimistic, wellness- and productivity-based perspective of aging be realized, one that champions the later years as a natural part of the developmental life span.

It is important for health care professionals to appreciate their influence upon these other factors and the opportunity, if not obligation, to educate the public about the facts of aging. This likely will result in a reduction of general stereotypes of aging and decrease the fear often associated with growing older. With appropriate innovation of programs within each of the factors listed above, the new paradigm of aging might be realized. An argument can be made to address issues of aging early in life

PAUL DAVID NUSSBAUM • Aging Research and Education Center, Lutheran Affiliated Services, Mars, Pennsylvania 16046; and Department of Neurology, University of Pittsburgh School of Medicine, Pittsburgh, Pennsylvania 15261.

before general stereotypes become entrenched. Similarly, training and education of our physicians and clinicians can be enhanced by emphasizing normal aging, enhancing preventative models of care, and integrating interdisciplinary practices of care for the older adult.

Health care for the older adult is likely to continue its transition from the acute care setting to the community, a trend that should be welcomed given the fact that older adults suffer from chronic illness, not acute illness. Physicians and clinicians will also make the transition from traditional medical/academic hospital settings to community-based geriatric care campuses. The continuum-of-care model will continue to gain popularity for the expanding older adult population, and managed care will enroll more and more seniors. These new models of health care will succeed if they are integrated, interdisciplinary, and framed within the new paradigm espoused above.

As we enter the "information age" of the 21st century, integration of health care and advanced technologies represents a new horizon that can enhance quality of life for seniors. Use of clinical software to promote case management, design of technologically advanced residential settings, creation of alternative extended care models, rapid distribution of information on aging across the worldwide market, and promotion of the older adult as an active participant in self-care represent but a few of the challenges for health care and society.

Current models of care that tend to be bureaucratically entrenched, slow to develop, rigid in philosophy, and outdated in approach must be replaced by more efficient, innovative, and integrated systems.

This handbook capitalizes on a traditional educational modality to promote the importance of understanding the aging process. Further, the handbook alerts the health care system of its inadequacies to address the rapidly developing demands that older adults present. This conclusion, however, is meant to advance a critical debate with regard to the current attitude of aging that exists in America. It is argued that a more comprehensive and integrated understanding of growing older is needed, one that results in enhanced quality of life and decreased ageism. The role of health care in this paradigm shift deserves critical thought, particularly with regard to alteration of the traditional disease-based approach championed by current clinical models. Neuropsychology and other health care disciplines have an opportunity to lead the paradigm shift. This will occur only with fundamental changes of the current education, academic, and clinical systems. It is argued that such changes will result in parallel changes in the social, educational, religious, political, and familial factors noted above. Ultimately, this comprehensive paradigm shift will result in enhanced appreciation of aging across the life span and improved clinical care for seniors with chronic illness.

Index

ISBN 0-306-45460-2

90000

9 780306 454608